Nailing the Written Emergency Medicine Board Examination

Bobby Desai • Brandon R. Allen
Editors

Nailing the Written Emergency Medicine Board Examination

Springer

Editors
Bobby Desai, MD, FACEP
Department of Emergency Medicine
University of Florida College of Medicine
Gainesville, FL
USA

Brandon R. Allen, MD
Department of Emergency Medicine
University of Florida College of Medicine
Gainesville, FL
USA

ISBN 978-3-319-30836-4 ISBN 978-3-319-30838-8 (eBook)
DOI 10.1007/978-3-319-30838-8

Library of Congress Control Number: 2016946055

Printed on acid-free paper

This Springer imprint is published by Springer Nature
The registered company is Springer International Publishing AG Switzerland

For my wife Katie and children Nila and Owen

–Brandon R. Allen

For Alpa, Jayden, Dylan, and Shayan
Your support in this endeavor has been incredible

–Bobby Desai

Contents

Cardiovascular Emergencies 1
Bobby Desai

Pulmonary Emergencies 131
Michael R. Marchick and Bobby Desai

Gastroenterology 185
Brandon R. Allen and Bobby Desai

Nephrology and Urology 261
Bobby Desai

Hematologic and Oncologic Emergencies 309
Bobby Desai

Disorders Affecting the Skin 349
Bobby Desai

Endocrine/Metabolic/Electrolytes 389
Bobby Desai

Ears, Nose, and Throat 467
Bobby Desai

Environmental Emergencies 517
Michael R. Marchick and Bobby Desai

Neurologic Emergencies 555
Michael R. Marchick and Bobby Desai

Obstetrics and Gynecology 617
Bobby Desai and Alpa Desai

Ophthalmology 637
Bobby Desai

Toxicologic Emergencies 675
Matthew Ryan and Bobby Desai

Orthopedic Emergencies 735
Bobby Desai

Trauma 813
Henry Young II and Bobby Desai

Index 869

Contributors

Brandon R. Allen, MD Department of Emergency Medicine, University of Florida College of Medicine, Gainesville, FL, USA

Alpa Desai, DO Community Health and Family Medicine, University of Florida College of Medicine, Gainesville, FL, USA

Bobby Desai, MD, MEd Department of Emergency Medicine, University of Florida, Gainesville, FL, USA

Michael R. Marchick, MD Department of Emergency Medicine, University of Florida College of Medicine, Gainesville, FL, USA

Matthew Ryan, MD, PhD Department of Emergency Medicine, University of Florida, Gainesville, FL, USA

Henry Young II, MD Department of Emergency Medicine, UF Health at the University of Florida, Gainesville, FL, USA

Cardiovascular Emergencies

Bobby Desai

Contents

Acute Coronary Syndrome 2
Other Causes of Acute Coronary Syndrome 4
Stable and Unstable Angina 6
Acute Myocardial Infarction 7
Arteries and Affected Areas 9
Inferior MI Specifics 13
Right Ventricular Infarction 15
Cardiac Markers 16
Reperfusion in AMI 18
Complications in AMI 22
Congestive Heart Failure 24
Valvular Emergencies 31
Mitral Regurgitation 33
Mitral Valve Prolapse 35
Aortic Stenosis 37
Causes of Aortic Regurgitation 39
Infective Endocarditis 42
Rheumatic Heart Disease 48
Cardiomyopathies (CM) 50
Myocarditis 56
Pericarditis 59
Cardiac Tamponade 62
Abdominal Aortic Aneurysm 64
Aortic Dissection 67

B. Desai, MD, MEd
Department of Emergency Medicine, University of Florida,
Gainesville, FL, USA
e-mail: bdesai@ufl.edu

B. Desai, B.R. Allen (eds.), *Nailing the Written Emergency Medicine Board Examination*,
DOI 10.1007/978-3-319-30838-8_1

Hypertension ... 72

Pulmonary Hypertension ... 76

Syncope ... 77

Deep Venous Thrombosis and Pulmonary Embolism ... 79

Acute Limb Ischemia ... 87

Pacemakers ... 89

Left Ventricular Assist Devices (LVAD) ... 94

EKG Changes Related to Electrolytes and Metabolic Conditions ... 96

EKG Changes Related to Medications ... 100

Dysrhythmias ... 102

Heart Blocks ... 118

Miscellaneous ... 127

Acute Coronary Syndrome

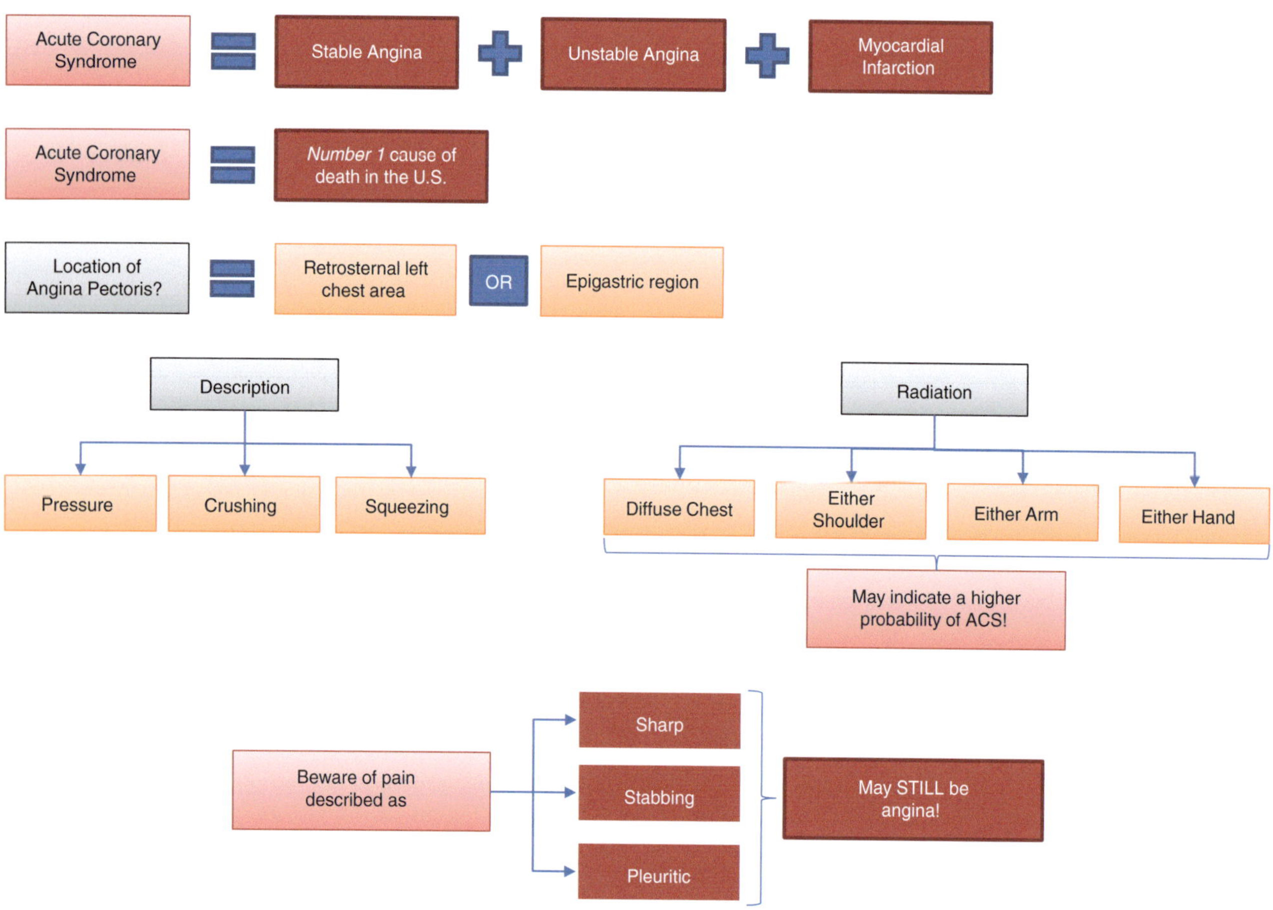

Angina Pectoris

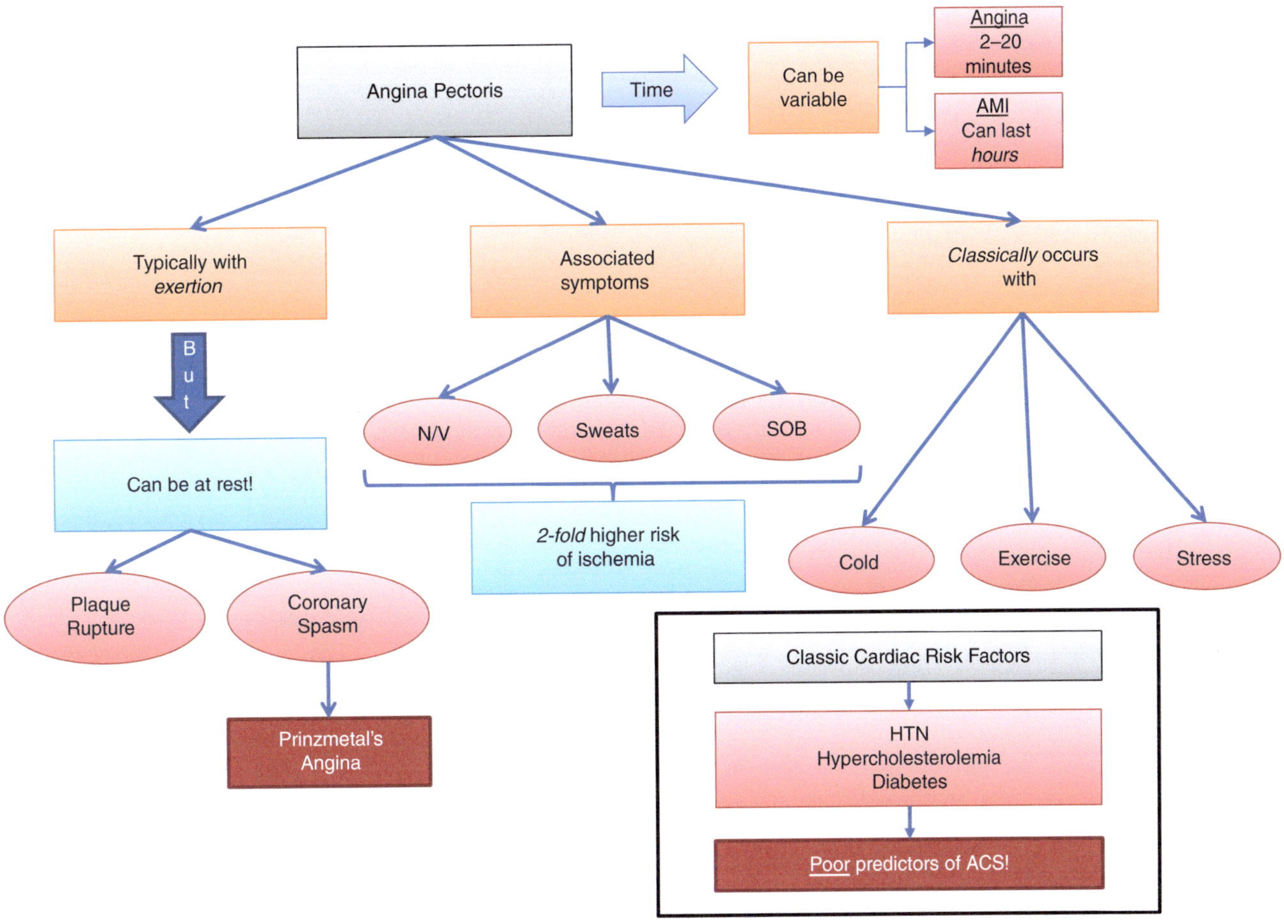

ACS Physical Exam

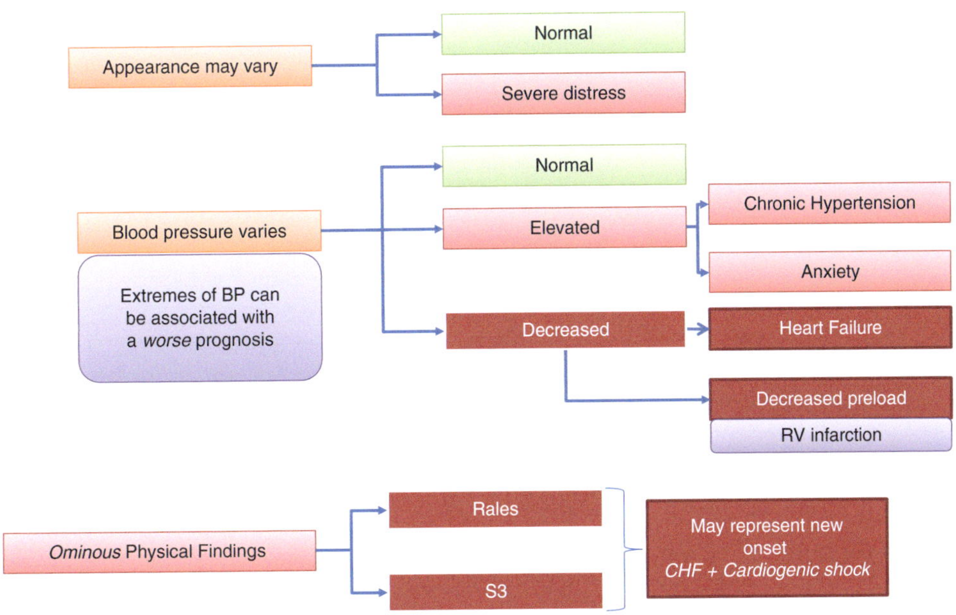

Pathophysiology

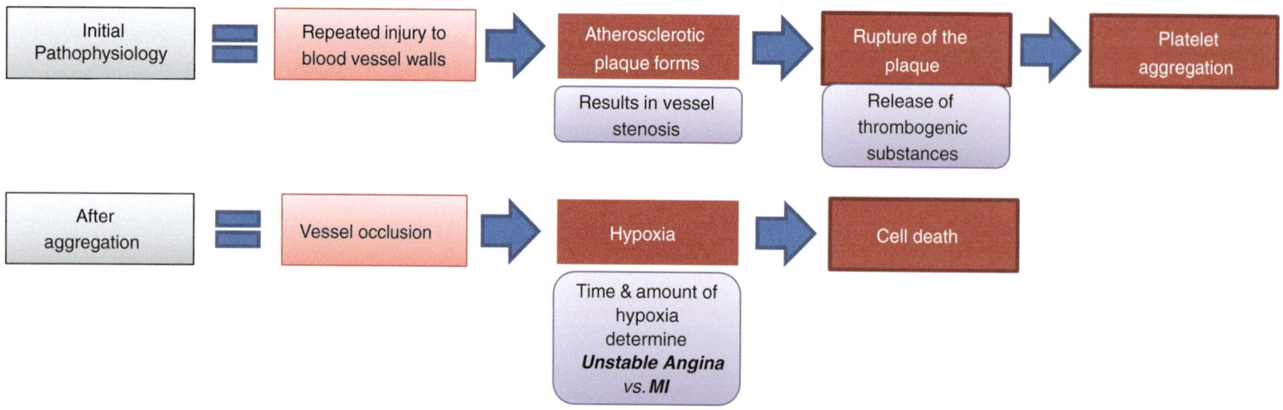

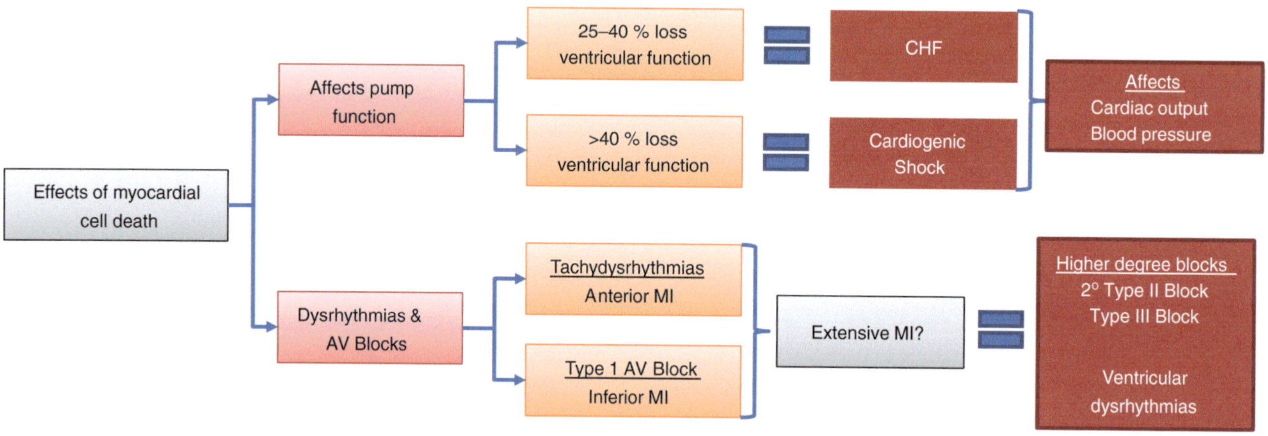

Other Causes of Acute Coronary Syndrome

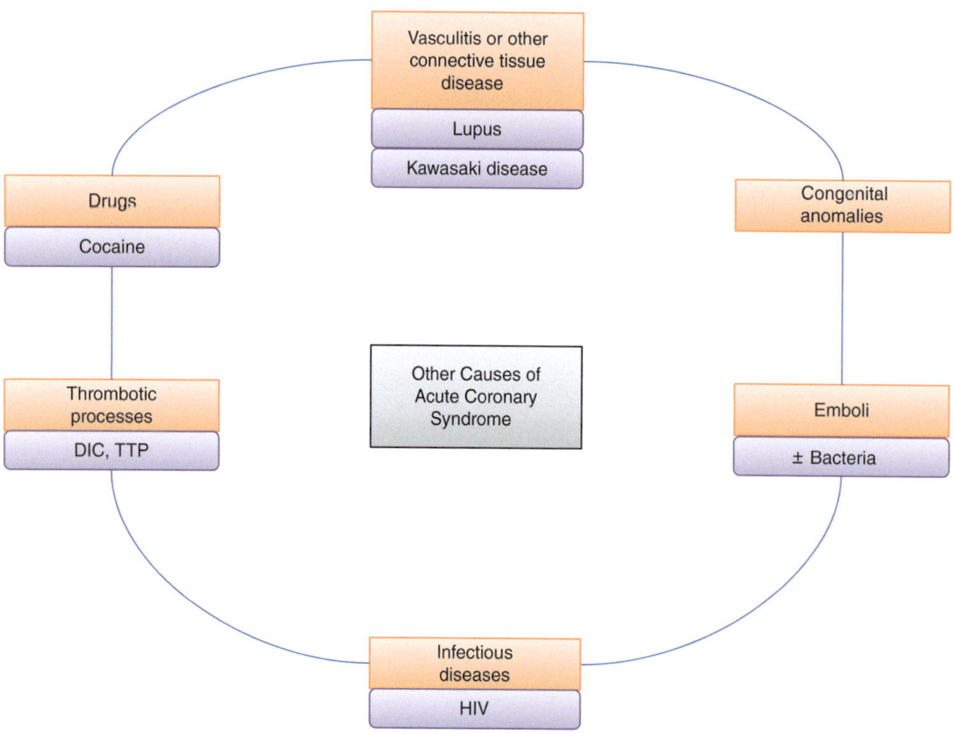

Cocaine and Chest Pain

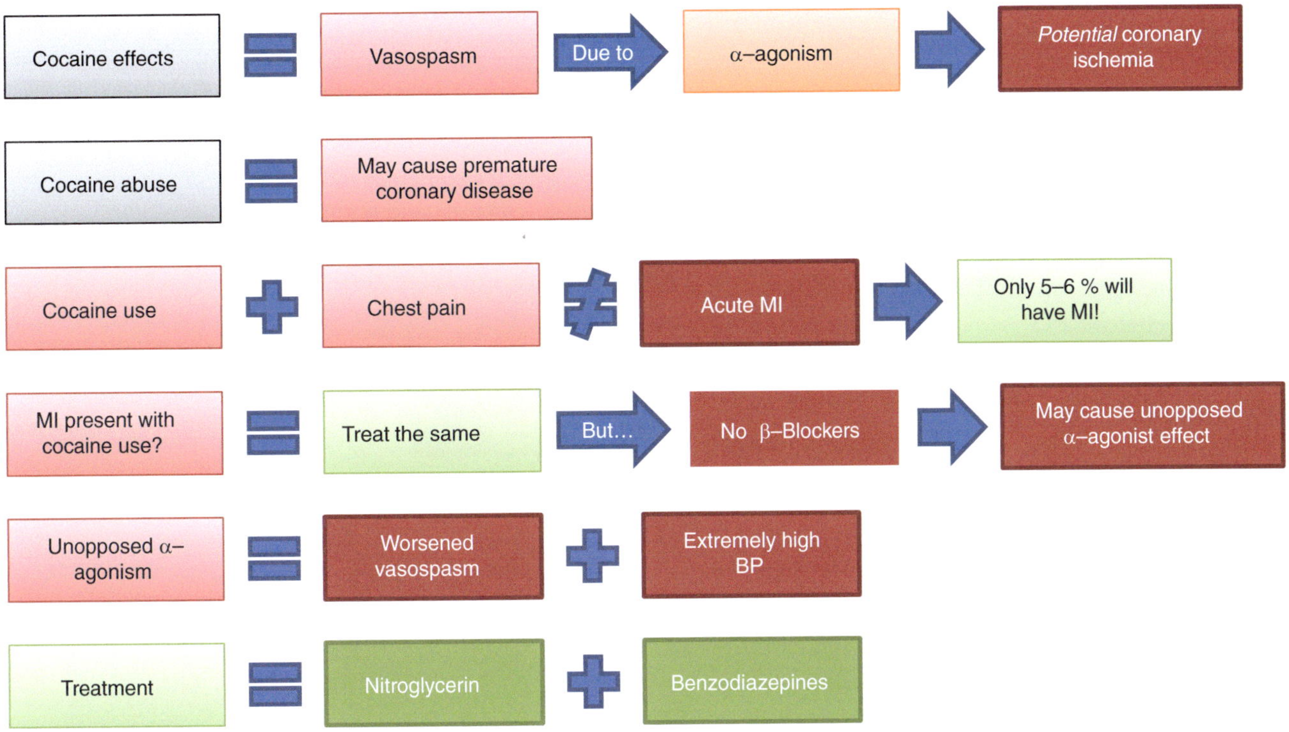

Atypical Chest Pain

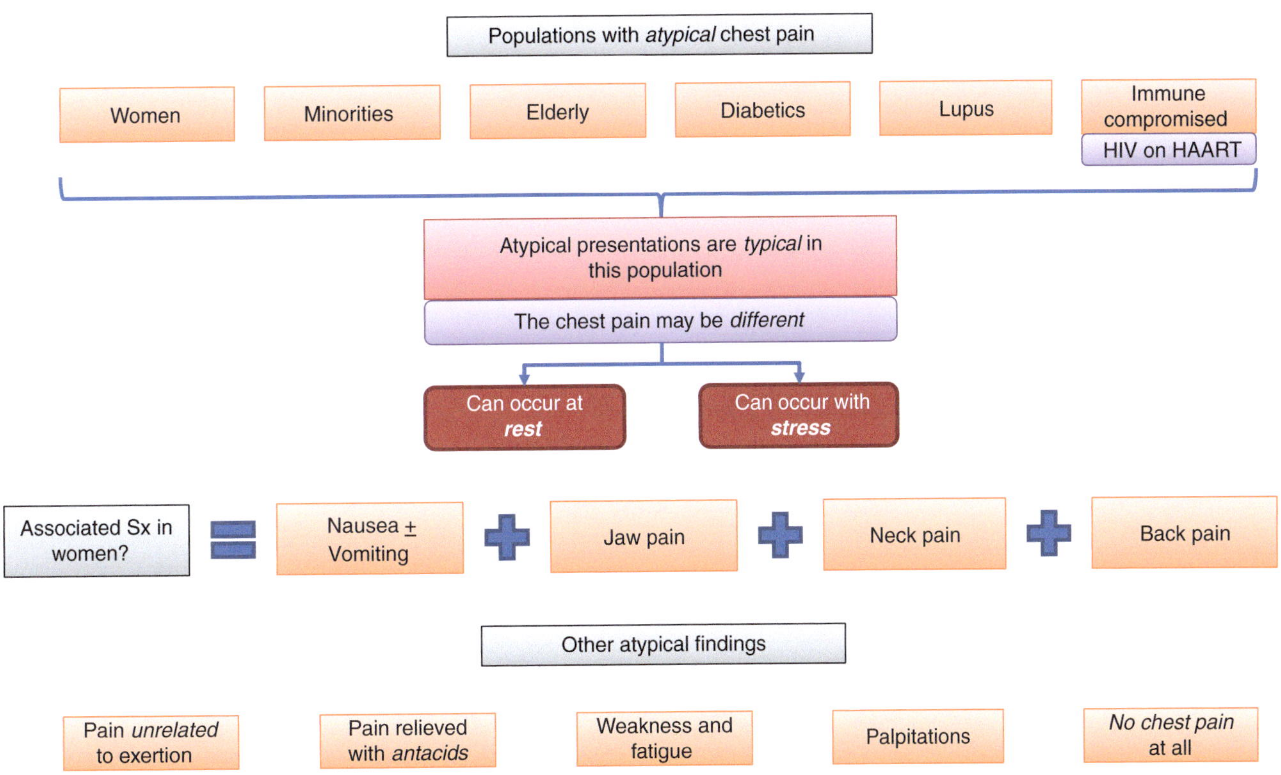

Stable and Unstable Angina

Stable angina = *Fixed* plaque

Pain of stable angina? = Exertional → *Crescendo-Decrescendo* pattern

Relieved by? = Nitroglycerin ± Rest

Pitfall of stable angina? = May progress to ***Unstable Angina*** & ***Myocardial Infarction***

Unstable angina = *Unstable* plaque → *Change* in chest pain → *Frequency, Intensity, Duration*

New-onset chest pain? = *Unstable angina*

Pain of unstable angina? = Exertional OR Rest → NOT Palliated by nitroglycerin or rest

Pain duration? = Greater than 20 minutes

Pitfall of unstable angina? = Have high risk of ***Myocardial Infarction*** & ***Death***

Prinzmetal's or Variant Angina

Prinzmetal's Angina

- Coronary artery spasm
- Occurs at rest
- *ST-elevation* occurs
- May *NOT* have evidence of coronary disease at catheterization

EKG = Similar to STEMI EKG

What Factors Predict Prinzmetal's Angina?

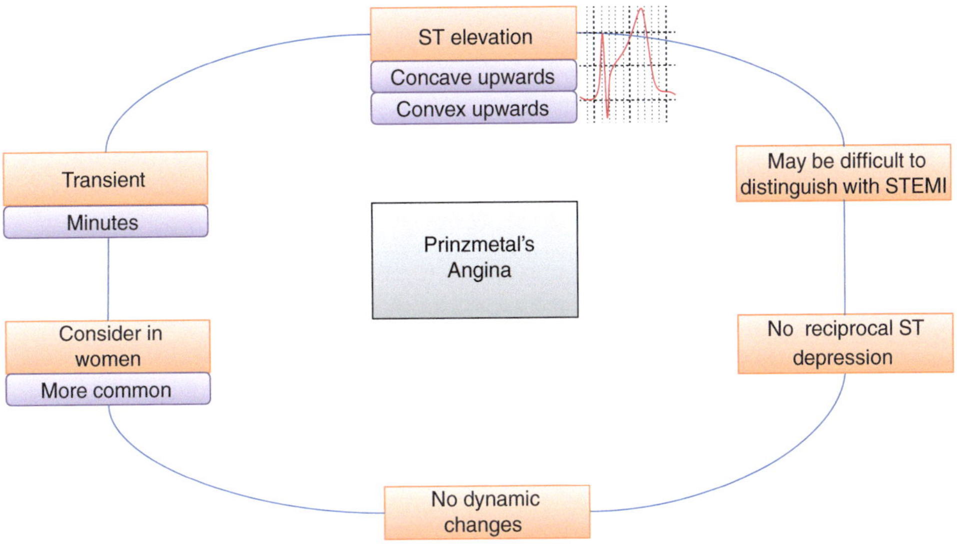

Acute Myocardial Infarction

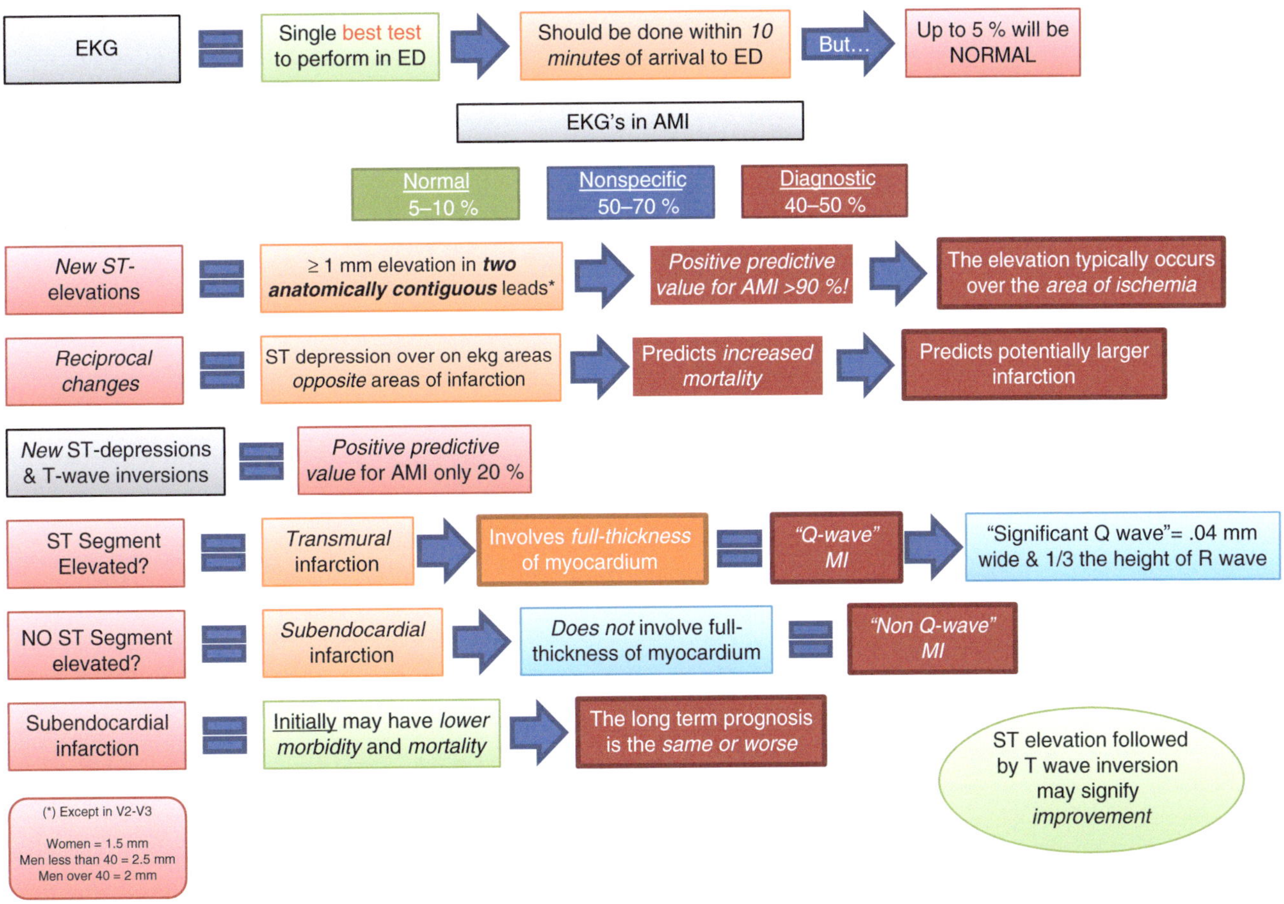

How Is the EKG Helpful?

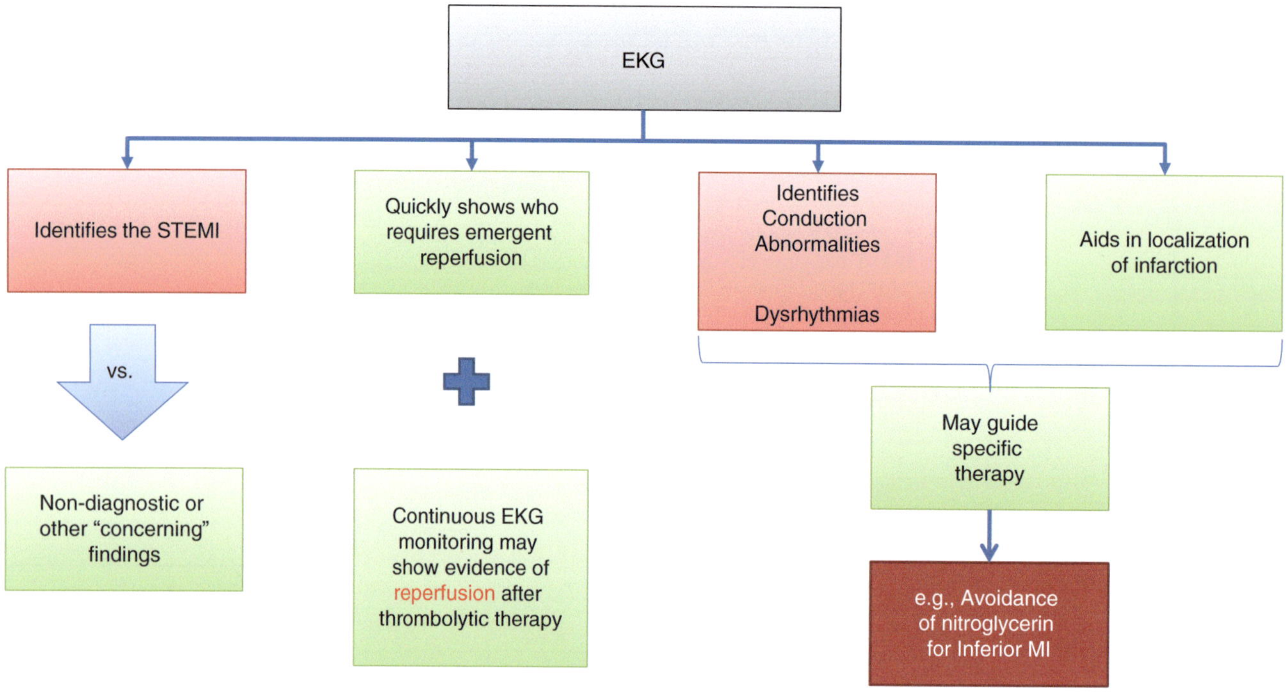

The EKG in Acute Myocardial Infarction

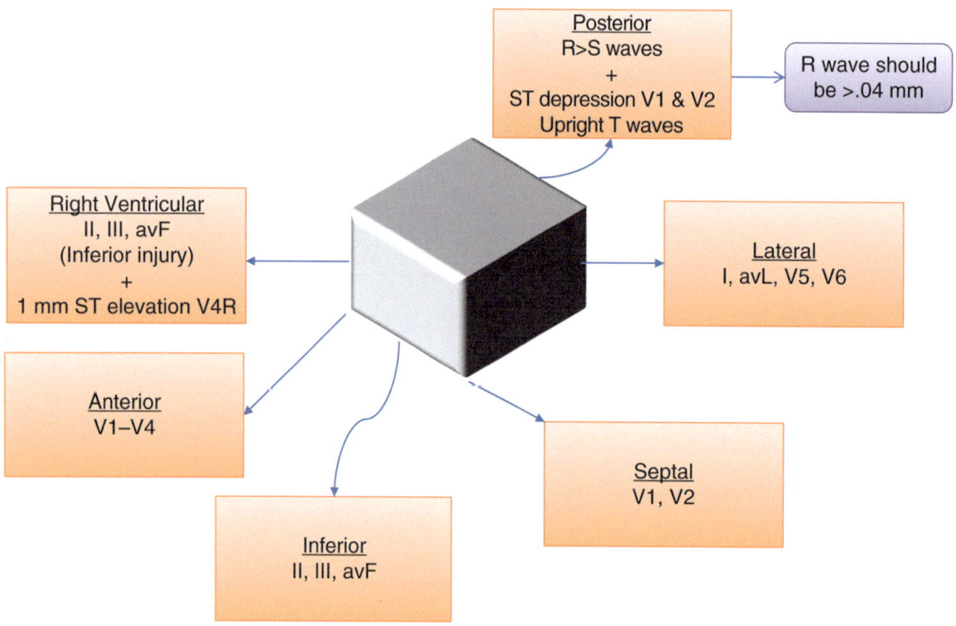

Causes of ST-Segment Elevation

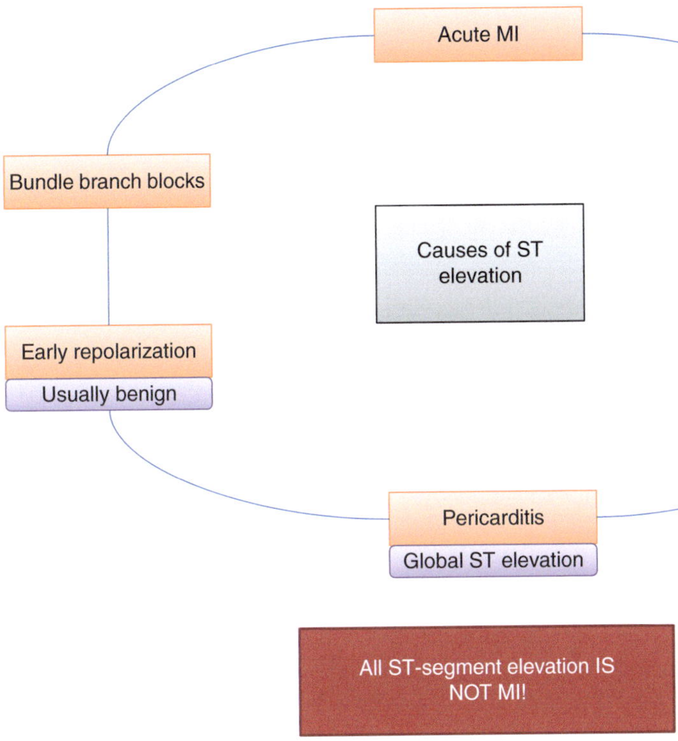

Arteries and Affected Areas

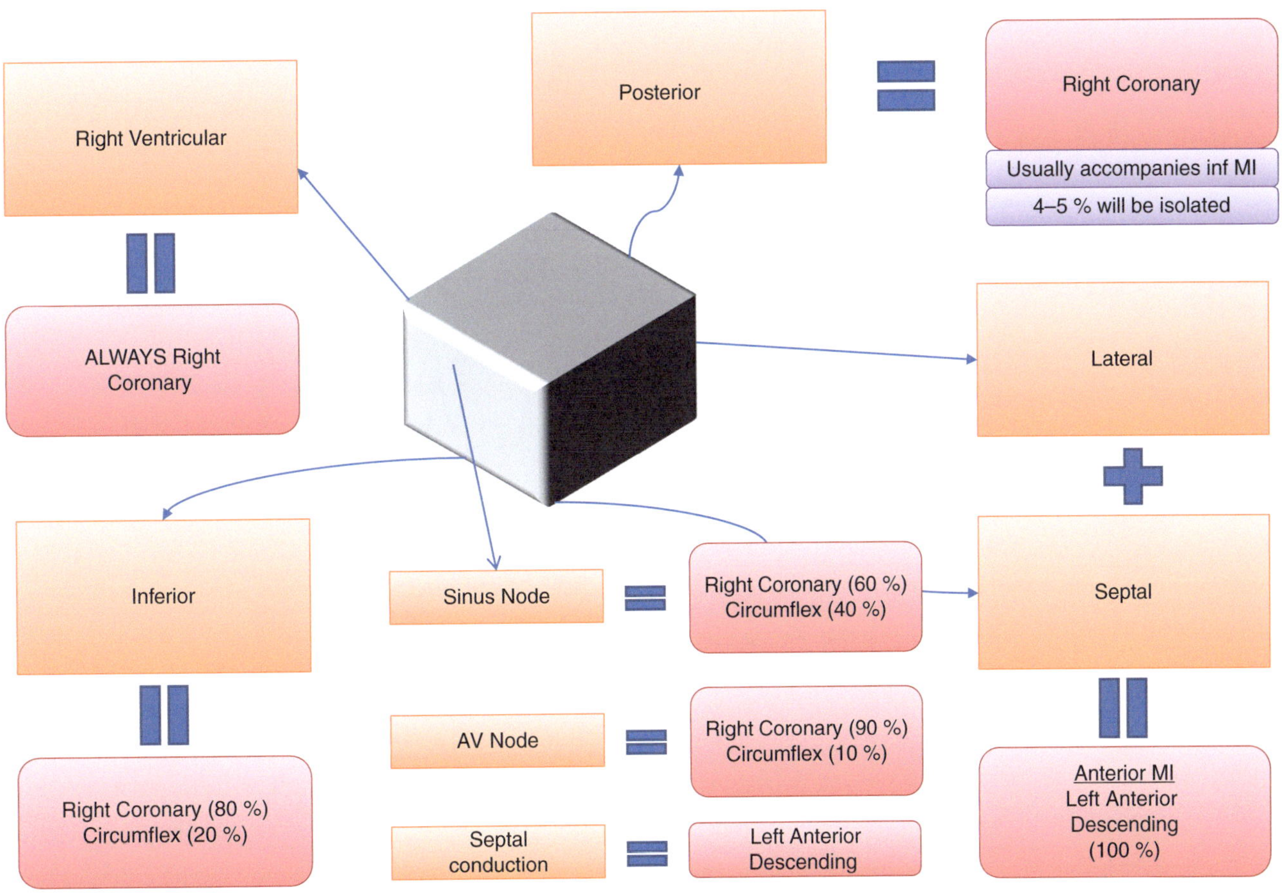

Anterior MI

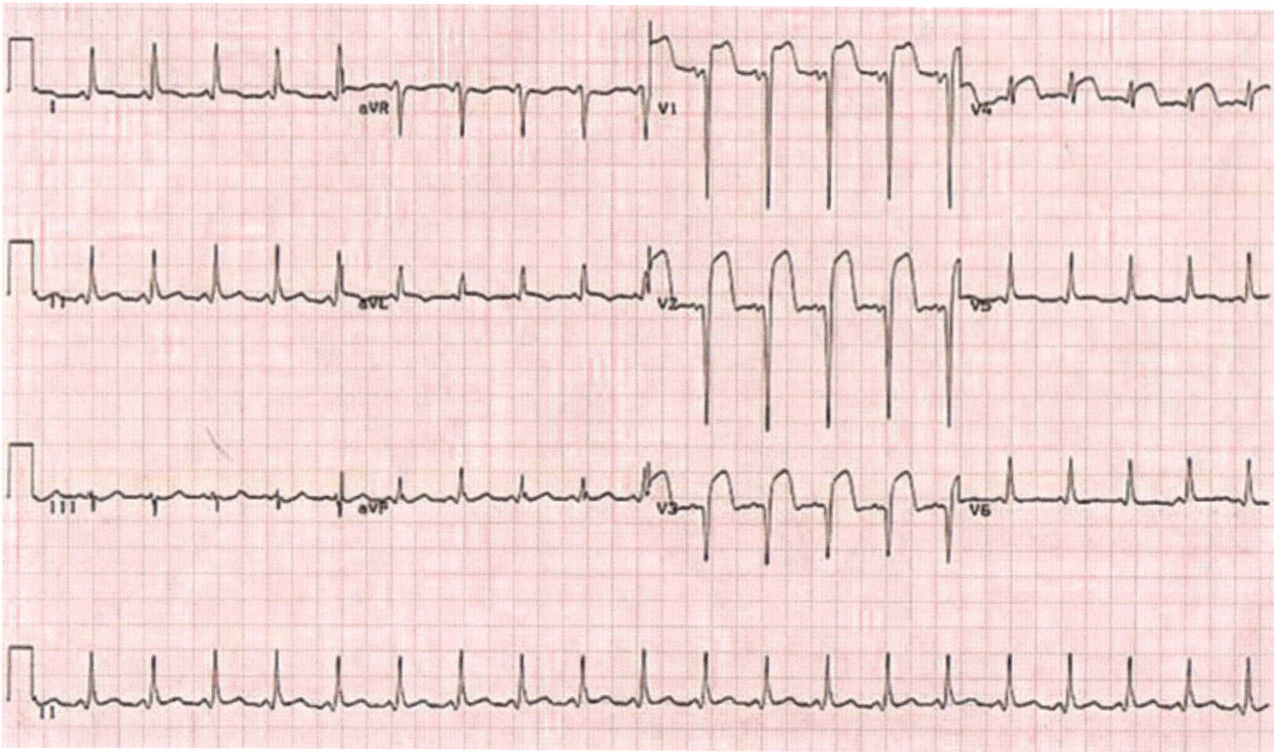

Center image (Reprinted from Davies A, Scott A. Acute coronary syndromes. In: Davies A, Scott A, editors. Starting to read ECGs (The basics). New York: Springer Science; 2013. p. 147–59. With permission from Springer Science + Business Media)

Hyperacute T Waves

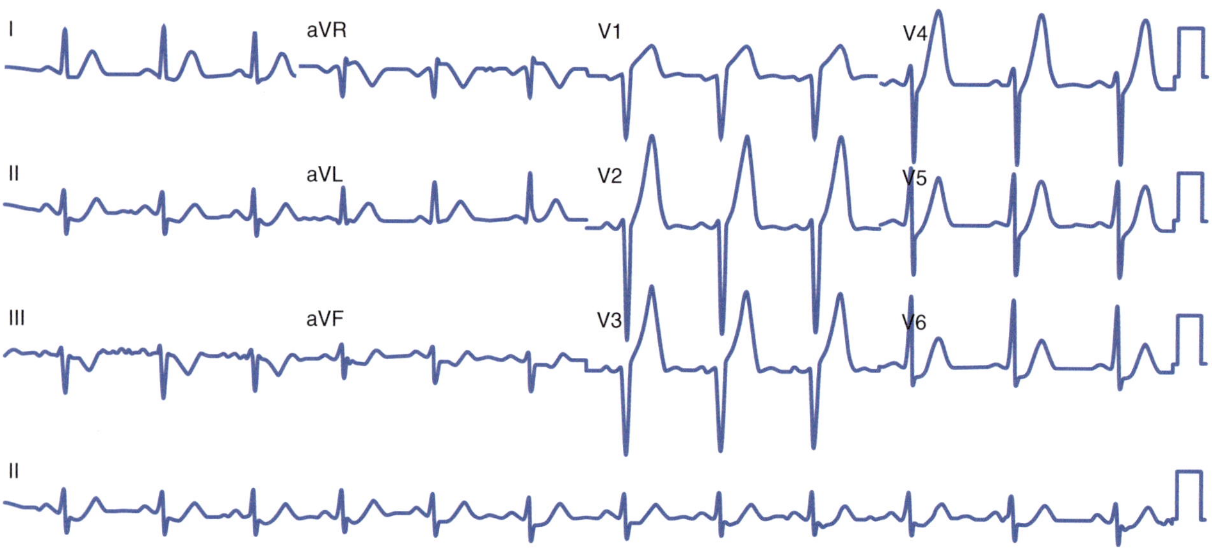

What Factors Predict MI on the EKG?

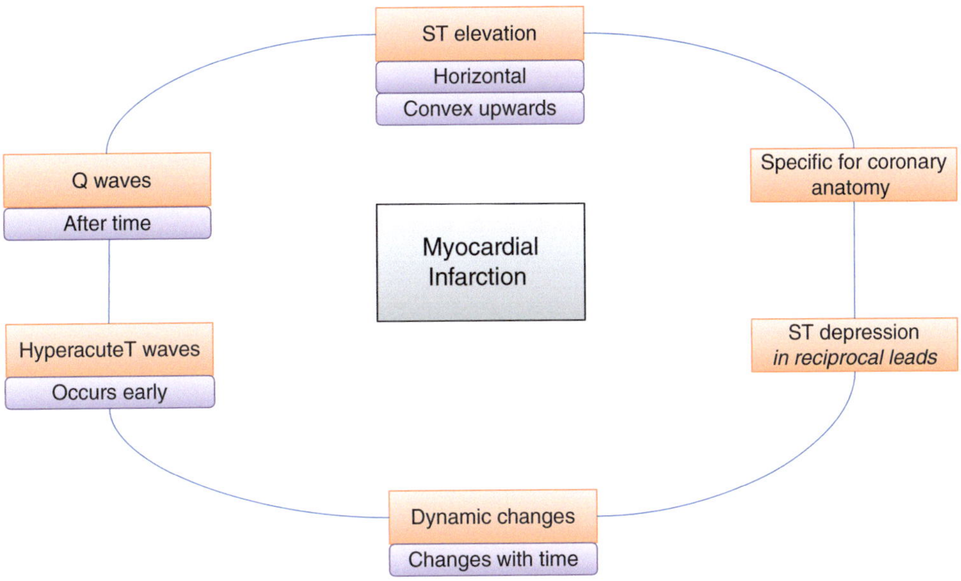

What Factors Predict Early Repolarization?

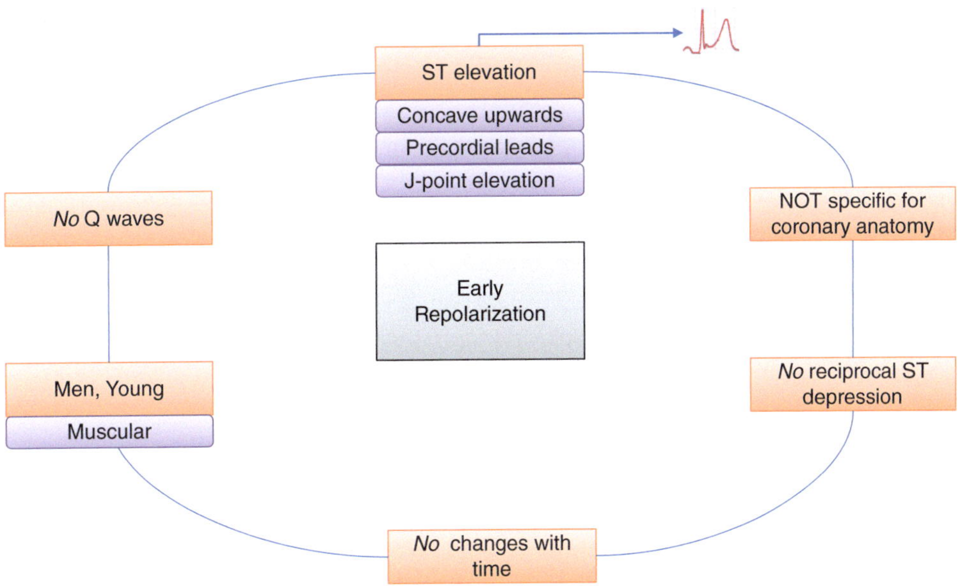

Anterior MI Specifics

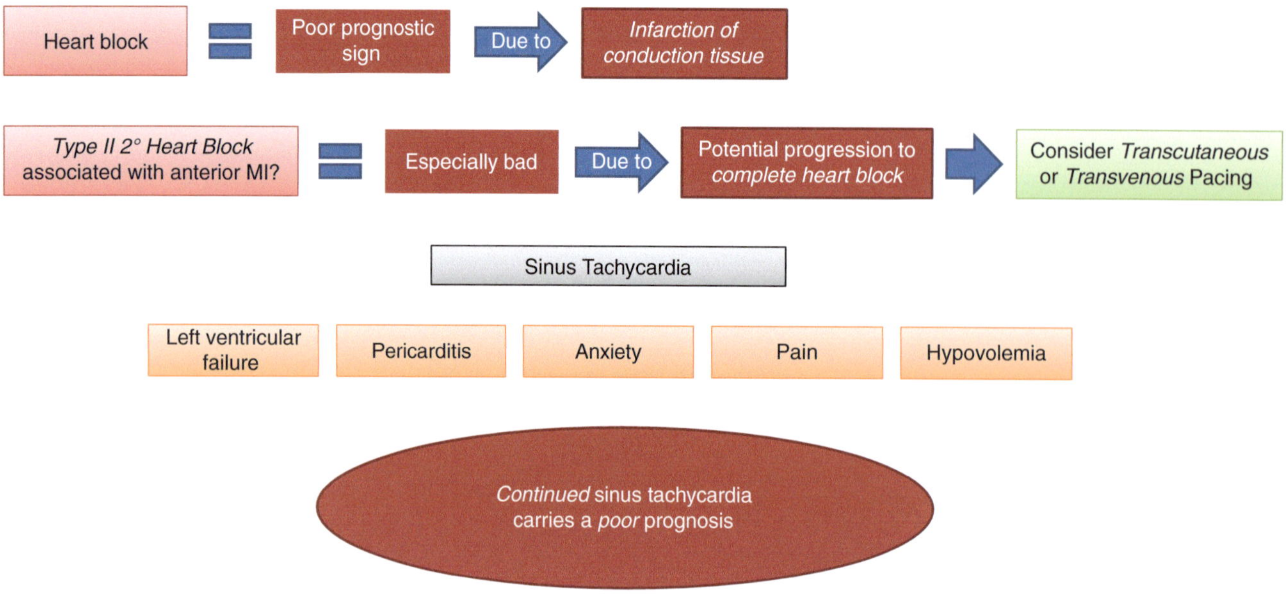

The EKG and Emergent Reperfusion

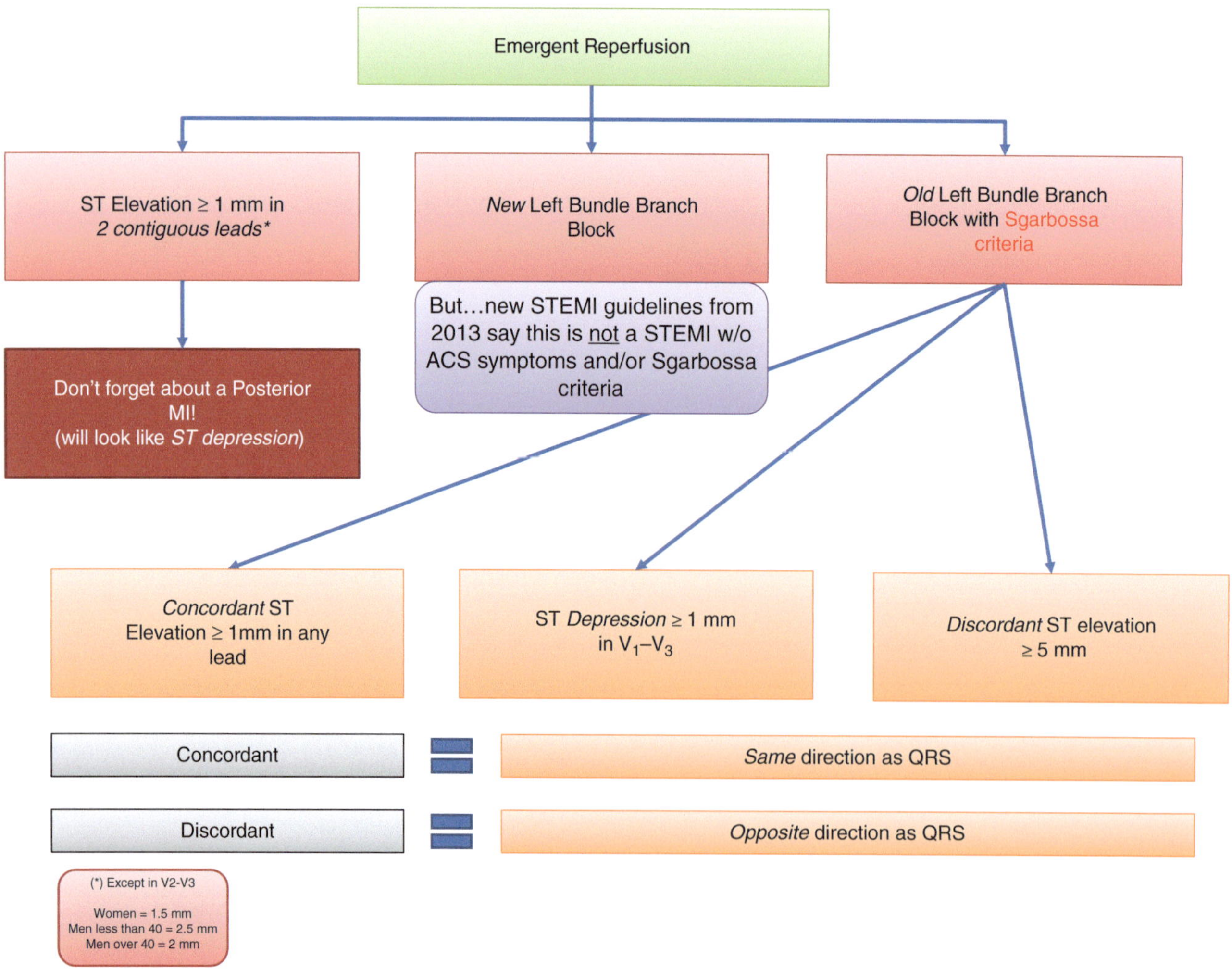

Sgarbossa Criteria

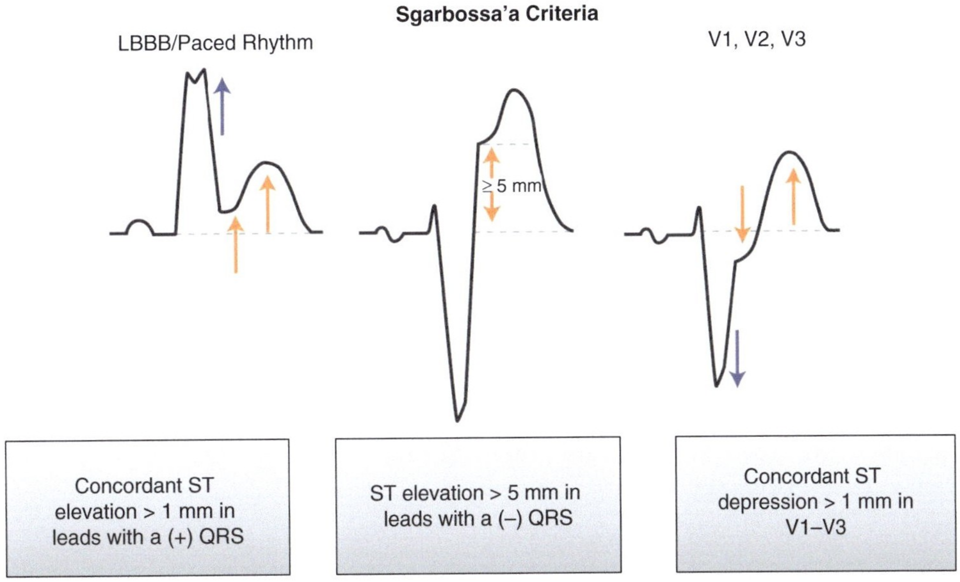

Center image (Reprinted from Allen B, Ganti L, Desai B. Cardiology. In: Allen B, Ganti L, Desai B, editors. Quick hits in emergency medicine. New York: Springer Science; 2013. p. 71–82. With permission from Springer Science + Business Media)

Inferior MI Specifics

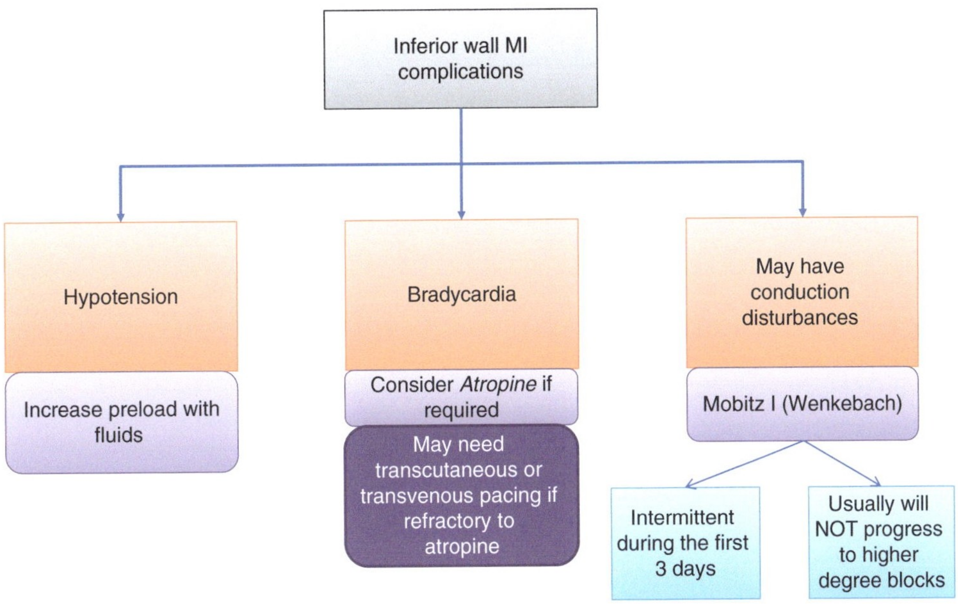

Inferior MI

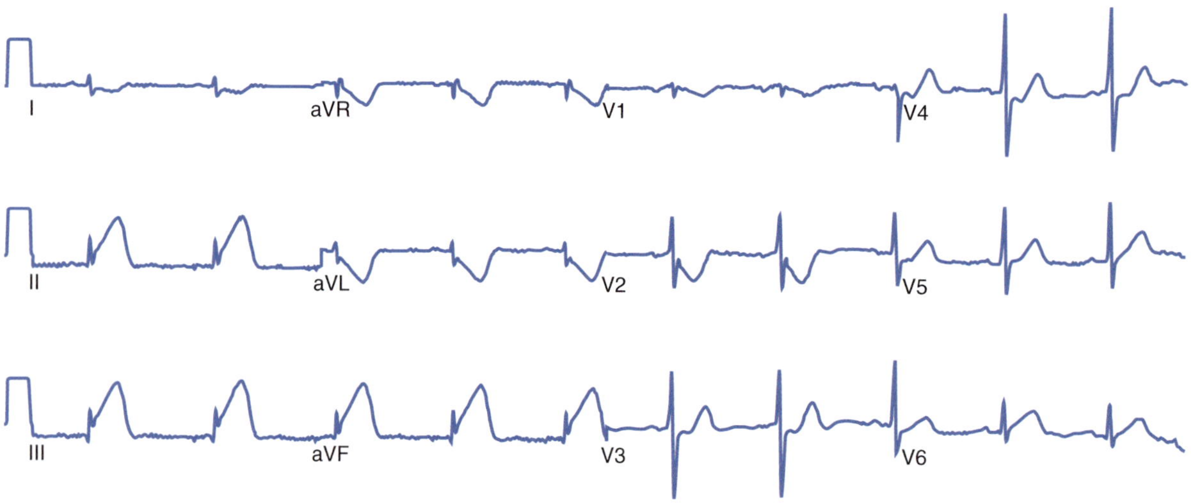

Inferior-Posterior MI

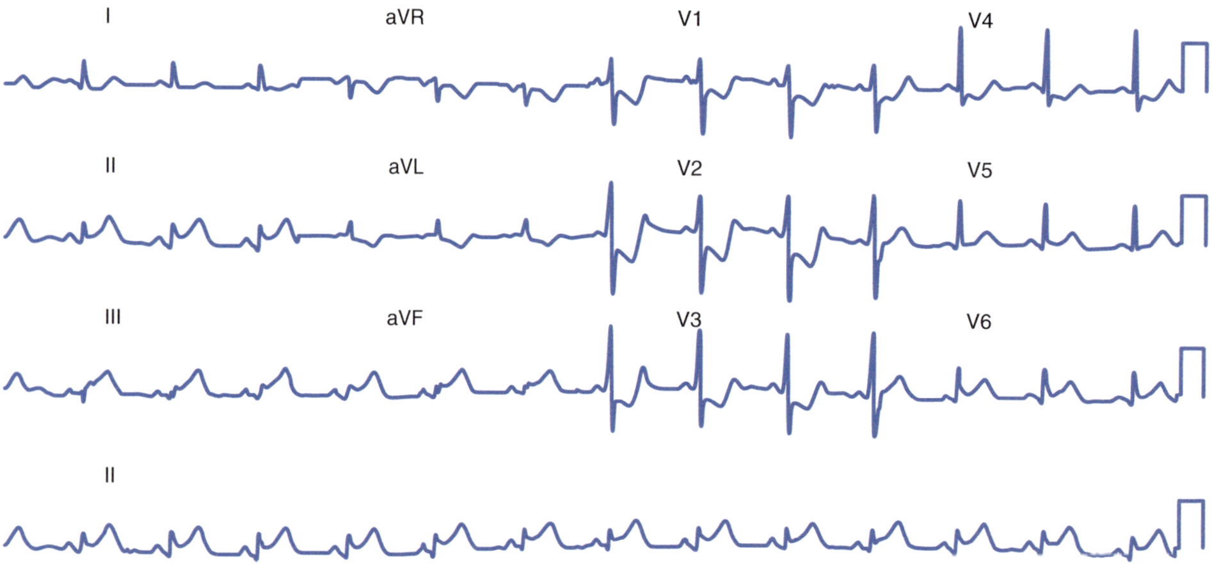

Right Ventricular Infarction

Right ventricular infarction = Complicates up to 40 % of inferior MI → Isolated RV infarction is extremely uncommon

Right ventricular infarction = *Very preload sensitive* → Can develop **severe hypotension in response to nitrates** or other preload-reducing agents → Treated with fluids

EKG in RV Infarction? = **ST elevation in V1** → V1 is the only standard EKG lead that looks directly at the right ventricle

Other EKG Tidbits? = **ST elevation in lead III > lead II** → Lead III is more "rightward facing" than lead II & more sensitive to the injury current produced by the right ventricle

Highly specific EKG changes for RV MI? = If the magnitude of ST elevation in V1 exceeds the magnitude of ST elevation in V2 + If the ST segment in V1 is isoelectric and the ST segment in V2 is markedly depressed

Confirmation of RV Infarction? = **Presence of ST elevation in the right-sided leads (V3R–V6R)** → The most useful lead is V4R → Sensitivity of 88 %, specificity of 78 % and diagnostic accuracy of 83 %

Right Ventricular Infarction

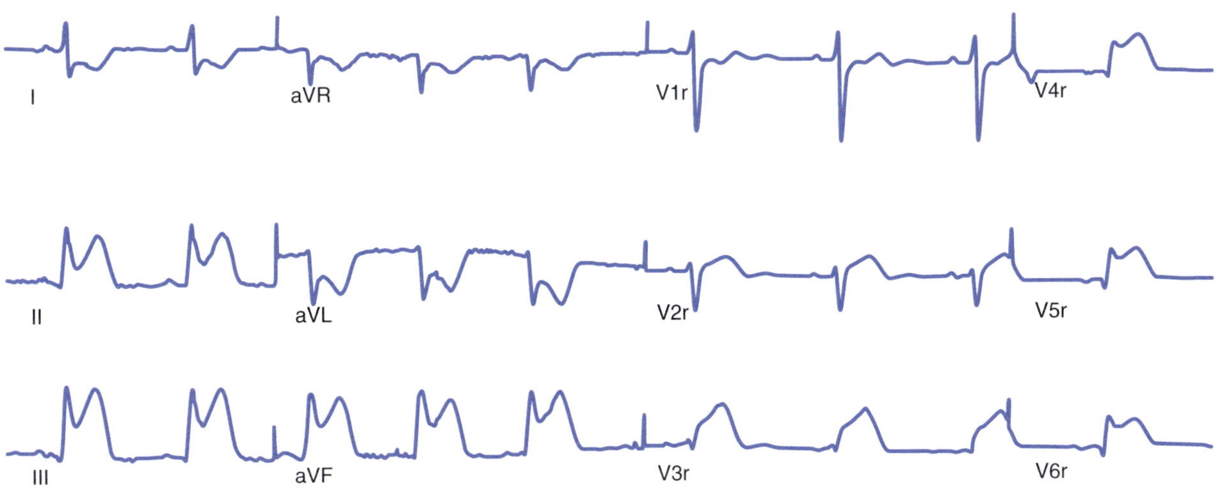

Posterior Infarction

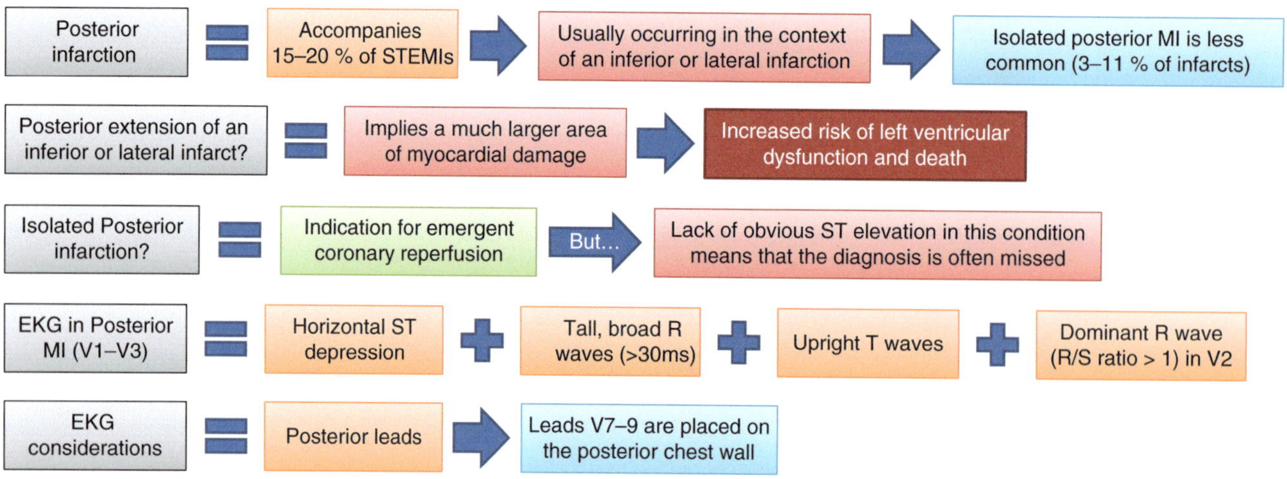

Cardiac Markers

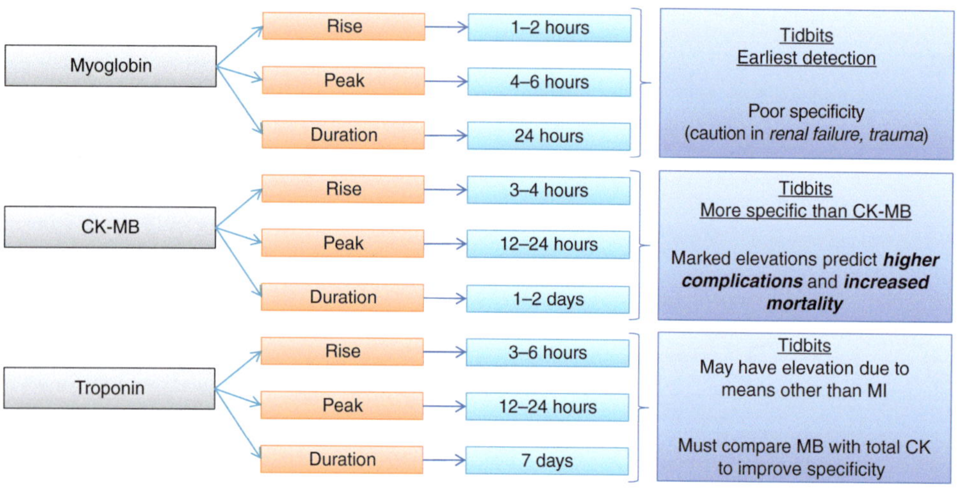

Other Reasons for Troponin Elevation

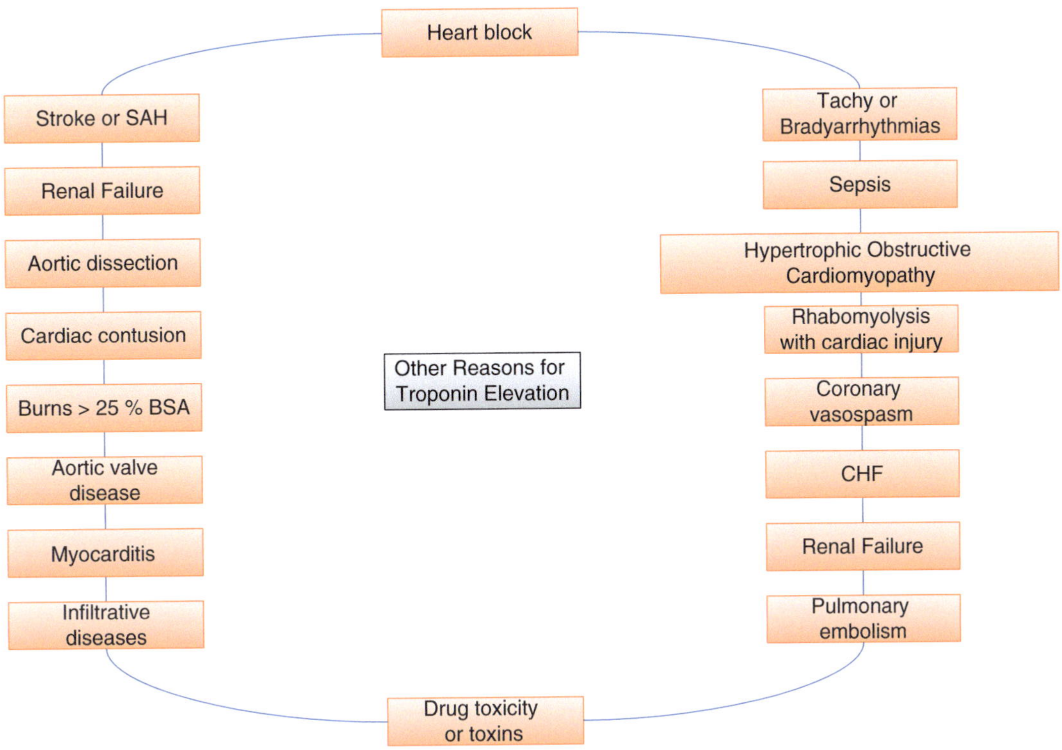

Initial Therapy for ACS

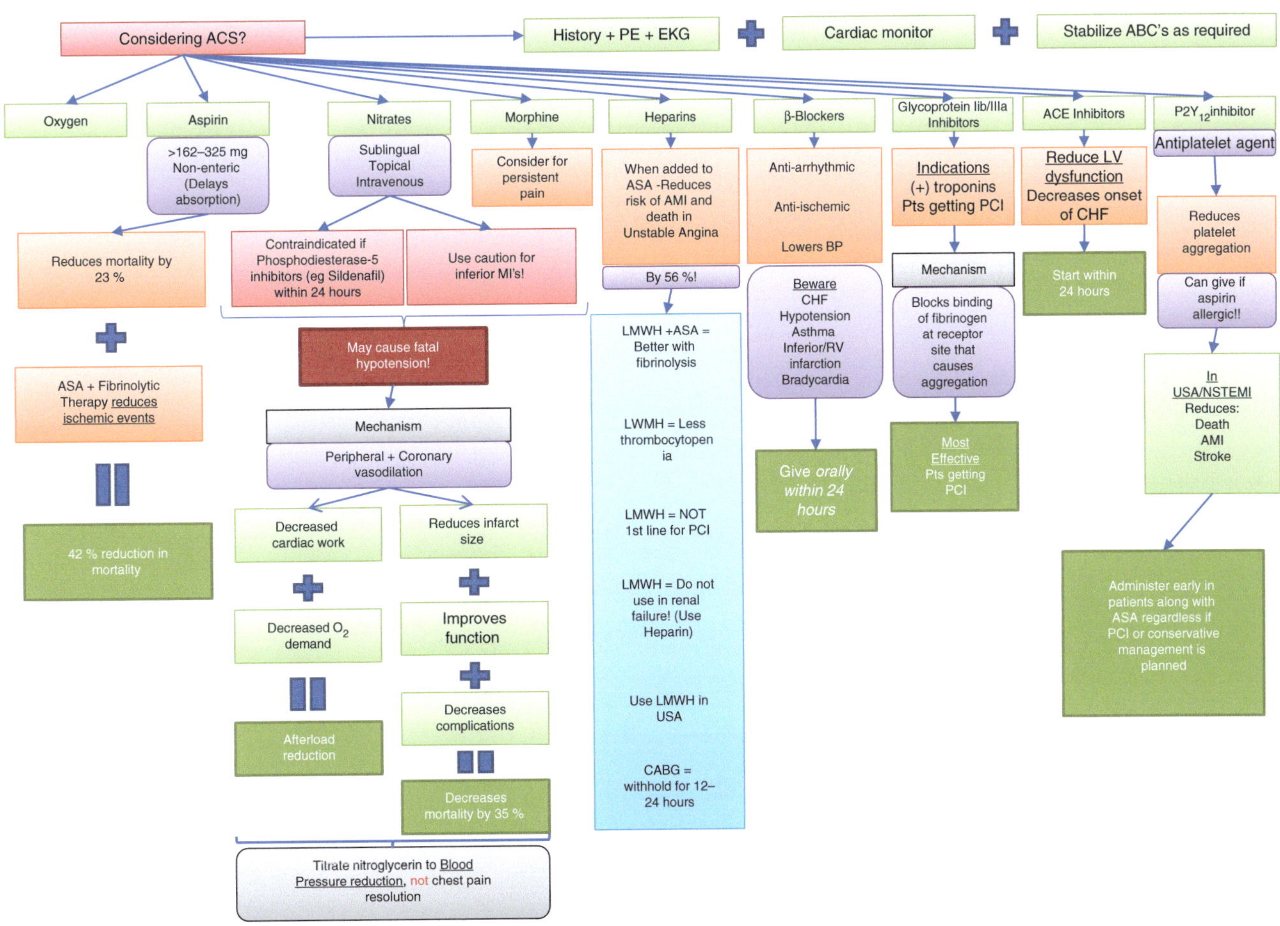

Reperfusion in AMI

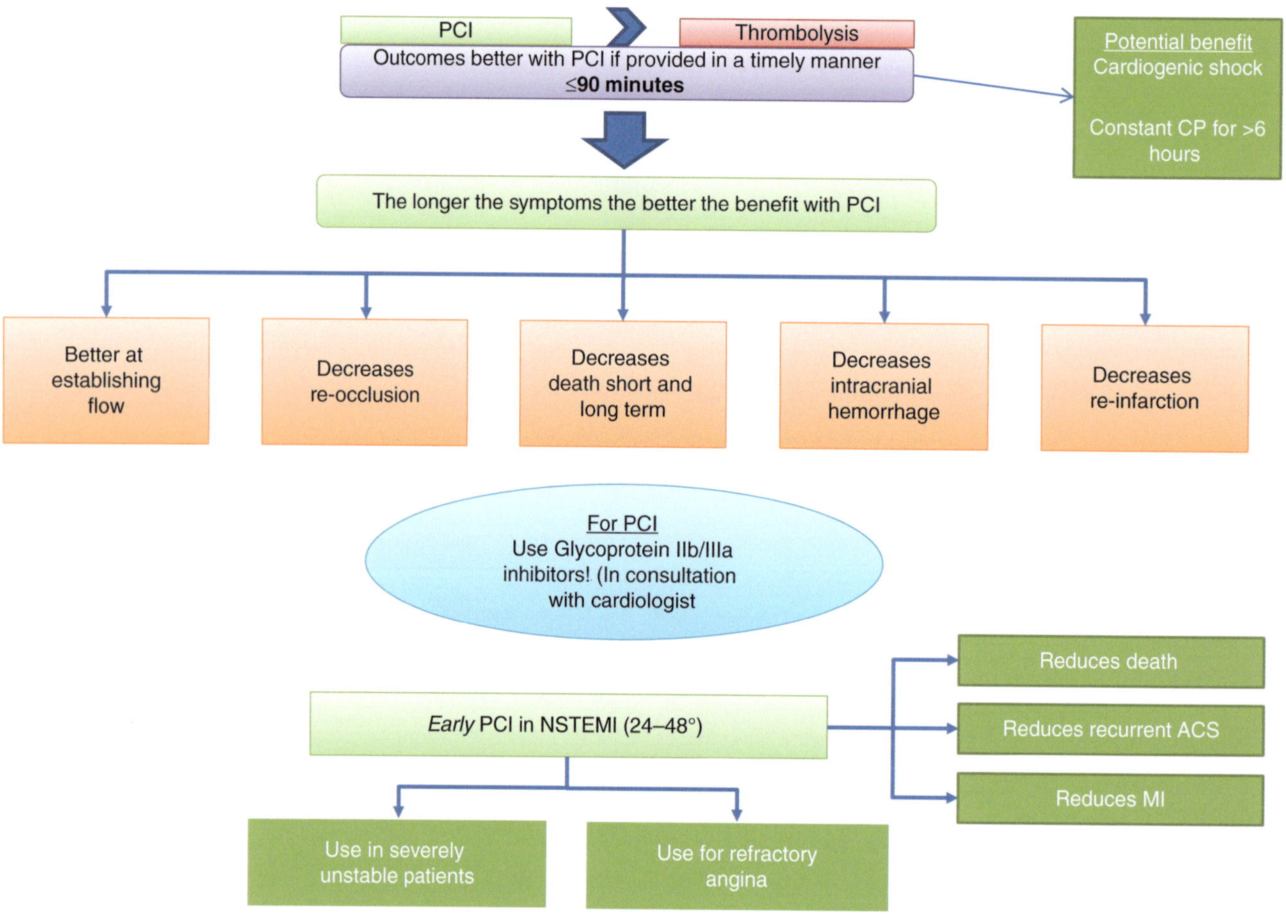

Reperfusion in AMI (2)

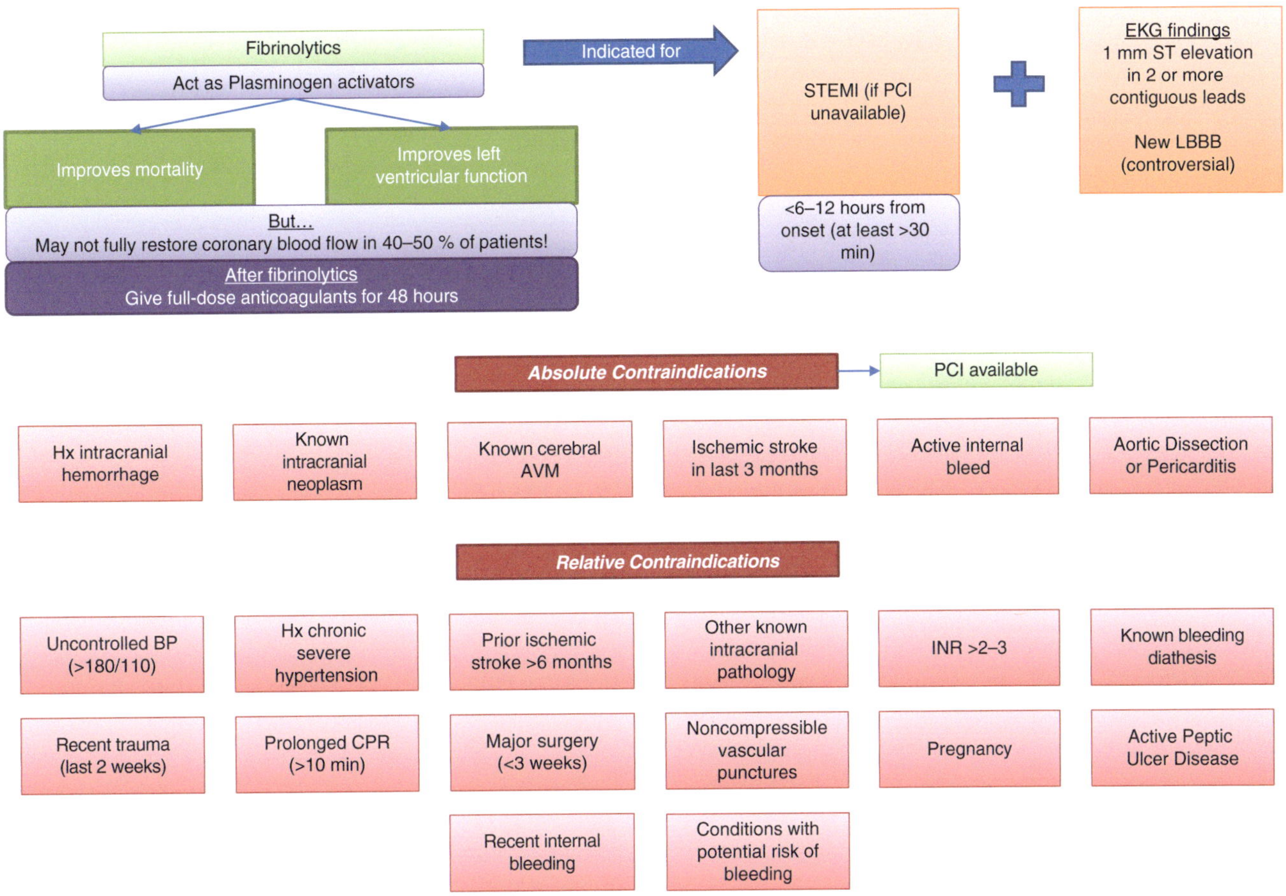

Thrombolytic Therapy Complications

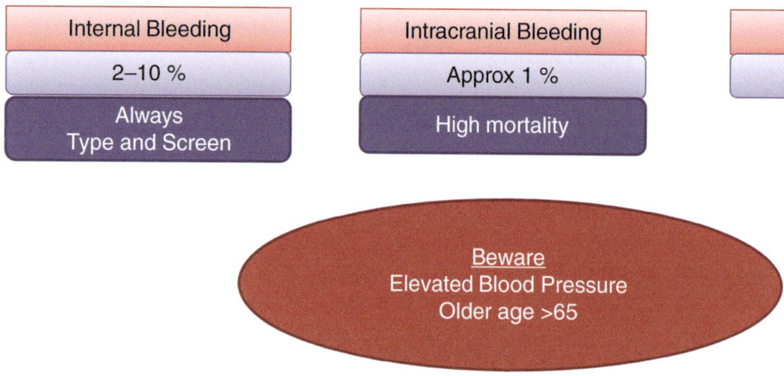

Successful Thrombolytic Therapy

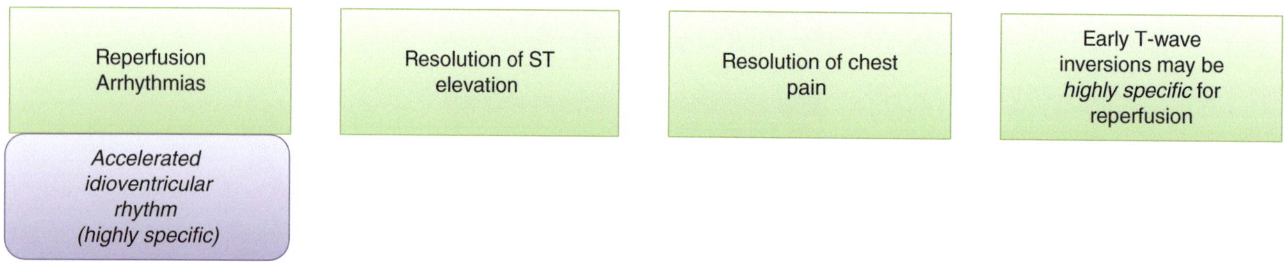

Successful Thrombolytic Therapy

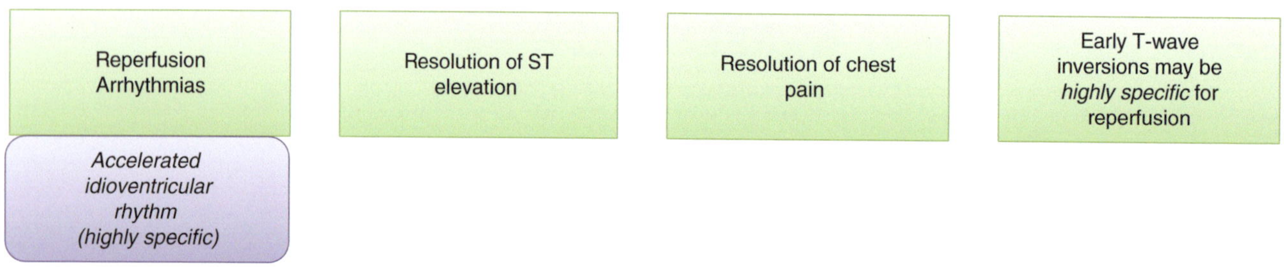

Accelerated Idioventricular Rhythm (AIVR)

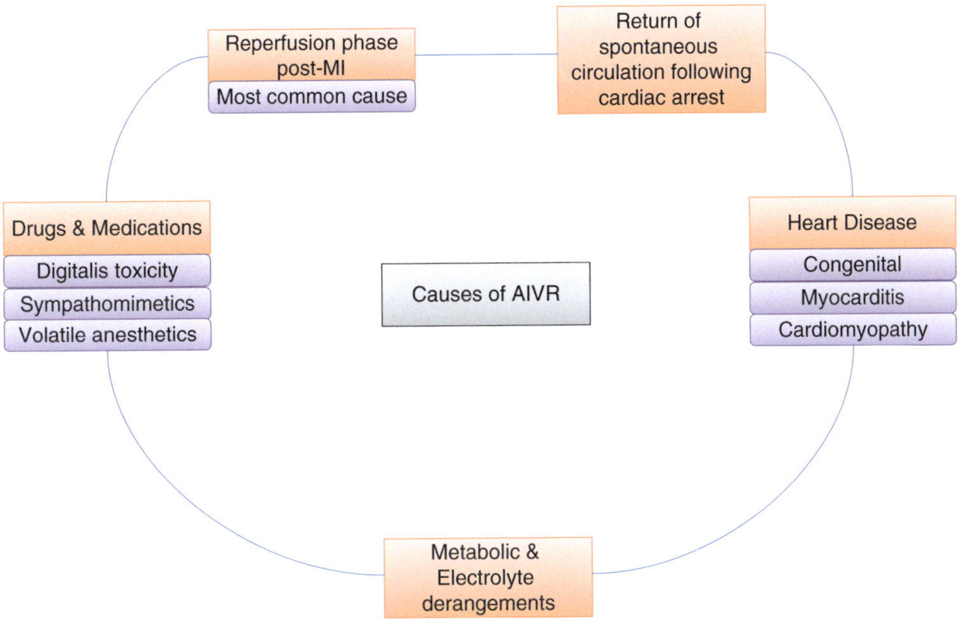

AIVR: EKG Changes

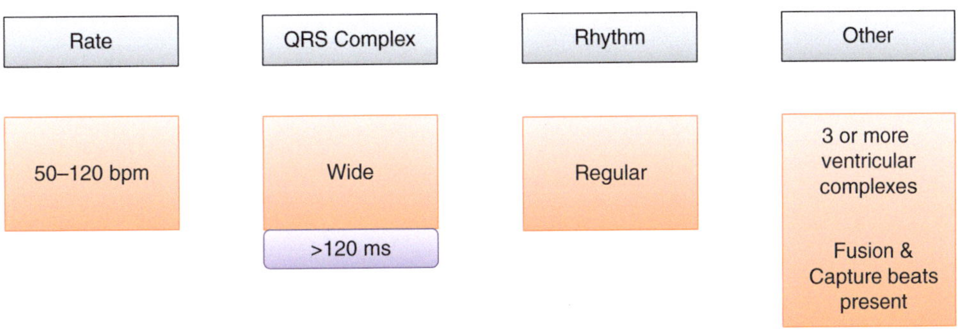

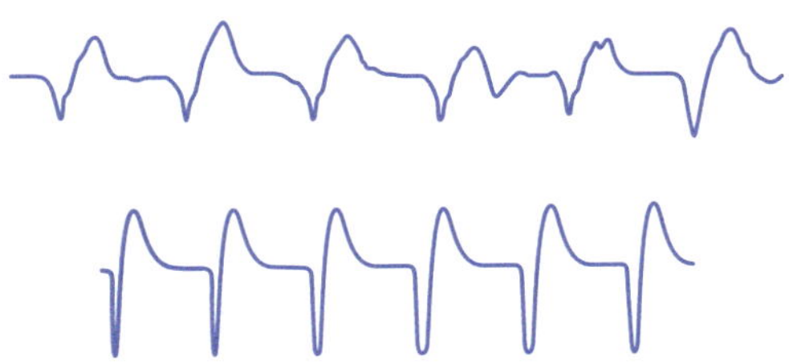

AIVR Treatment

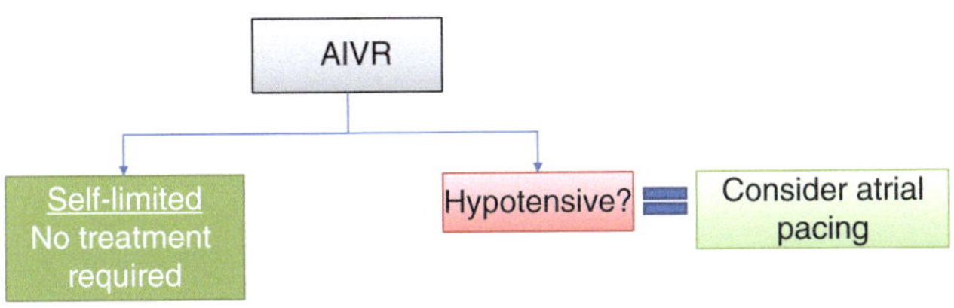

Complications in AMI

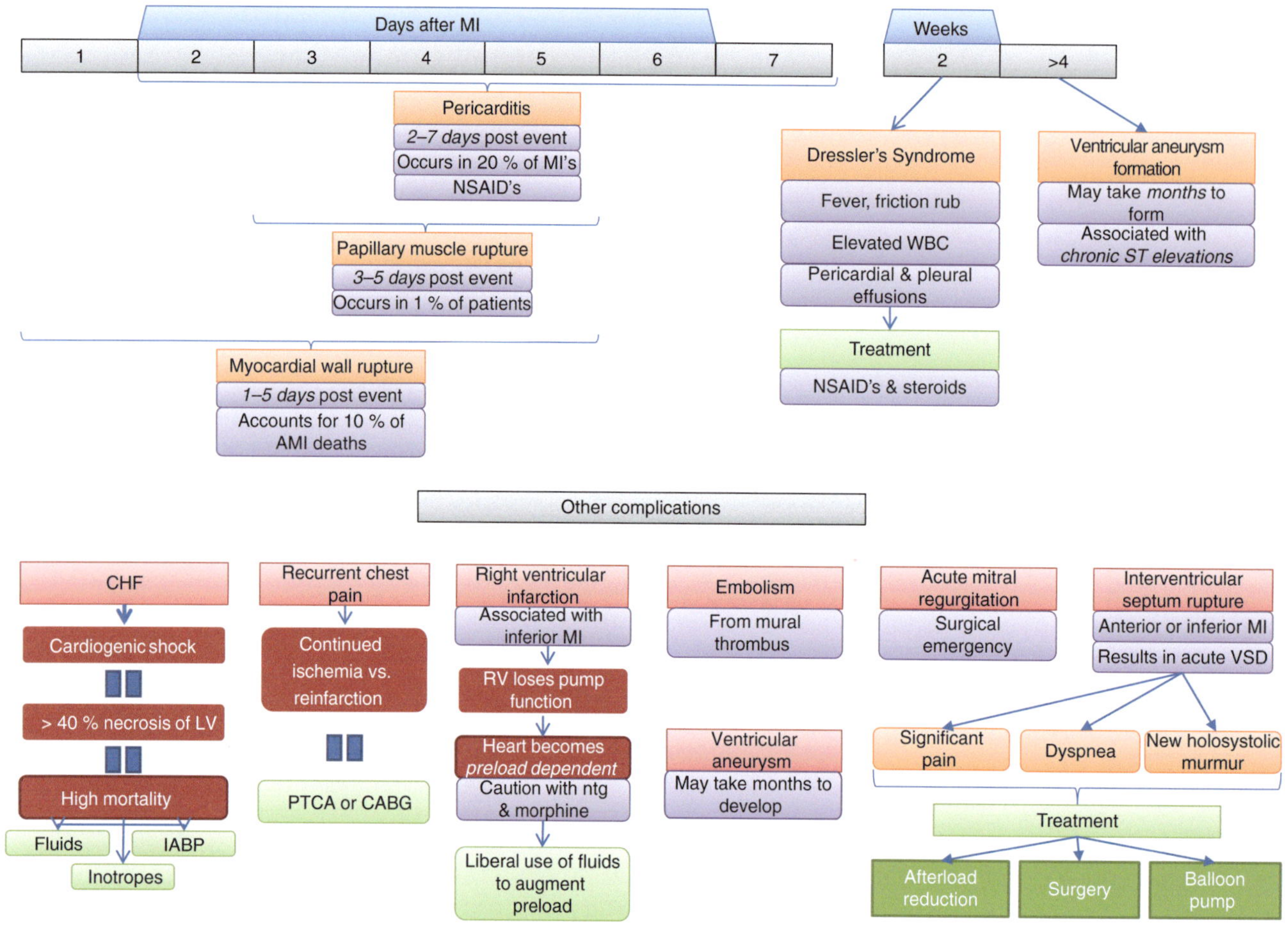

What Factors Predict Ventricular Aneurysm on EKG?

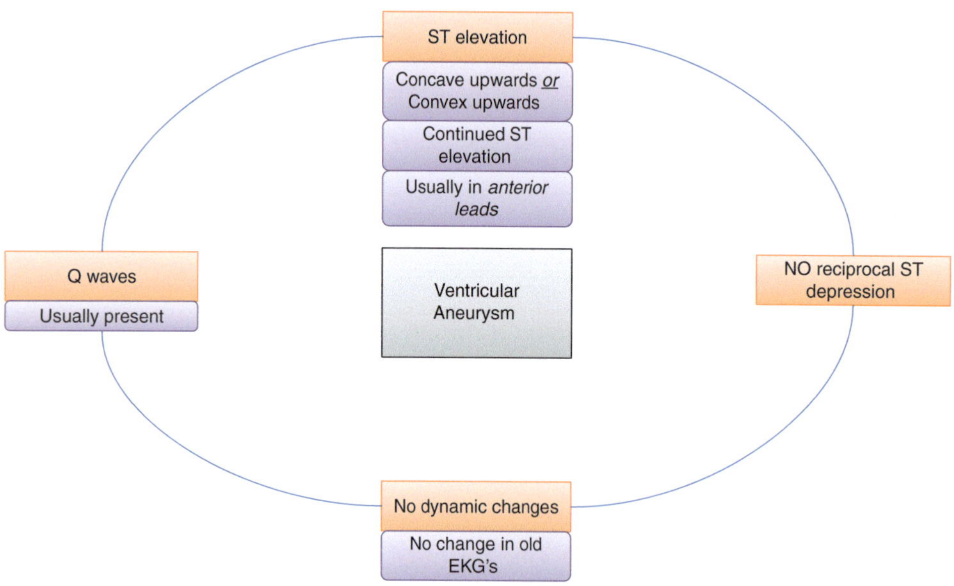

Rhythm Abnormalities in AMI

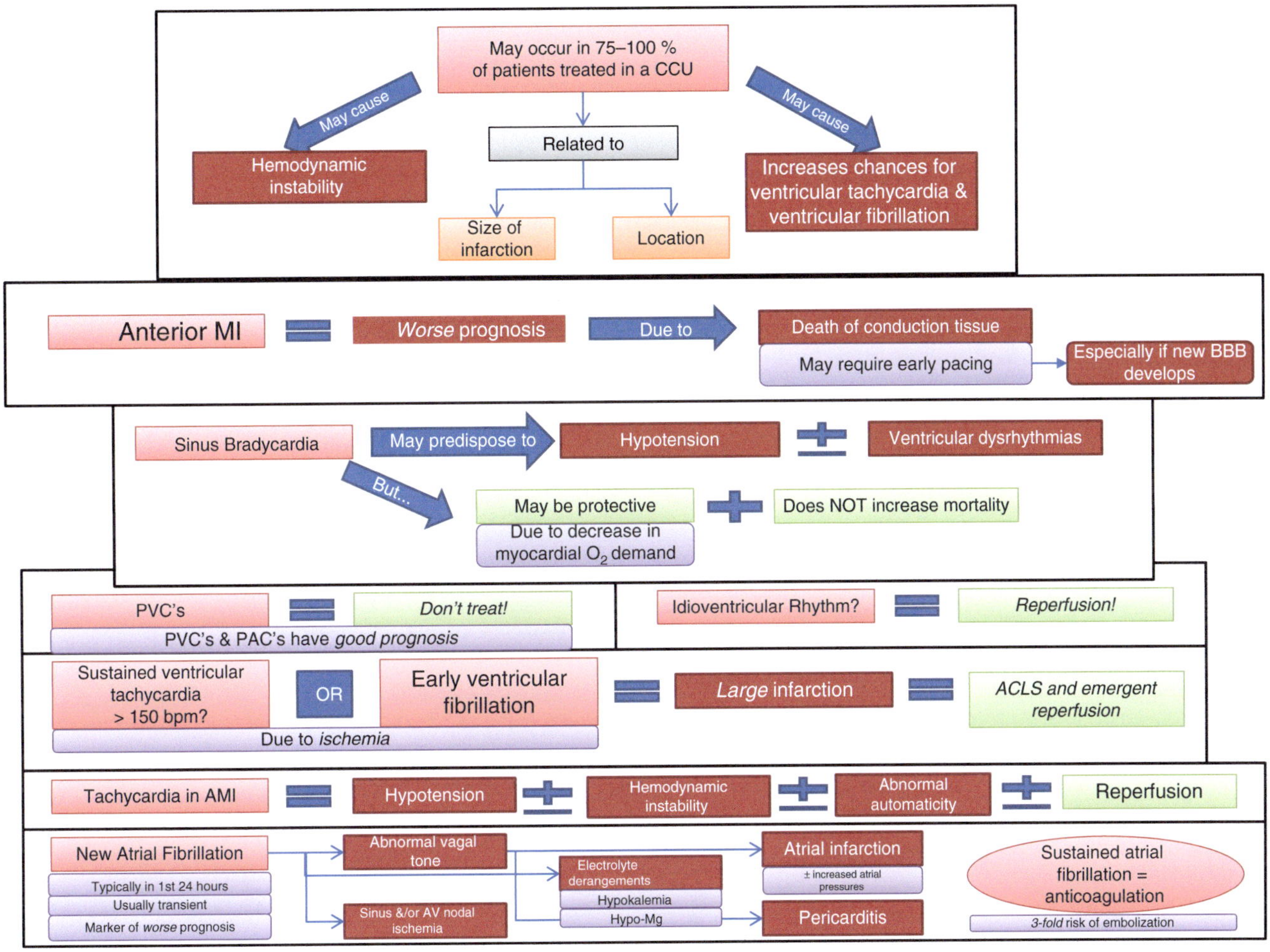

Conduction Disturbances in AMI

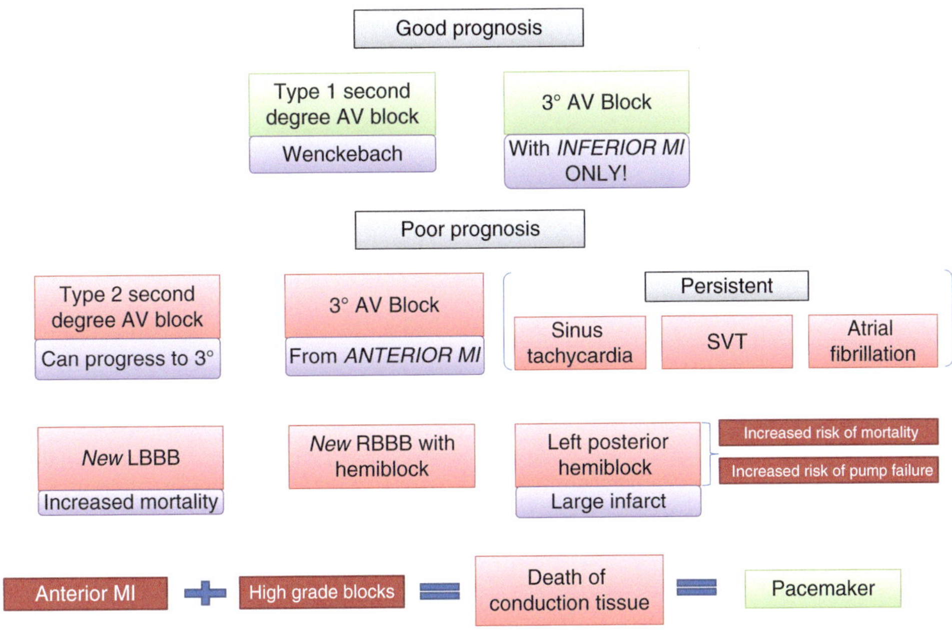

Congestive Heart Failure

Heart Failure Pathophysiology

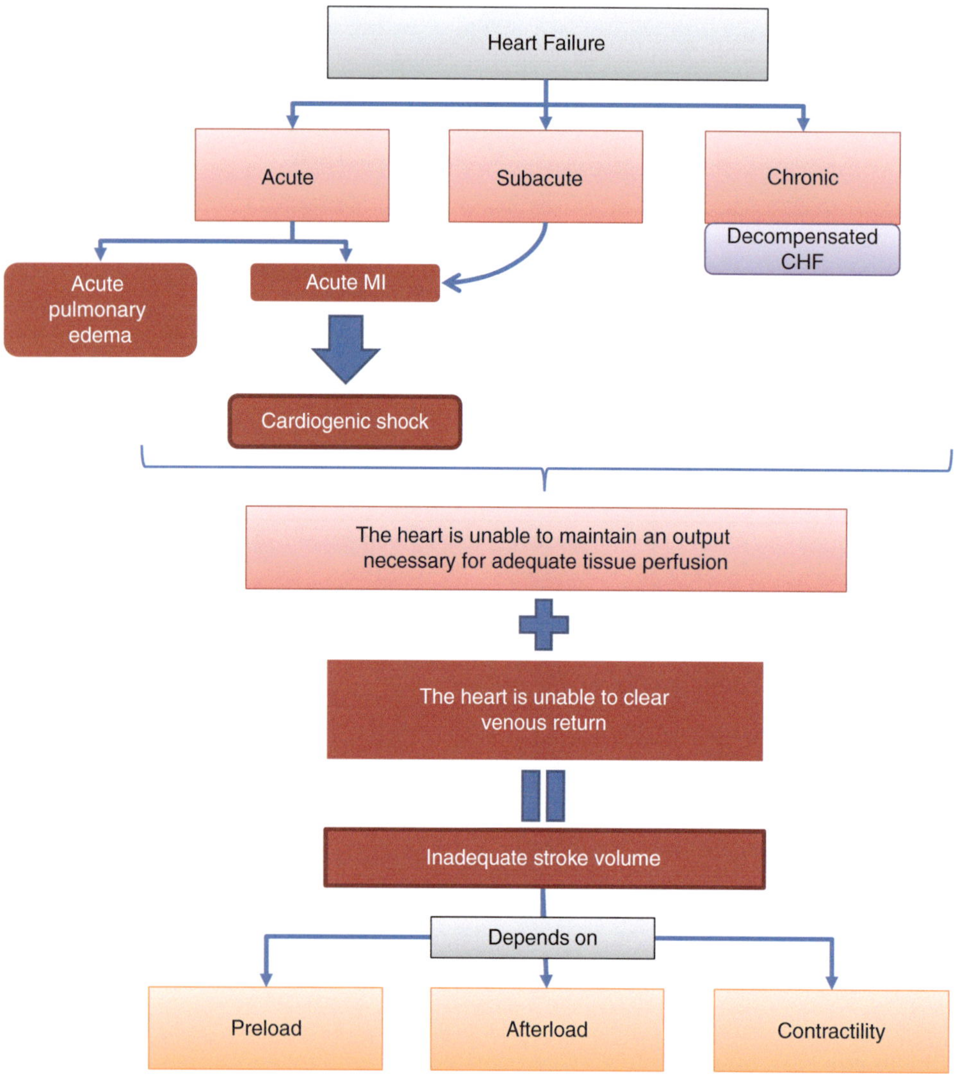

Causes of Heart Failure

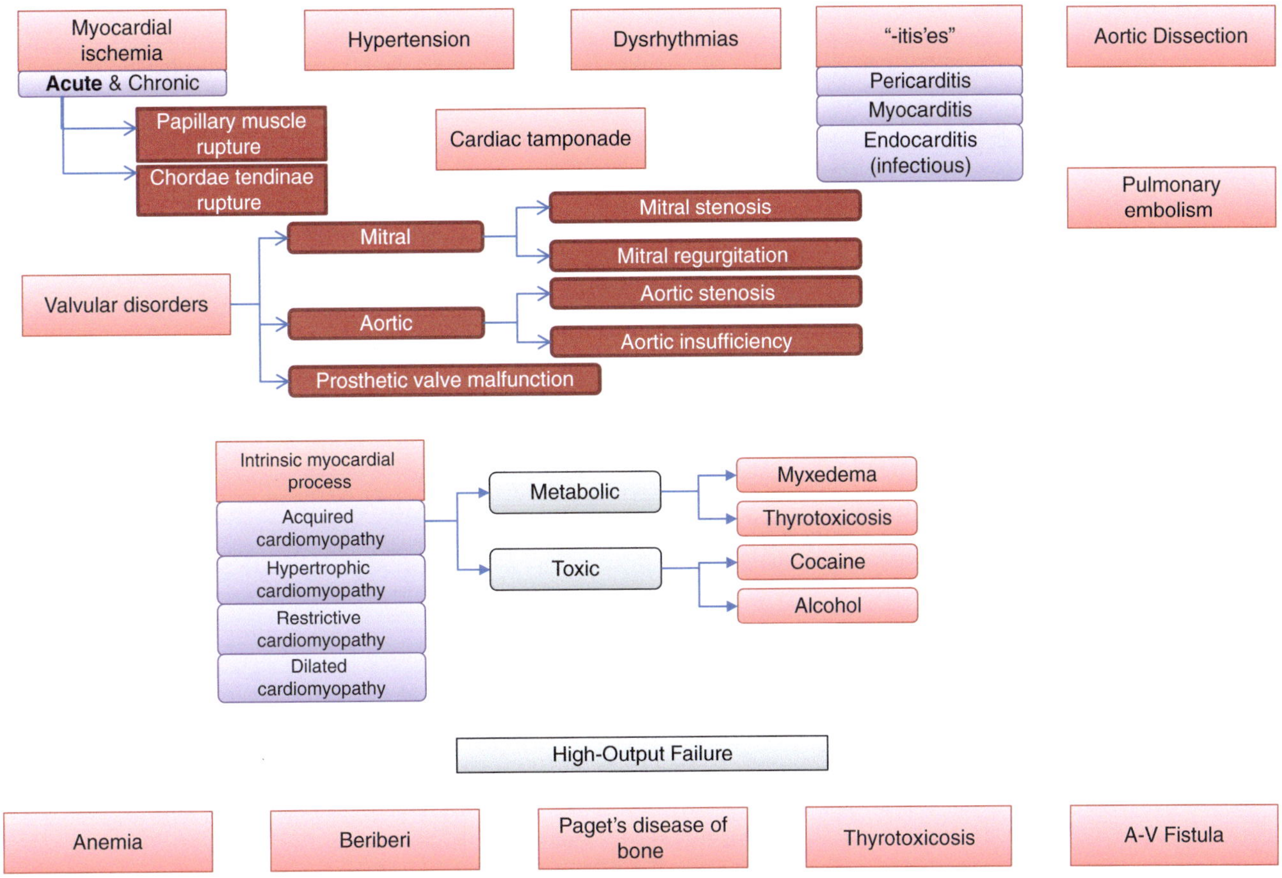

Systolic Heart Failure (Heart Failure Reduced Ejection Fraction)

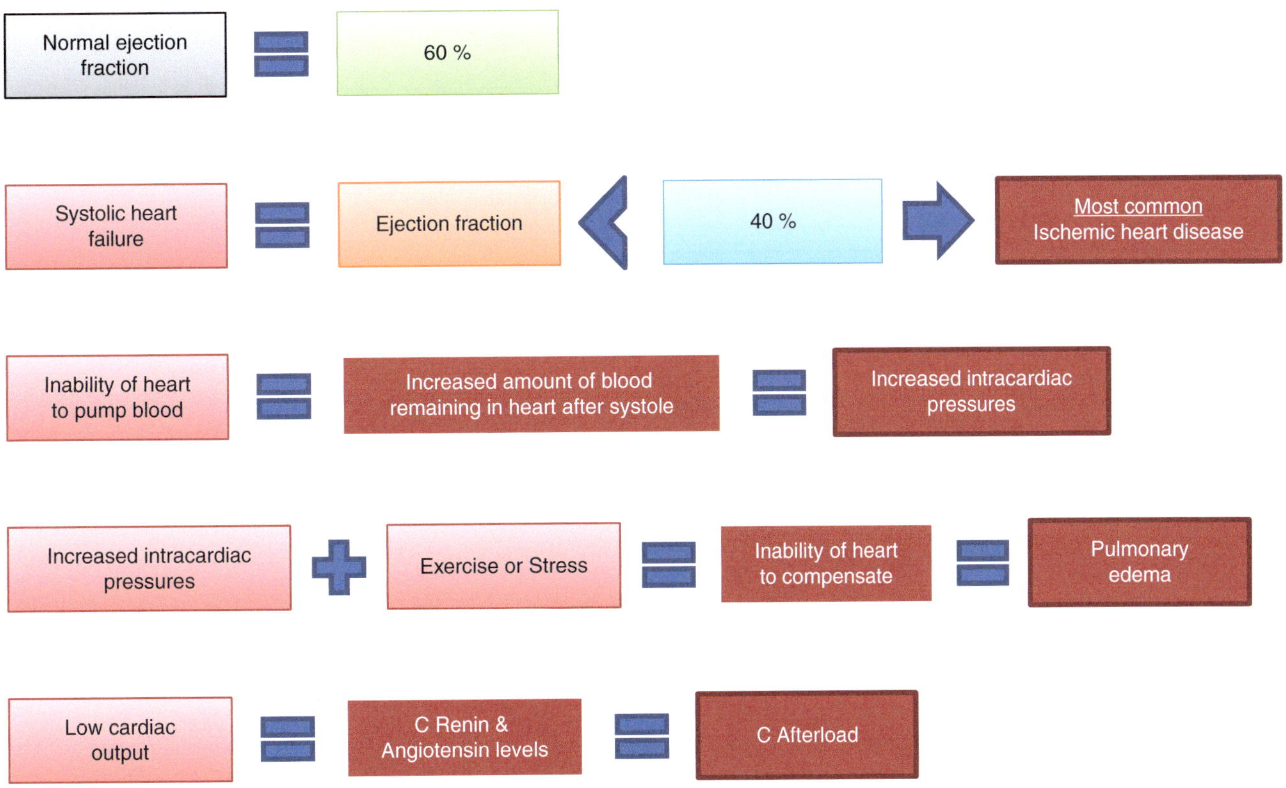

Diastolic Heart Failure (Heart Failure Preserved Ejection Fraction)

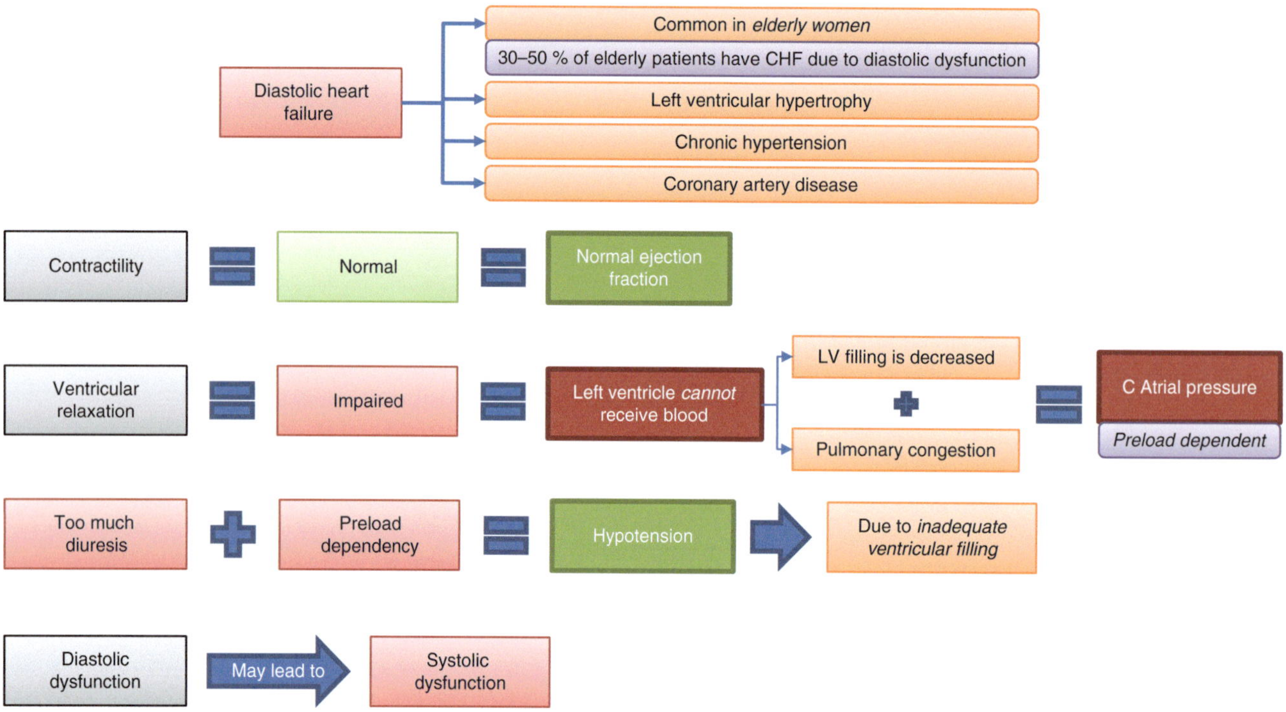

Left Versus Right Heart Failure

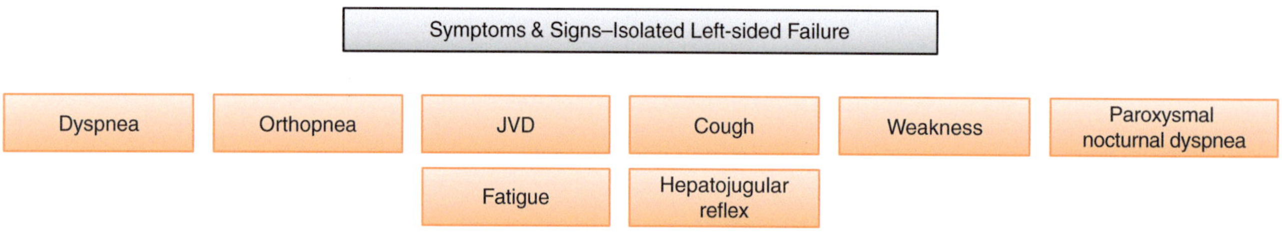

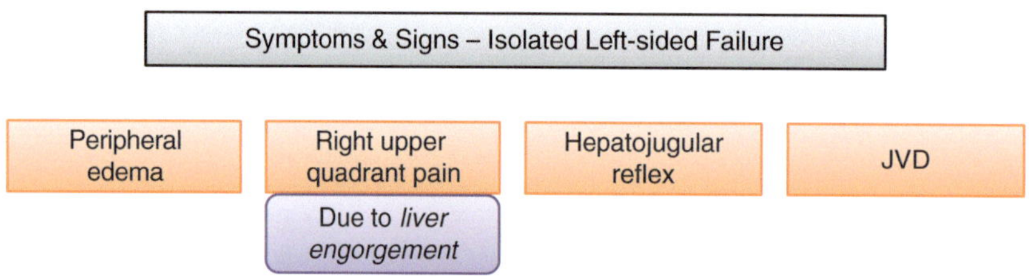

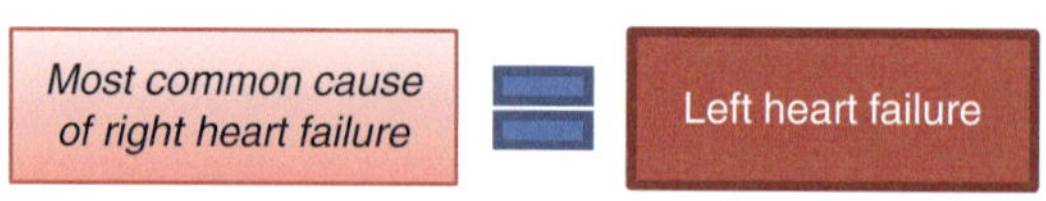

Heart Failure Clinical Features and Presentation

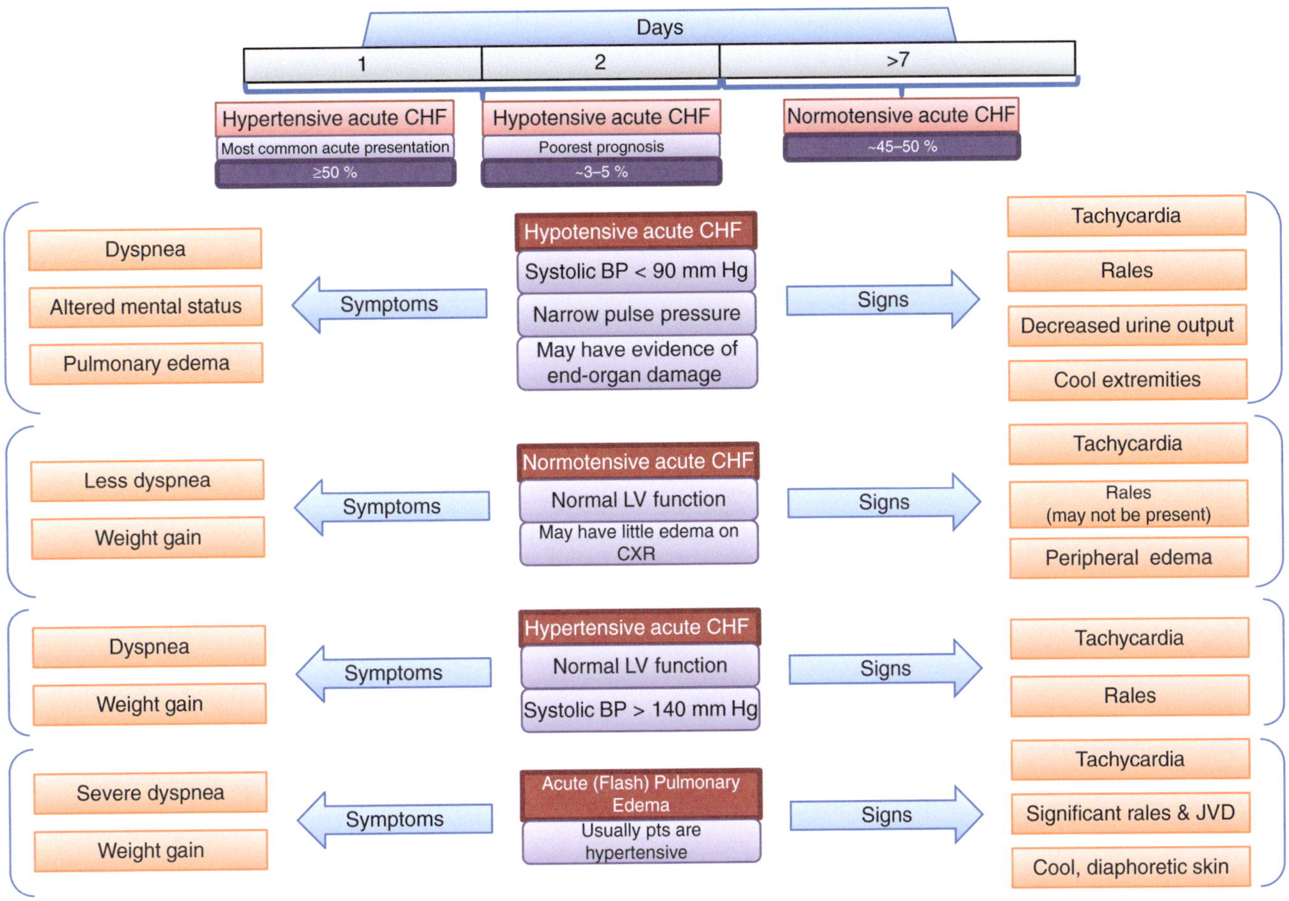

CHF Diagnosis

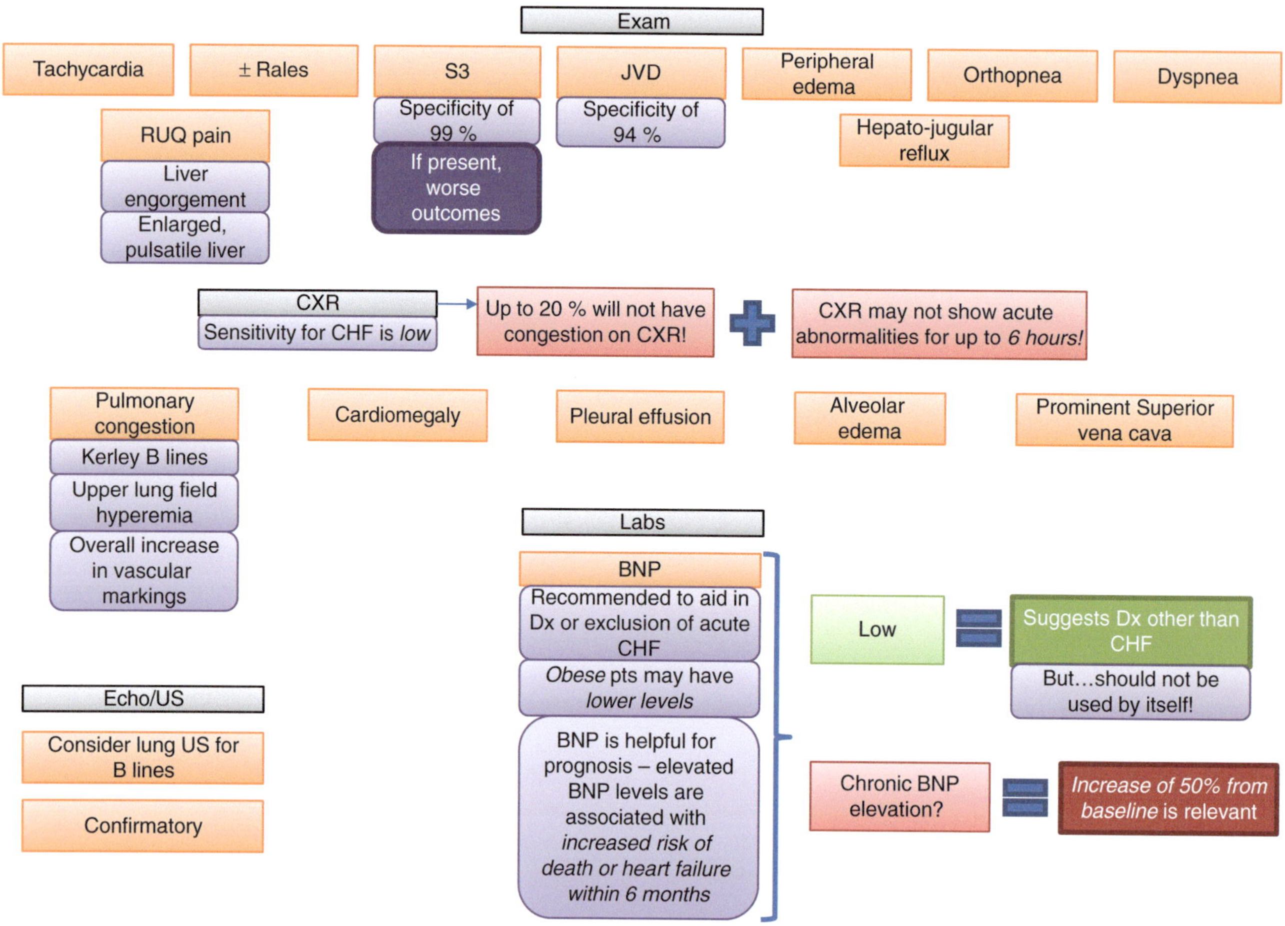

CHF Treatment: General

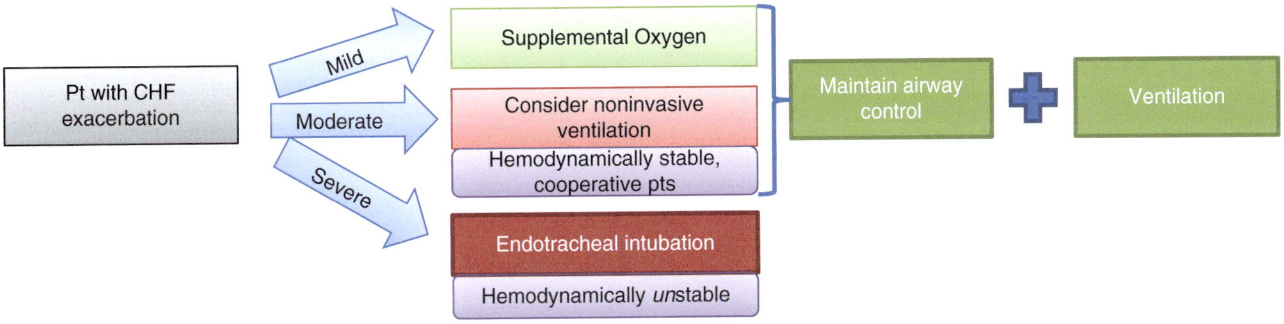

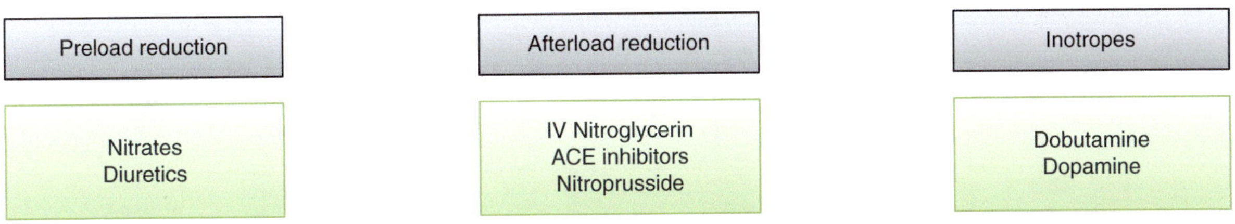

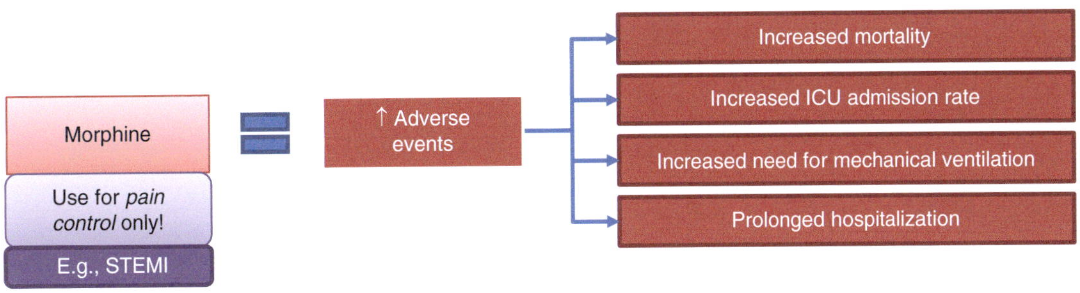

CHF Treatment: Specific

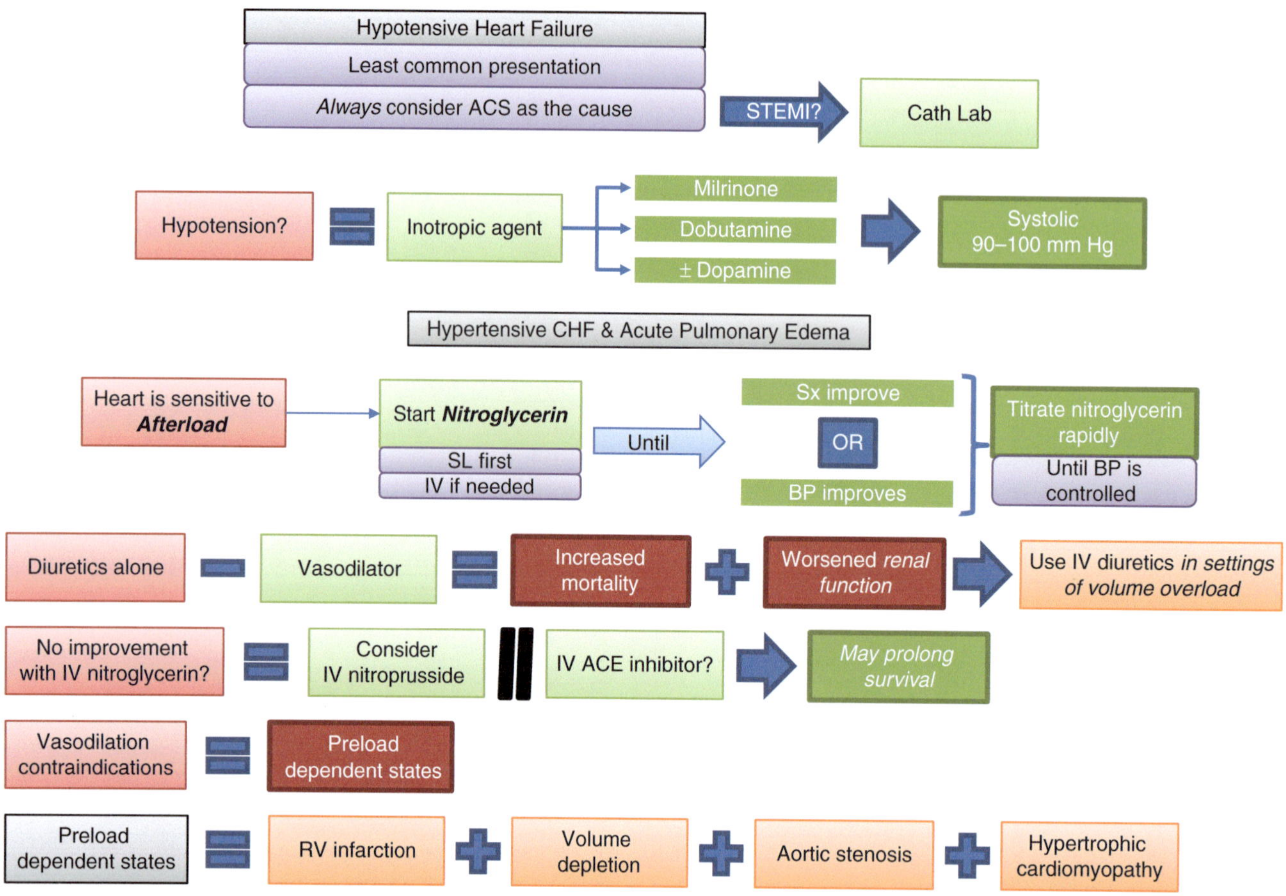

Non-cardiogenic Pulmonary Edema

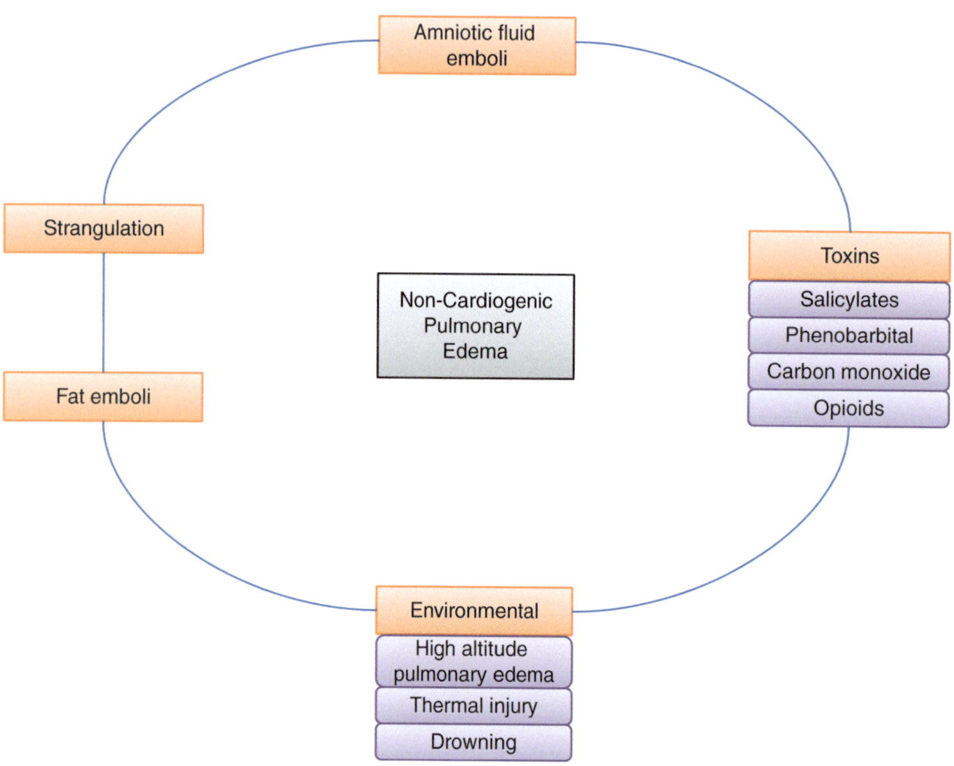

Valvular Emergencies

New Murmur

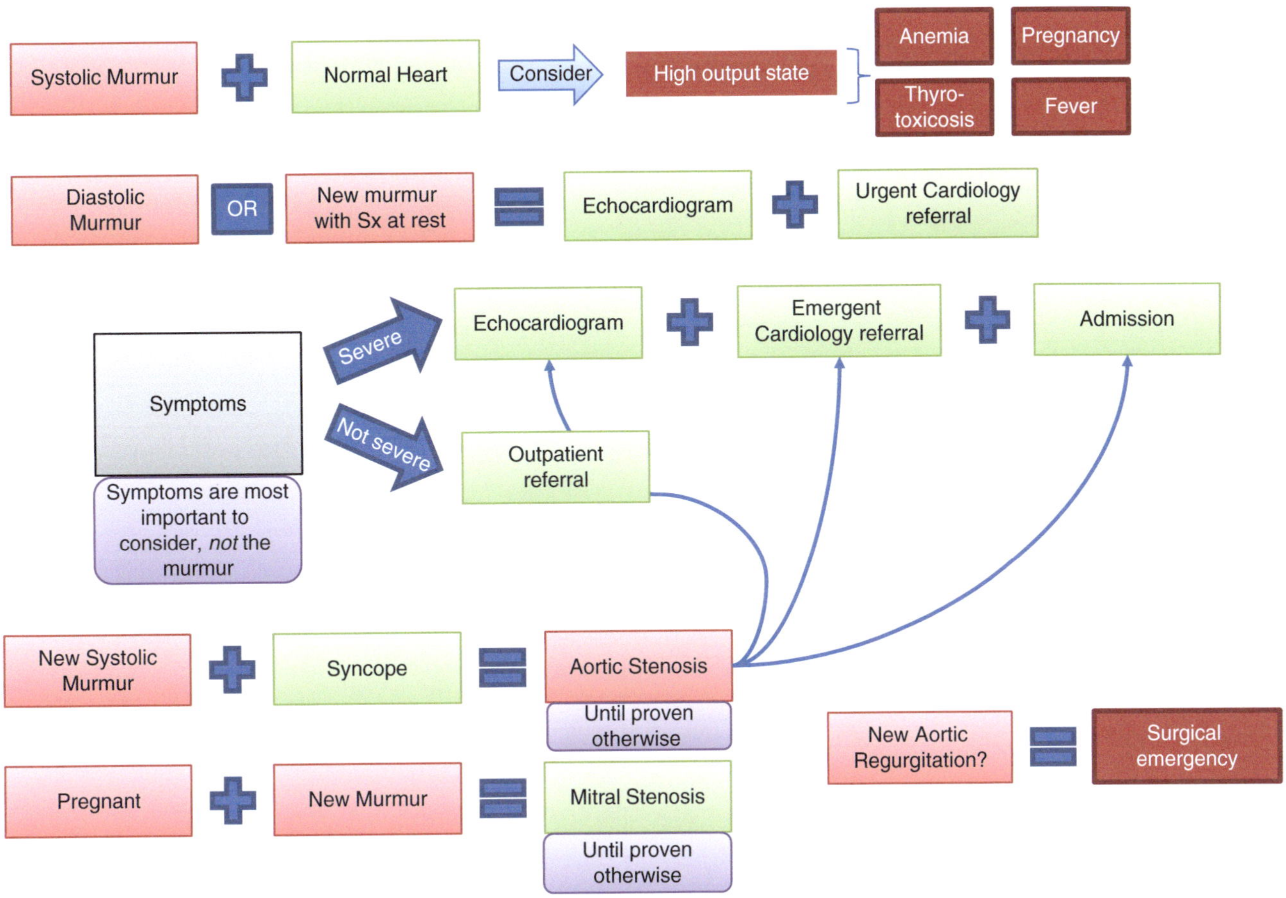

Mitral Stenosis

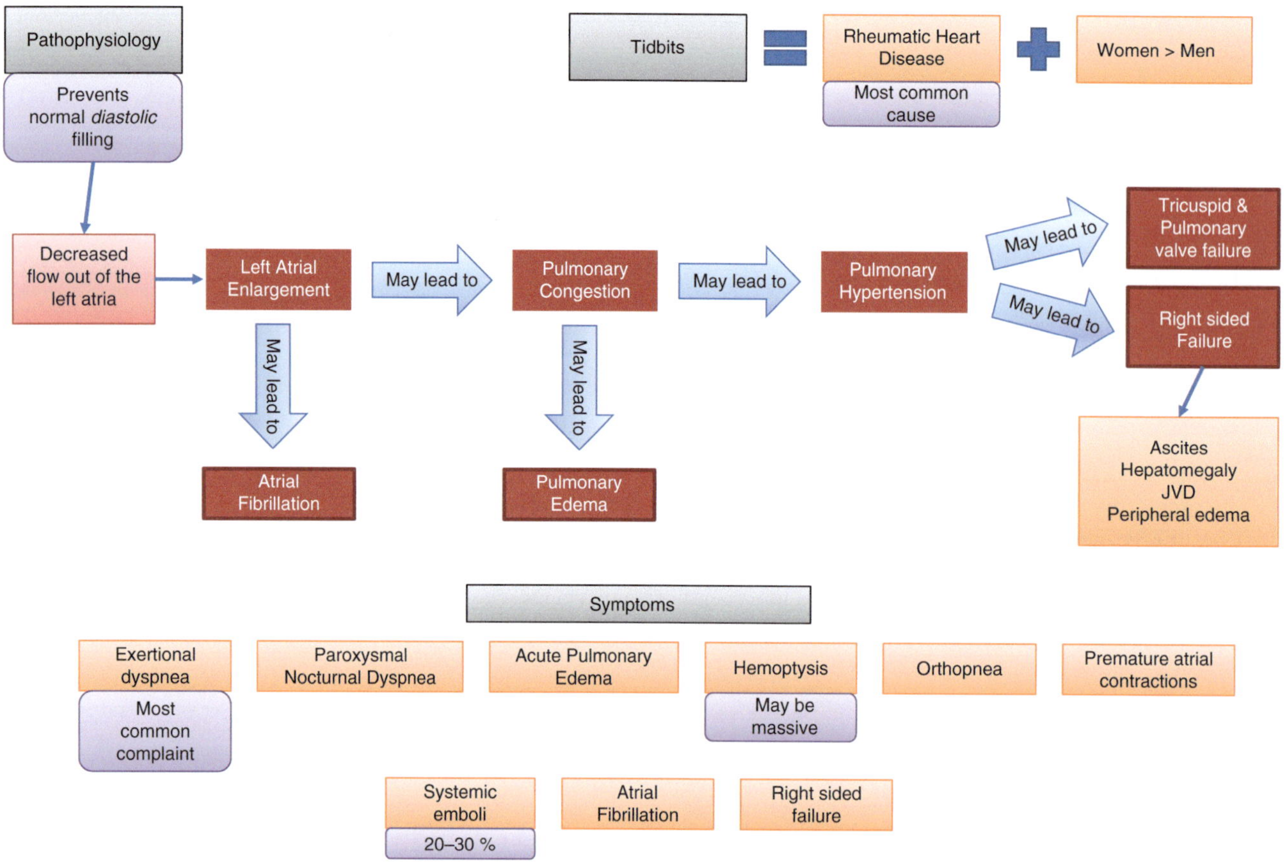

Mitral Stenosis Diagnosis

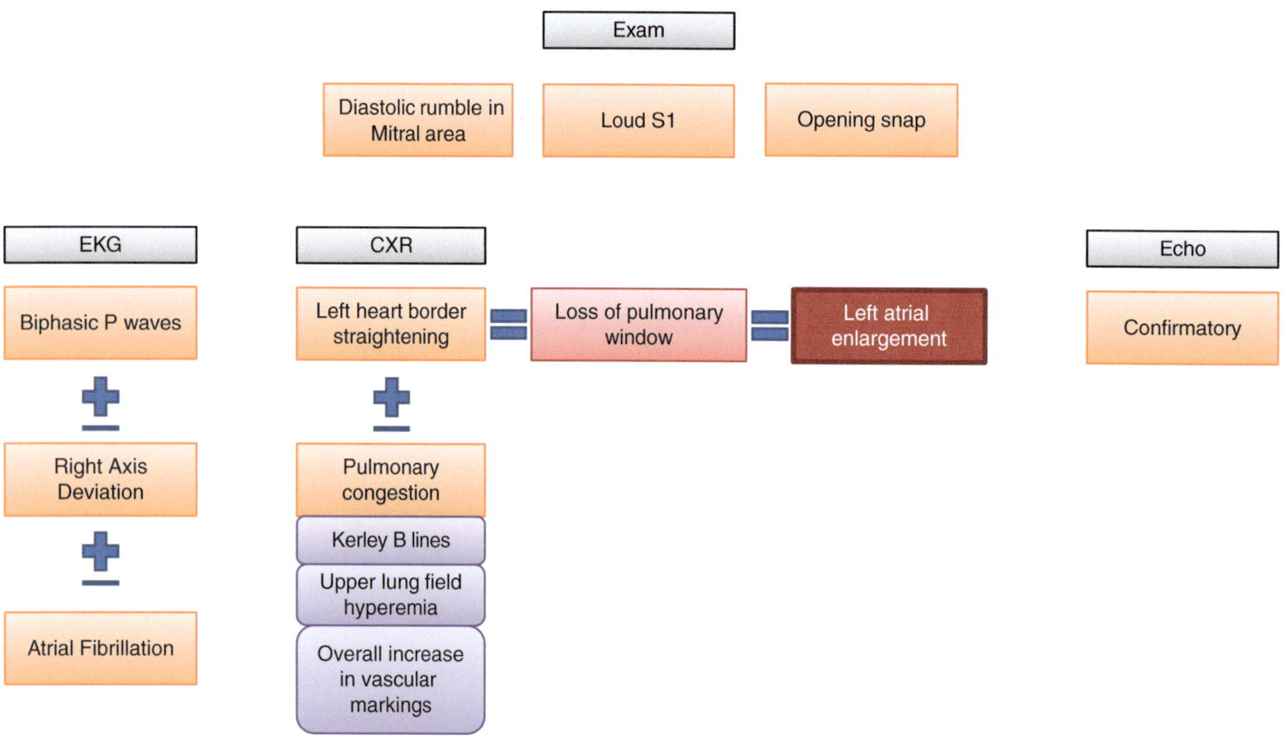

Mitral Stenosis Treatment

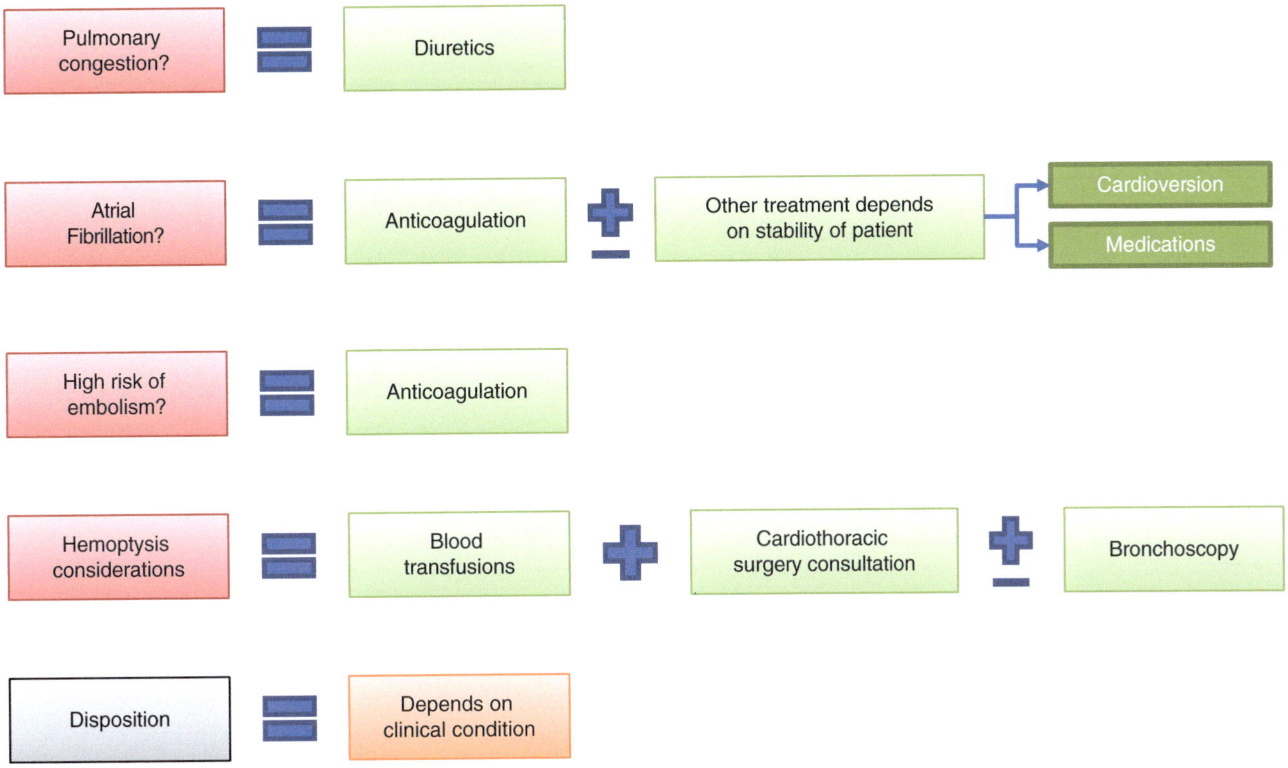

Mitral Regurgitation

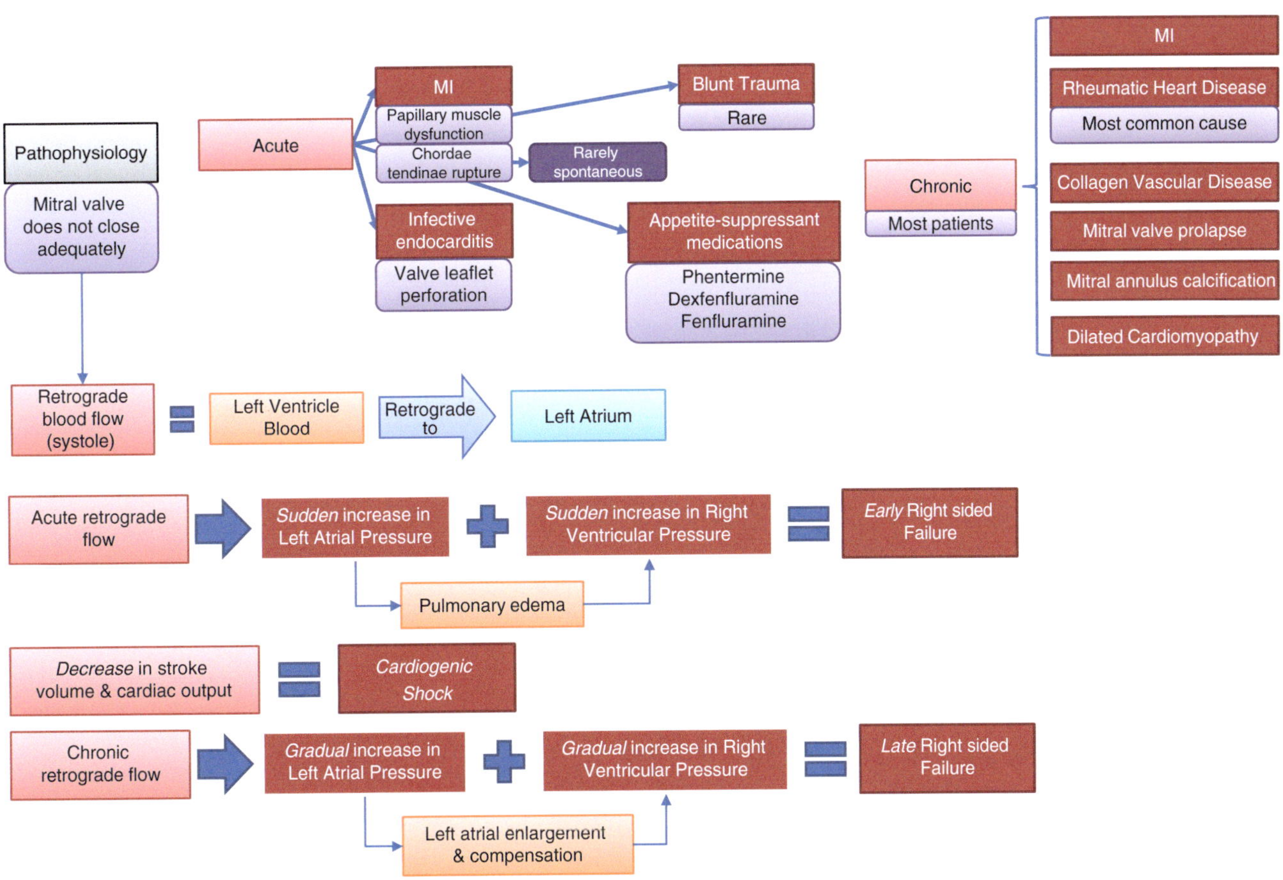

Mitral Regurgitation Symptoms

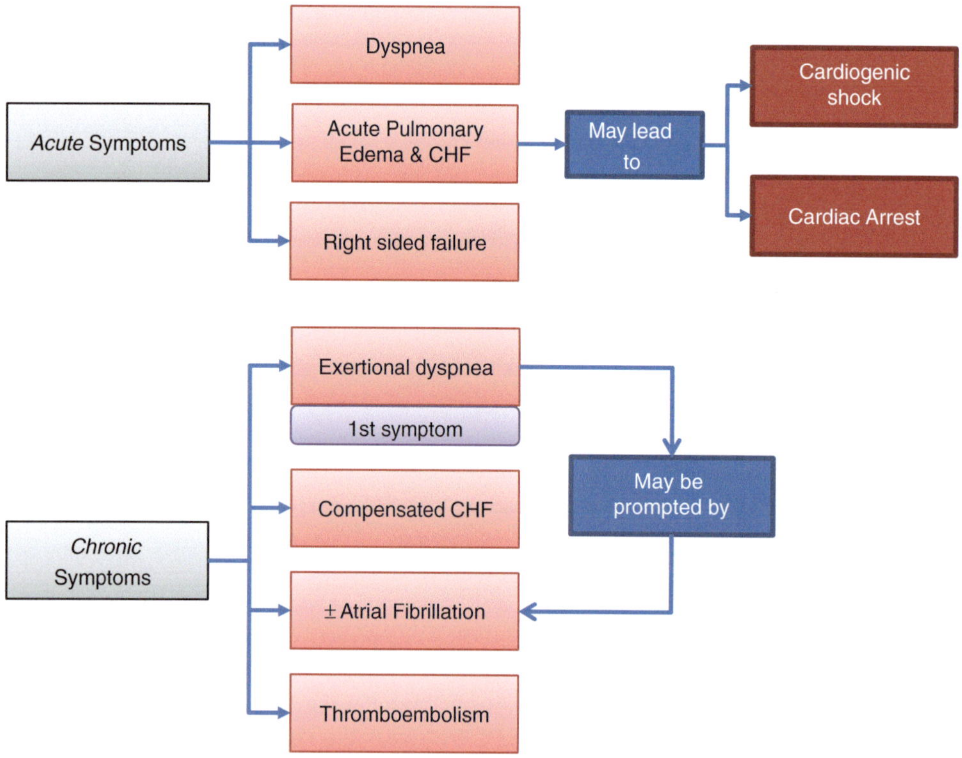

Mitral Regurgitation Diagnosis

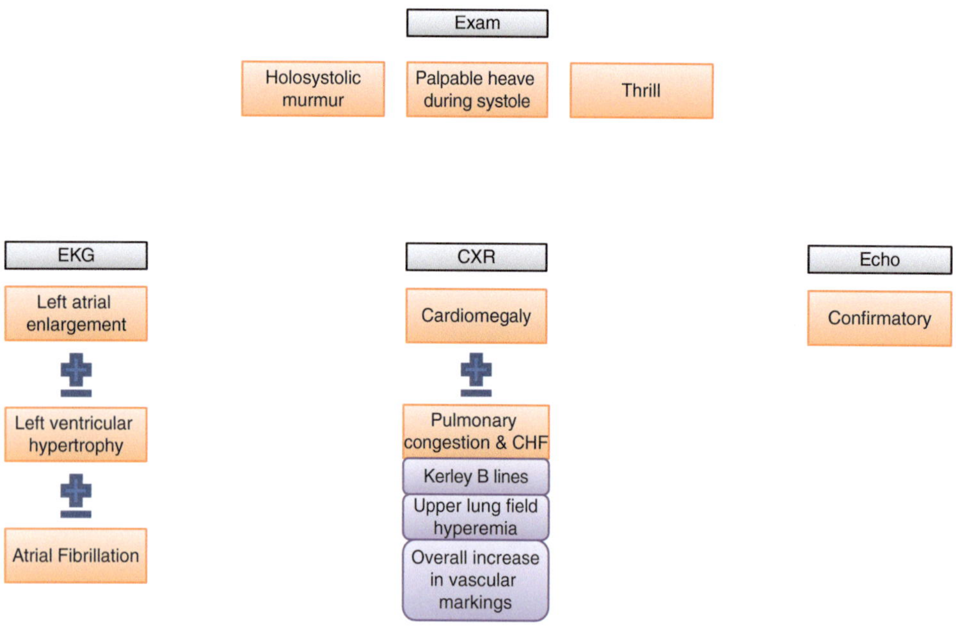

Mitral Regurgitation Treatment

Severe acute MR? = Afterload reduction + ICU admission + Balloon pump + Emergency surgery

Chronic MR? = Treat CHF + Treat Atrial Fibrillation → Disposition = Depends on clinical condition

New onset Atrial Fibrillation? = Anticoagulation ± Other treatment depends on stability of patient → Cardioversion / Medications

High risk of embolism? = Anticoagulation

Mitral Valve Prolapse

Mitral Valve Prolapse = Women > Men → The most common valvular disorder in developed countries → Most have no issues

Pathophysiology = Idiopathic myxomatous degeneration of mitral valve leaflets + Displacement of thickened leaflets into left atrium (During systole)

Higher rate of complications? = Male ± > 45 ± Mitral regurgitation

Pitfalls = There is a increased incidence of *arrhythmias* + There is a possibility of *thromboembolic disease*

Symptoms

- Most are asymptomatic
- Palpitations
- *Atypical* Chest Pain
- Dyspnea (Not exertional)
- Weakness
- Fatigue

Mitral Valve Prolapse Diagnosis

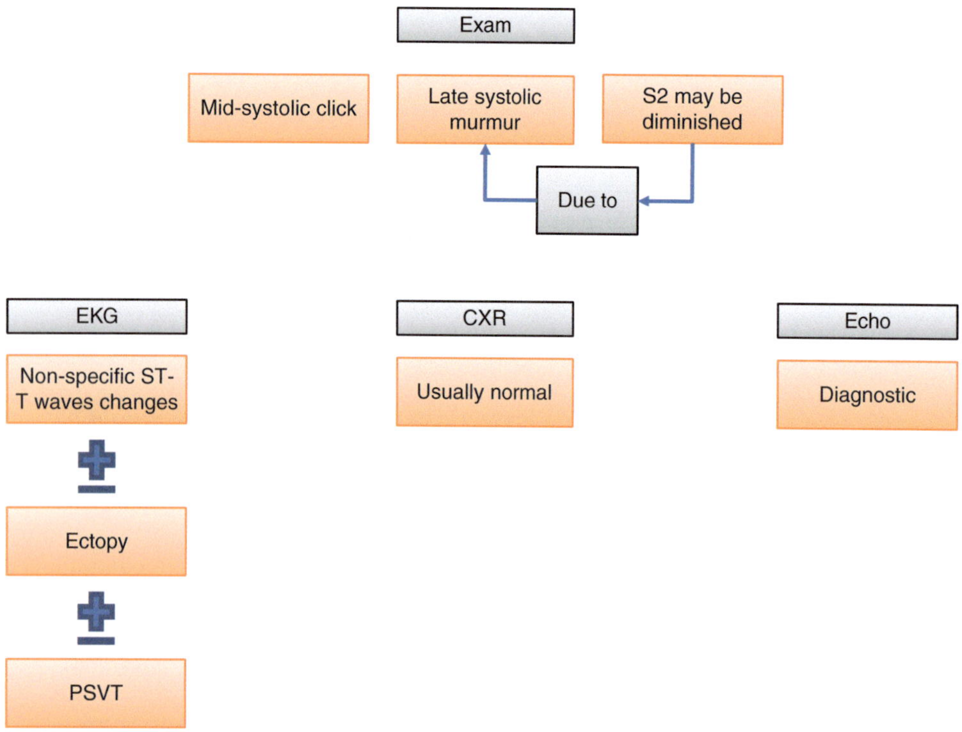

Mitral Valve Prolapse Treatment

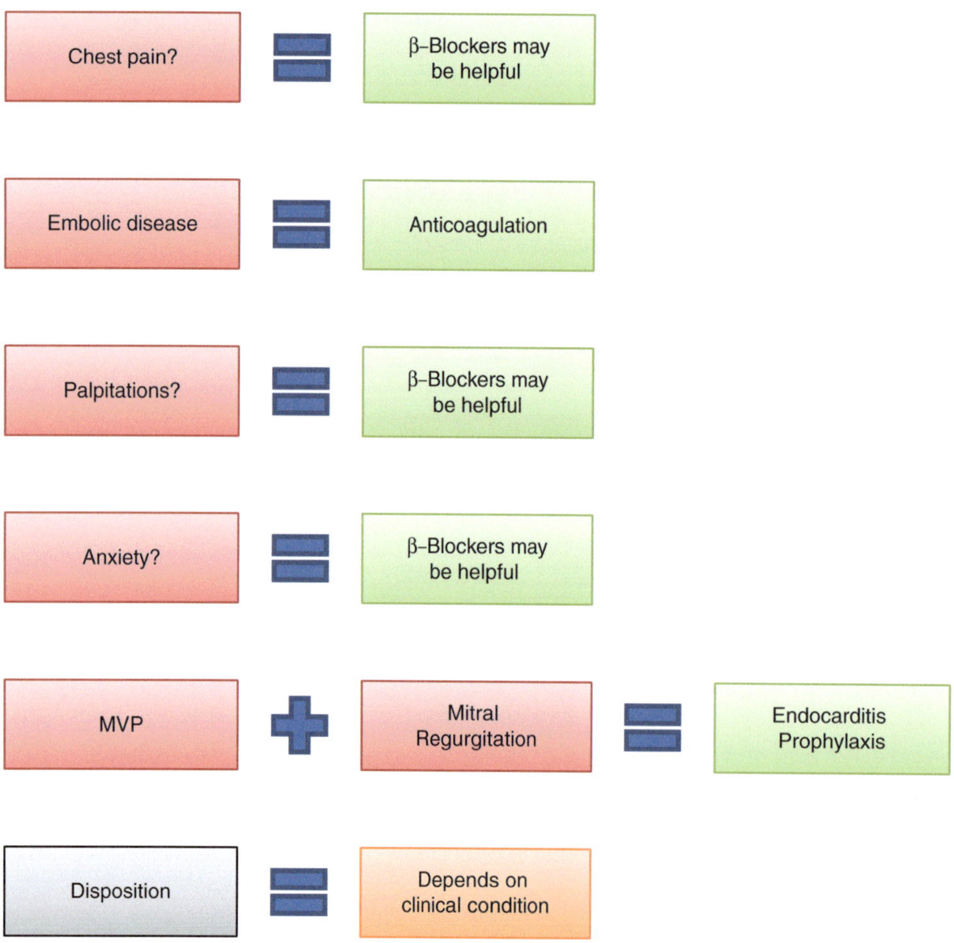

Aortic Stenosis

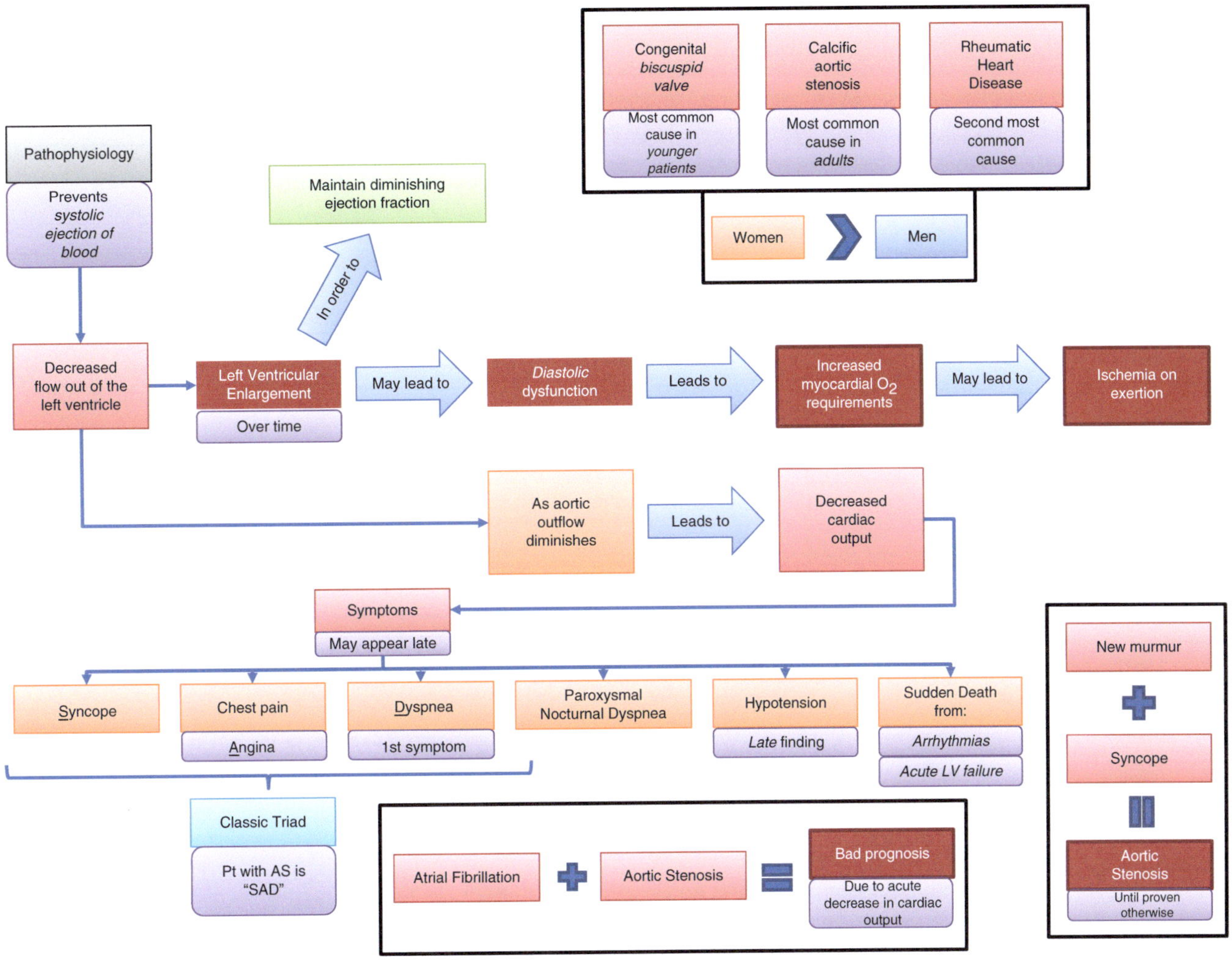

Aortic Stenosis Diagnosis

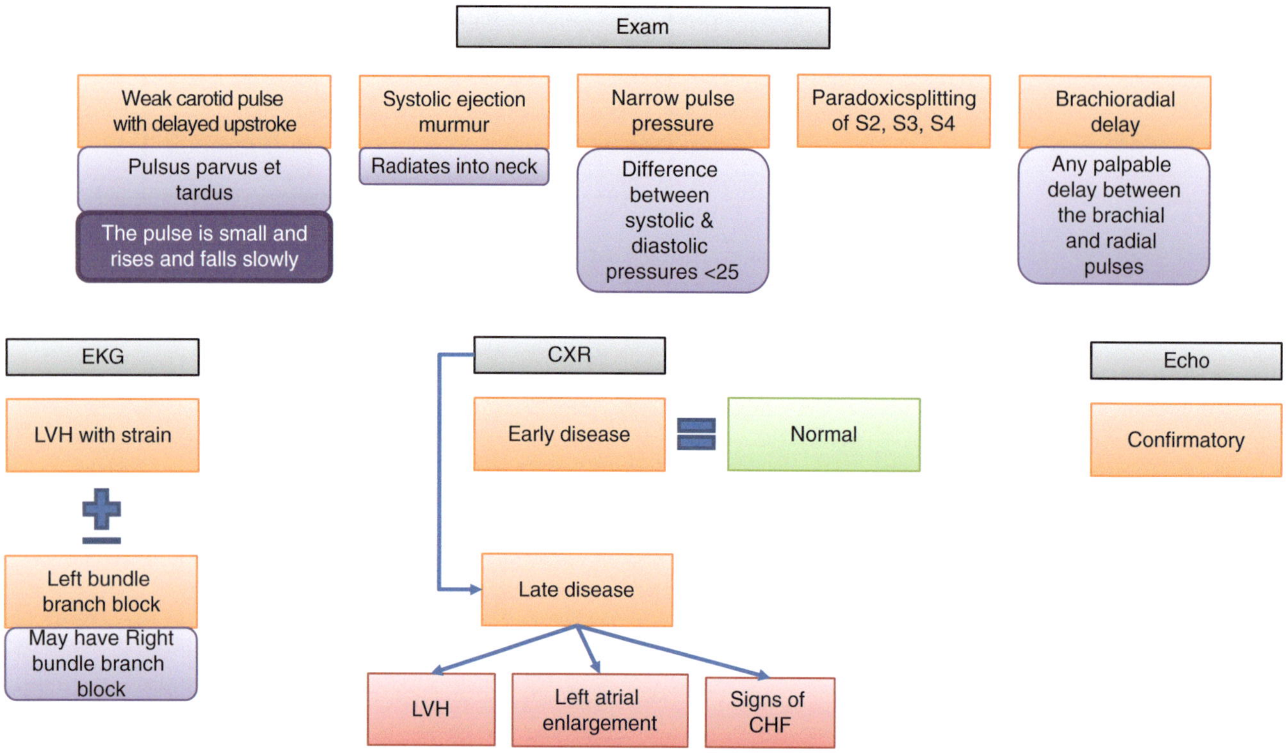

Aortic Stenosis Treatment

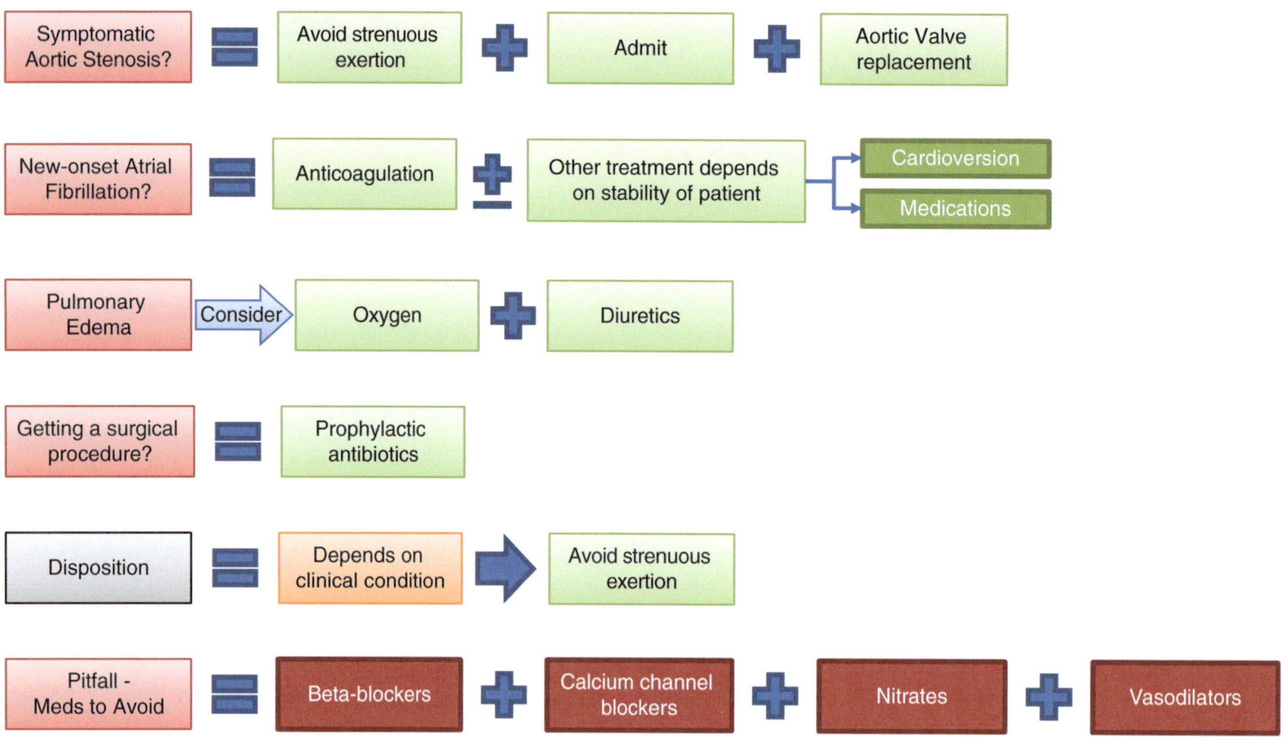

Causes of Aortic Regurgitation

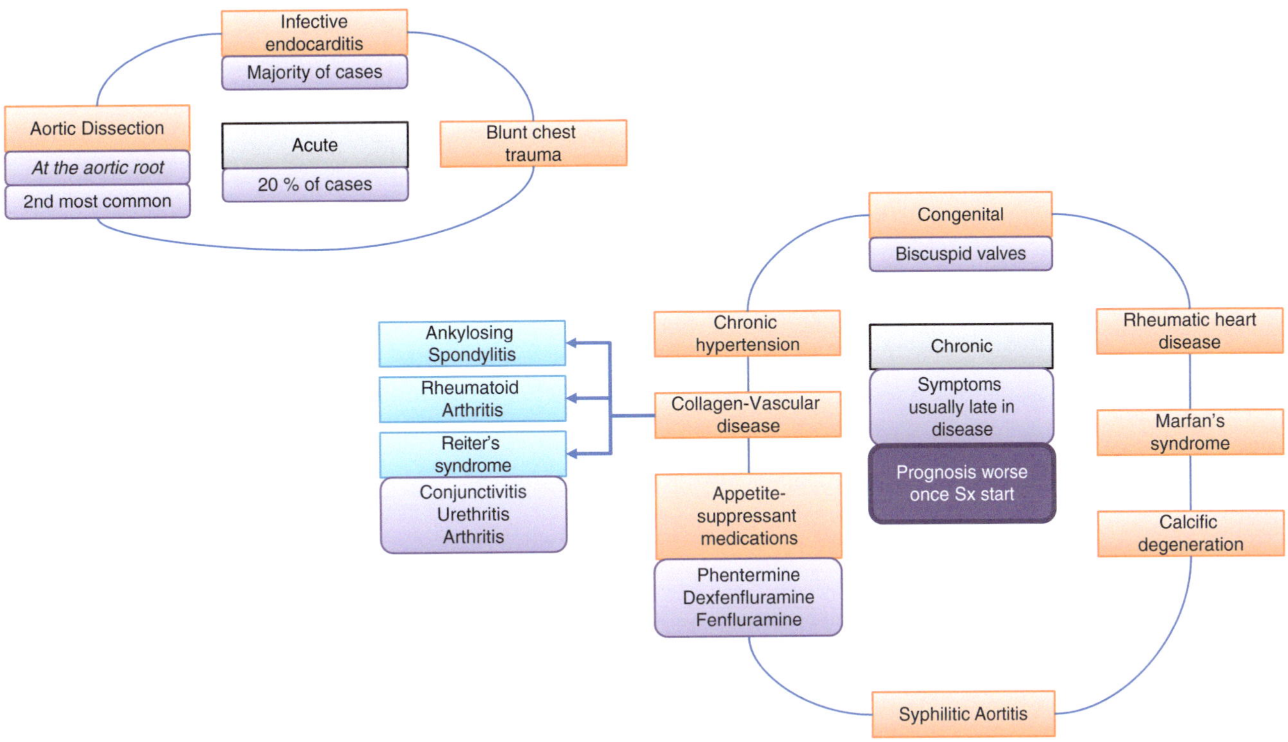

Aortic Regurgitation

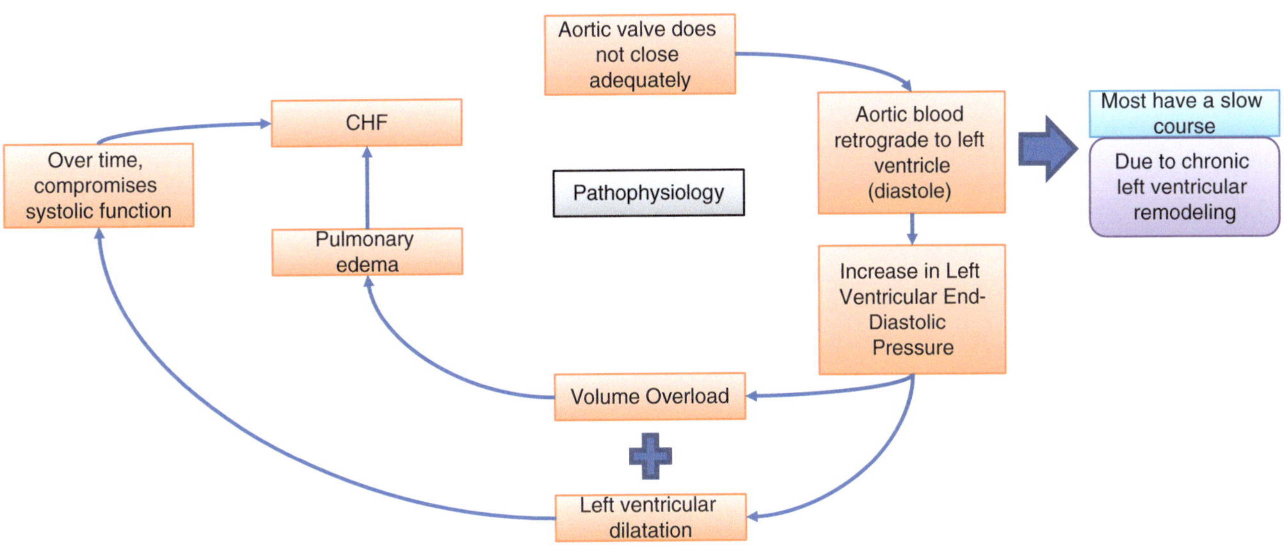

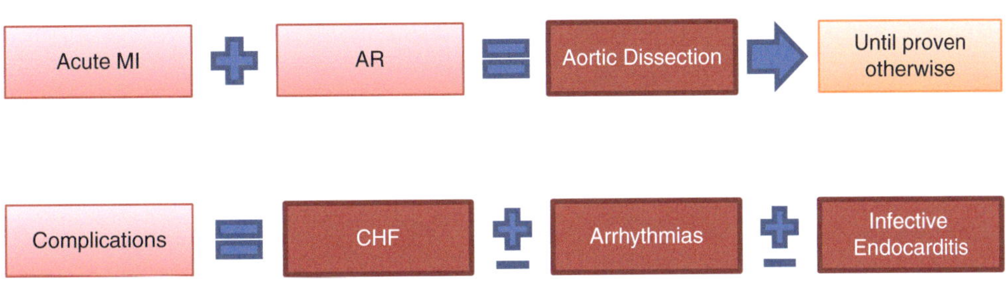

Aortic Regurgitation Symptoms

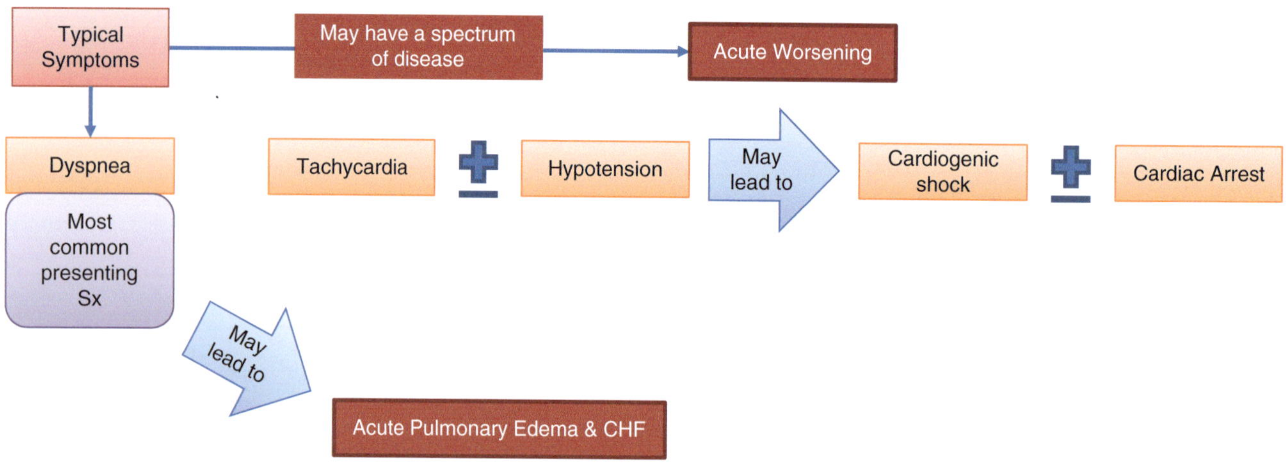

Aortic Regurgitation Diagnosis

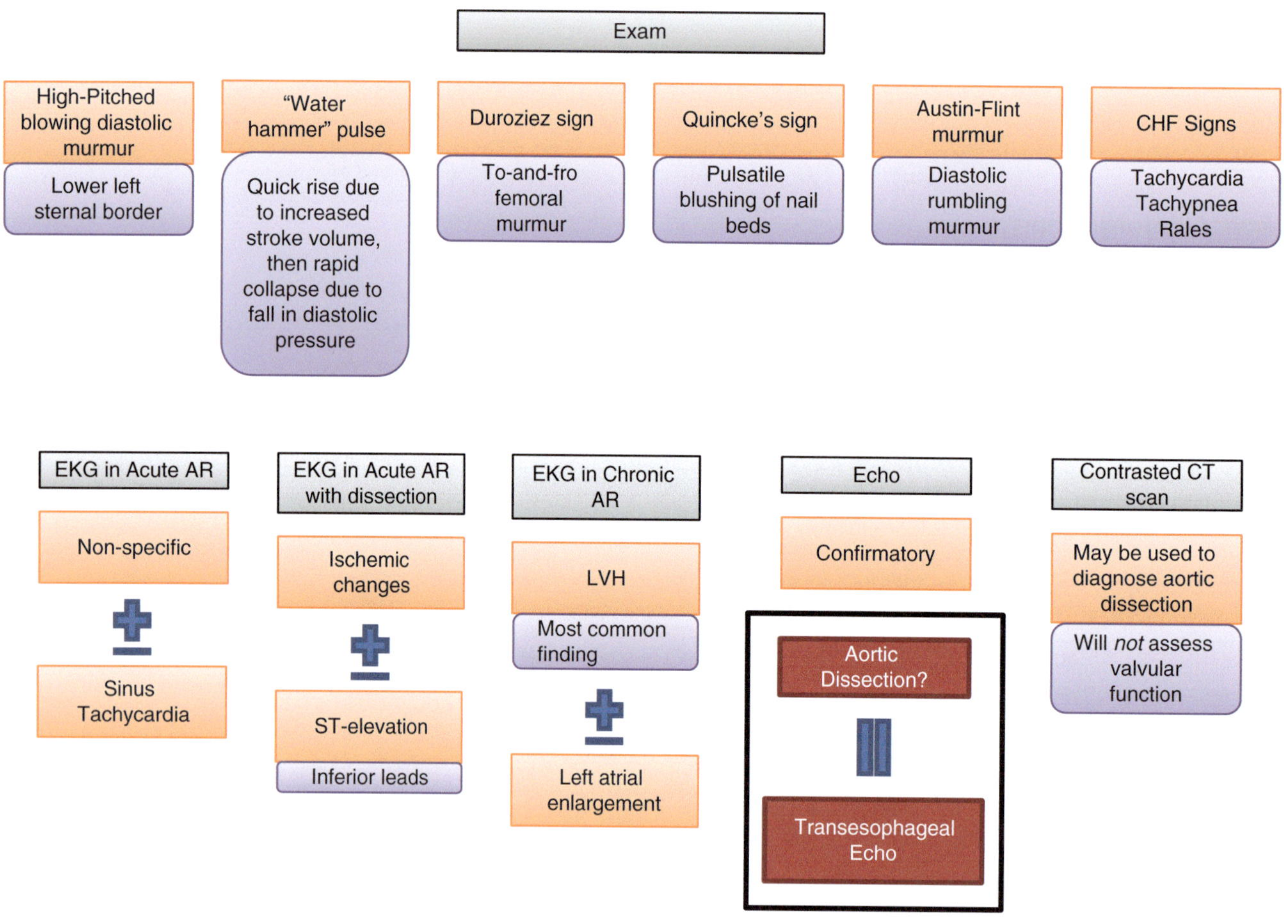

The CXR in Aortic Regurgitation

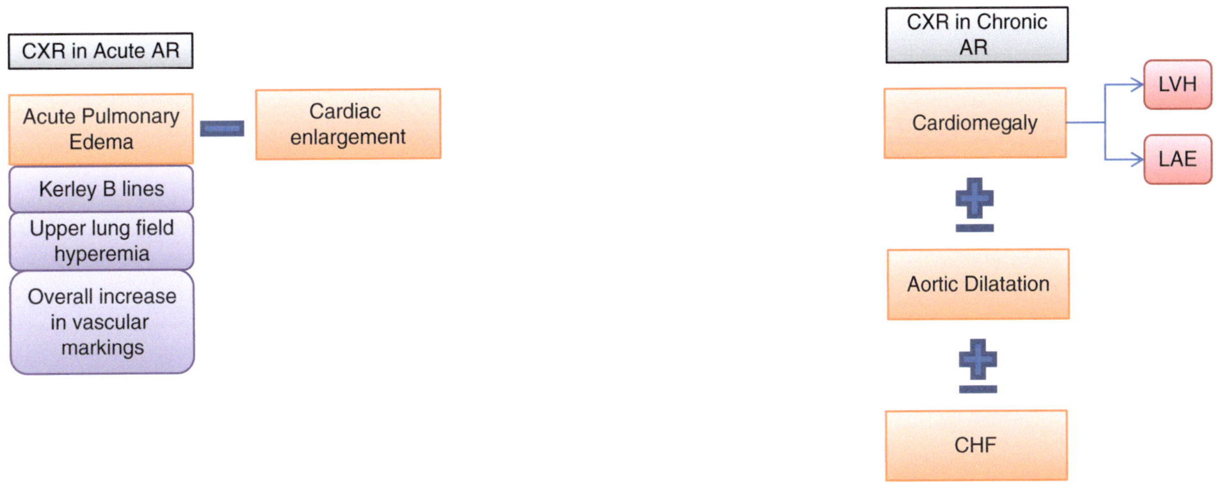

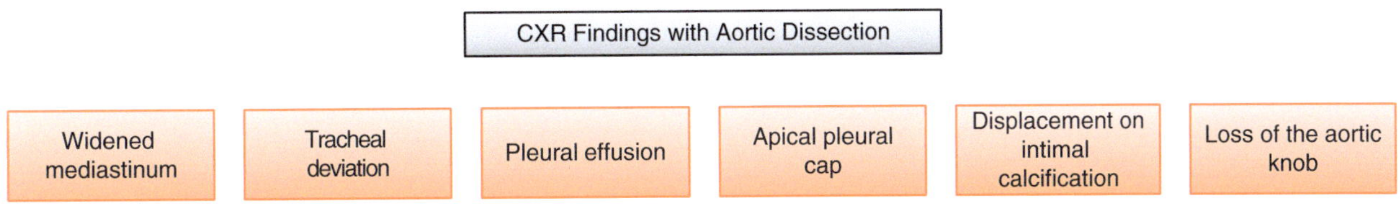

Aortic Regurgitation Treatment

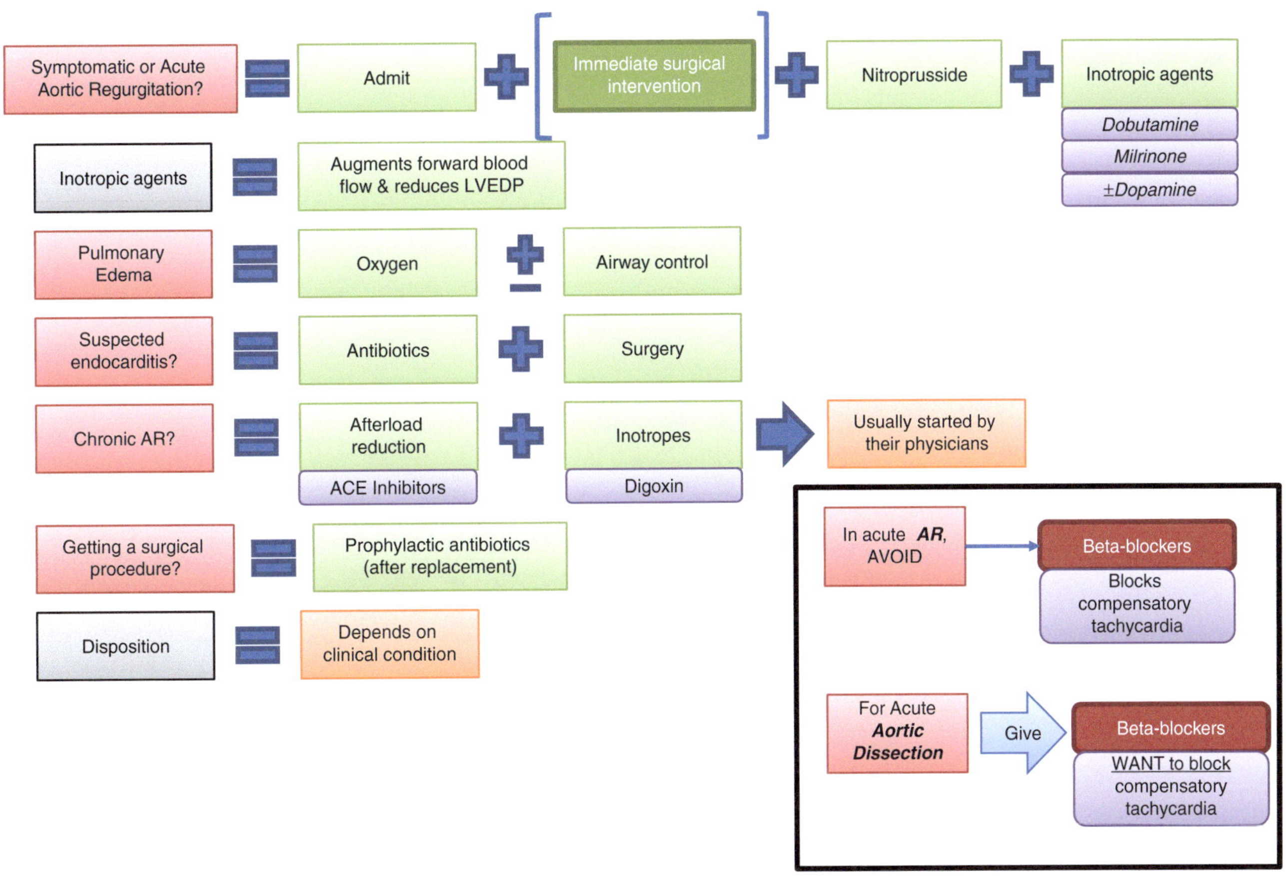

Infective Endocarditis

Introduction

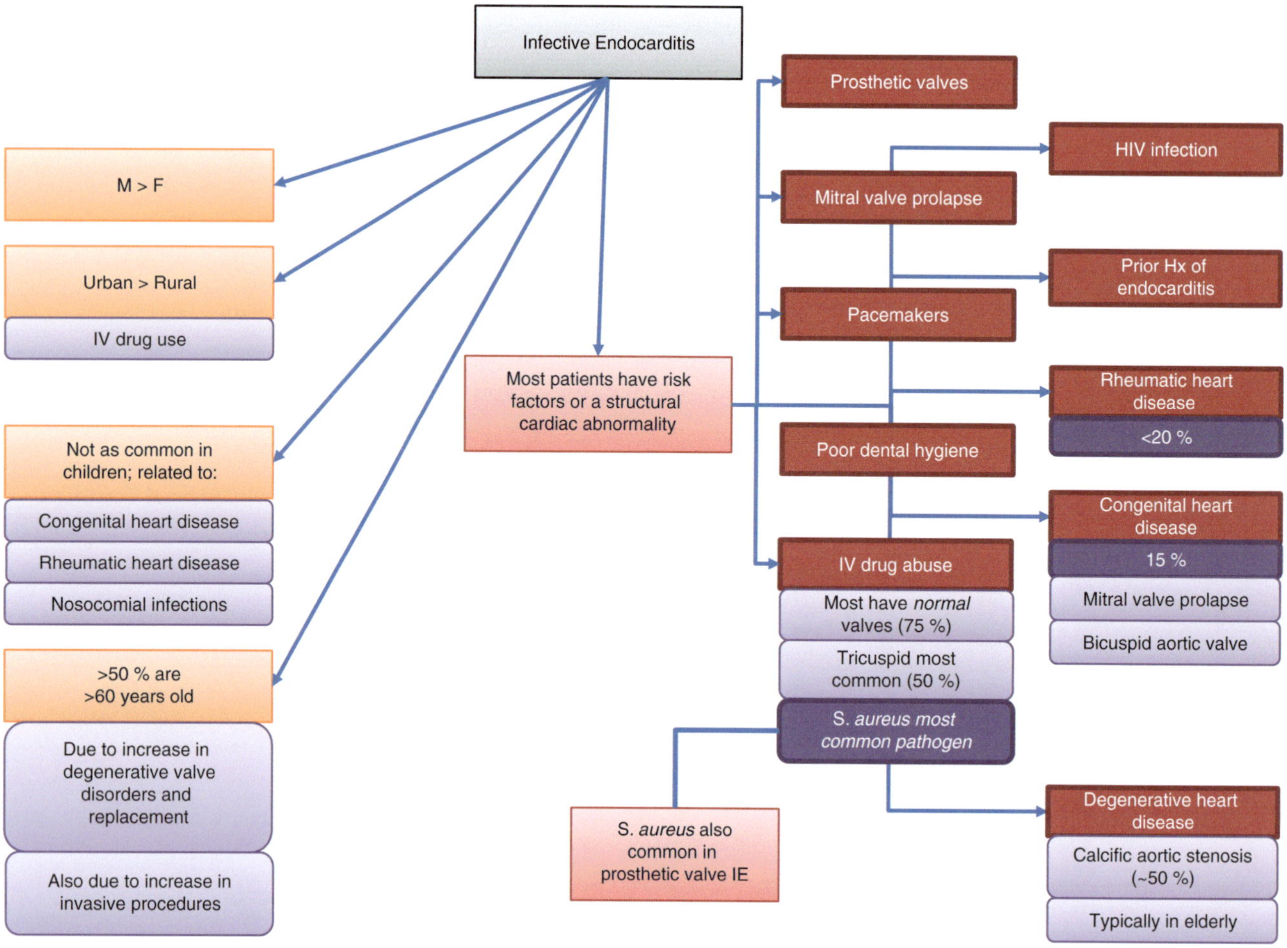

Introduction (2)

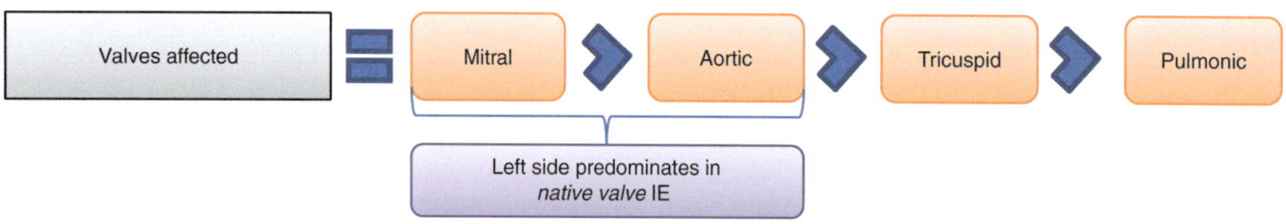

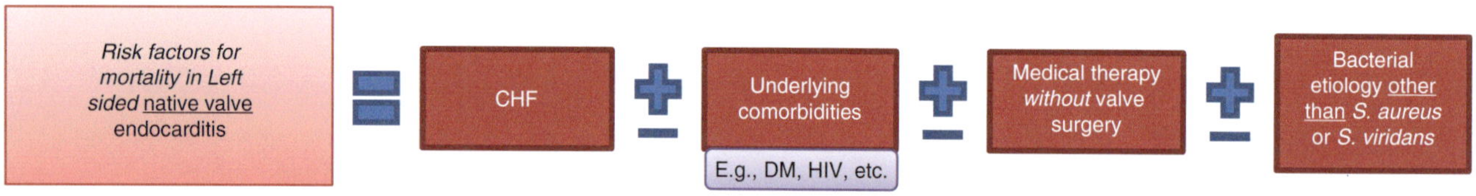

Pathophysiology

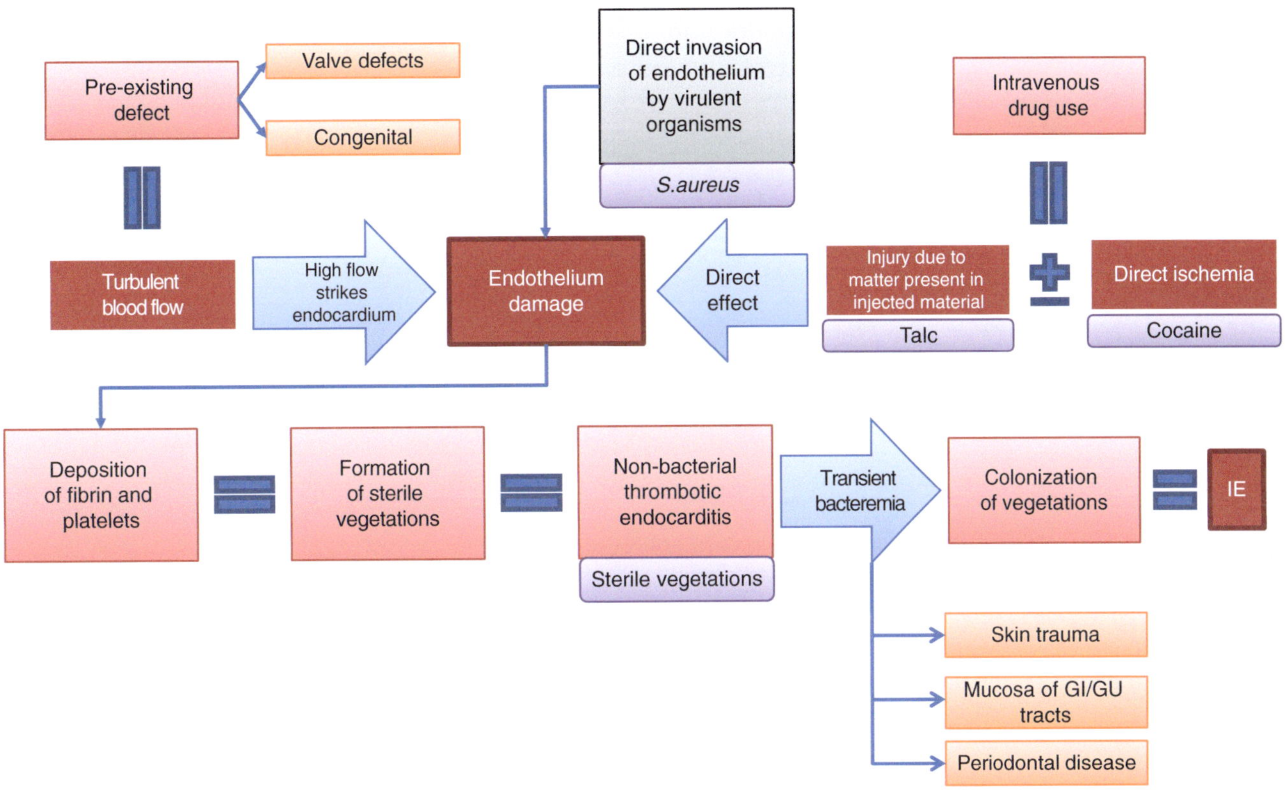

Acute Versus Subacute Endocarditis

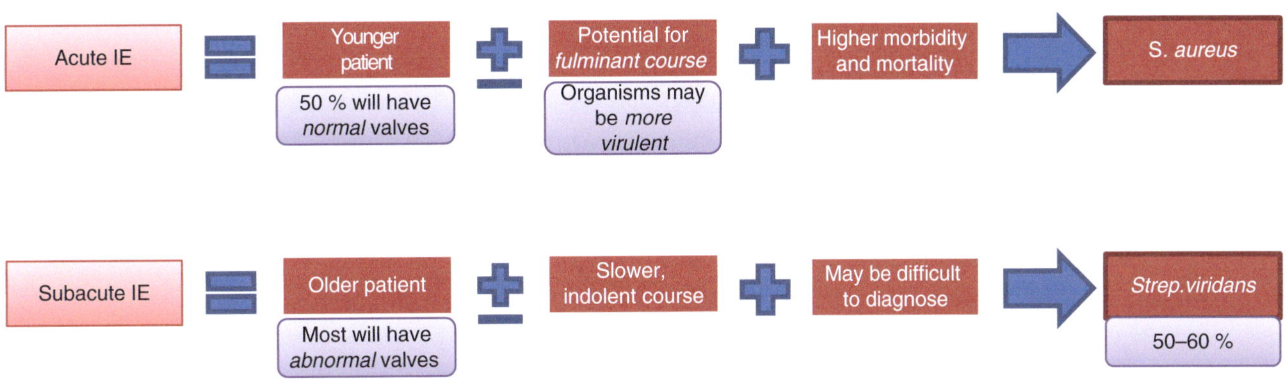

Left-Sided Versus Right-Sided Endocarditis

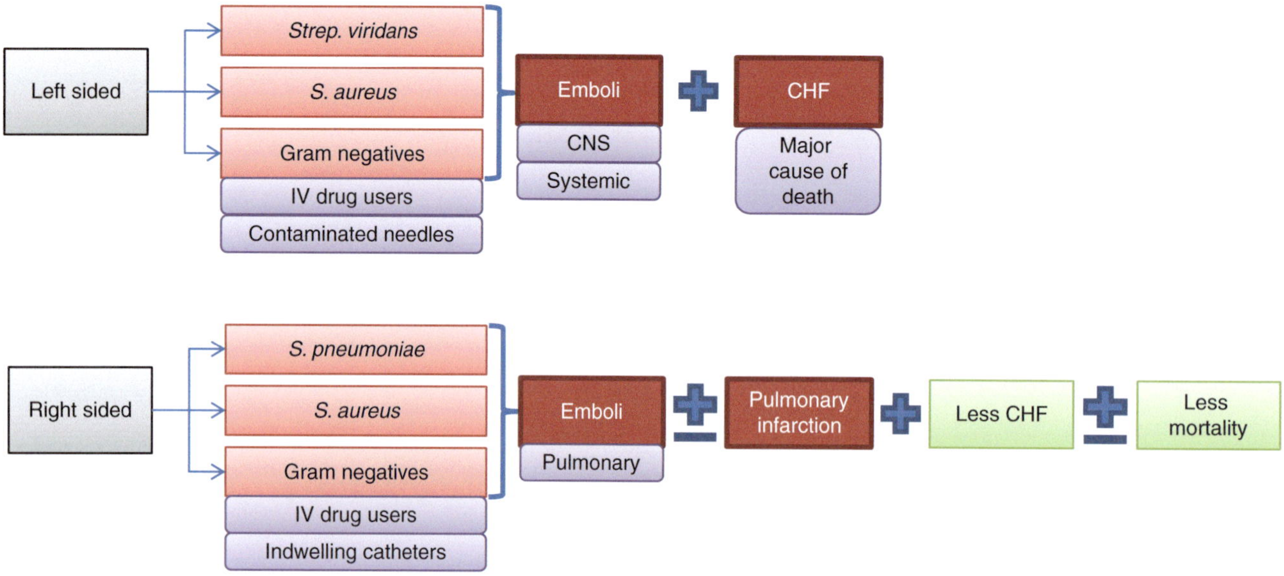

Organisms

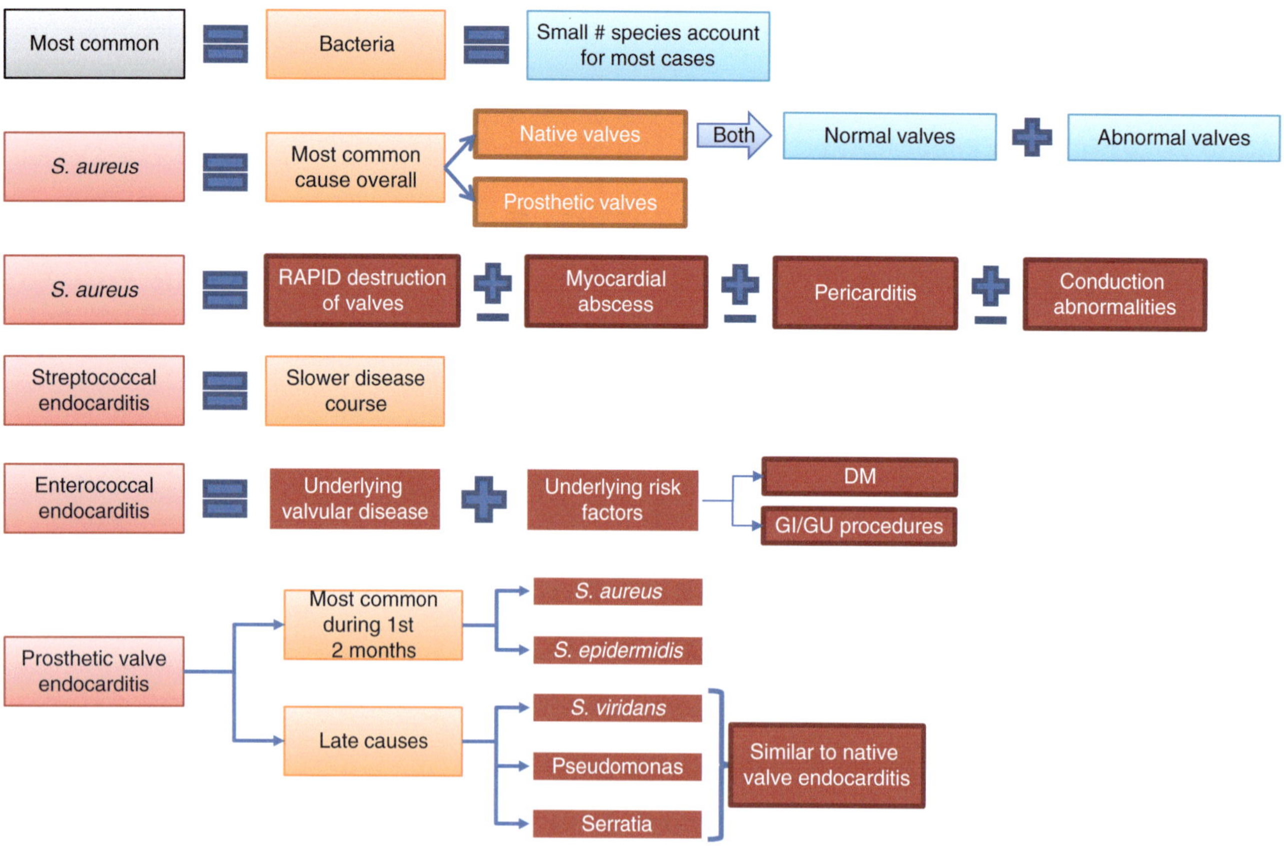

Organisms (2)

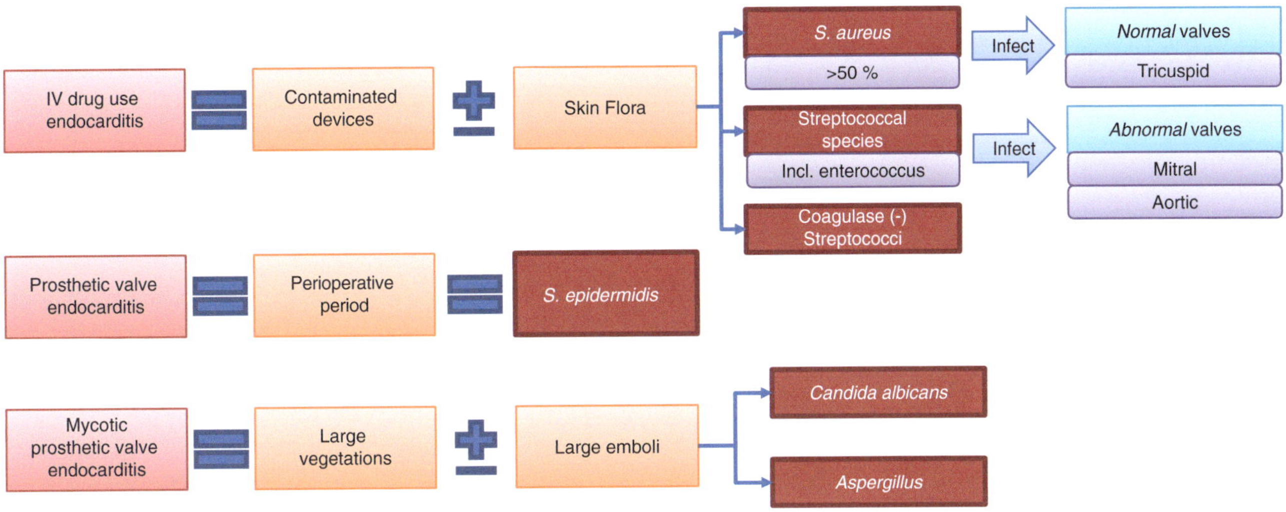

Clinical Findings

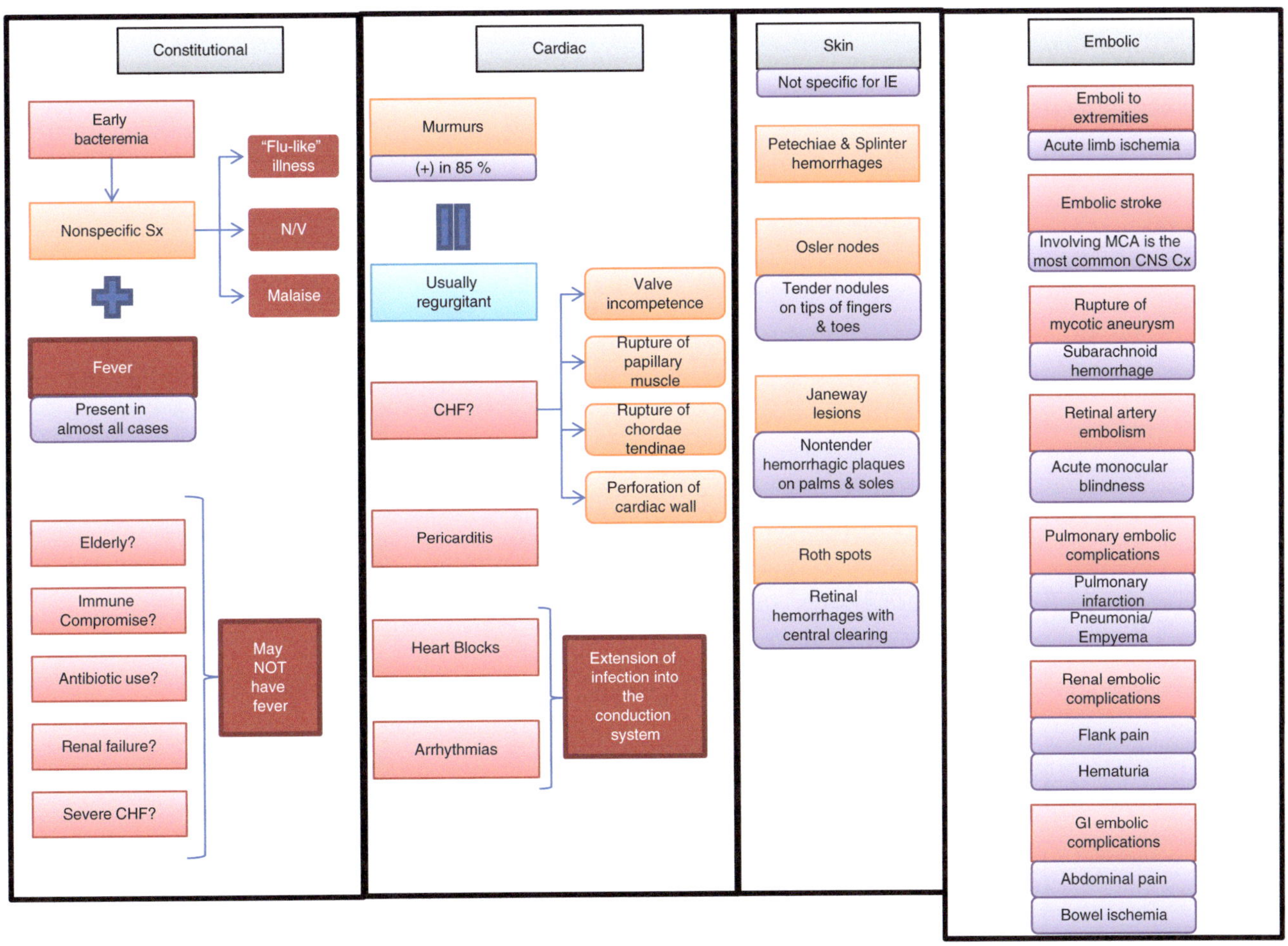

Diagnosis

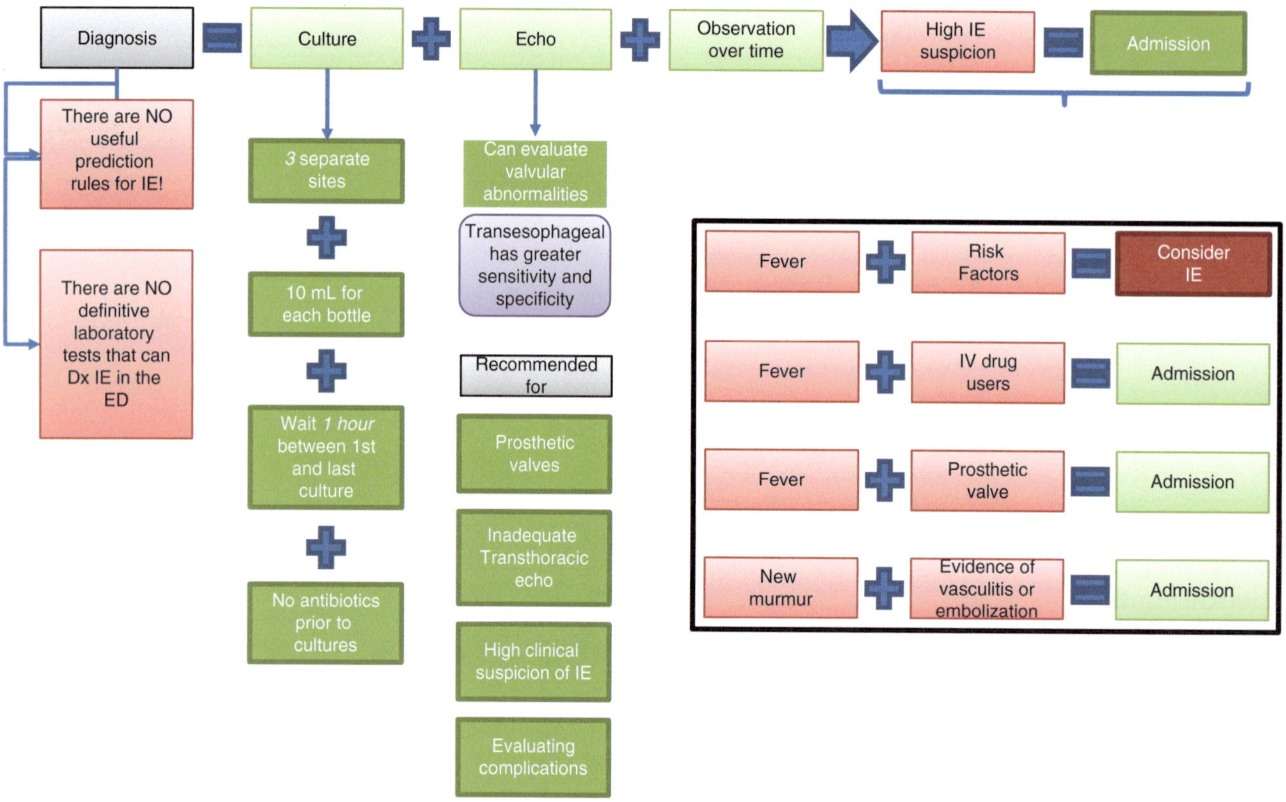

Treatment

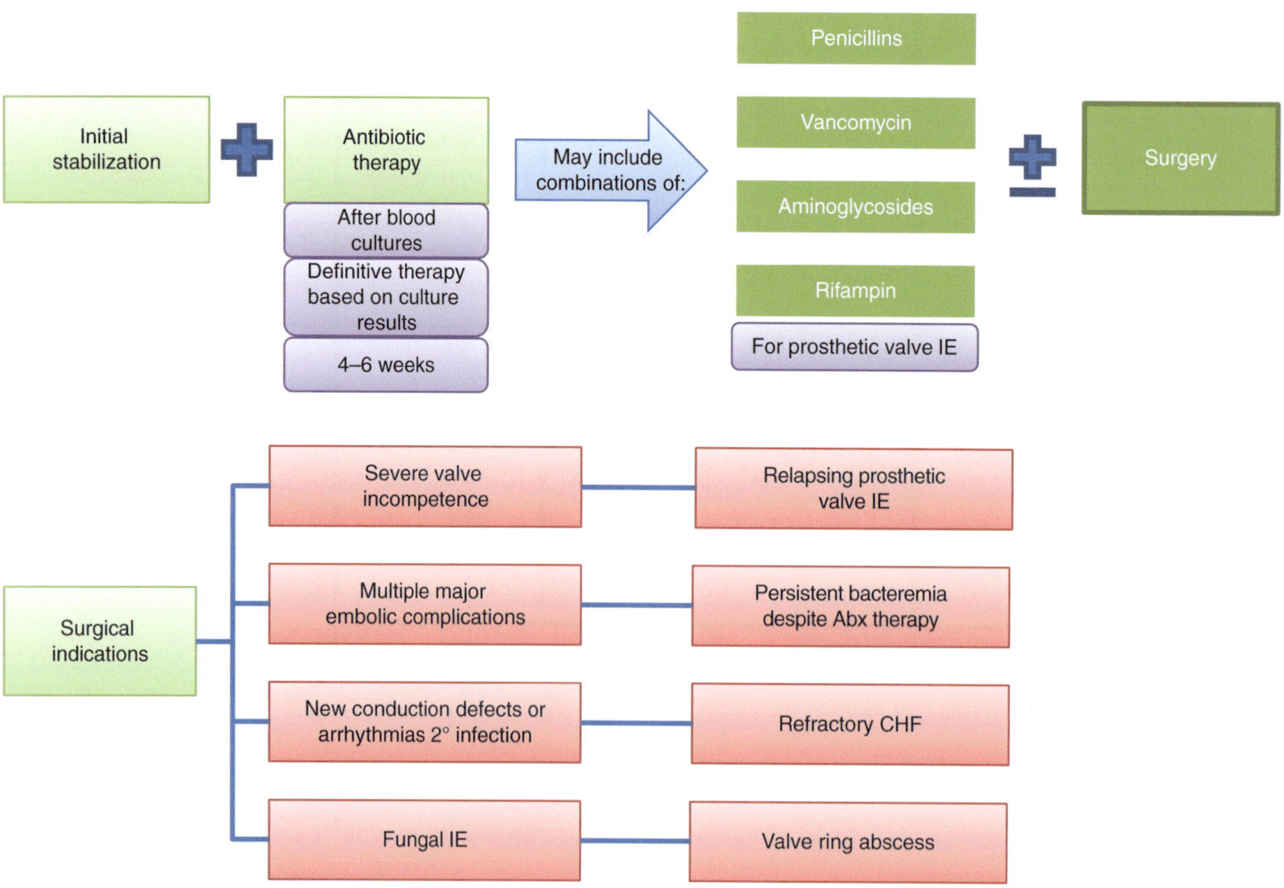

Endocarditis Prophylaxis

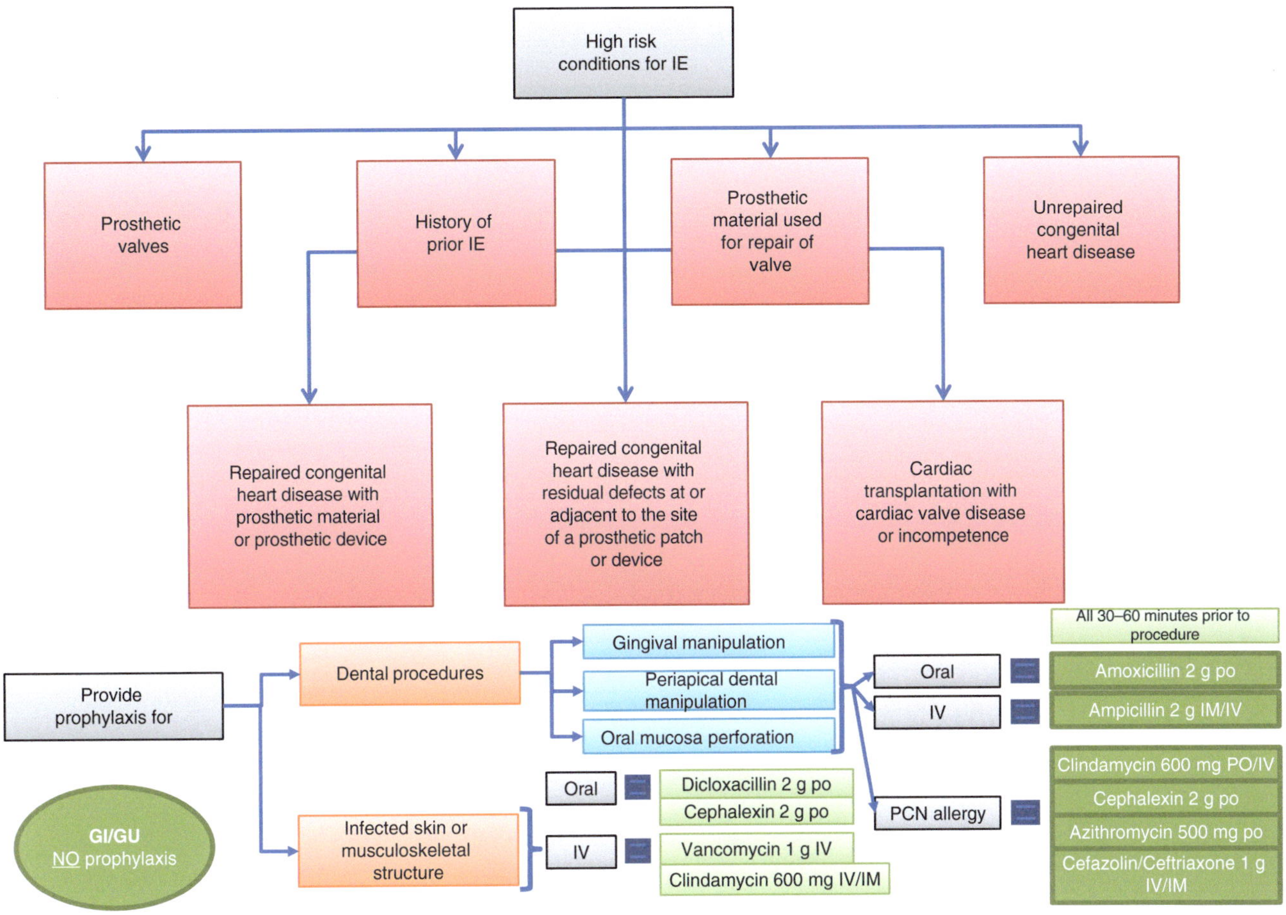

Endocarditis Prophylaxis NOT Indicated

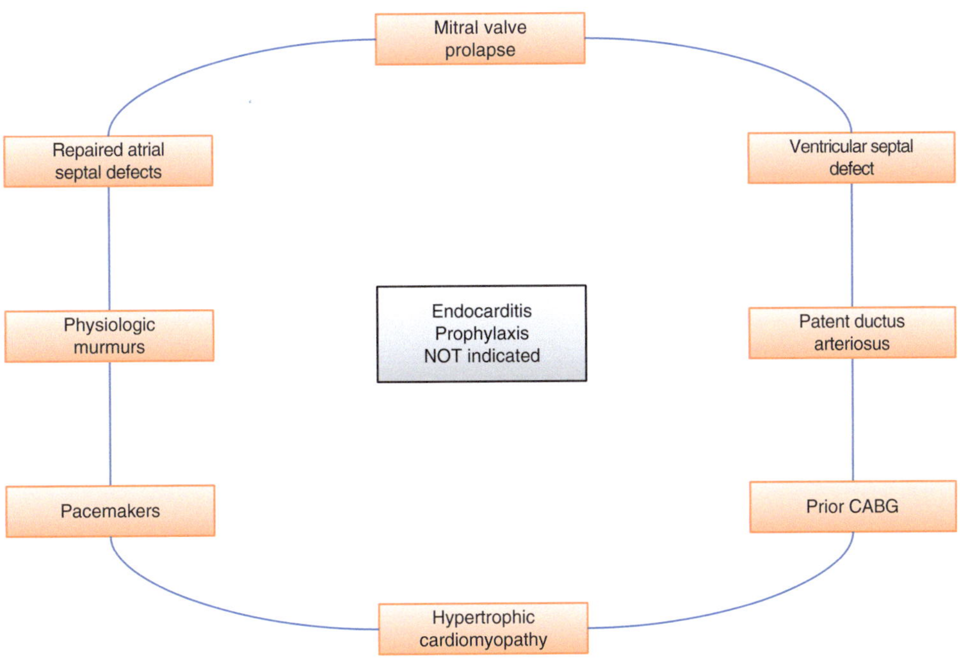

Rheumatic Heart Disease

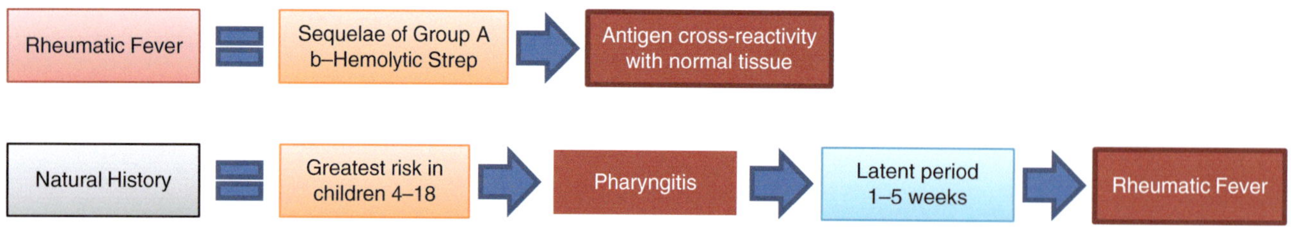

Rheumatic Heart Disease: Diagnosis

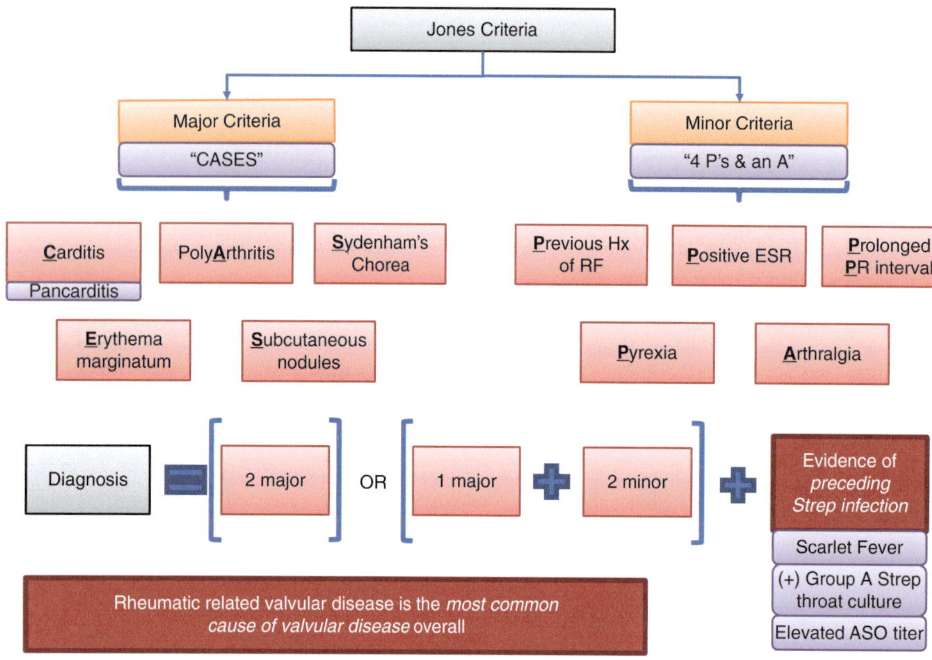

Rheumatic Heart Disease: Treatment

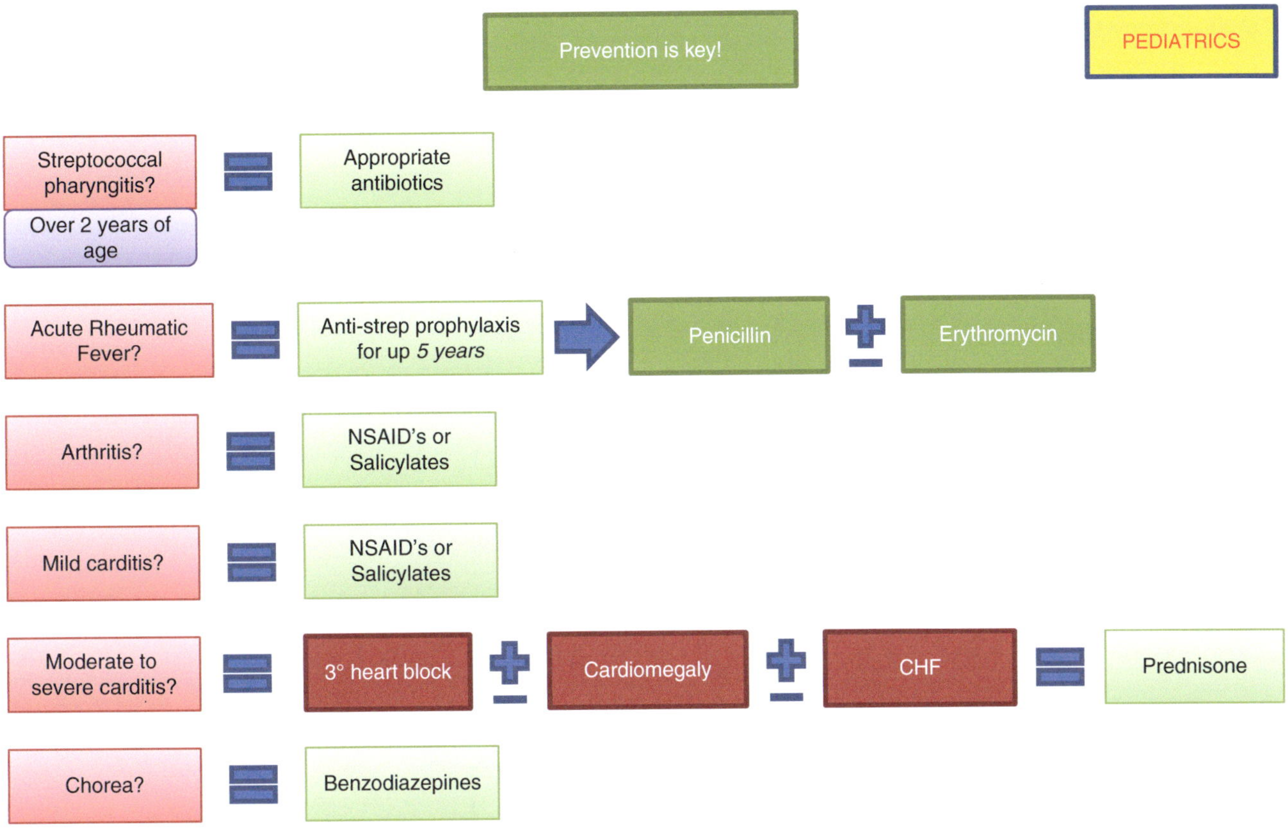

Cardiomyopathies (CM)

Cardiomyopathy: General

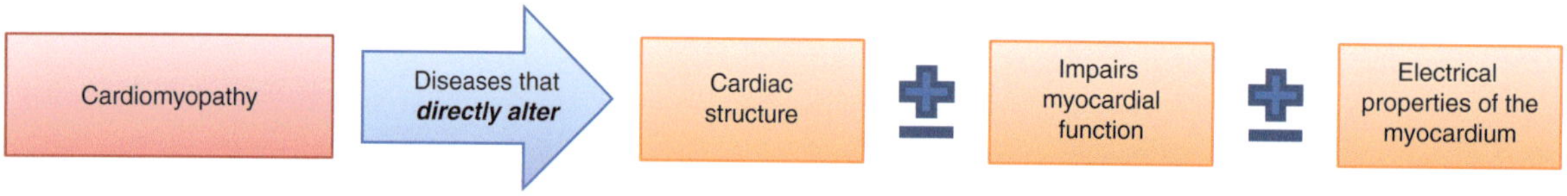

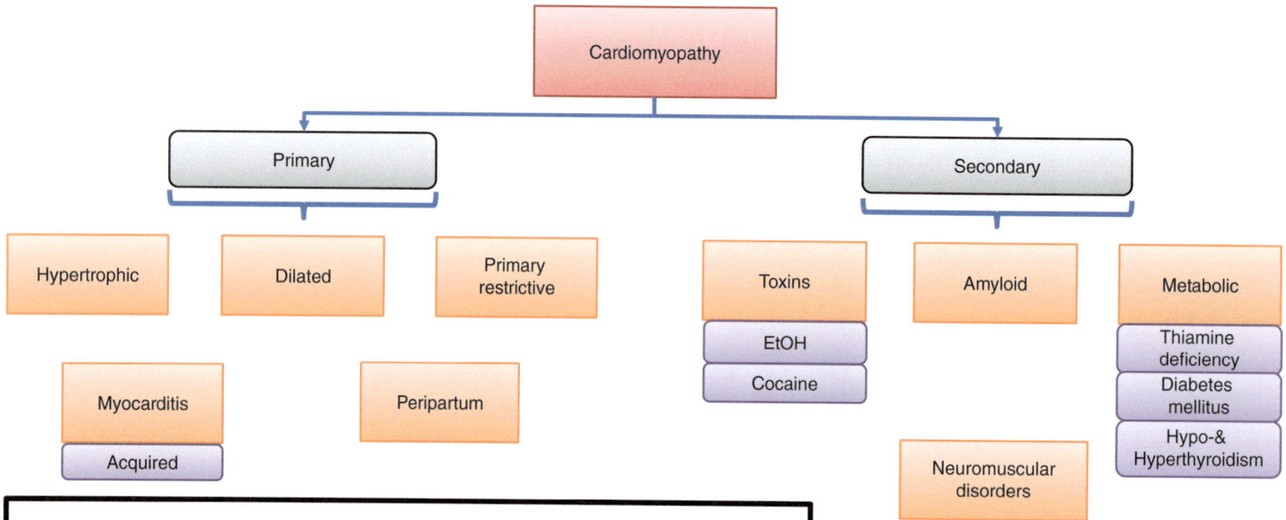

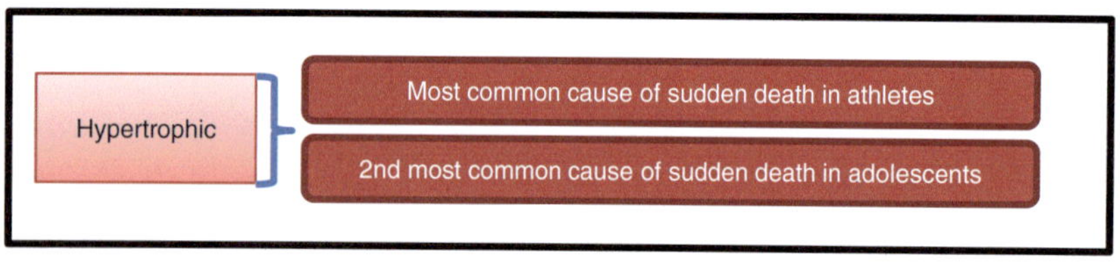

Dilated Cardiomyopathy

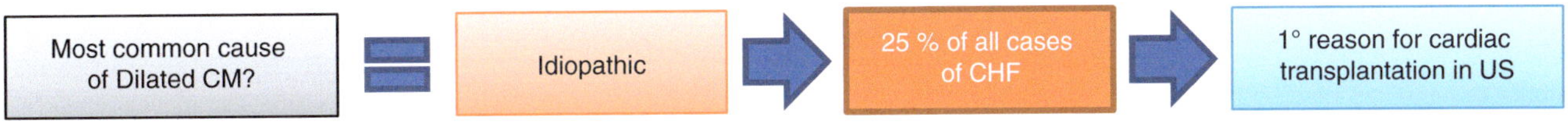

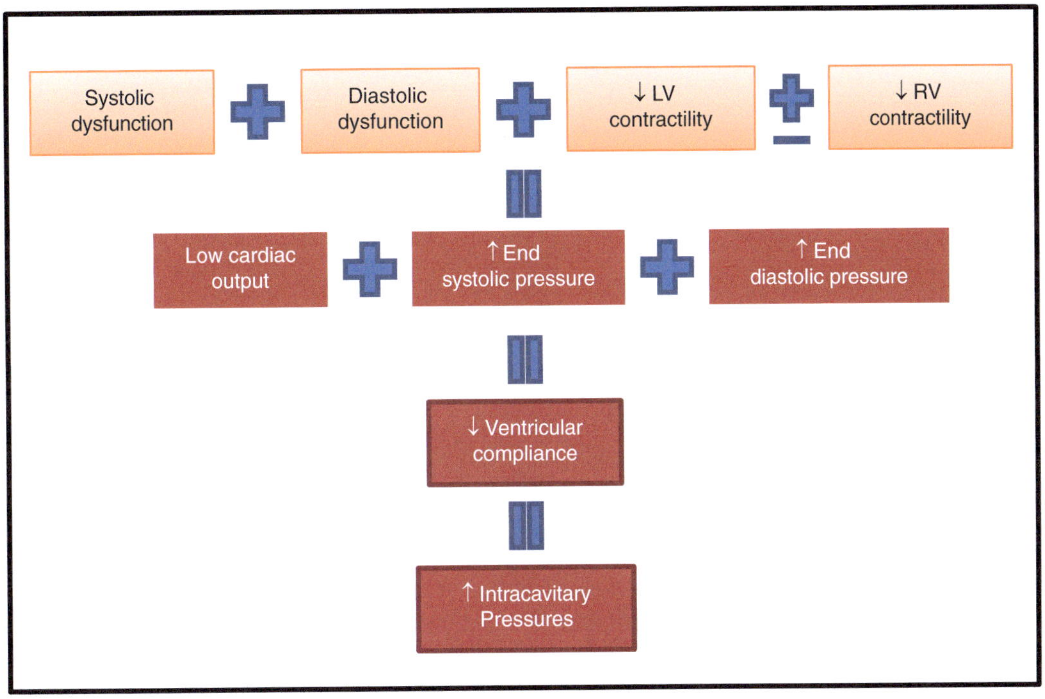

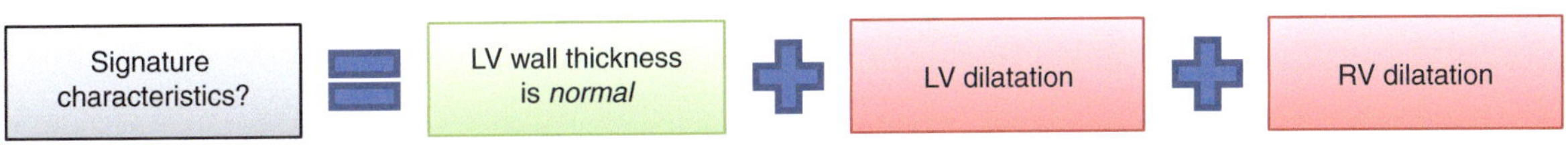

Dilated Cardiomyopathy: Clinical Features

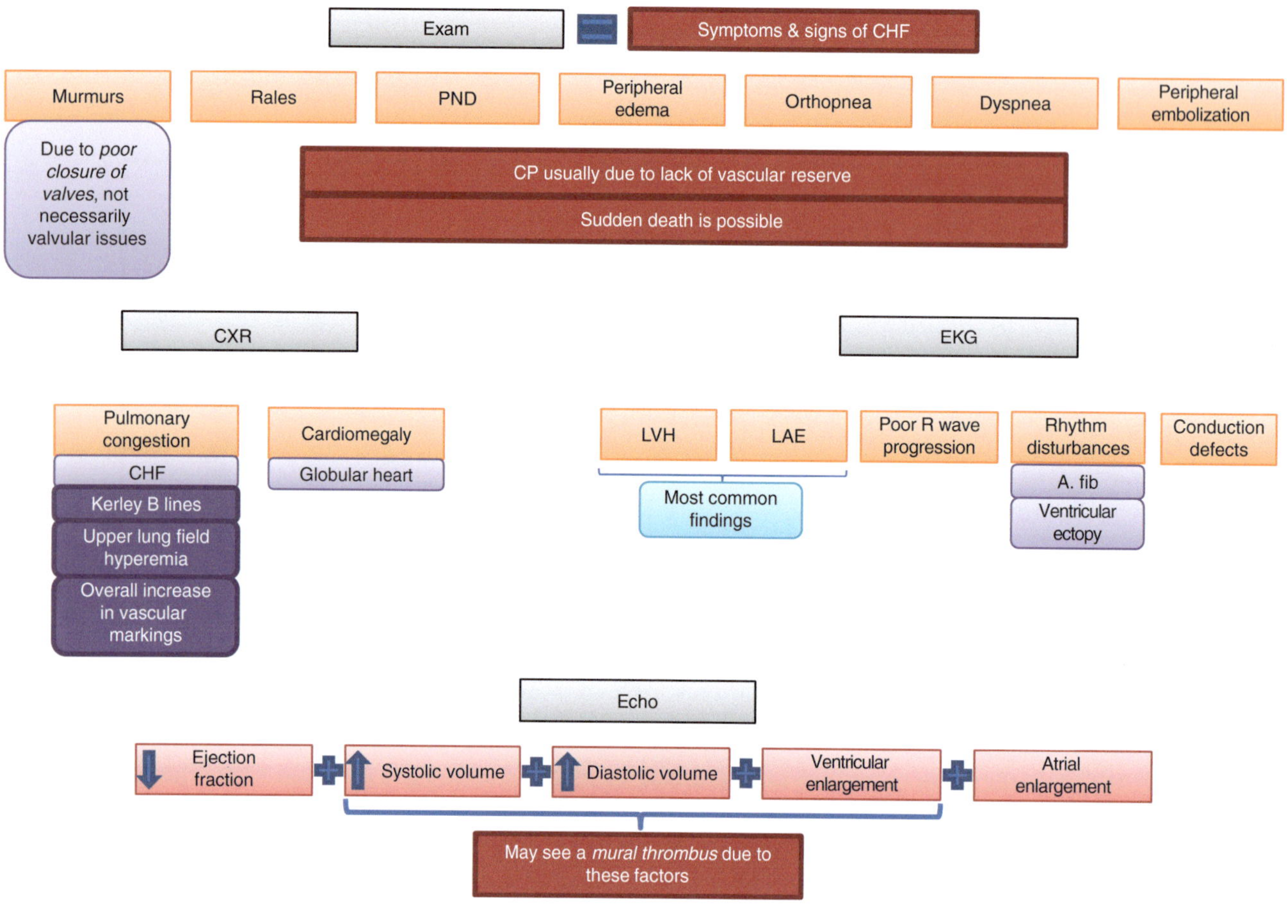

Dilated Cardiomyopathy: Treatment

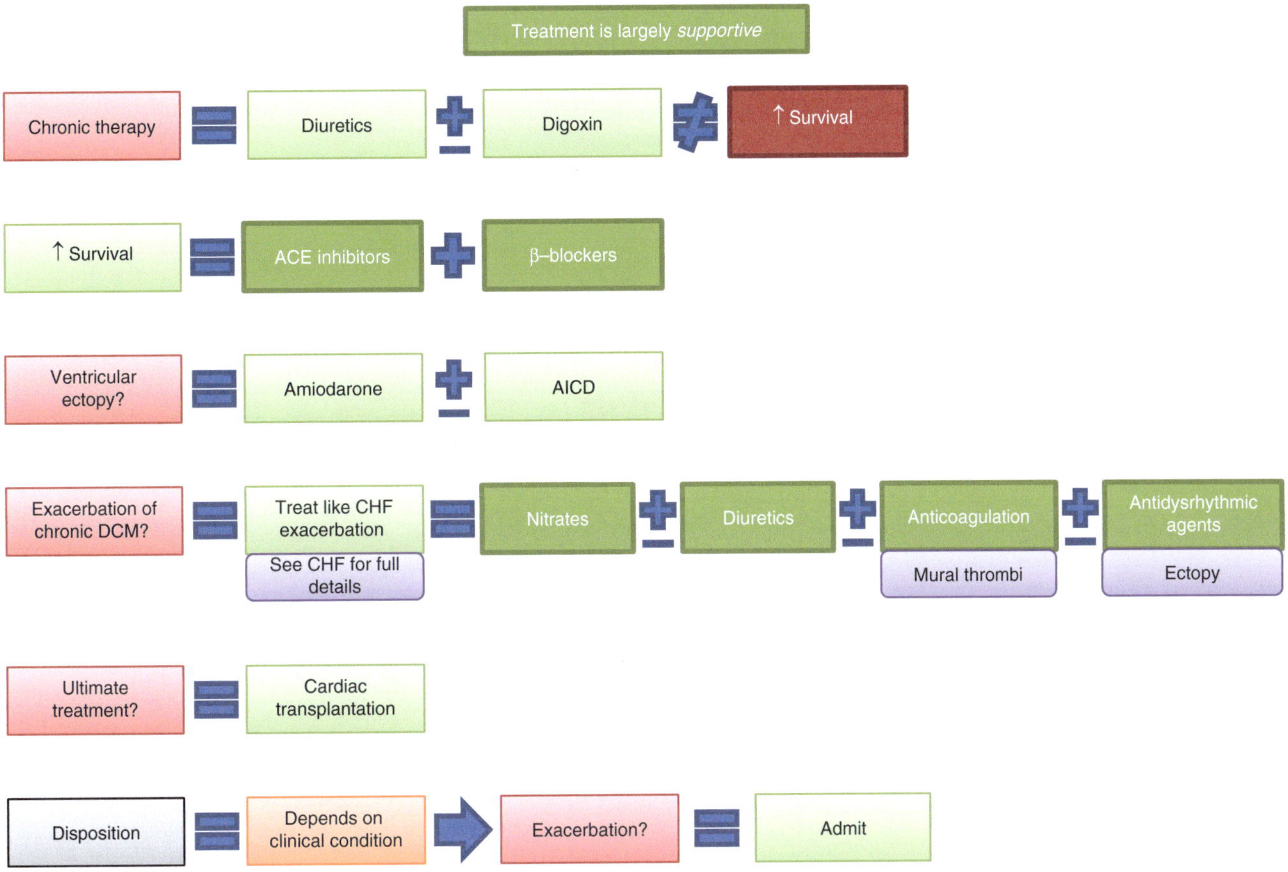

Hypertrophic Cardiomyopathy

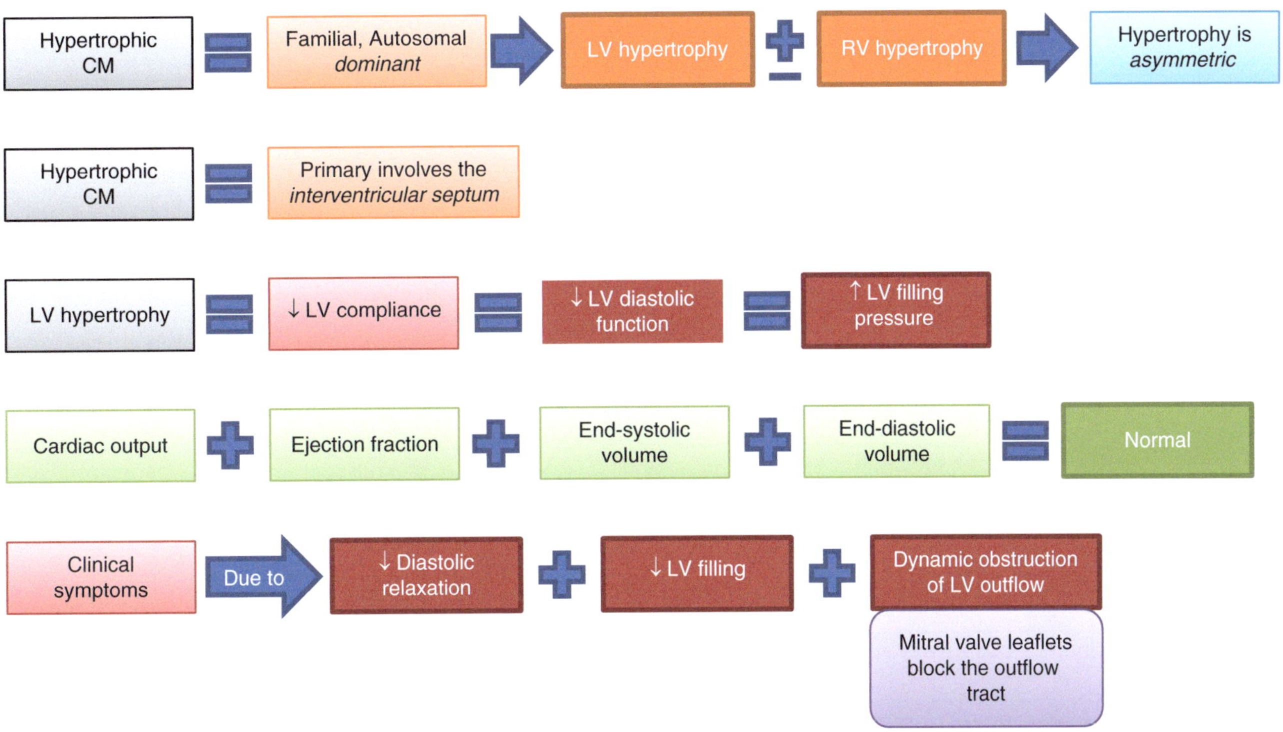

Hypertrophic Cardiomyopathy: Clinical Features

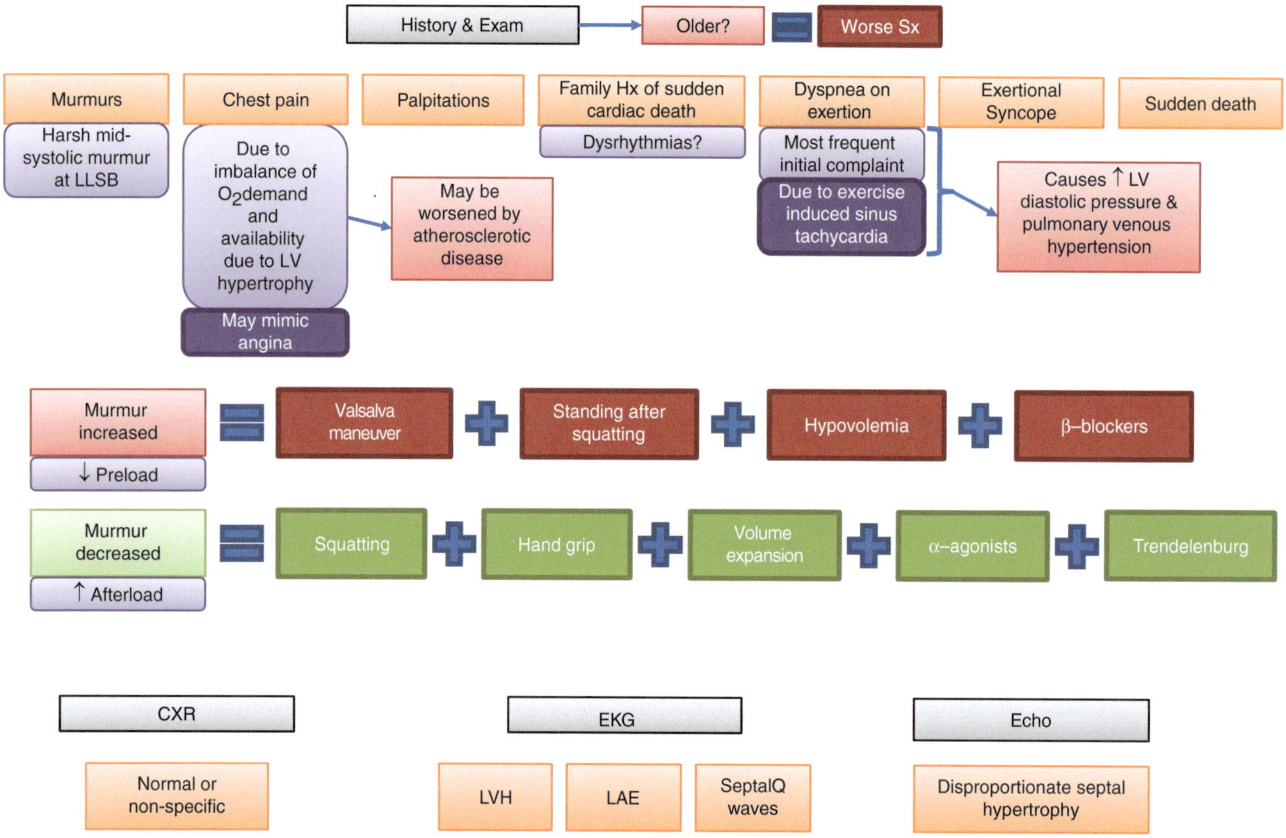

Hypertrophic Cardiomyopathy: Treatment

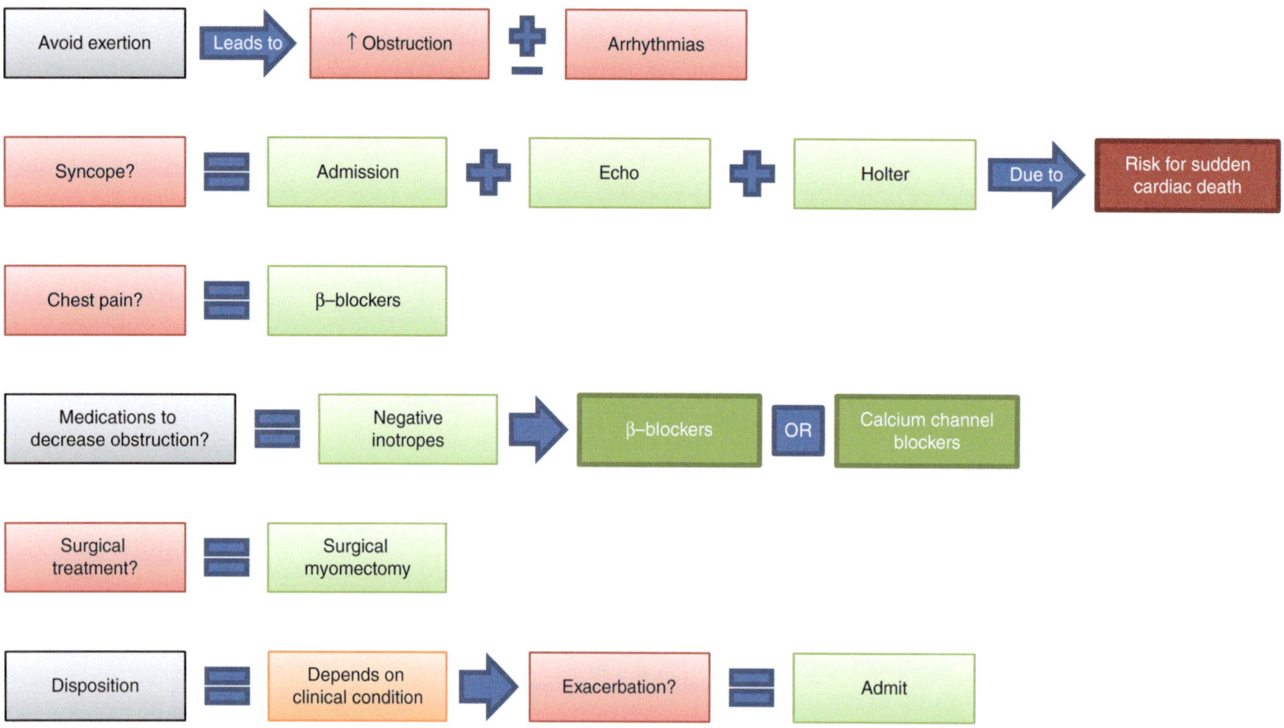

Restrictive Cardiomyopathy

Most common cause of Restrictive CM? = Idiopathic → May be familial *Autosomal dominant* + Multiple other causes:
- Sarcoid
- Amyloid
- Scleroderma
- Hemochromatosis

Restrictive CM = Systolic function is usually *normal* But… → Normal or decreased filling of one or both ventricles ± Ventricular wall thickness may be normal or increased

Restrictive CM = ↑ LV end diastolic pressure + ↑ RV end diastolic pressure + Normal LV systolic function (EF ≥ 50 %) + Early diastolic pressure has a decrease followed by a rapid rise & plateau

Restrictive Cardiomyopathy: Clinical Features

Exam = Symptoms & signs of CHF
- JVD
- Rales
- PND
- Peripheral edema
- Orthopnea
- Dyspnea
- Right sided CHF
  - Hepatomegaly
  - RUQ pain
  - Ascites
- CP uncommon
  - Except in *amyloidosis*

CXR
- Pulmonary congestion
  - CHF
    - Kerley B lines
    - Upper lung field hyperemia
    - Overall increase in vascular markings
- ***Normal*** heart size

EKG
- Nonspecific ST-T changes
- Low voltage may be seen
- A. Fib may be seen

Echo
- Confirmatory

Restrictive Cardiomyopathy: Treatment

Treatment is largely *supportive* & depends on type of RCM

Diastolic dysfunction? = Calcium channel blockers OR β–blockers

Medical management (Less effective) = Diuretics ± ACE inhibitors

Sarcoid? = Steroids

Hemochromatosis? = Chelation therapy

Disposition = Depends on clinical condition → Exacerbation? = Admit

Myocarditis

Introduction

Myocarditis = Form of & common cause of *dilated cardiomyopathy*

Causes of Myocarditis = Idiopathic + Infectious + Connective tissue disorders + Chemotherapy

Myocarditis = Inflammation of heart muscle → But… Systolic function is usually *normal*

Myocarditis tidbits = Many episodes are *mild* → Thus many cases are not diagnosed + Myocarditis may be accompanied by ***Pericarditis***

Natural History = Most recover

Complications of Myocarditis = Sudden Cardiac Death ± Dilated cardiomyopathy

Infectious Causes of Myocarditis

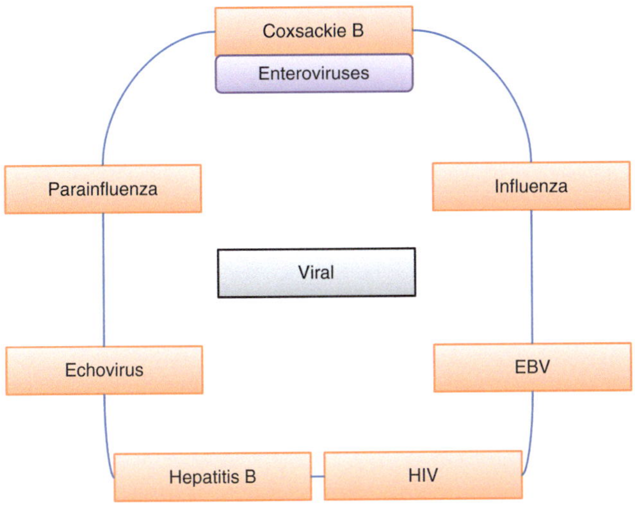

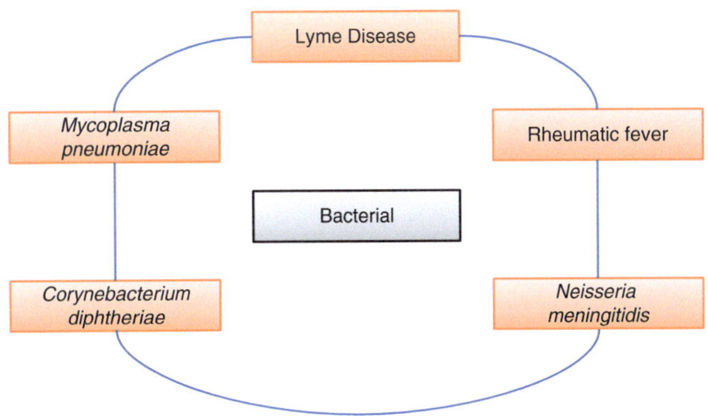

Myocarditis: Clinical Features

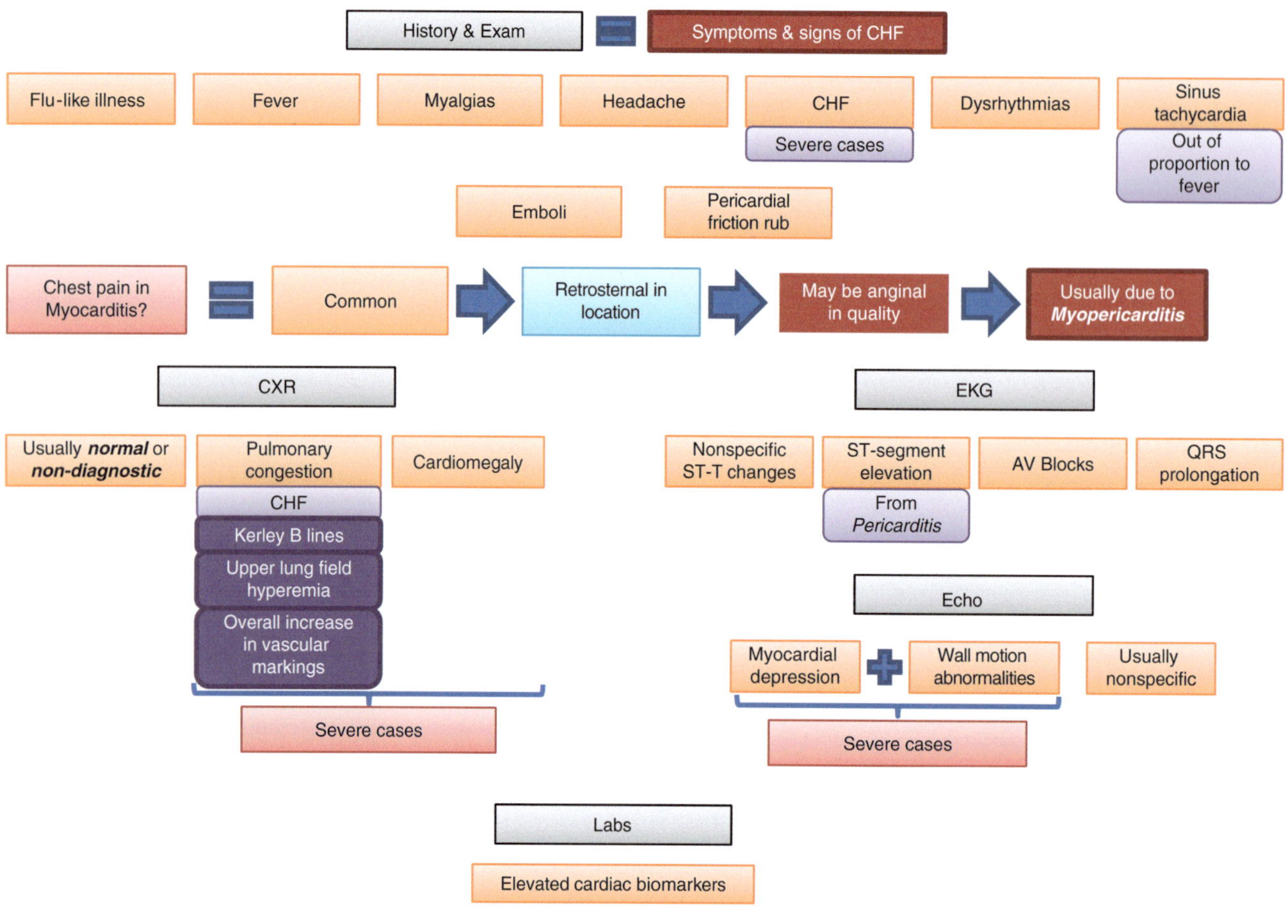

Myocarditis: Treatment

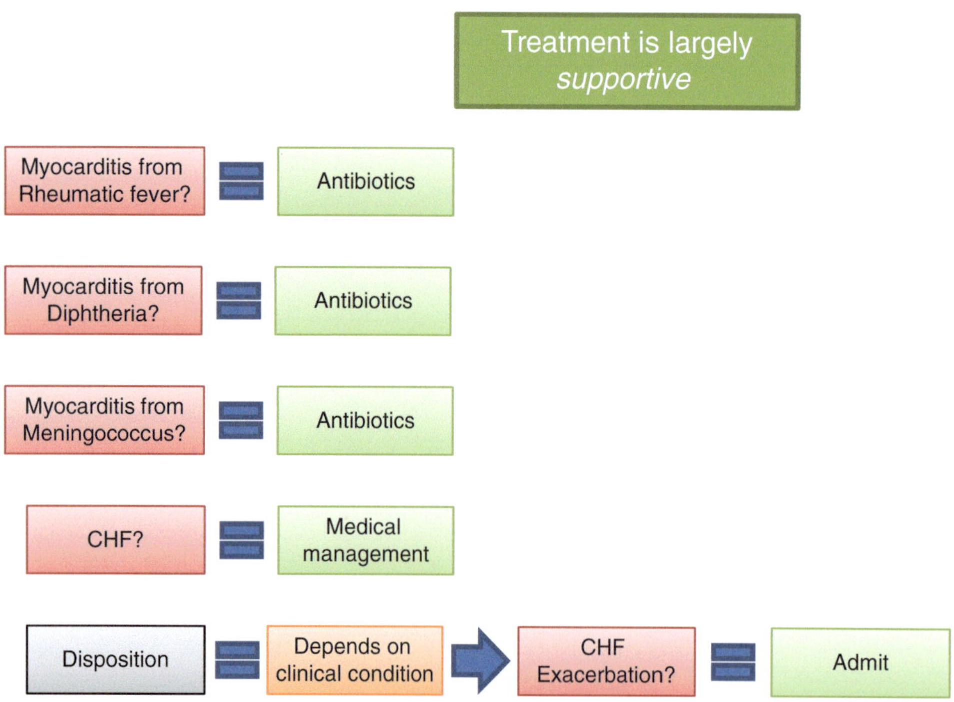

Pericarditis

Causes of Pericarditis

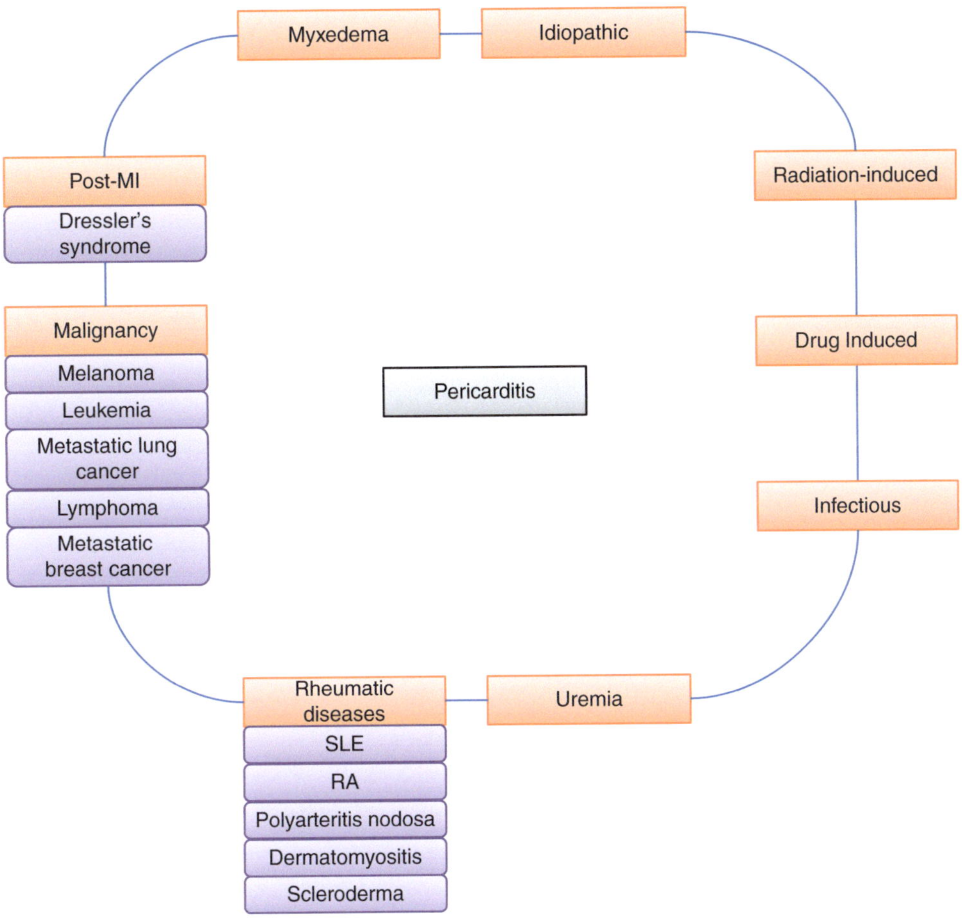

Infectious Causes of Pericarditis

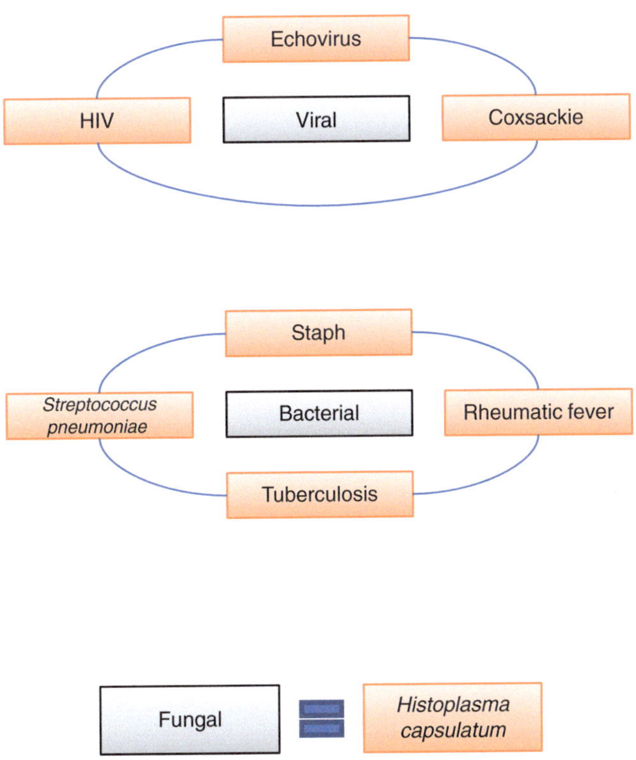

Pericarditis: Clinical Features and Diagnosis

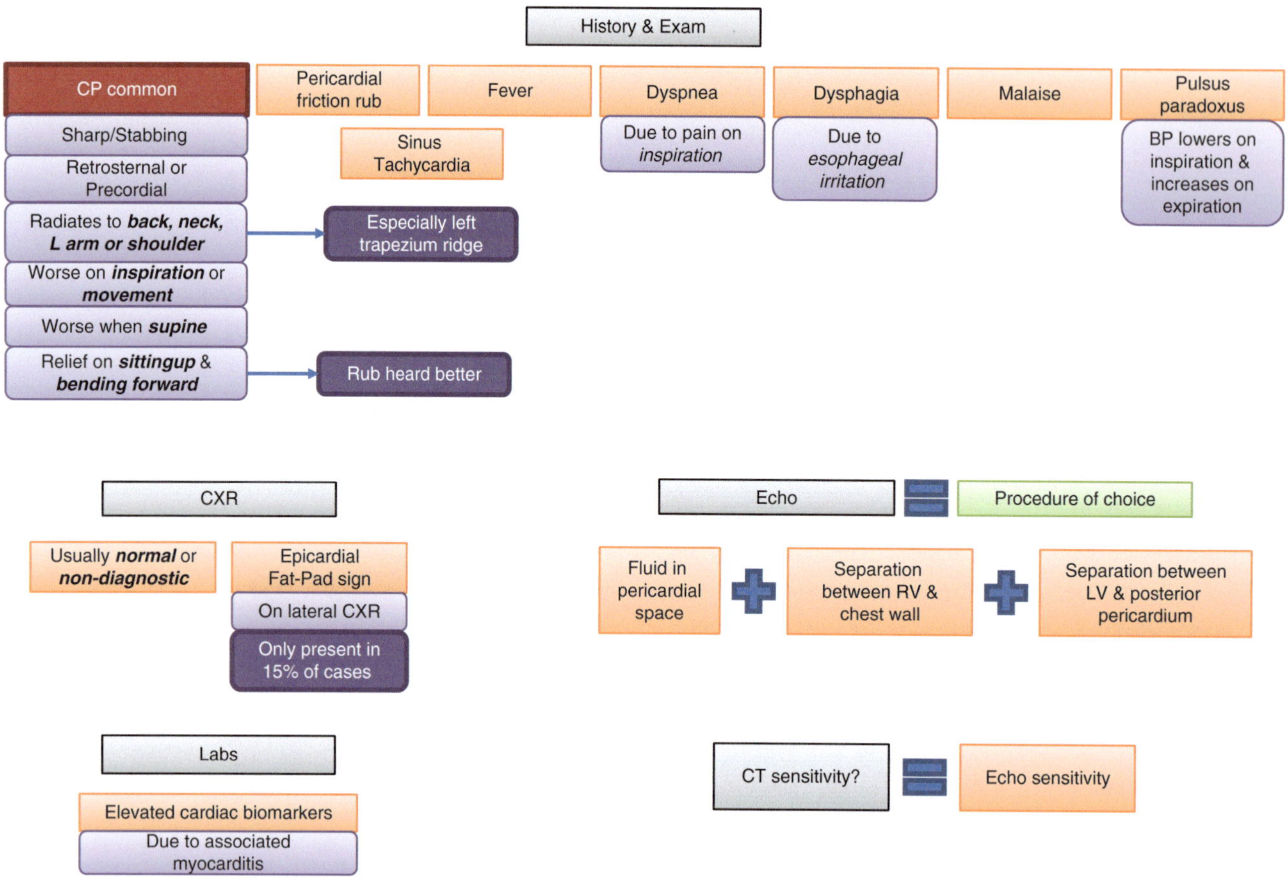

Pericarditis: EKG Changes

Stage	PR Segment	ST Segment	T wave
1	**Depression,** especially in II, aVF& V4–V6	**Diffuse elevation** (does not correlate with coronary distribution)	N/A
2	Returns to baseline	Returns to baseline	N/A
3	N/A	Isoelectric	**Inversions**, especially in I, V5, V6
4	N/A	Isoelectric	Normal

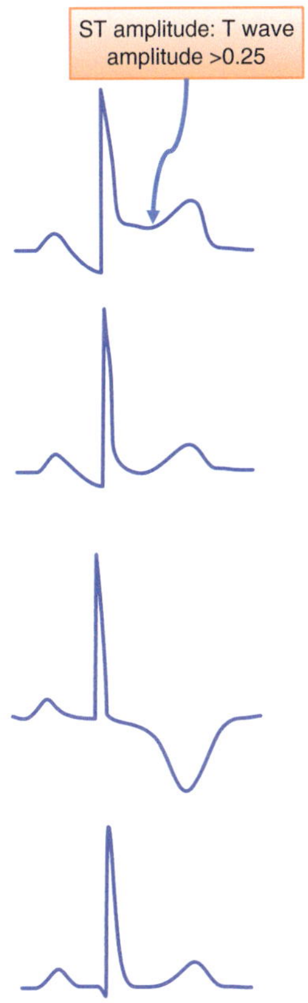

Large pericardial effusion = Low-voltage QRS complexes (Due to attenuation of electrical signals) + Electrical Alternans (Due to pendular motion of heart within fluid filled pericardium)

Pericarditis: Treatment

Treatment depends on cause

Viral pericarditis? = NSAID's → Course is benign

T > 38°C? + Immune-compromised? + Hx of oral anticoagulant use? + Large pericardial effusion? + Onset over weeks? + Associated myocarditis? → Poor prognostic signs

Disposition = Depends on clinical condition → Hospitalization usually not necessary → But… Poor prognostic signs = Admit

Cardiac Tamponade

Introduction

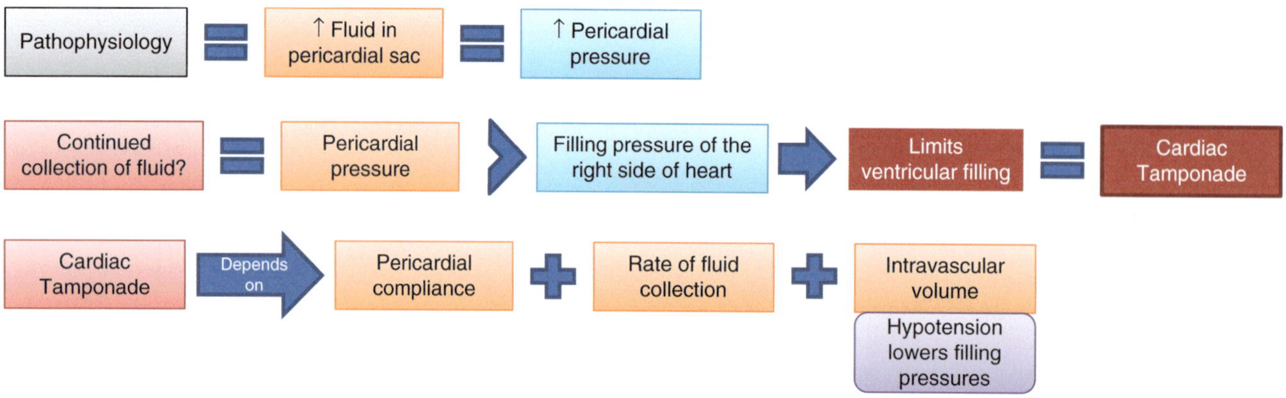

Causes of Cardiac Tamponade

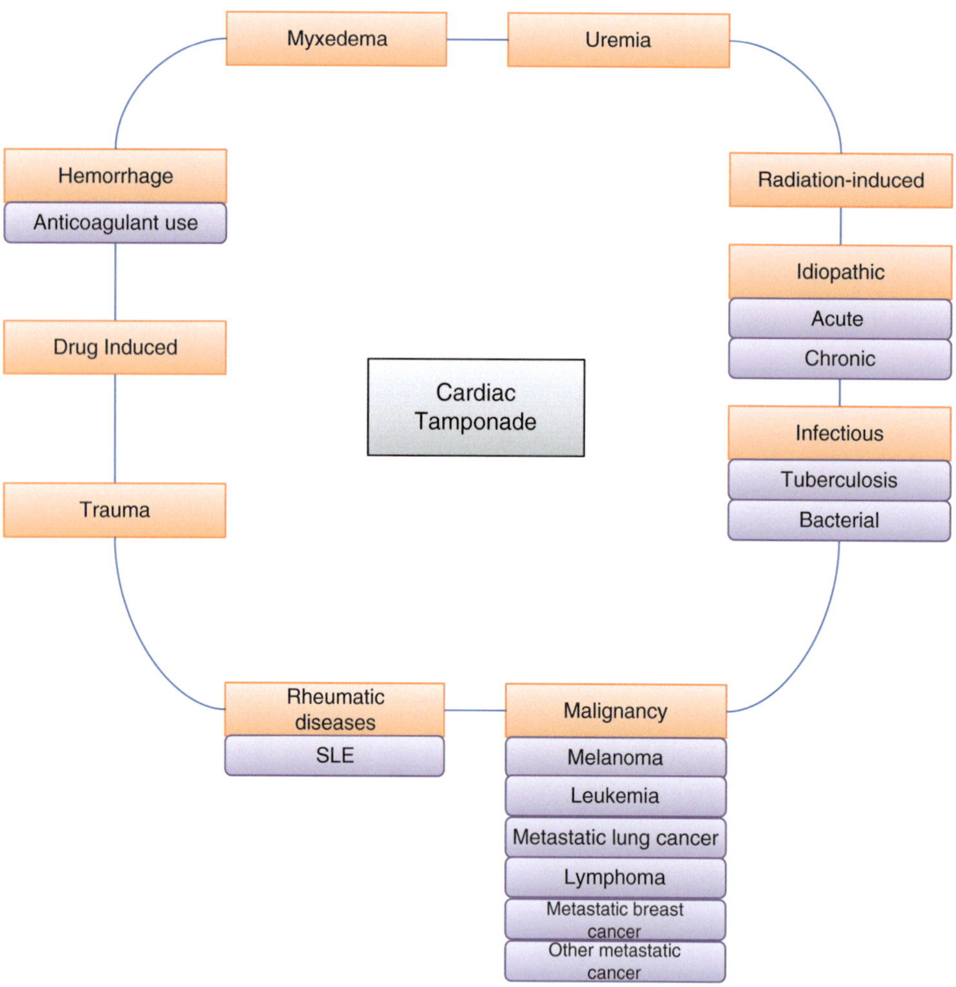

Cardiac Tamponade: Clinical Features

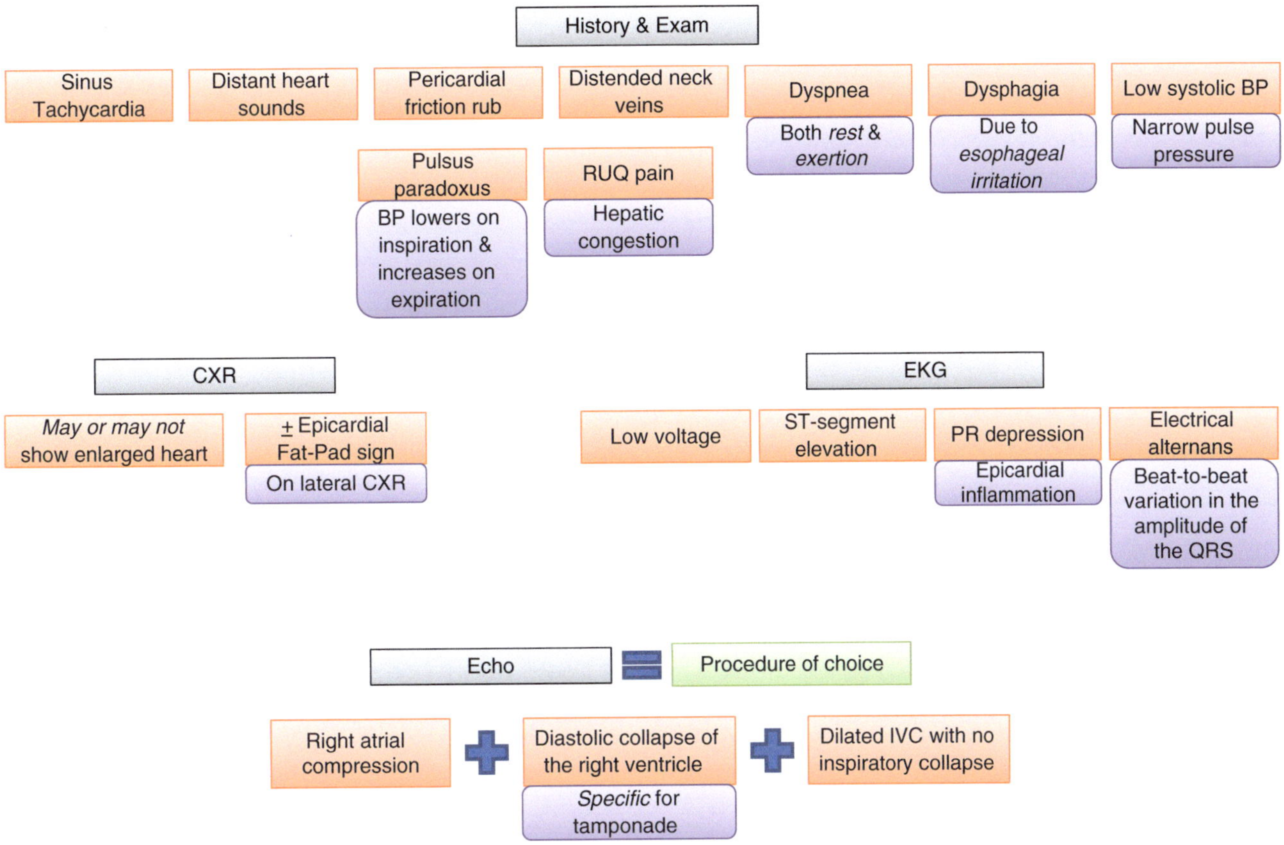

Cardiac Tamponade: Treatment

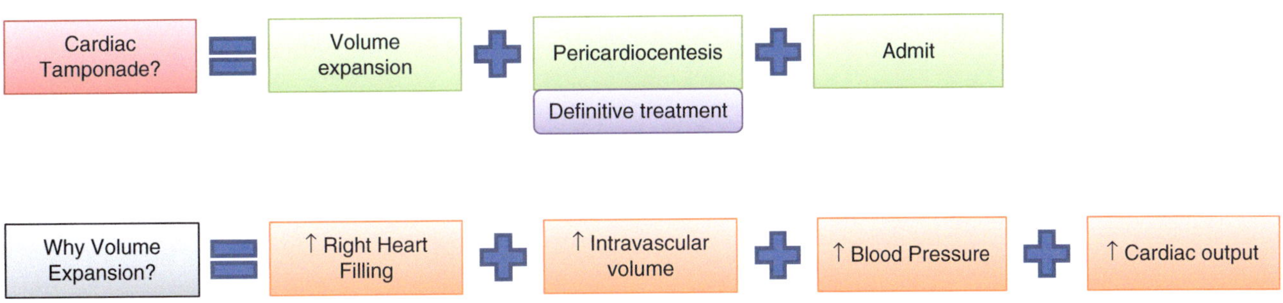

Abdominal Aortic Aneurysm

Introduction

Aneurysms = Dilatation of arterial wall → > 1.5 times normal diameter → Due to *Medial degeneration* → Usually atherosclerotic

True Aneurysms = *All* layers of vessel wall

Risk Factors for True Aneurysms = Family Hx + Connective tissue disorders + Atherosclerosis

*Pseudo*aneurysm = *Some* layers of vessel wall + Fibrous tissue formation

Causes of Fibrous tissue formation = Prior surgery + Prior catheterization + Trauma + Infection

Mycotic aneurysm = Develops due to *infection in vessel wall* → Due to → Direct extension of neighboring infection OR Embolization from endocarditis

Abdominal Aortic Aneurysm: General

Abdominal Aortic Aneurysm = Aneurysm >3.0 cm in diameter

AAA Tidbits = M > F + Majority are *infrarenal* + 18 % of patients with 1st degree relative with AAA have a AAA of their own

Risk Factors = Atherosclerosis + Hypertension + Connective tissue diseases

Abdominal Aortic Aneurysm >5.0 cm? = Consider repair → Due to → Increased risk of rupture

Symptomatic Abdominal Aortic Aneurysm of any size? = Emergent repair

Pt with Peripheral arterial disease? = Higher risk for AAA

Aneurysms elsewhere? = Higher risk for AAA

Abdominal Aortic Aneurysm: Symptoms

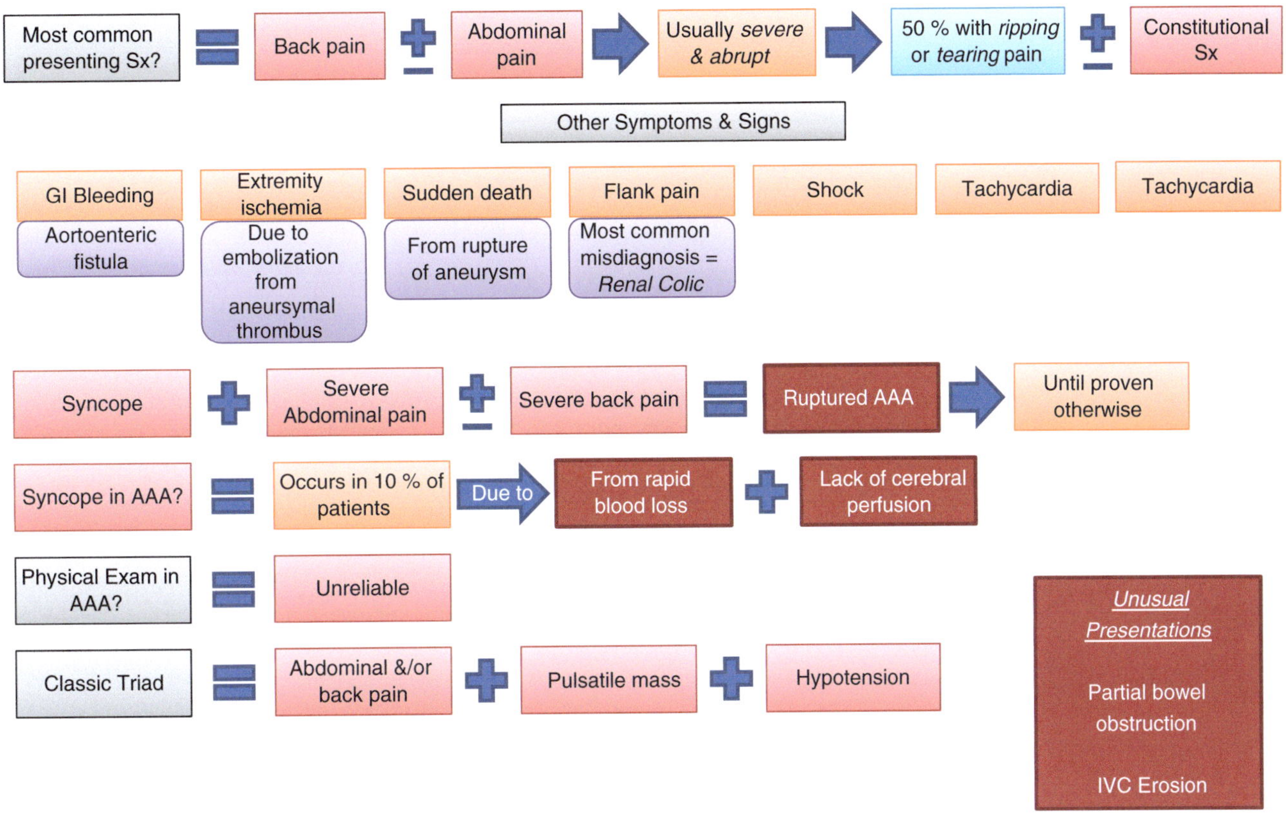

AAA Signs

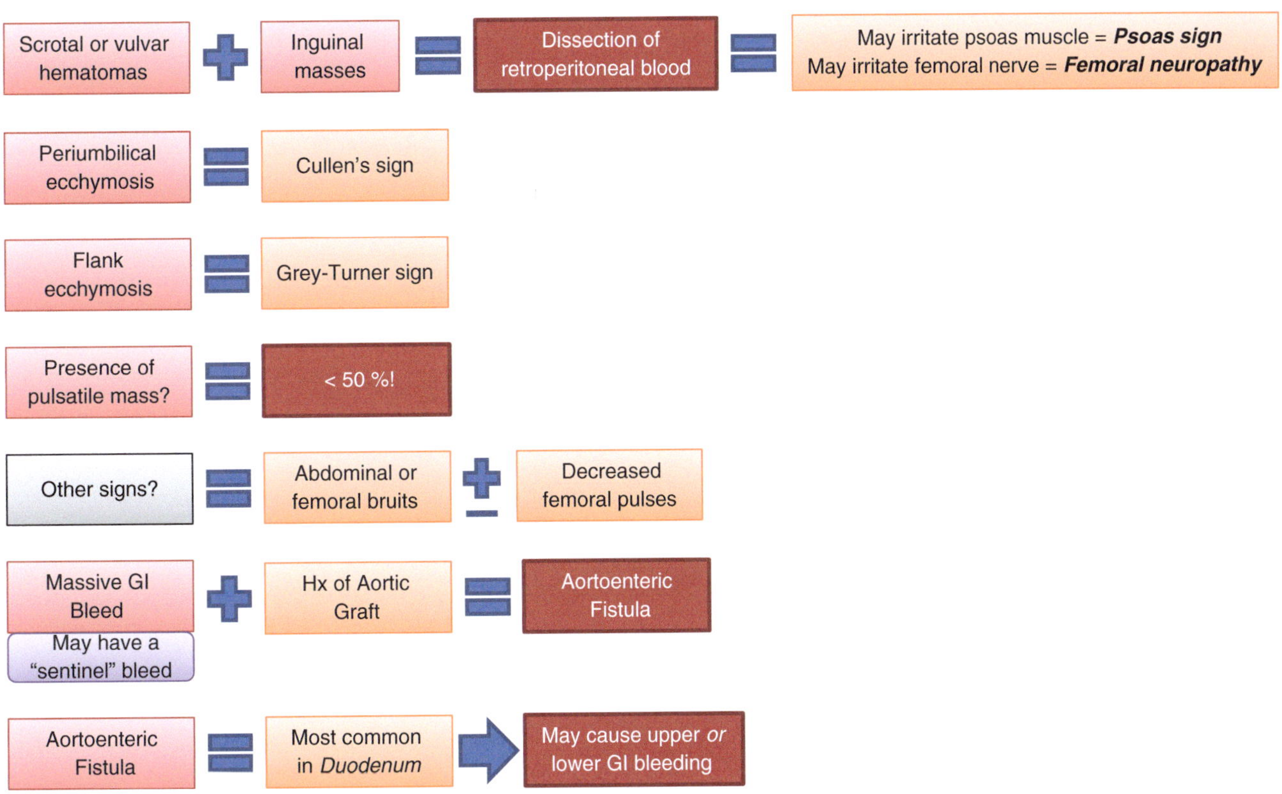

Diagnosis

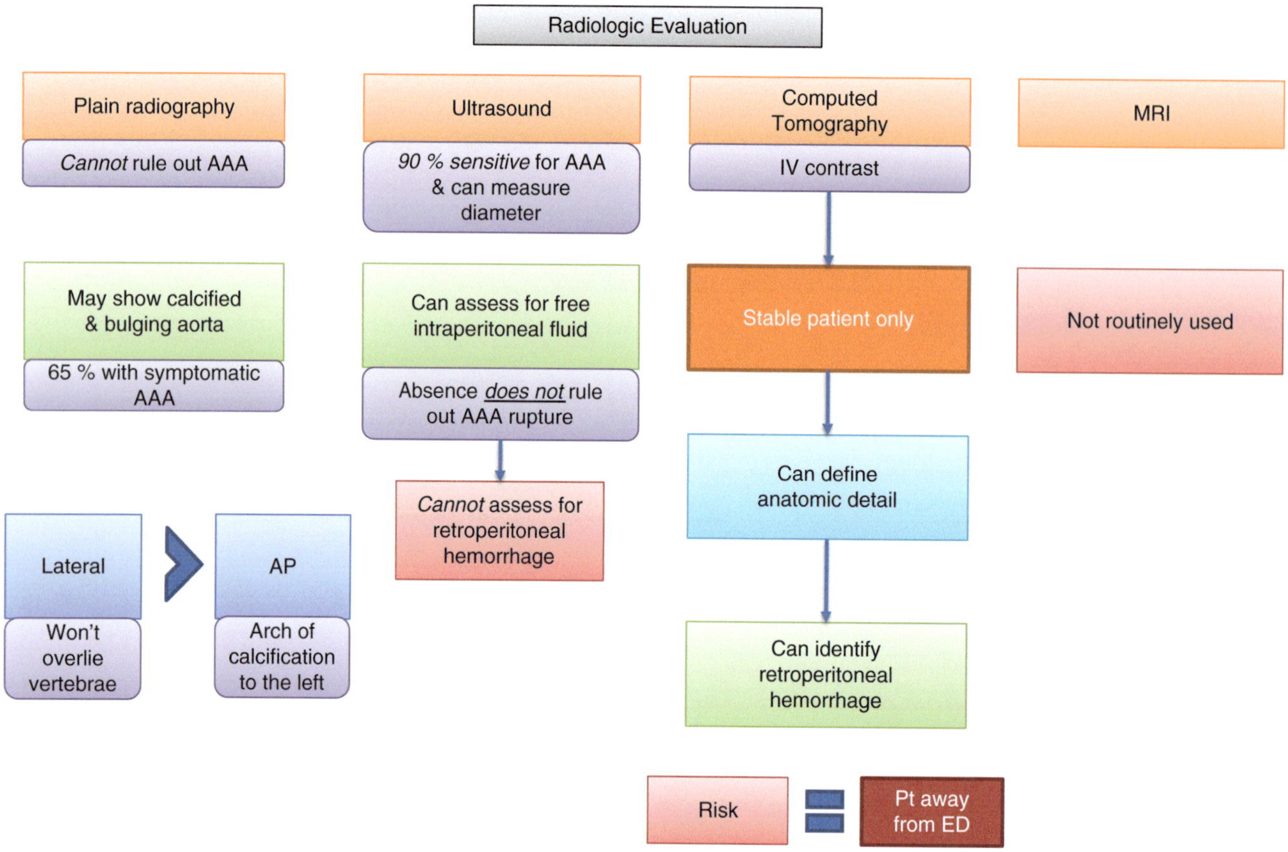

Treatment

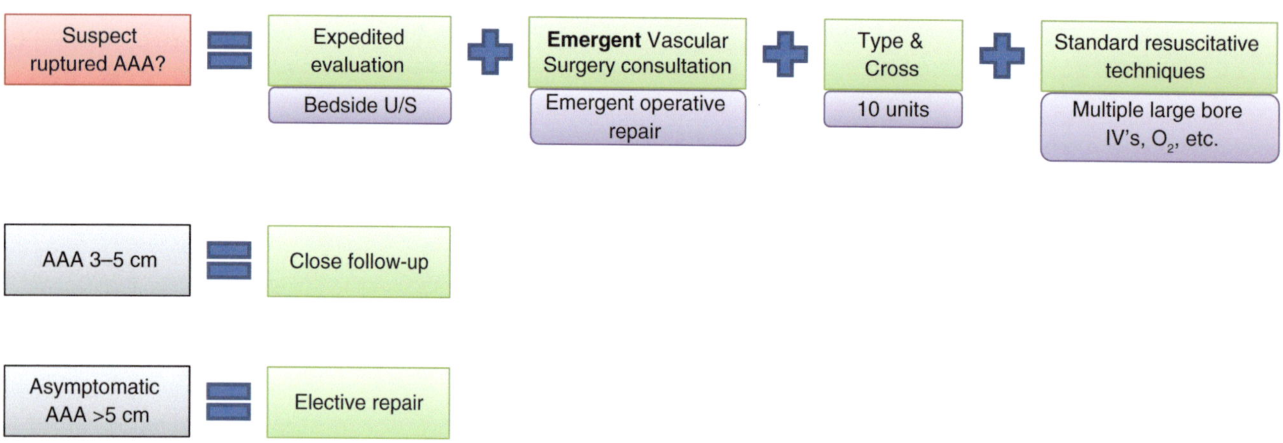

Aortic Dissection

Introduction

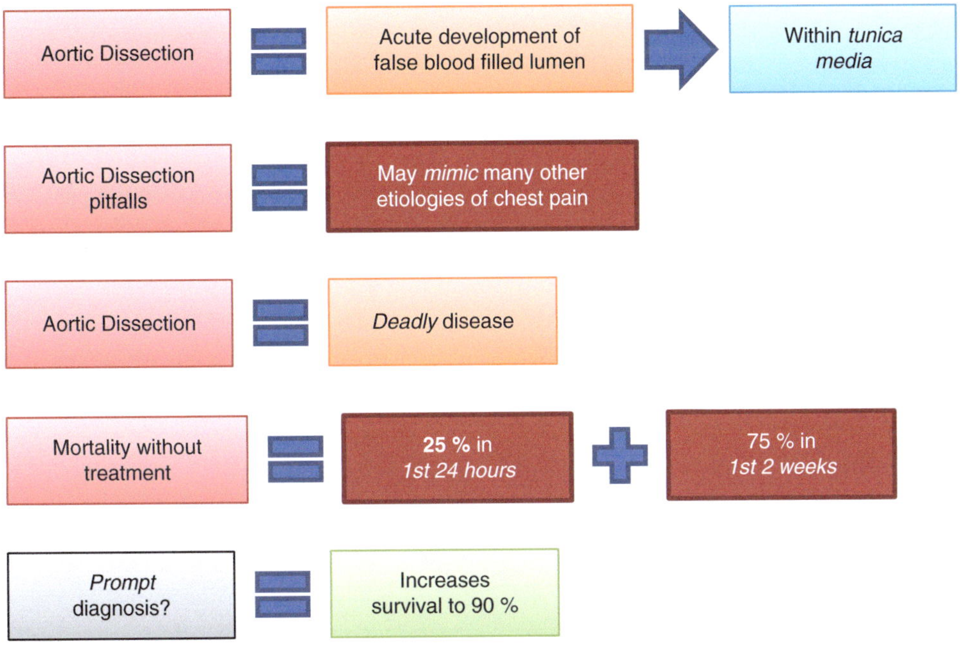

Anatomy

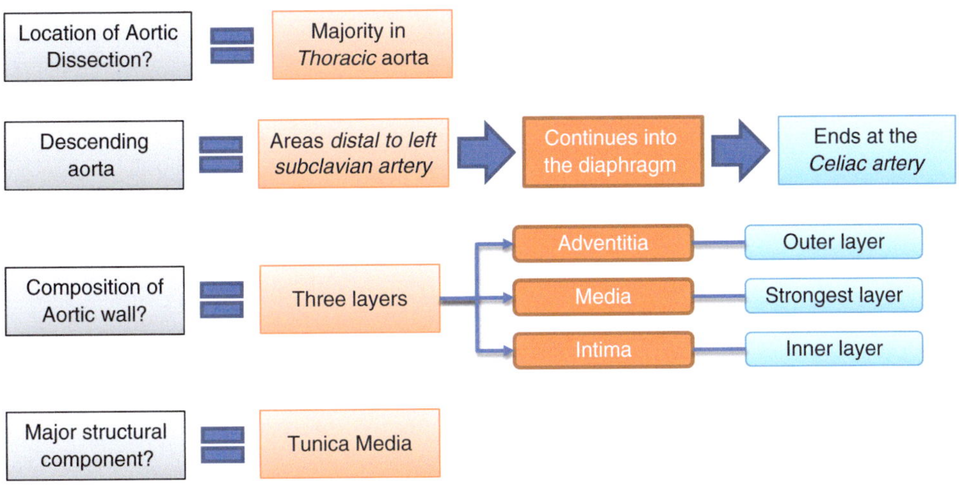

Aortic Dissection Risk Factors

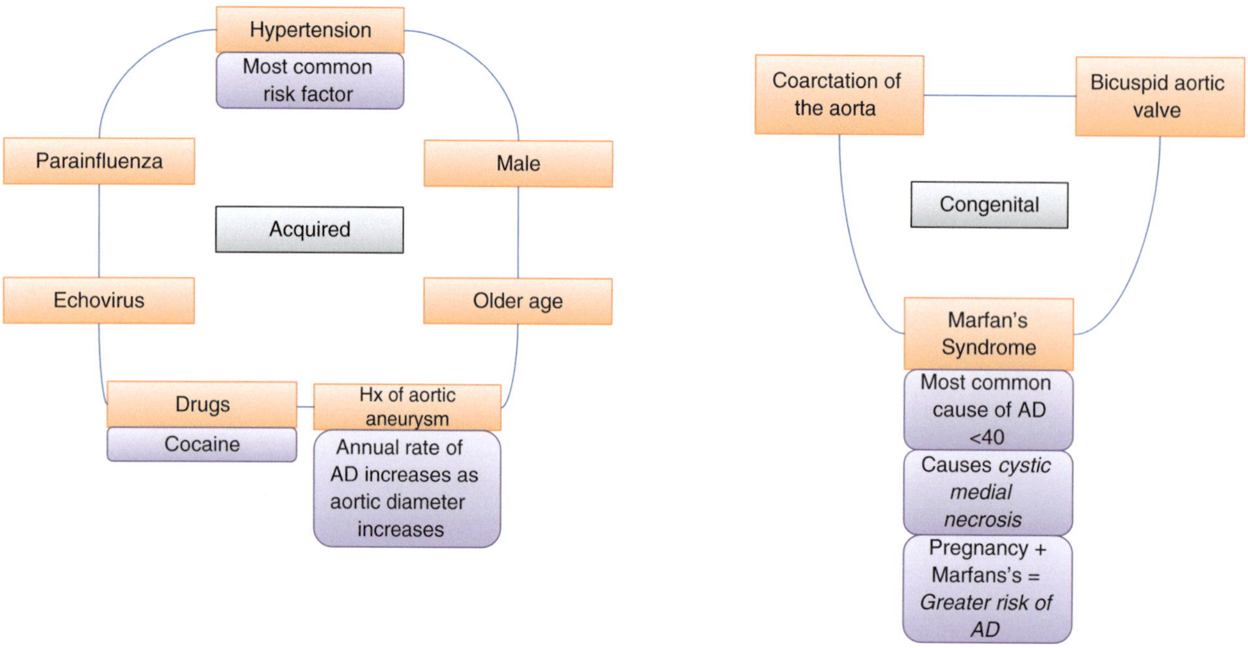

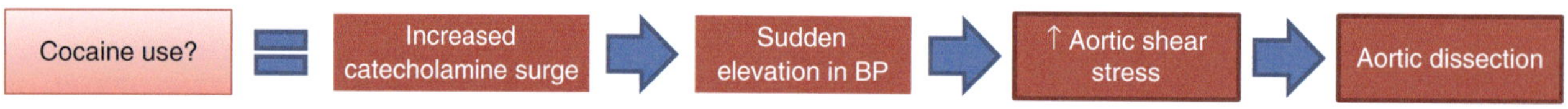

Aortic Dissection Pathophysiology

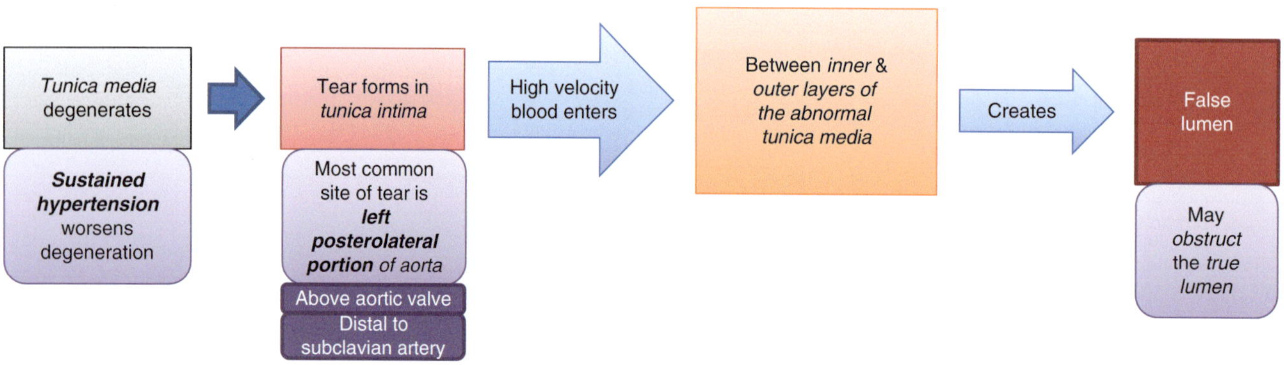

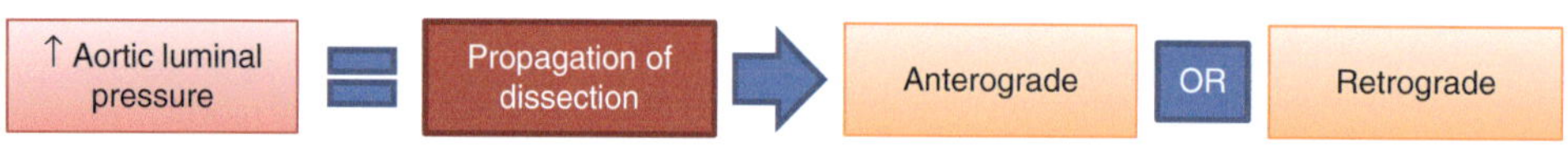

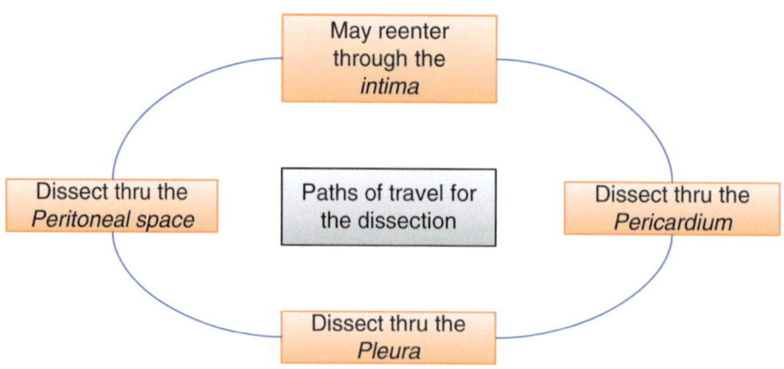

Aortic Dissection Classification

- Ascending = 60 %
- Aortic arch = 10 %
- Descending = 30 %

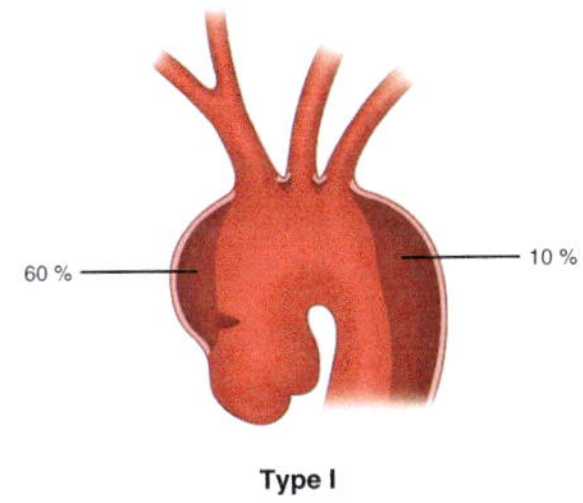

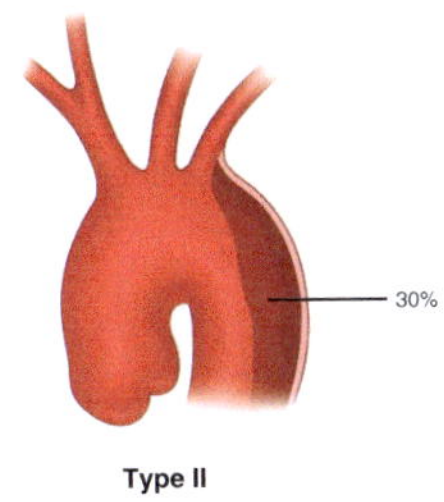

Anatomy and Classification of Aortic Dissection

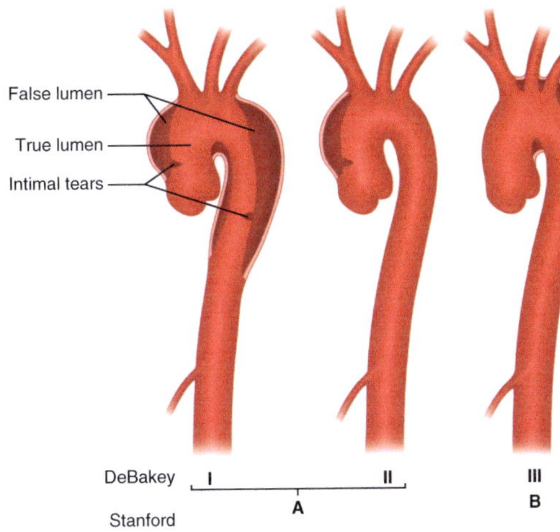

A = 62 % | B = 38 %

Aortic Dissection: Clinical Features

History

- **CP common**
  - Abrupt, Sharp/Stabbing
  - Anterior = Ascending
- **Back Pain**
  - Abrupt & stabbing
- **Radiation pain to *neck, jaw, throat***
  - Aortic arch
- **Radiation pain to *abdomen, back, intrascapular region***
  - Descending

All pain may *migrate*

Others: Feeling of impending doom; Diaphoresis; Syncope; N/V

Symptoms & Signs

- Myocardial Infarction
- Stroke
- Neurologic findings
- Syncope
- Limb Ischemia
- Hyper-or hypotension
- Aortic regurgitation
- Pulse deficit between extremities
- Renal infarction
- Mesenteric ischemia
- Tamponade
- Asymmetric pulses

Myocardial Infarction = 5 % of Type A Dissections → ***RCA*** most commonly involved → Leads to *Inferior* wall MI

Aortic Dissection Diagnosis

CXR

- *Abnormal* in 80–90 % with AD
  - 12 % with *normal* CXR
  - Findings are often non-specific
- Mediastinal widening
  - Most common finding
  - Seen in 63 % with Type A
  - Seen in 56 % with Type B
- Calcium sign
  - Separation of the intimal calcification from the outer aortic soft tissue border by 10mm
- *Left* pleural effusion
  - More common with ***descending aorta***
- Obliteration of aortic knob
- Loss of paratracheal stripe
- Depression of *left* mainstem bronchus
- Tracheal deviation

EKG

- 31 % are ***normal***
- Ascending AD involving RCA
  - Inferior wall MI
  - Will have same signs & symptoms

CT Angiography

- Diagnostic test of choice
- Sensitivity 95–100 %
- Specificity 98 %

Findings →

- Main Findings
  - Dilation of the aorta
  - Intimal flap identification
  - Presence of true & false lumen
- Other Findings
  - Pleural effusion
  - Pericardial effusion
  - Aortic rupture
  - Branch vessel involvement

Transthoracic Echocardiography

- *Lacks sensitivity 77–80 %*
- CAN identify → Pericardial effusions + Valvular abnormalities
- CANNOT fully visualize → Aortic arch + Descending aorta

Transesophageal Echocardiography

- Diagnostic test of choice in the *unstable patient*
- Sensitivity 98 %
- Specificity 95 %
- Can image most of the thoracic aorta
- CAN identify → Pericardial effusions + Valvular abnormalities
- → Identifies the *mobile intimal flap* that separates the true & false lumen

Angiography

- The "gold standard"
- Sensitivity varies – up to 85 %
- Very specific - 98 %
- Logistically difficult
- May have *false negatives* due to *false lumen thrombosis*
- Being replaced (or has been replaced by CT)

Findings →

- Main Findings
  - Site of origin of the original dissection
  - Branch artey involvement
  - Aortic regurgitation
  - Coronary artery involvement

→ Almost always requires further imaging

MRI

- Limited use in the ED
- Highest Sensitivity 98 %
- Highest specificity 98 %

Labs

- Of little value
- Do not use D-dimer to exclude dissection
- Type & cross if going to OR

Aortic Dissection Management

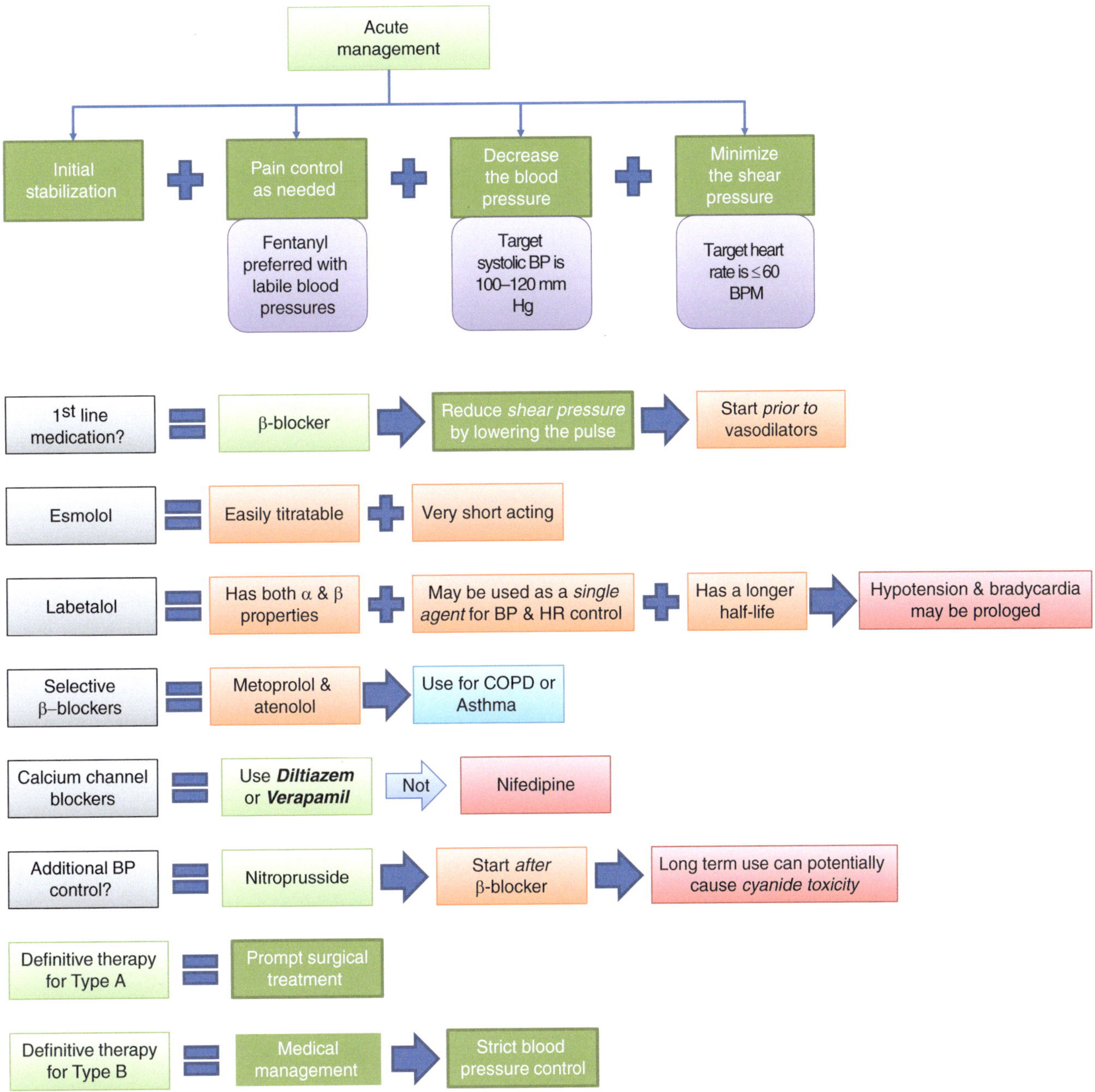

Aortic Dissection Special Circumstance

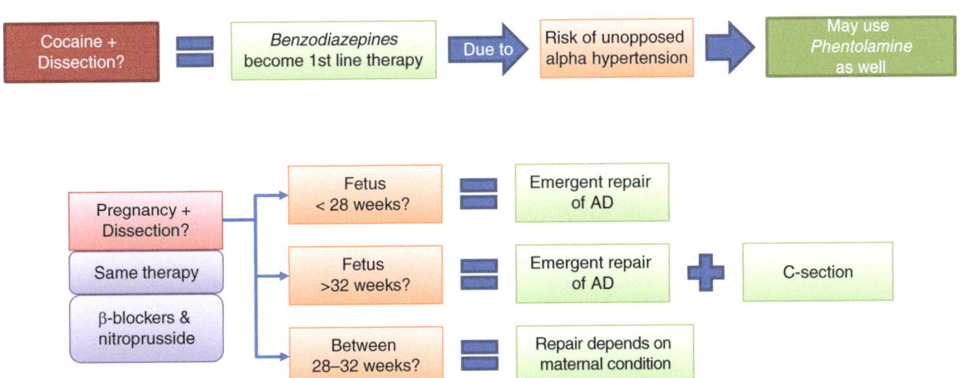

Hypertension

Blood Pressure Definitions

	Systolic BP (mm Hg)		Diastolic BP (mm Hg)
Normal	<120	&	<80
Prehypertension	120–139	OR	80–89
Stage 1	140–159	OR	90–99
Stage 2	≥160	OR	≥100

Hypertensive Urgency = Severe elevation in BP (**Arbitrary** BP ≥ 180/120) + NO signs or symptoms of end organ damage = Initiate therapy + Modify behavior

Hypertensive Emergency = Severe elevation in BP (No specific BP level!!) + Signs or symptoms of *end organ damage* = Emergent BP reduction

End Organs = Heart + Aorta + Brain + Eyes + Kidney

Hypertensive Emergencies

Hypertensive emergency? OR Malignant hypertension? = Reduce **M**ean **A**rterial **P**ressure **(MAP)** → 30 % in 30 minutes

MAP = DBP + (SBP-DBP) ÷ 3

End Organ and Other Syndromes Related to Hypertension

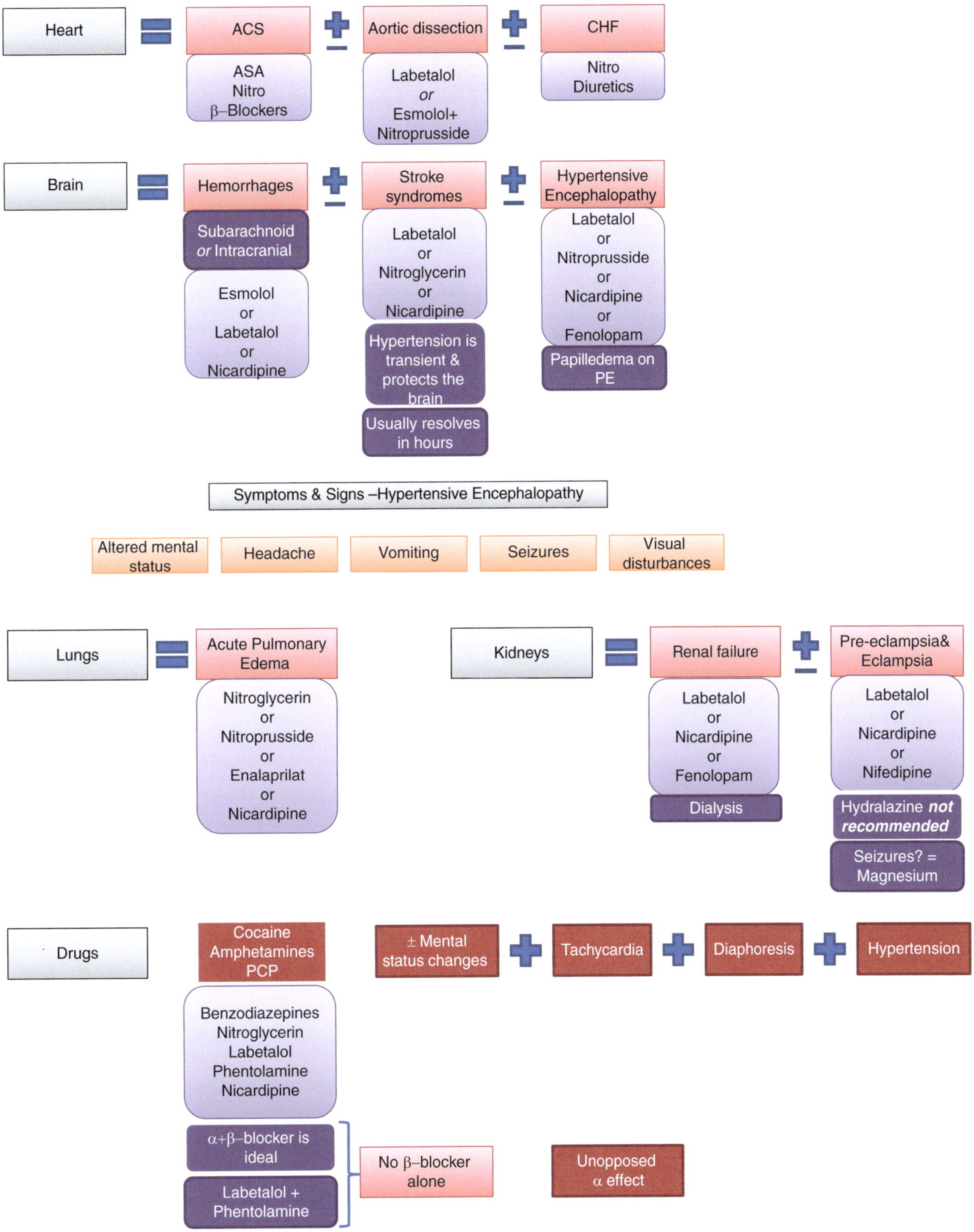

Adrenals = Catecholamine crisis ± Pheochromocytoma
Labetalol + Phentolamine
α+β–blocker is ideal

Pheochromocytoma = Headache + Flushing + Alternating periods of hypertension and normal BP

Eyes = Exudates ± Hemorrhages = Treat associated syndromes

Medication Effects and Side Effects

Medication	Effects	Side Effects & Cautions
Nitroglycerin	Arterial, venous, coronary vasodilator Onset = immediate	Reflex tachycardia Headache
Nitroprusside	Arterial & venous vasodilator Onset = 1-2 min	Reflex tachycardia Use with β-blocker ↑ Increased ICP Long term use Cyanide toxicity
Labetalol	α+β–blocker Onset = 2-5 min	No reflex tachycardia Do not use in *AV blocks*, *CHF*, or *bronchospasm*
Esmolol	β–blocker Onset = immediate	Do not use in *bradycardia*, *CHF*, *bronchospasm*

Medication	Effects	Side Effects & Cautions
Nicardipine	Selective for *cerebral* & *coronary* arteries Onset = 5–10 min	Do not use in *CHF*
Phentolamine	α_1 & α_2 blocker Onset = 5–10 min	Cerebrovascular occlusion MI
Enalaprilat	ACE Inhibitor Onset = 5–10 min	Avoid in *pregnancy* Dizziness Headache
Hydralazine	Arteriolar vasodilator May be used in Pediatric nephritis **Not recommended** Pregnancy-induced hypertension Onset = 10 min	Reflex tachycardia Chronic use = "Lupus-like" syndrome

Evaluation of Severe Asymptomatic Hypertension

Completely depends on patient condition, history, and review of systems

Commonly ordered investigations

- EKG
- Basic metabolic panel
- CXR
- Urinalysis

Disposition = Depends on clinical condition

Pulmonary Hypertension

Introduction

Pulmonary Hypertension = Dx cannot be made in the ED!

Time between symptom start and diagnosis = 2 years due to lack of specificity

Pulmonary Hypertension = ↑ Pulmonary vascular pressure → Causing → ↓ Right ventricular function

Acute Sx in pts Dx with PH = Worsening of underlying condition ± Complications of medication administration ± Adverse effects of drugs ± Rebound effects due to drug stoppage

Symptoms

- Dyspnea
  - Most common Sx
  - On rest or exertion
- Chest pain
  - Poor coronary blood flow
- Fatigue
- Syncope
  - Poor cardiac output
- Sx of underlying disease
- Peripheral edema
  - RV failure

Exam may include

- Increase in pulmonary component of 2nd heart sound
- Murmur of tricuspid regurgitation
- Murmur of Pulmonary insufficiency
- Ascites
- Peripheral edema
- Hepatic congestion
- Sternal heave
  - RV hypertrophy
- JVD
  - Severe cases

Diagnostic Studies

CXR

- Use to show any signs of pulmonary disease

EKG

- RVH
- Incomplete RBBB
- RBBB with right axis deviation

Confirmatory

- Transthoracic echocardiography
- Cardiac catheterization
- PFT's

Goal of Treatment

Treatment goals = Decrease symptoms + Improve exercise tolerance + Prolong survival → Consult your pulmonologist for definitive Rx

Syncope

Introduction

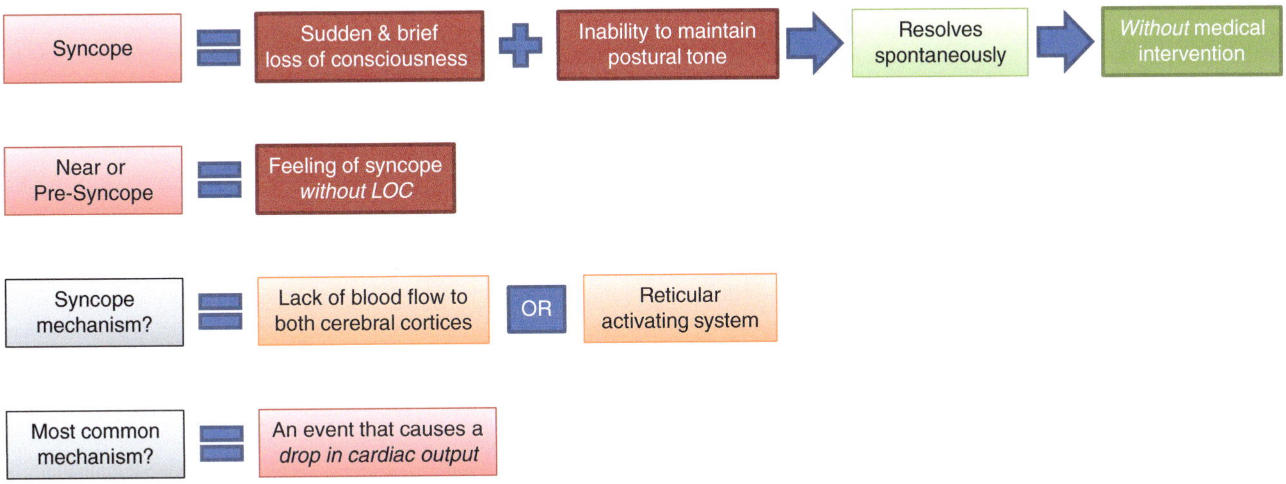

Causes of Syncope

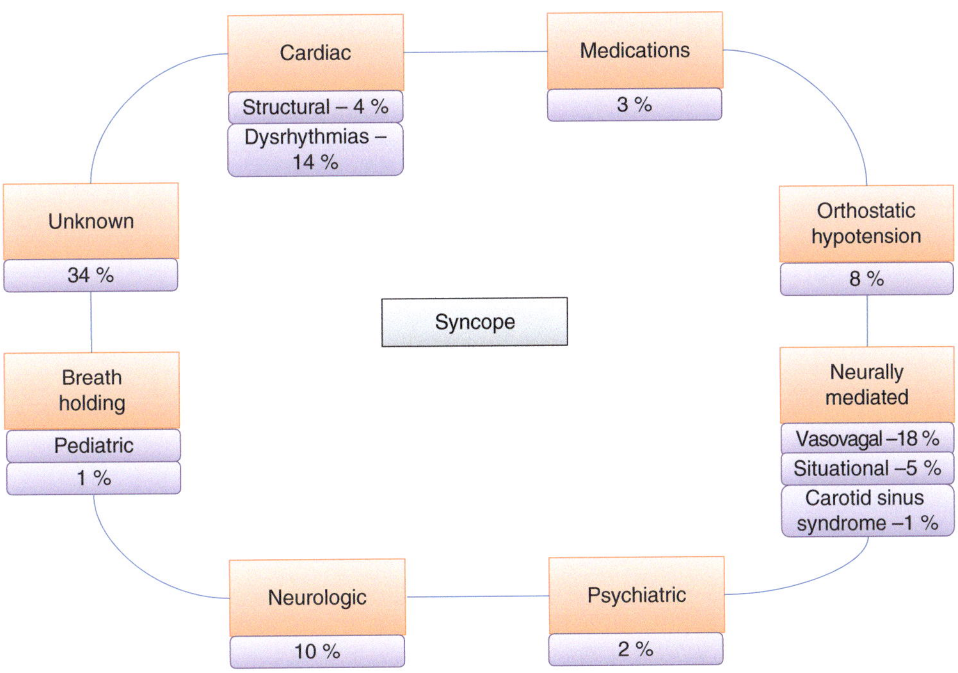

Cardiac Syncope

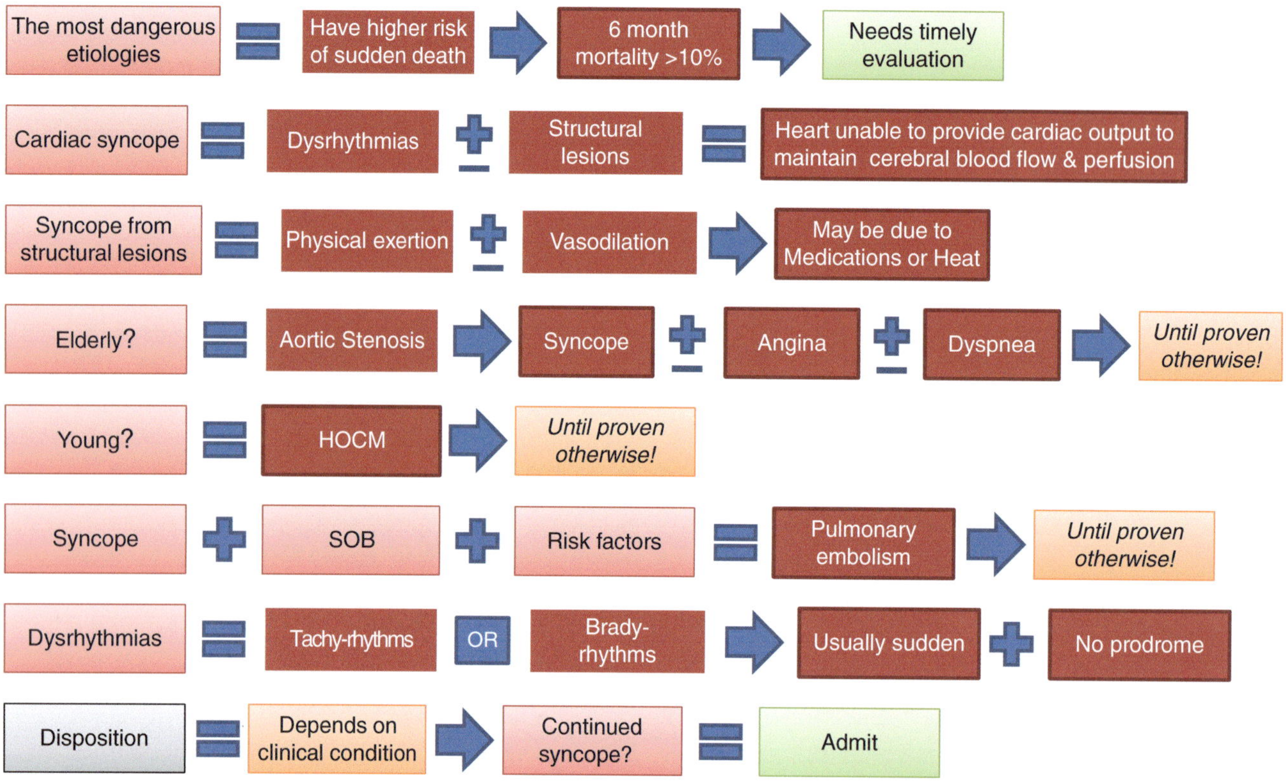

Vasovagal and Orthostatic Syncope

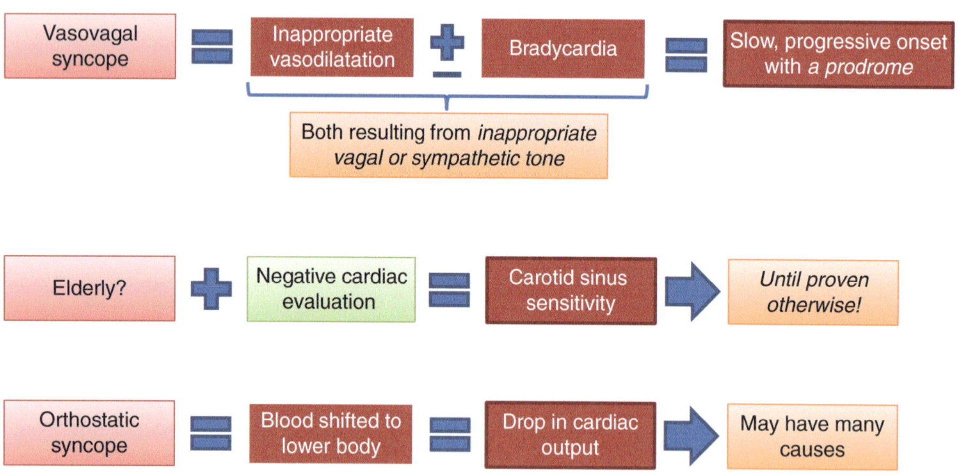

Evaluation of Syncope

Completely depends on patient condition, history, and review of systems

Disposition = Depends on clinical condition

Deep Venous Thrombosis and Pulmonary Embolism

Introduction

Pulmonary embolism = Thrombi formation → Usually form near venous valves (Due to slow blood flow) → Portion of venous clot breaks off → Lodges in Pulmonary arteries (Pre-capillary)

Veins in which clots can form: Popliteal, Pelvic, Axillary, Jugular, Great veins, Superficial Femoral

PE symptoms = Pulmonary vessels 20–30 % occluded

Obstruction of pulmonary blood flow = ↑ Ventilation ↓ Perfusion = Alveolar dead space

Hypoxemia in PE? – *Unpredictable* Due to → Shunting of blood flow

Risk Factors for Thromboembolism

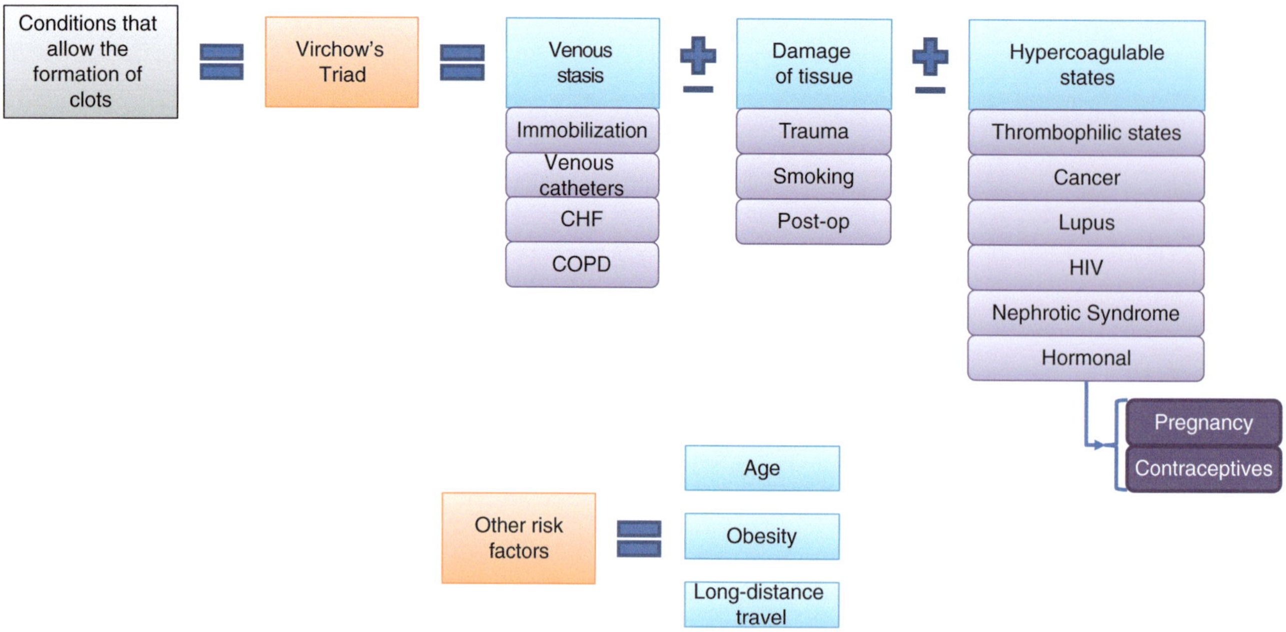

PE: Clinical Features

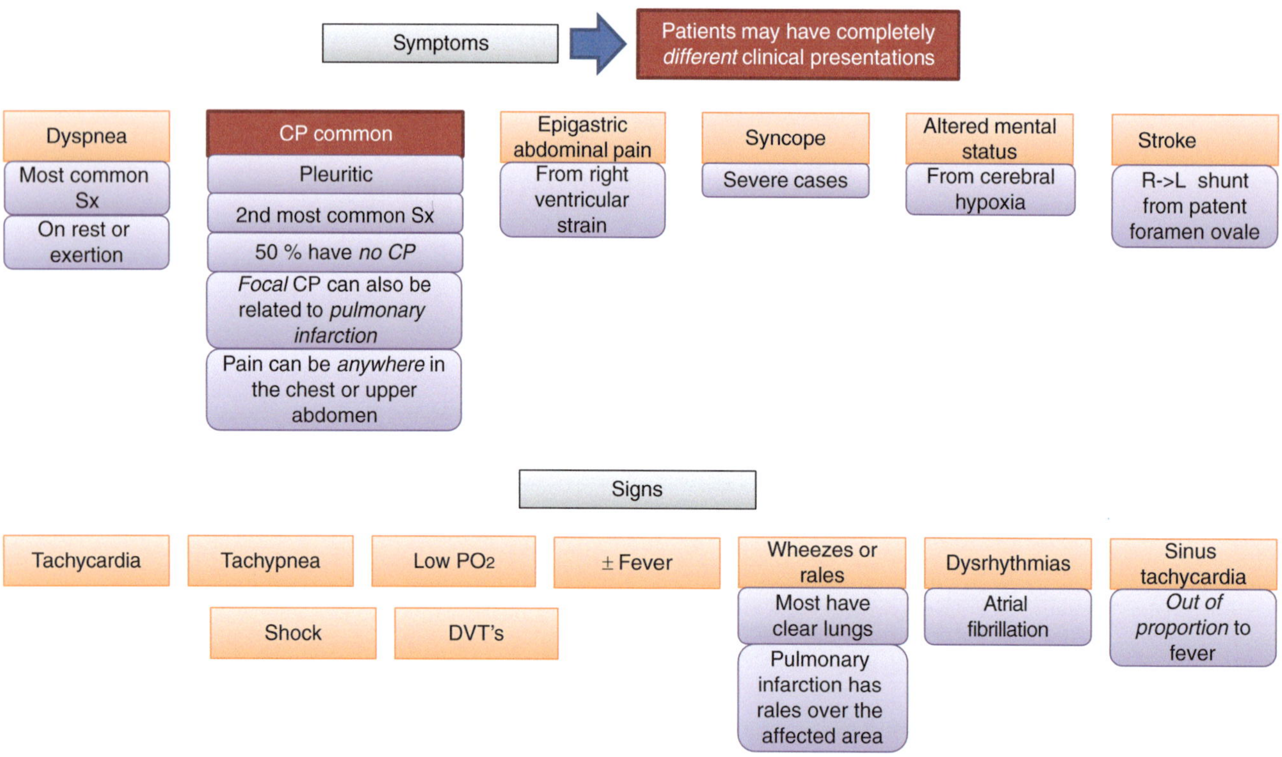

DVT: Clinical Features

Symptoms

- Extremity pain
- Swelling — Unilateral
- Cramping
- Erythema
- ± Fever

Signs

- Venous insufficiency — Hyperpigmentation; Skin ulcers
- Erythema
- U/L swelling
- ± Fever
- Homan's sign — Not sensitive or specific — Calf pain when passively dorsiflexing the affected foot

Massive ileofemoral DVT = Phlegmasia cerulean dolens → Cyanotic congested extremity + Phlegmasia alba dolens → Pale swollen extremity

Phlegmasia alba dolens associations = Pregnancy + Has associated arterial spasm

Pitfalls of both = ↑ Compartment pressure + Possible ischemia → Requiring Thrombectomy or Thrombolysis ± Surgery for compartment syndrome

Diagnosis

Pitfalls for PE Diagnosis = Routine testing usually shows ***nonspecific findings***

Diagnostic approach? = Depends on ***Pre-test probability*** → ↑ Pre-test probability = More aggressive workup But… → No perfect test exists

Determination of Pre-test probability? = Clinician's training & experience + History + Physical exam ± Scoring system — Well's score

Well's Score		
PE Unlikely < 4	OR	Low < 2
PE Likely > 4		Moderate = 2–6
		High > 6

- PE is leading diagnosis or equally likely — 3 points
- Signs and symptoms of DVT — 3 points
- HR > 100 bpm — 1.5 points
- Prior PE or DVT — 1.5 points
- Immobilization within 4 weeks — 1.5 points
- Active malignancy — 1 point
- Hemoptysis — 1 point

Using Pretest Probability in the Diagnosis of PE

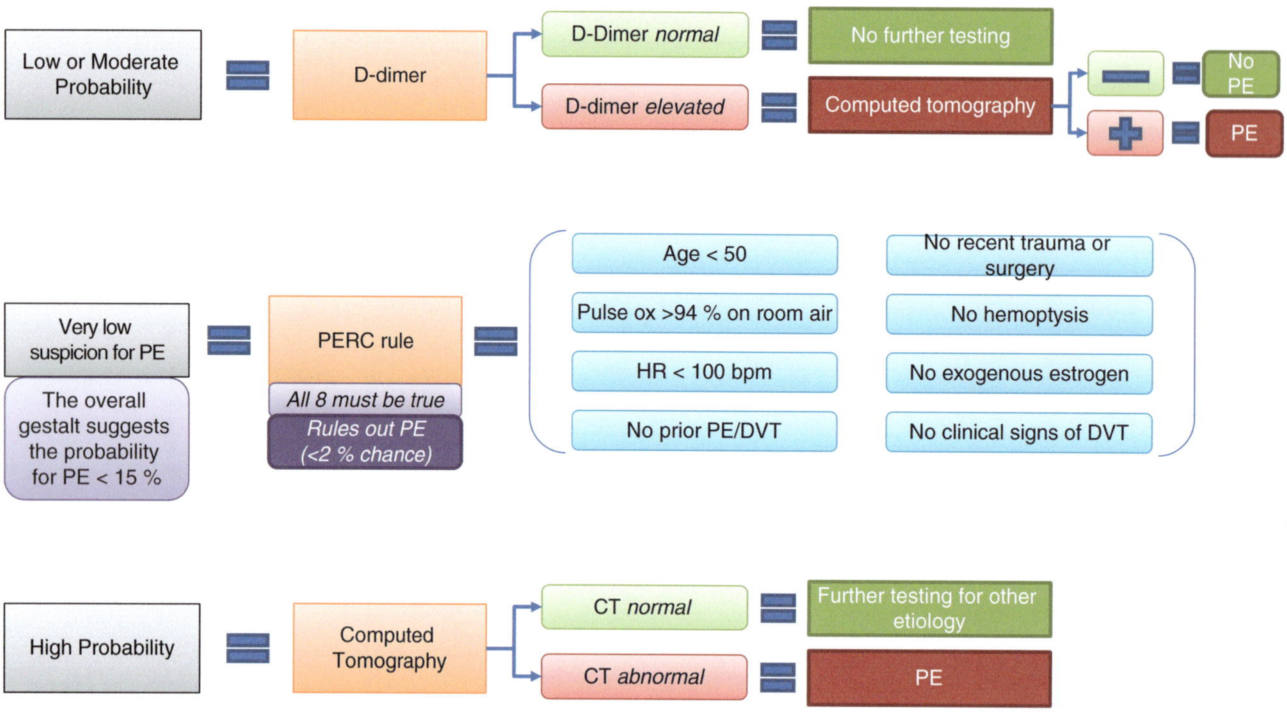

Other Basic Tests

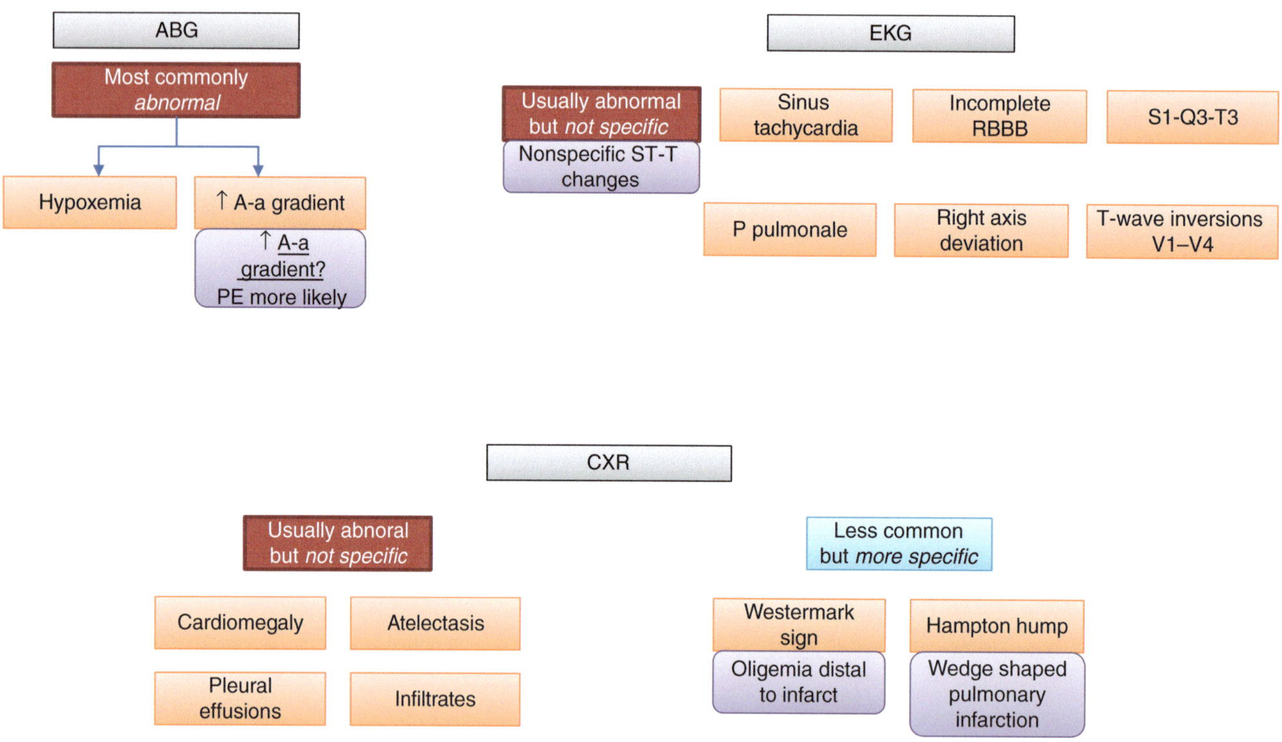

D-Dimer

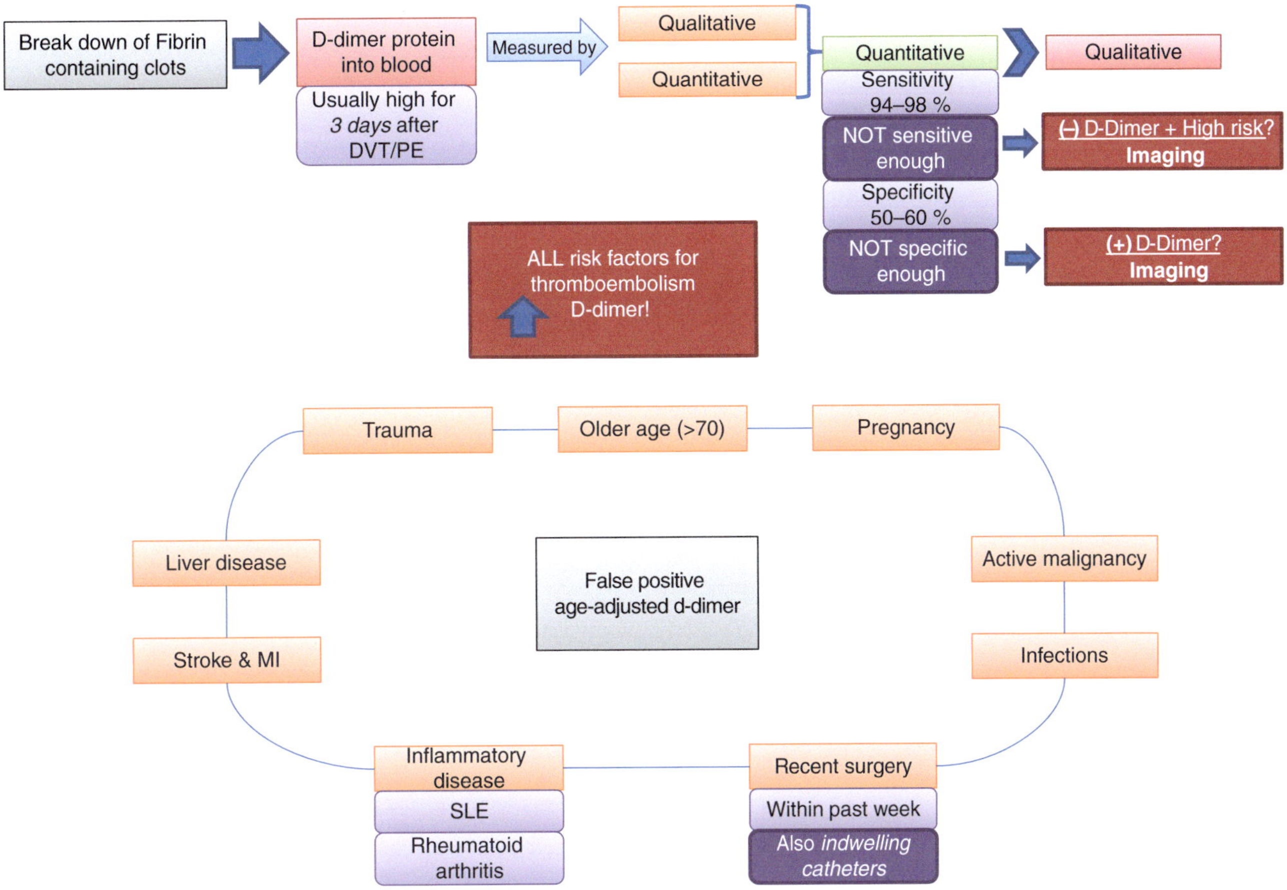

PE Imaging: CT Angiography

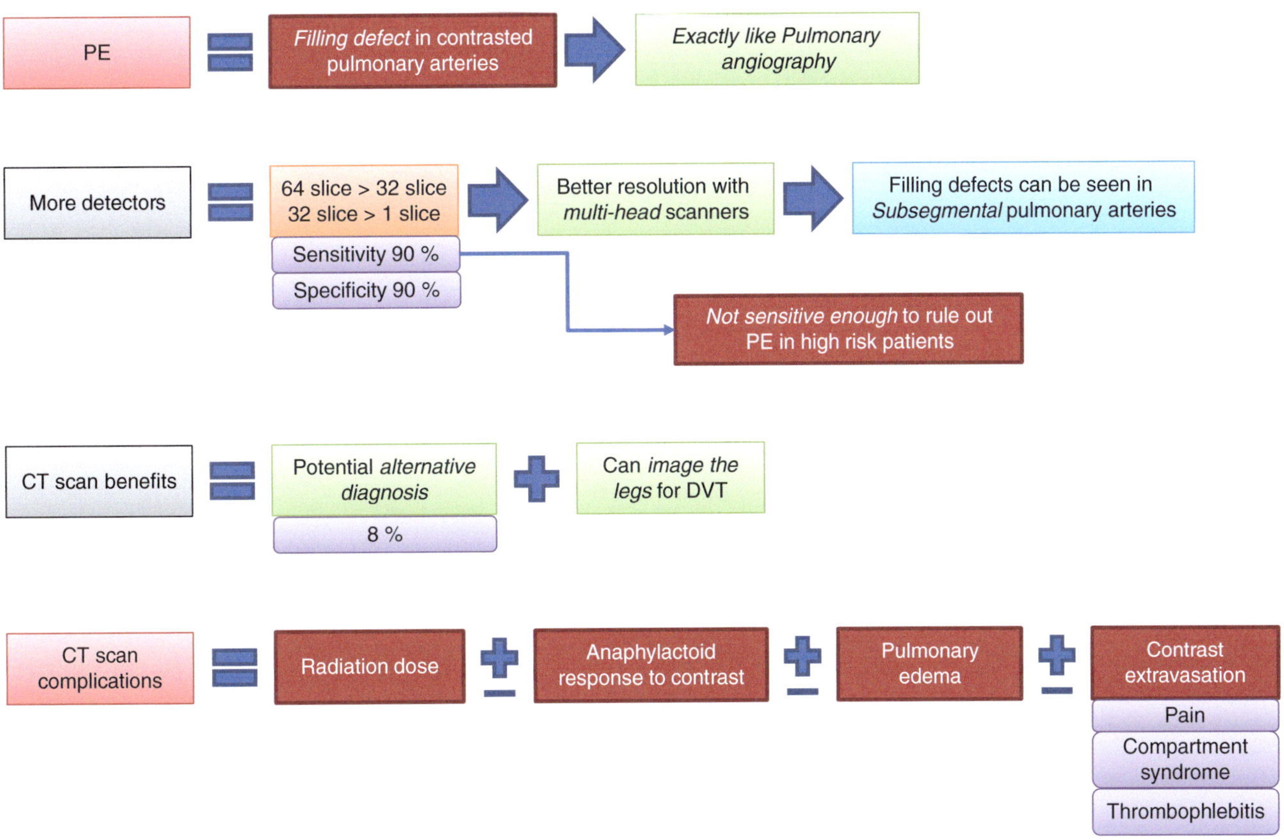

PE Imaging: Pulmonary Angiography

Angiography benefits = Direct treatment of PE (Lysis of clots; IVC filter placement) ± Can measure *pulmonary artery pressures* ± Can see *filling defects in ≥ 3 mm vessels*

Angiography complications = Not consistently available ± Contrast complications ± Cardiac or pulmonary artery perforation ± Arrhythmias ± Radiation exposure

PE Imaging: VQ Scanning

Normal V/Q = *Sensitive enough* to rule out PE (Even in high risk patients!)

All other V/Q findings = *Nondiagnostic*

Venous Ultrasound

Ultrasound benefits = Readily available + No radiation + ↑ Sensitivity & Specificity (for DVT) (Sensitivity = 90–95 %; Specificity = 95 %; Need experienced sonographers)

DVT diagnosis? = *Non-compressible veins*

Ultrasound Pitfalls = Lack of experienced sonographers ± Difficult in obese patients ± Pain ± Prior Hx of DVT + non-compressible vein (New vs. old clot)

Venography

Indirect = From CT angiography = *Filling defect* in contrasted veins

Direct ("Gold standard"; Rarely used) = Injection of contrast material into foot vein = *Filling defect* in contrasted veins → Complication: *Phlebitis*

Treatment: Anticoagulation

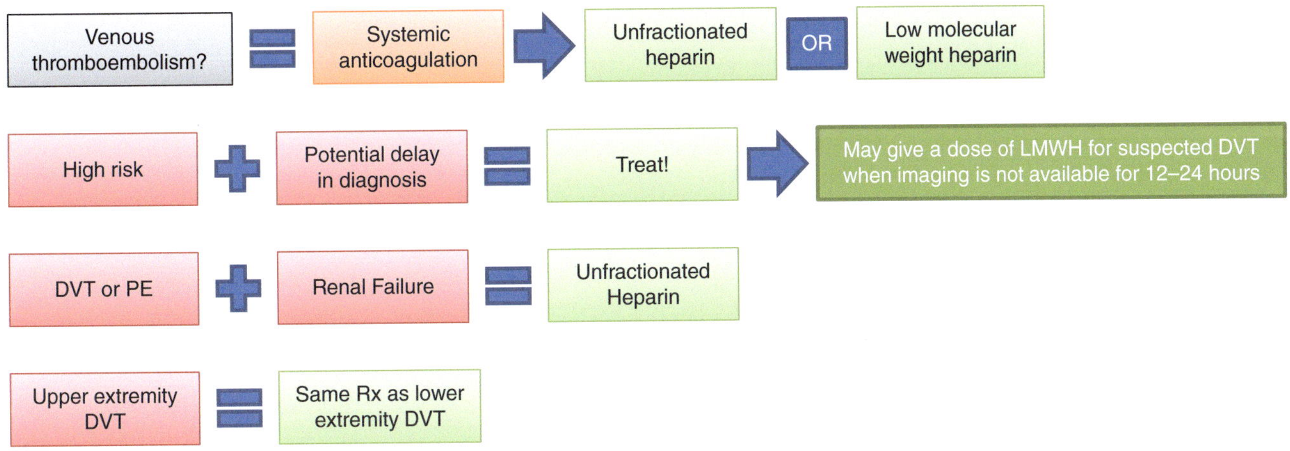

PE Tidbits

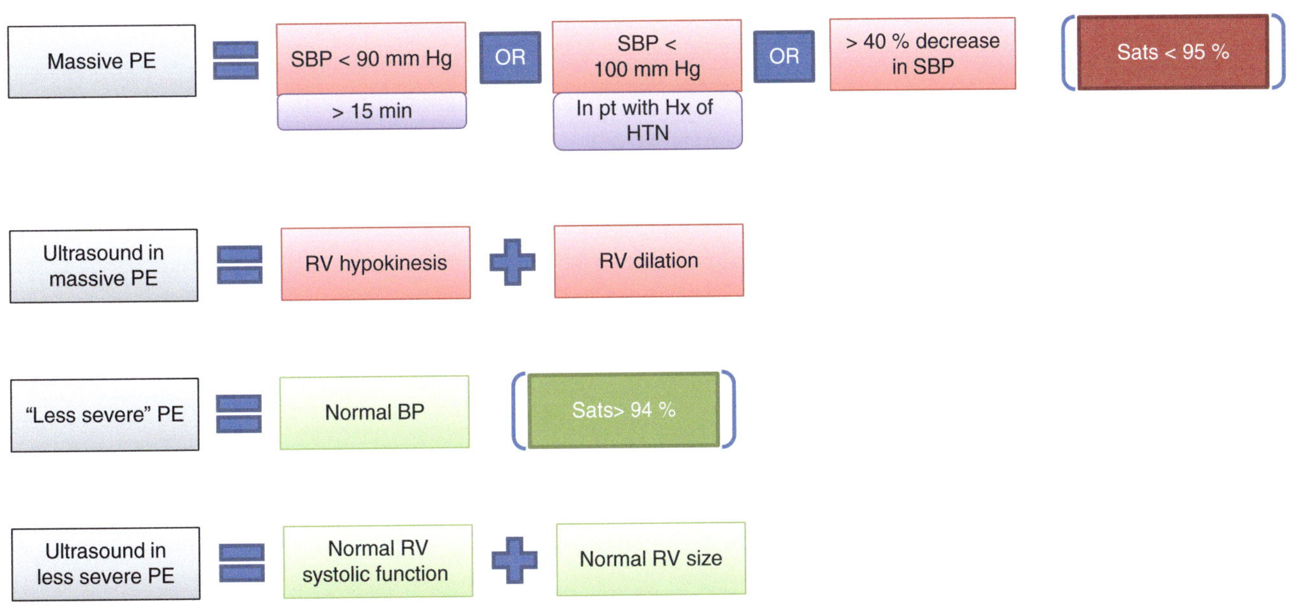

Treatment: Fibrinolysis

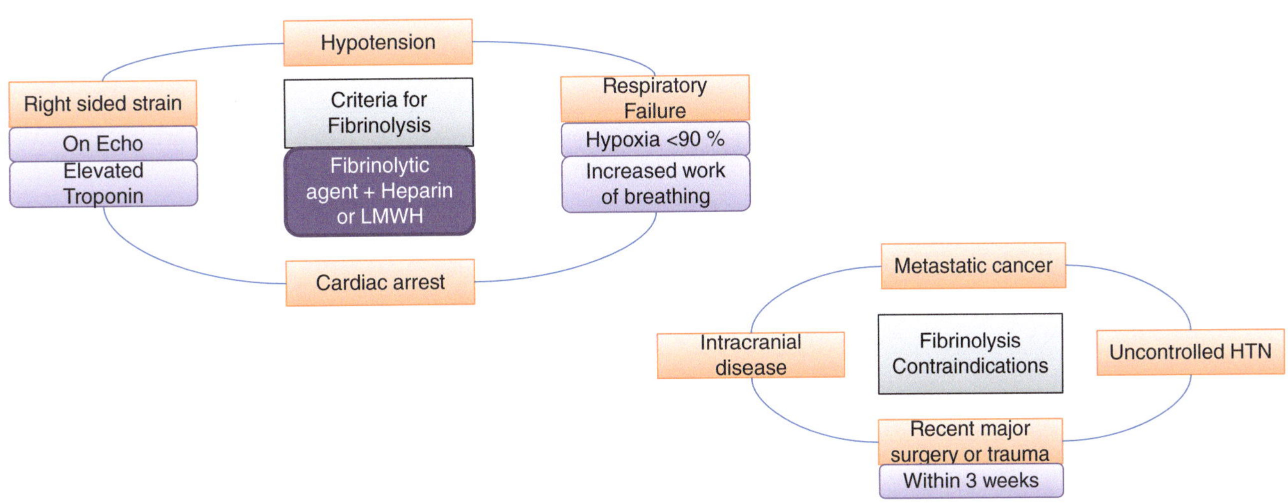

Treatment: Embolectomy

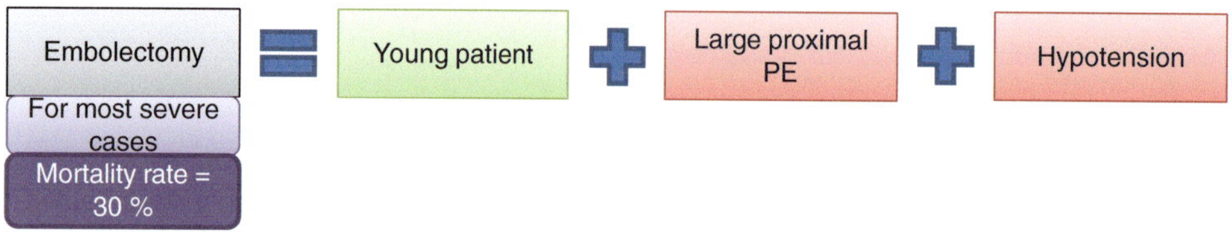

Disposition

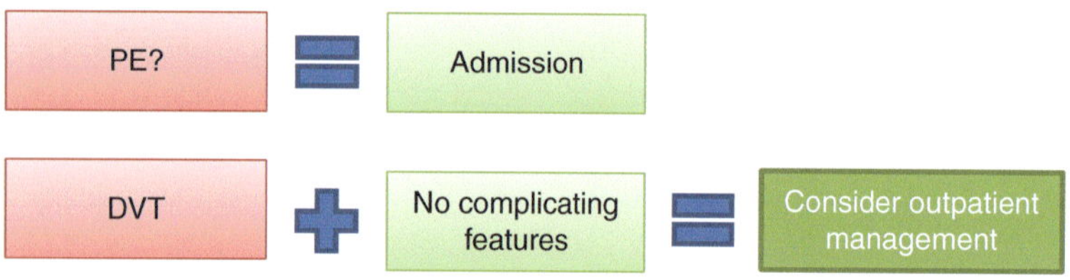

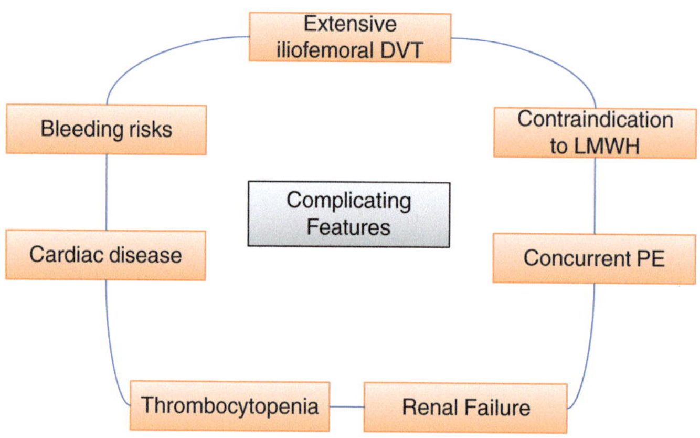

Acute Limb Ischemia

Introduction

Acute Limb Ischemia = Medical emergency

Acute Limb Ischemia Tidbits = *Smoking* & *Diabetes* are most important risk factors + Men > Women

Acute Limb Ischemia = Lack of blood flow to an affected extremity → With passage of time have irreversible cell death → Usually within ***6 hours*** but can occur sooner due to lack of collateral flow

Thrombosis? = Most common → Typically due to atherosclerosis → Has a slow onset

Embolism? = Usually cardiac in origin → *Atrial fibrillation* → Rapid onset

Reperfusion injury = Complete or partial restoration of blood flow → Formation of oxygen radicals

Reperfusion injury = Related to time → Peripheral muscle infarction + Myoglobinemia + Renal Failure

Lab abnormalities in Reperfusion injury = Myoglobinemia + ↑ K+ + ↑ CK + Metabolic acidosis

Clinical Features

Symptoms & Signs

Pain	Paralysis	Pallor	Pulselessness	Paresthesias	Polar	Muscle weakness
Severe & Constant	With continued ischemia	Early	Severe cases			
Earliest Sx		Later = Mottled				
		Latest = Necrosis				

Symptoms & Signs = The ***"6 P's"*** → May not manifest all Sx → In diseased arteries, collateral blood flow may prevent abrupt Sx

Ischemic neuropathy = Hypoesthesia OR Hyperesthesia

Preservation of light touch? = Tissue is *probably viable*

Claudication = Crampypain with exertion → Relieved with rest → **Femoral + Popliteal disease** Calf pain

Neurogenic claudication = Worsened with erect posture + Inconsistent response to exercise

Clinical Diagnosis

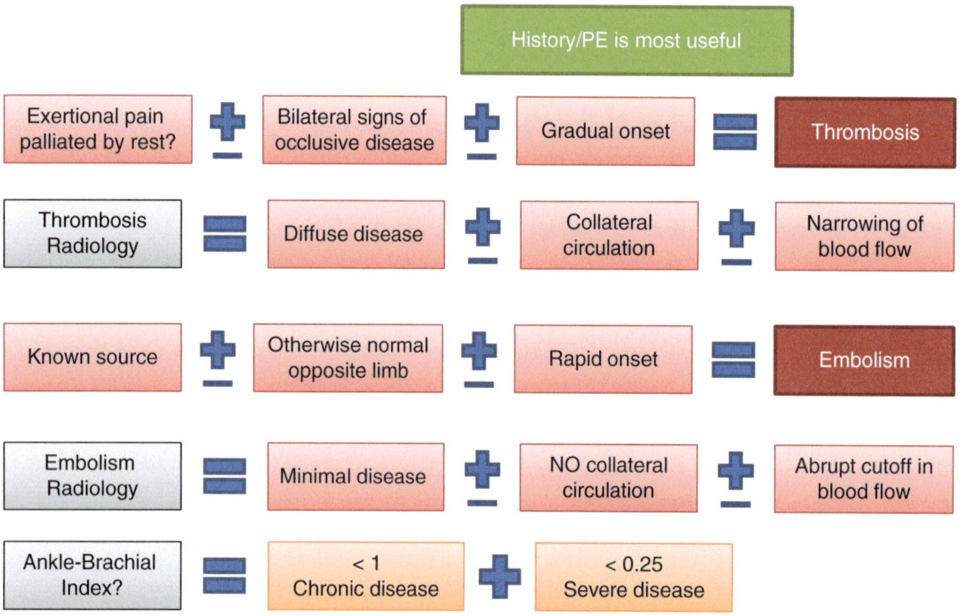

Diagnosis

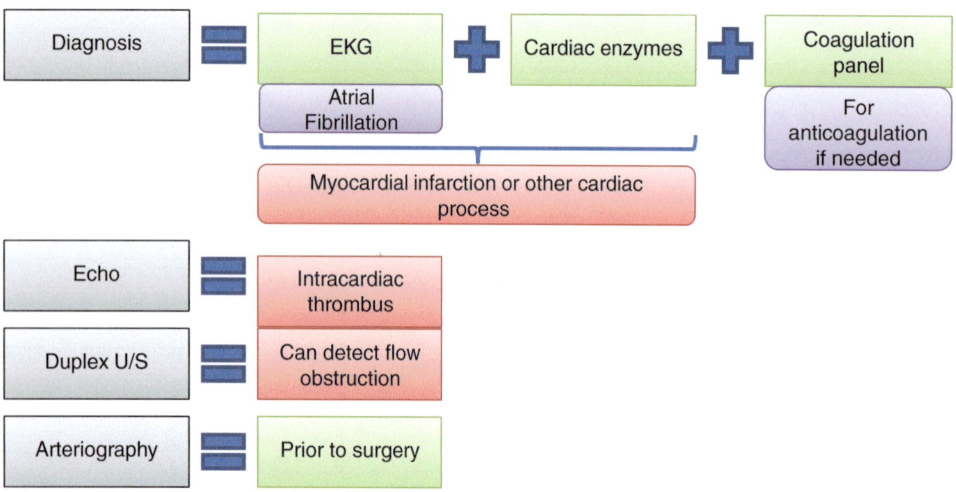

Treatment

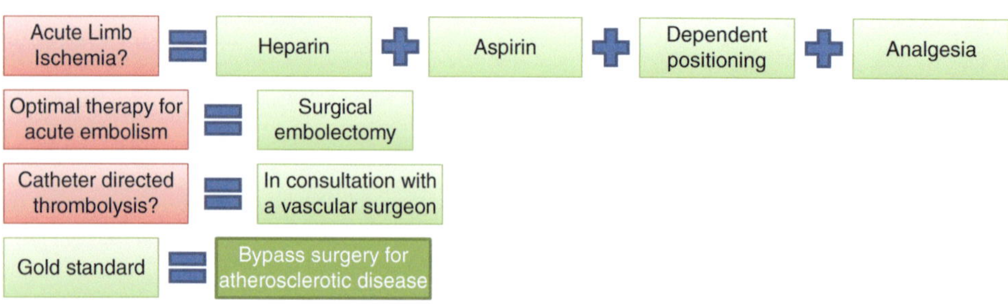

Pacemakers

Emergency Pacing

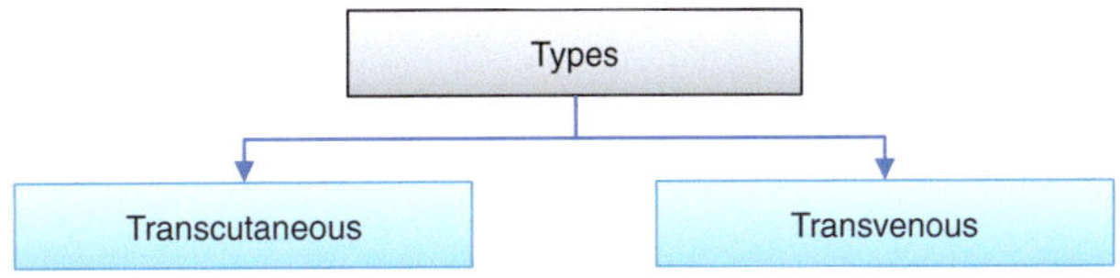

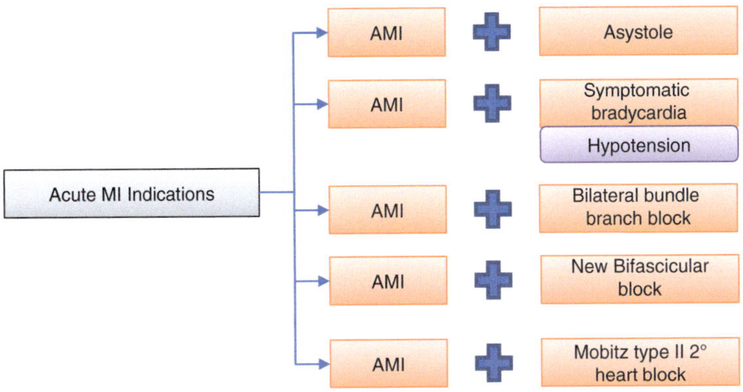

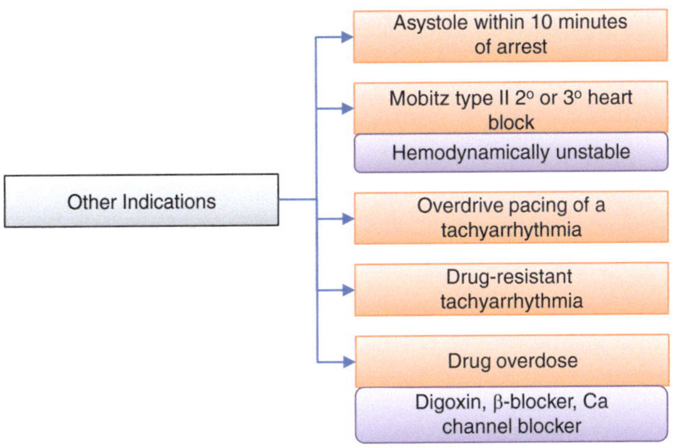

Pacemaker Nomenclature

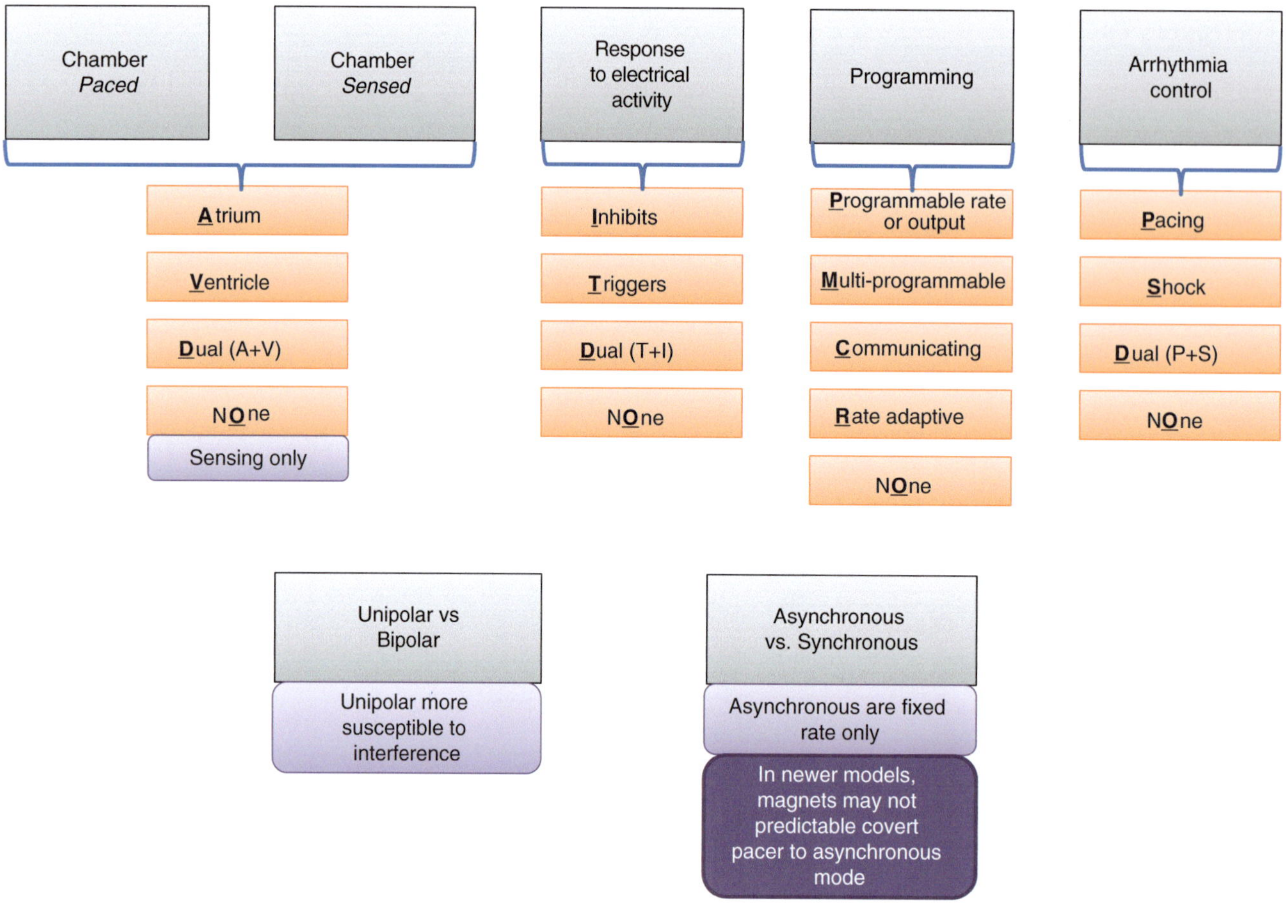

Automatic Implantable Cardioverter: Defibrillator Nomenclature

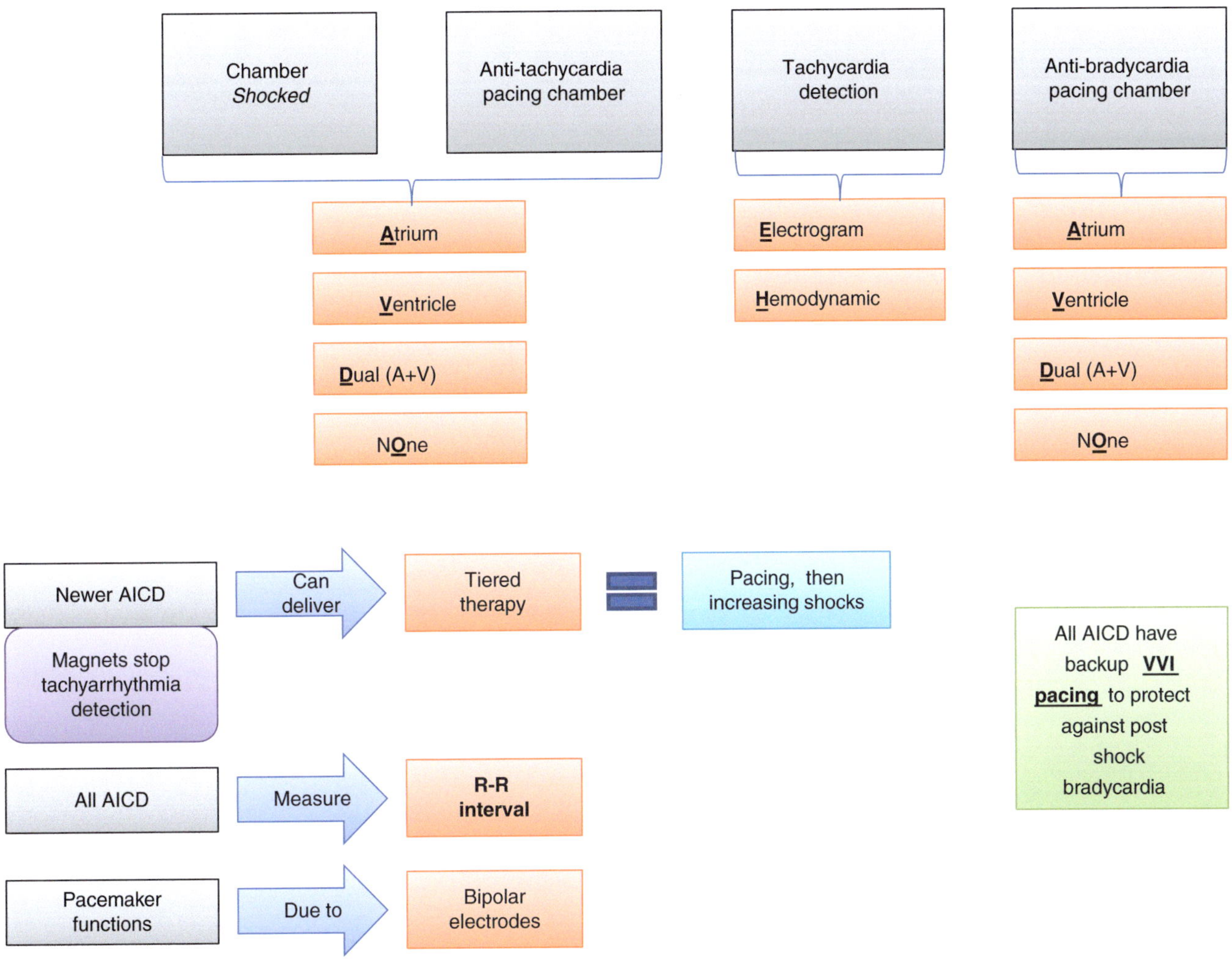

Specific Pacemaker Malfunctions

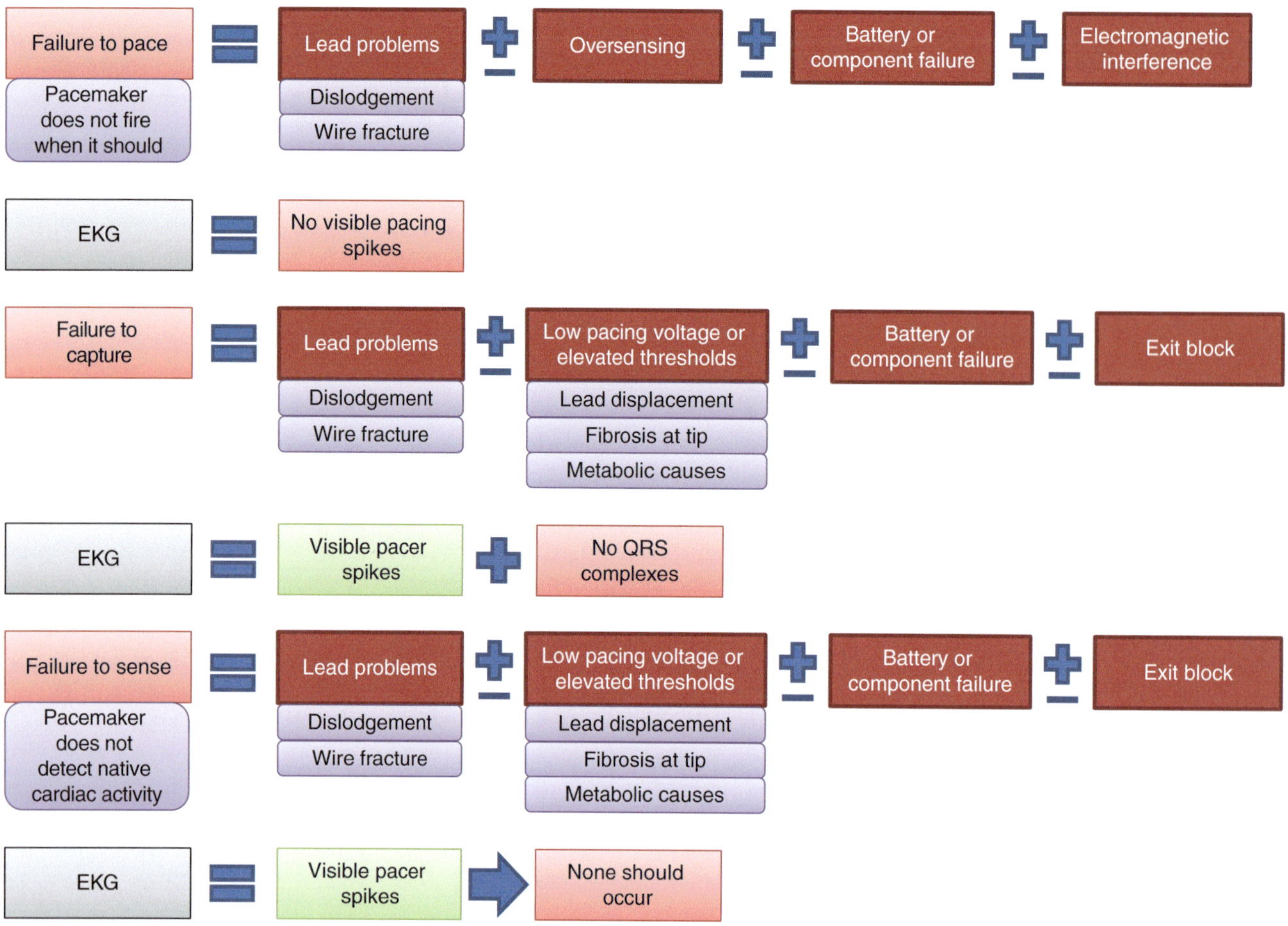

Pacemaker Failure

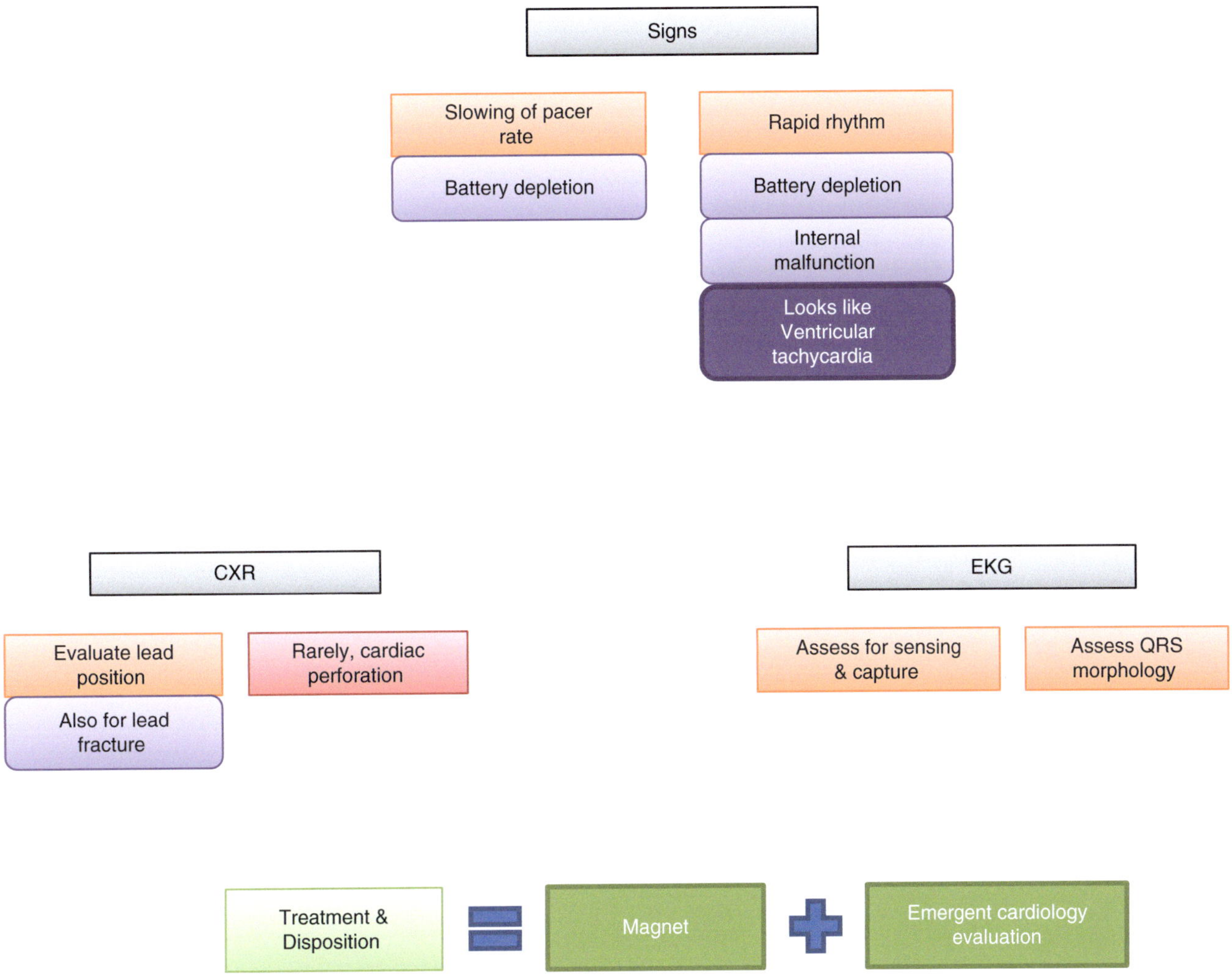

Left Ventricular Assist Devices (LVAD)

Introduction

LVAD = Bridge to transplant + Improves quality of life for those not eligible for transplant

Stable patients = May have no pulse at baseline!

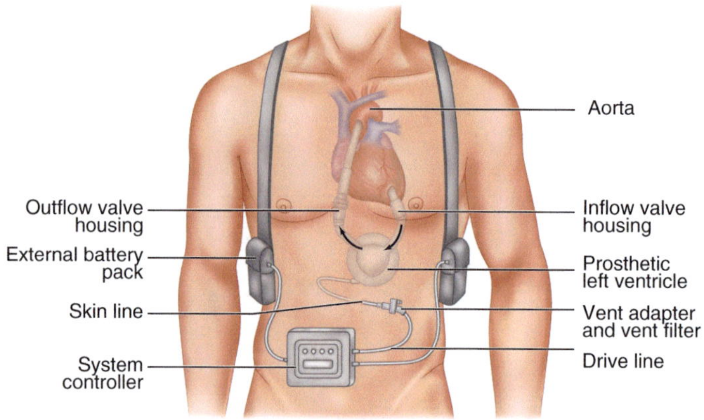

LVAD Emergencies

Pt in extremis

- LISTEN for humming sound from machine
- Check battery
  - Pt should have travel bag with extra batteries
- Check the lines
- Check the alarm
  - Will be flashing
- Use the hand pump back up
  - 60-90 bpm

LVAD: Patient Assessment

Check MAP → Ideally >65 → Use *manual BP* or *Doppler*

↓ Preload? = Fluids ± Blood

↑ Afterload? = Nitrates or Anti-hypertensives

Coding with LVAD

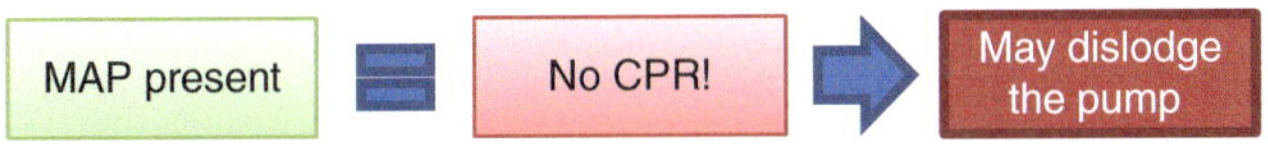

LVAD Complications

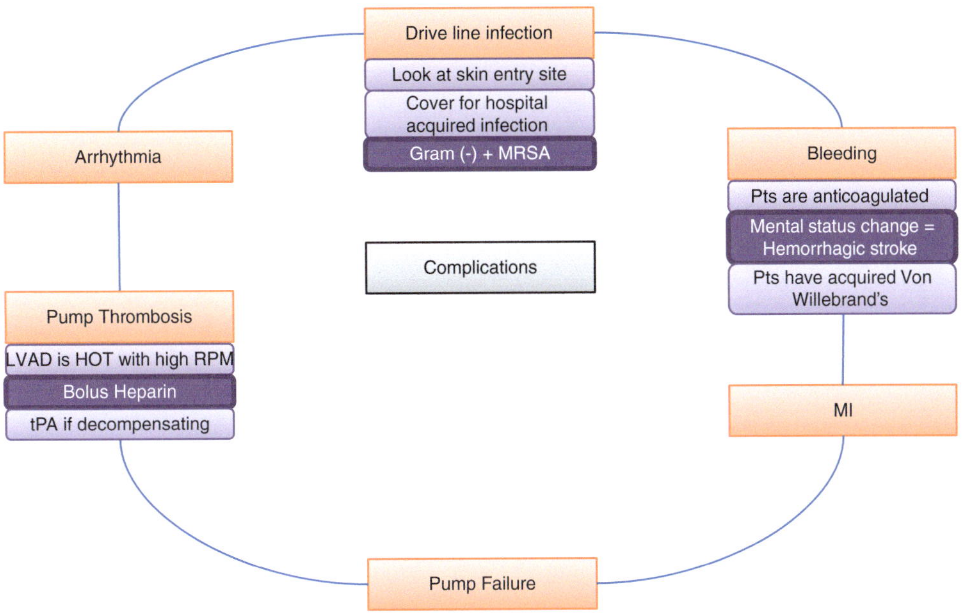

Echo Findings

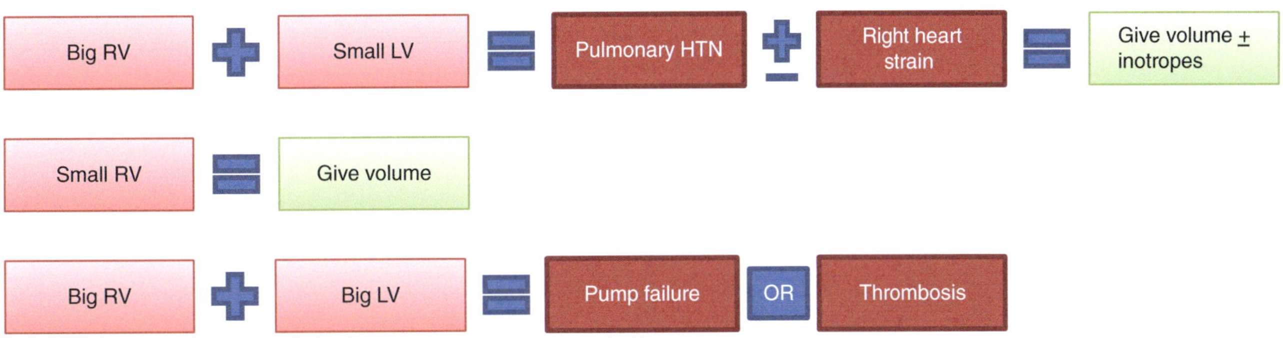

EKG in LVAD

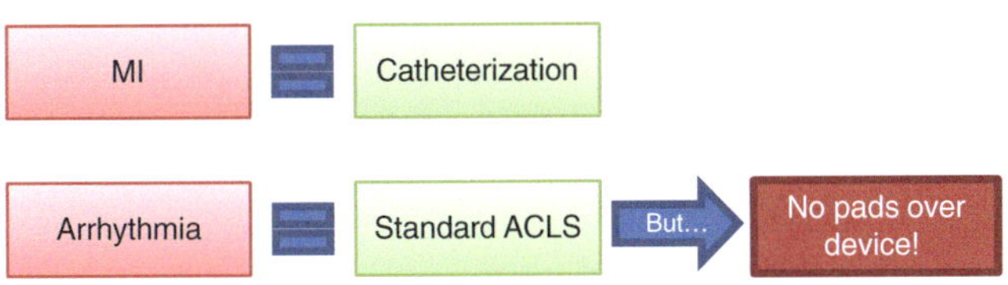

EKG Changes Related to Electrolytes and Metabolic Conditions

Hypothermia: EKG Changes

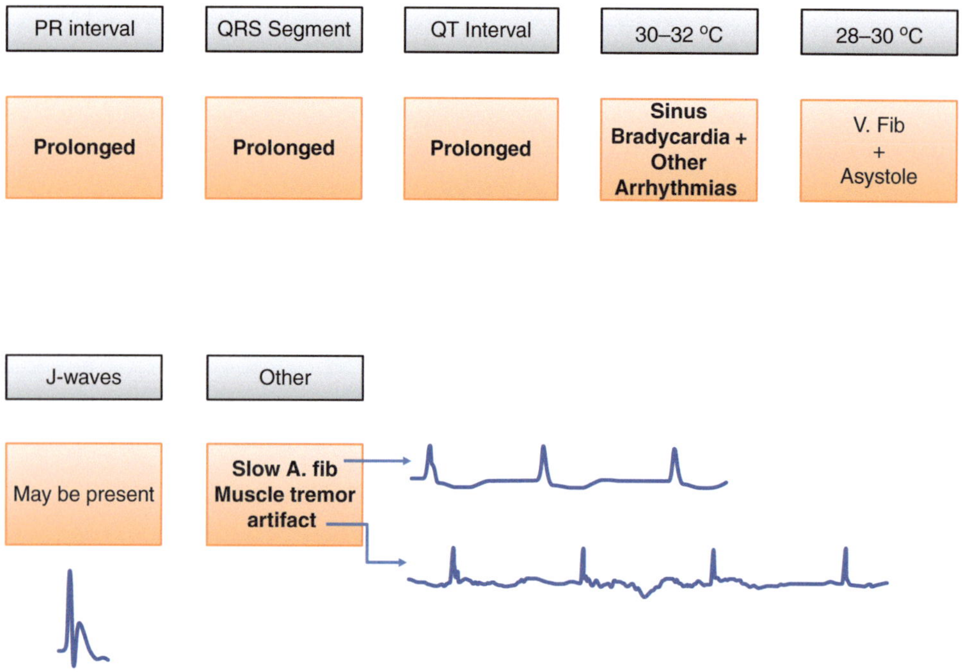

Hypokalemia: EKG Changes

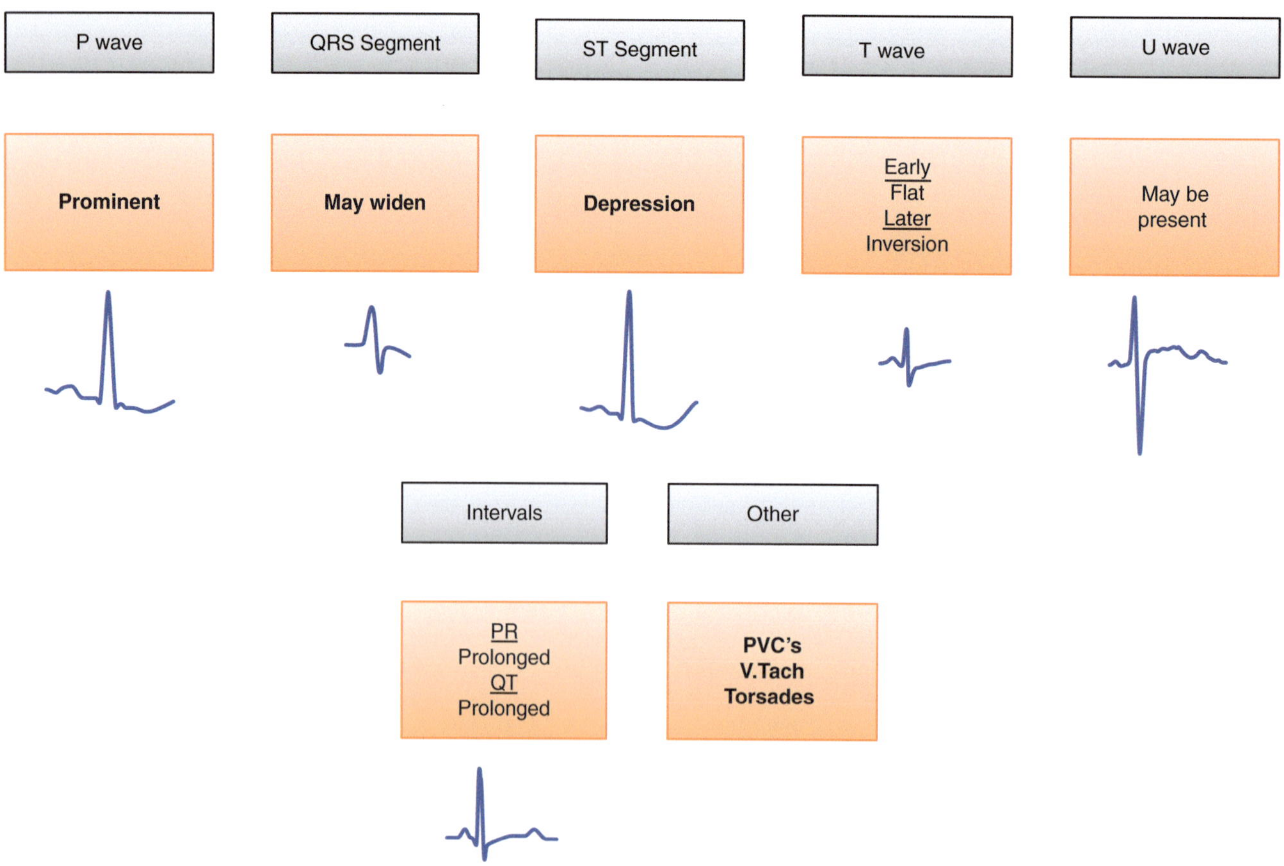

Hyperkalemia: EKG Changes

P wave	QRS Segment	ST Segment	T wave
Flat or Absent	**Wide**	**May be elevated**	Early Hyperacute" Later QRS + T = Sine wave
7.5–8.0 mEq/L	7.5–8.0 mEq/L		Early: 6.5–7.5 mEq/L

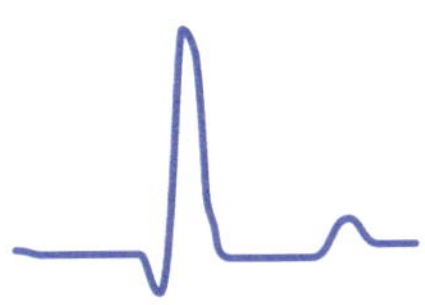

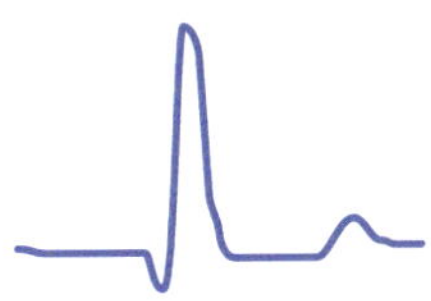

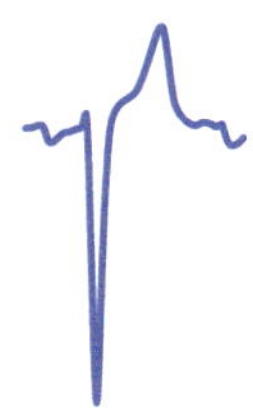

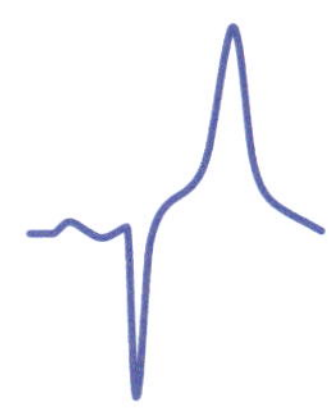

Intervals	Rhythms	Blocks
PR Prolonged QT Shortened	Bradycardia V. Fib Sine Wave	**AV Blocks**
6.5–7.5 mEq/L	10–12 mEq/L	

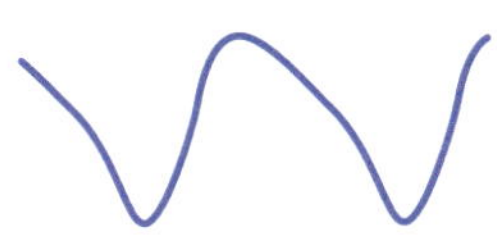

Hypocalcemia: EKG Changes

Intervals	Rhythms	T wave
QT Prolonged	Ventricular dysrhythmias Torsades	**Inversions**

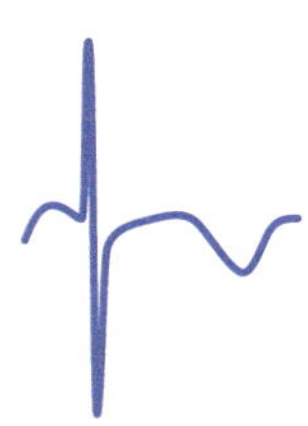

Hypercalcemia: EKG Changes

QRS Segment	ST Segment	Intervals
May be wide	**May be depressed**	<u>PR</u> Prolonged <u>QT</u> Shortened

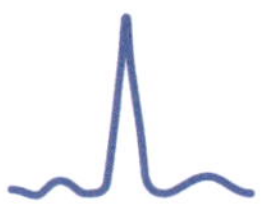

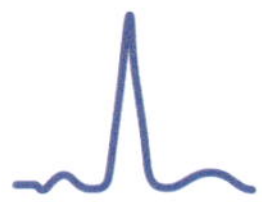

Hypomagnesemia: EKG Changes

Intervals	QRS Segment	ST Segment	T wave	Other
<u>PR</u> Prolonged <u>QT</u> Prolonged	**Wide**	**Not normal**	Flat or inverted	**PVC's V.Tach Torsades V. fib**

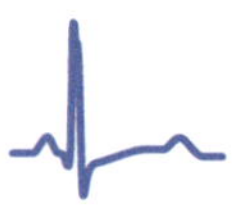

QT

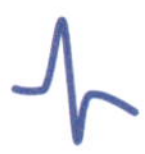

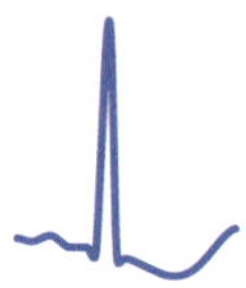

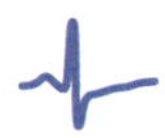

<u>QT prolongation</u>
*Hypo*kalemia
*Hypo*calcemia
*Hypo*magnesemia
*Hyper*phosphatemia

<u>Hypomagnesemia</u>
Usually in association with
hypokalemia ± *hypocalcemia*

Torsades De Pointes

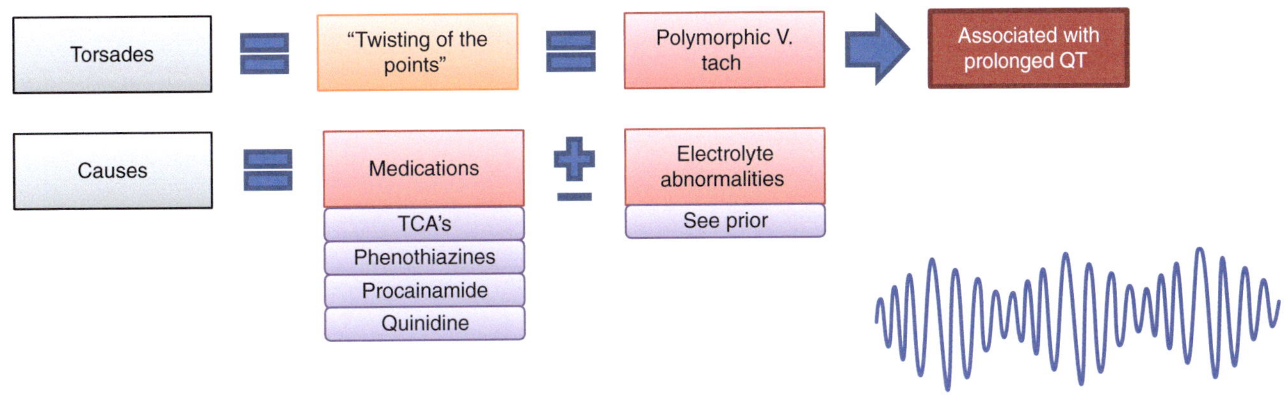

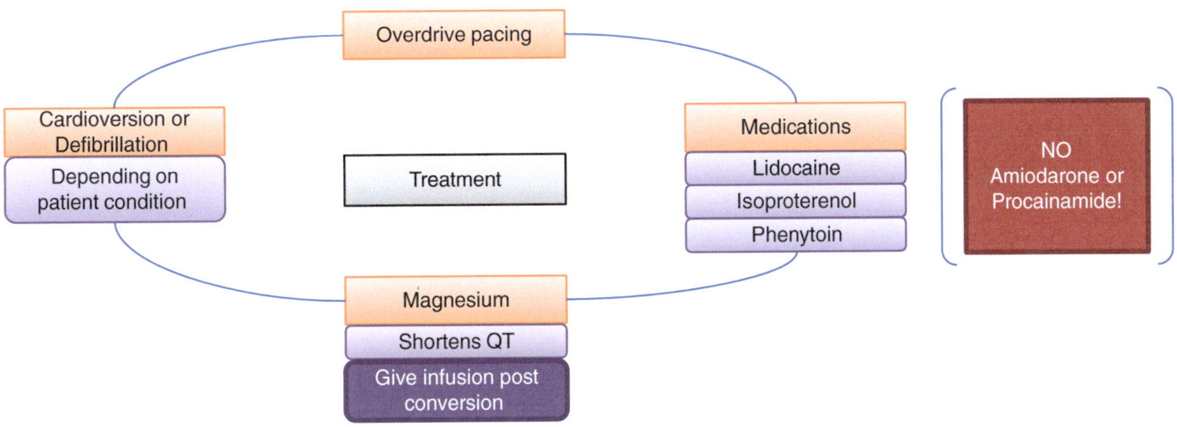

EKG Changes Related to Medications

Digitalis: EKG Changes

Intervals

PR
Prolonged
QT
Shortened

ST Segment

Sagging, Concave upwards (dig effect and may be normal)

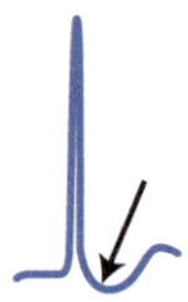

T wave

Flat or inverted

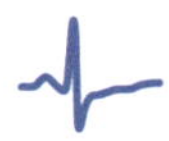

Rhythms & Blocks

PVC's (most common)
AV dissociation
PAT with blocks
Sinus bradycardia
SA blocks
AV blocks
Bidirectional V.tach
Slow A. Fib
Junctional tachycardia
Sinus Arrest

PAT with block

Pathognomonic

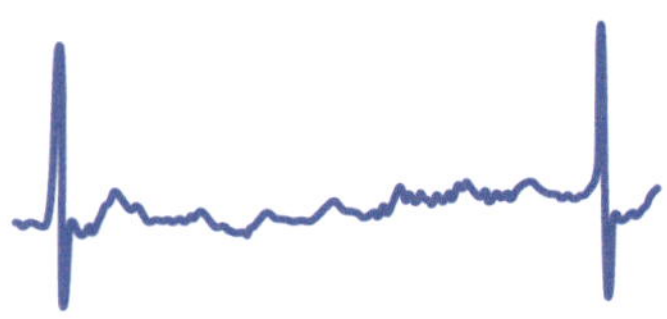

Bidirectional V. Tach

Rare but suggests Digitalis toxicity

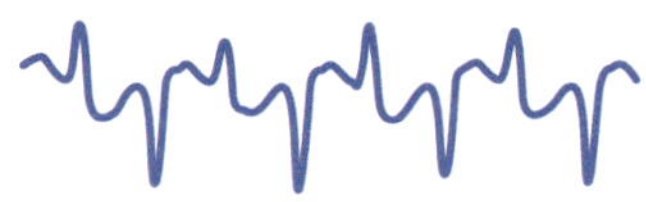

Tricyclic Antidepressants: EKG Changes

Axis

Right axis deviation

- Terminal R wave >3mm in aVR
- R/S ratio >0.7 in aVR

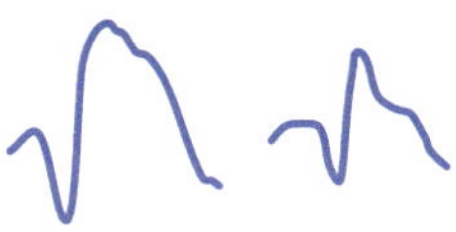

QRS Segment

Wide >100 ms

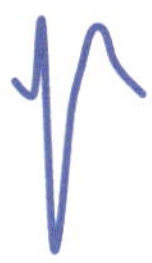

QT Interval

Prolonged

Rhythms

Sinus tachycardia (most common)

Blocks

May be present

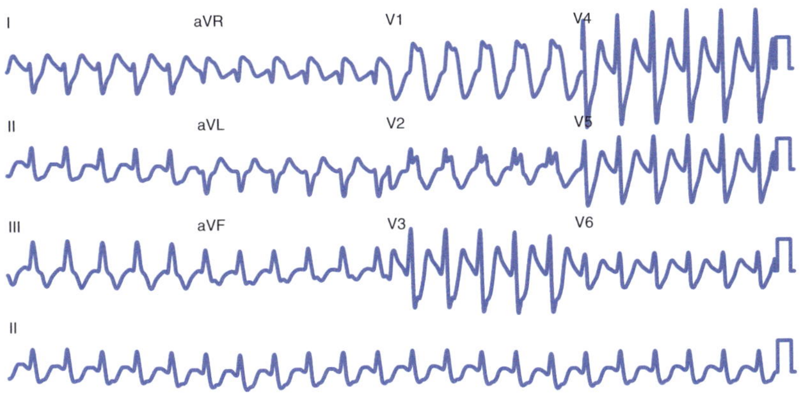

Same effect with other *Sodium channel blocking agents*

Quinine
Propranolol
Antimalarials
(Chloroquine)
Local anesthestics
(Bupivacaine)
Type 1a antiarrhythmics
(Quinidine, Procainamide)
Type 1c antiarrhythmics
(Flecainide, Encainide)

Dysrhythmias

Junctional Escape Rhythm (JER)

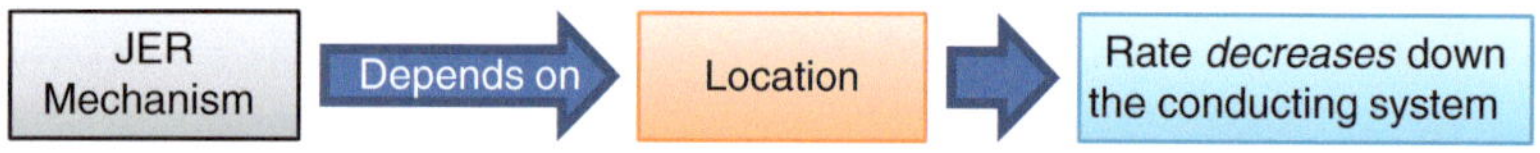

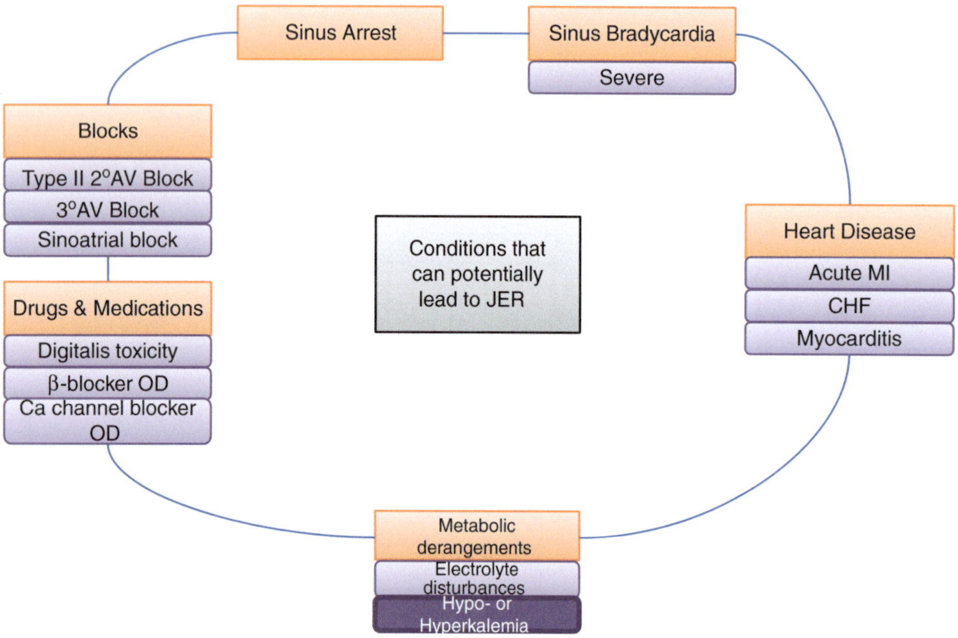

JER: EKG Changes

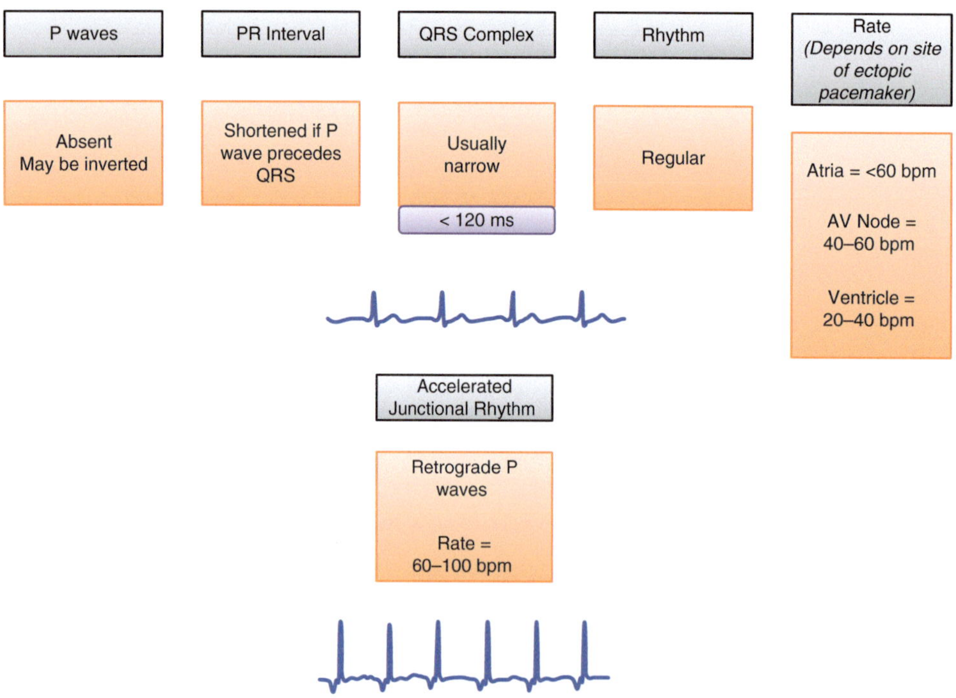

JER Treatment

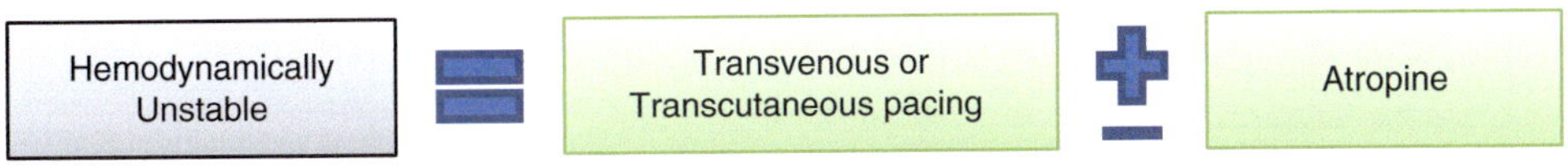

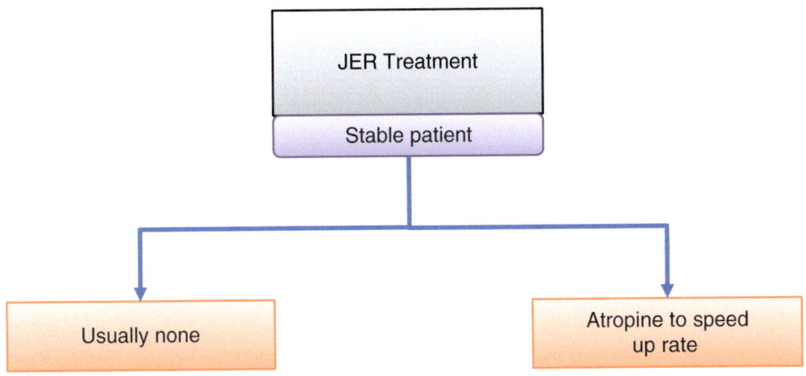

Supraventricular Tachycardia (SVT)

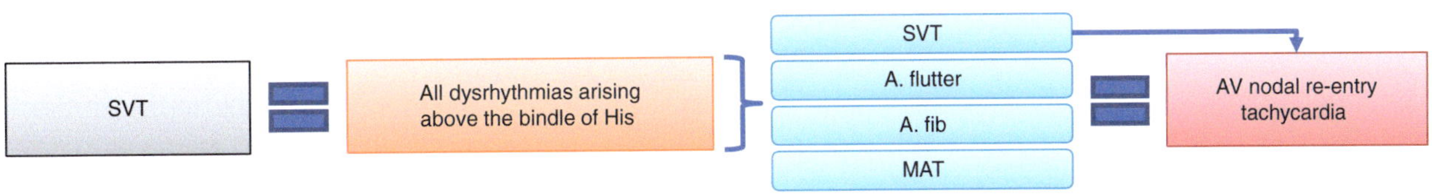

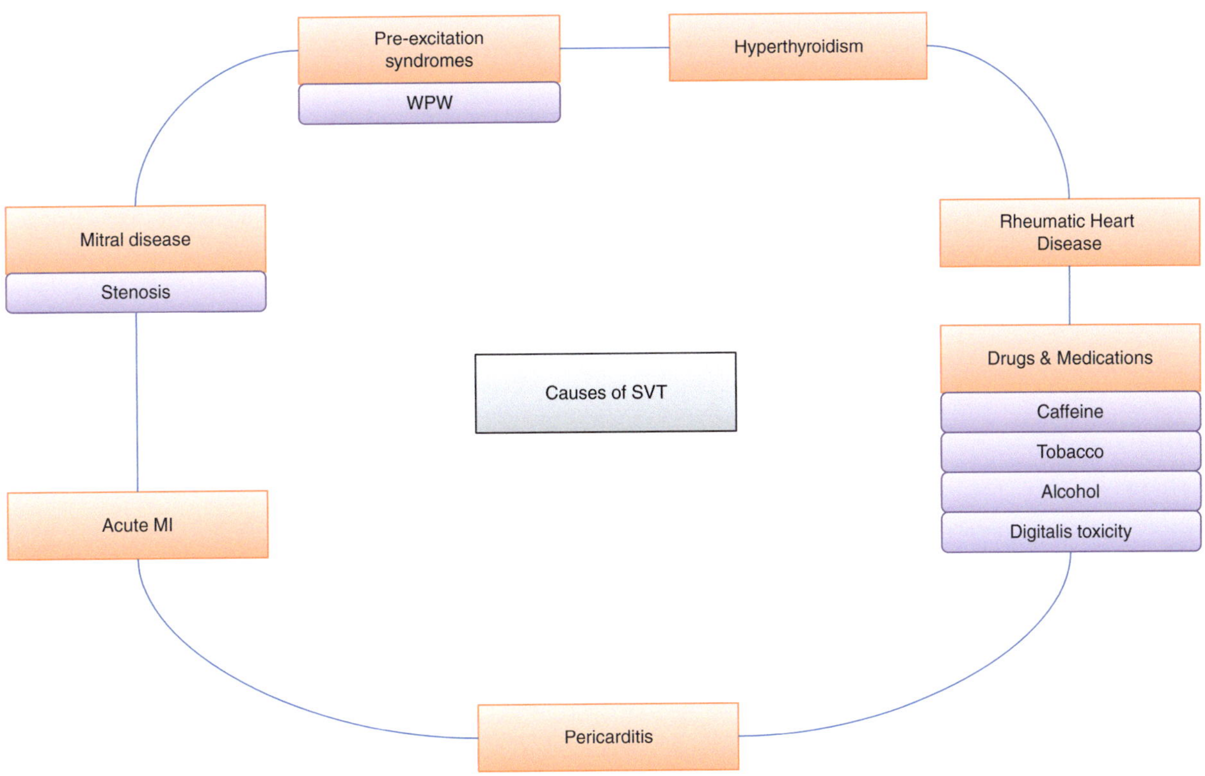

SVT: EKG Changes

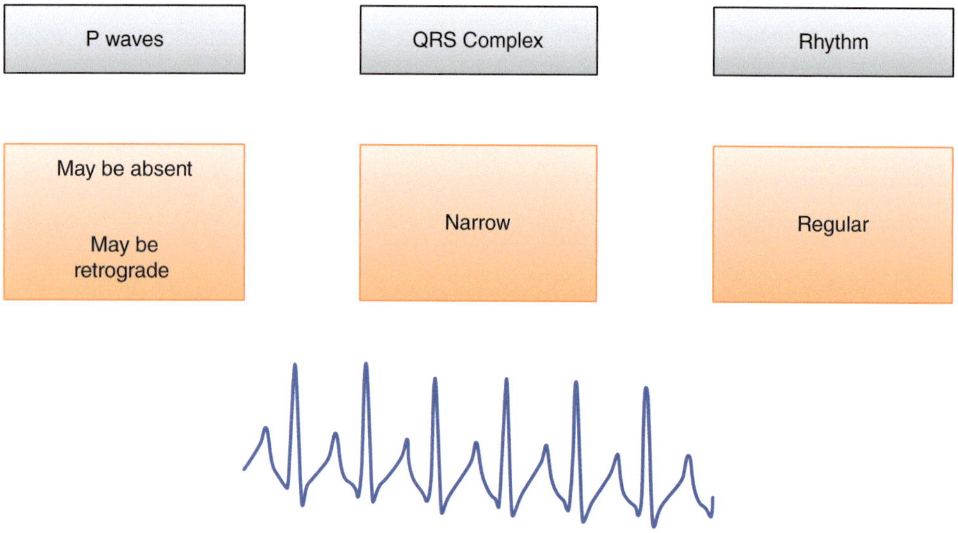

SVT Treatment

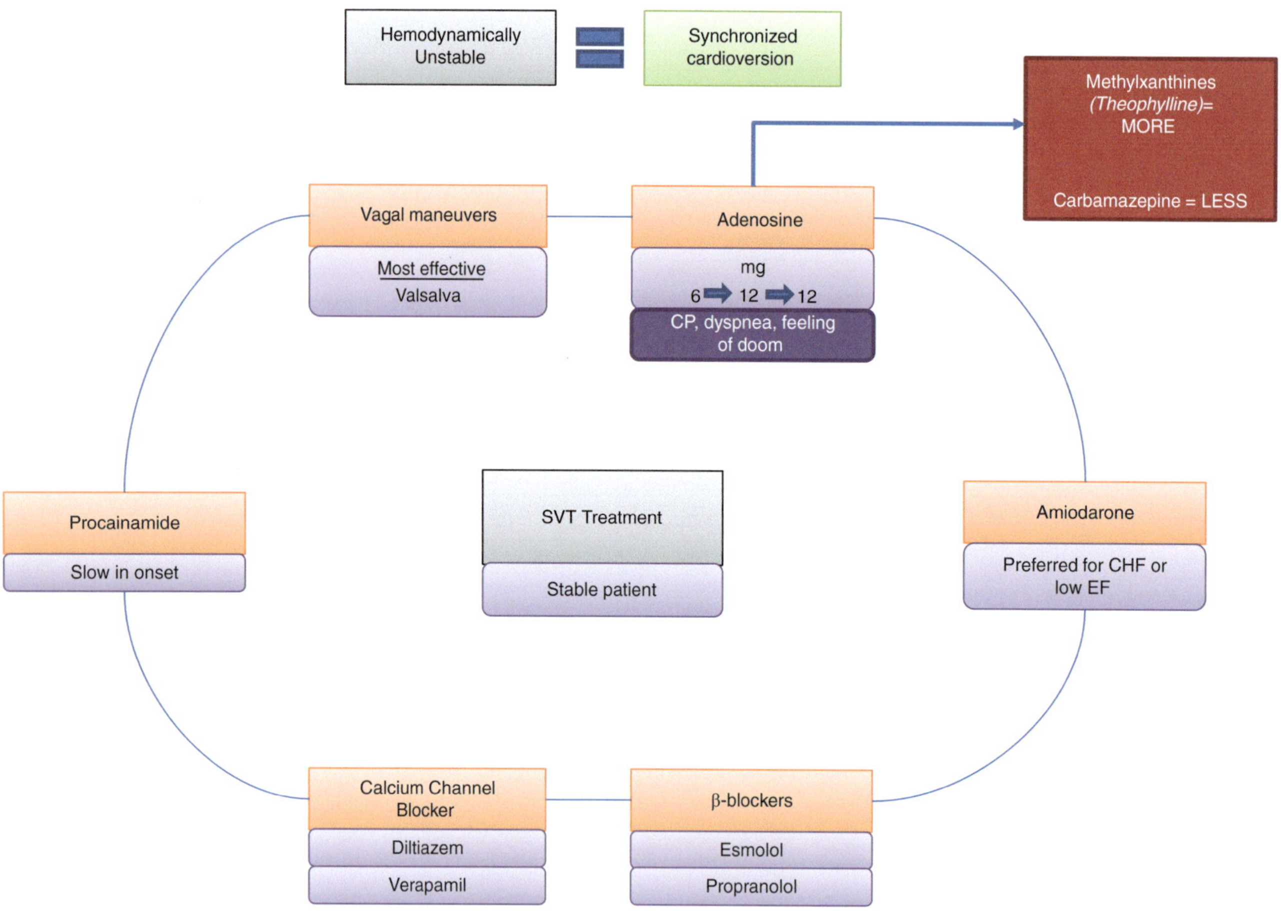

Other Choices for SVT Treatment

SVT 2° Thyrotoxicosis? = Propranolol

SVT 2° Digoxin Toxicity? = Consider Digibind + Magnesium ± Lidocaine ± Phenytoin + Slow correction of hypokalemia

Other agents? = Procainamide ± Amiodarone

Disposition = Depends on clinical condition

Atrial Fibrillation (AF) and Atrial Flutter (AFL)

AF = Most common supraventricular arrhythmia

Causes of AF/AFl

- Pre-excitation syndromes
  - WPW
- Thyrotoxicosis
- Heart Disease
  - Acute MI
  - Rheumatic HD ± Valvular HD
  - Hypertension
  - Dilated cardiomyopathy
  - HOCM
- COPD
- Metabolic derangements
  - Electrolyte disturbances
  - Acid-base disturbance
- Pericarditis
- Drugs & Medications
  - Digitalis toxicity
  - Sympathomimetics
- Pulmonary Embolism

AF: EKG Changes

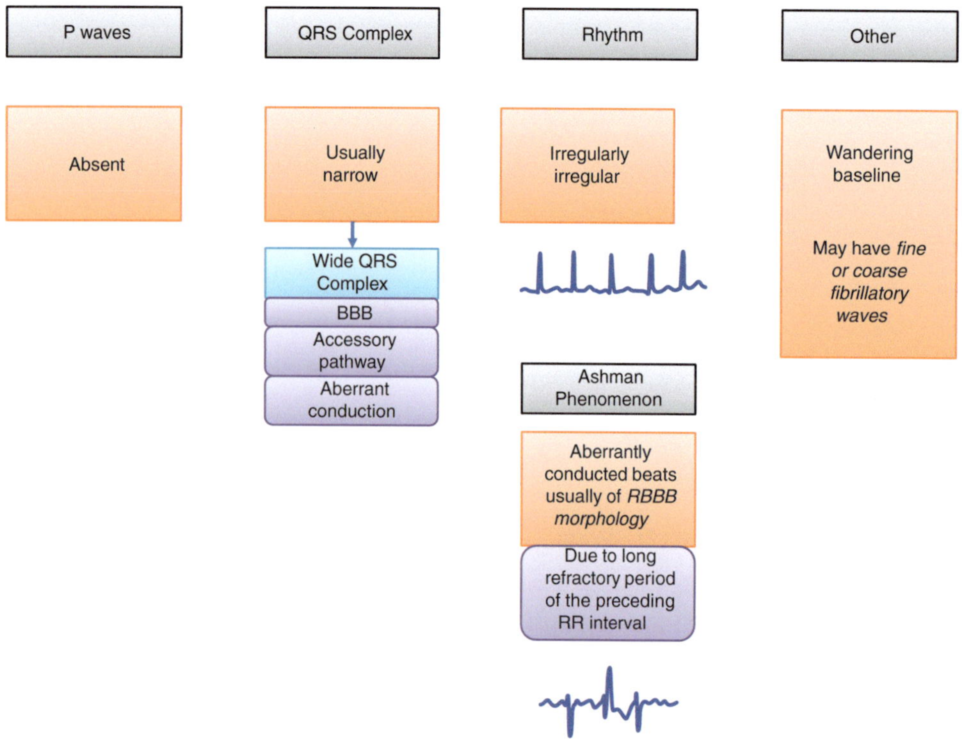

Atrial Flutter: EKG Changes

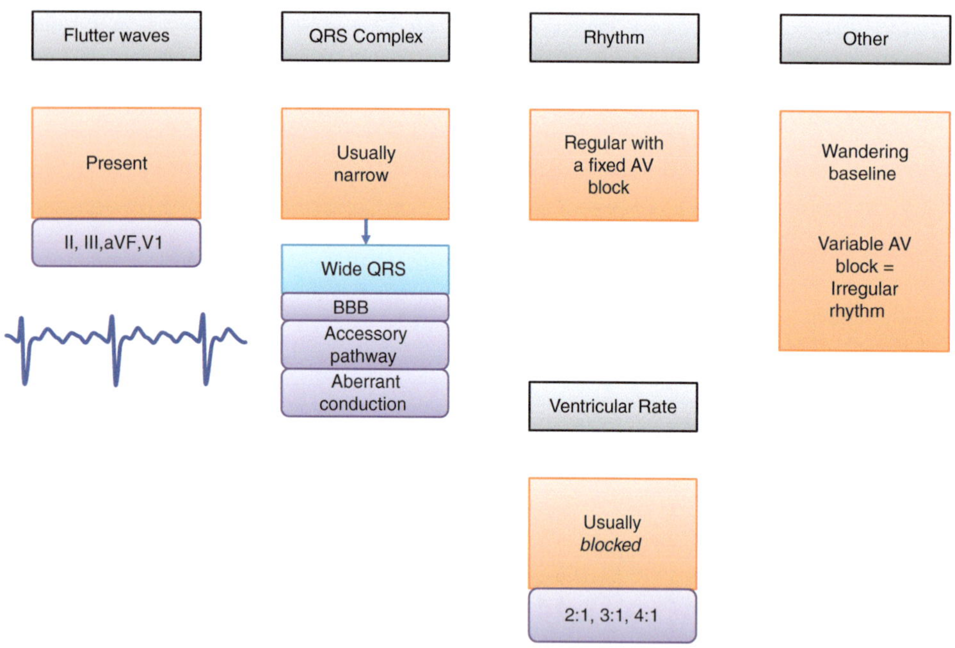

AF/AFL Treatment

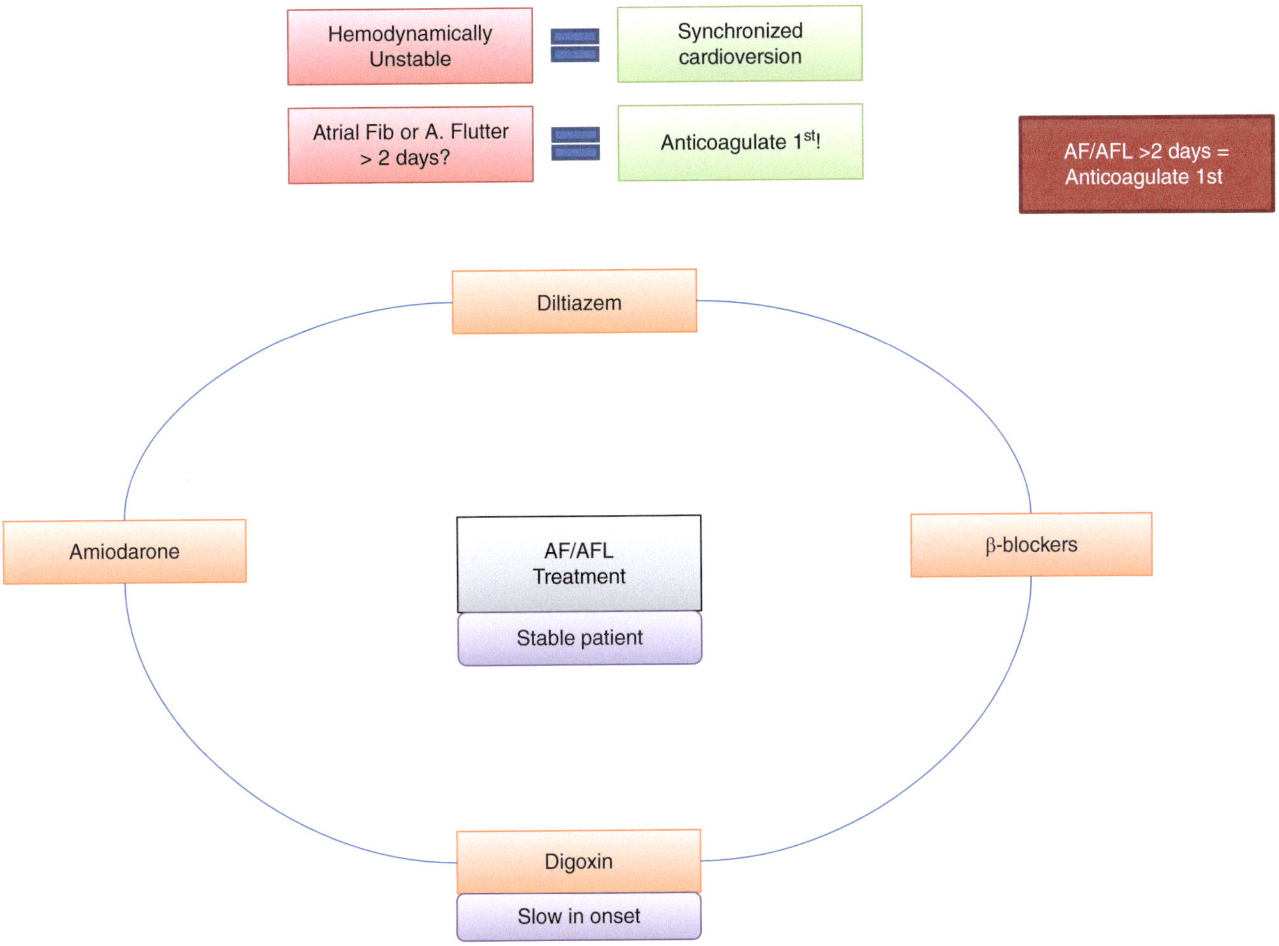

Other Tidbits Concerning AF/AFL

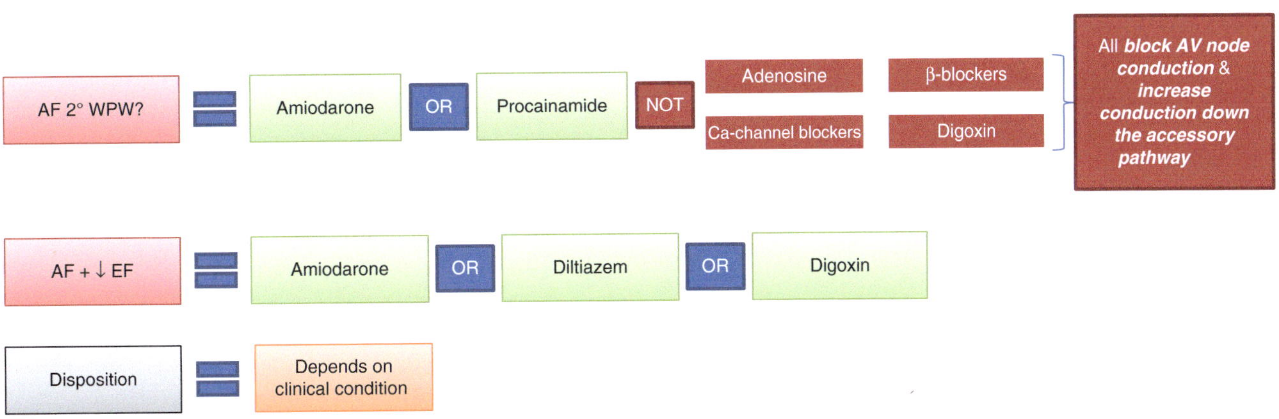

Multifocal Atrial Tachycardia (MAT)

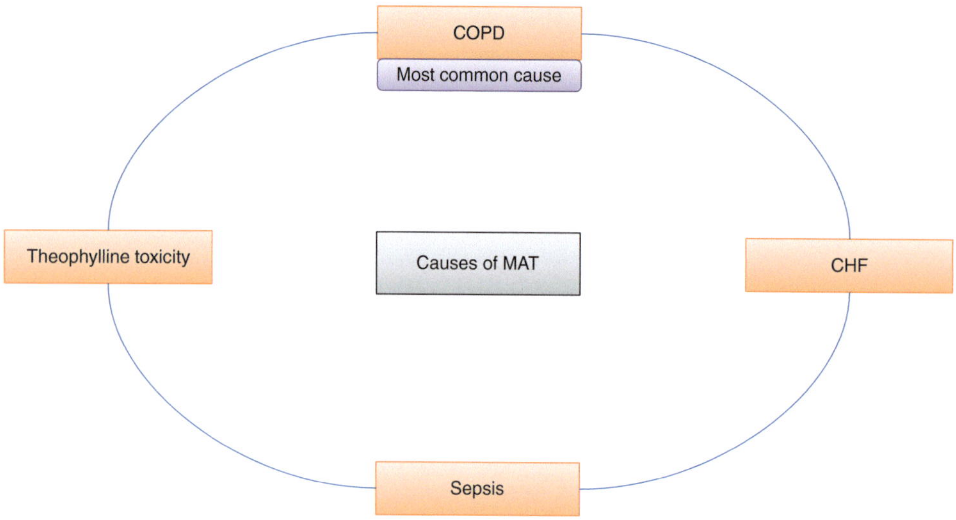

MAT: EKG Changes

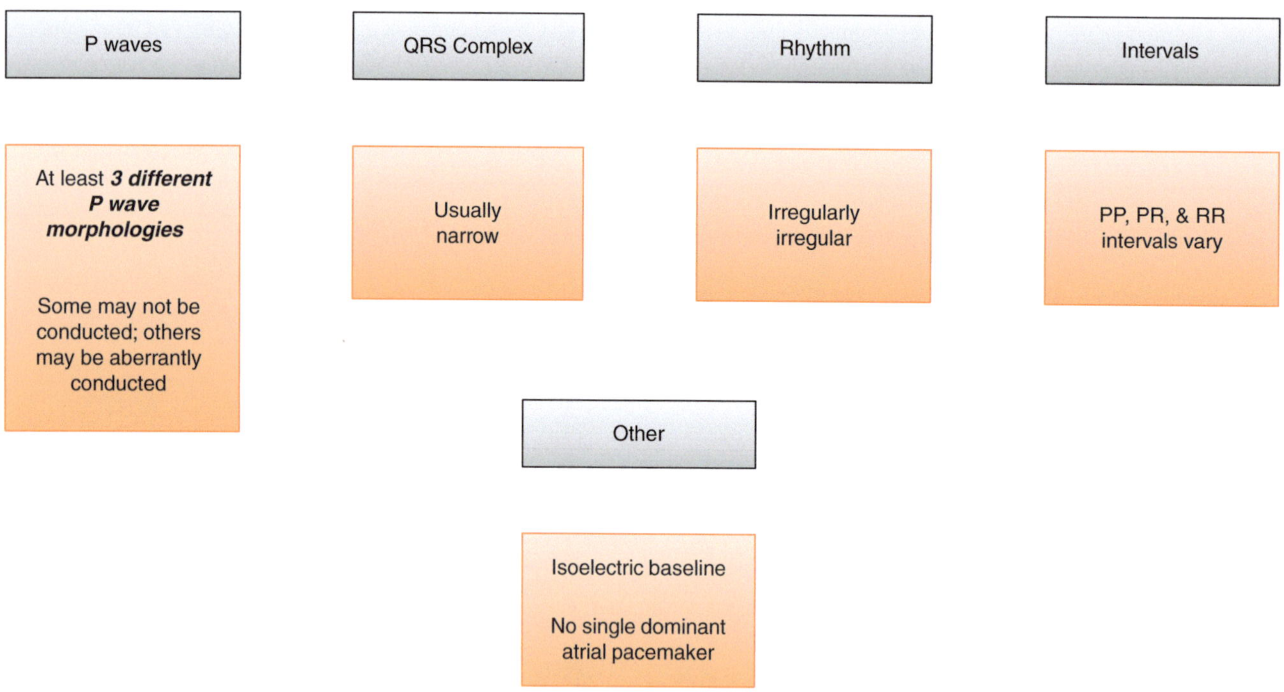

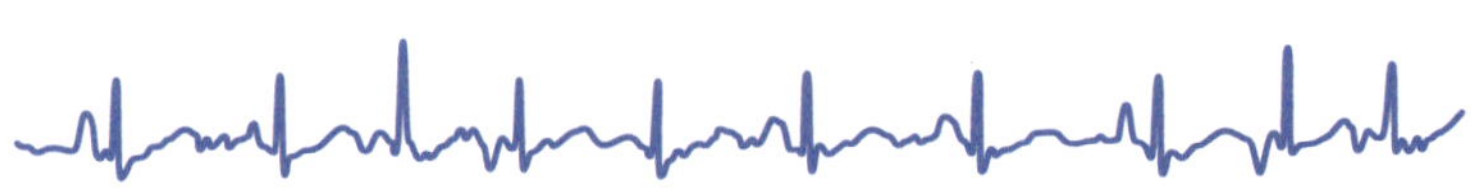

MAT Treatment

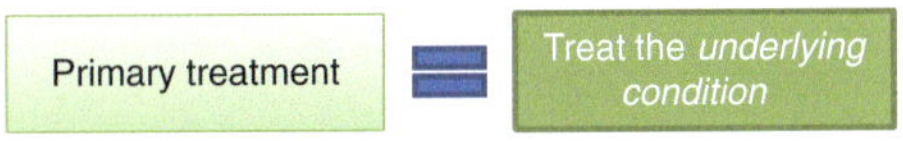

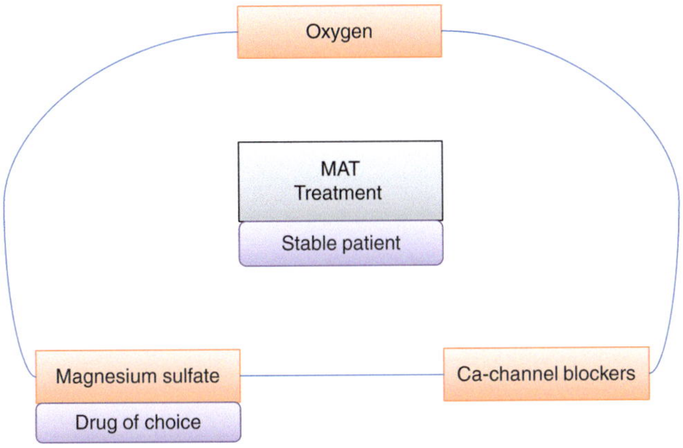

Premature Ventricular Contractions

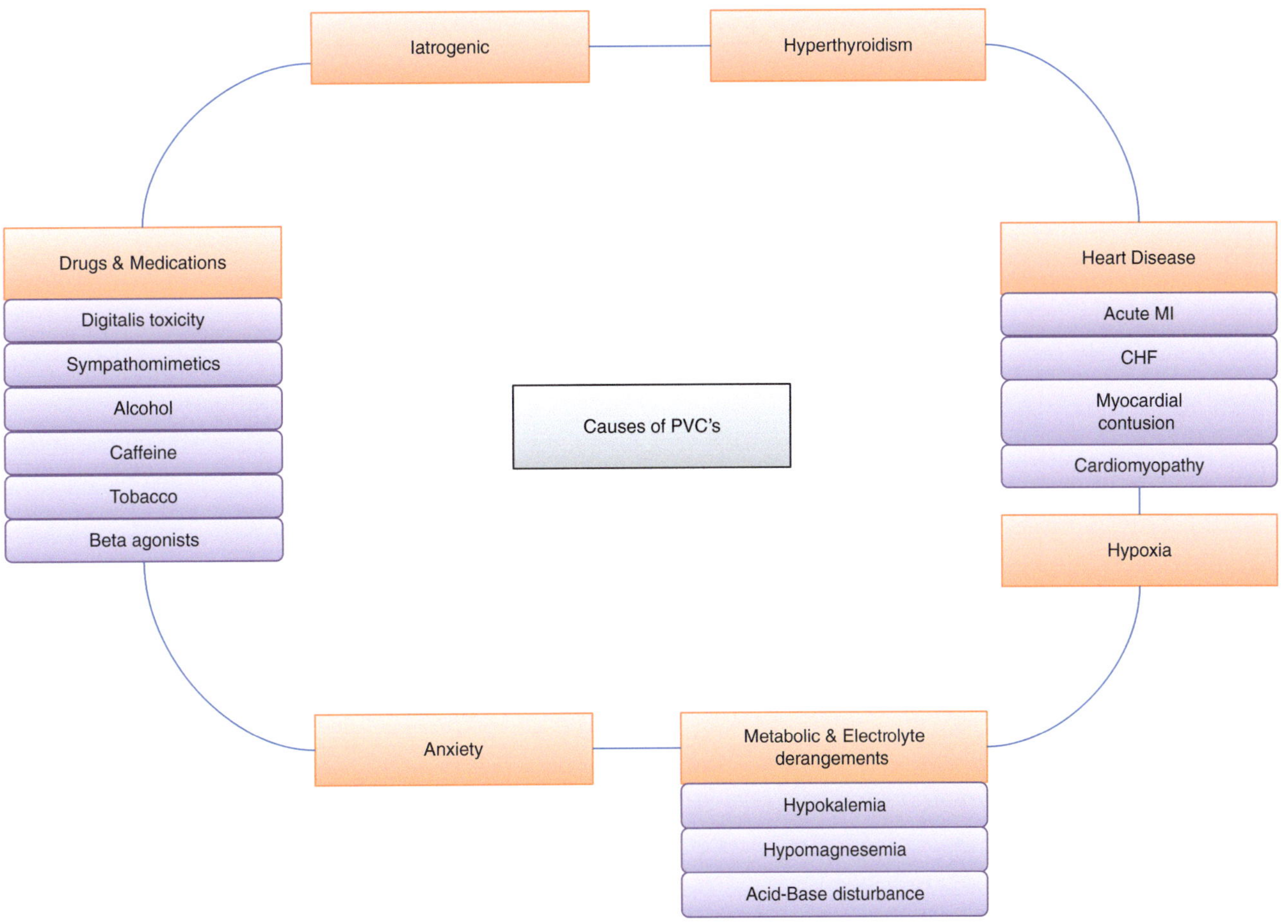

PVCs: EKG Changes

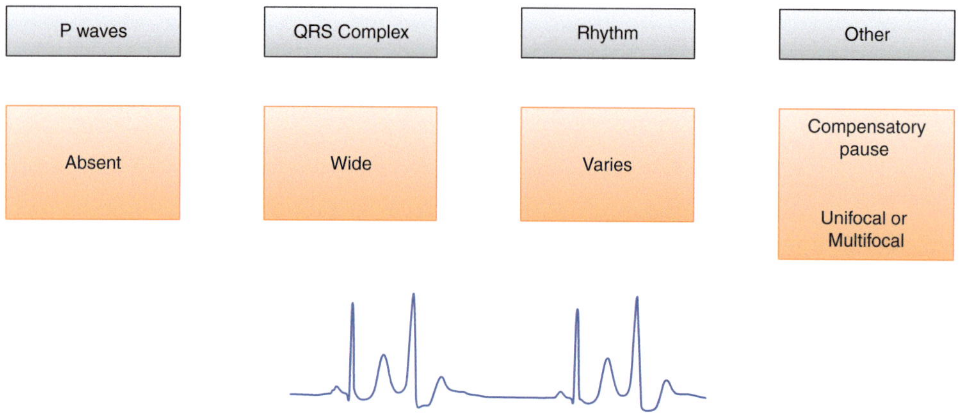

PVC Treatment

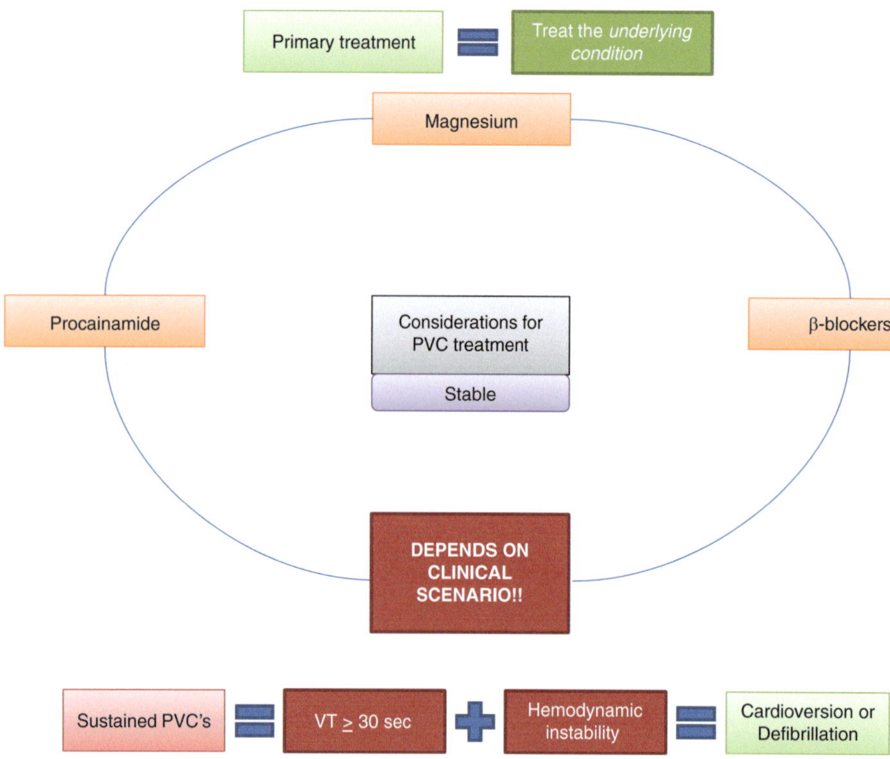

Wolff-Parkinson-White (WPW) Syndrome

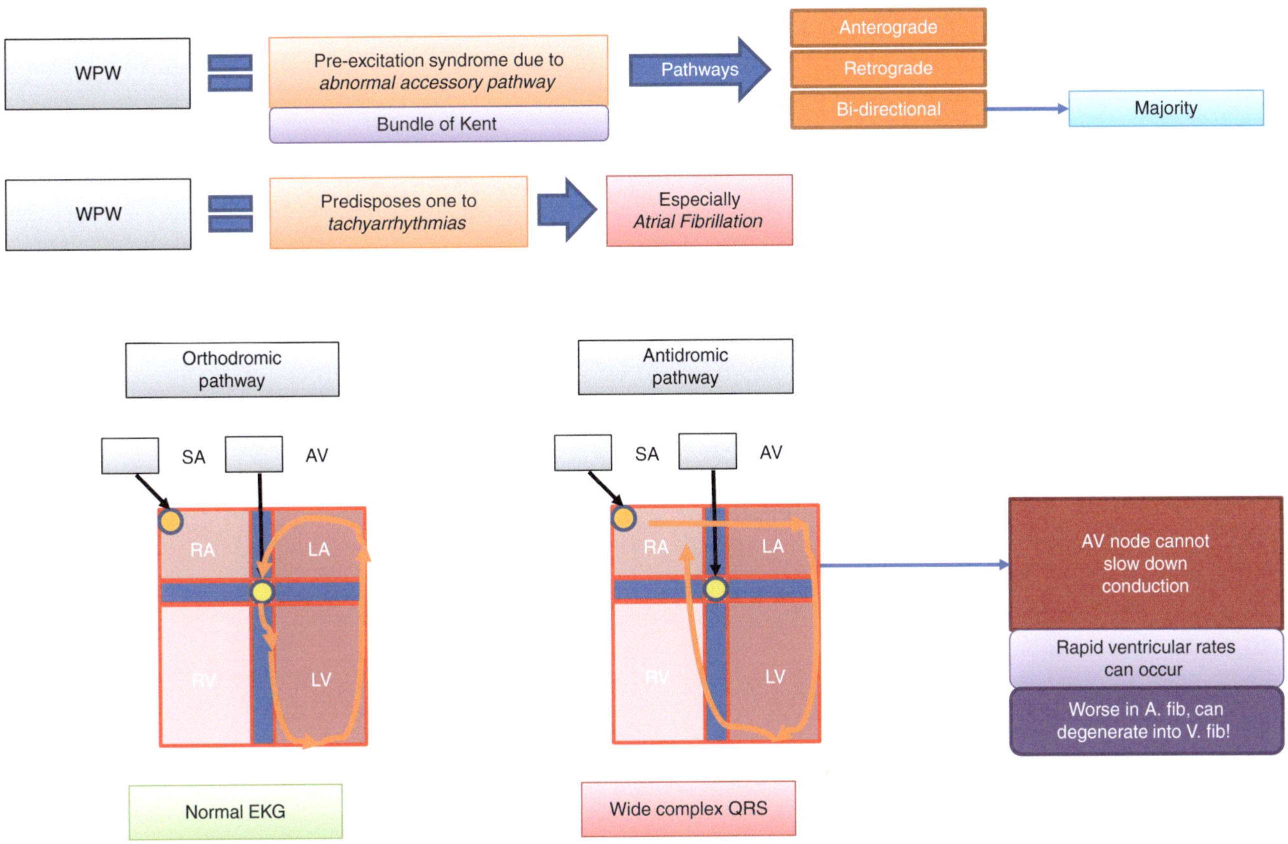

WPW: EKG Changes in Sinus Rhythm

PR interval
- Shortened
- <120 ms

QRS Complex
- Wide
- ≥ 100 ms

Delta wave
- Slurred initial upstroke of QRS may be present
- May not be seen in tachyarrhythmias

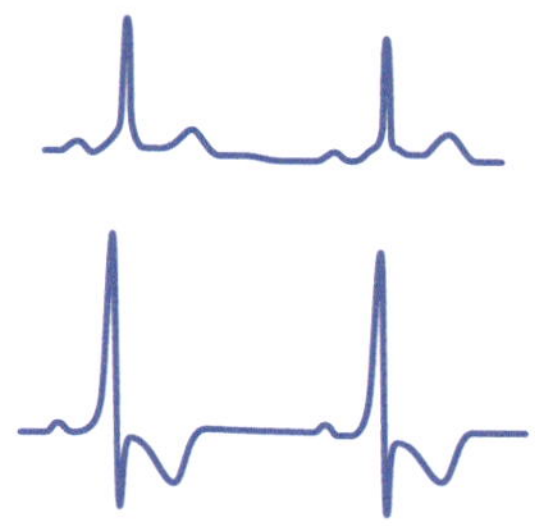

ST segment
- ST segment & T wave may show discordant changes

Pseudo-Infarction
- Delta waves are negatively deflected in anterior & inferior leads
- Pseudo Q waves
- Prominent R waves in V1–3
- Mimicks posterior infarction

Atrioventricular Reentry Tachycardias (AVRT): RD

AVRT = Type of SVT

→ Has a reentry circuit that allows for circus movement

→ During tachyarrhythmias pre-excitation features are *lost*

→ Direction of reentry determines shape of QRS

→ AVRT with orthodromic (left) & antidromic (right) AV nodal conduction

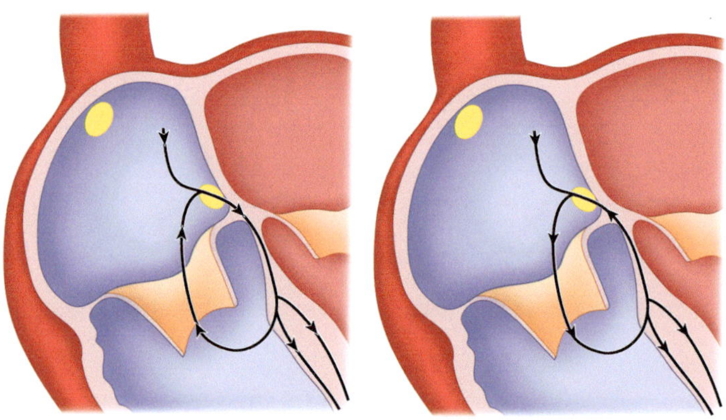

AVRT: EKG Changes

P waves	QRS Complex	T waves	ST segment	Rate
Buried in QRS or Retrograde	Orthodromic: Normal Antidromic: Wide ≤ 120 ms	May be inverted	Depression	200–300

Orthodromic =

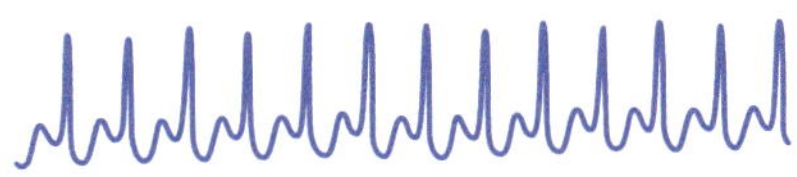

Antidromic =

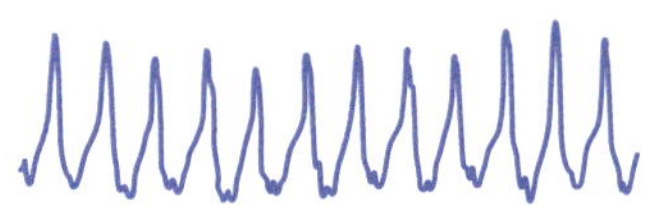

Atrial Fibrillation/Flutter in WPW: EKG Changes

Rate	Rhythm	QRS Complex	Axis
>200 bpm	Irregular A. Flutter = Regular	Wide May change in shape	Stable

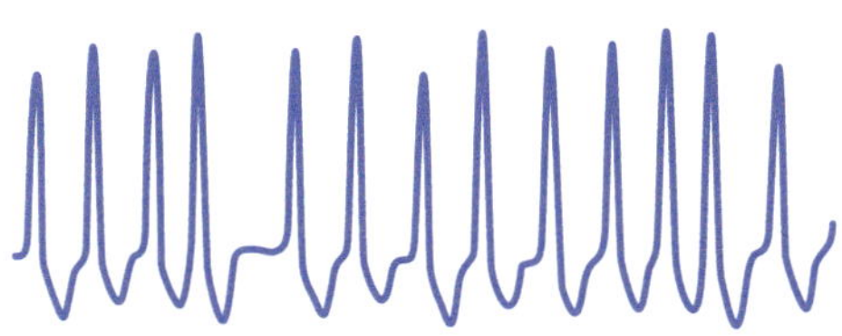

WPW Treatment: Narrow QRS Complex: Stable

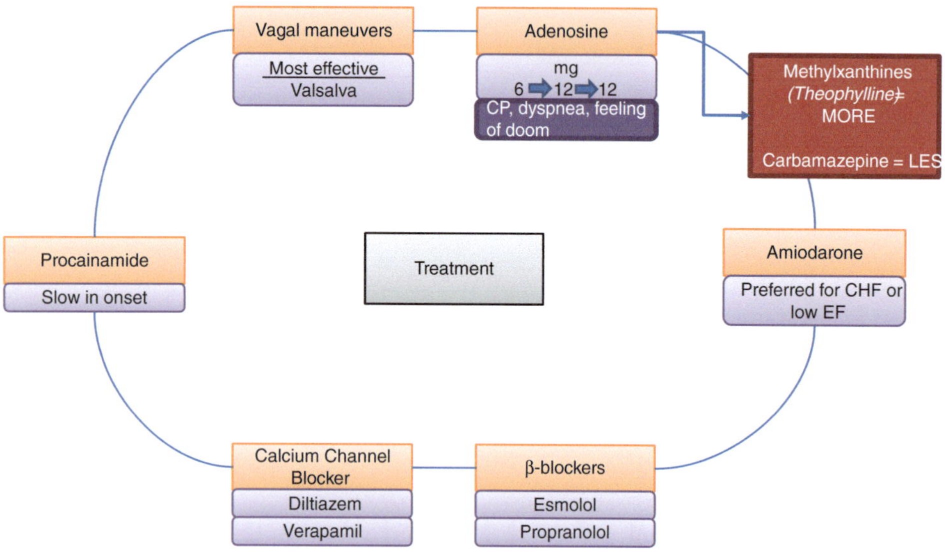

WPW Treatment: Unstable: Any Size QRS Complex

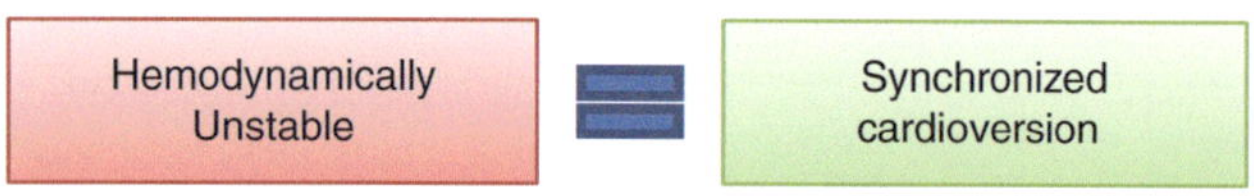

WPW Treatment Atrial Fibrillation or Flutter: Stable

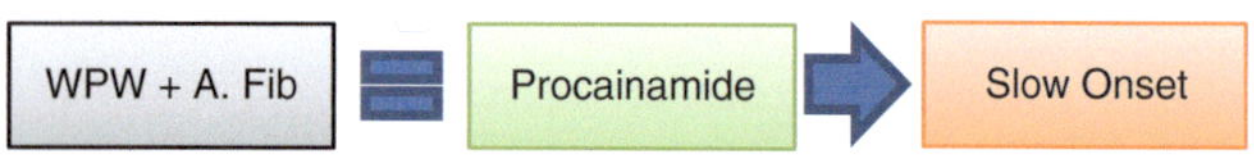

WPW Treatment Wide QRS Complex: Stable

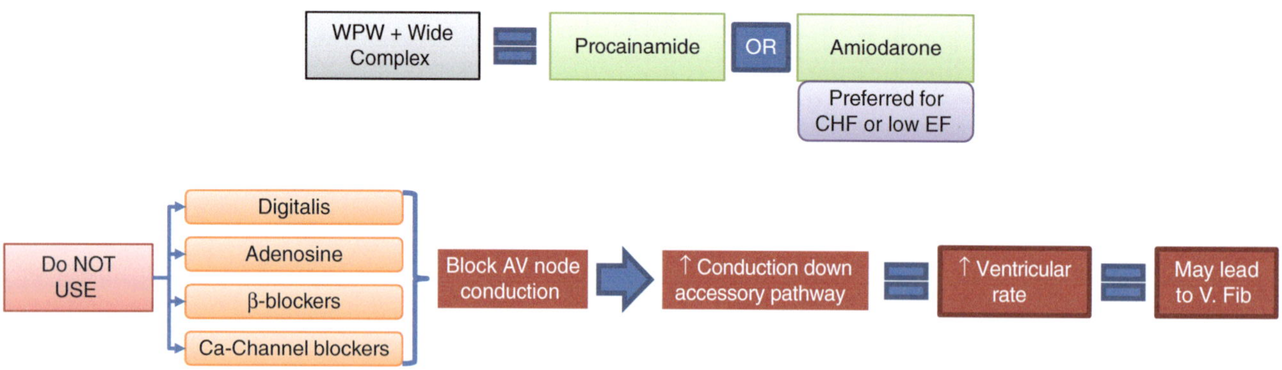

Ventricular Tachycardia (VT)

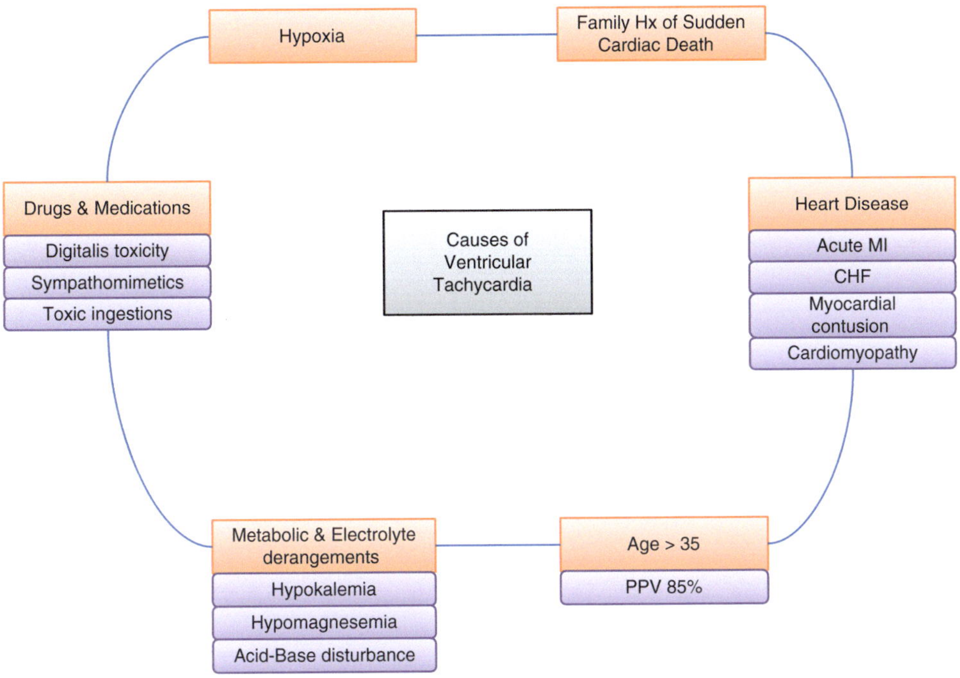

Ventricular Tachycardia: EKG Changes

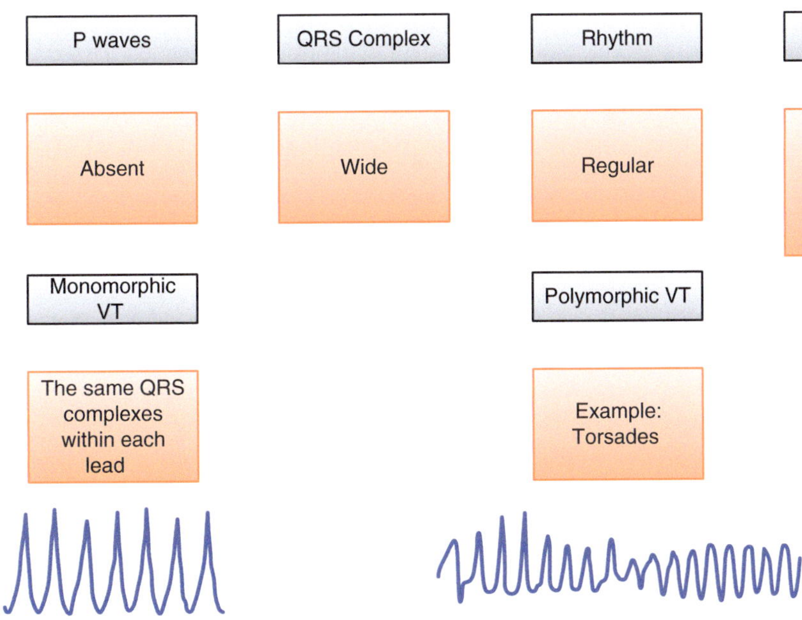

Other EKG Features of VT

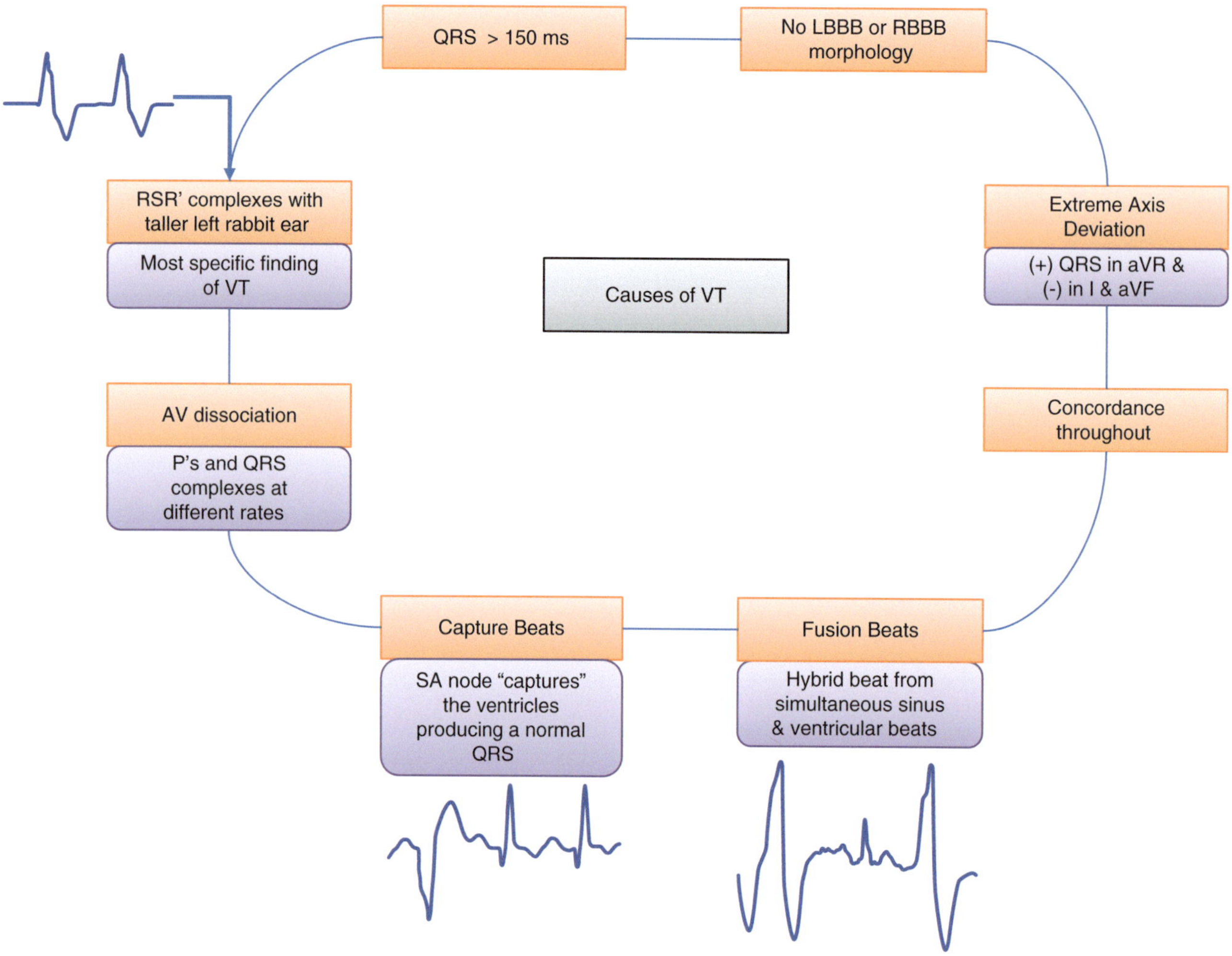

VT Treatment

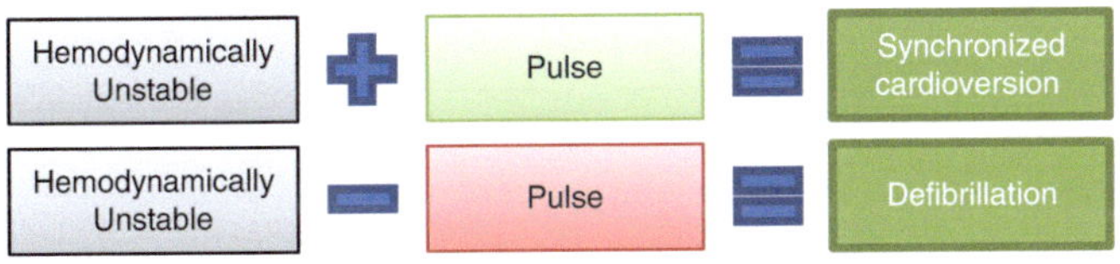

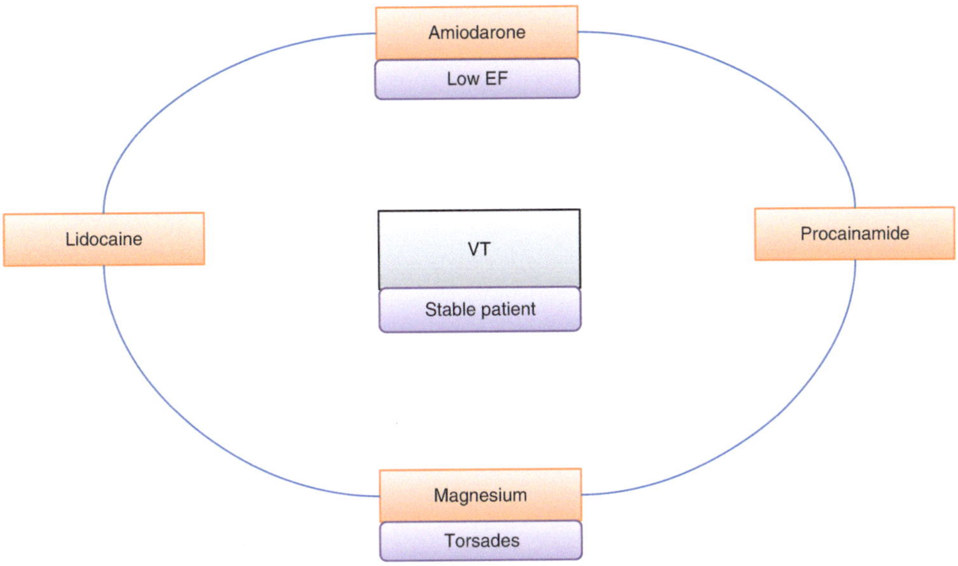

Ventricular Fibrillation (VF)

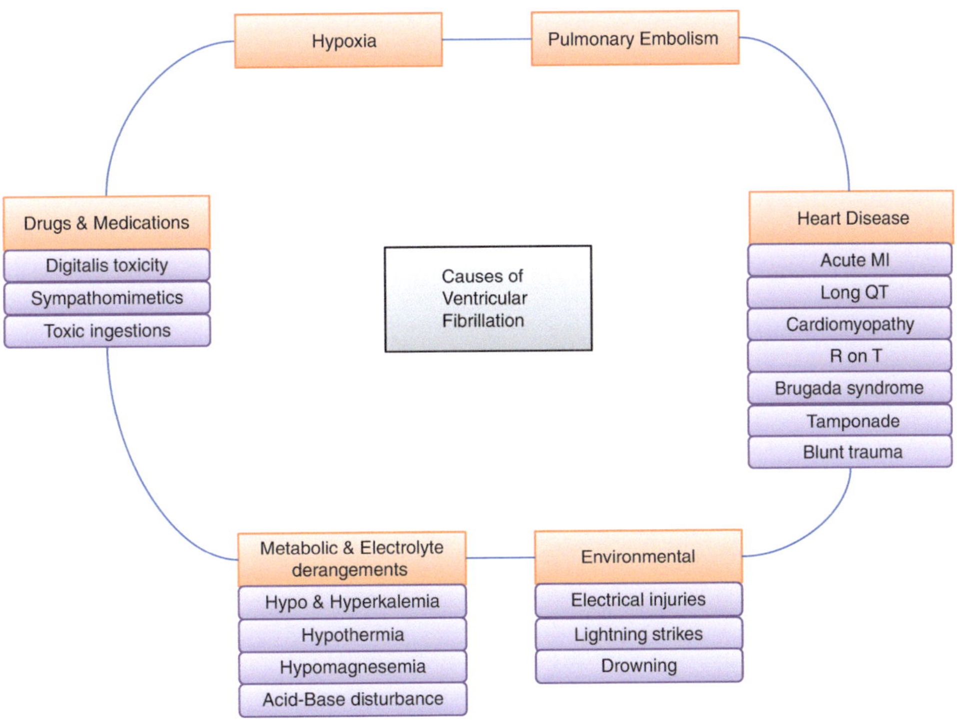

Ventricular Fibrillation: EKG Changes

P waves	QRS Complex	T waves	Rhythm	Rate
Absent	Absent	Absent	Chaotic	150–500 per minute

Other

- Amplitude decreases with duration
  - Coarse to Fine

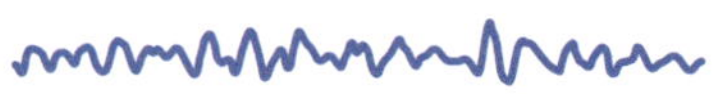

Heart Blocks

Left Bundle Branch Block (LBBB)

Causes of LBBB

- Aortic stenosis
- Ischemic Heart disease
- Anterior MI
- Hypertension
- Electrolyte derangements
  - Hyperkalemia
  - Hypermagnesemia
- Dilated Cardiomyopathy
- Primary cardiac fibrosis of the conducting system
- Drugs & Medications
  - Digitalis toxicity

LBBB: EKG Changes

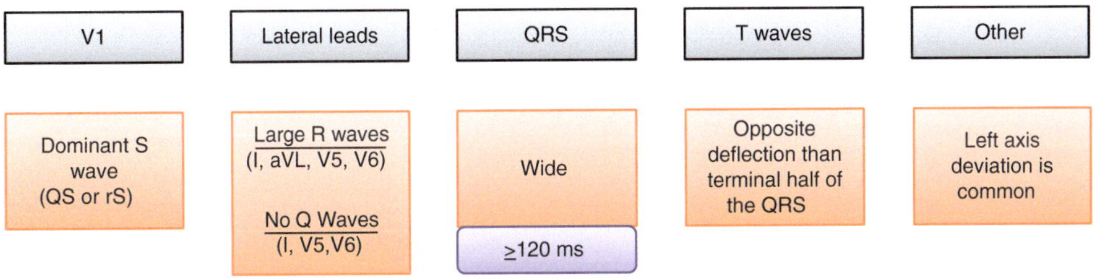

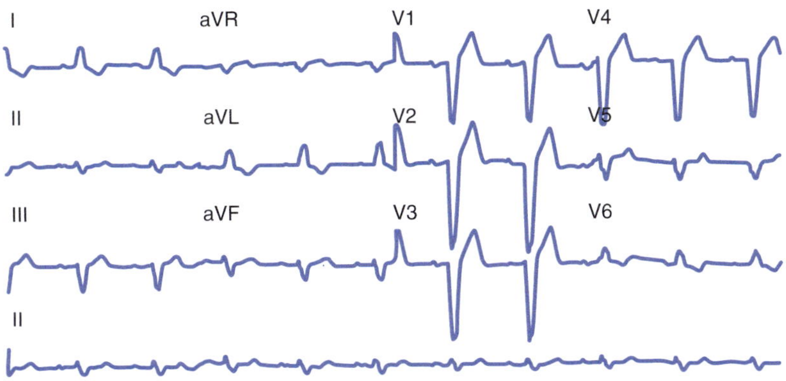

Right Bundle Branch Block (RBBB)

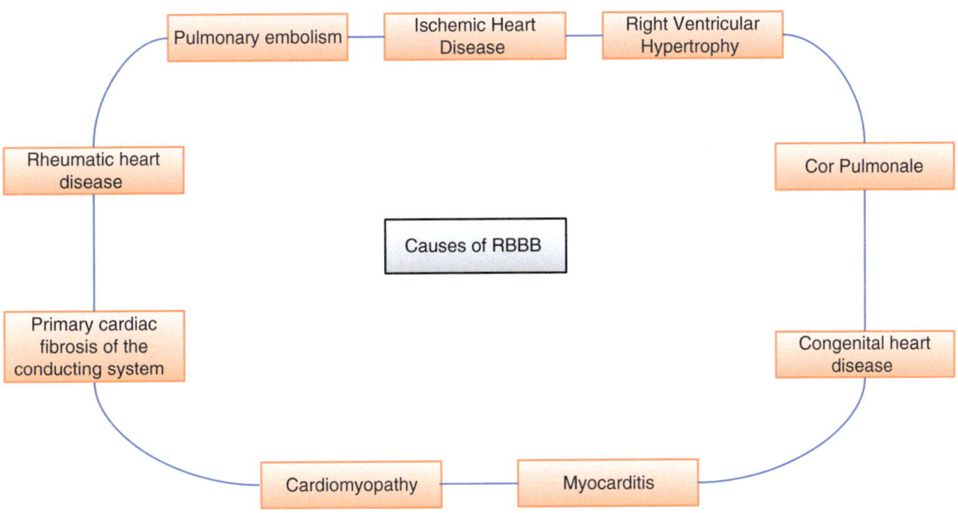

RBBB: EKG Changes

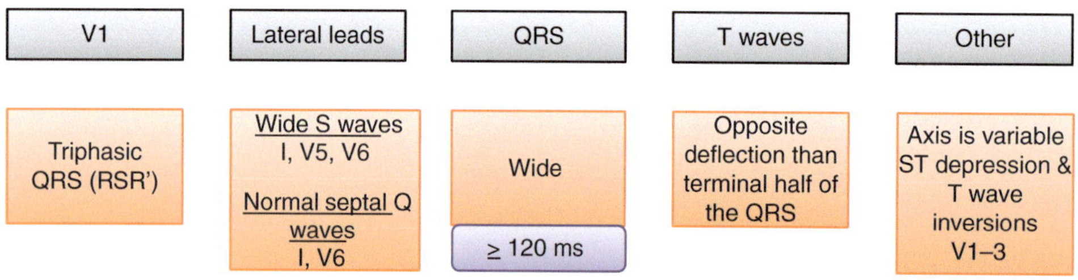

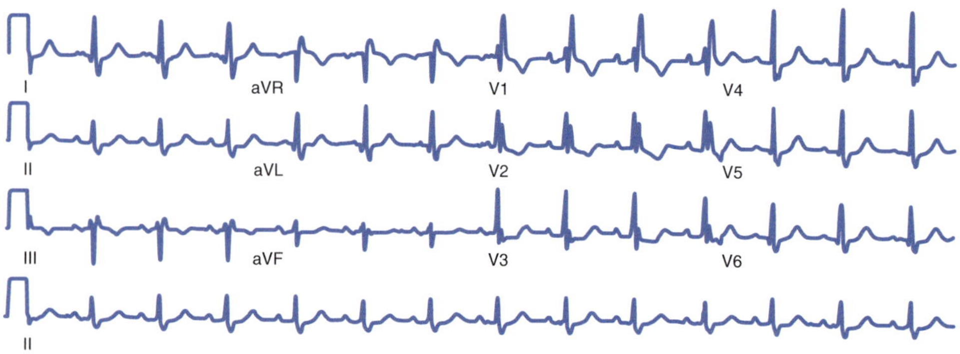

First-Degree Heart Block (1° HB)

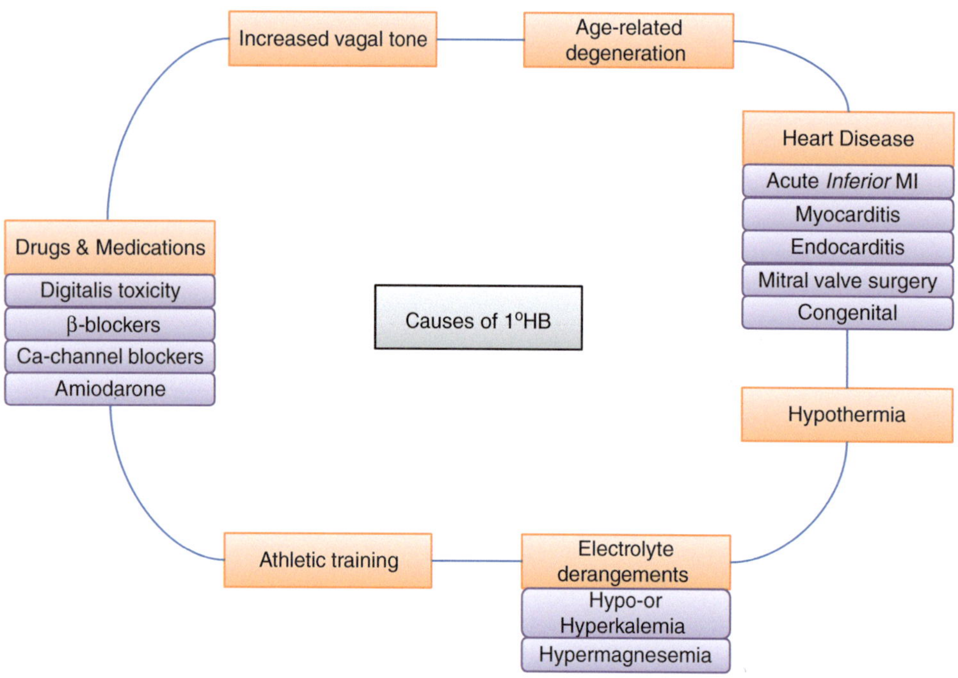

1° HB: EKG Changes

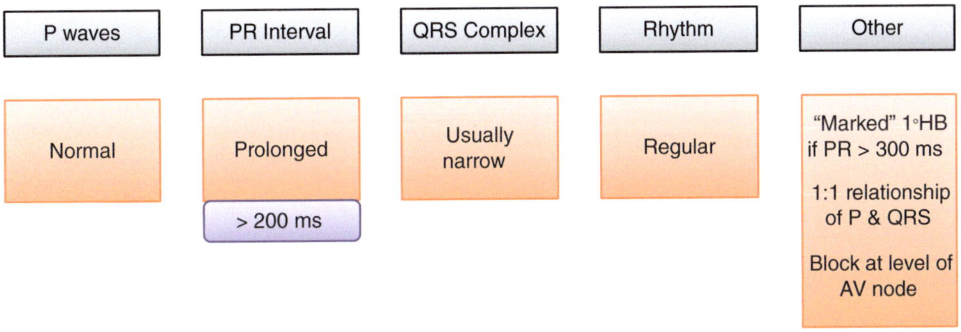

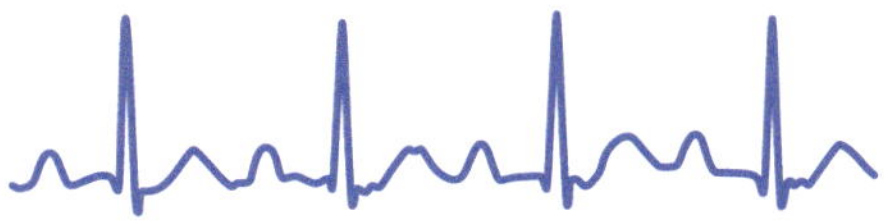

1° HB Treatment

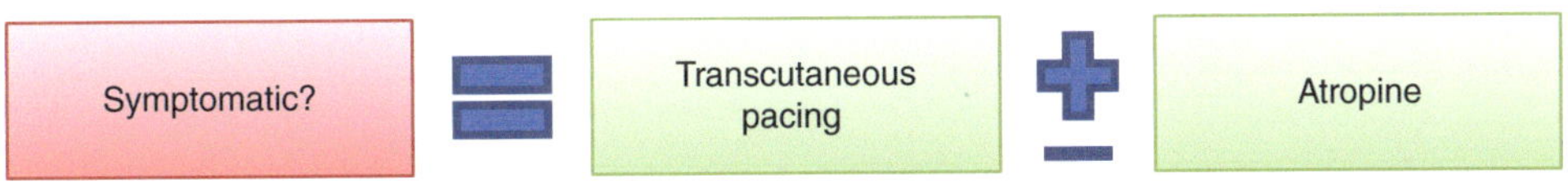

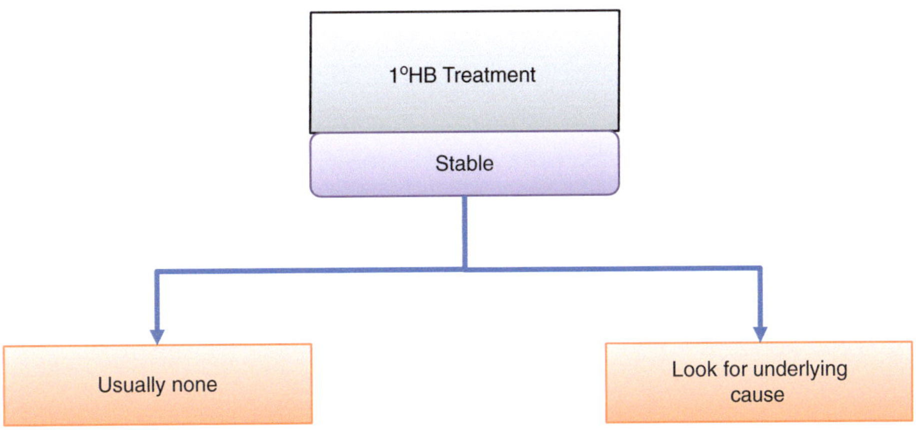

Second-Degree Type 1 Heart Block (2° Type 1 HB)

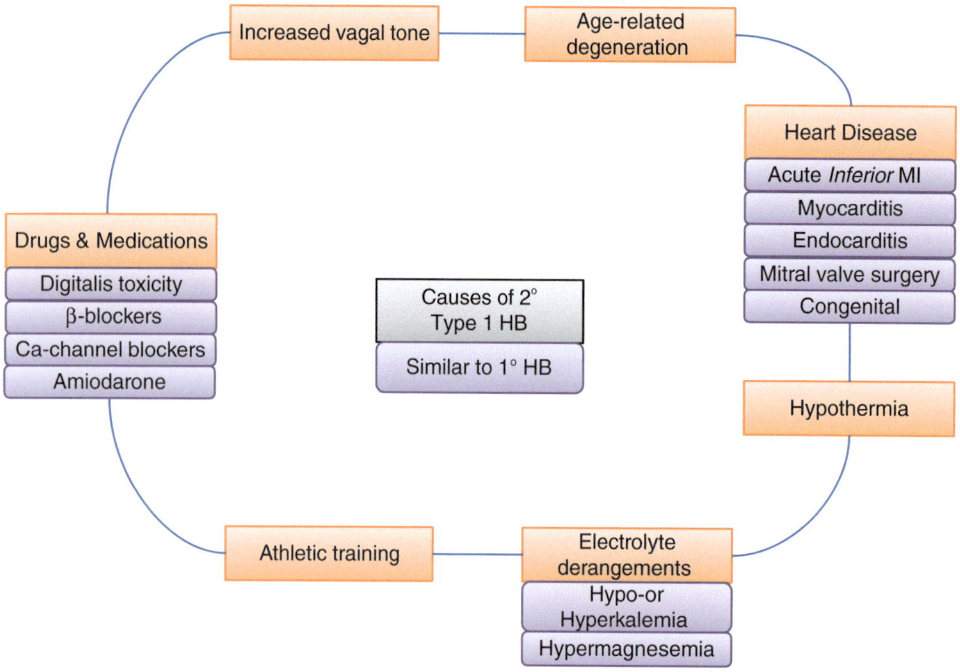

2° Type 1 HB: EKG Changes

P waves	PR & RR Intervals	QRS Complex	Rhythm	Other
Normal	**PR** Progressively lengthens **RR** Progressively shortens Until a beat is dropped	Usually narrow	Regular	"Marked" 1°HB if PR > 300 ms 1:1 relationship of P & QRS Block at level of AV node

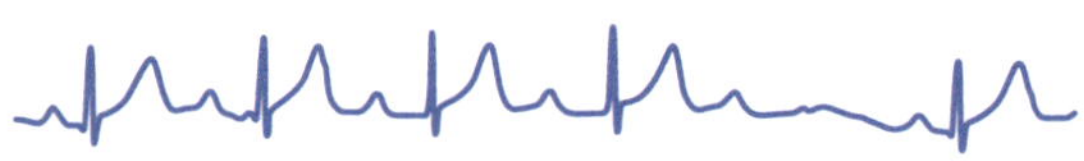

2° Type 1 HB Treatment

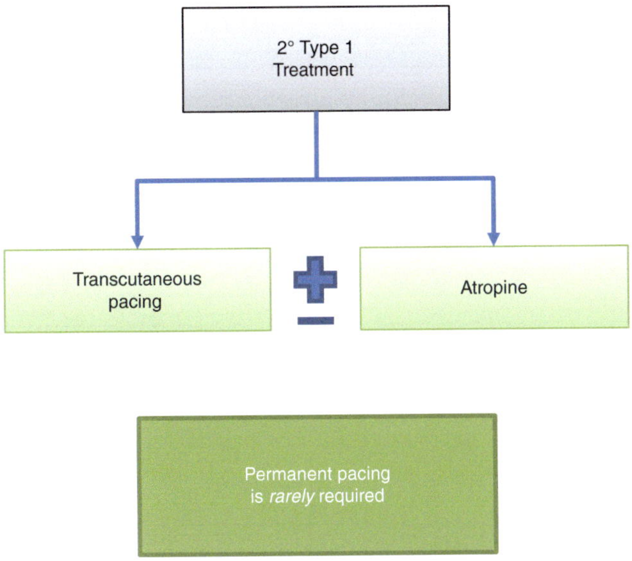

Second-Degree Type 2 Heart Block (2° Type 2 HB)

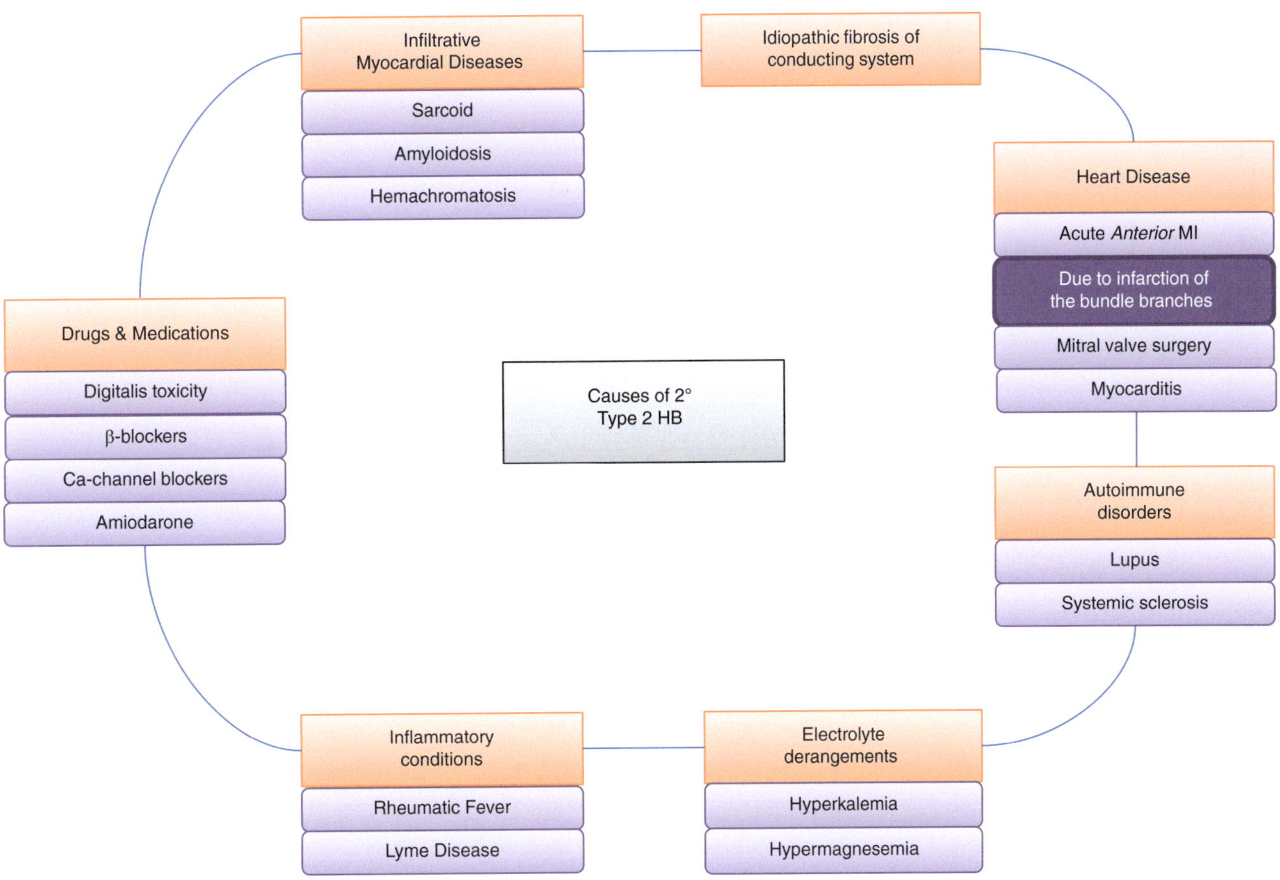

2° Type 2 HB: EKG Changes

P waves	PR Intervals	QRS Complex	Dropped Beats	Other
Normal	When they occur are of the same duration	Usually wide	Present	Block below AV node Typically with pre-existing LBBB or bifascicular block

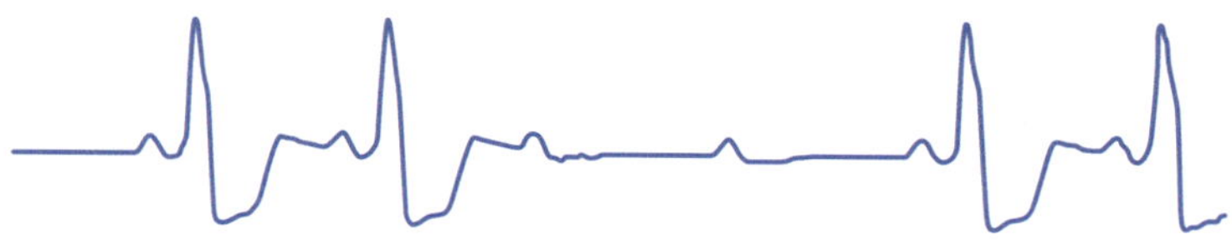

2° Type 2 HB Treatment

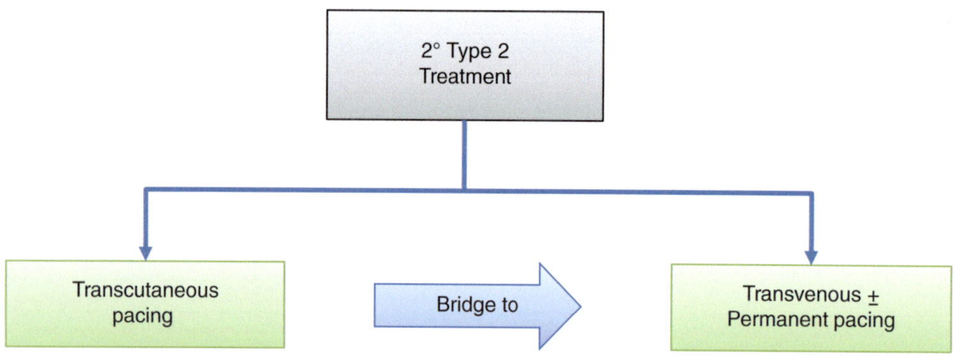

Permanent pacing *may* be required

Other Tidbits Concerning 2° Type 2 HB

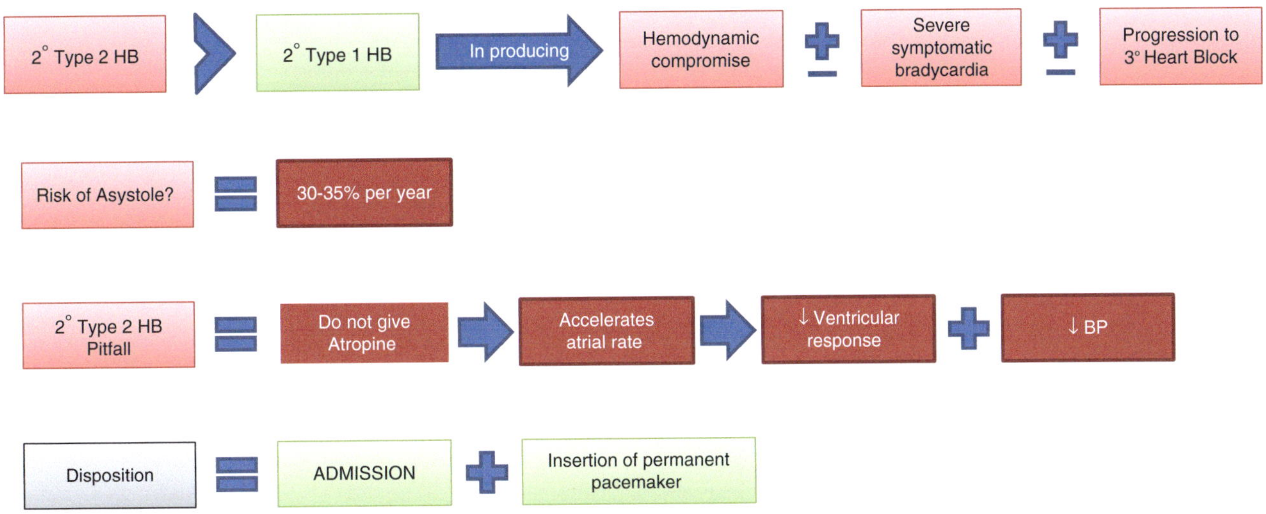

Third-Degree Heart Block (3° HB)

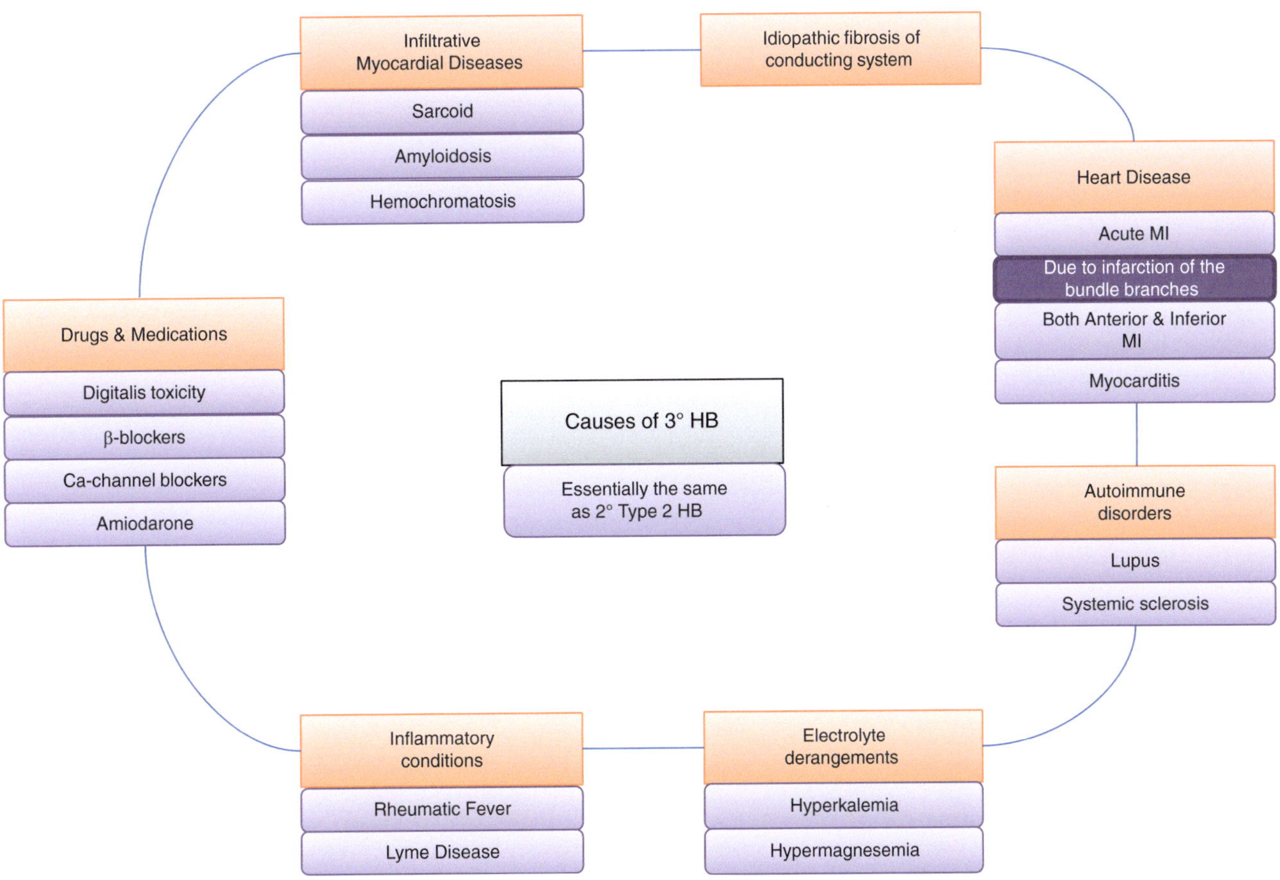

3° HB: EKG Changes

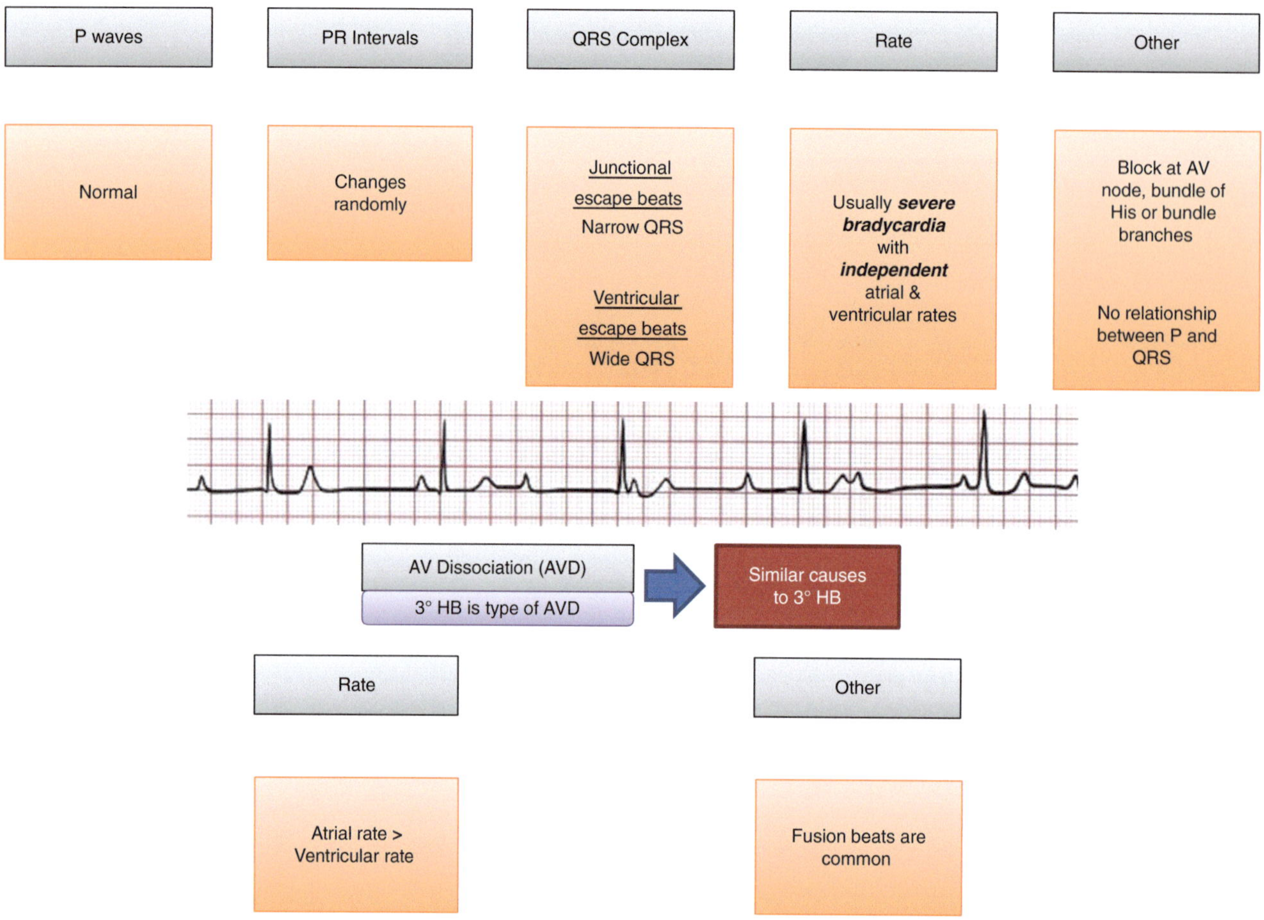

3° HB Treatment

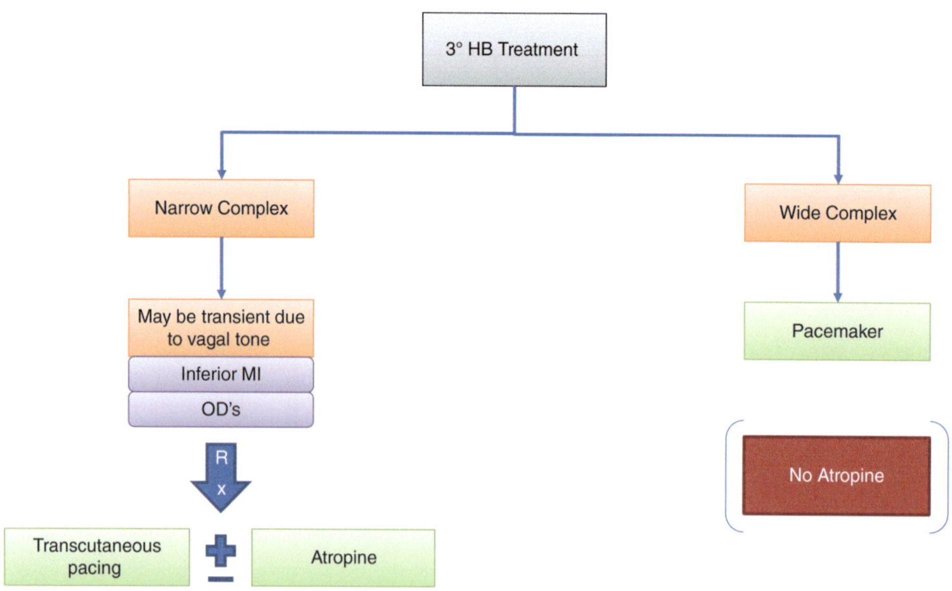

Miscellaneous

Brugada Syndrome Introduction

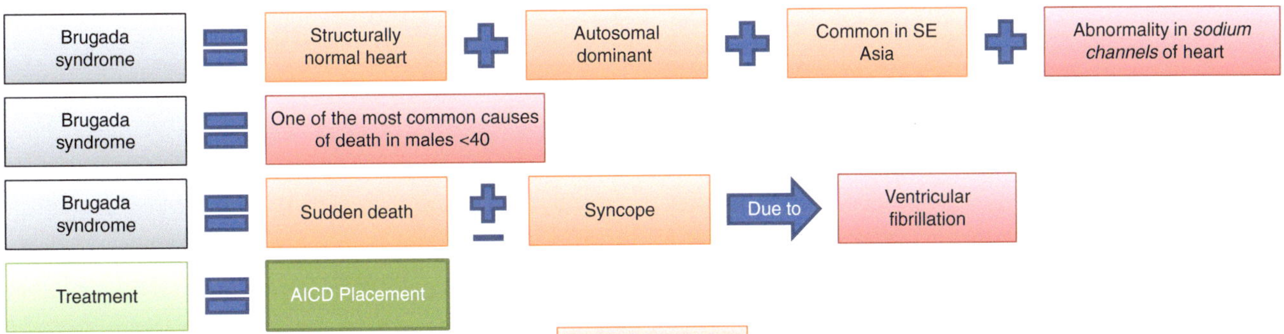

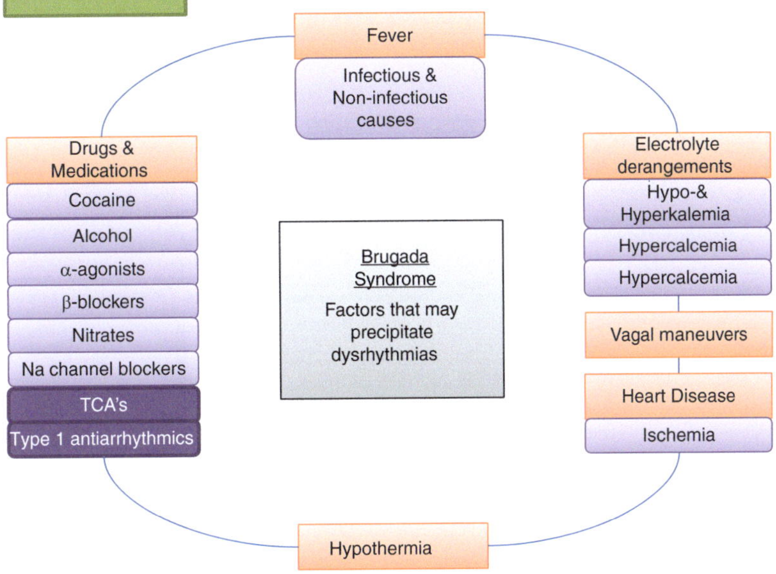

Brugada Syndrome: EKG Changes

ST segments	Brugada Sign Type 1	Type 2	Type 3
Elevated in V1 & V2	Coved ST segment elevation > 2mm in V1-3 (only need 1 lead) followed by a (-) T wave	ST elevation resembling a saddle > 2mm	Morphology of Type 1 or 2, but <2 mm ST elevation
	"Pseudo RBBB"		

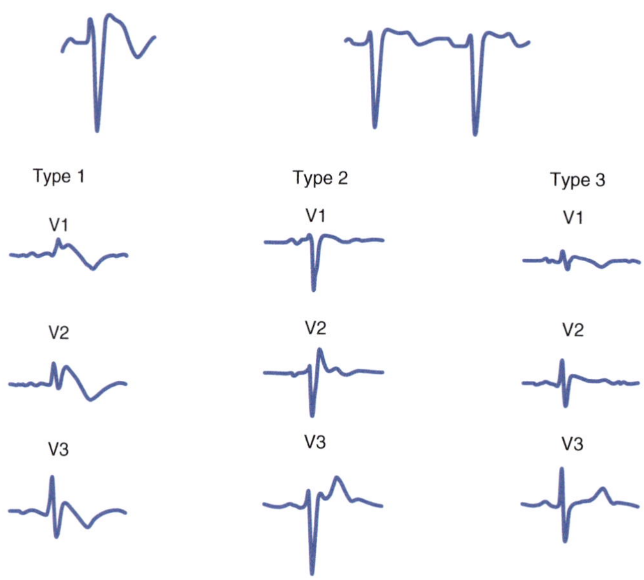

Tetralogy of Fallot

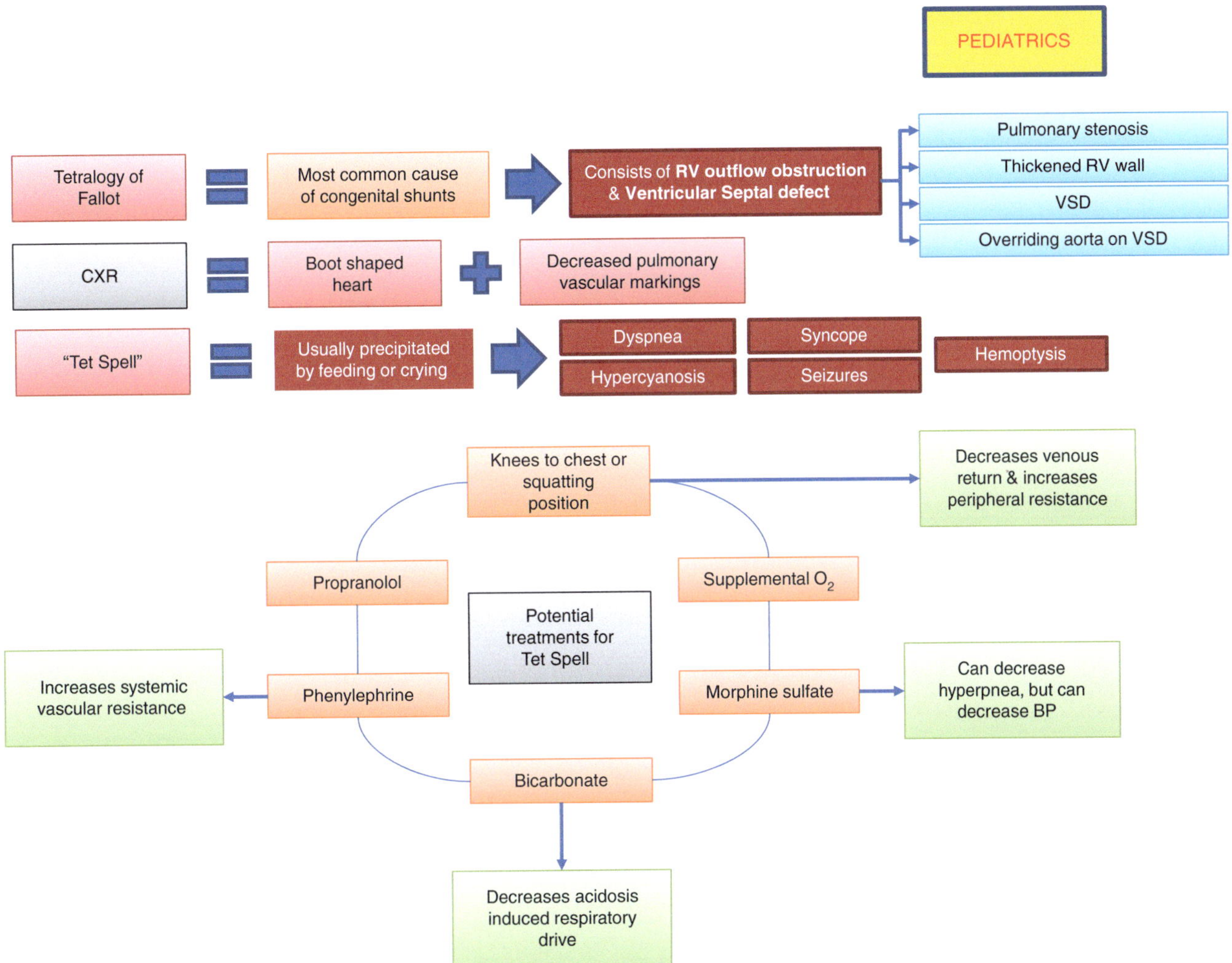

Pulmonary Emergencies

Michael R. Marchick and Bobby Desai

Contents

Definitions and Clinical Presentations 132
Pneumothorax 135
Asthma 138
Chronic Obstructive Pulmonary Disease 143
Bronchiolitis 150
Pertussis 152
Pneumonia 153
Tuberculosis 168
Lung Abscess 172
Acute Respiratory Distress Syndrome 172
Pleural Effusions 173
The Airway 179
General Pediatrics 181

M.R. Marchick, MD
Department of Emergency Medicine,
University of Florida College of Medicine,
Gainesville, FL, USA

B. Desai, MD, MEd (✉)
Department of Emergency Medicine,
University of Florida, Gainesville, FL, USA
e-mail: bdesai@ufl.edu

B. Desai, B.R. Allen (eds.), *Nailing the Written Emergency Medicine Board Examination*,
DOI 10.1007/978-3-319-30838-8_2

Definitions and Clinical Presentations

Hypoxemia

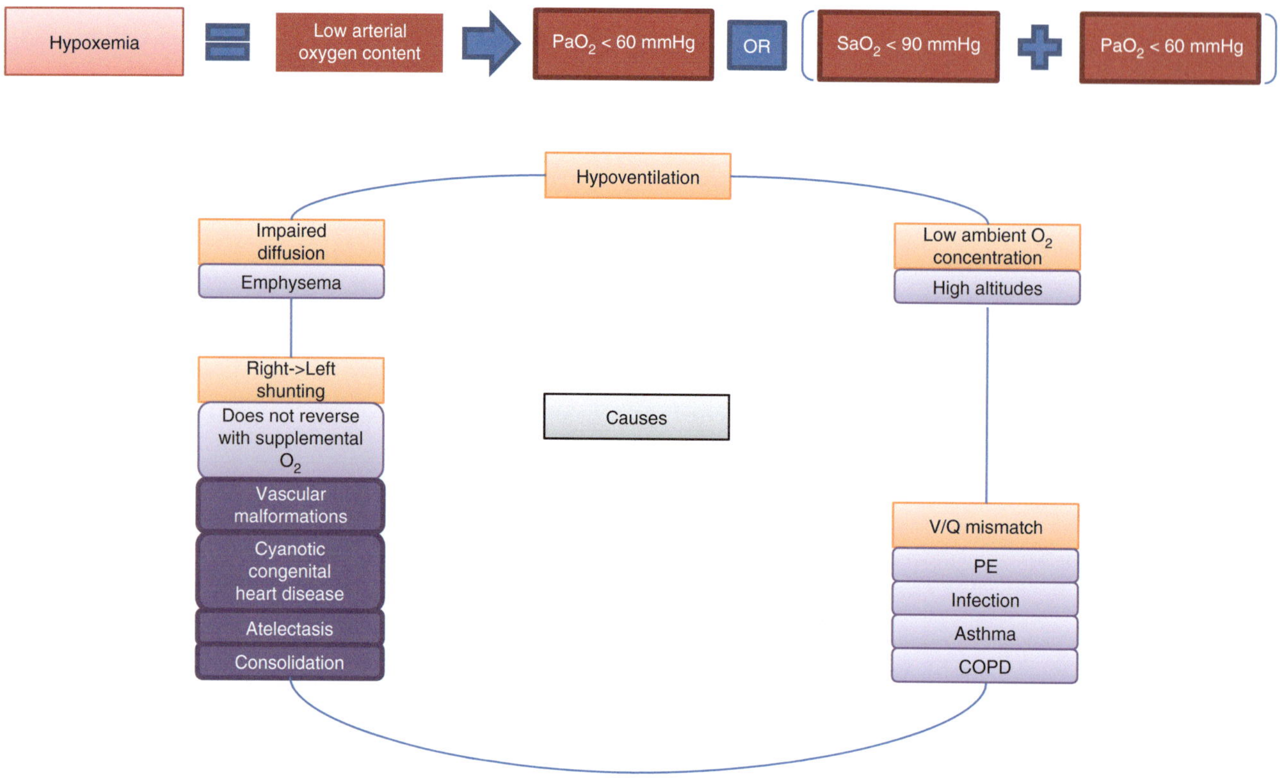

Hypoxia

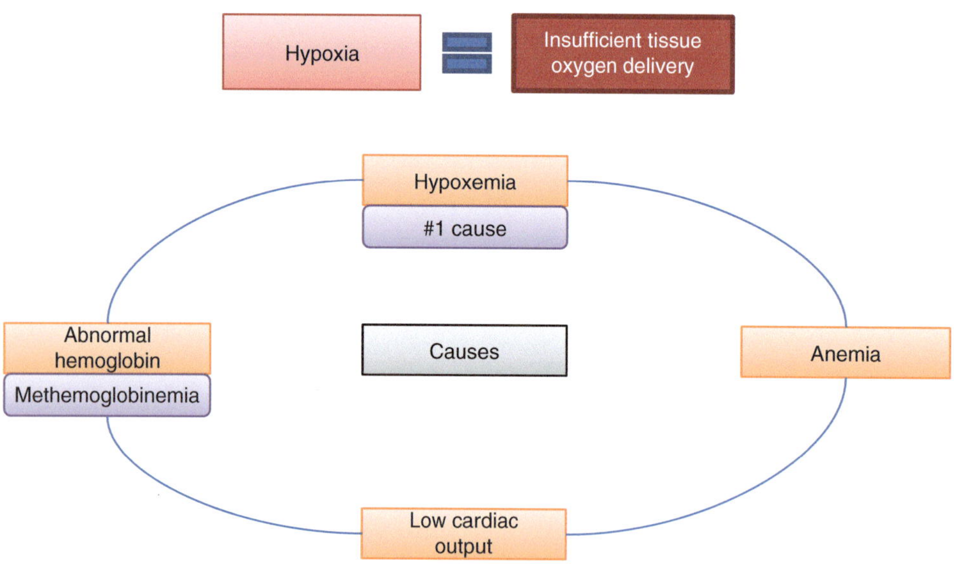

Hypercapnia

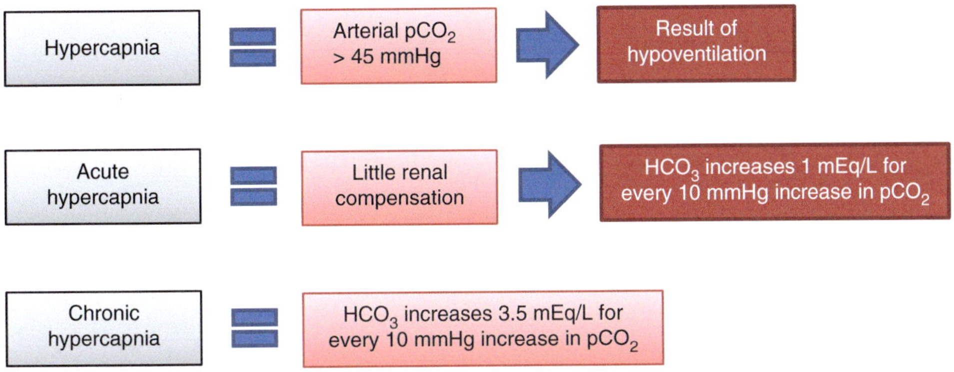

Arterial-Alveolar Gradient

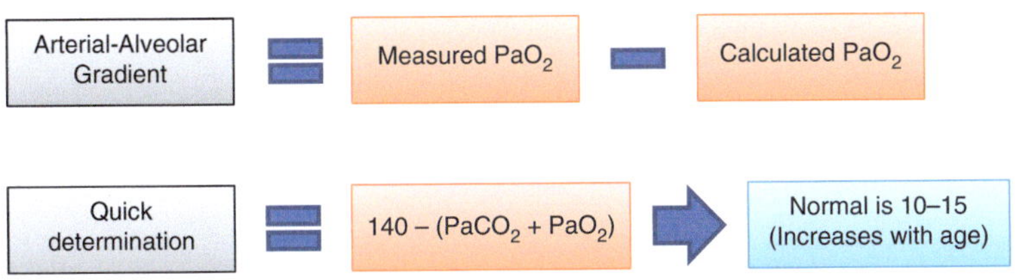

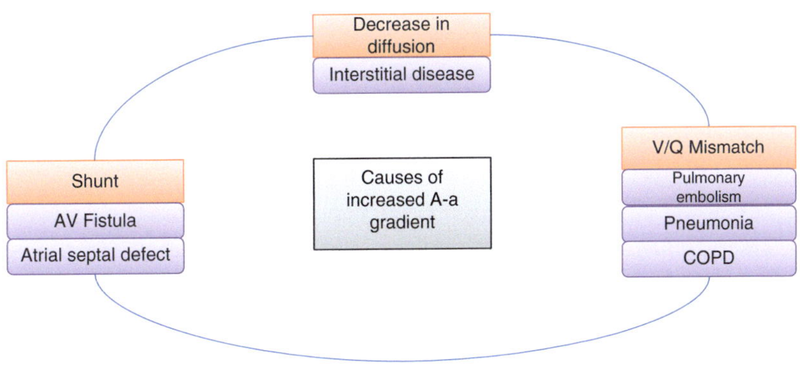

Cyanosis

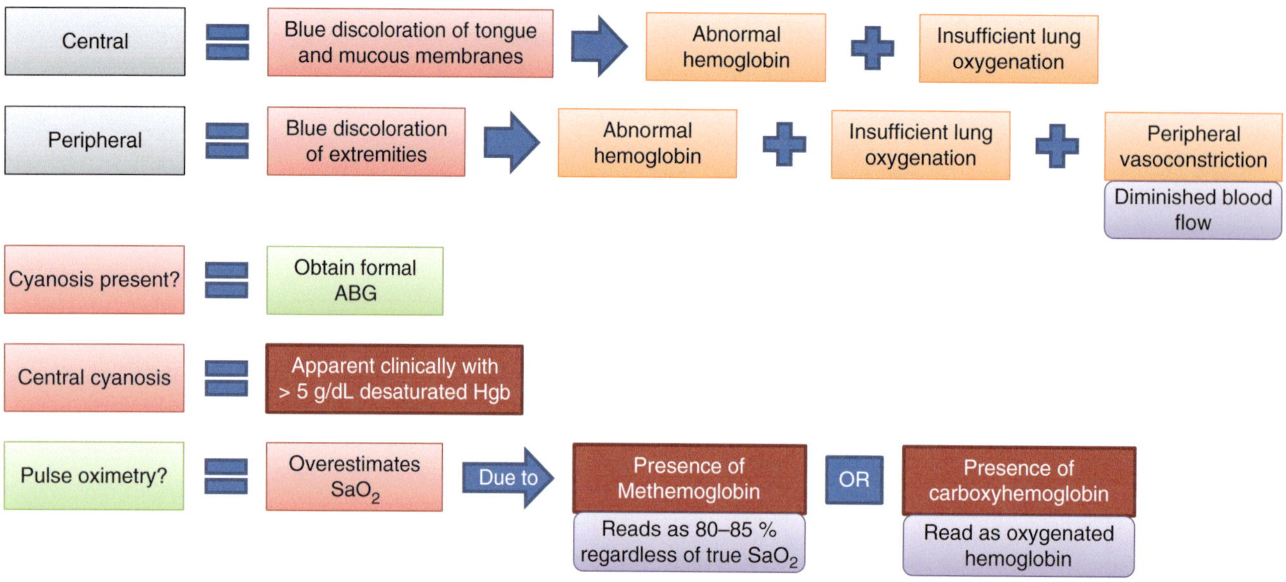

Hemoptysis

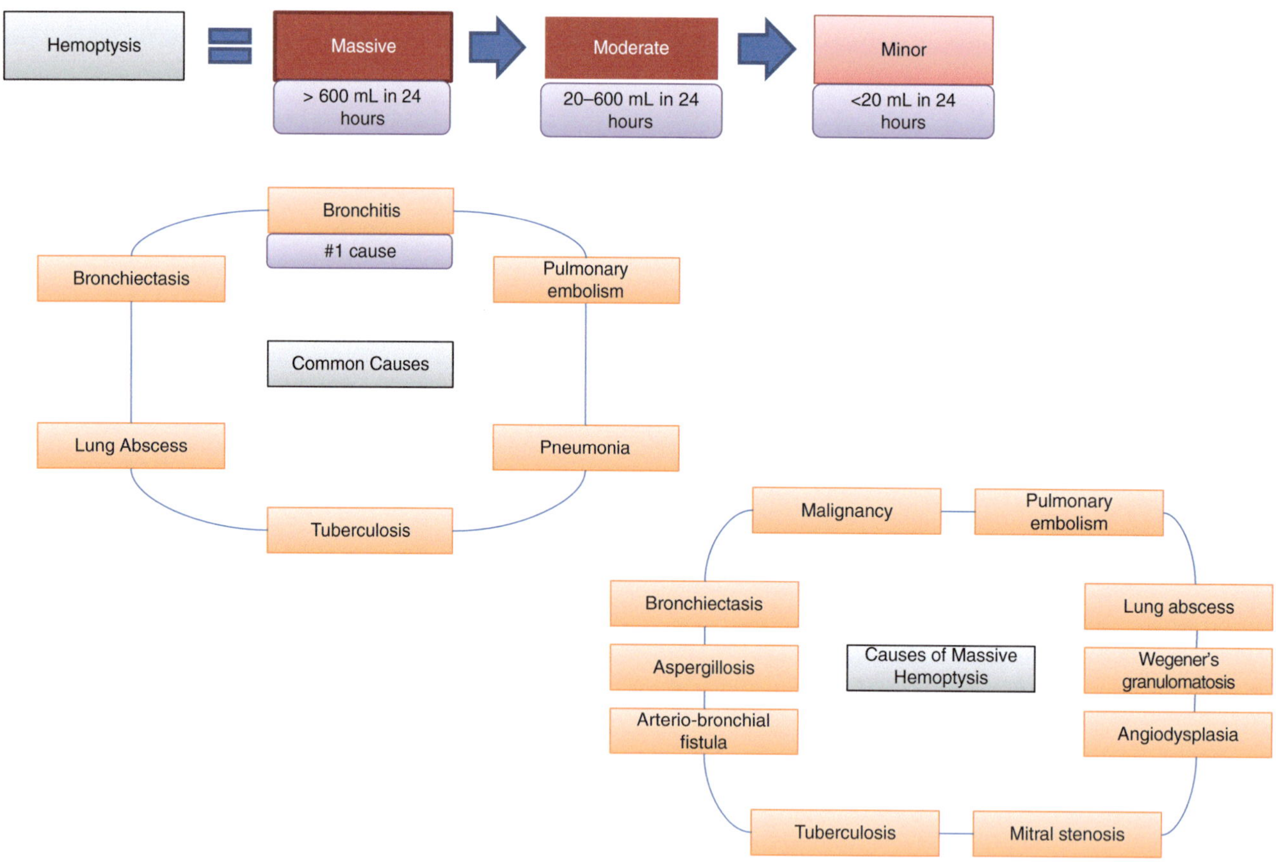

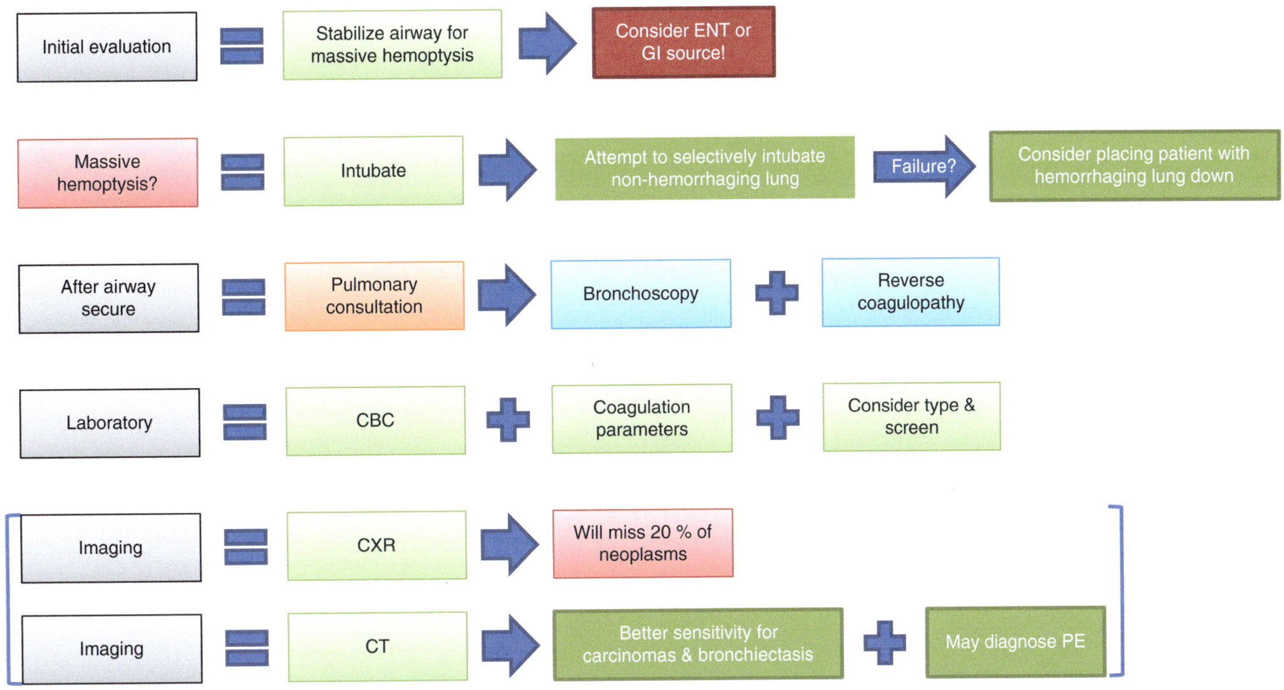

Pneumothorax

Spontaneous Pneumothorax

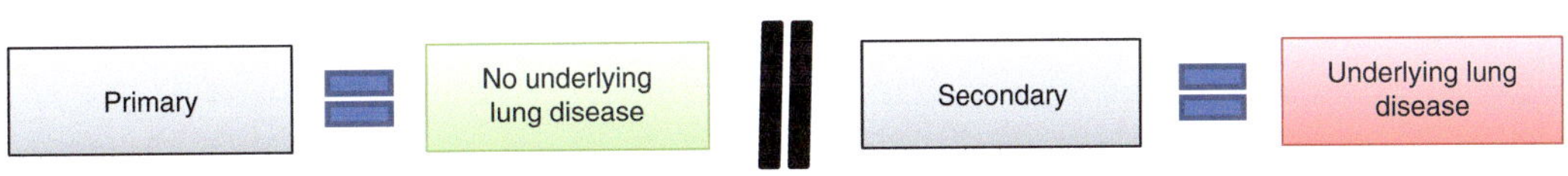

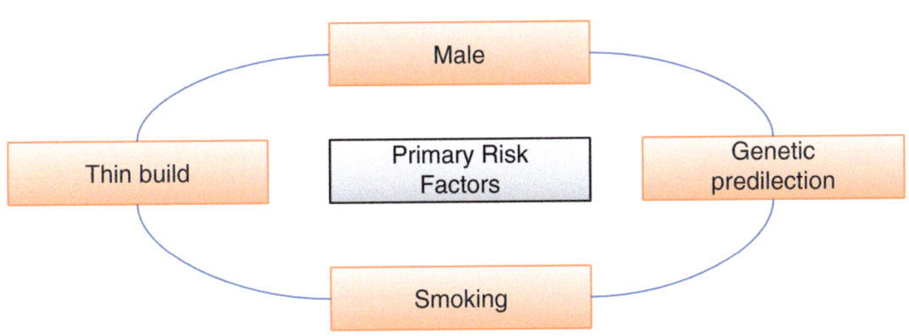

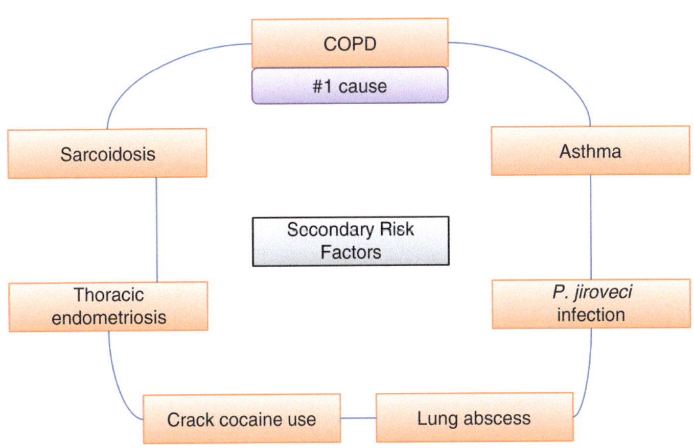

Pneumothorax Diagnosis and Management

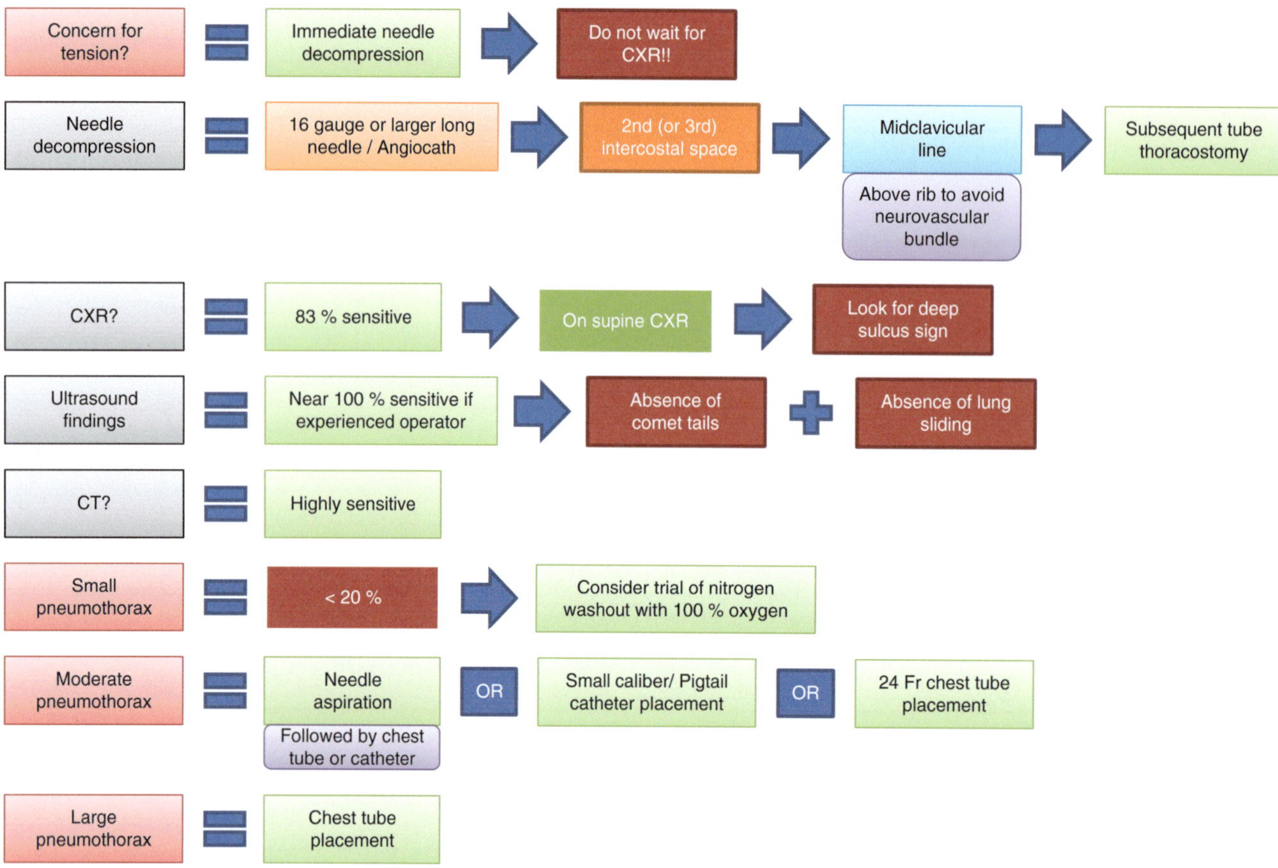

Iatrogenic PTX

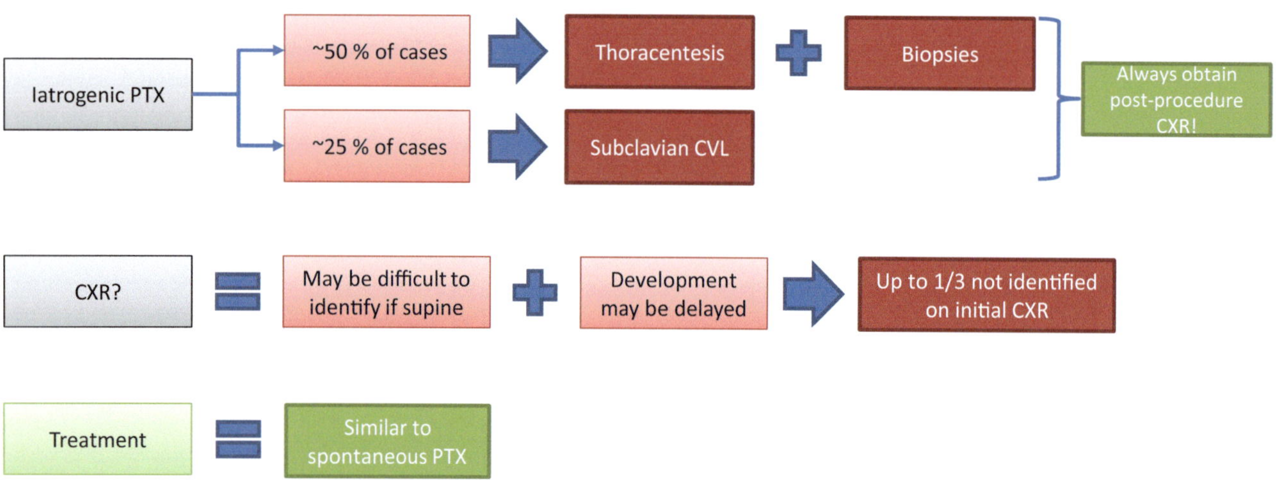

Pneumomediastinum

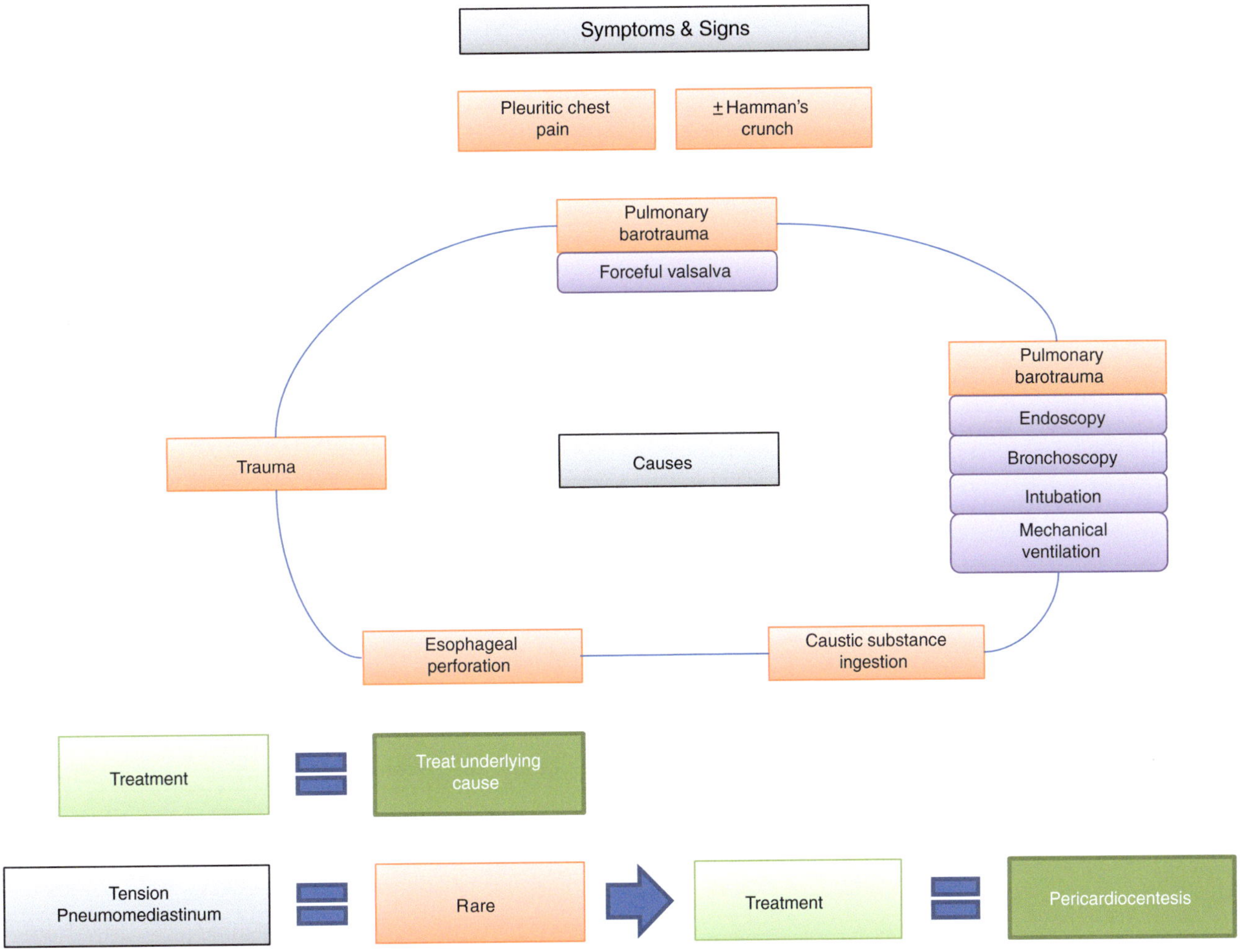

Asthma

Introduction

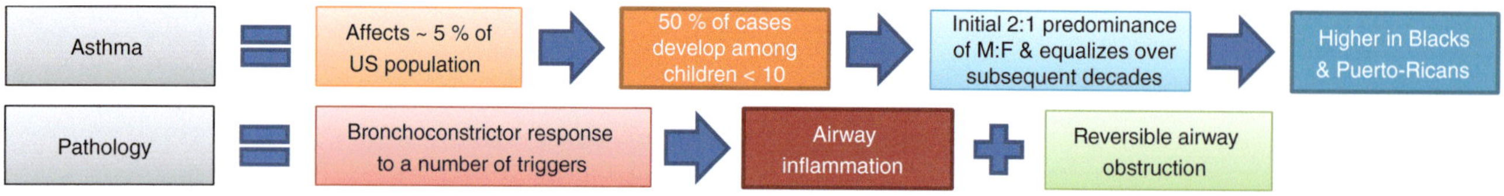

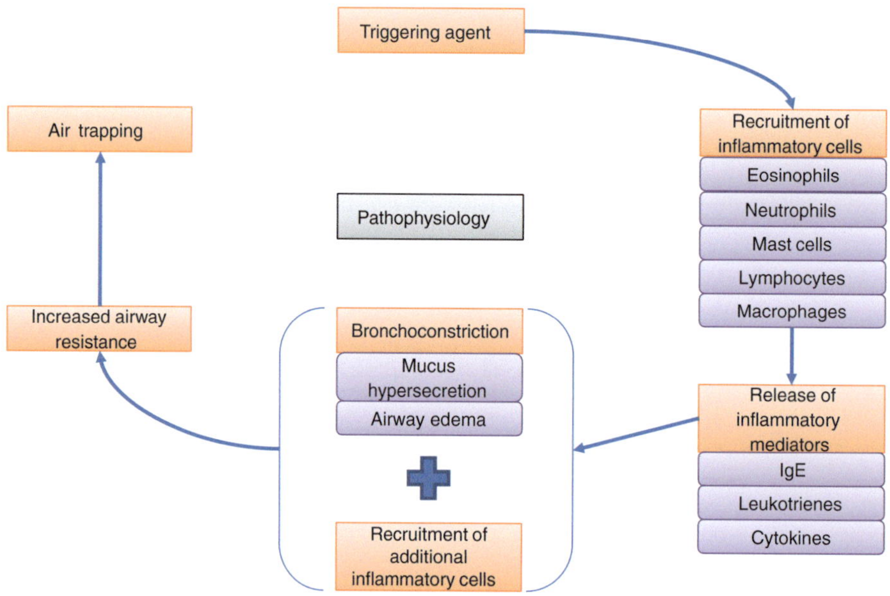

Triggering Agents

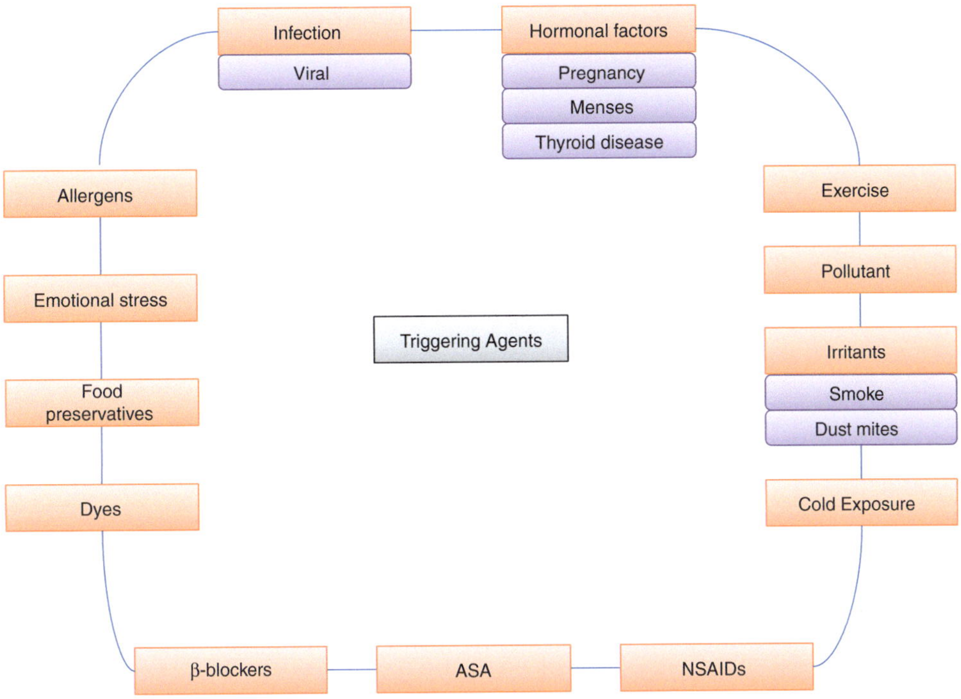

Clinical Features

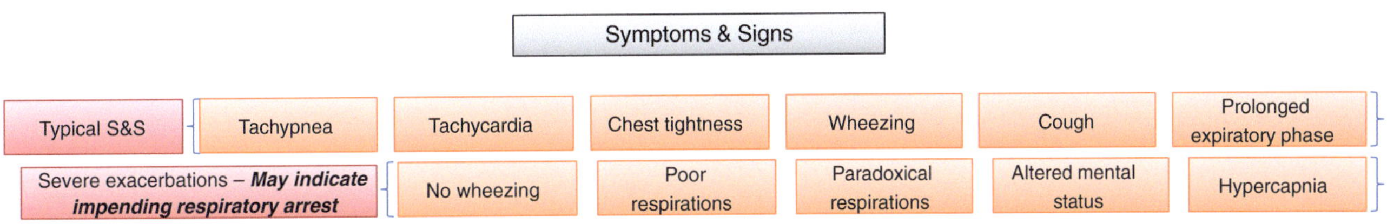

Risk Factors for Death

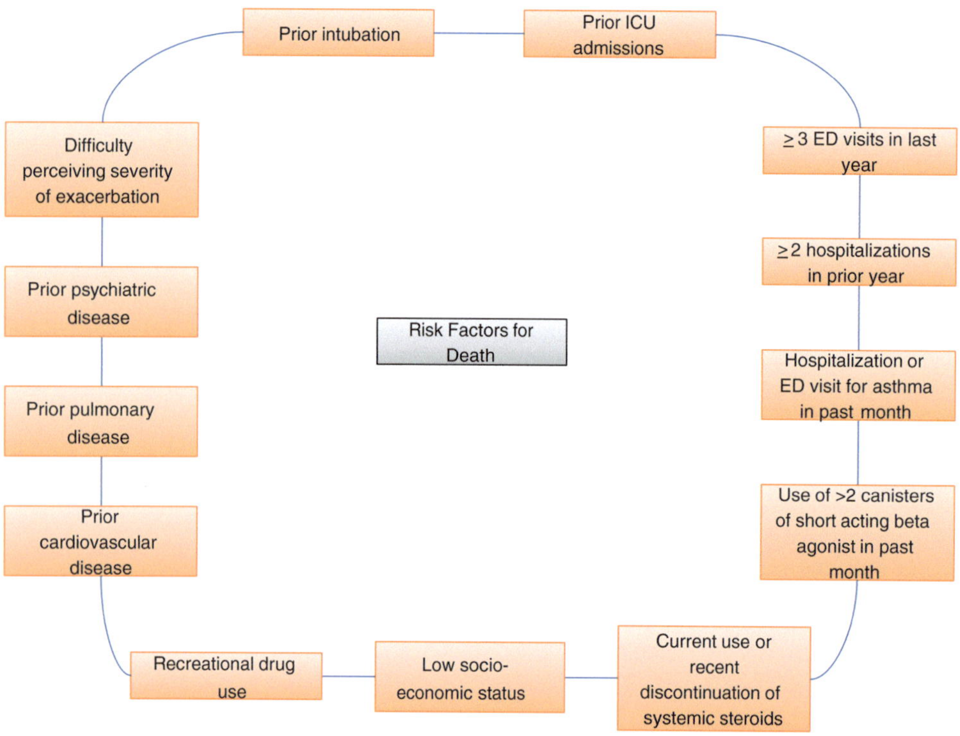

Peak Flow

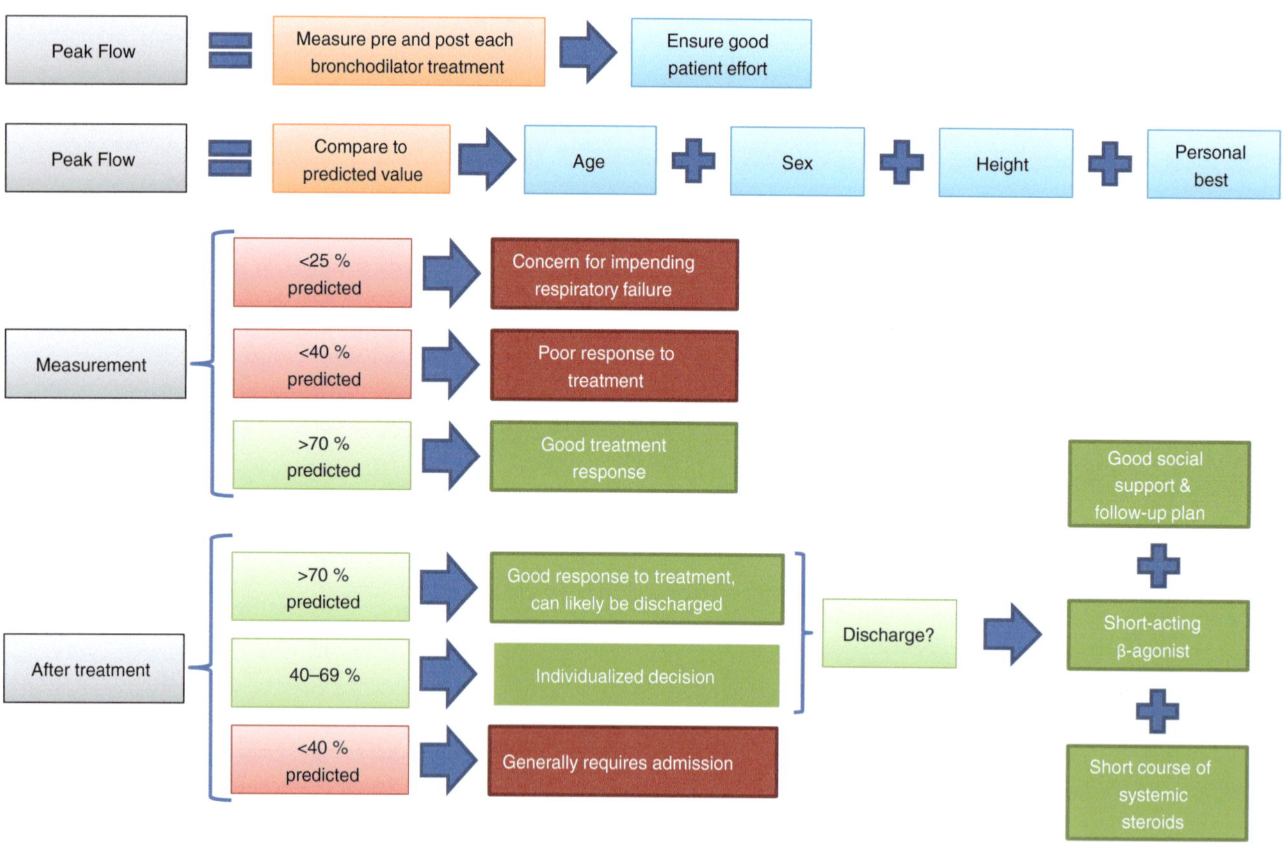

β-Agonists and Anticholinergics

β-2 adrenergic agonists = Primarily dilate small, peripheral airways → Short acting agents have rapid onset → Long acting agents have slow onset = *Not* indicated for acute sx

β-2 adrenergic agonists = Stimulate adenyl cyclase → Increase cyclic AMP → Decreased intracellular Ca++ → Smooth muscle relaxation

Side effects = Tremor (#1) + Tachycardia + HTN + Anxiety + Rare arrhythmias, e.g., MAT / Seen with ***theophylline***

Systemic β-agonists = No advantage over inhaled → Unless unable to deliver via inhalation ‖ IV infusions = More side effects

Subcutaneous epinephrine = 0.2–0.5 mL 1:1000 solution → *Not* β-2 selective → Increased cardiovascular side effects → Via β-1 receptors

Terbutaline = 0.25 mg SC → β-2 selective

Anticholinergics = Inhibits parasympathetic reflex bronchoconstriction + Decrease respiratory secretions → Primarily affect large airways

Ipratropium = Poorly absorbed from airways → Minimal systemic side effects → Slower onset of action → Less potent action than β-2 agonists / *Not* appropriate for monotherapy

Ipratropium + β-blockers → Work synergistically → Commonly given together in 3 stacked doses early in ED

Steroids, Methylxanthines, Magnesium, and Leukotriene Modifiers

Corticosteroids = Reduce recruitment & activation of inflammatory cells + Reduce release of pro-inflammatory mediators → Increase responsiveness of β-adrenergic receptors + Onset of action 4-8 hours

Methylxanthines = Theophylline → Bronchodilatory effects + Anti-inflammatory effects → Occasionally used for chronic management

Methylxanthines = Narrow therapeutic window → Significant arrythmogenic potential + CNS side effects → Check level on all patients taking theophylline

Leukotriene modifiers = Modulate inflammatory response → Useful for chronic management → *Not* indicated for ED use

Magnesium = Relaxes bronchial smooth muscle + Stabilizes mast cells & T-lymphocytes → Indicated only in *severe* exacerbations → 25–75 mg/kg up to 2 g IV over 30 minutes

Magnesium side effects = Respiratory depression + Flushing + Nausea + Hypotension + ↓Reflexes + Muscle weakness

Severe Asthma Management

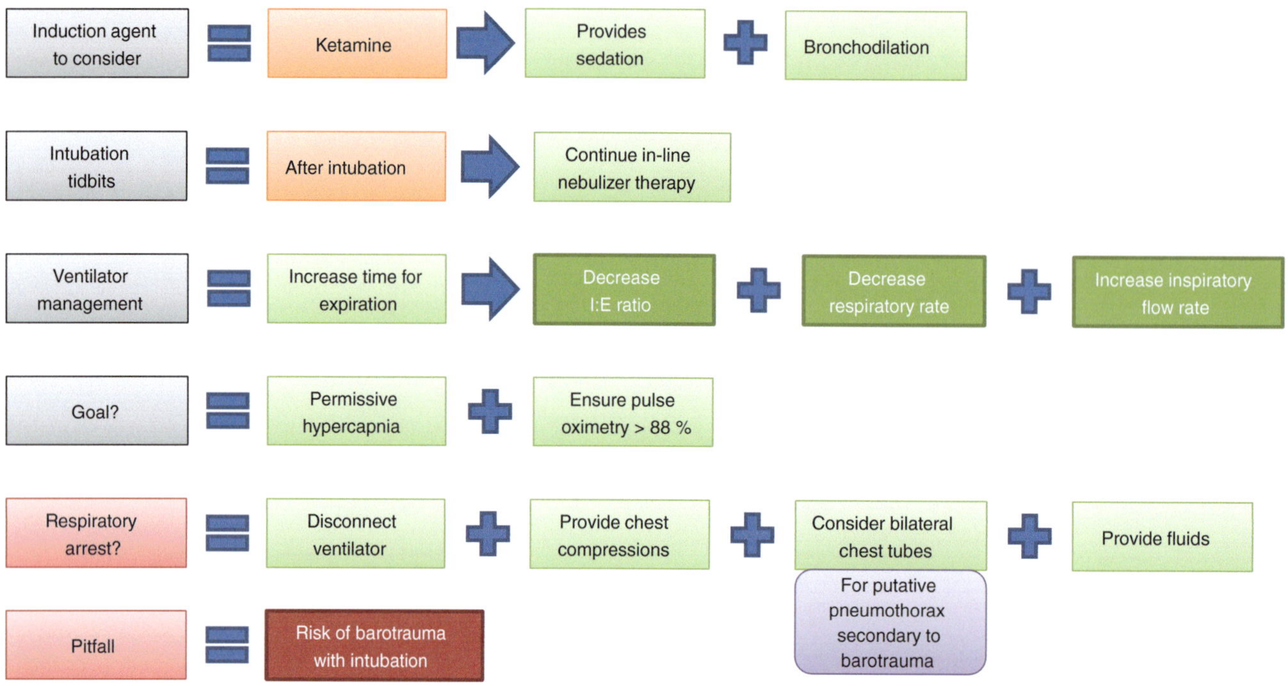

Chronic Obstructive Pulmonary Disease

Introduction

COPD = 4th leading cause of death in US → Increasing prevalence in women → Only major cause of death which is increasing → Insidious onset typically over decades

Clinical definition = FEV_1/FVC< 70 % + FEV_1 < 80 % predicted → FEV_1 Forced expiratory volume in 1 sec || FVC Forced vital capacity

More severe COPD? = Further diminishment in FEV_1 vs. predicted value

COPD = Chronic bronchitis + Emphysema + Bronchiectasis → Common overlap of these conditions

Chronic bronchitis "blue bloater" = Clinical diagnosis → Productive cough for ≥ 3 months in 2 consecutive years without other apparent cause

Emphysema "pink puffer" = Pathologic diagnosis → Destruction of small pulmonary airspaces

Risk factors = Cigarette smoking (#1 risk factor) + Indoor air pollutants + Occupational dust exposure + Long-term passive smoking + α-1 antitrypsin deficiency (Very rare)

Cigarette smoking = COPD develops in ~15 % smokers

Interventions which improve disease progression = Smoking cessation + Long-term O_2 therapy || Consider pneumococcal vaccination for all COPD patients

COPD Pathophysiology

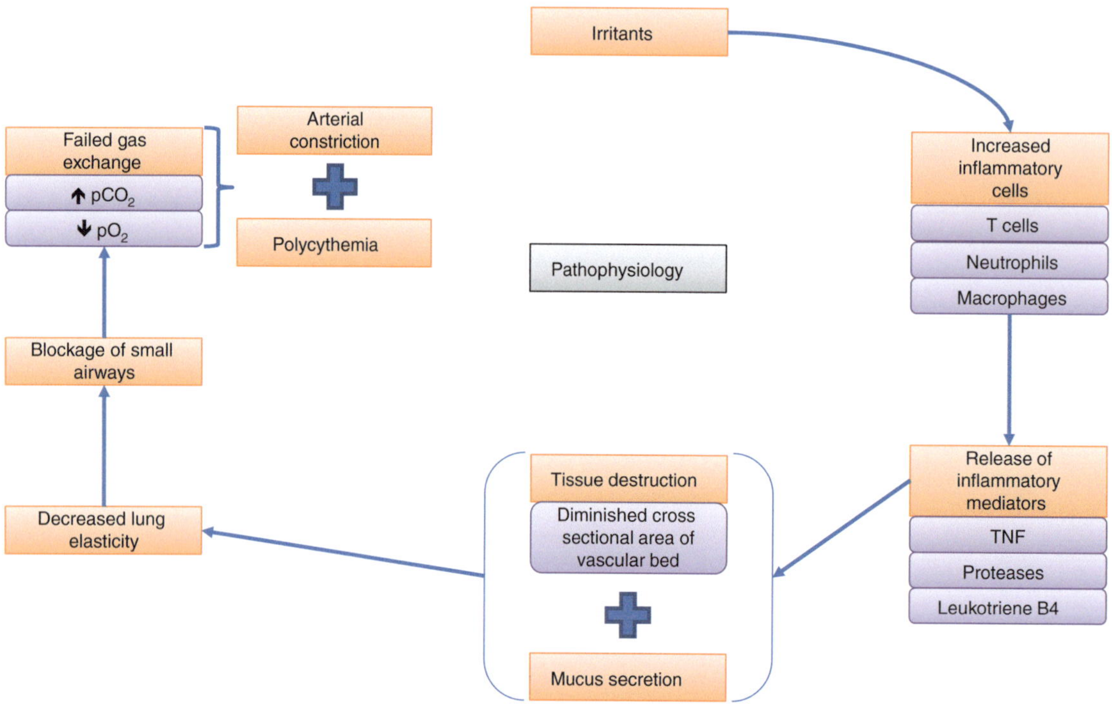

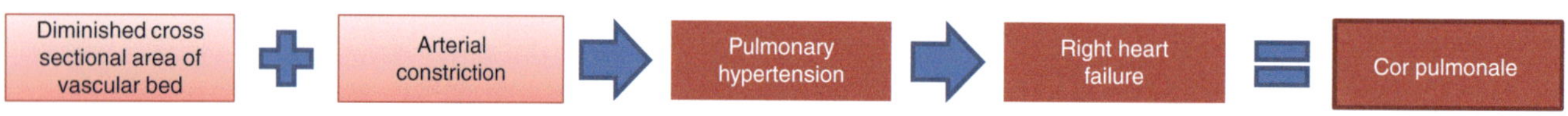

Acute COPD Exacerbation Causes

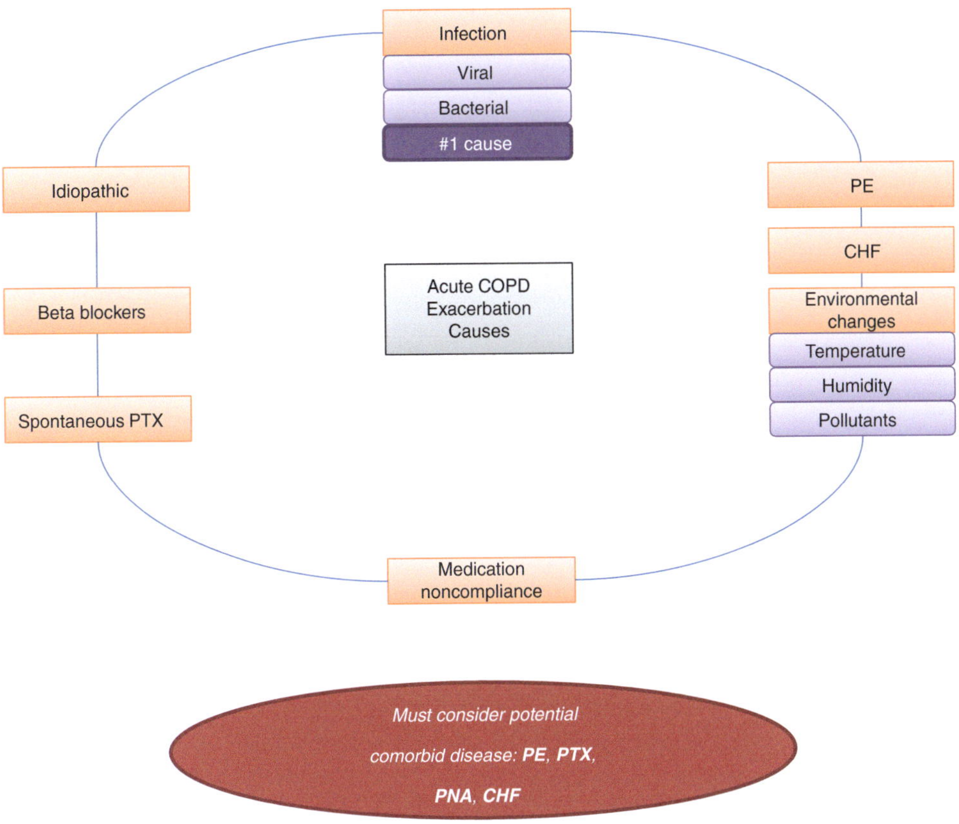

Diagnostics

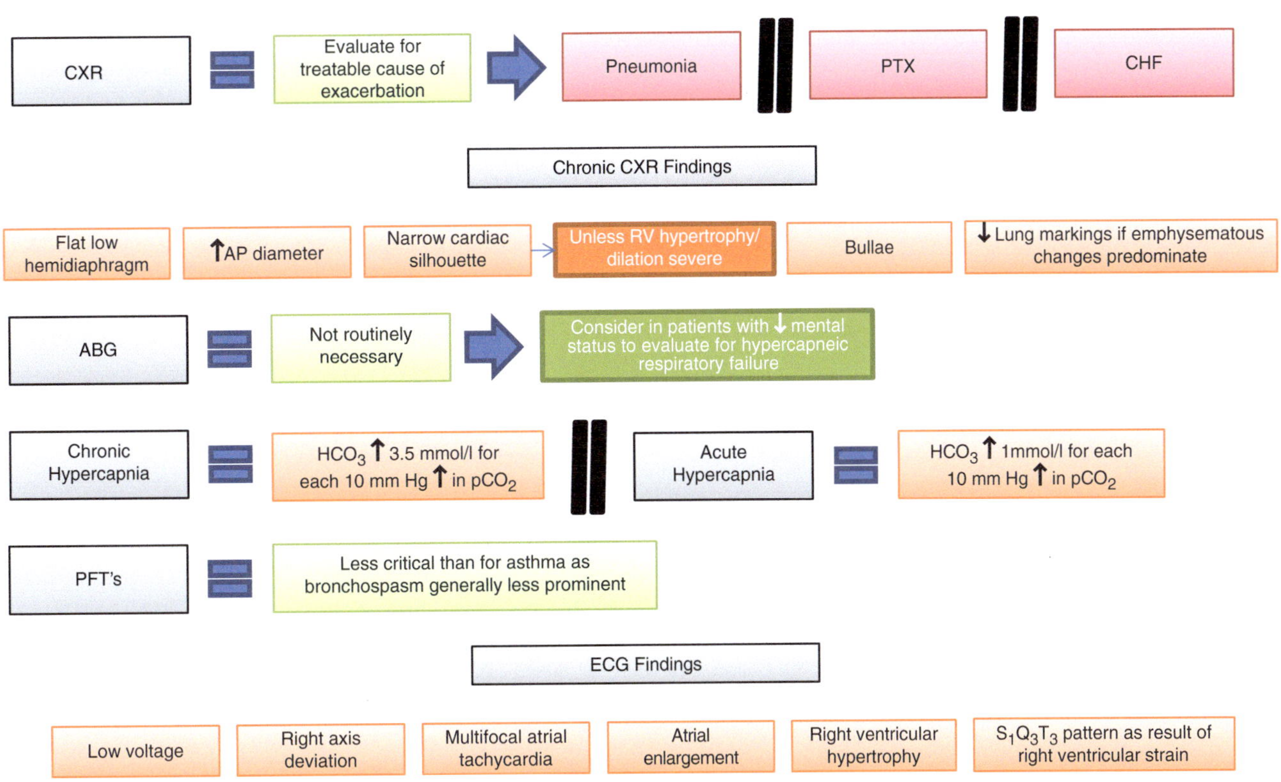

COPD Exacerbation Management

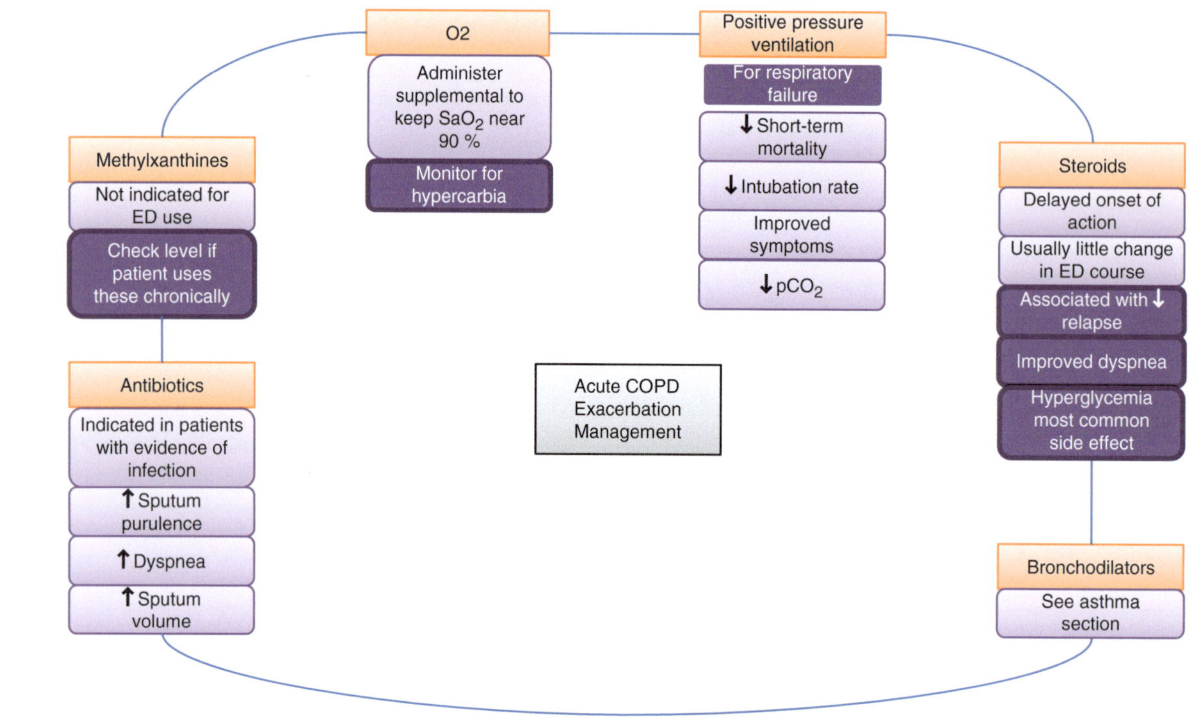

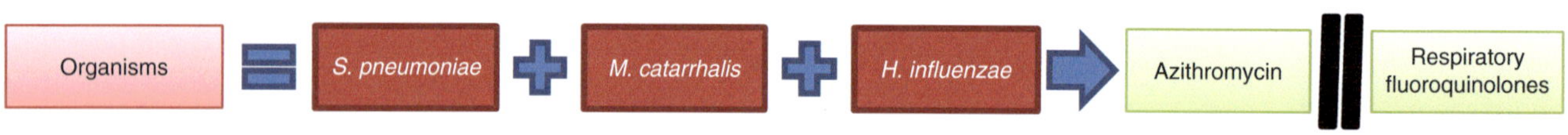

NIPPV Indications and Contraindications

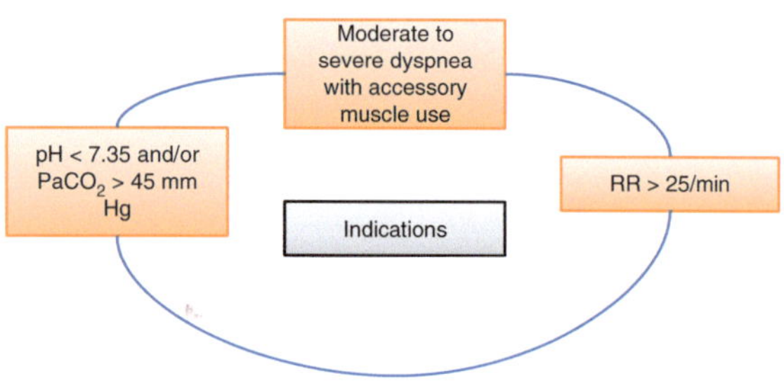

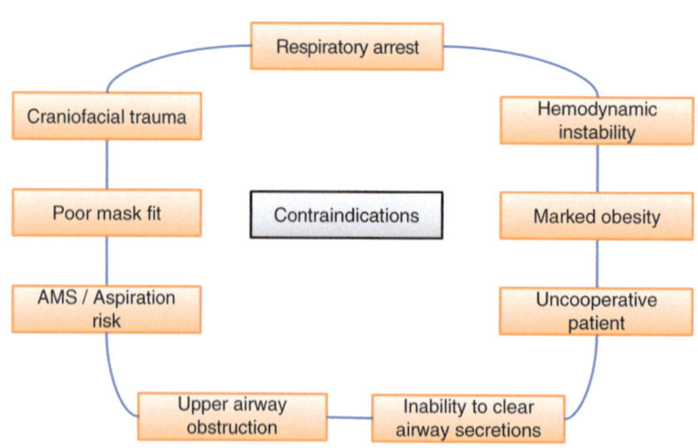

Indications for Intubation

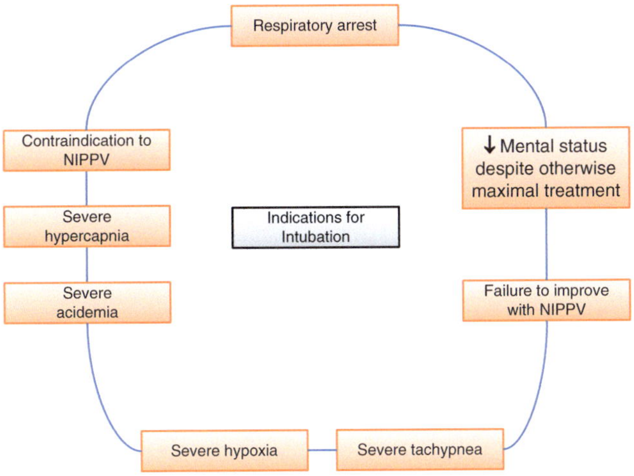

COPD Ventilator Management and Pitfalls

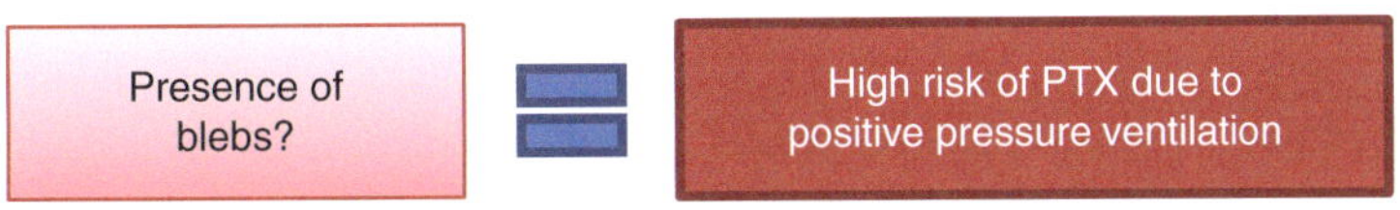

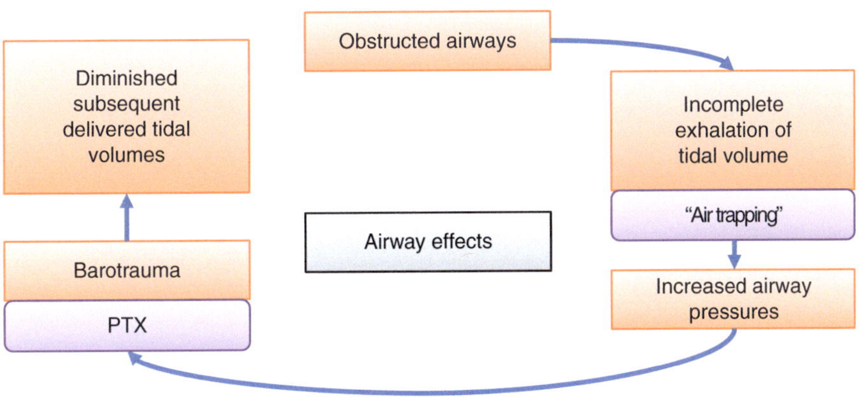

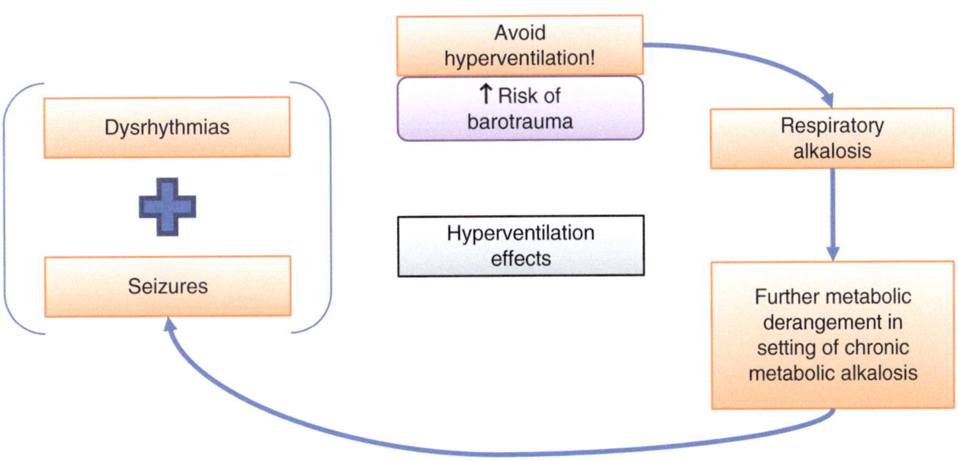

Permissive Hypercapnia

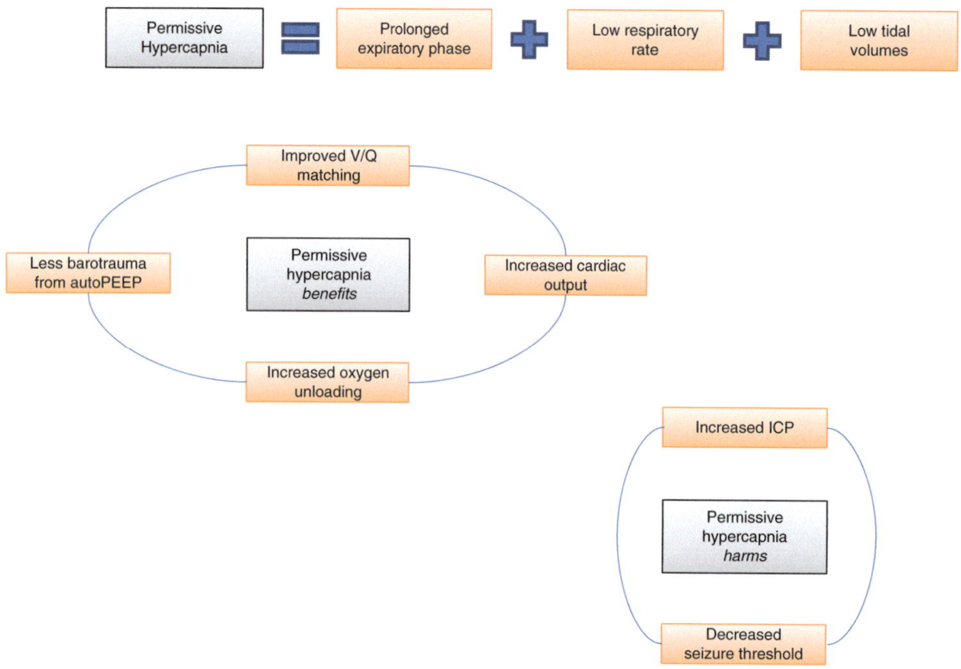

COPD Exacerbation Disposition

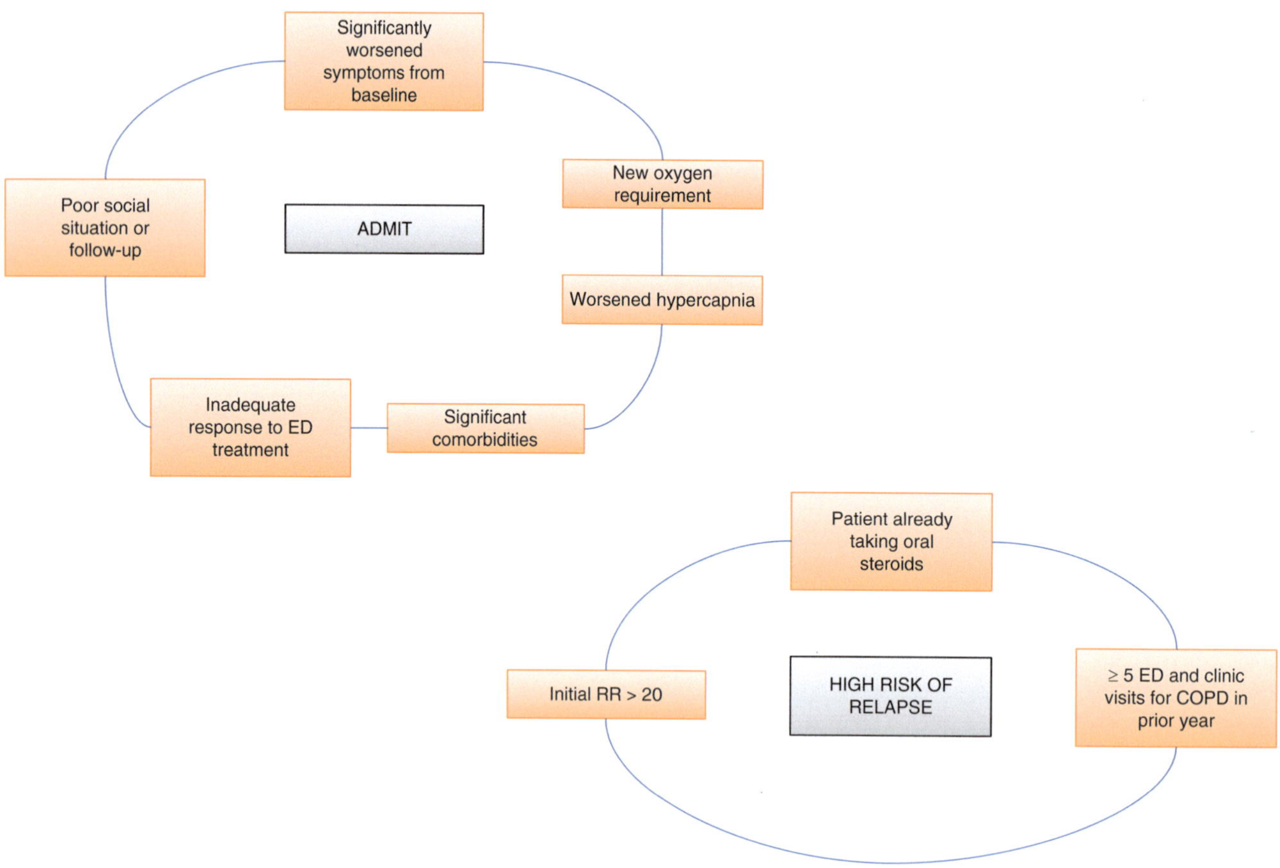

Acute Bronchitis

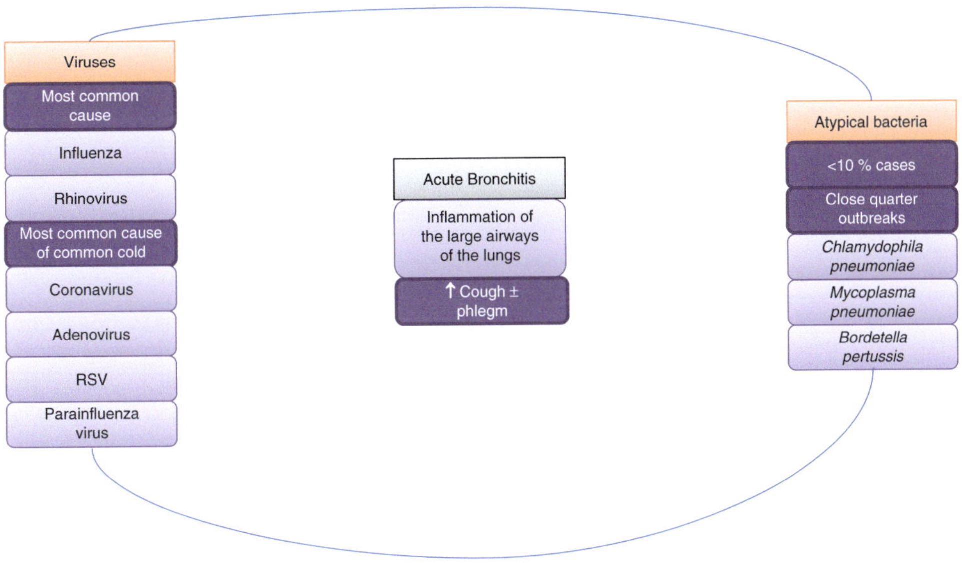

Acute Bronchitis Management

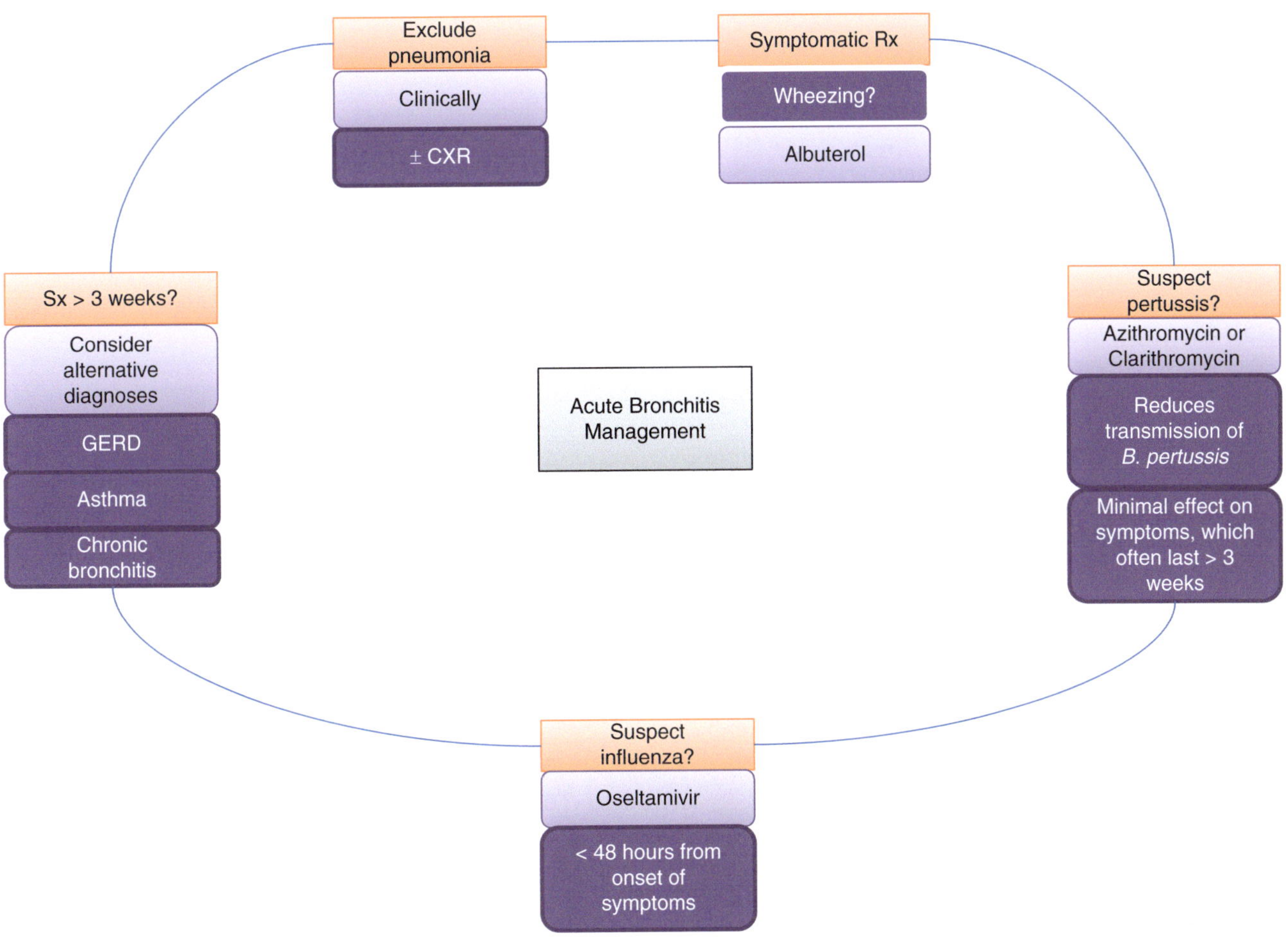

Bronchiolitis

Bronchiolitis

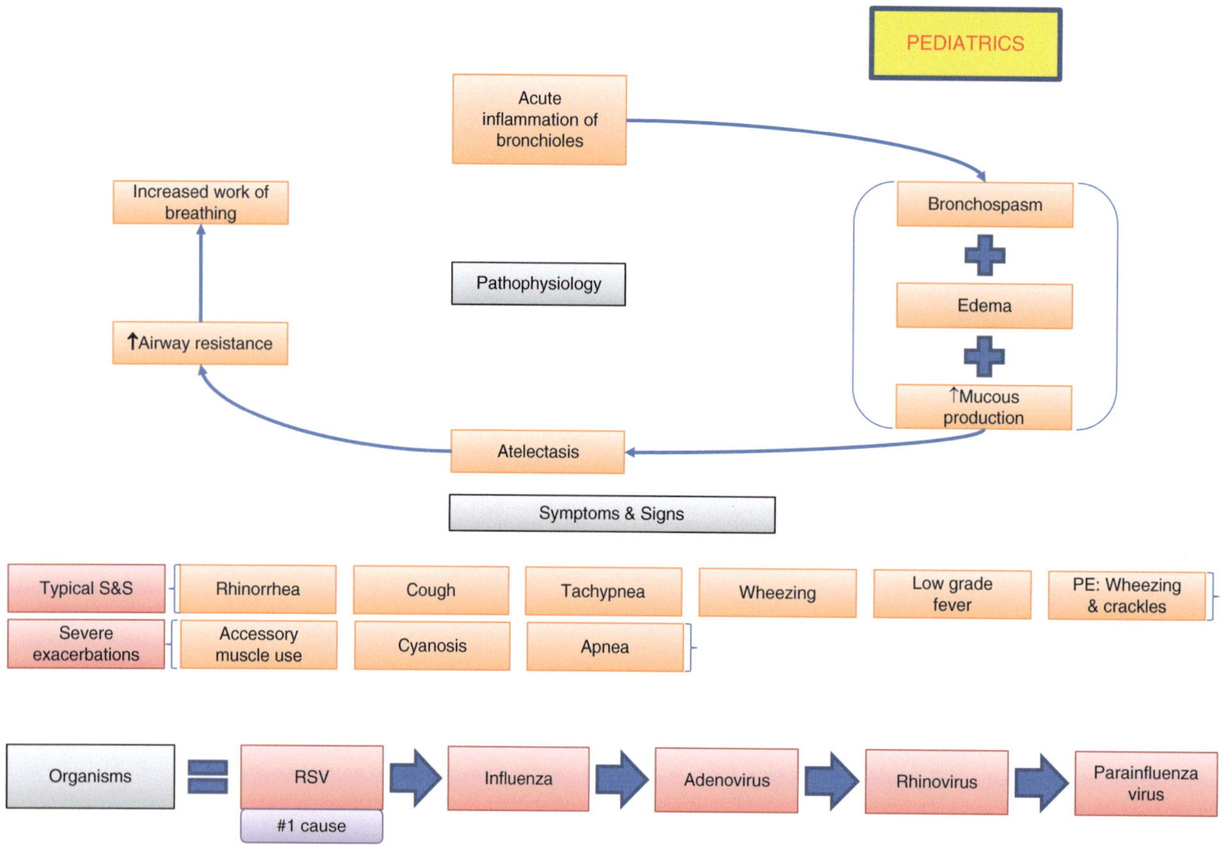

RSV Management

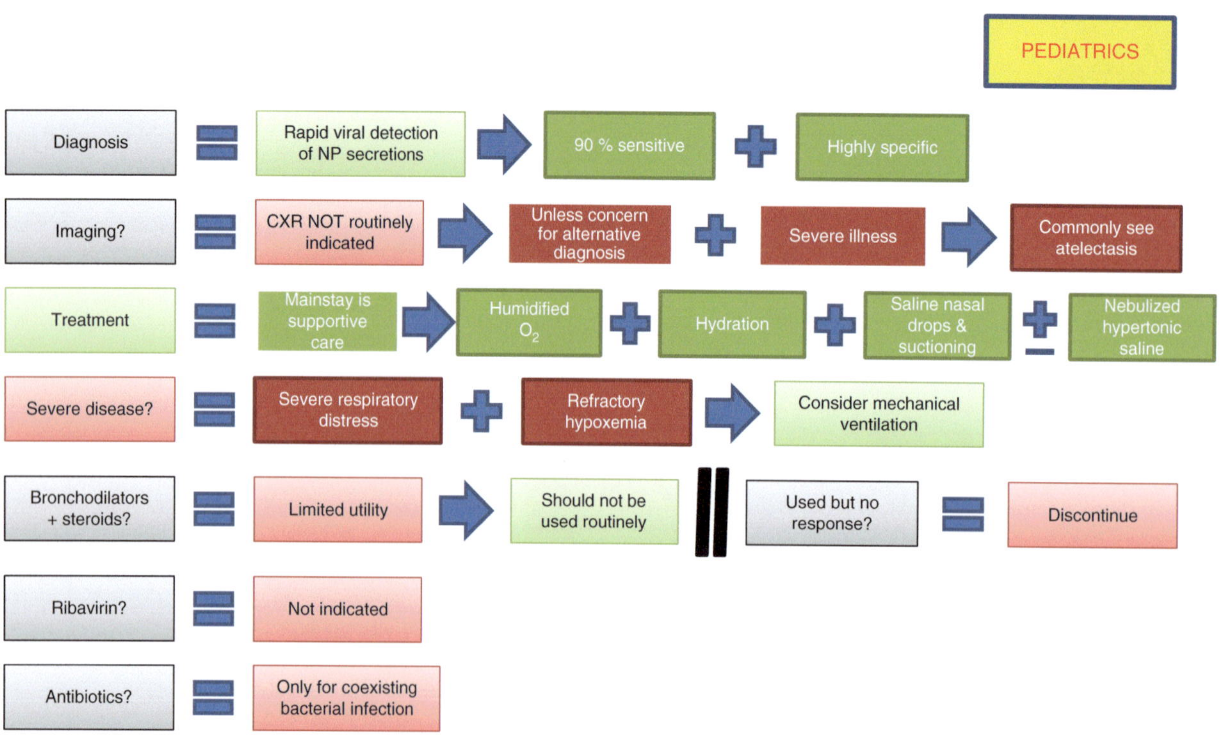

Bronchiolitis Disposition

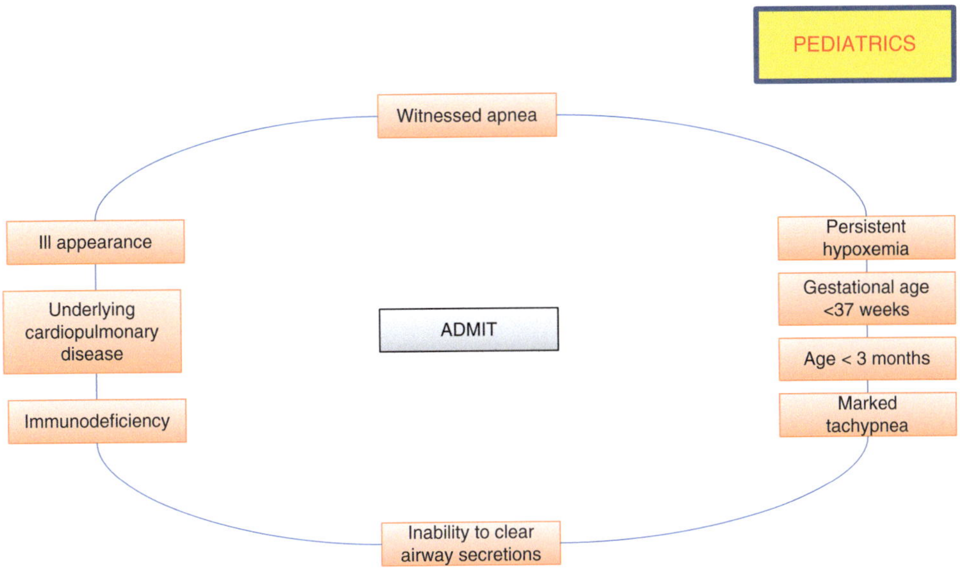

Bronchopulmonary Dysplasia

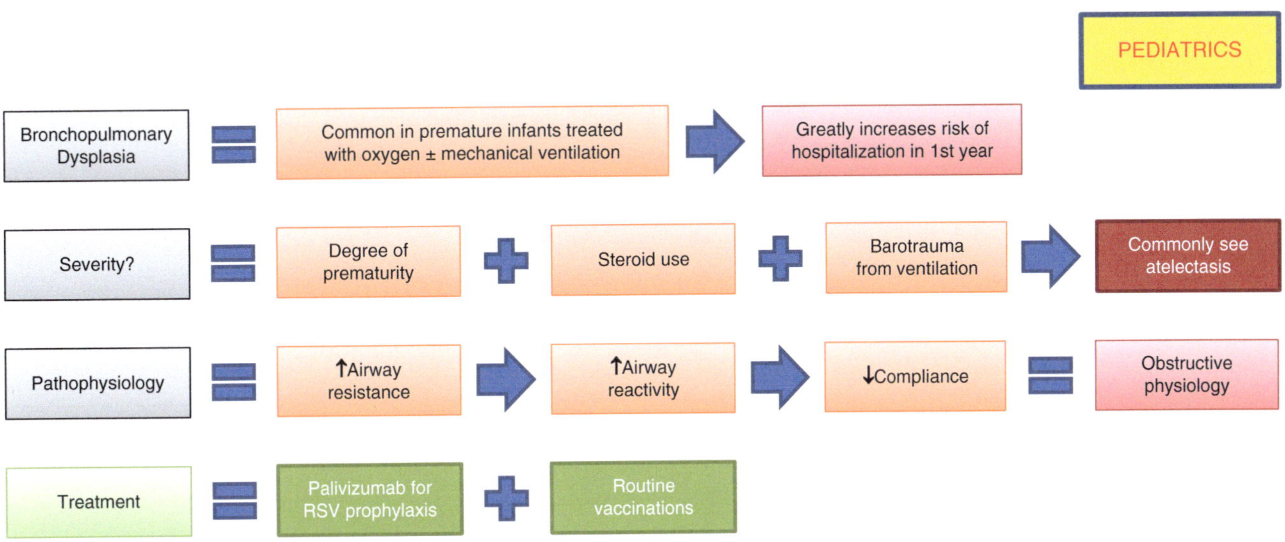

Pertussis

Introduction

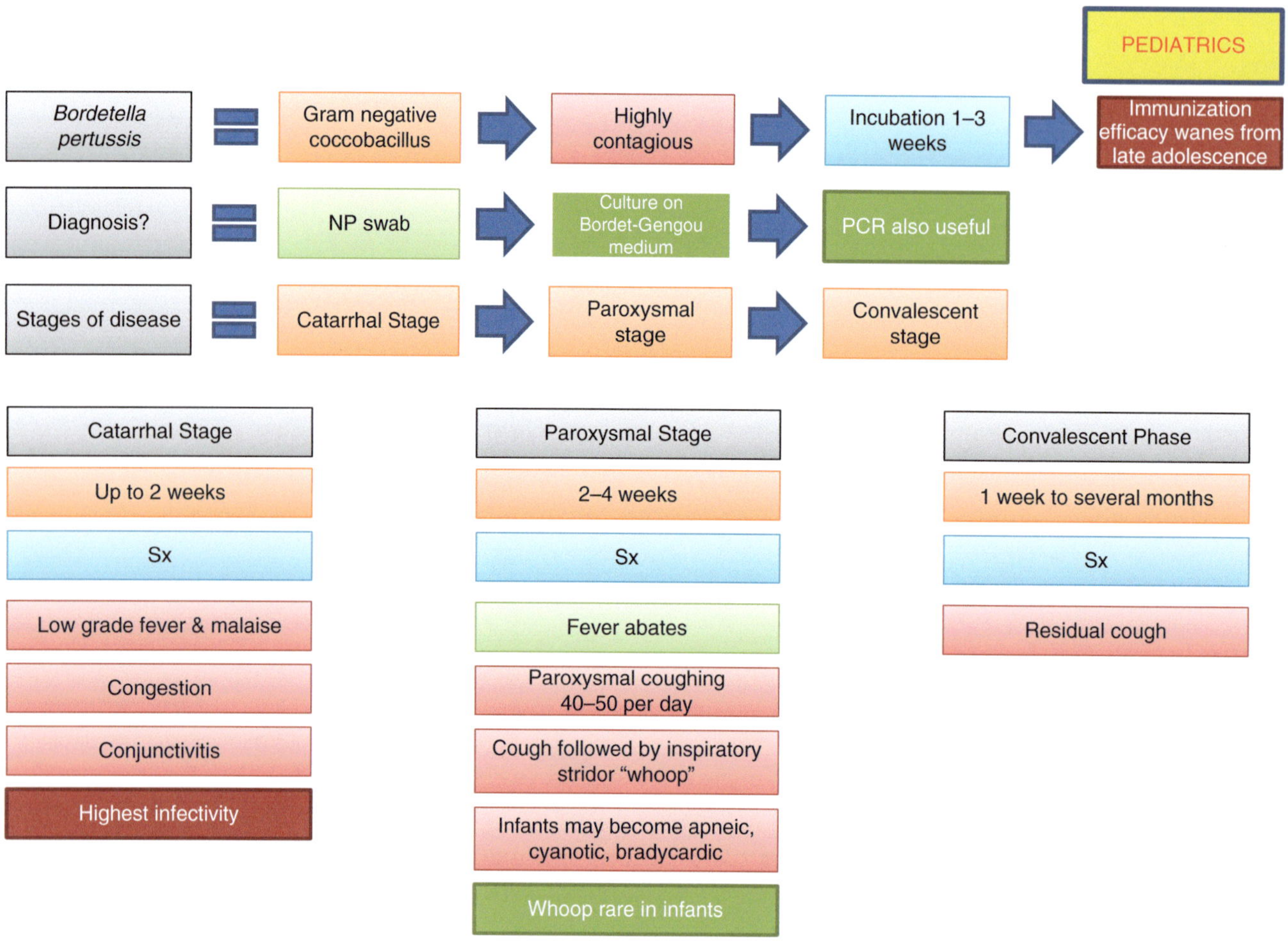

Pertussis Complications

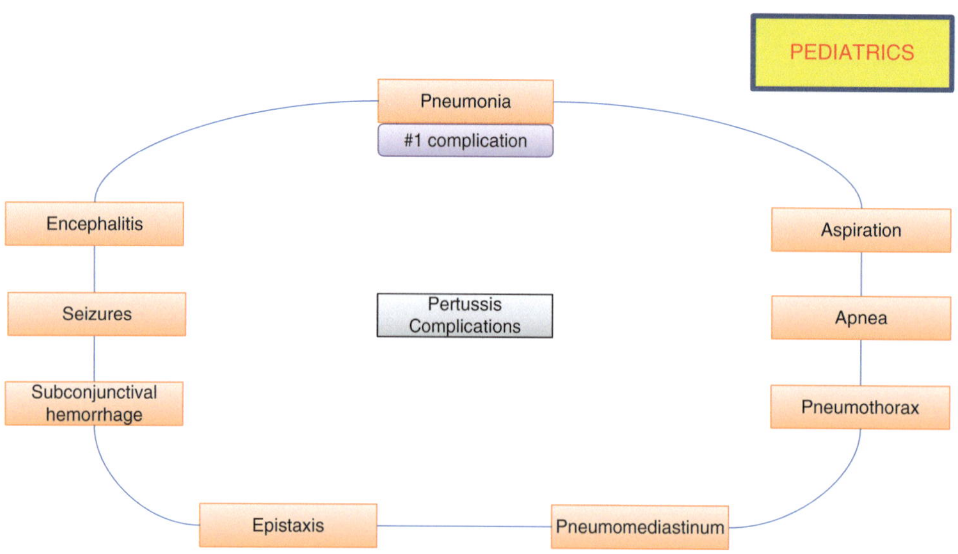

Pertussis Treatment

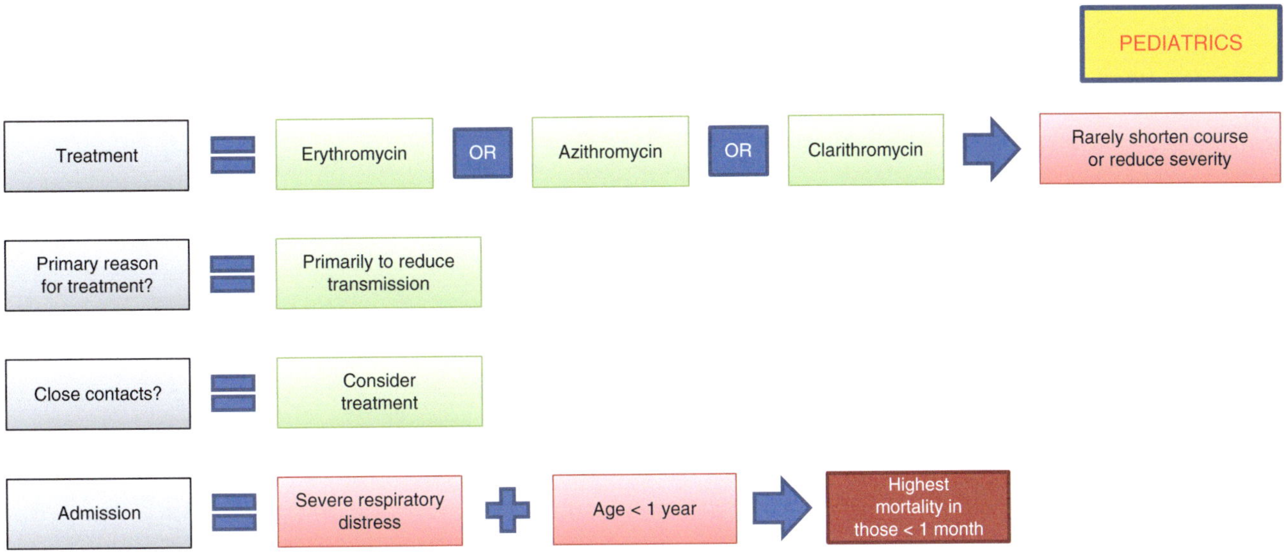

Pneumonia

Pneumonia Classification

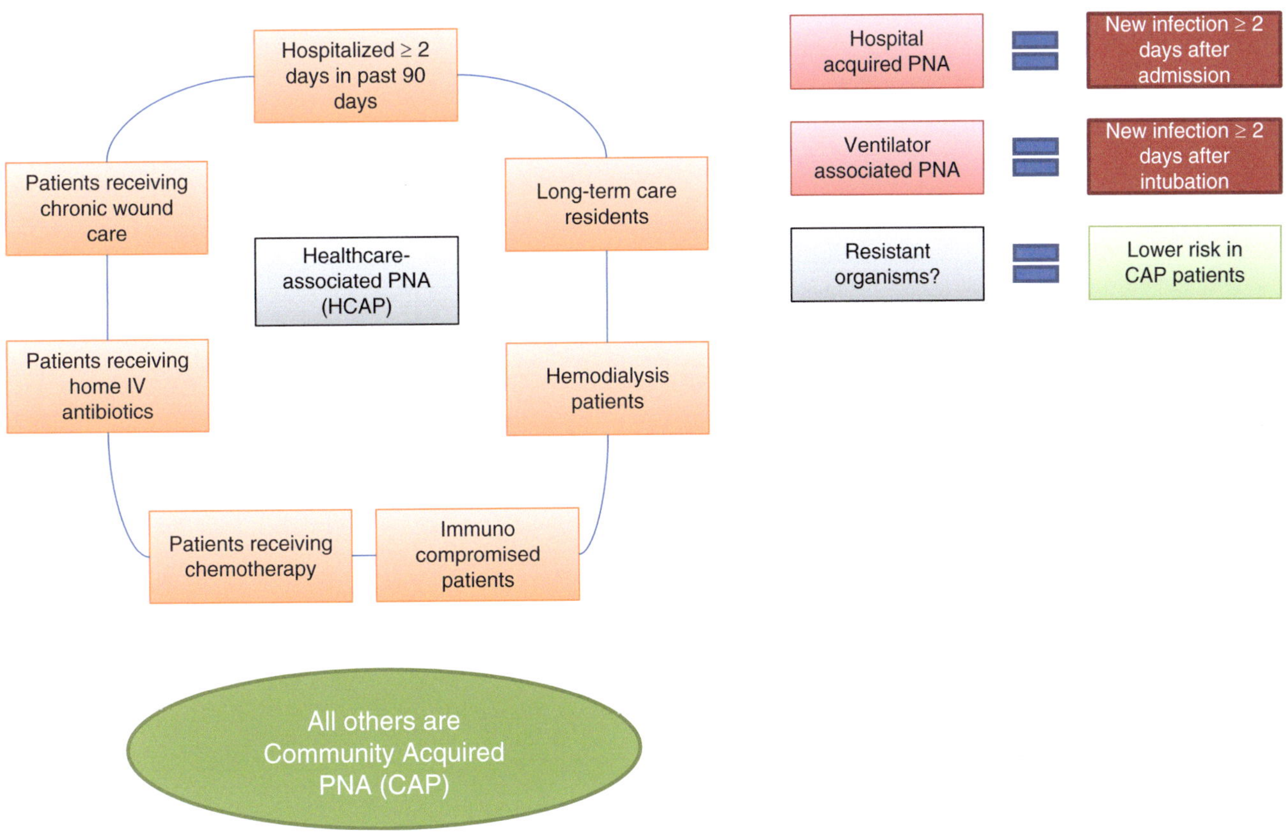

Pneumonia Pathophysiology

Pneumonia Pathophysiology = Pathogens inhaled or aspirated into respiratory tract → Overwhelm the lung's typically robust defense mechanisms

Diminished host defenses = Impaired cough/gag + Impaired mucociliary transport + Chronic underlying disease OR Immune disease

Impaired cough/gag = AMS + Seizure + CVA

Impaired mucociliary transport = Smoking + COPD + Pre-existing viral infection

Chronic underlying disease = Alcoholism + AIDS + Cystic fibrosis + Hepatic failure + Cancer + ESRD

Hematogenous seeding = *Pseudomonas* + *S. aureus* → Otherwise uncommon

Atypical agents? = Less intense inflammatory response = More indolent course, mild symptoms

Pneumonia Treatment

Patient Type	Organisms	Treatment
Outpatient Previously healthy No Abx within 3 months	*S. pneumoniae* *H. influenza* *Mycoplasma pneumonia* *Chlamydophila pneumoniae*	Macrolide (preferred) *or* Doxycycline
<u>Comorbidities</u> Chronic heart, lung, liver, renal disease, DM, Alcoholism, Malignancies, Immune disease	Same as above	Respiratory fluoroquinolone *or* β-lactam + Macrolide
Inpatients Non-ICU	Same as above + *Legionella* species Aspiration	Respiratory fluoroquinolone *or* β-lactam + Macrolide
Inpatients ICU	*S. pneumoniae* *Staph aureus* *Legionella* species Gram (-) bacilli *H. influenza*	β-lactam + <u>either</u> Azithromycin or Respiratory fluoroquinolone (substitute Aztreonam for the β-lactam if penicillin allergy)

Special Considerations

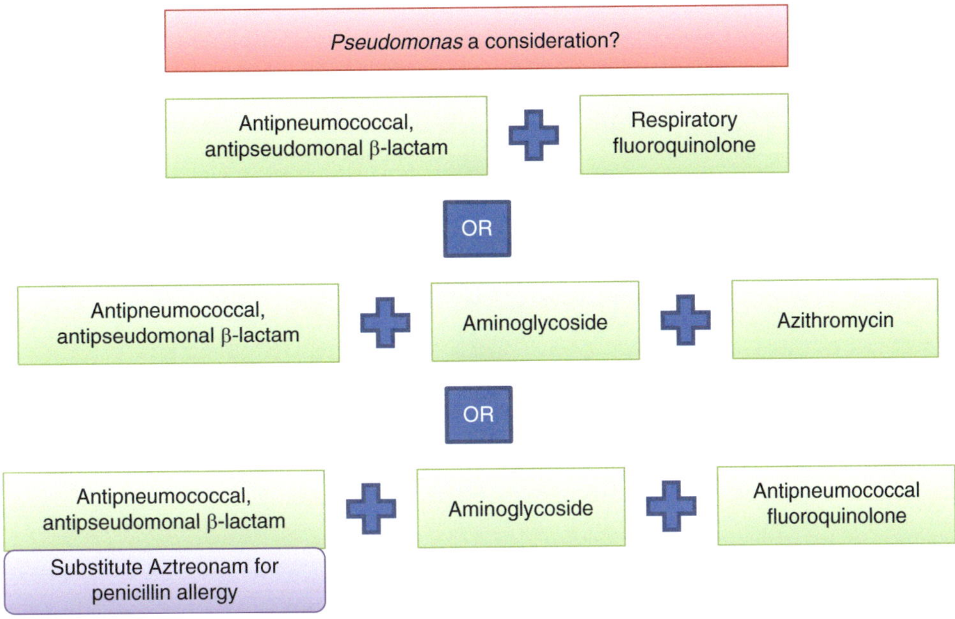

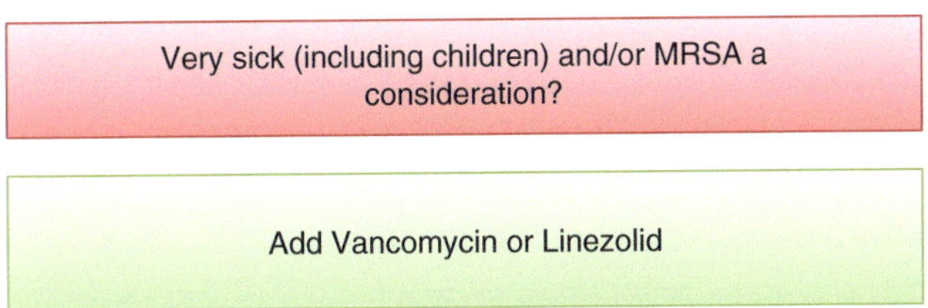

Pediatric Pneumonia Tidbits and Treatment

PEDIATRICS

Patient Age	Organisms	Treatment
Birth – 3 weeks	Group B Streptococcus *E. coli* *Listeria monocytogenese*	Ampicillin + Gentamicin *or* Cefotaxime
3 weeks – 3 months	*S. pneumoniae* *Bordetella pertussis* *Chlamydia trachomatis* *H. influenza* Viral – RSV/Parainfluenza	Erythromycin *or* Cefotaxime
4 months – 4 years	Viruses *S. pneumoniae* *Mycoplasma pneumoniae*	Same as above
5 years – 15 years	*Mycoplasma pneumonia* *S. pneumoniae*	Erythromycin (Doxycyline if >8) *or* Cefotaxime

Group B streptococcus = Most common cause → Acquired in utero → Results in a rapid fulminant disease process

Symptoms & Signs –> 3 weeks – 3 months – Typical bacteria

- Decreased feeding
- Fever
- Tachypnea
- Nasal flaring
- Intercostal retractions
- Grunting
- Severe irritability

Symptoms & Signs –> Chlamydia

- Afebrile
- Staccato cough: Short sudden bursts of cough
- Tachypnea
- Conjunctivitis
- Lung hyperinflation

Streptococcus pneumoniae

Streptococcus pneumoniae = Most commonly identified pathogen (Even in HIV) + Encapsulated Gram (+) diplococci

Symptoms & Signs

- Sudden onset chills
- Fever
- Chest pain
- Hemoptysis
- May have more indolent presentation

CXR = Lobar infiltrate ± Parapneumonic effusion

High risk groups = Elderly (especially unvaccinated) + Children <2 + HIV + Sickle cell disease

Functional or surgical asplenia OR Immunosuppressed patients = Potential rapid development of septic shock

Haemophilus influenzae

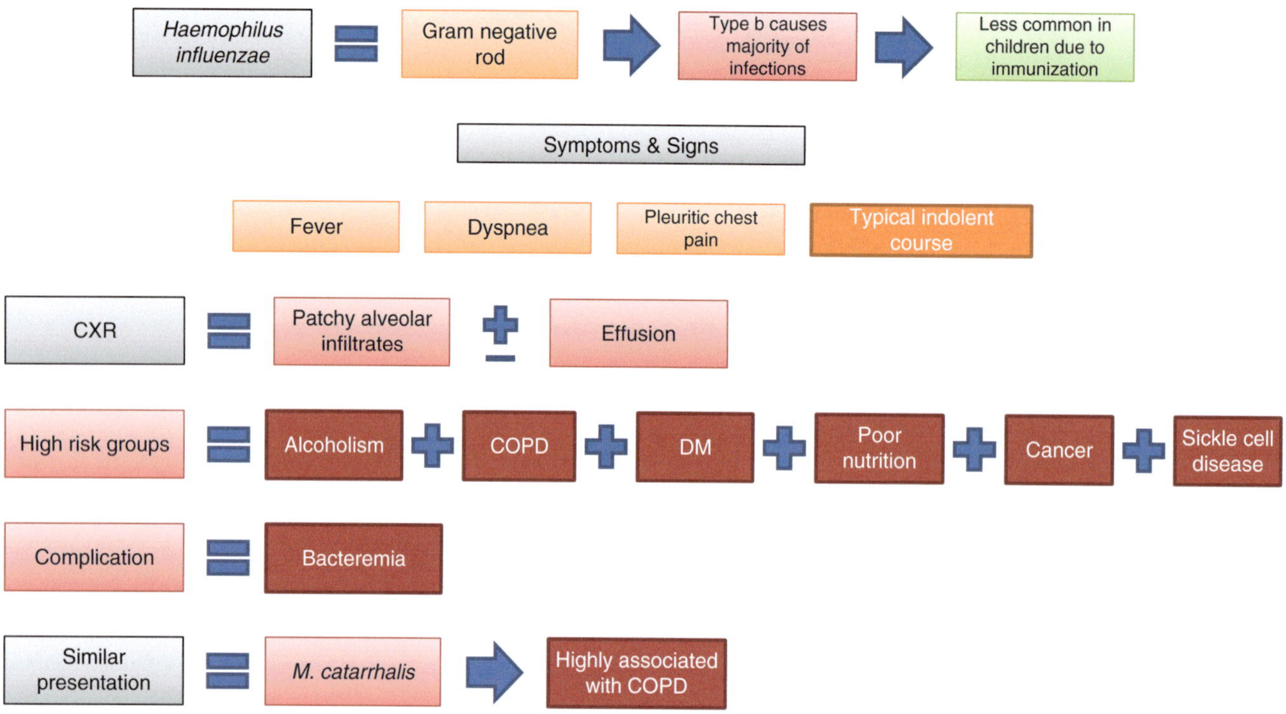

Pseudomonas aeruginosa

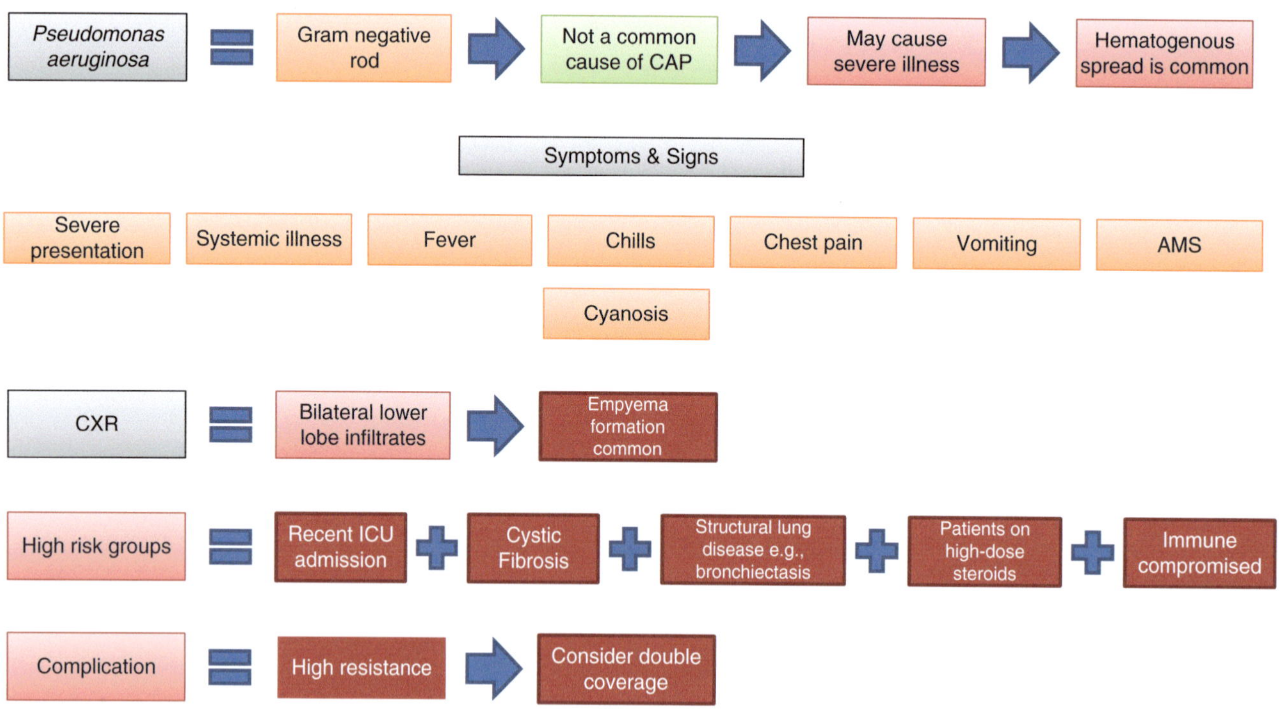

Klebsiella pneumoniae

Klebsiella pneumoniae = Gram negative rod

Symptoms & Signs

Abrupt onset fever; Rigors; Chest pain; "Currant jelly sputum" → Necrotizing infection → High incidence of empyema formation

CXR = Lobar pattern ± Abscess formation

High risk groups = Alcoholics + Elderly + History of aspiration + Pre-existing lung disease

Complication = Necrotizing infection → Due to → Common producer of extended spectrum β-lactamases = Antibiotic resistance

Staphylococcus aureus

Staphylococcus aureus = Large gram (+) cocci in pairs and clusters → Uncommon cause of CAP → Incidence increasing (MRSA) → High association with concomitant influenza infection

Symptoms & Signs

Insidious onset of Sx; Often necrotizing; Fever; Chills; Chest pain

CXR = Patchy, multilobar infiltrate common → But… → Cavitation + Pneumatocele formation = Necrotizing infection

High risk groups = IVDA + Nursing home residents + Aspiration + Immuno-suppression + Laryngeal CA history

Complication = Hematogenous spread

Chlamydophila and *Mycoplasma pneumoniae*

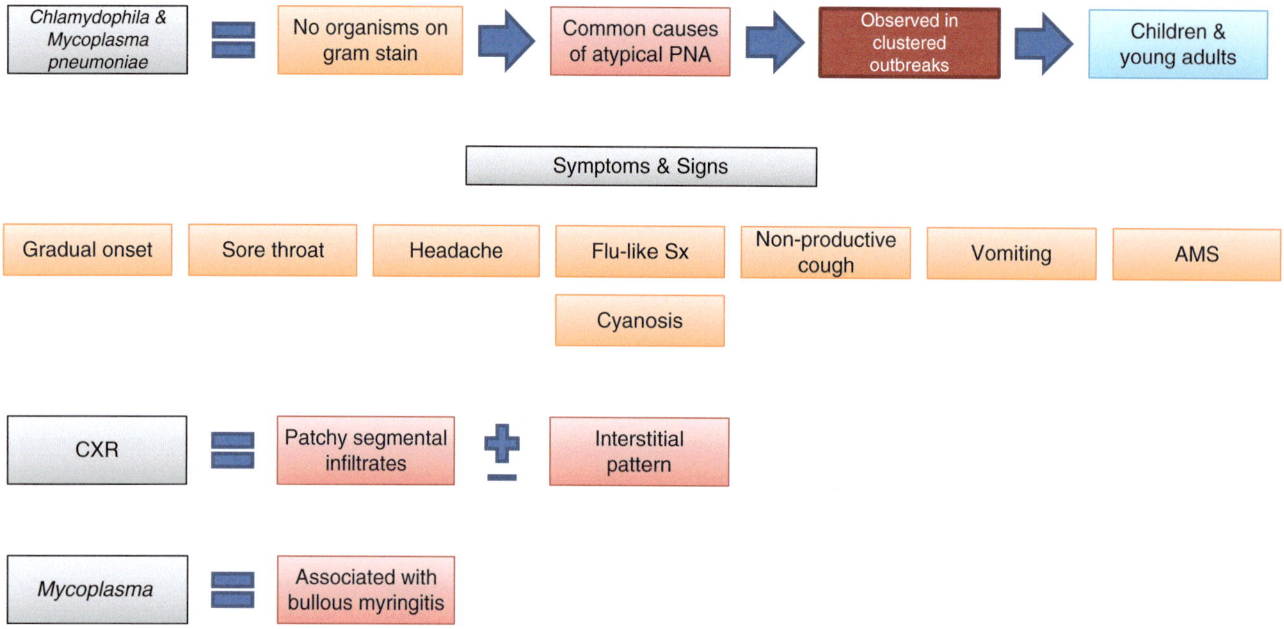

Legionella

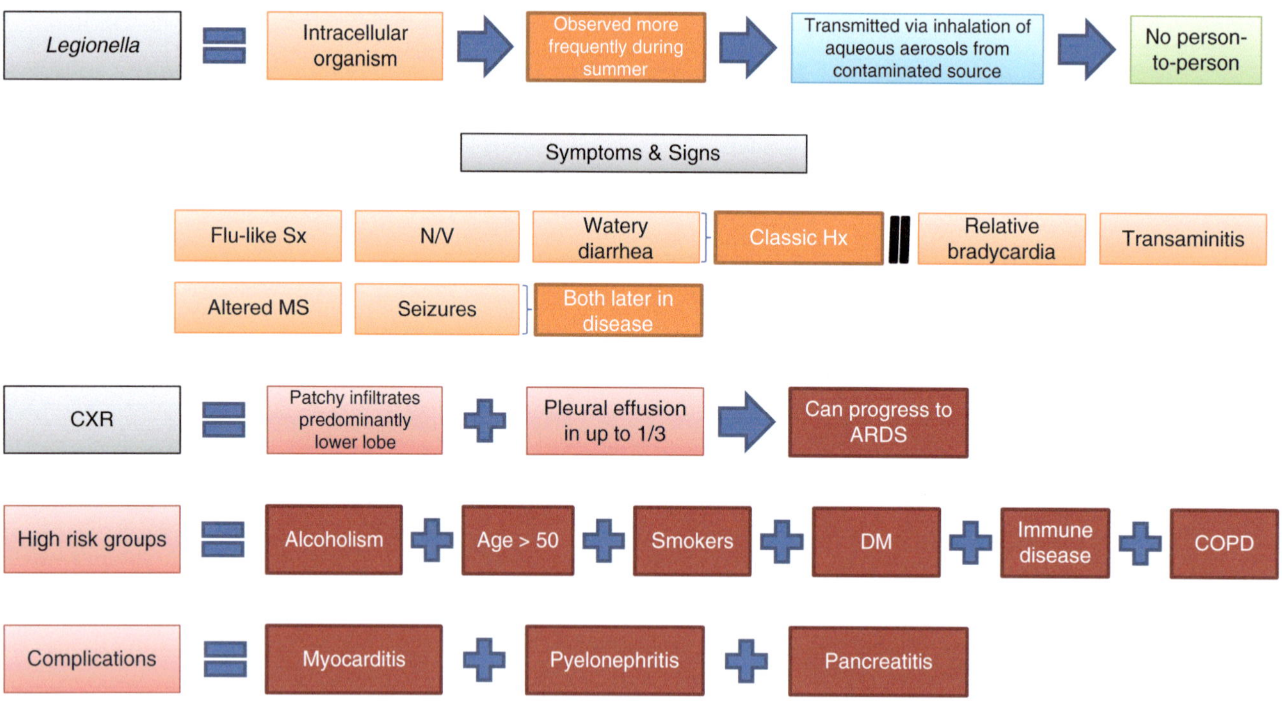

Zoonotic PNA Etiologies

Tularemia = Direct contact with → Infected animal tissue (Rabbits) OR Post-tick bite → Onset of high fever, cough, adenopathy, ulcerated skin lesion

Q-fever = *Coxiella burnetti* → Inhalation of dust contaminated with tissue or excretions → From infected sheep, cattle, goats

Psittacosis = *Chlamydia psittaci* → Inhalation of droplets/dust from infected birds

Hantavirus = Inhalation of aerosols from rodent feces or urine (Most cases in the Southwest) → Bilateral pulmonary infiltrates + Respiratory distress → Often fatal, No treatment (Cardiac failure; Renal failure)

Pneumocystis jirovecii (Formerly PCP)

Pneumocystis jirovecii = Fungal etiology → But… But does not respond to antifungals! → Predisposed patients → HIV; Immune compromise

Symptoms & Signs

General malaise | Dyspnea | Fever | Non-productive cough | Weight loss | Night sweats

CXR Appearance varies! = Bilateral interstitial pattern with hilar prominence (Most common) + Pleural effusion + Lobar consolidation + Hilar adenopathy + Risk of PTX

Diagnosis = Serum lactate dehydrogenase often elevated → Confirm with silver staining or immunofluorescence assay of sputum or bronchial washings

Treatment = High dose TMP-SMX first line → 21 days if HIV + OR Pentamidine can be used if allergic to TMP-SMX → But… High incidence of severe side effects

Steroids? = Indicated if HIV(+) + ABG on room air with PaO_2 <70 mm Hg OR Alveolar-arterial gradient > 35 mm Hg → Initiate early!

Pathogens in HIV

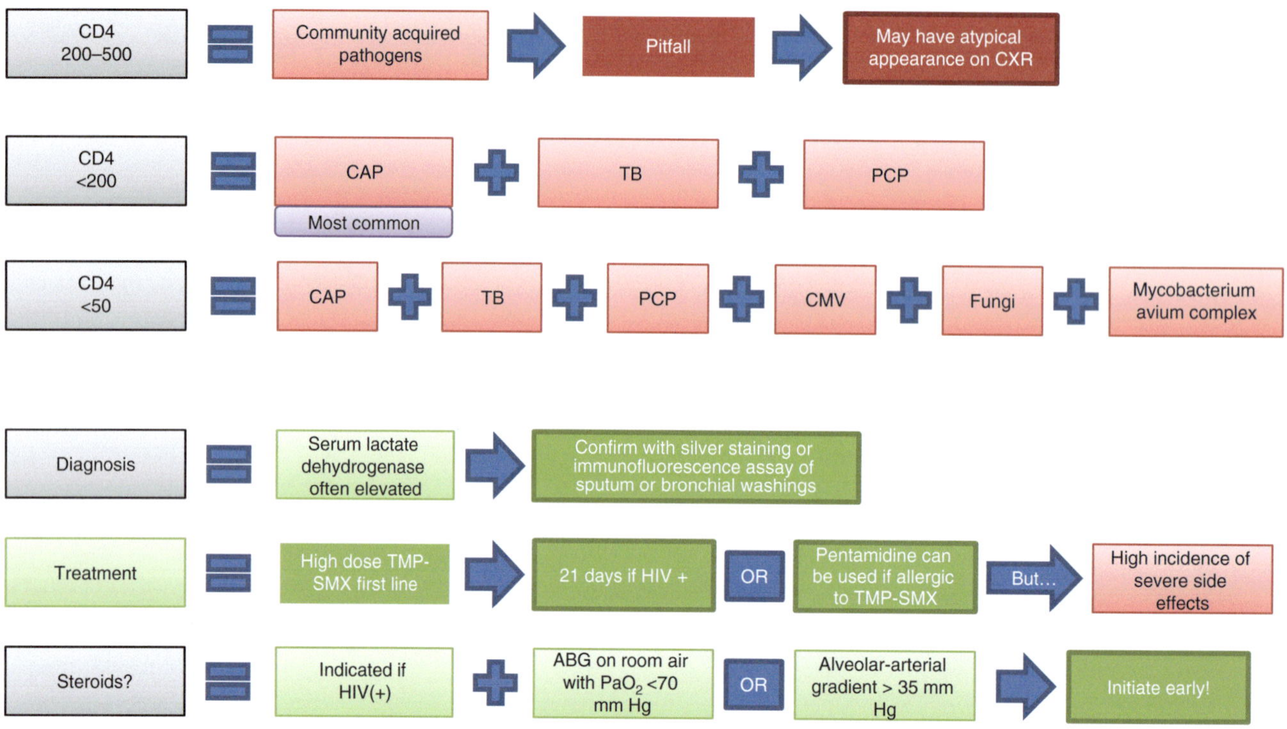

Fungal PNA Etiologies

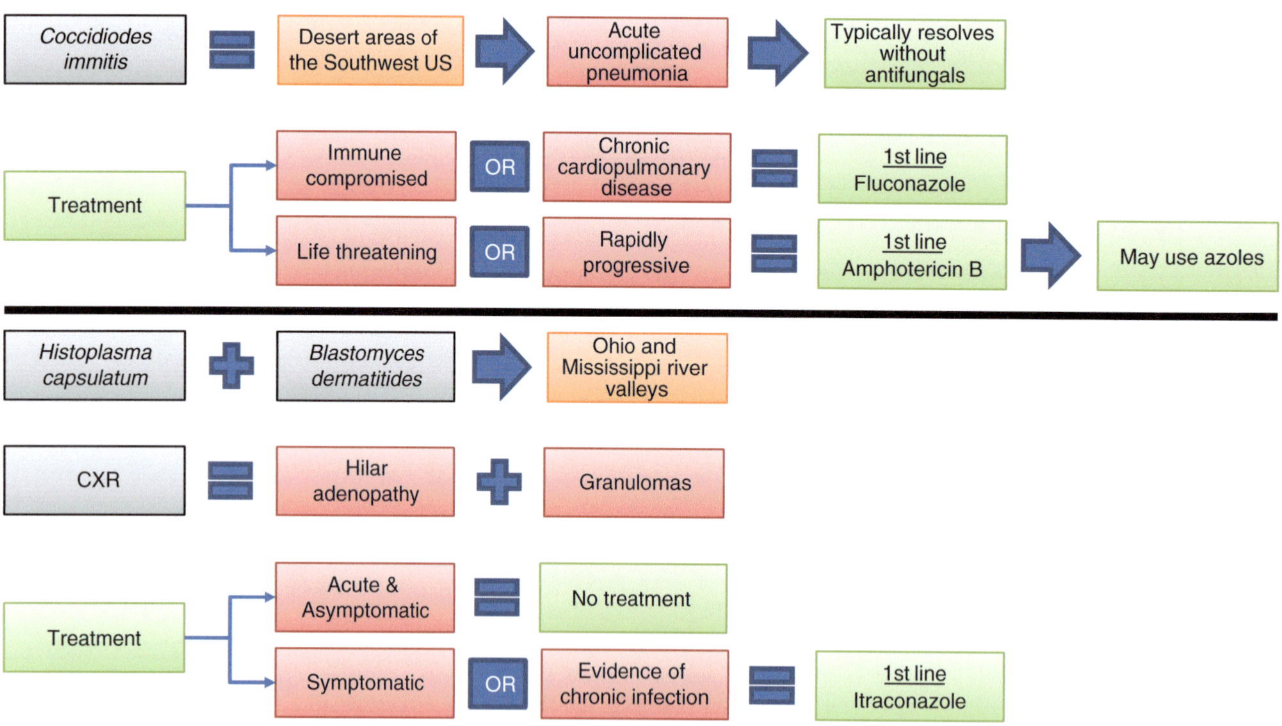

Disposition

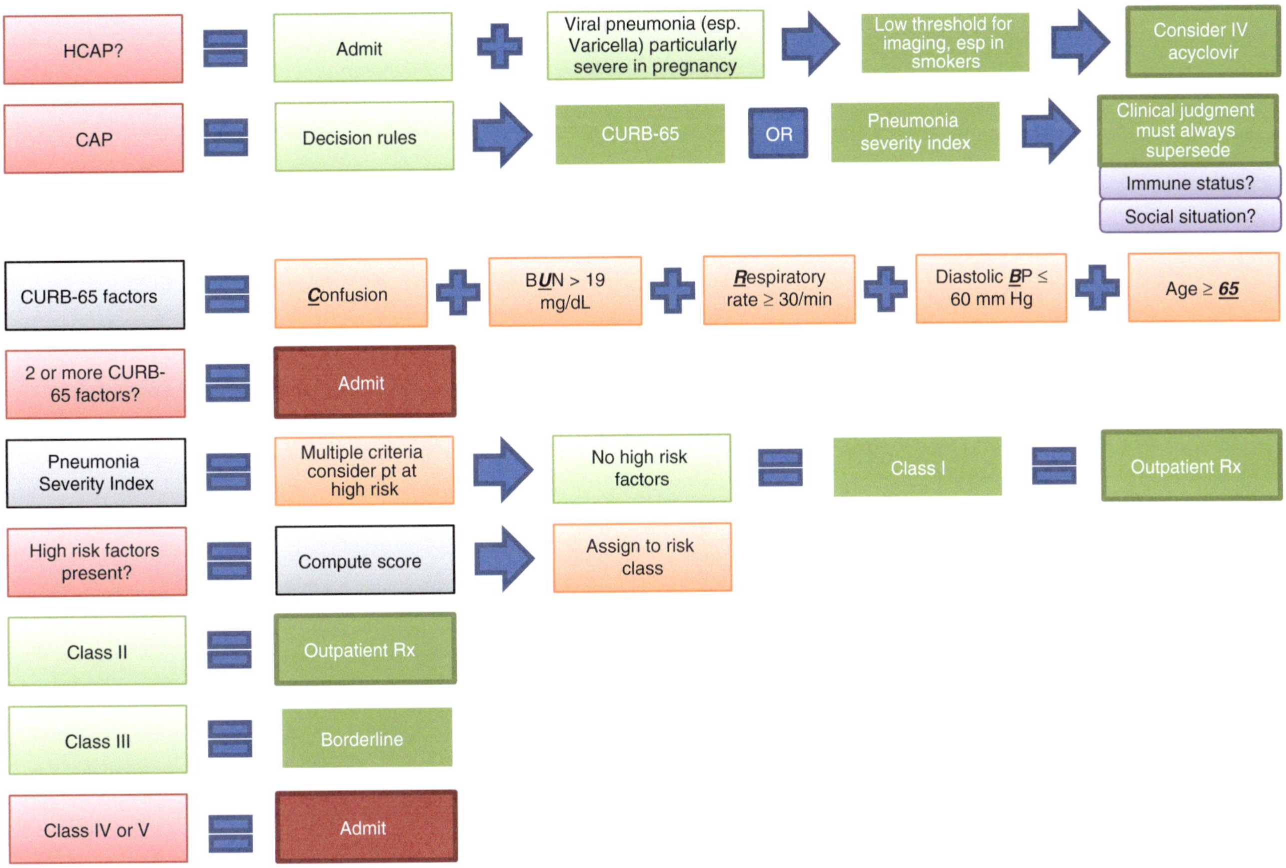

Cultures and Treatment

- Cultures = If indicated, obtain prior to antibiotics
- Blood cultures? = ICU Pts + Abscess formation + Pleural effusions + Immune compromise (Asplenia, Liver Dz) + Alcoholics
- Sputum culture? = Similar indications to blood cultures → Limited utility due to inability to produce adequate sample
- Urine Legionella antigen? = ICU patients + Alcoholics + Other high risk populations

---

- Outpatient CAP? = Respiratory fluoroquinolone OR Azithromycin/Clarithromycin OR Doxycycline → Least preferred - less *S. pneumoniae* activity
- Inpatient CAP? = Respiratory fluoroquinolone OR Ceftriaxone + Azithromycin
- ICU CAP? = 3rd or 4th gen. cephalosporin, i.e., ceftriaxone + Vancomycin + Respiratory fluoroquinolone
- HCAP? = Antipseudomonal cephalosporin, β-lactam, or carbapenem + Respiratory fluoroquinolone (or Aminoglycoside) + Vancomycin (or Linezolid)

Pneumonia in Special Patients

- Pregnancy = Bacterial pneumonia similar to that in non-pregnant + Viral pneumonia (esp. Varicella) particularly severe in pregnancy → Low threshold for imaging, especially in smokers → Consider IV acyclovir

---

- Transplant patients = Heart, liver, lung at greatest risk
- Organisms within 3 months of transplant (Poor prognosis) = *K. pneumoniae* + *E. coli* + *S. aureus* + *Pseudomonas* + *Legionella* + Fungi
- Organisms within 6 months of transplant = CMV + *P. jirovecii* + Fungi → Especially *Aspergillus*
- Organisms > 6 months of transplant = Ordinary CAP pathogens → Better prognosis

Cystic Fibrosis

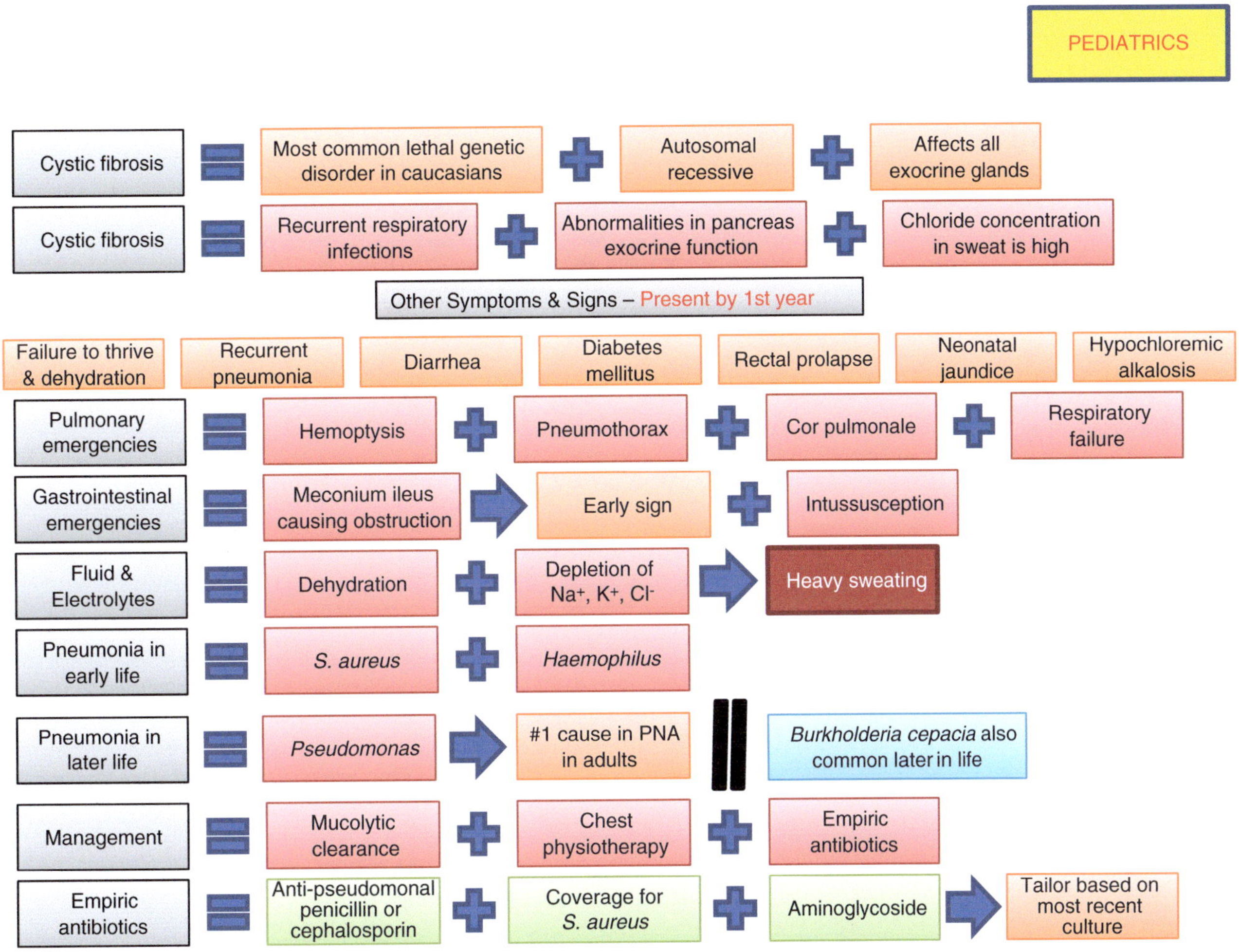

Aspiration

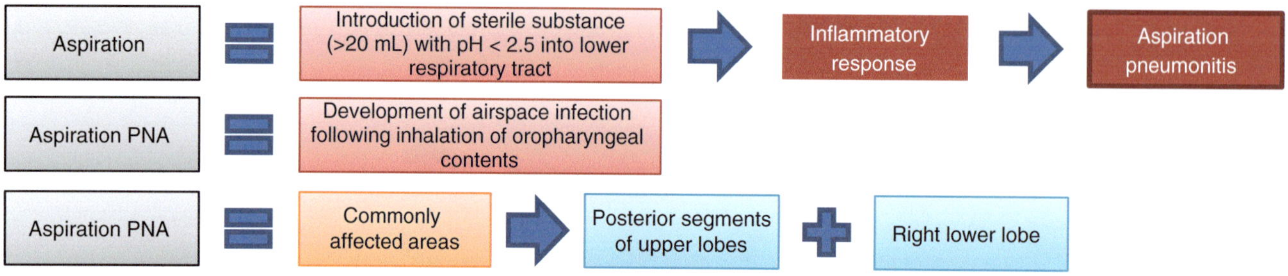
Aspiration
Introduction of sterile substance (>20 mL) with pH < 2.5 into lower respiratory tract
Inflammatory response
Aspiration pneumonitis
Aspiration PNA
Development of airspace infection following inhalation of oropharyngeal contents
Aspiration PNA
Commonly affected areas
Posterior segments of upper lobes
Right lower lobe

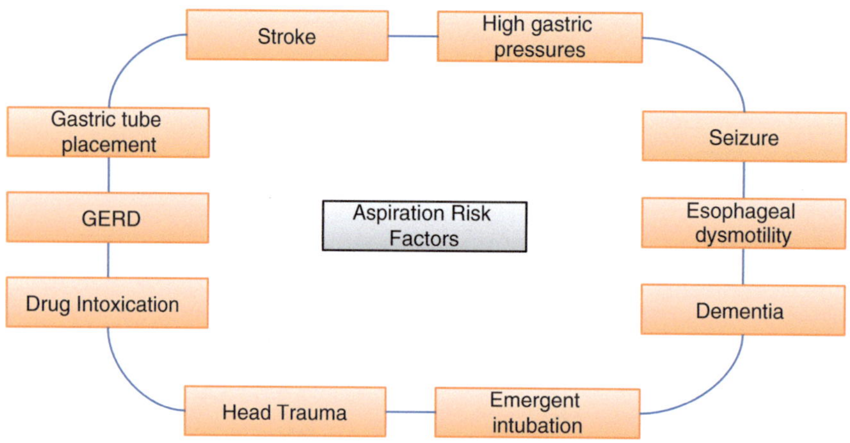
Aspiration Risk Factors
Stroke
High gastric pressures
Seizure
Esophageal dysmotility
Dementia
Emergent intubation
Head Trauma
Drug Intoxication
GERD
Gastric tube placement

Aspiration Management

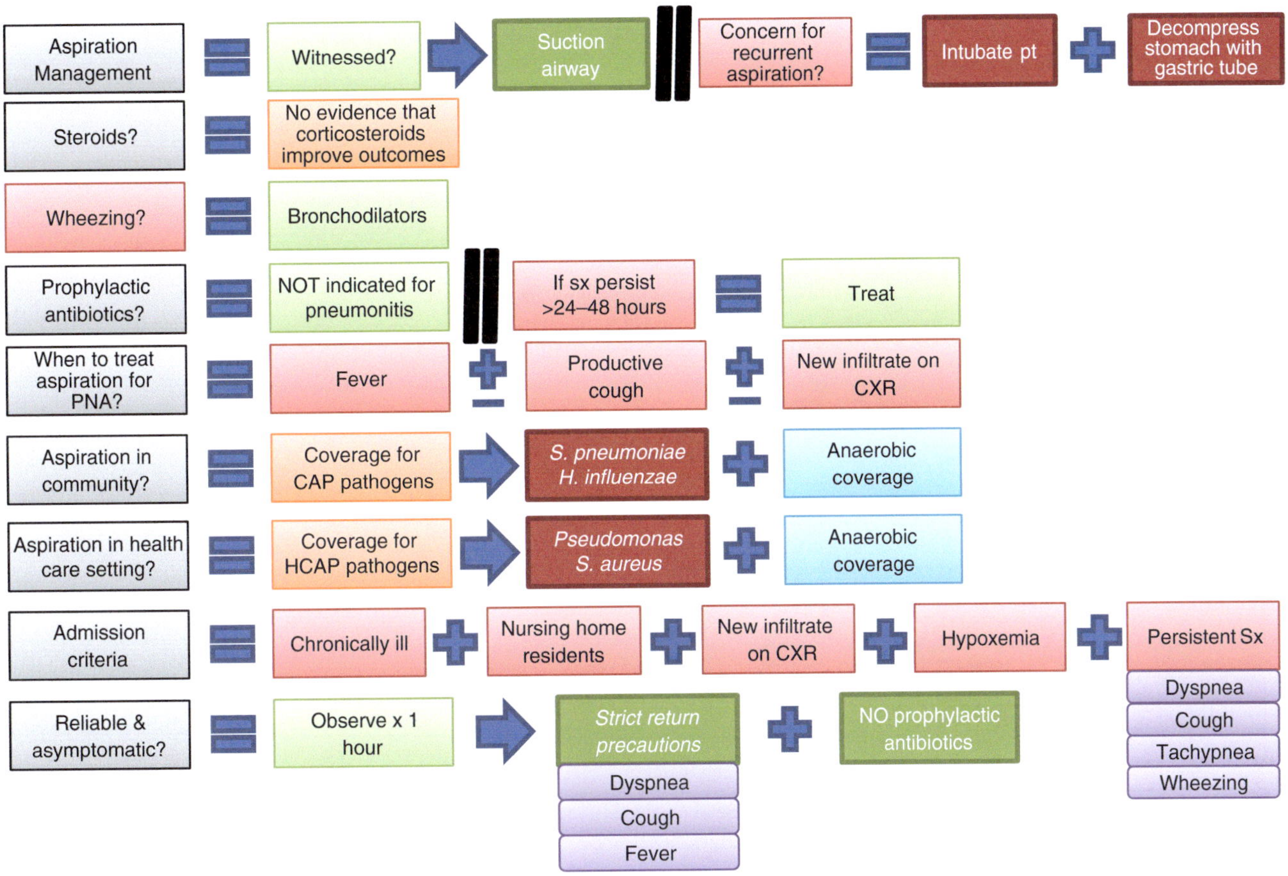

Tuberculosis

TB Tidbits

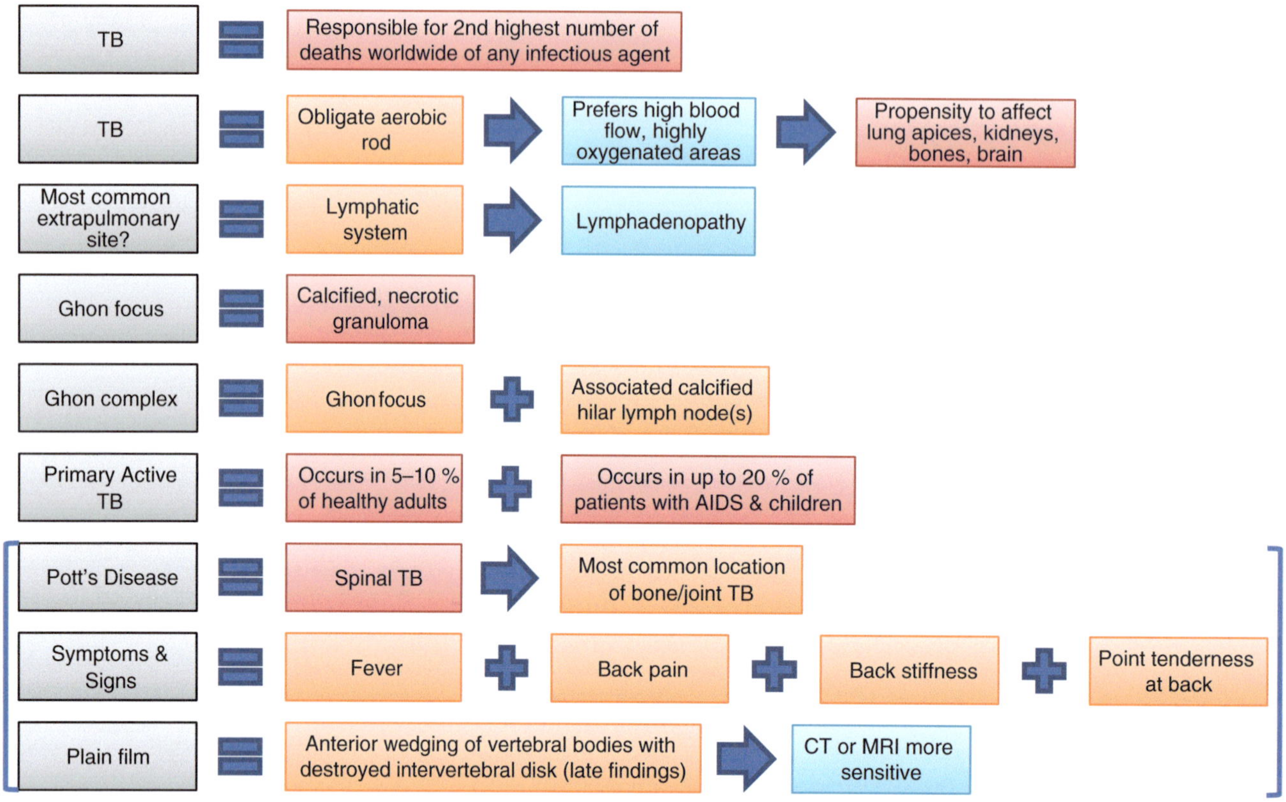

TB Pathophysiology

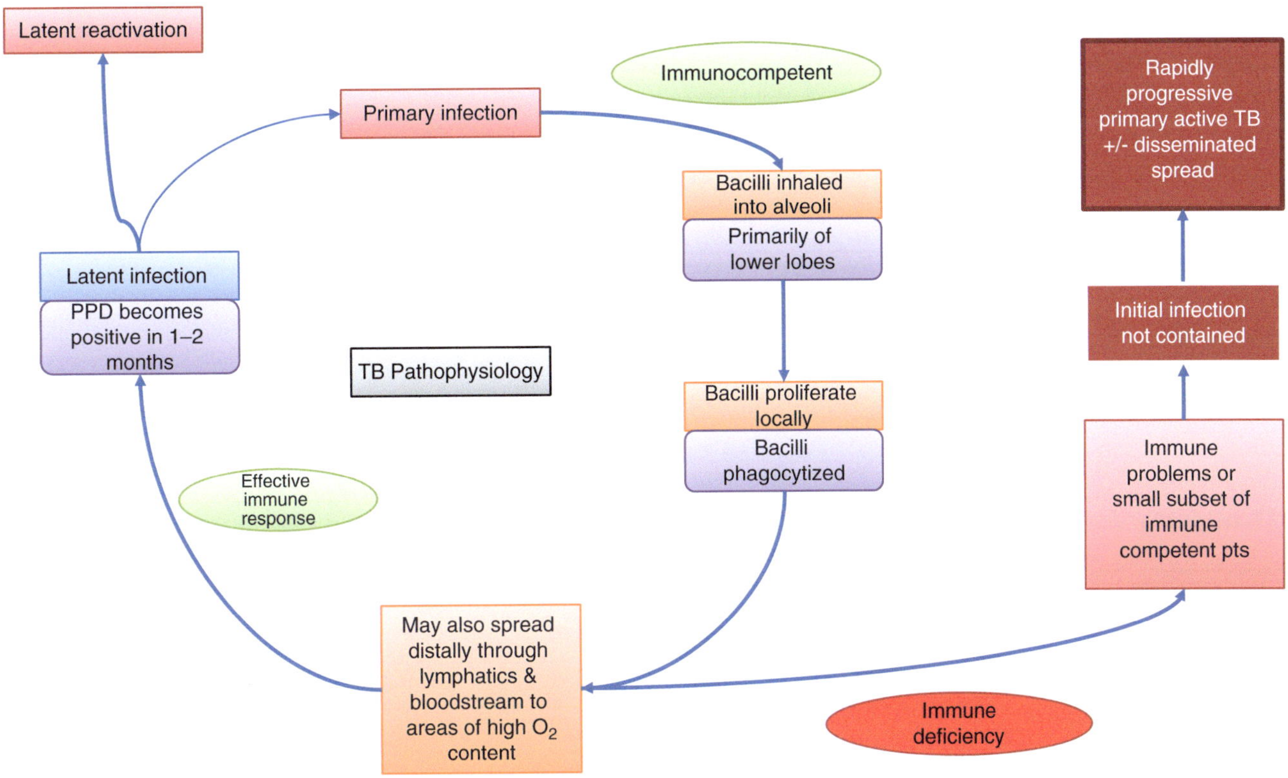

Reactivation TB

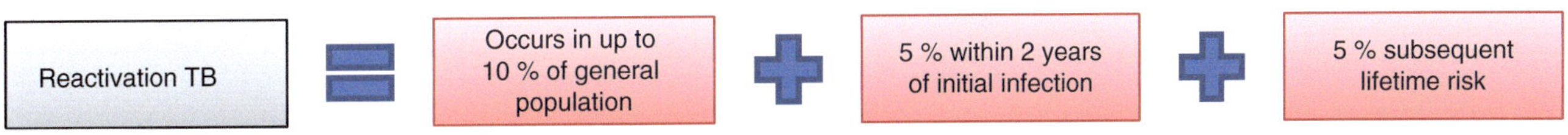

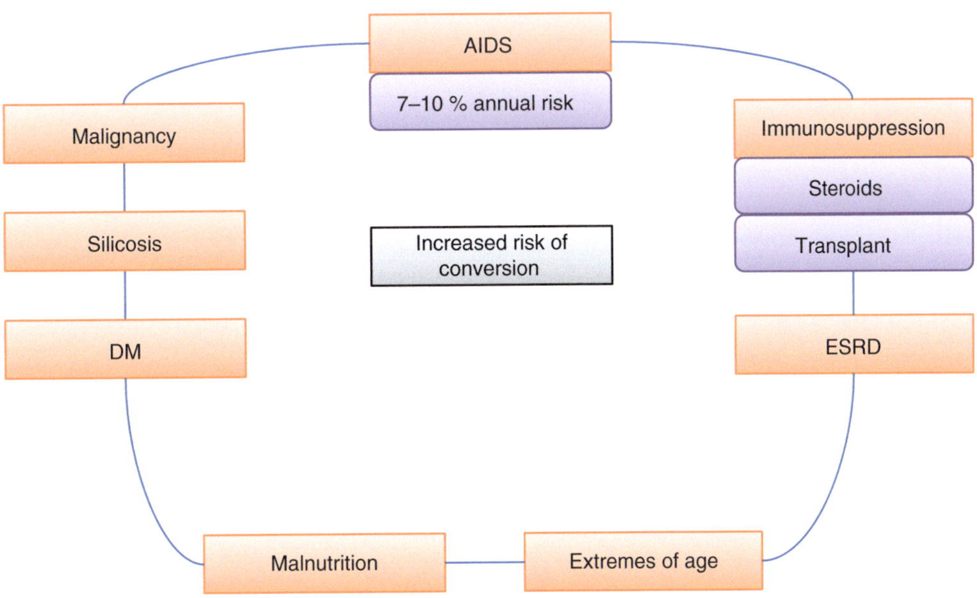

TB Presentation

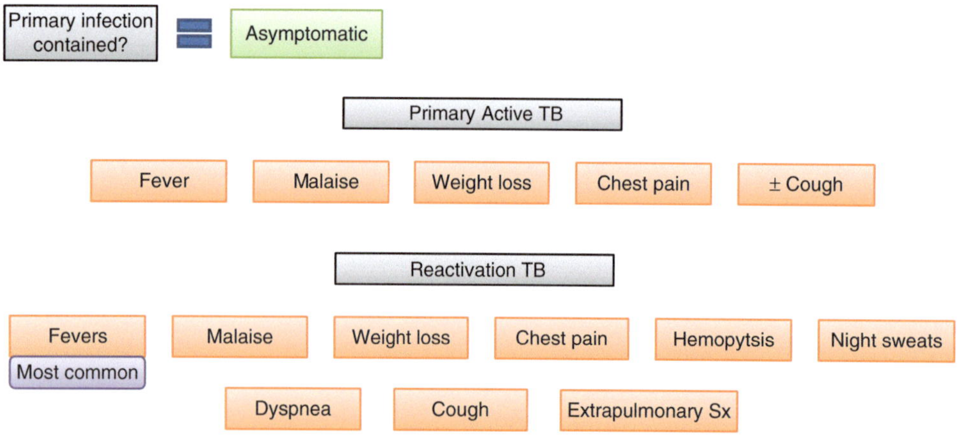

TB Initial Evaluation: PPD and CXR

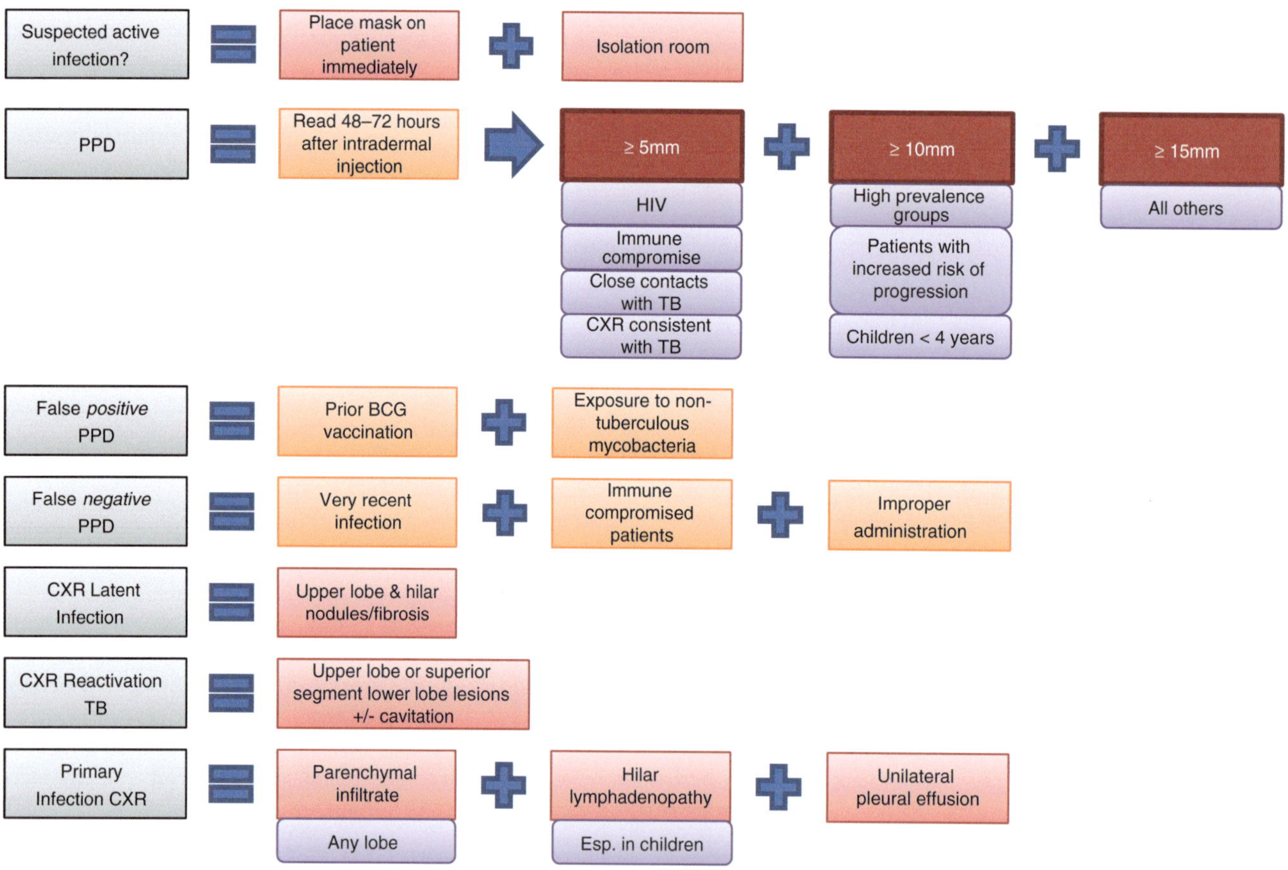

TB Diagnosis

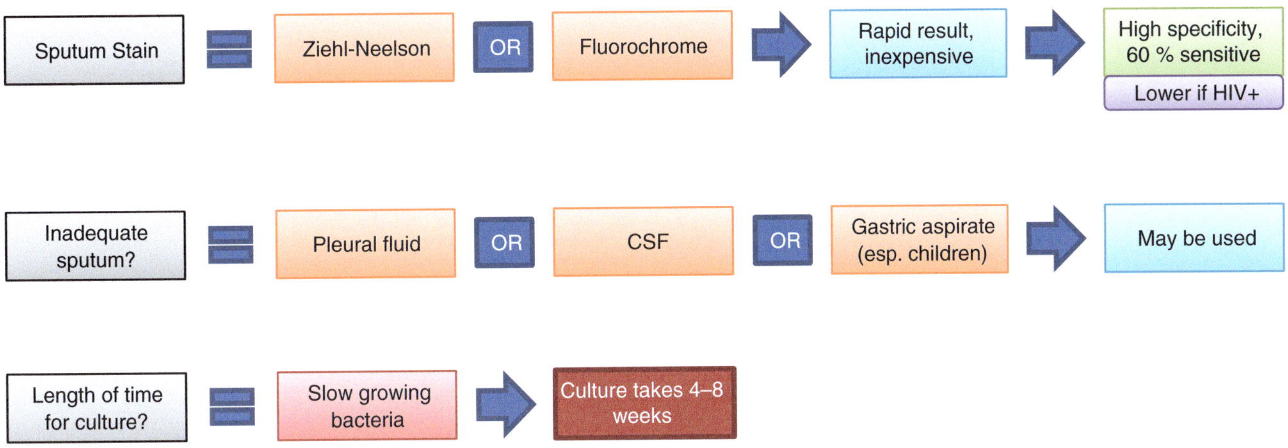

Tuberculosis Treatments and Side Effects

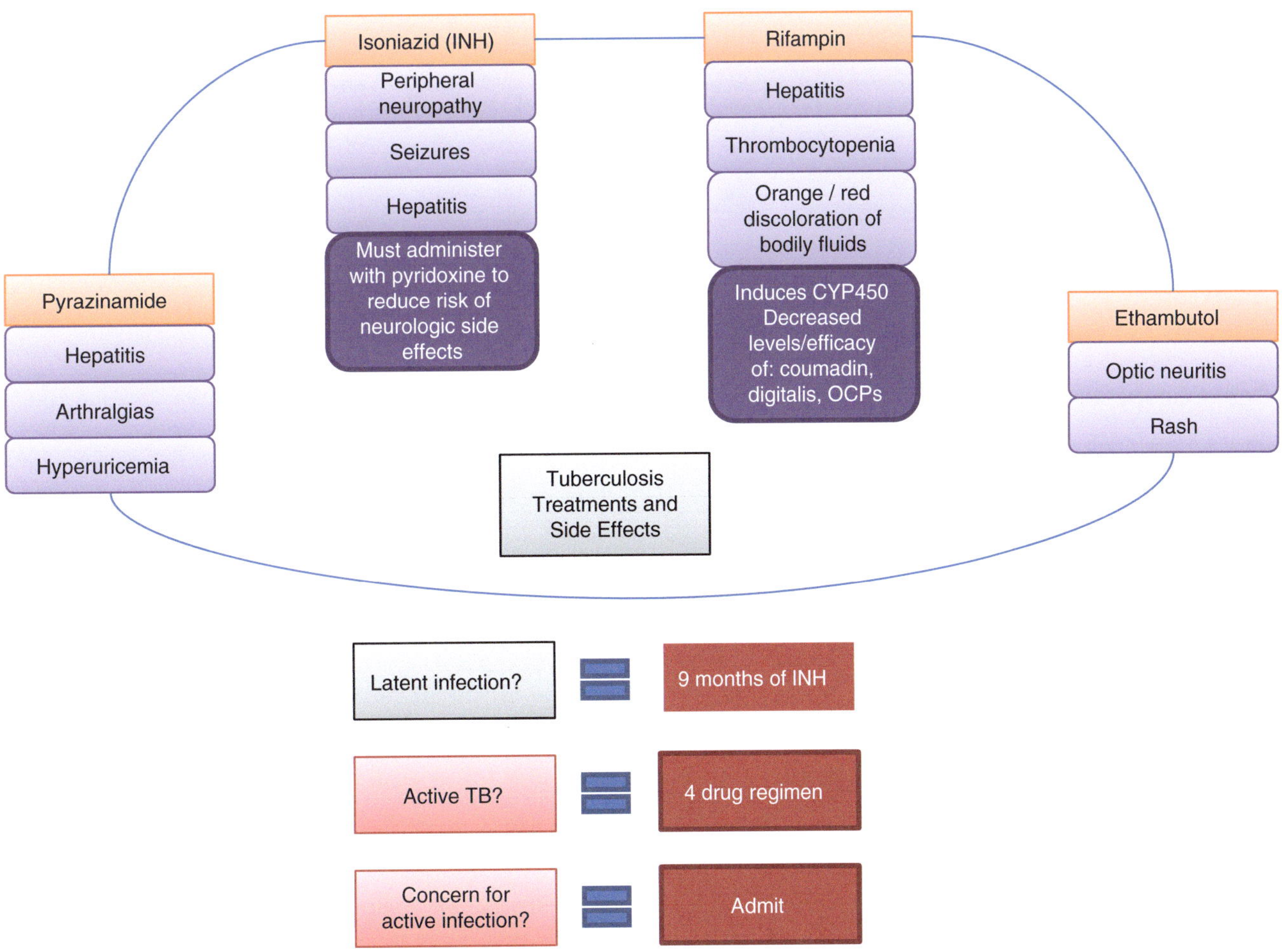

Lung Abscess

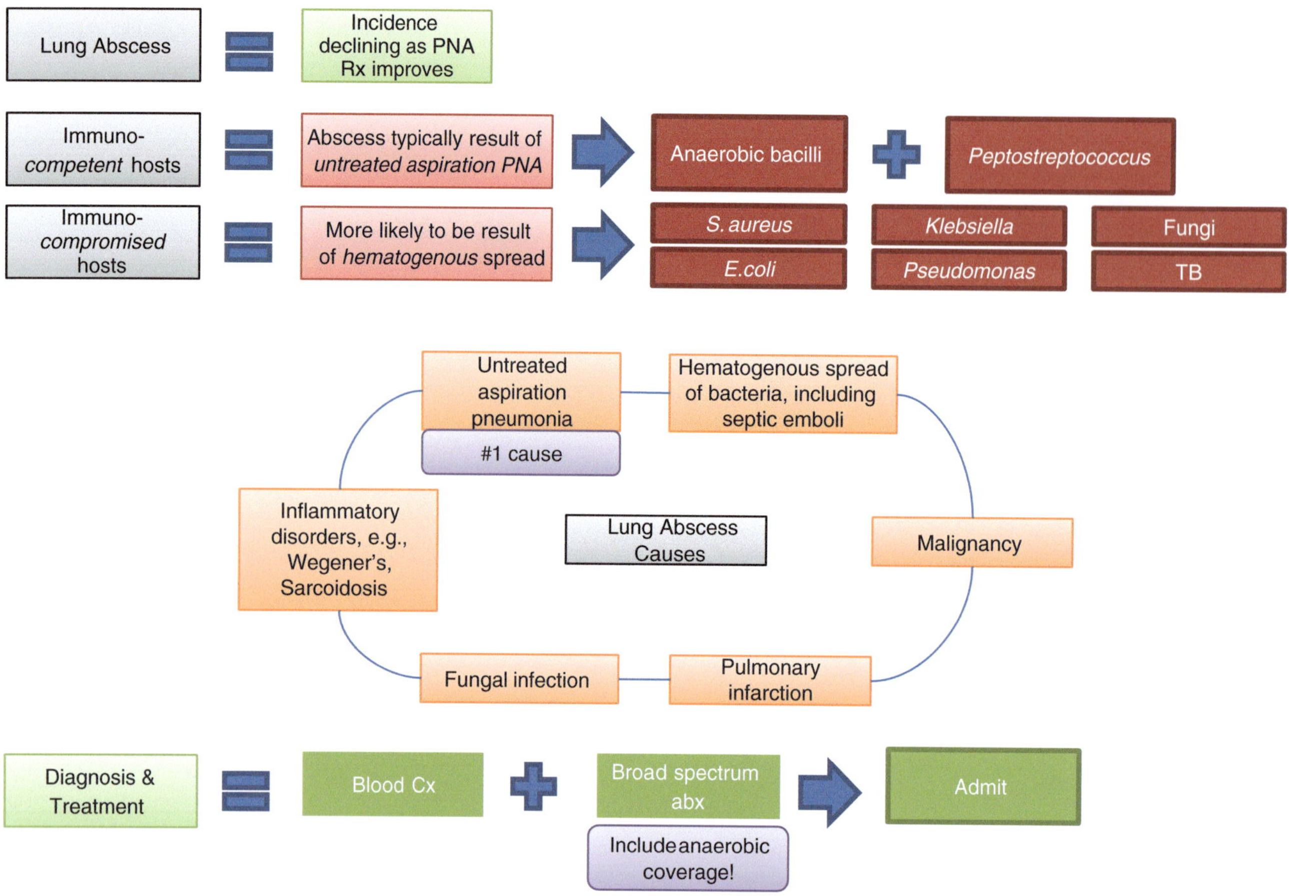

Acute Respiratory Distress Syndrome

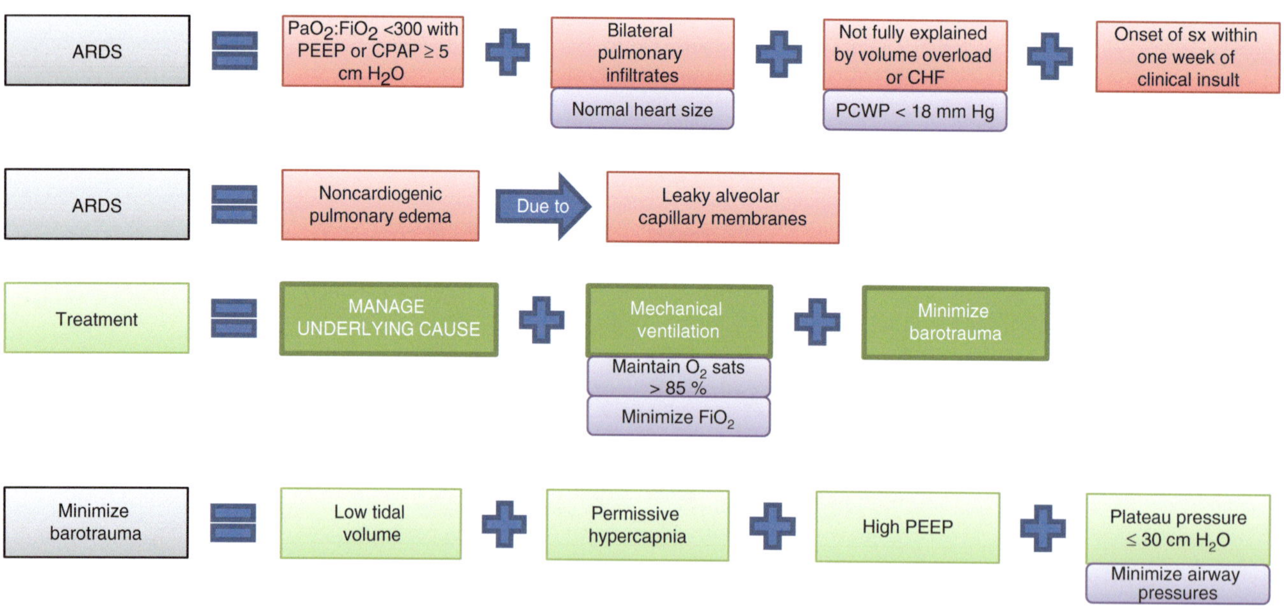

ARDS Causes

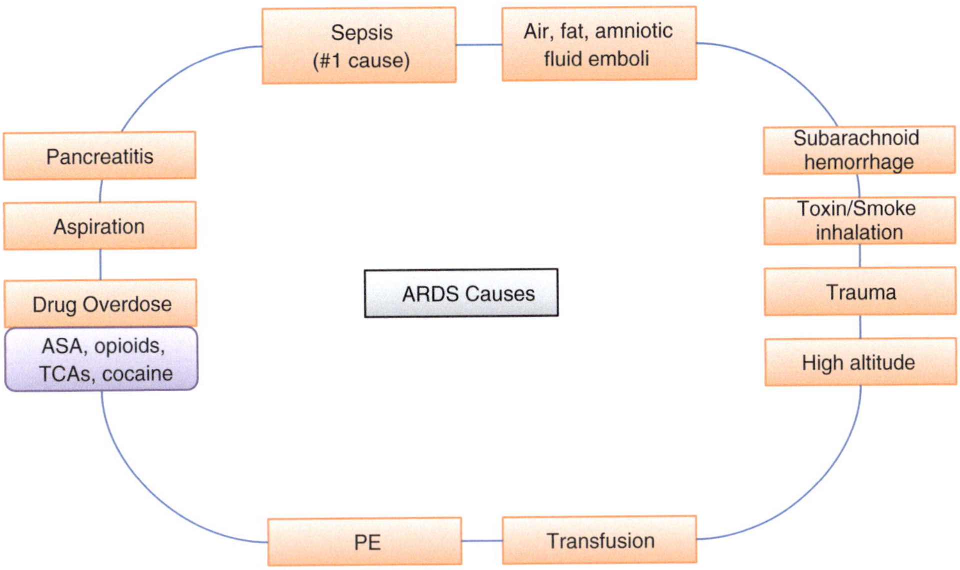

Pleural Effusions

Introduction

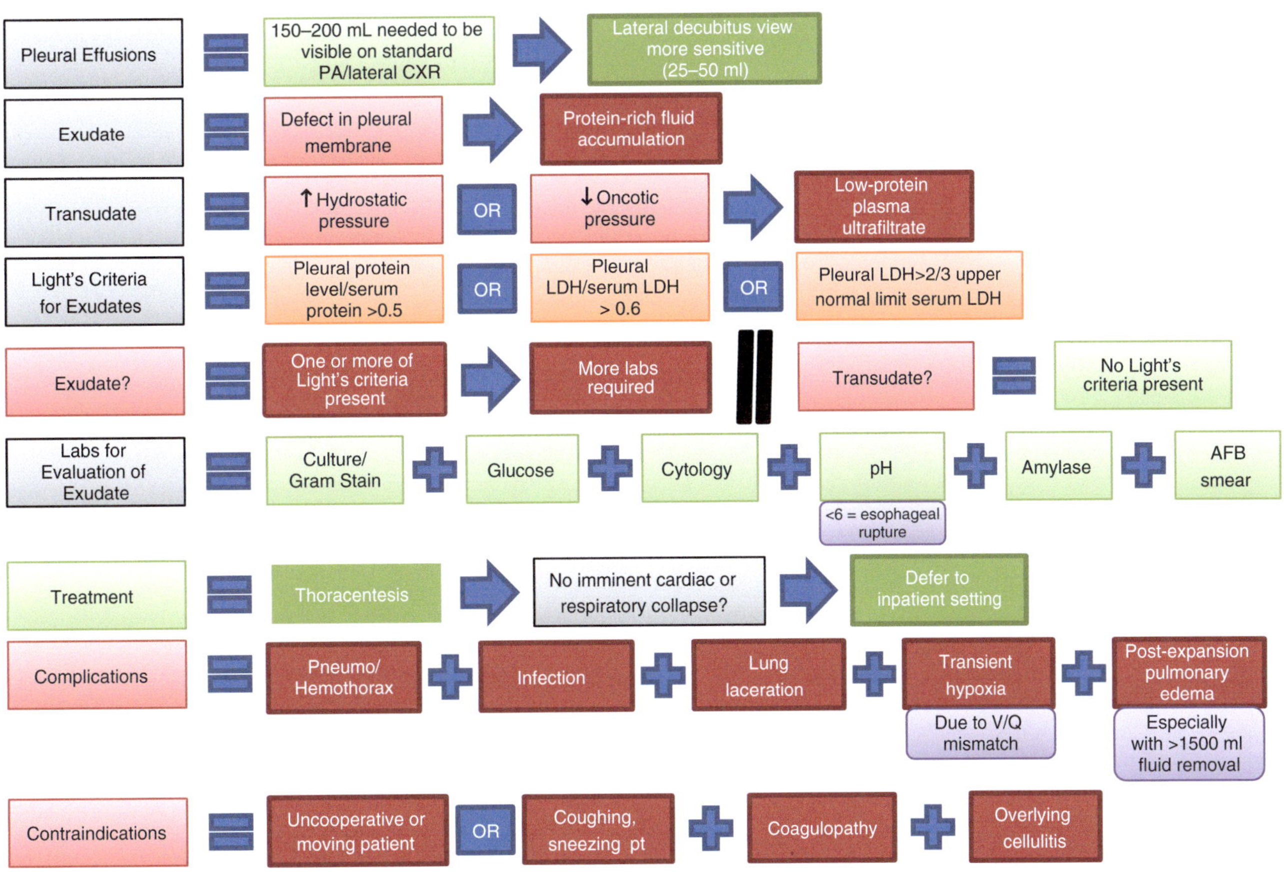

Transudates

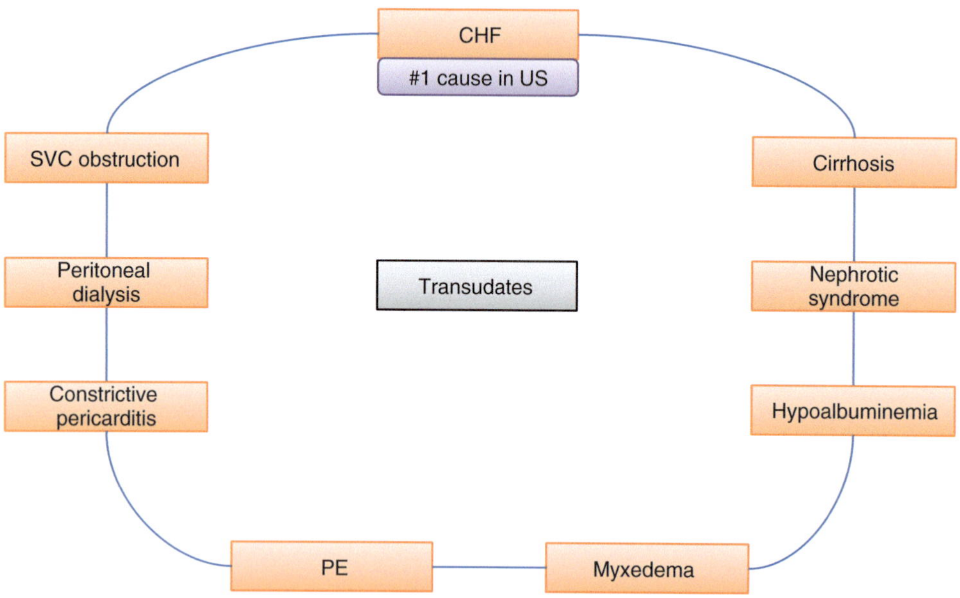

Exudates

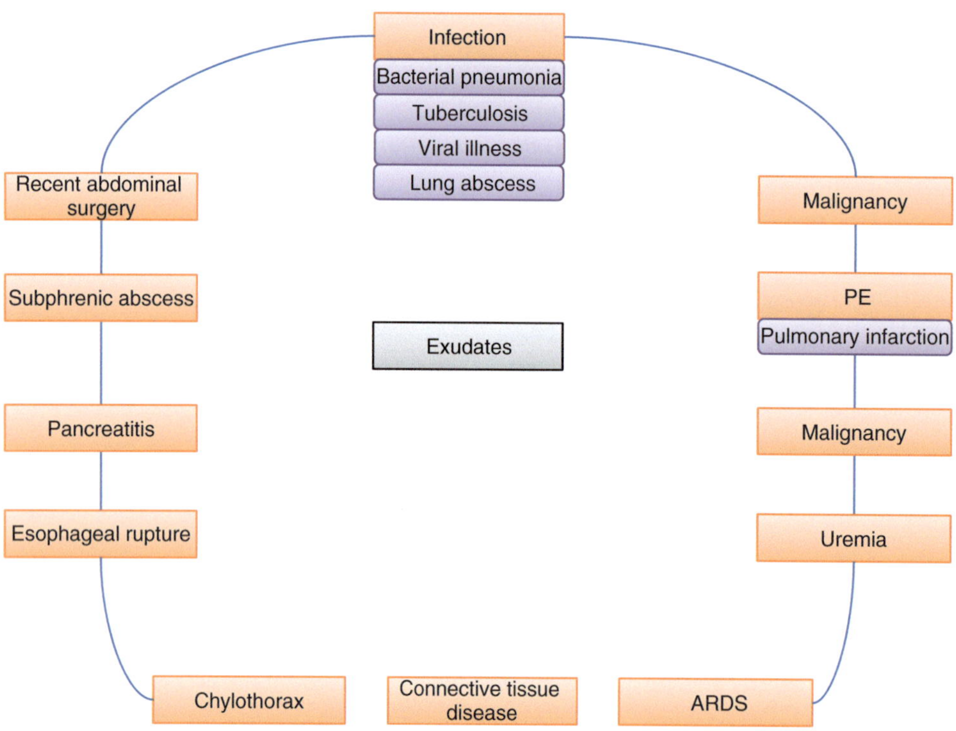

Empyema

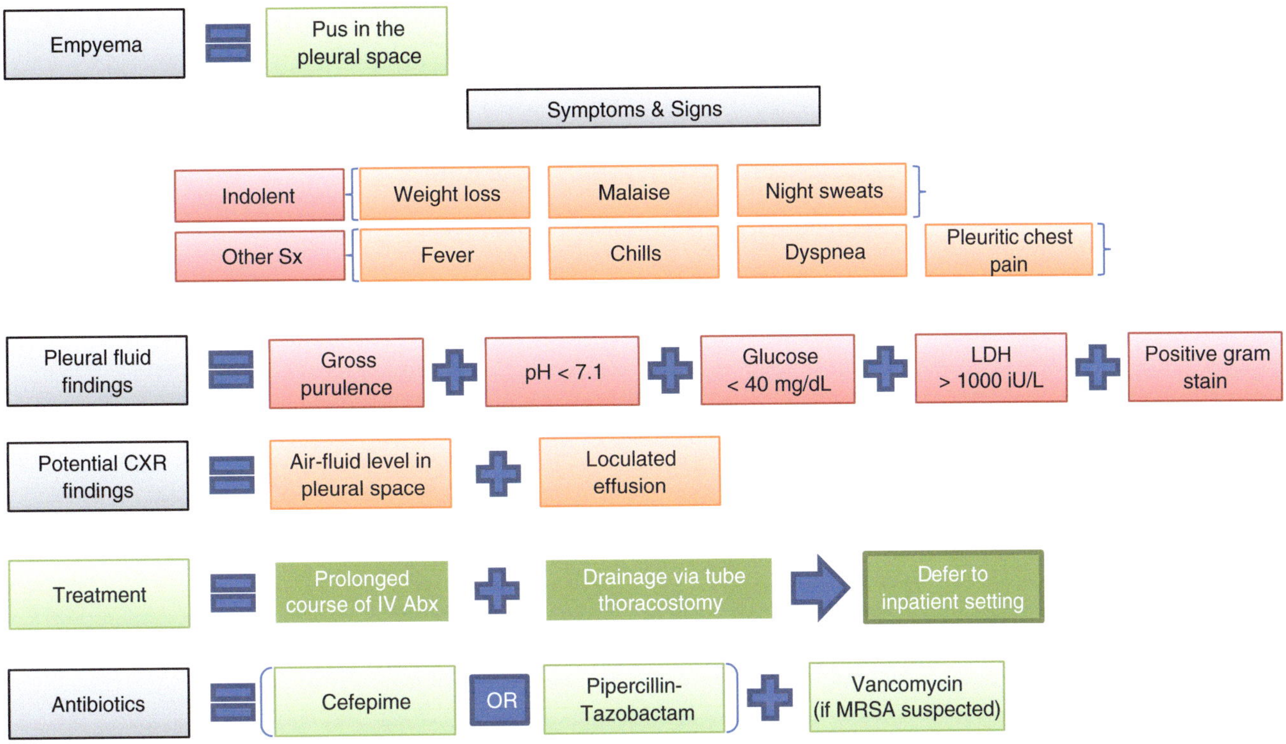

Causes of Empyema

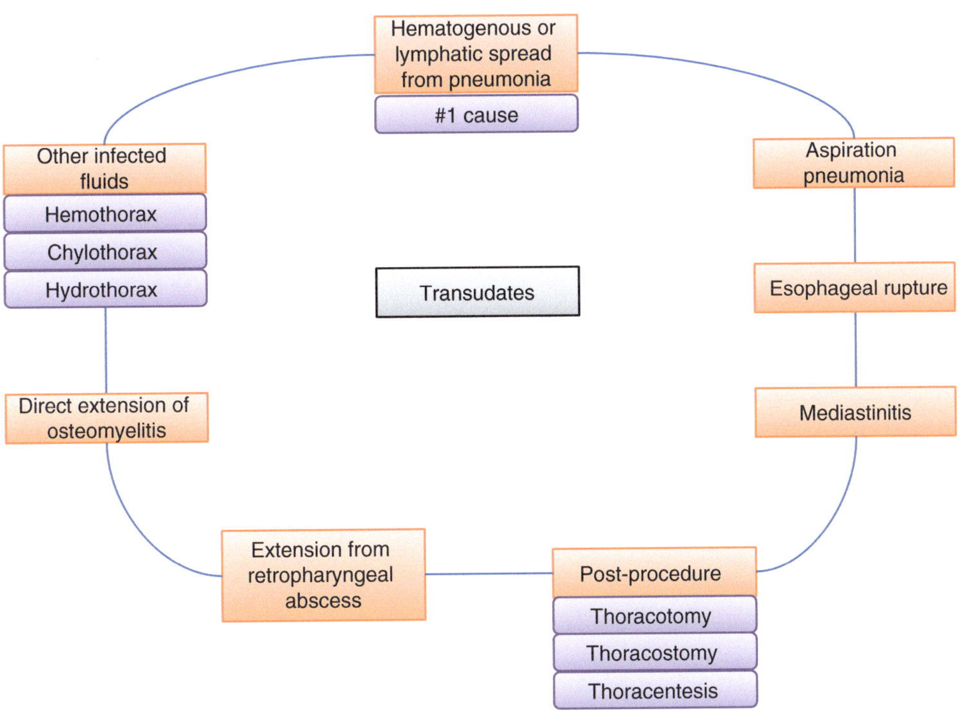

Mediastinitis

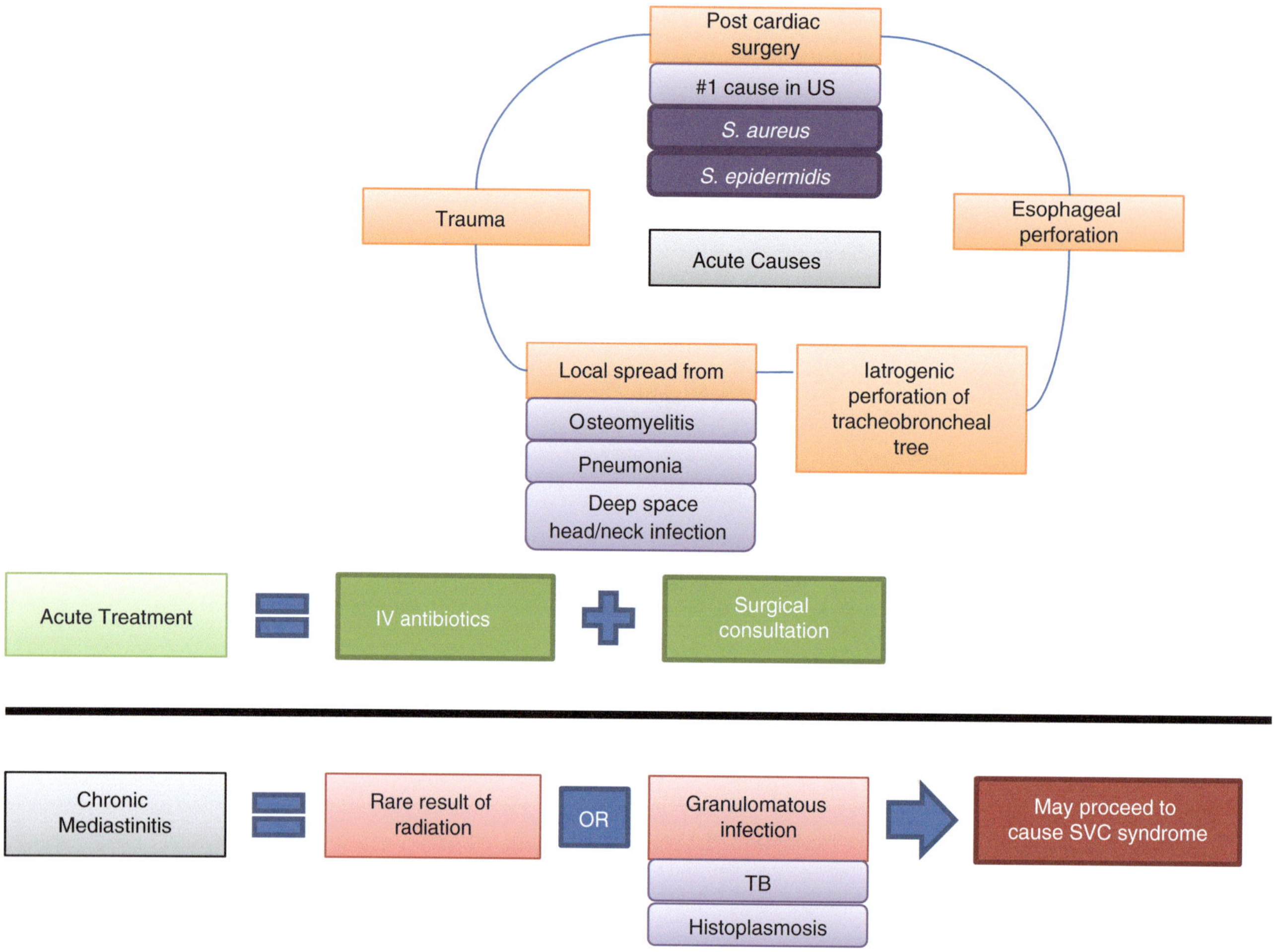

Hiccups

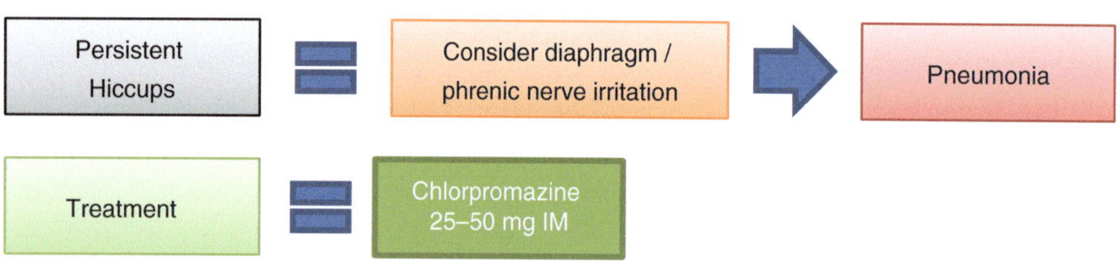

Pneumoconioses

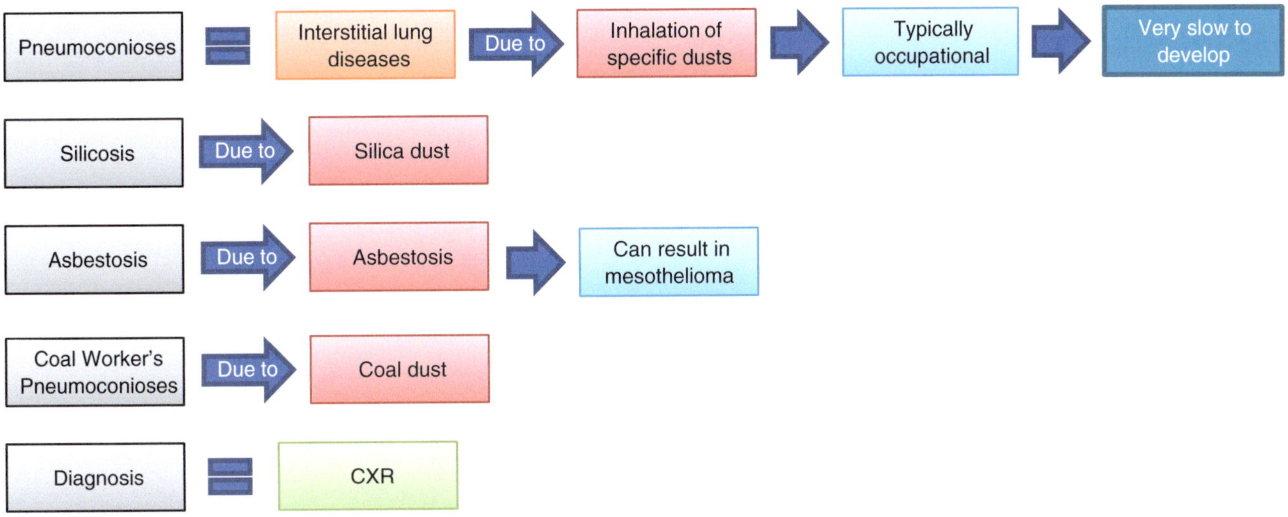

Sarcoid

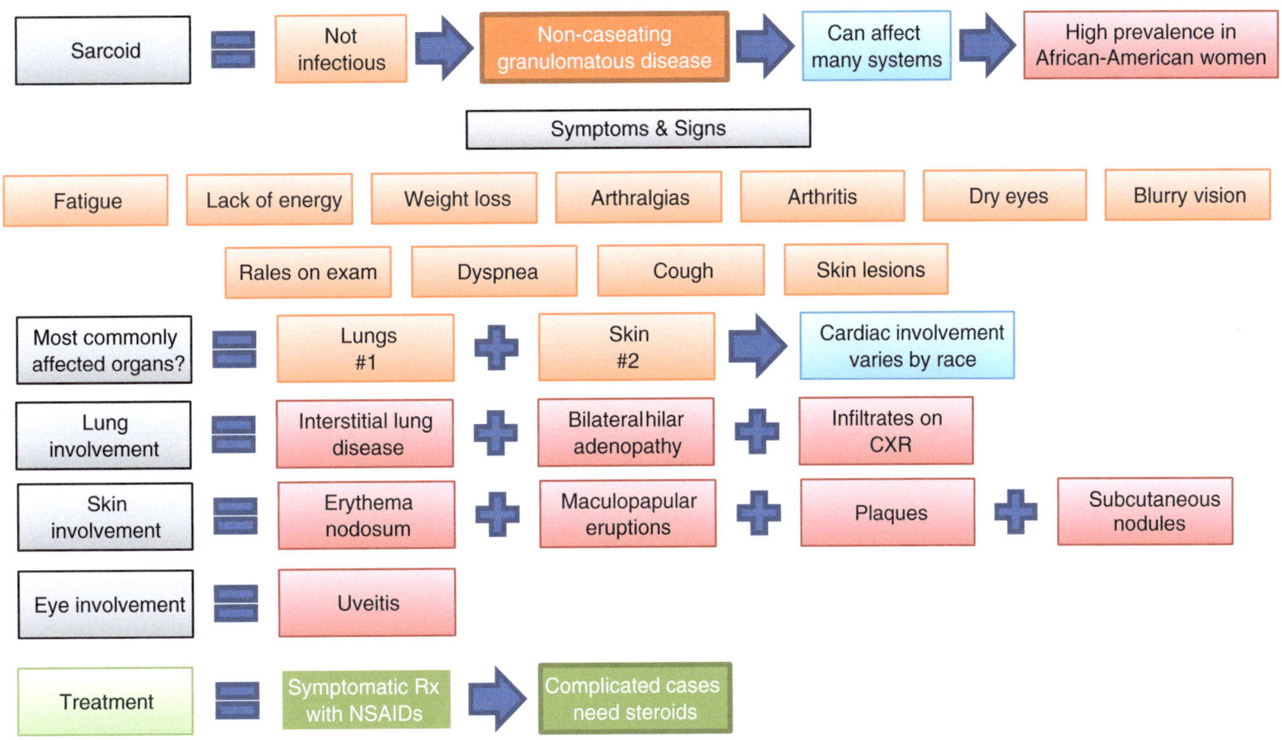

Superior Vena Cava (SVC) Syndrome

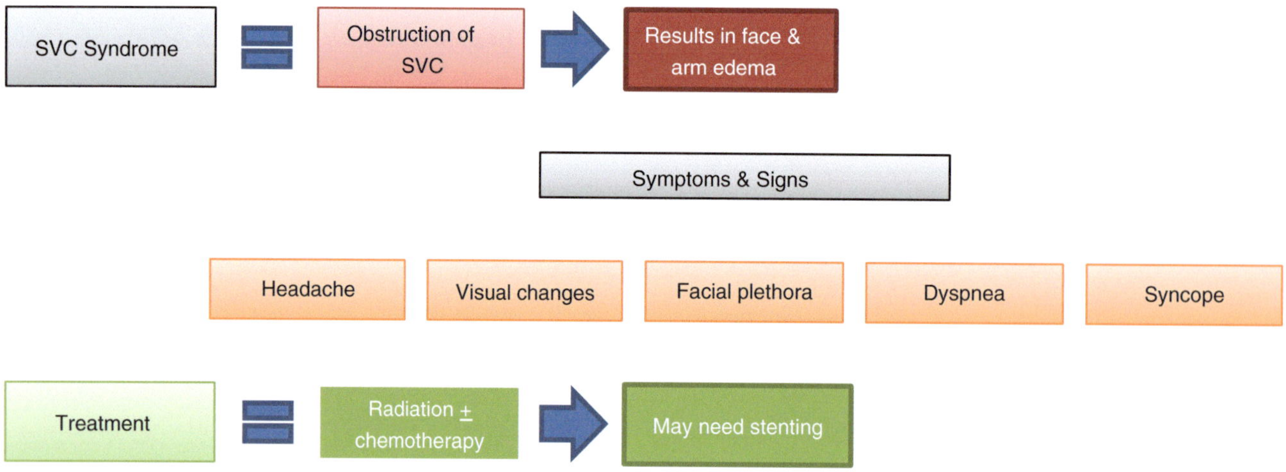

Mediastinal Masses

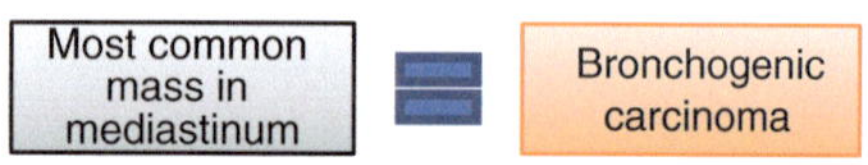

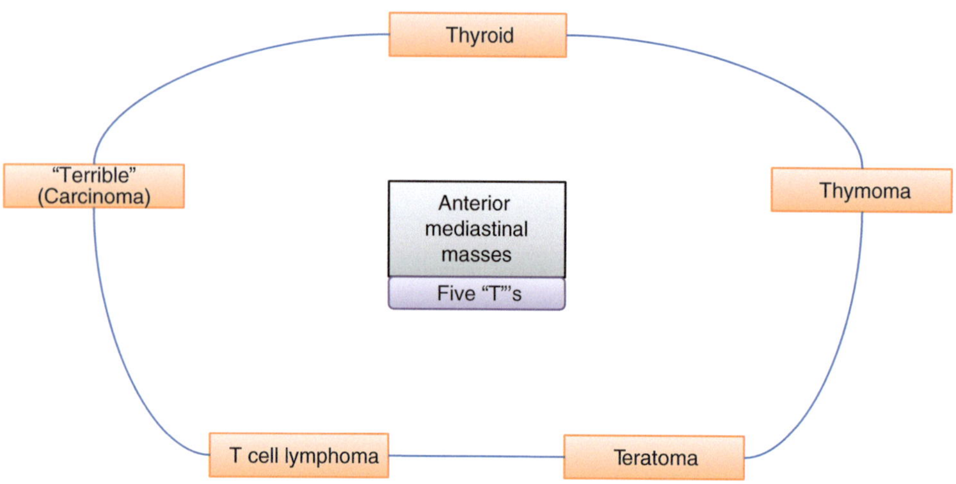

The Airway

Rapid Sequence Intubation

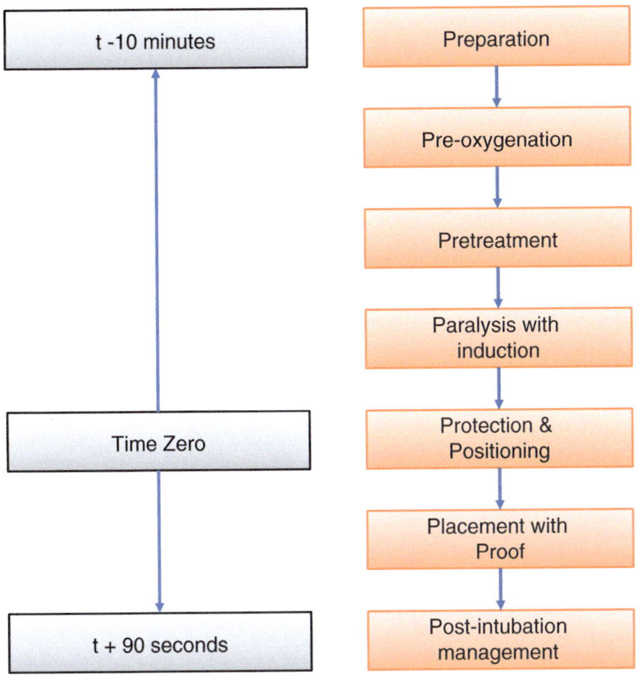

Airway Tidbits

3-3-2 Rule

Opening of mouth = 3 fingers
Hyoid-chin distance = 3 fingers
Distance from thyroid cartilage to floor of mouth = 2 fingers

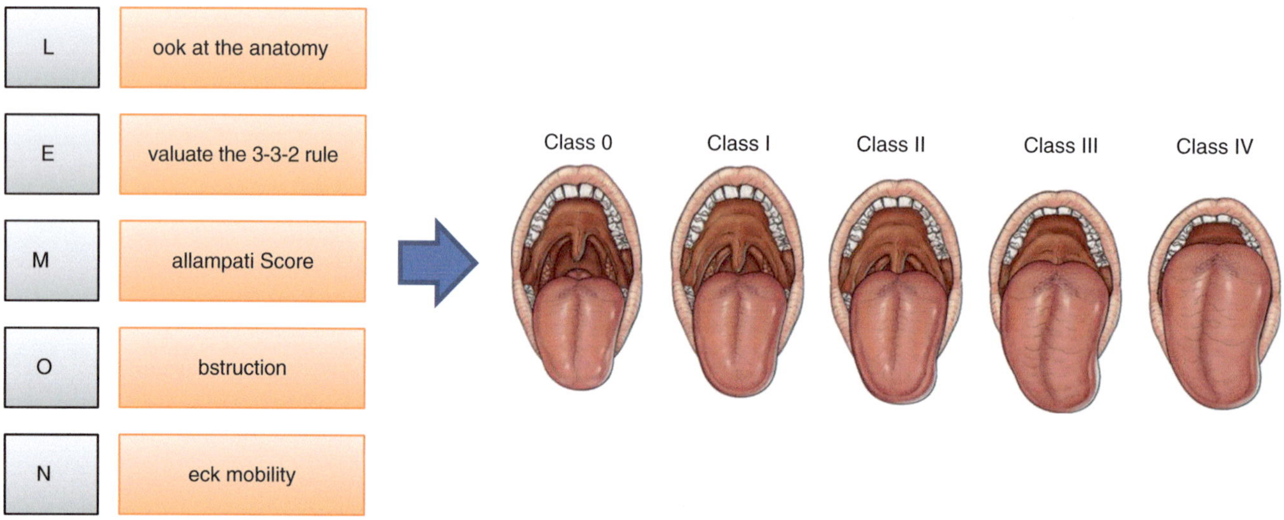

Tracheostomy and Respiratory Distress

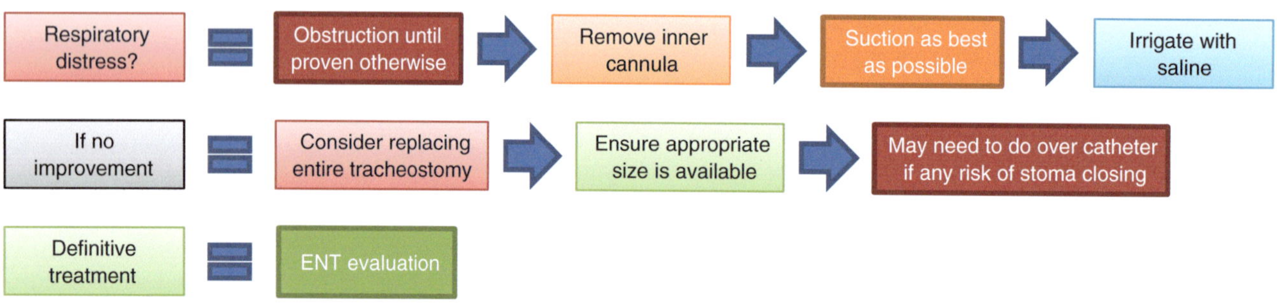

(Reprinted from Ramachandran SK, Kheterpal S. The expected difficult airway. In: Glick DB, Cooper RM, Ovassapian A, editors. The difficult airway: an atlas of tools and techniques for clinical management. New York: Springer Science; 2013. p. 11–32. With permission from Springer Science + Business Media)

Tracheostomy and Bleeding

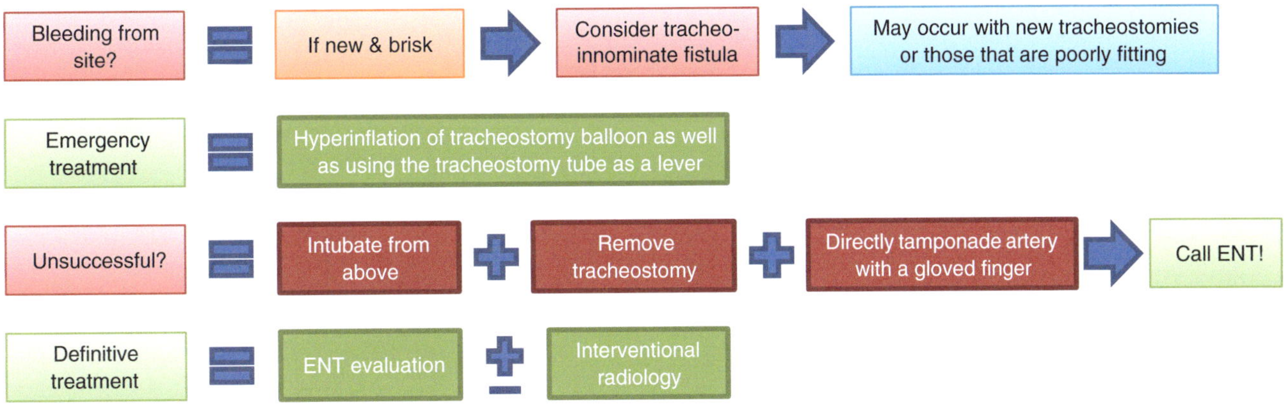

General Pediatrics

Apparent Life-Threatening Events (ALTE)

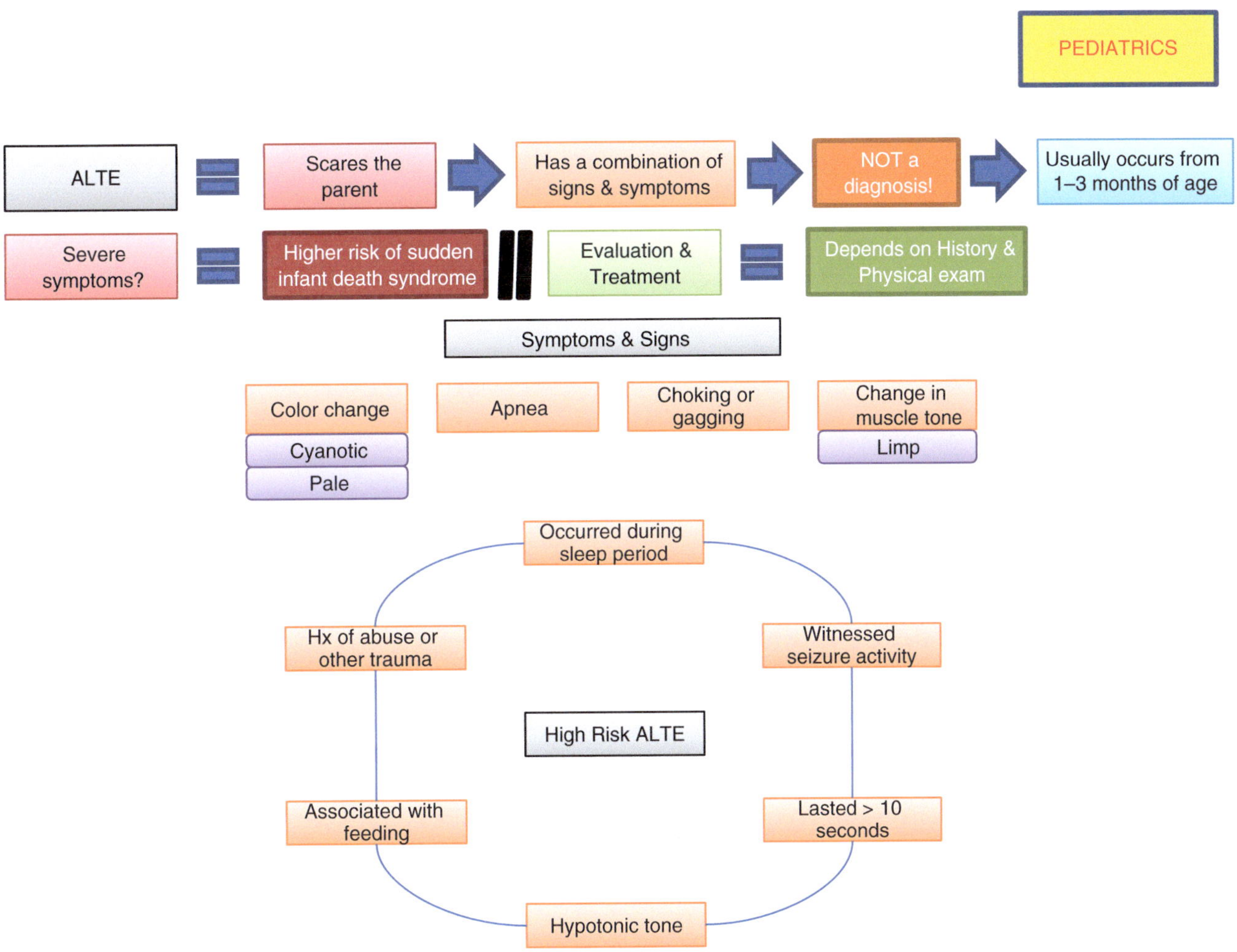

Selected Causes of ALTE

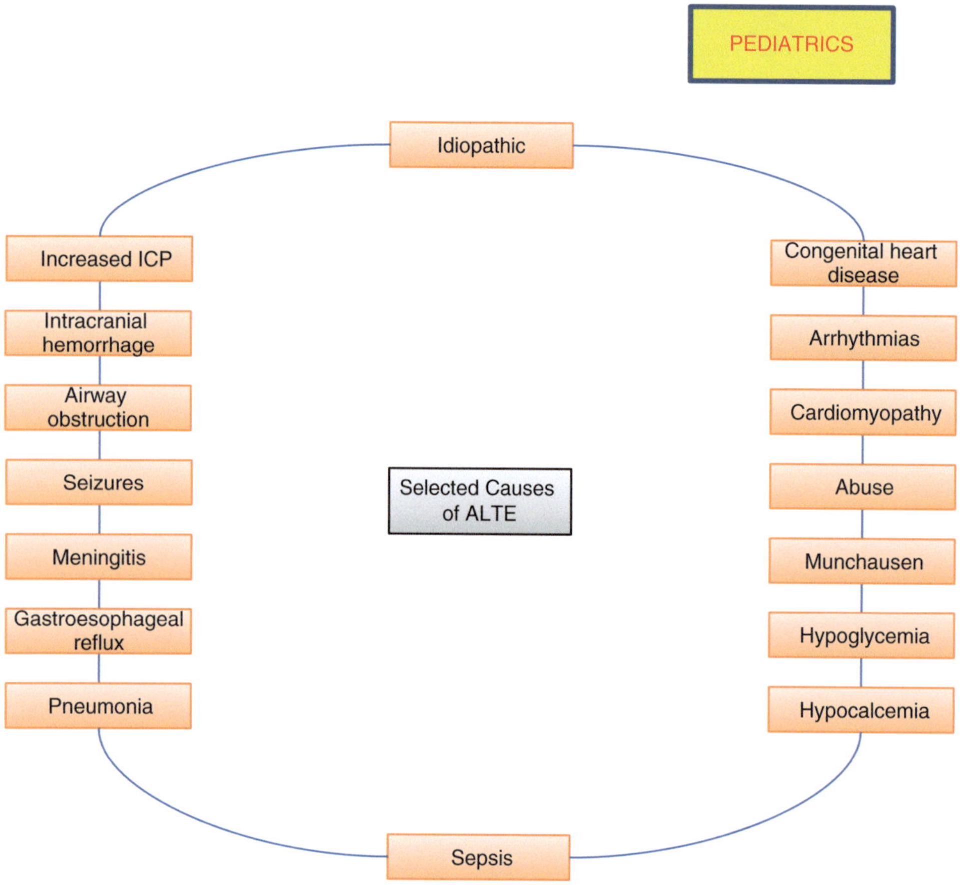

Sudden Infant Death Syndrome (SIDS)

PEDIATRICS

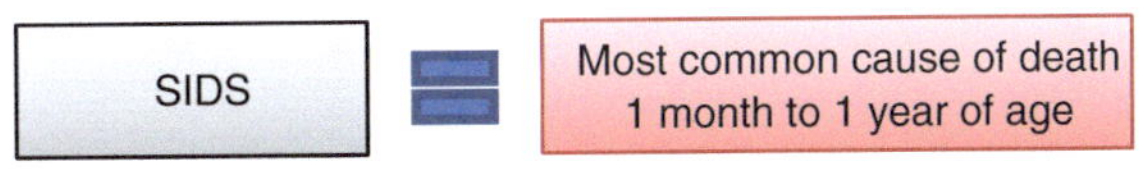

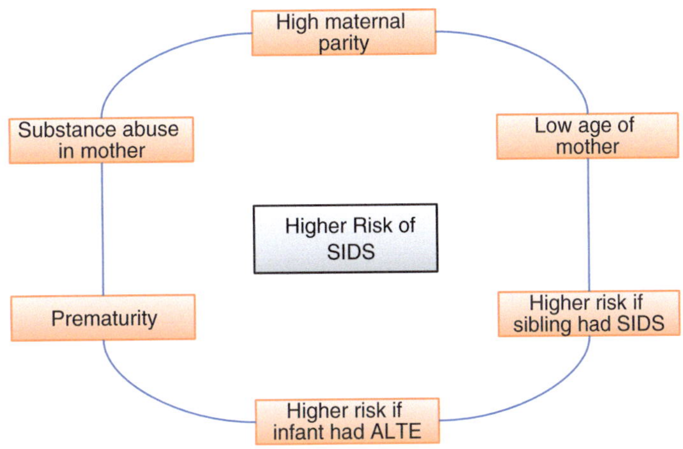

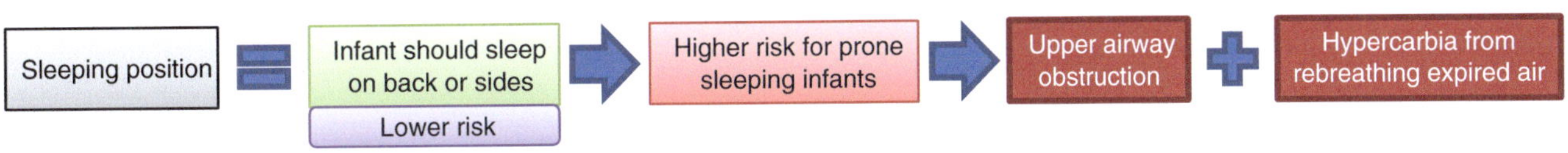

Gastroenterology

Brandon R. Allen and Bobby Desai

Contents

Pediatric Gastroenterology ... 186
Constipation ... 187
Diarrhea ... 189
Esophageal Emergencies ... 199
Esophageal Perforation ... 204
Esophageal Foreign Bodies ... 207
GERD ... 210
Peptic Ulcer Disease ... 212
GI Bleeding ... 214
Liver and Gallbladder ... 219
Pancreatitis ... 229
Ileus ... 233
Bowel Obstruction ... 234
Intussusception ... 236
Volvulus ... 240
Hernias ... 242
Bowel Perforation ... 245
Acute Appendicitis ... 246
Acute Diverticulitis ... 248
Mesenteric Ischemia ... 251
Crohn's Disease ... 253
Ulcerative Colitis ... 256
Irritable Bowel Syndrome ... 257
Miscellaneous Anorectal Emergencies ... 257

B.R. Allen, MD (✉)
Department of Emergency Medicine,
University of Florida College of Medicine, Gainesville, FL, USA
e-mail: brandonrallen@ufl.edu

B. Desai, MD, MEd
Department of Emergency Medicine, University of Florida,
Gainesville, FL, USA
e-mail: bdesai@ufl.edu

B. Desai, B.R. Allen (eds.), *Nailing the Written Emergency Medicine Board Examination*,
DOI 10.1007/978-3-319-30838-8_3

Pediatric Gastroenterology

Pediatric GI Tidbits: Vomiting

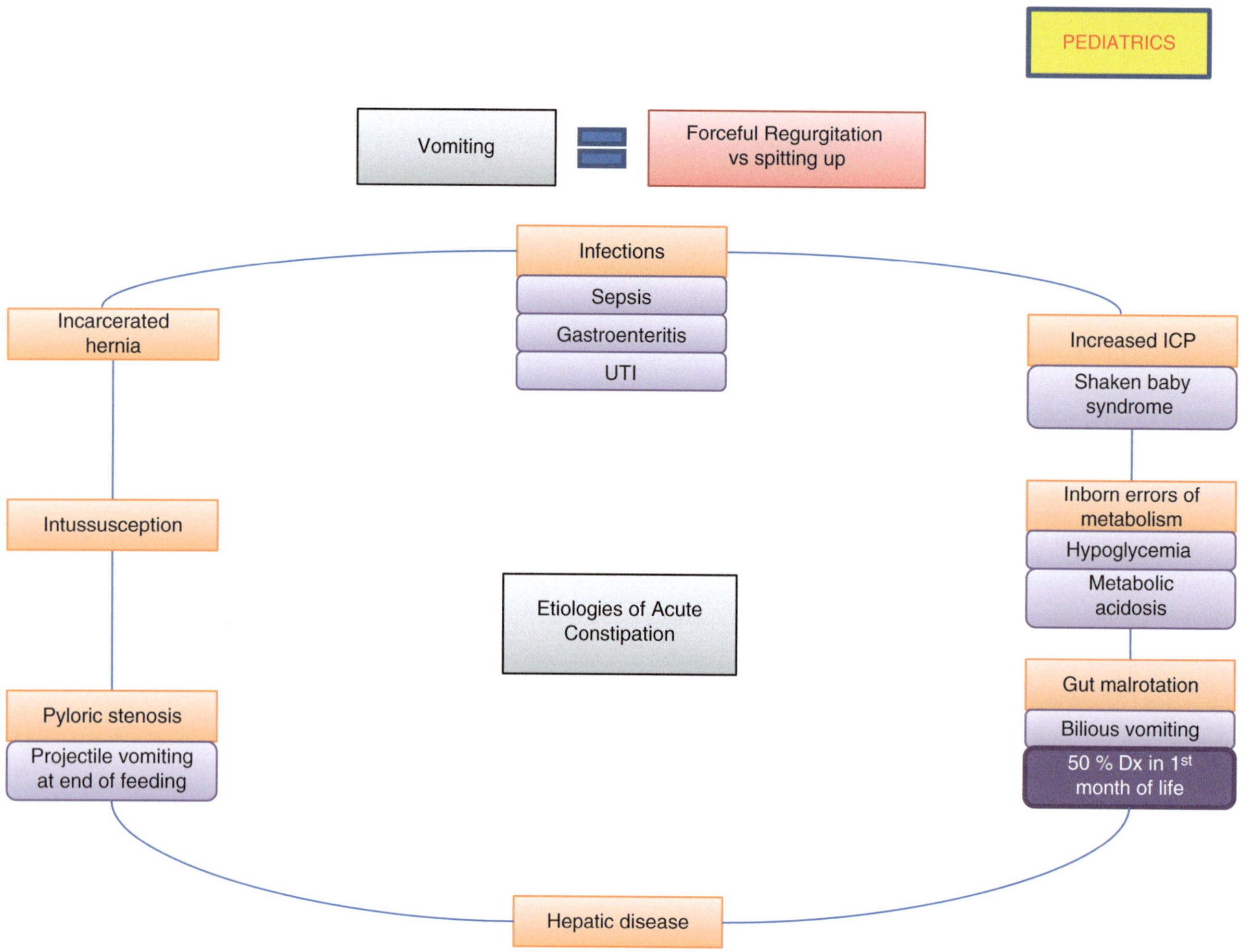

Necrotizing Enterocolitis

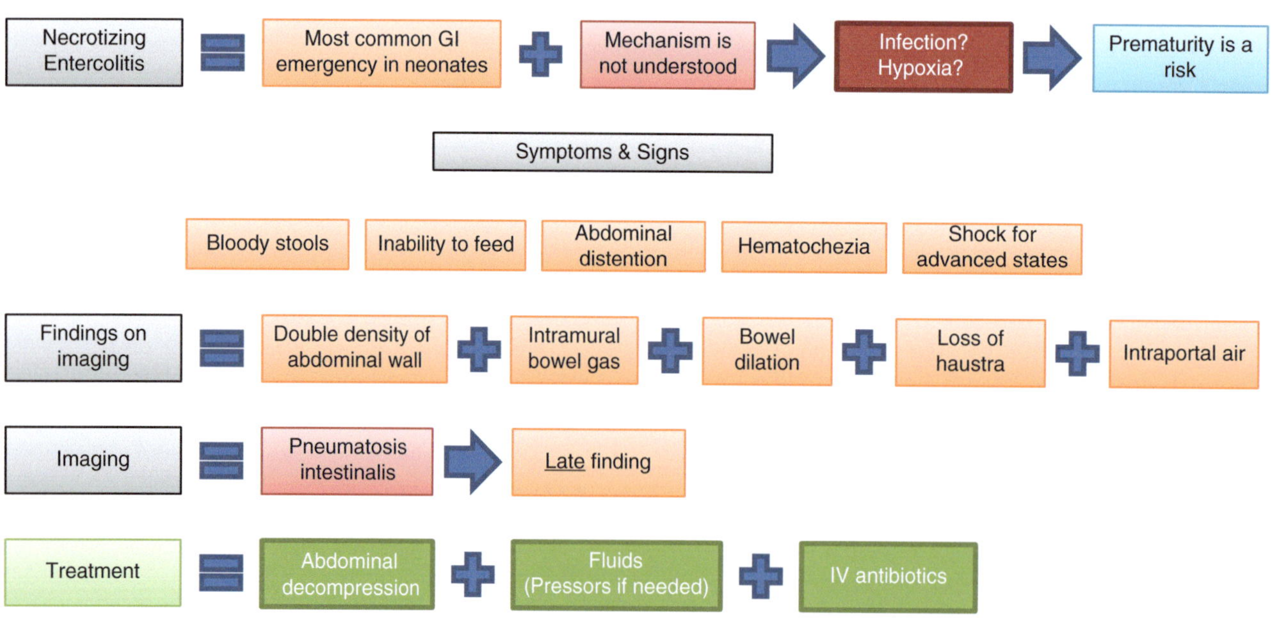

Constipation

Introduction

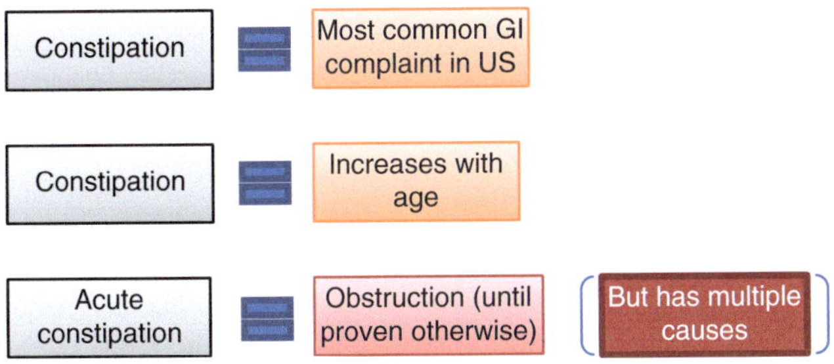

Symptoms and Signs

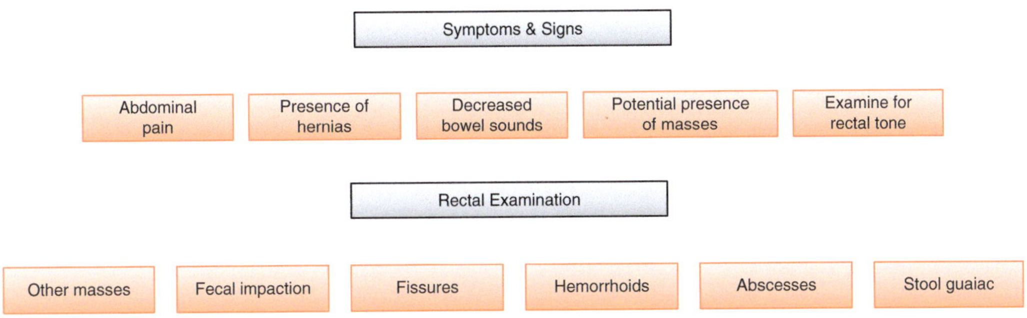

Etiologies of Acute Constipation

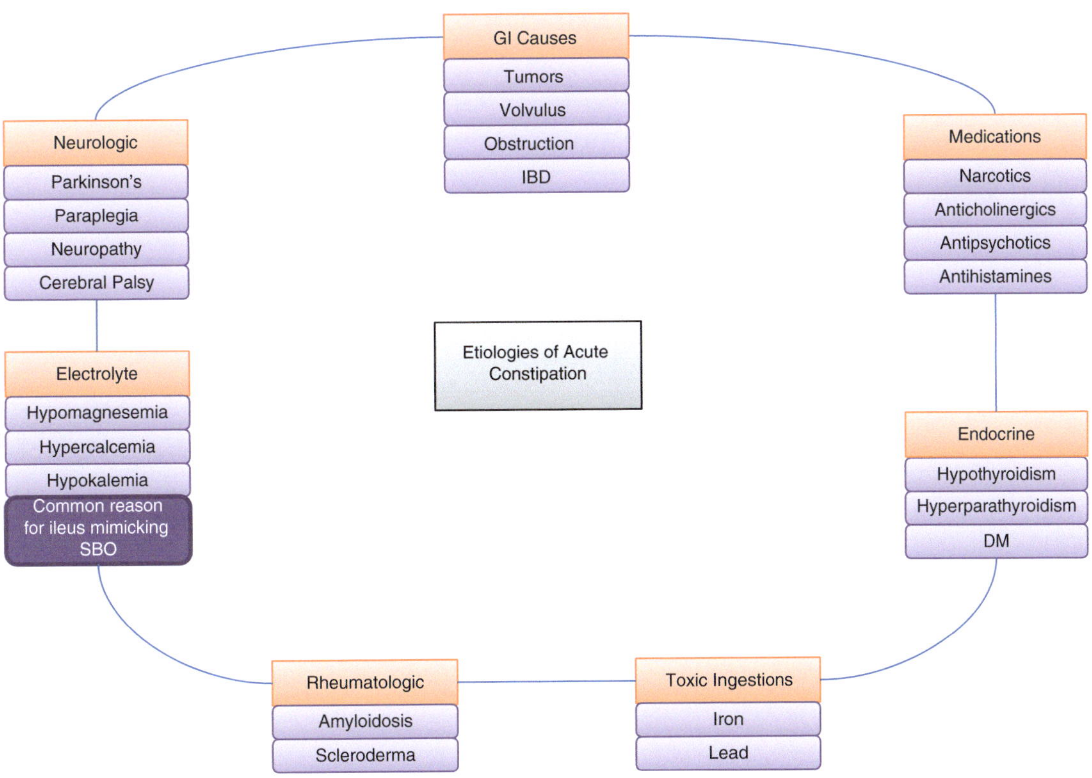

Etiologies of Chronic Constipation

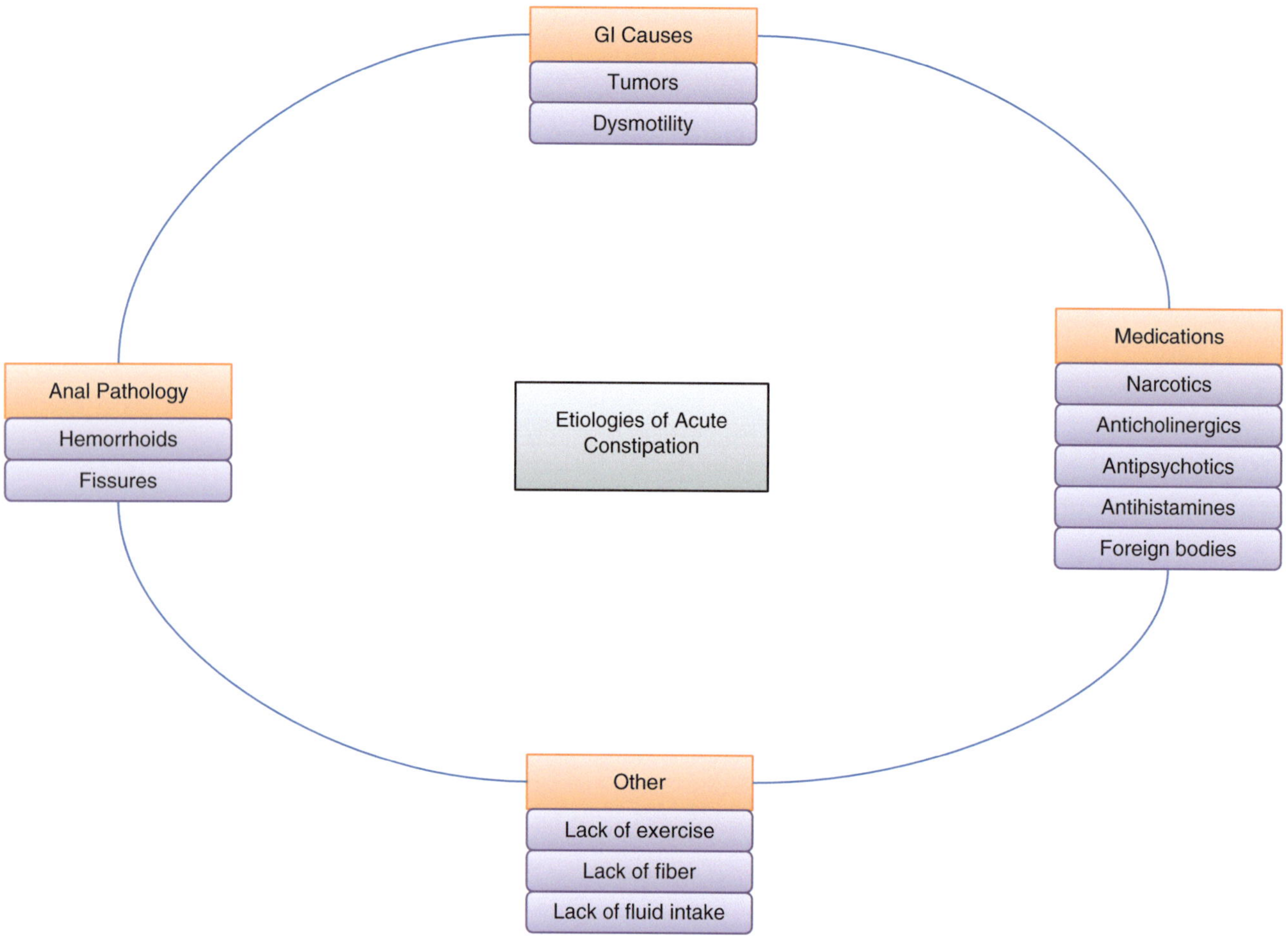

Diagnosis

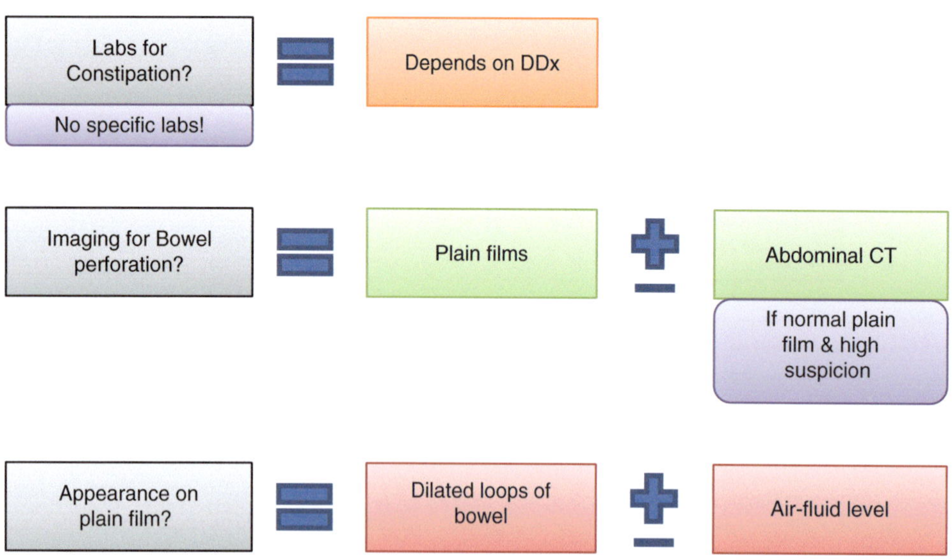

Treatment

Constipation? = Depends on etiology → Treat underlying cause ± Dietary changes ± Medical adjuncts (Enemas; Cathartics)

Diarrhea

Introduction

Acute Diarrhea = Increase in normal water content of stool = Increased frequency of stools of lesser consistency = A leading cause of death worldwide

Mechanisms of Diarrhea = Decreased intestinal absorption OR Increased intestinal secretion OR Abnormal motility OR Increased osmotic load

Diarrhea = Infectious 85 % + Non-infectious 15 %

Infectious diarrhea = Viruses (Vast majority) → Bacterial → Parasitic

Pediatric GI Tidbits: Diarrhea

PEDIATRICS

Blood in stool of infants? = Cow's milk intolerance + Swallowed maternal blood + Anal fissure

Viral causes = Rotavirus → Most common || Adenovirus → 2nd most common

Bacterial causes = Most common summer cause → Viruses more common in winter

Viral Diarrhea

Increased incidence of viral diarrhea = Winter & Spring + Children + Daycare

Specific viruses = Rotavirus + Adenovirus + Calcivirus + Enterovirus + Norwalk

Rotavirus = Most common cause of diarrhea in children

Norovirus (Norwalk-like) = Leading cause of gastroenteritis in the US

Viral diarrhea = No bloody stools + No WBC's in stool

Bacterial Diarrhea

Foreign travel = High likelihood of bacterial diarrhea → Potential consumption of contaminated food & drink = Most common cause of Traveler's diarrhea

Traveler's Diarrhea = *E. coli* → *C. jejuni* → *Shigella* → *Salmonella*

Consider bacterial diarrhea → Abdominal pain + Fever + Bloody stool

Consider bacterial diarrhea → (+) stool WBC (Also (+) stool lactoferrin) + Bleeding (Depending on pathogen)

Bloody stools = Invasive pathogens → *E. coli* O157:H7 + *Shigella* + *Campylobacter* + *Yersinia*

Non-invasive pathogens = Enterotoxin producing organisms → Usually food-borne infections

Diarrhea from toxins → Watery, copious diarrhea + Mild to No Fever − Bloody stool − WBC's in stool

Specific Bacterial Pathogens: *E. coli*

E. coli O157:H7 = Enterohemorrhagic *E. coli* = Bloody stool − WBC in stools

Causes of *E. coli* O157:H7 = Untreated water + Raw milk + Petting zoos + Undercooked meat

Complications of *E. coli* O157:H7 = Thrombotic Thrombocytic Purpura (Adults) + Hemolytic-Uremic Syndrome (Children) (Antibiotics may increase risk of HUS)

Traveler's Diarrhea = Enterotoxogenic *E. coli*

Traveler's diarrhea treatment? = Ciprofloxacin OR TMP-SMX + Bismuth salicylate + Antiperistaltic agents

Specific Bacterial Pathogens: *Shigella*

Shigella = High infectivity + 2–6 day incubation period

Symptoms of *Shigella* = Very high fever + Potential for ***febrile seizures*** + Bloody diarrhea (Dysentery)

Treatment = Ciprofloxacin

Specific Bacterial Pathogens: *Salmonella*

Salmonella = Very common pathogen + Not as infective as *Shigella*

Symptoms of Salmonella = Watery, mucoid stools

Reservoirs of *Salmonella* = Eggs + Chicken + Amphibians + Undercooked food

Complications of *Salmonella* = Osteomyelitis (Sickle cell disease)

Treatment = Ciprofloxacin

Specific Bacterial Pathogens: *Campylobacter*

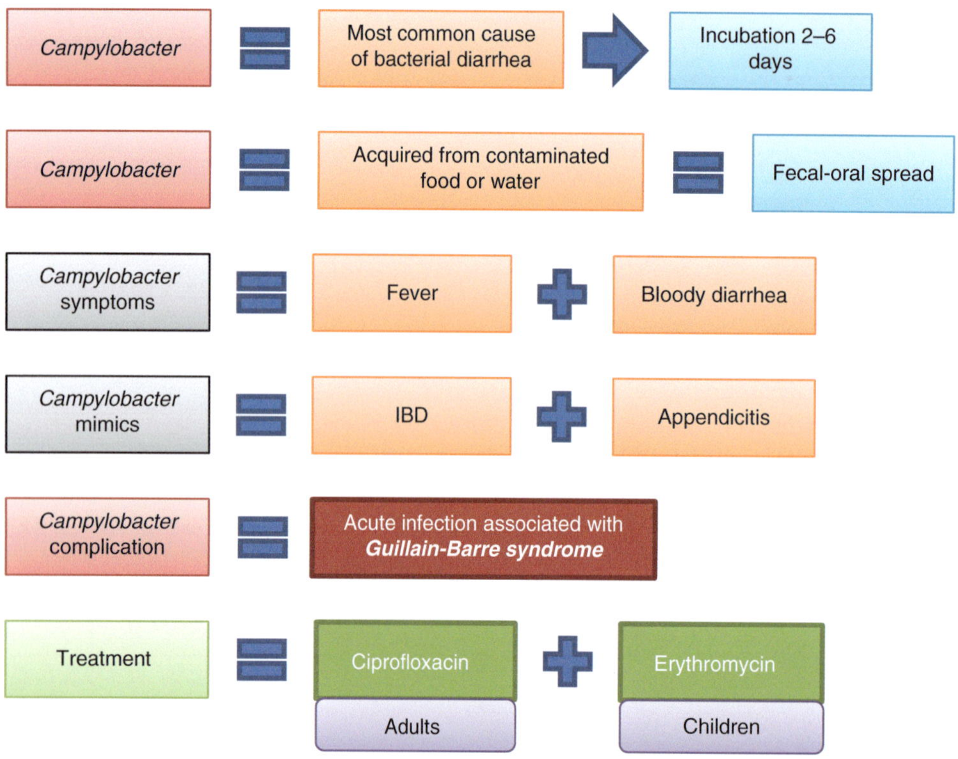

Specific Bacterial Pathogens: *Yersinia*

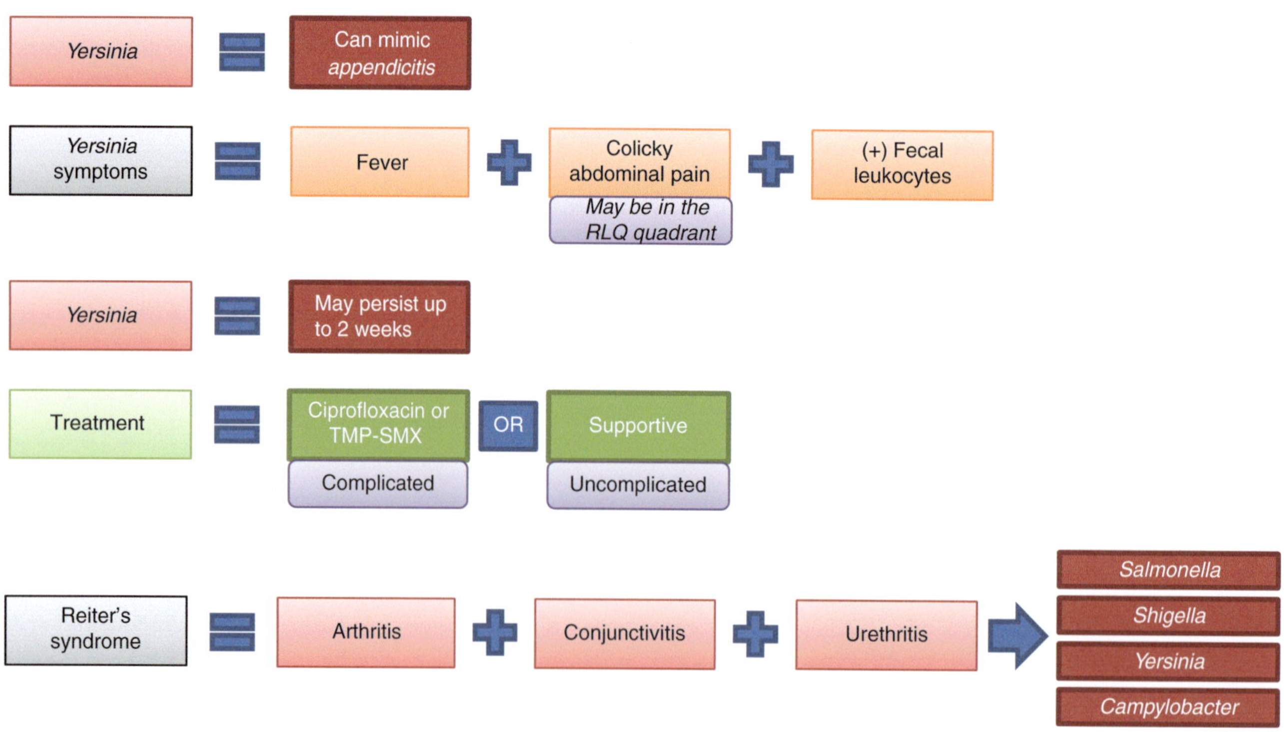

Specific Bacterial Pathogens: *Vibrio*

V. parahaemolyticus = Raw oysters + Clams + Shrimp

V. parahaemolyticus = 6–24 hour incubation

V. vulnificus = Raw oysters + Shellfish

V. cholera = Food or drink contaminated by feces of infected person

V. cholera sign = Rice water stool = Severe fluid & electrolyte disturbances = Potentially severe & fatal diarrhea

Treatment = Ciprofloxacin (Or TMP-SMX) + WHO rehydration

Specific Bacterial Pathogens: *Staphylococcus*

Staph = Most common cause of food-borne illness + Sx within 6 hours

Staph = Contaminated foods (Via pre-formed toxin) → Potato salad + Dairy & Eggs + Meats including poultry

Staph symptoms = N/V + Watery diarrhea − Fever

Treatment = No antibiotics!

Specific Bacterial Pathogens: *Clostridium perfringens*

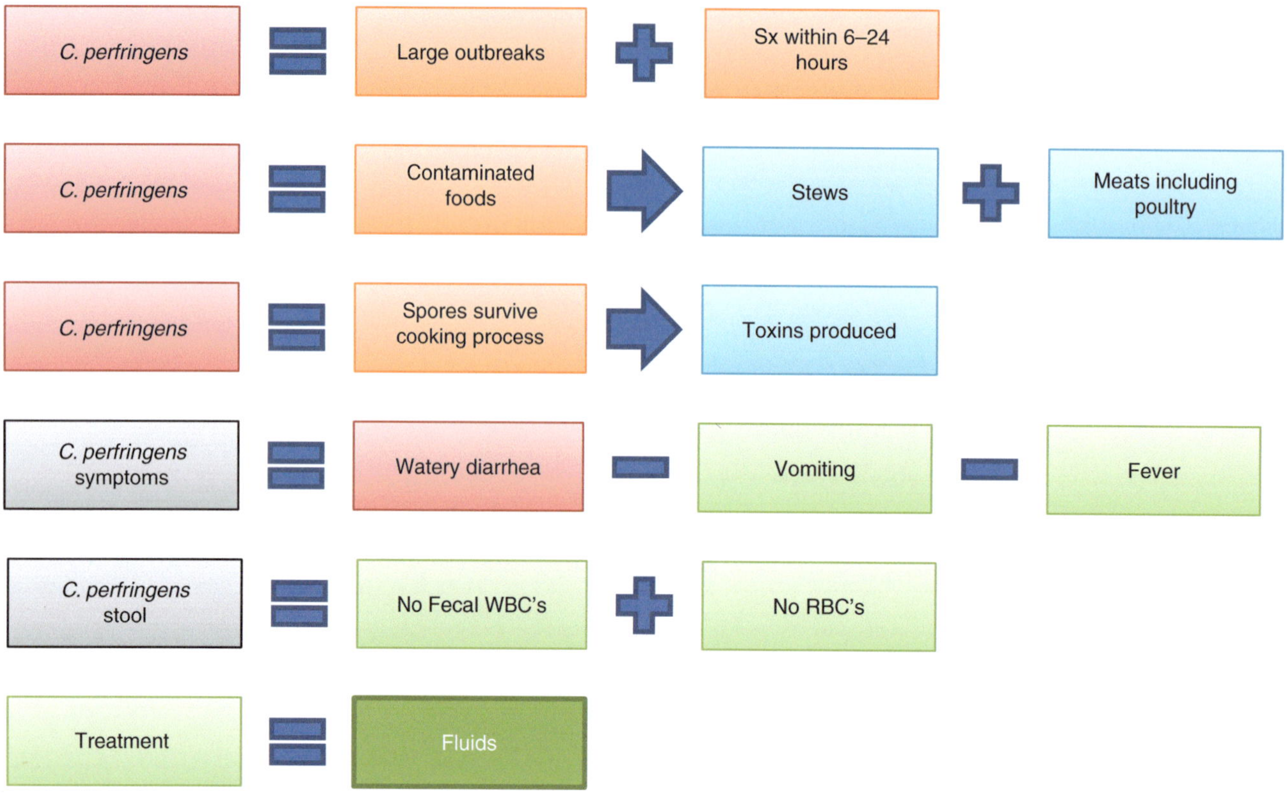

Specific Bacterial Pathogens: *Bacillus cereus*

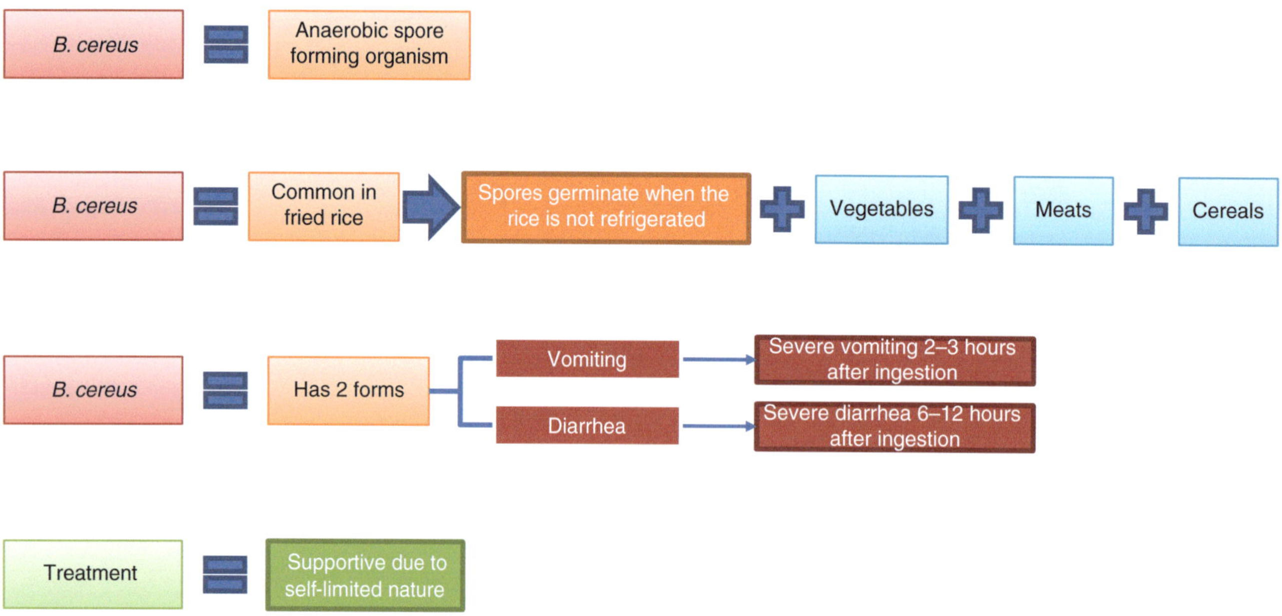

Specific Toxins: Scombroid

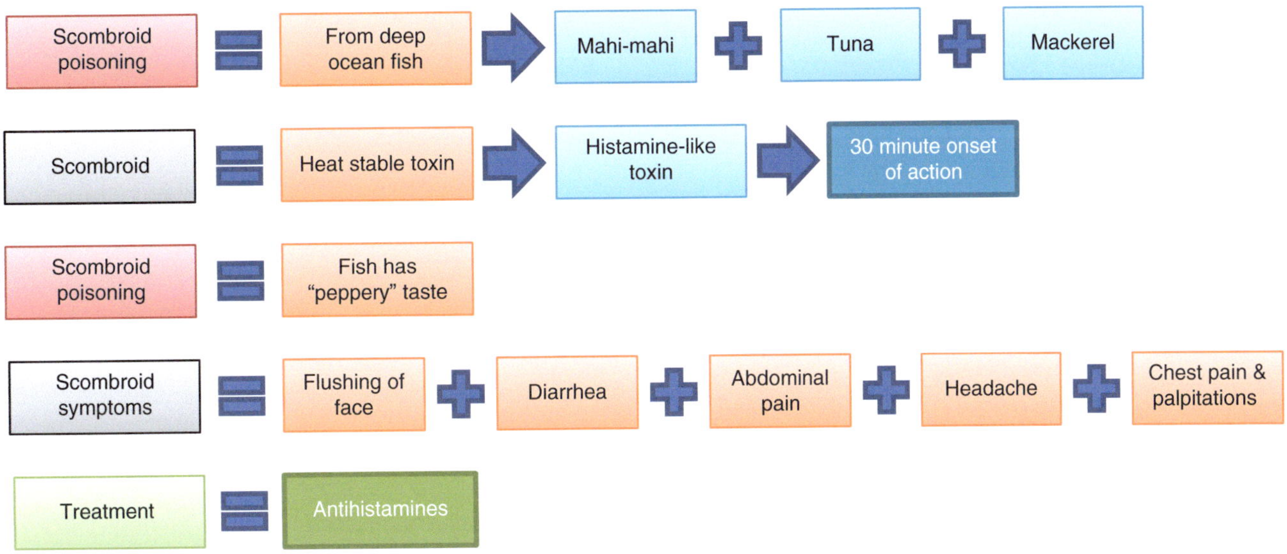

Specific Toxins: Ciguatera

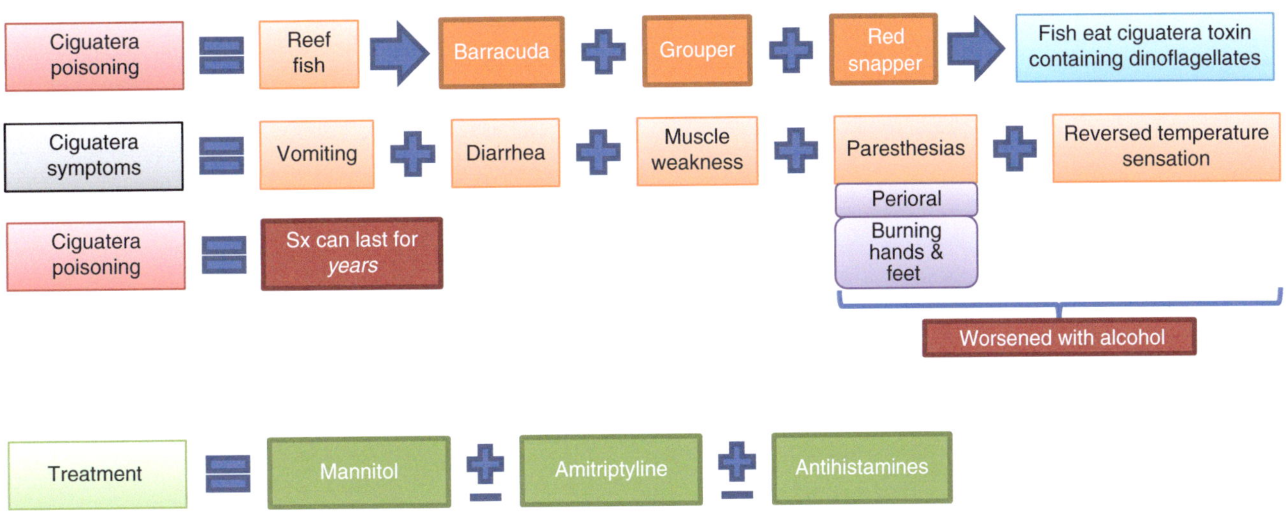

Specific Protozoan Pathogens: *Giardia*

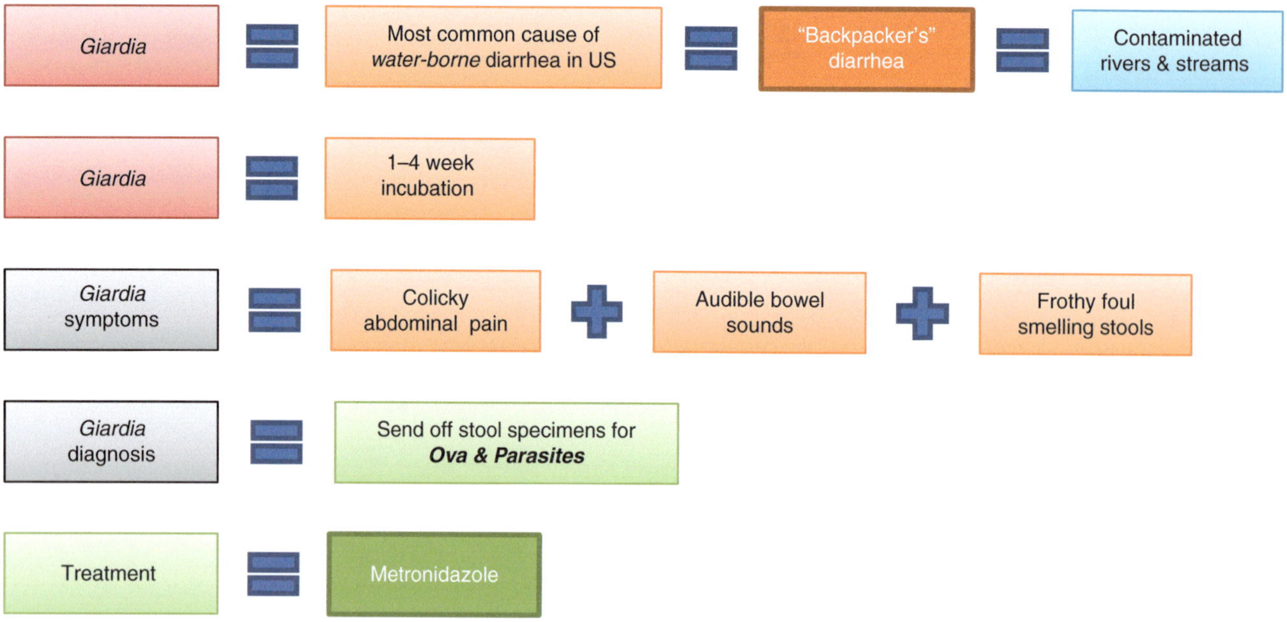

Specific Protozoan Pathogens: *Entamoeba histolytica*

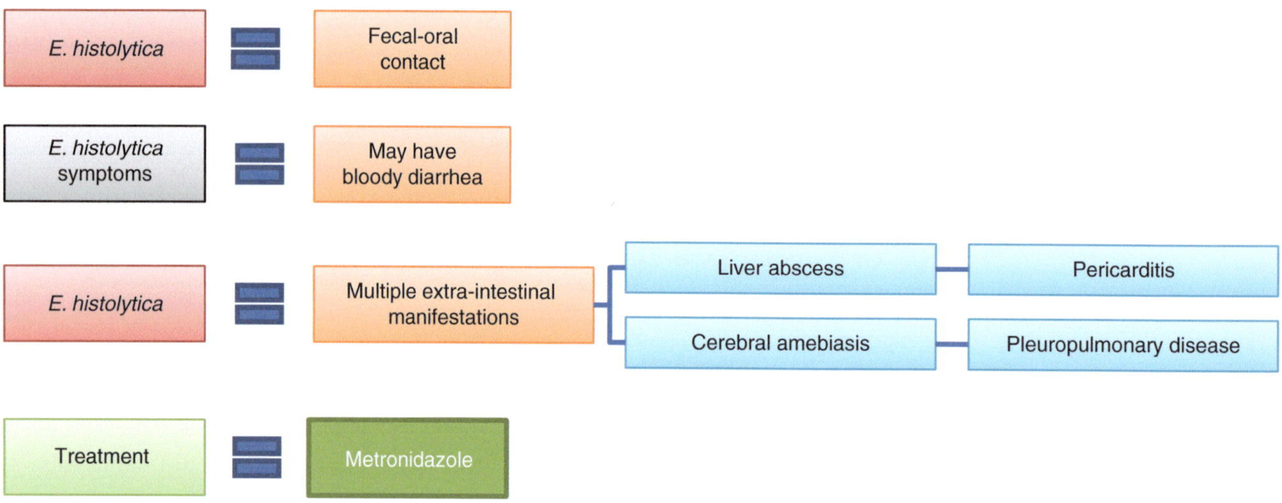

Specific Protozoan Pathogens: *Cryptosporidium*

Cryptospordium = Most common cause of chronic diarrhea in *AIDS* → From contaminated water

Cryptospordium = 1 week incubation

Cryptospordium symptoms = Abdominal pain + Watery diarrhea

Cryptospordium diagnosis = Send off stool specimens for *Ova & Parasites*

Treatment = Fluids + Nitazoxanide + Azithromycin

Antibiotic-Associated Diarrhea

Antibiotic Associated Diarrhea = Moderate diarrhea − Fever − Abdominal cramps − Fecal leukocytes

Antibiotic Associated Diarrhea = *C. difficile* (until proven otherwise)

Treatment = Stop offending antibiotic

Clostridium difficile and Pseudomembranous Enterocolitis

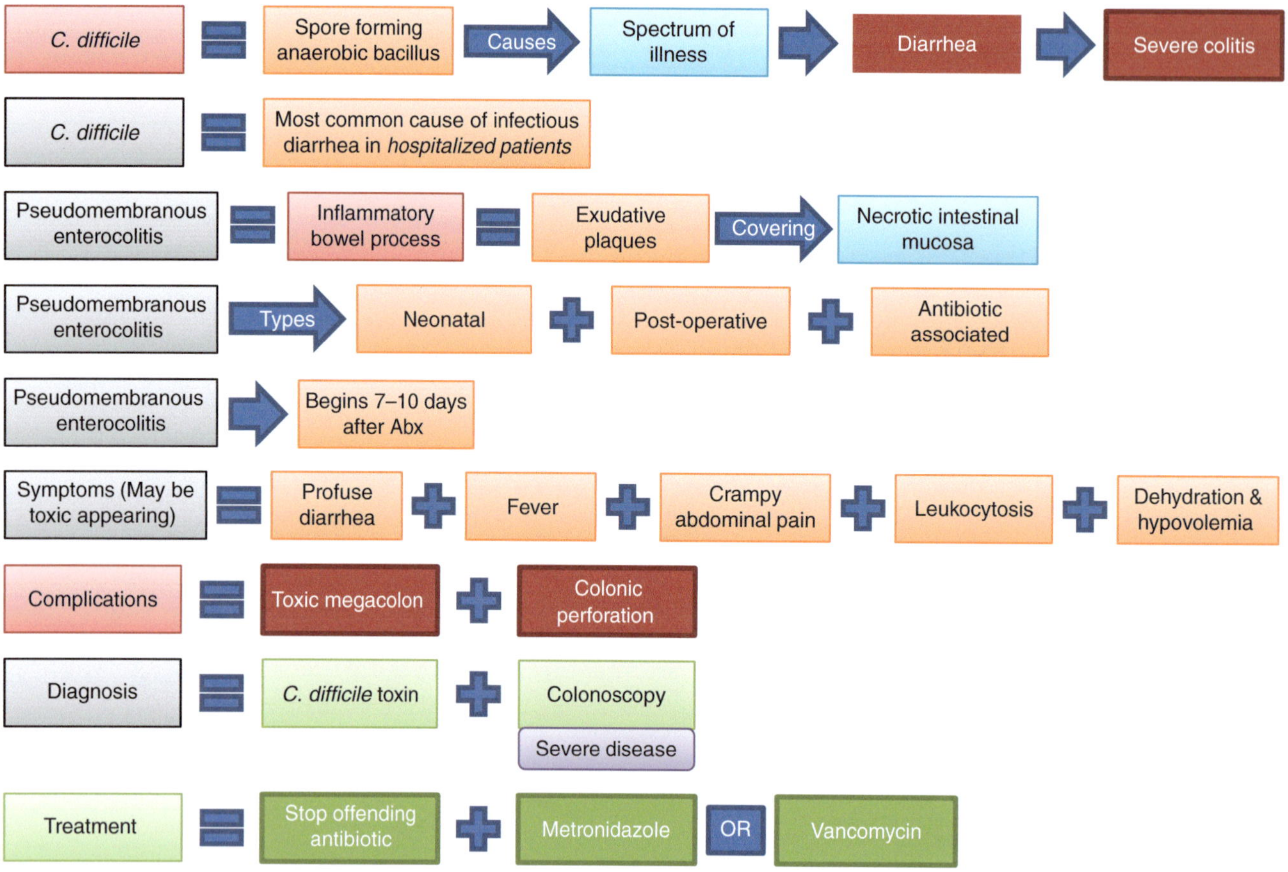

Esophageal Emergencies

Dysphagia

Dysphagia = Difficulty swallowing → Most patients have an *organic* etiology

Dysphagia = *Transfer* dysphagia OR *Transport* dysphagia

Transfer dysphagia = *Early* in swallowing = Difficulty in *initiating* swallowing = Neuromuscular disorder; Stroke

Transport dysphagia (Impaired movement of food) = *Later* in swallowing = Sensation of stuck food (May be localized by patient if in *upper 1/3* of esophagus)

Other classifications → *Functional* dysphagia (Intermittent) OR *Mechanical* dysphagia (Progressive; Solids then liquids)

Diagnosis = Usually made outside of ED

Transfer Dysphagia

Transfer Dysphagia = Pharynx → Transfer problems → Esophagus = ↑ Risk of Aspiration

Symptoms

- Coughing
- Gagging
- Regurgitation through nose
- Problems initiating a swallow

Signs

- Malnutrition
- Pneumonia
- Weight loss

Neuromuscular Causes of Transfer Dysphagia

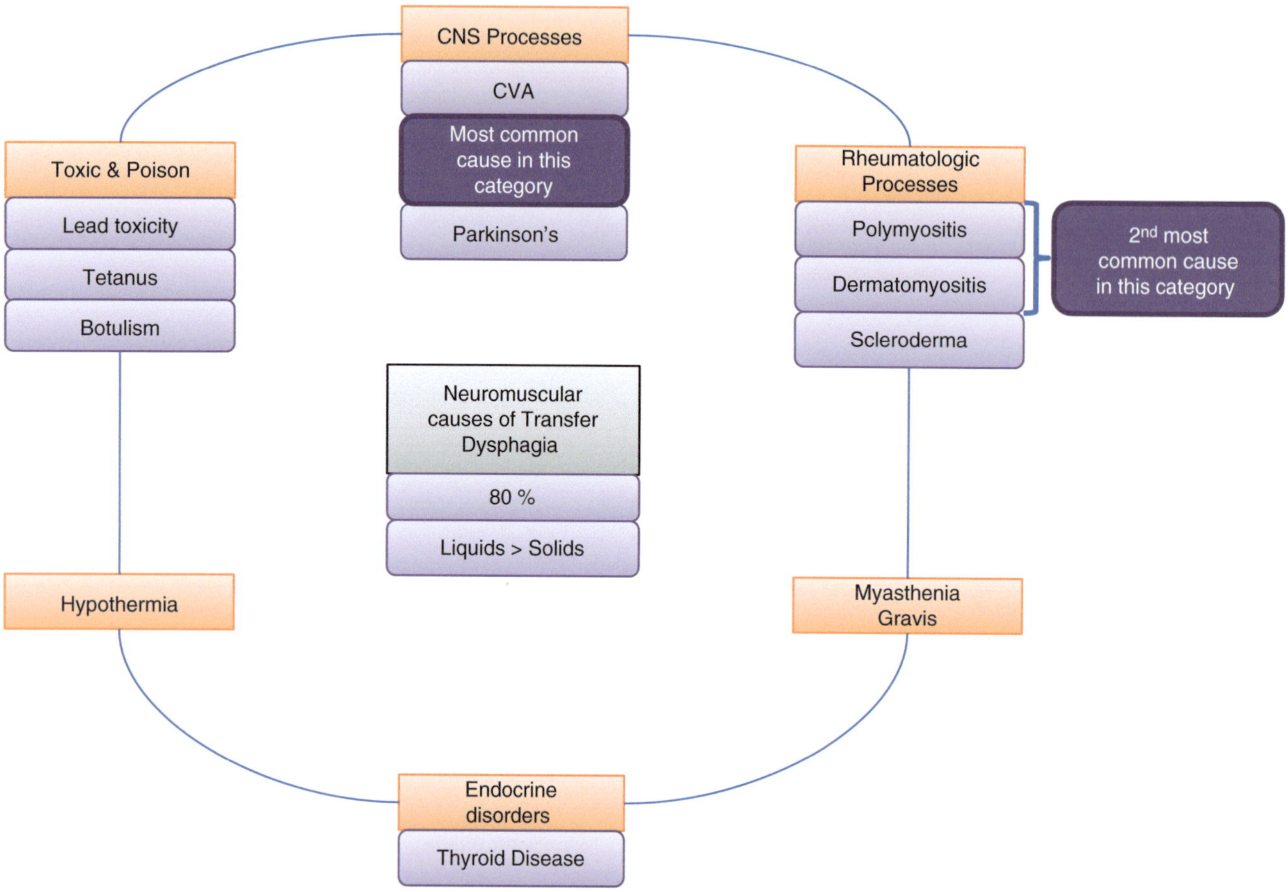

Localized Causes of Transfer Dysphagia

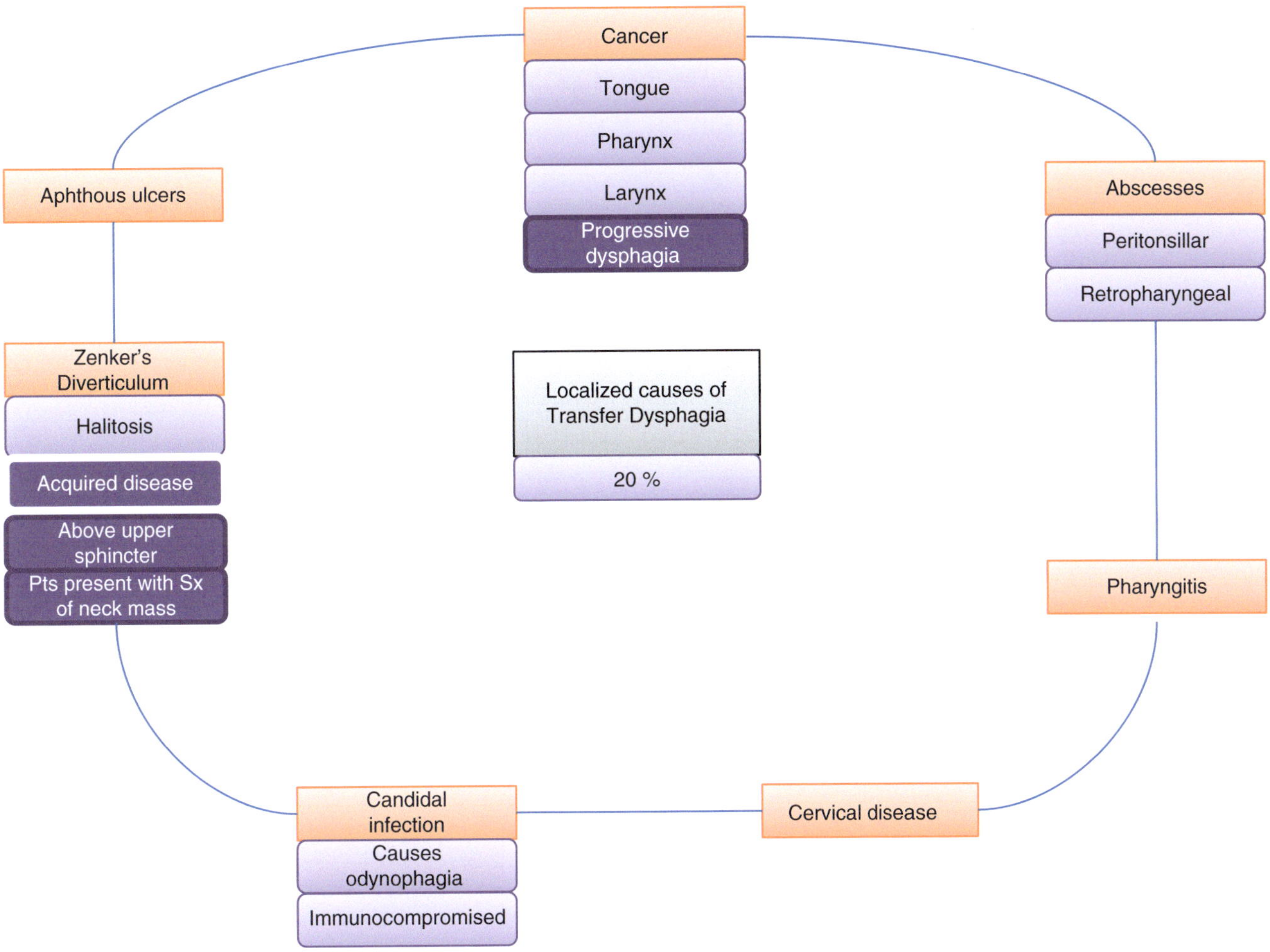

Transport Dysphagia

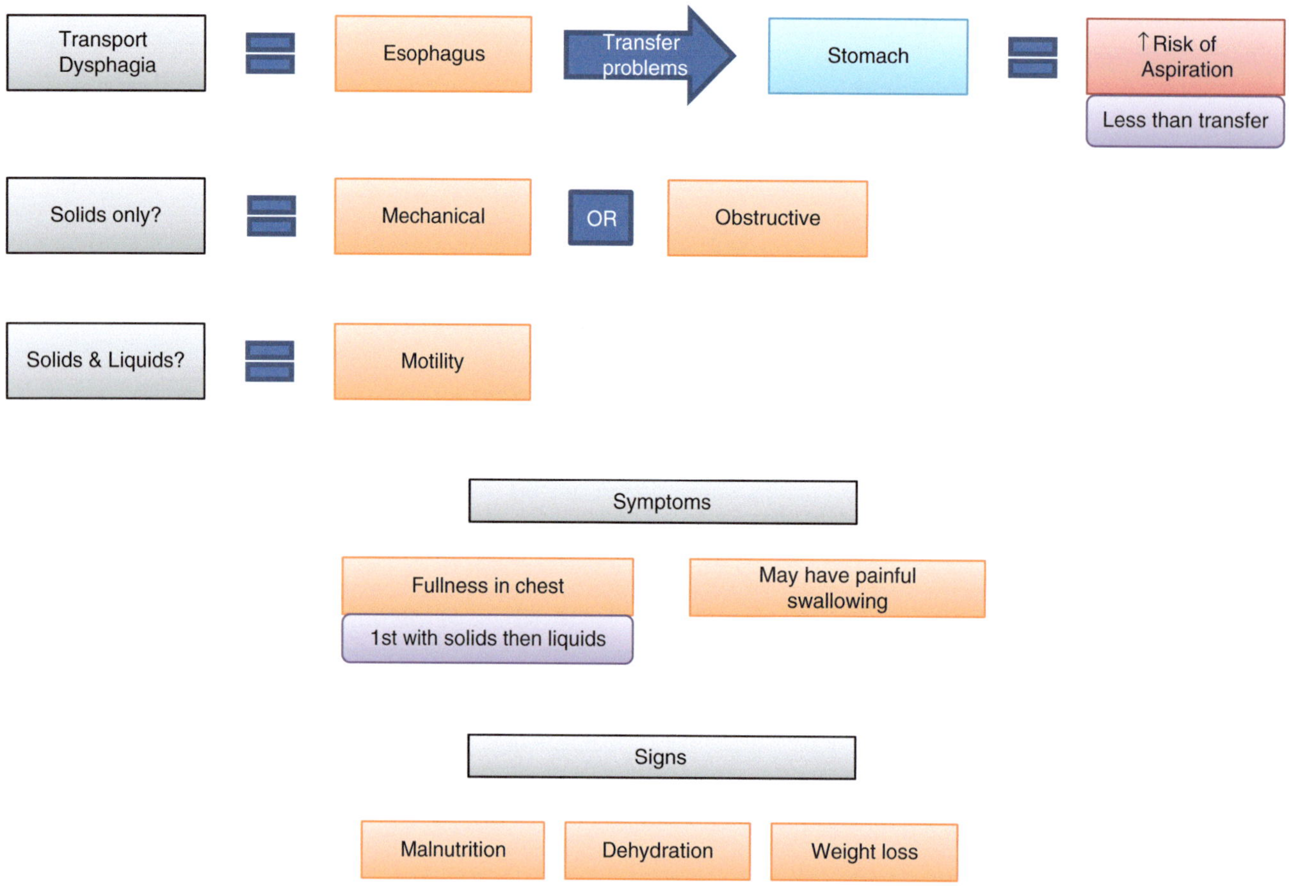

Obstructive Causes of Transport Dysphagia

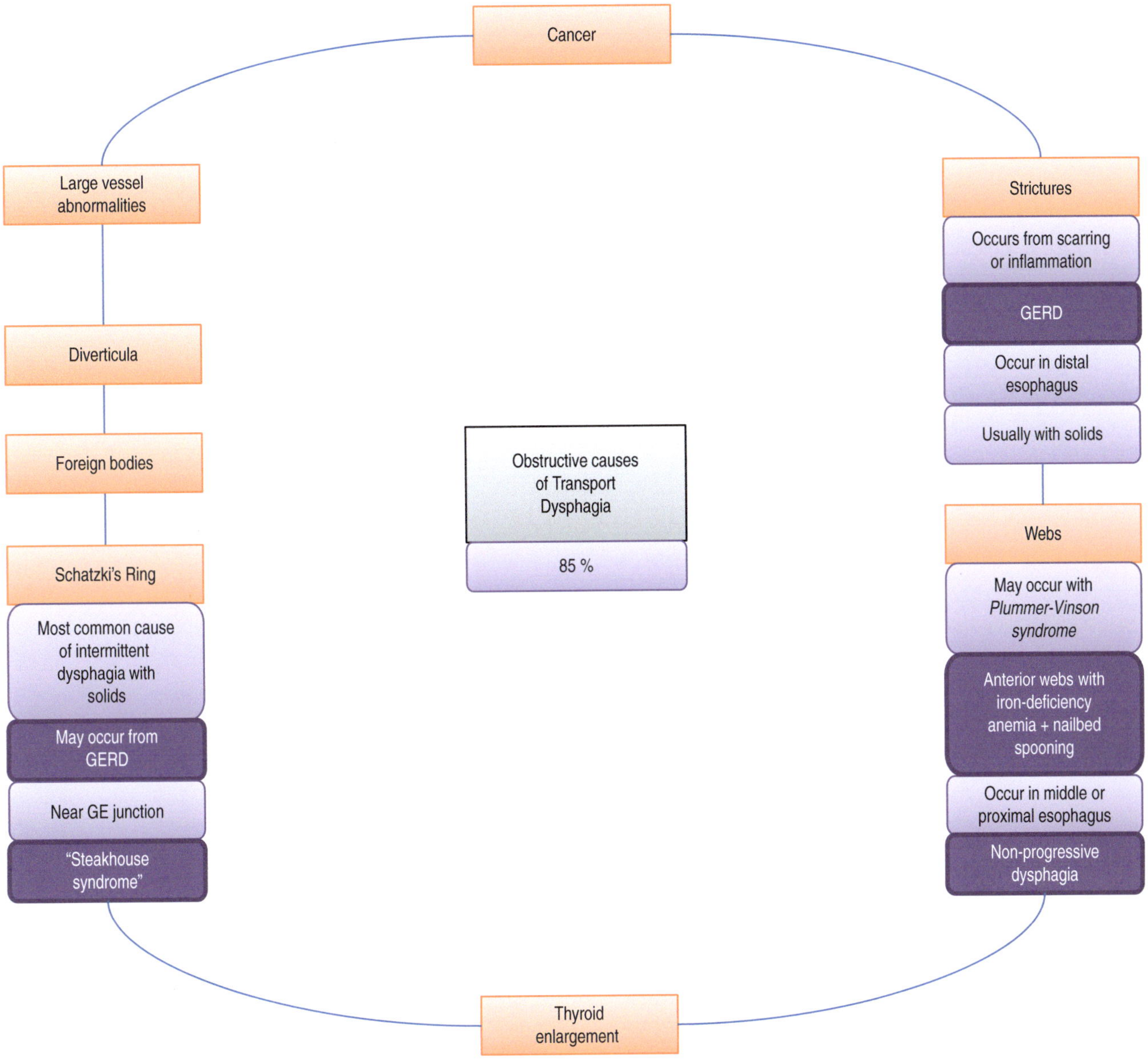

Motor Causes of Transport Dysphagia

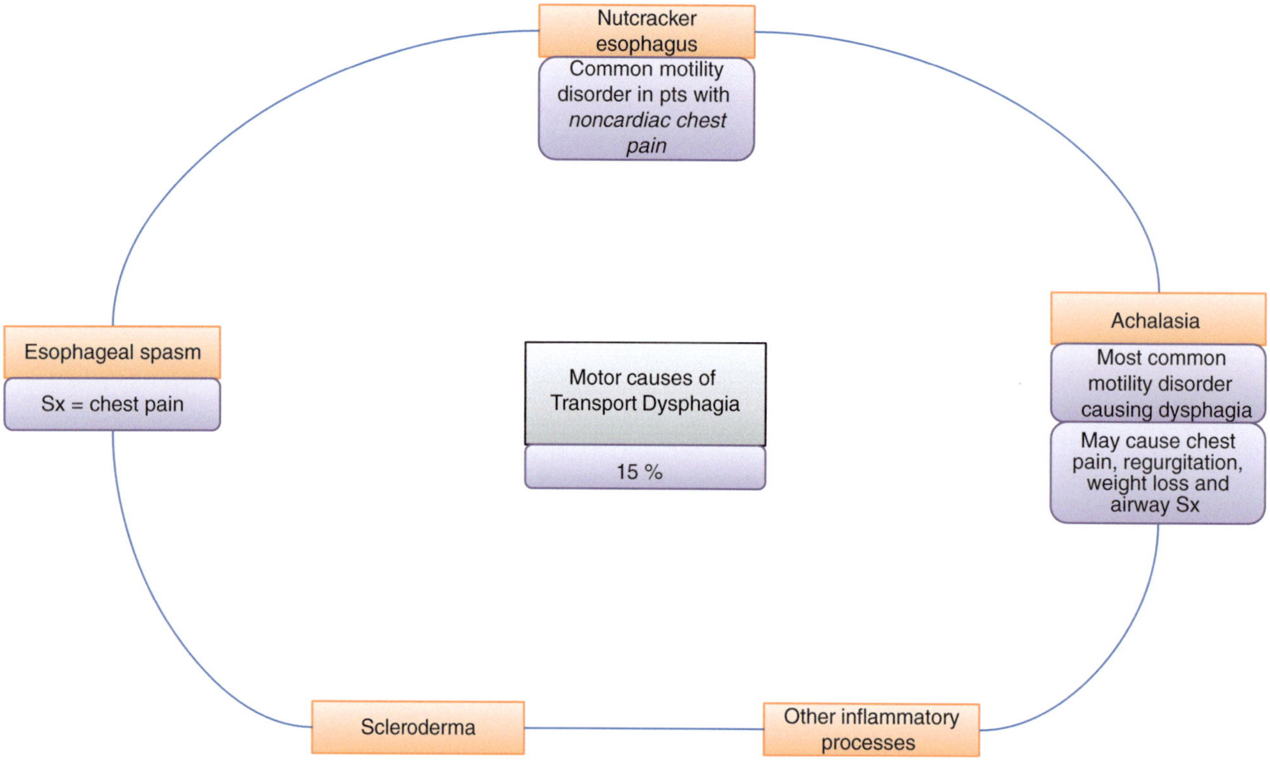

Esophageal Perforation

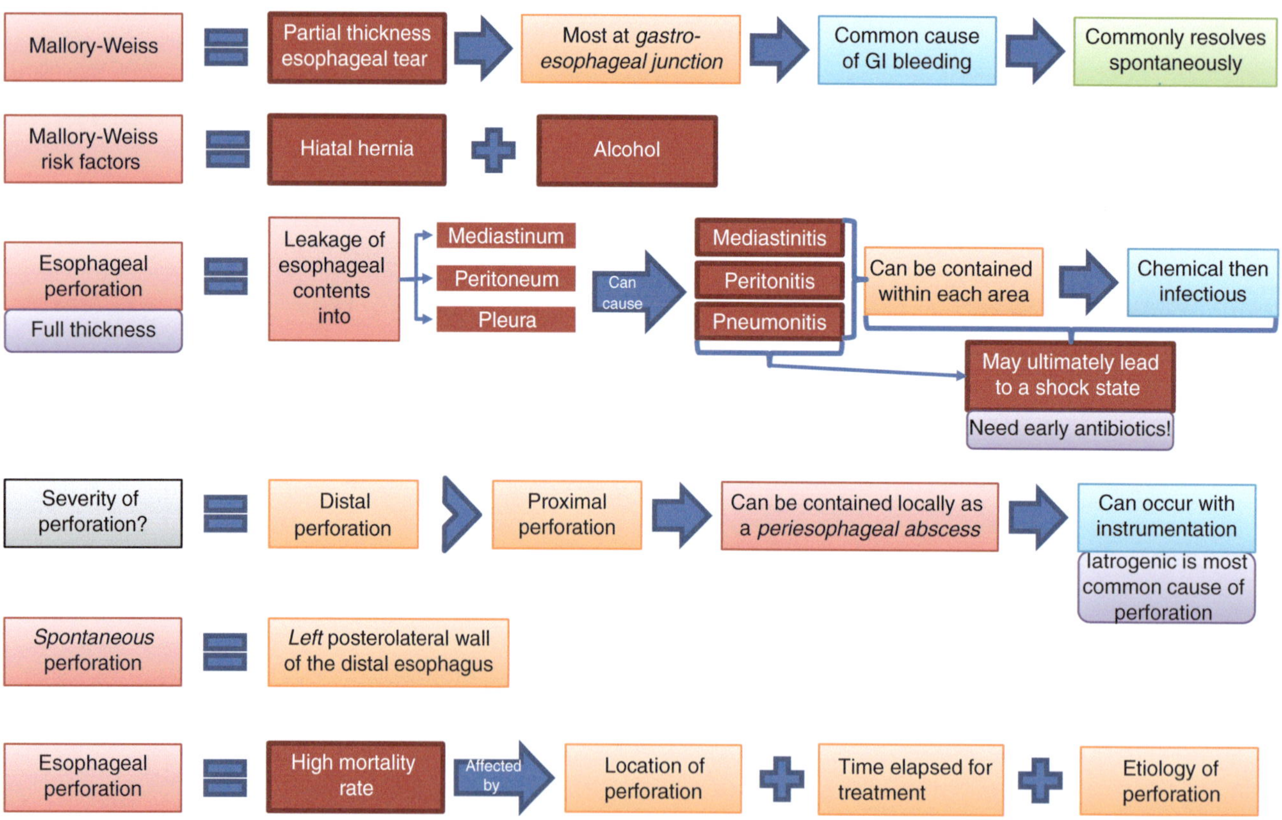

Causes of Esophageal Perforation

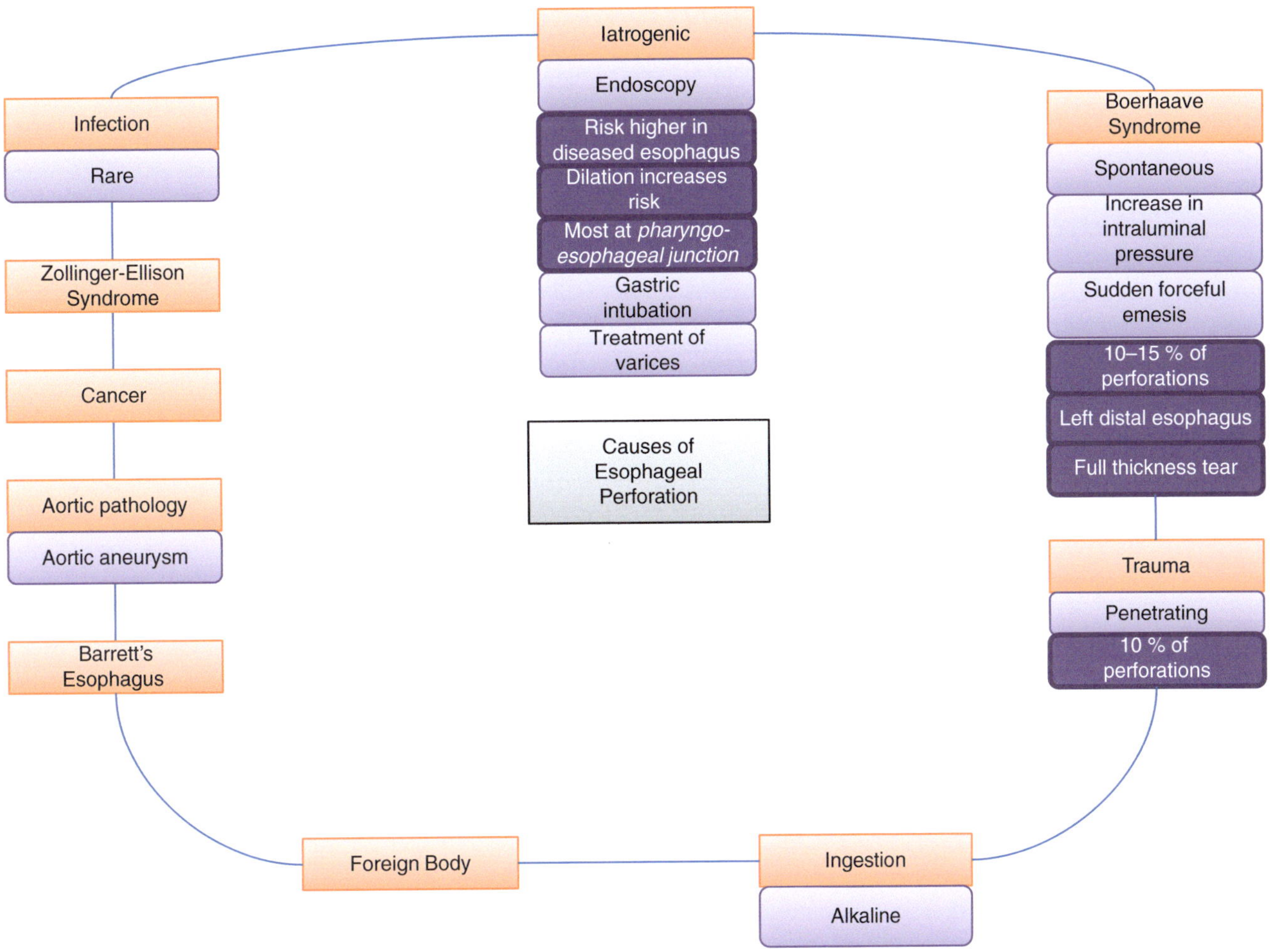

Esophageal Perforation Symptoms and Signs

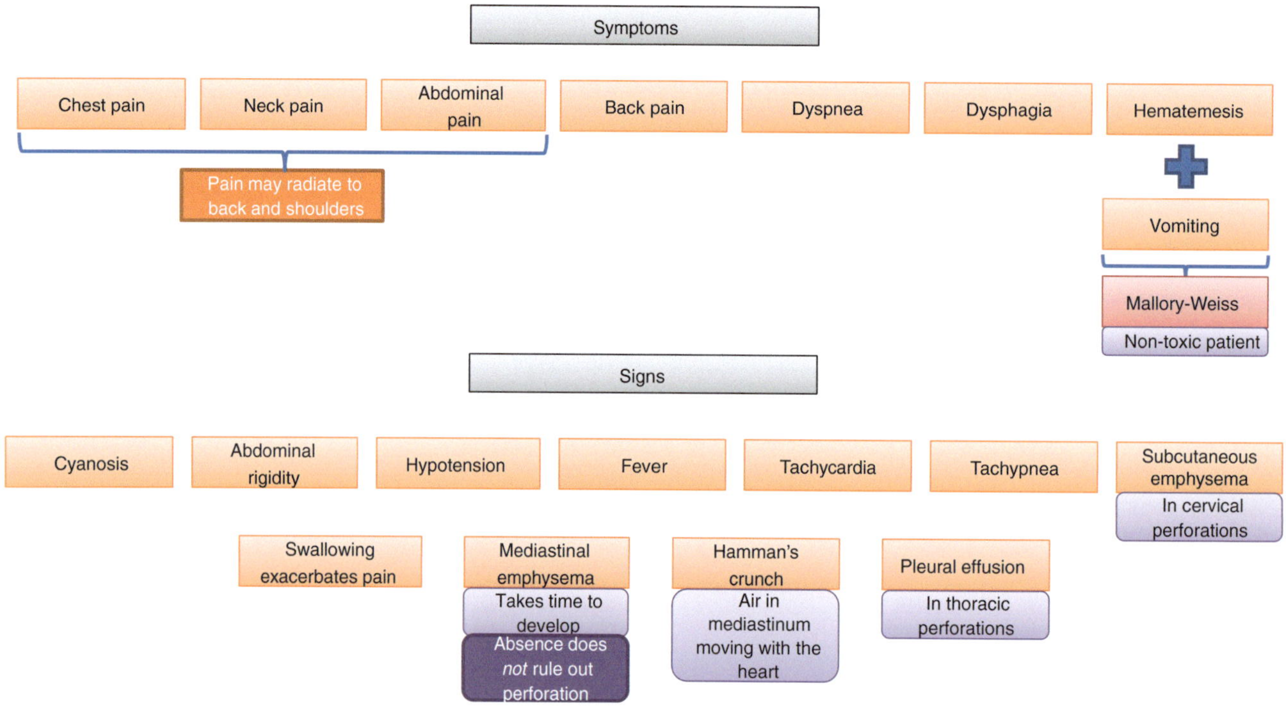

Diagnosis and Treatment

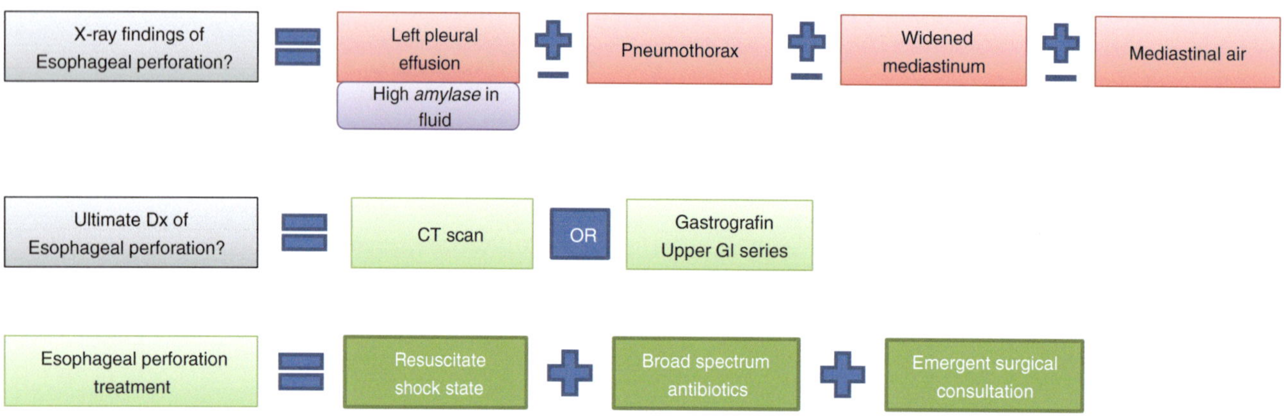

Esophageal Foreign Bodies

Children → Adults

- Children: 80 %. Small objects lodge in *proximal* esophagus
- Adults: Most impactions are *distal*

Levels of narrowing in esophagus

- **C6**: Cricopharyngeus muscle
- **T4**: Aortic arch
- **T6**: Tracheal bifurcation
- **T11**: Gastroesophageal junction

FB past the pylorus? = Usually continues through GI tract → Unless Sharp or irregular OR Long (> 6 cm) OR Wide (> 2.5 cm) = May become lodged distal to the pylorus. Requiring OR vs. endoscopy

FB Complications = Esophageal perforation OR Esophageal strictures OR Airway obstruction

Esophageal Foreign Body Symptoms and Signs

Center bottom image (Reprinted without modification from James Heilman https://commons.wikimedia.org/wiki/File:CoinAP.jpg. With permission from the Creative Commons License https://creativecommons.org/licenses/by-sa/3.0/deed.en)

Symptoms & Signs

- Chest pain
- Dysphagia
- Vomiting
- Choking or gagging
- Coughing
- Dysphagia
- Drooling
- Refusal to eat
- Neck pain
- Sore throat
- Vomiting

Especially in children = High index of suspiciion

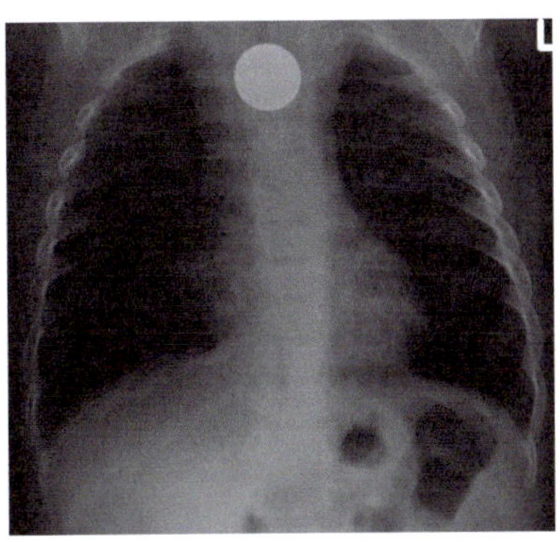

Diagnosis and Treatment of Esophageal Foreign Bodies

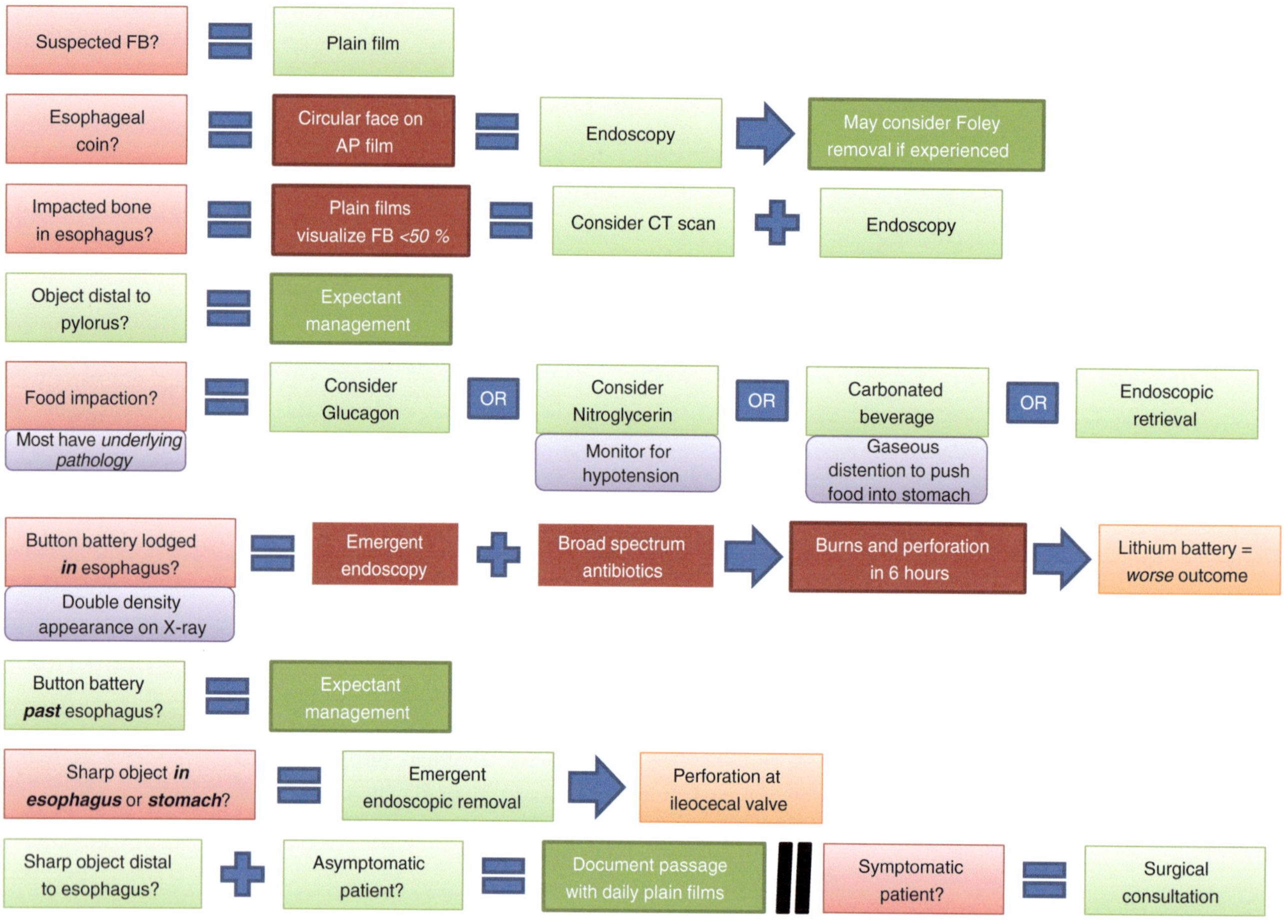

Caustic Ingestions

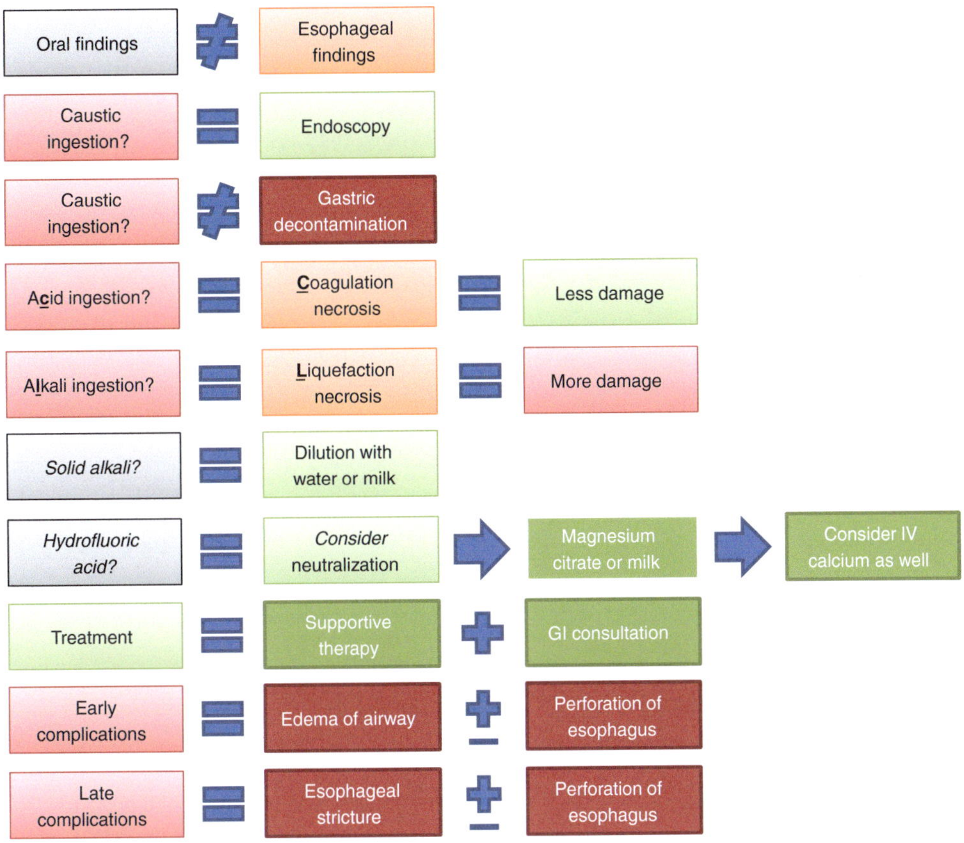

GERD

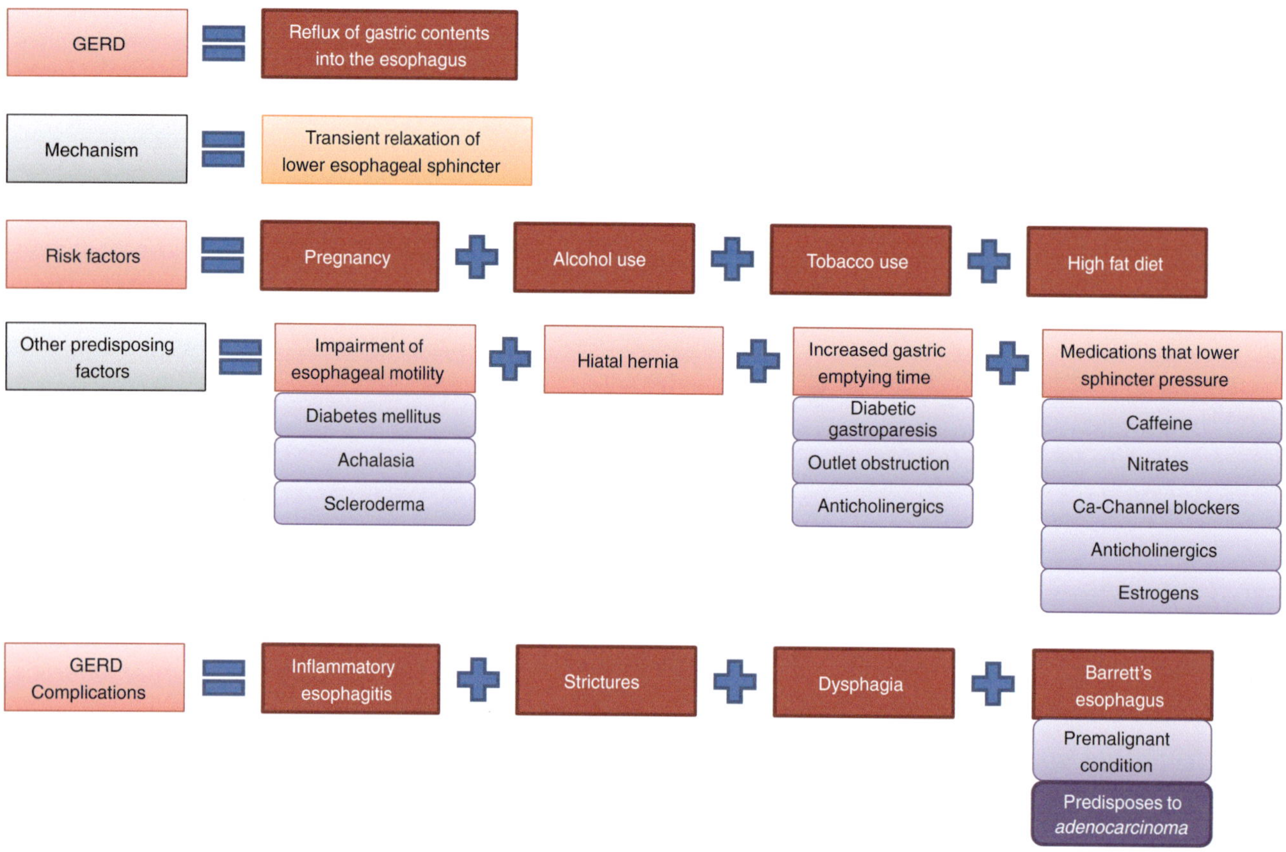

GERD Symptoms and Signs

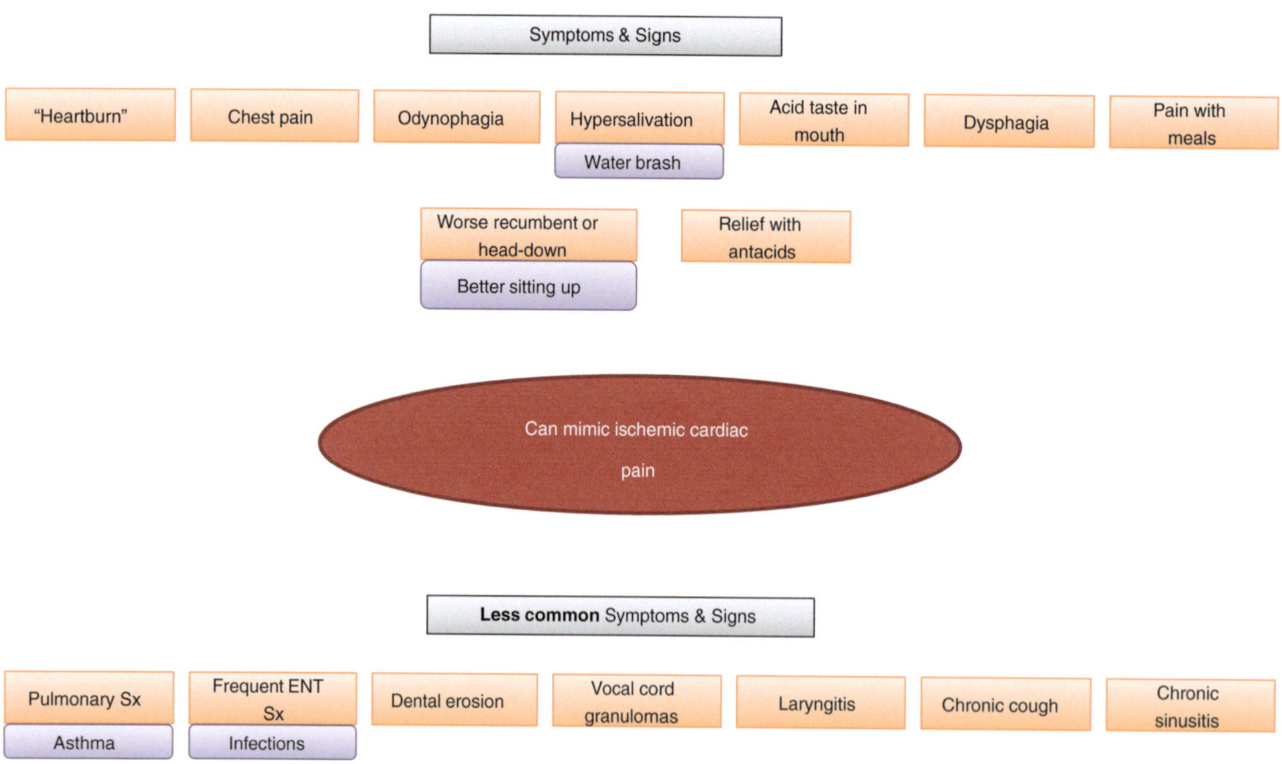

GERD Treatment

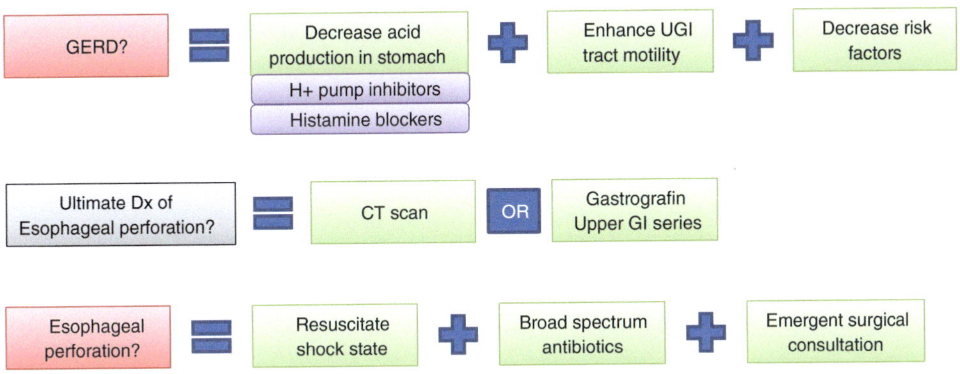

Esophagitis

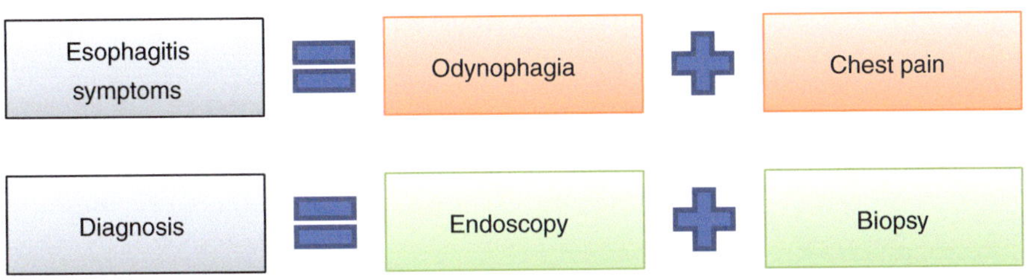

Causes of Esophagitis

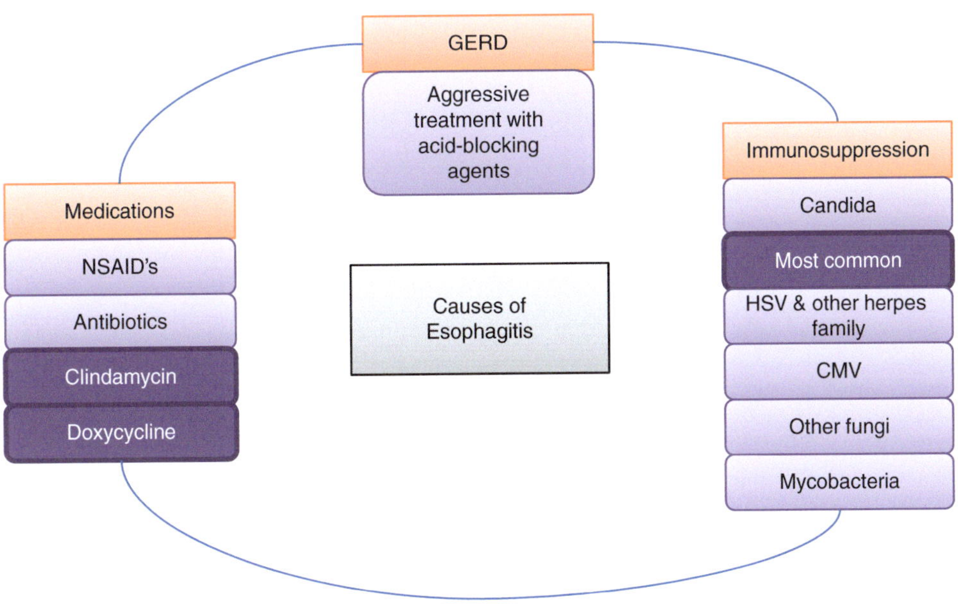

Peptic Ulcer Disease

Introduction

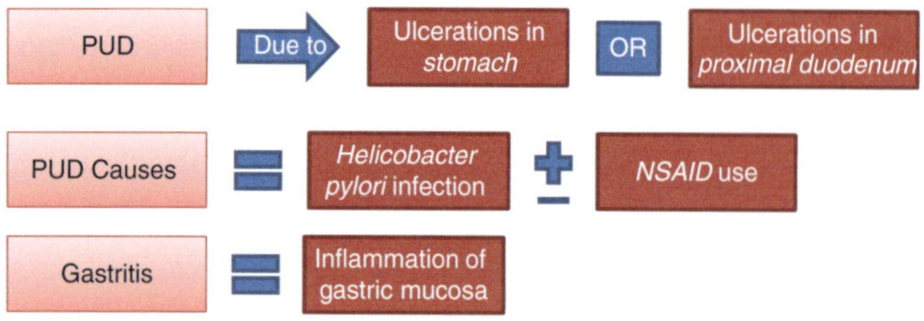

Pathophysiology

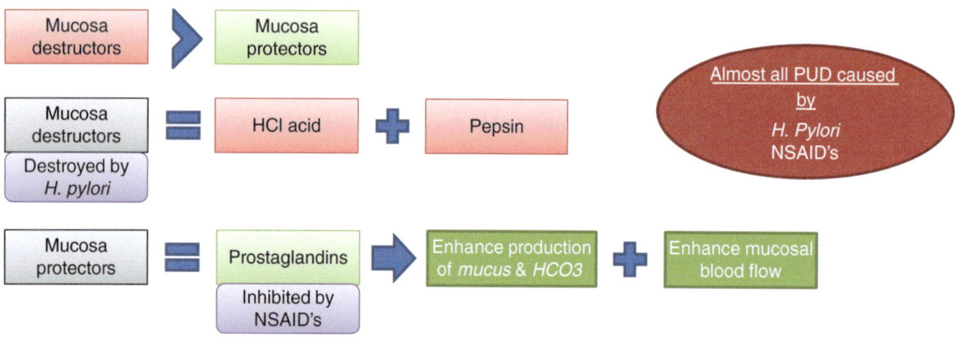

Causes of PUD and Gastritis

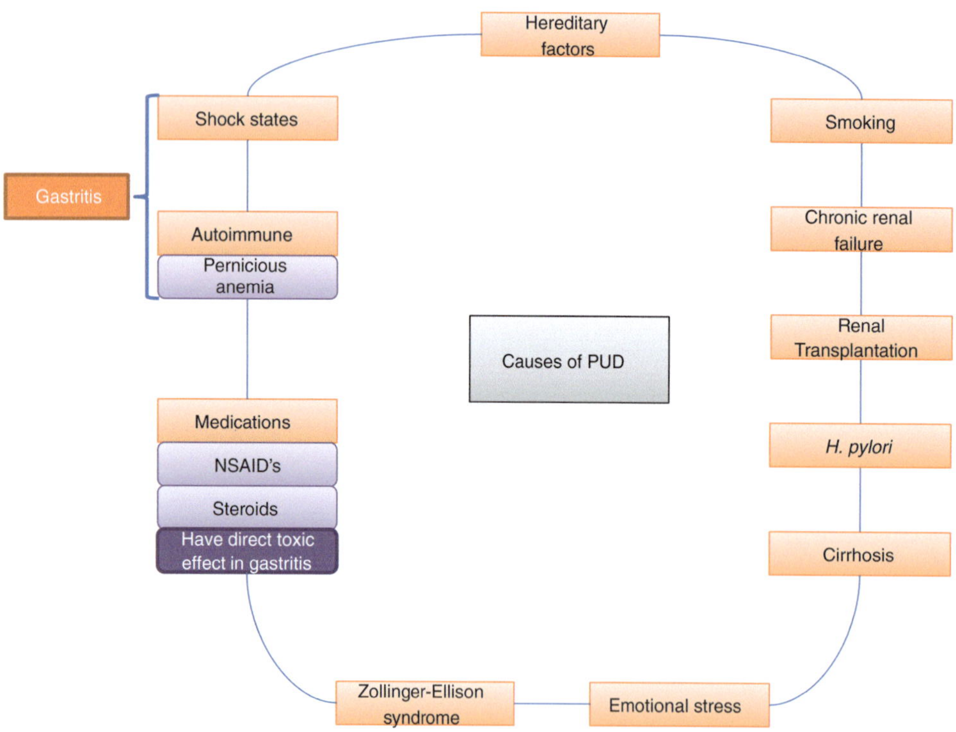

PUD Symptoms and Signs

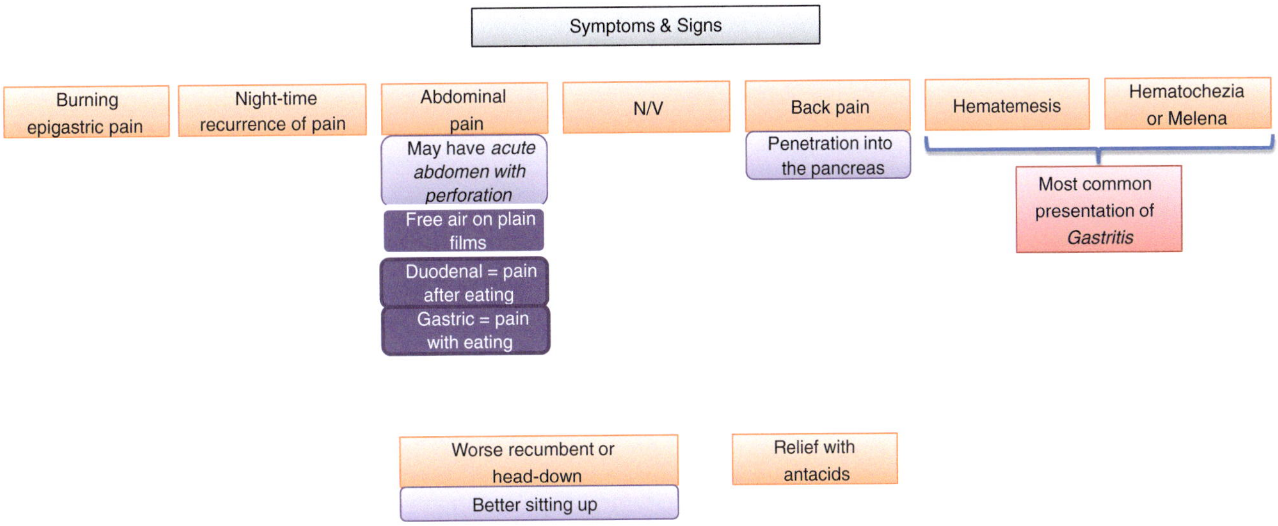

PUD Diagnosis and Treatment

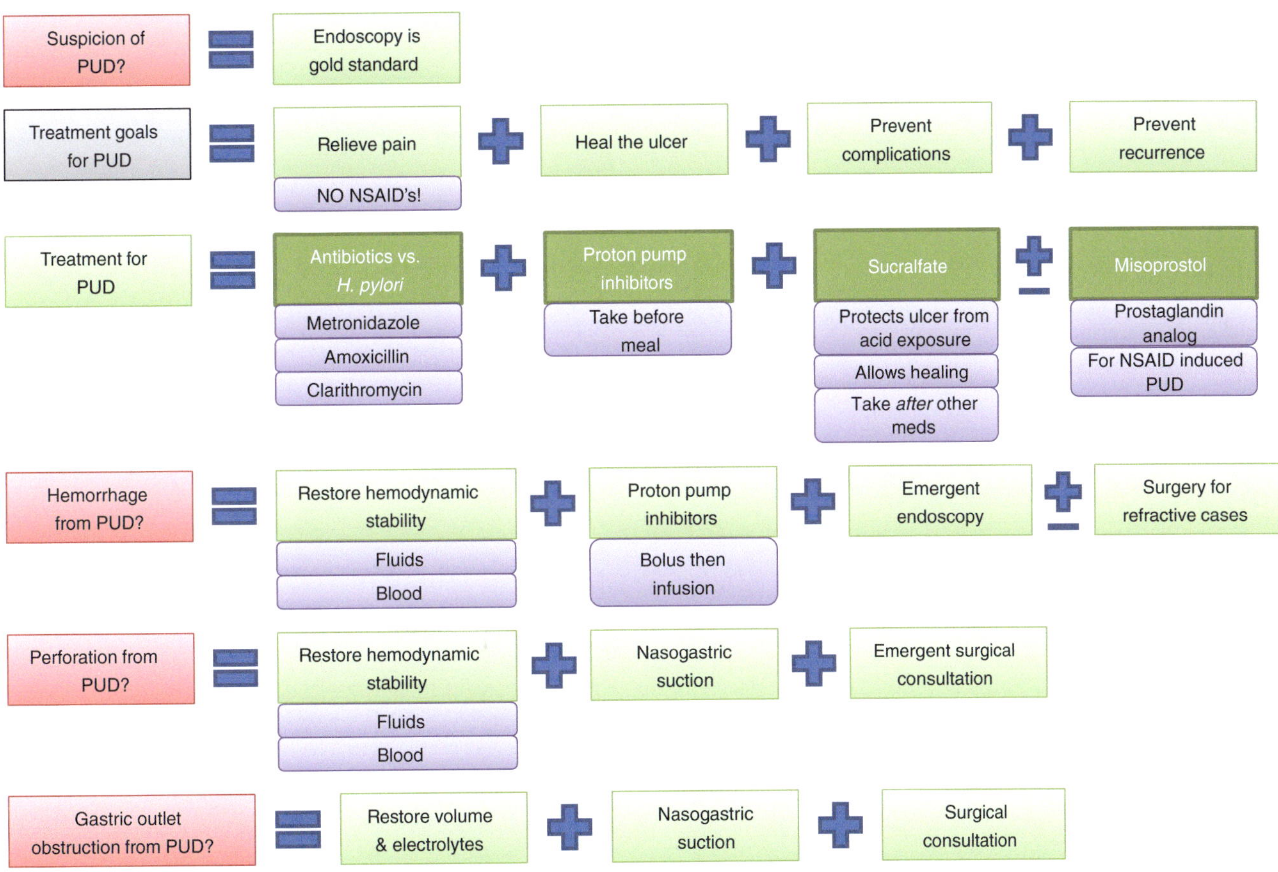

PUD Complications

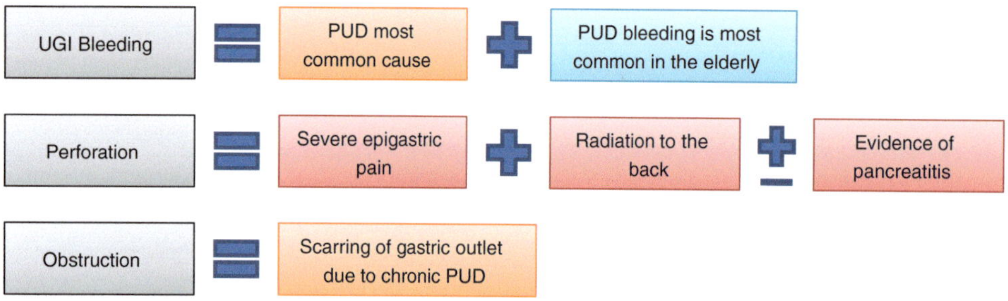

GI Bleeding

Terminology

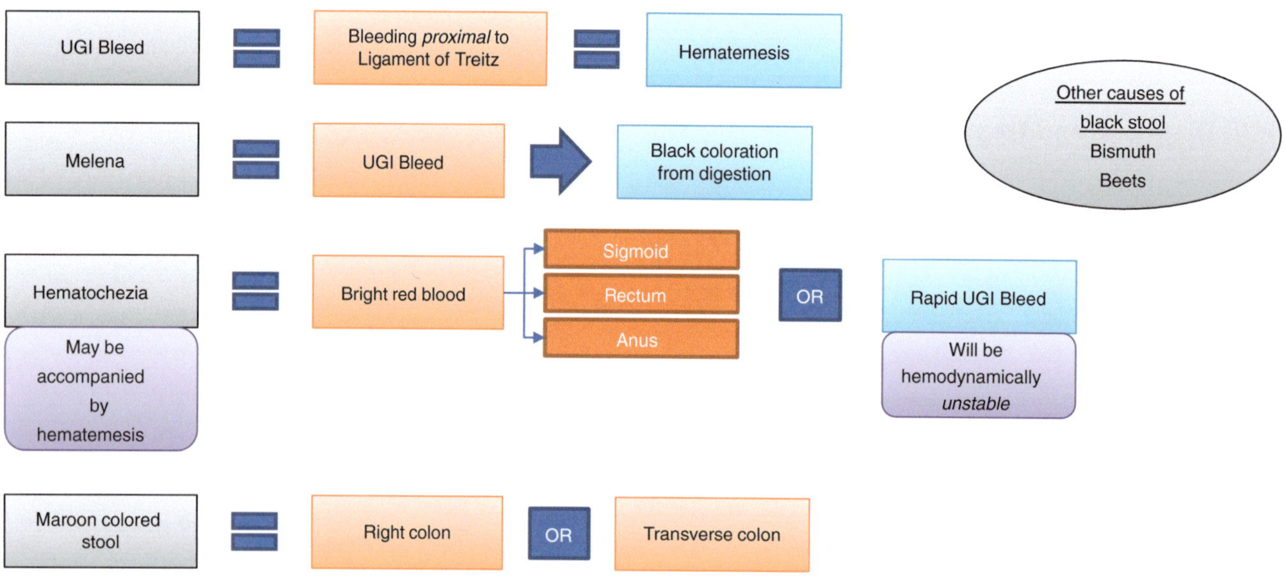

Introduction: Upper GI Bleeding (UGIB)

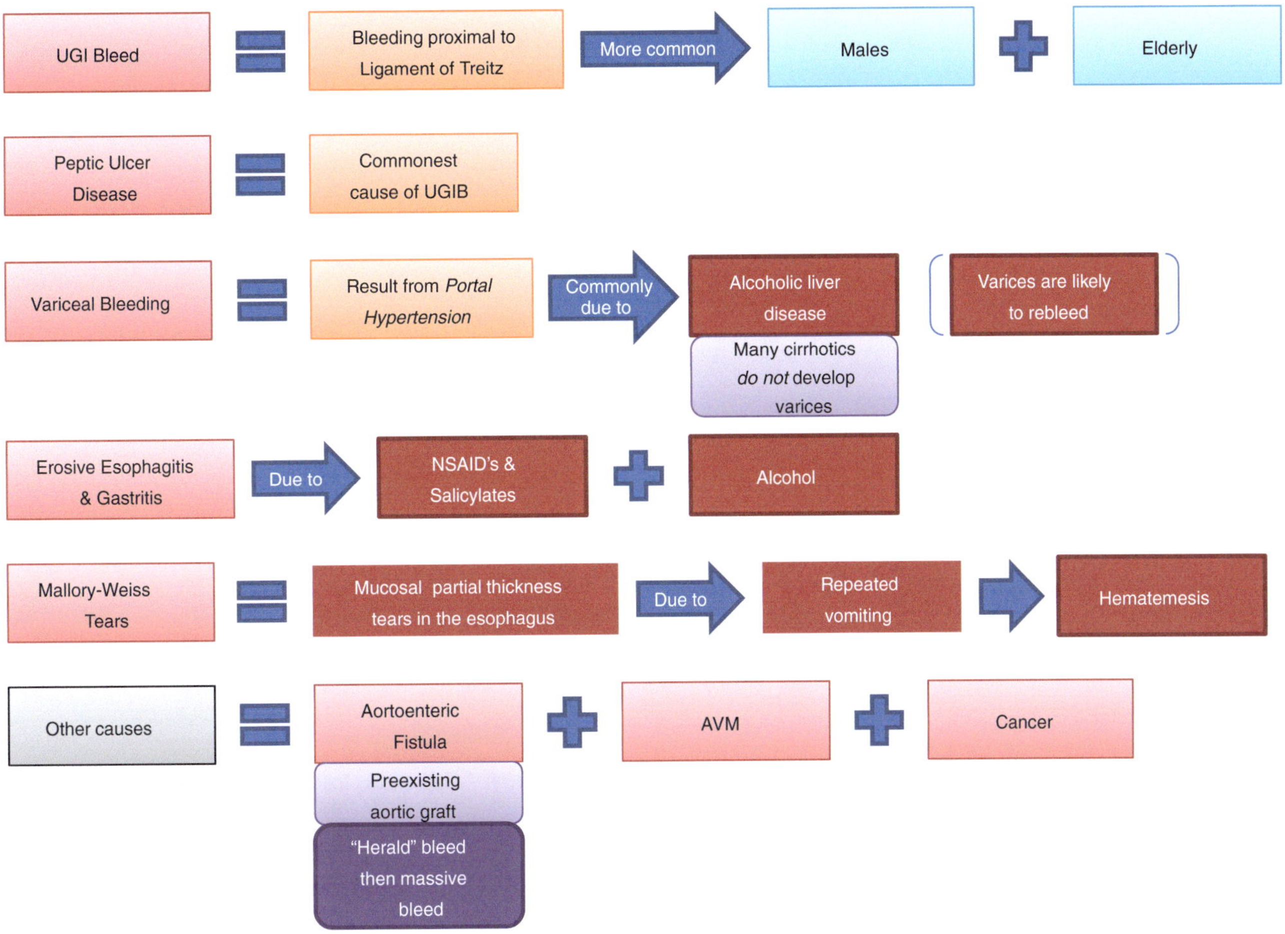

UGIB Symptoms and Signs

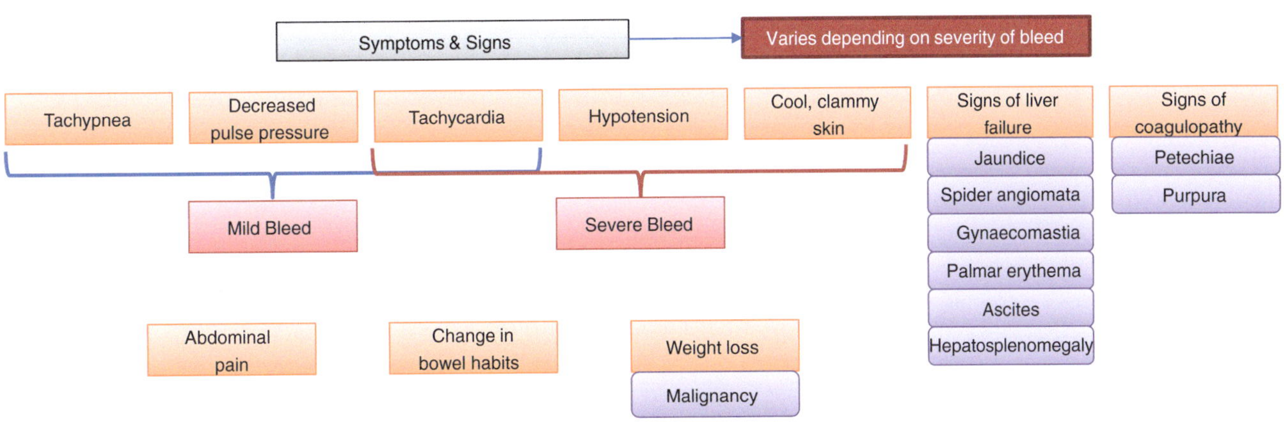

UGIB Diagnosis and Treatment

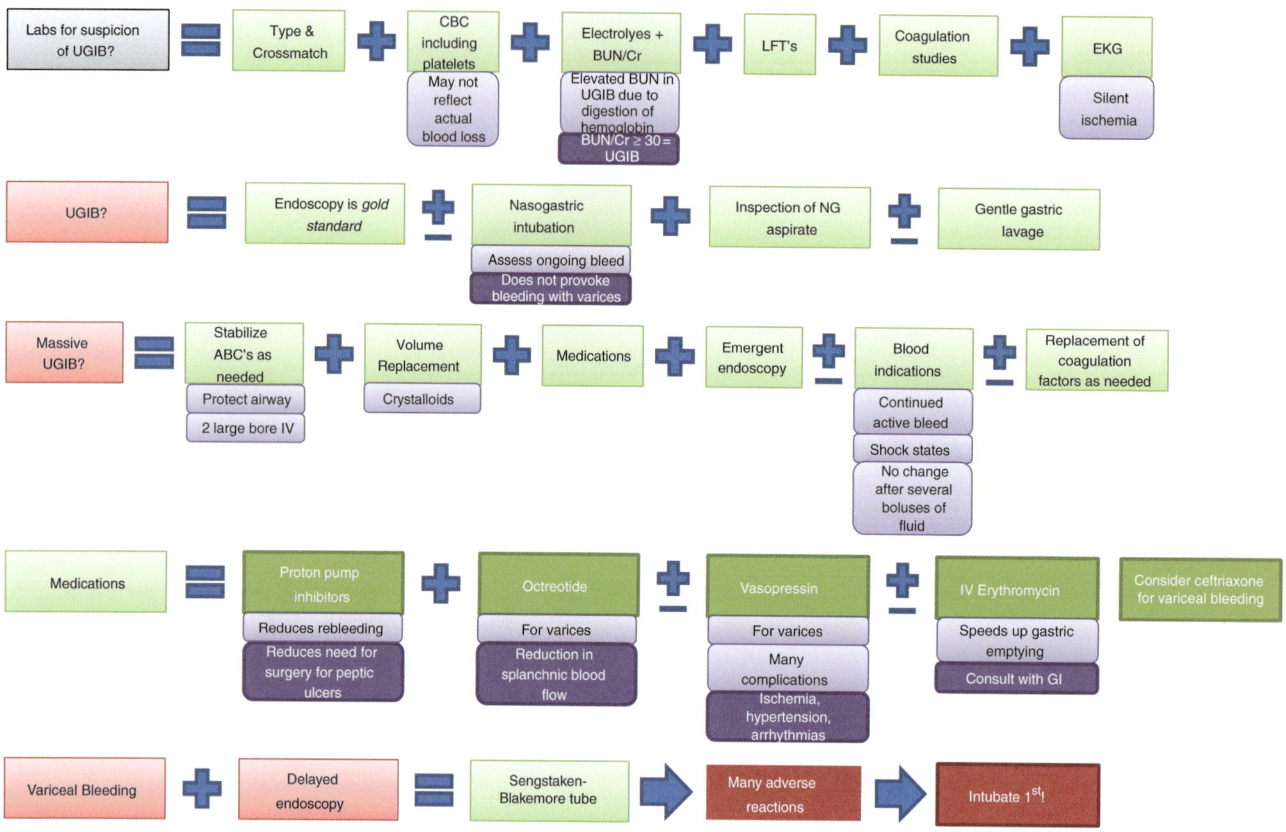

Disposition

Image just left of center (Reprinted from Allen B, Ganti L, Desai B. GI bleeding/hemorrhage. In: Allen B, Ganti L, Desai B, editors. Quick hits in emergency medicine. New York: Springer Science; 2013. p. 83–5. With permission from Springer Science + Business Media)

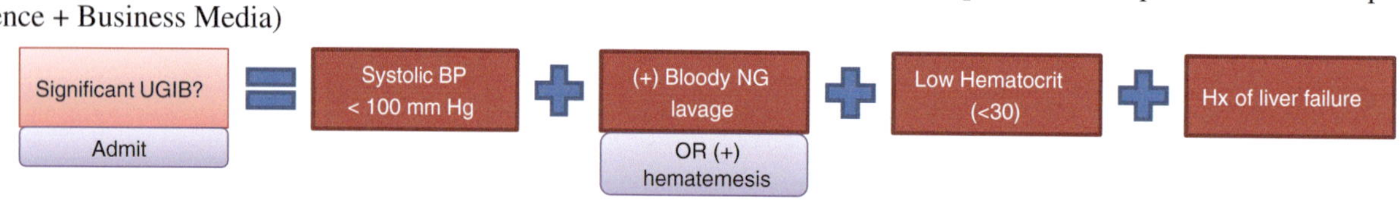

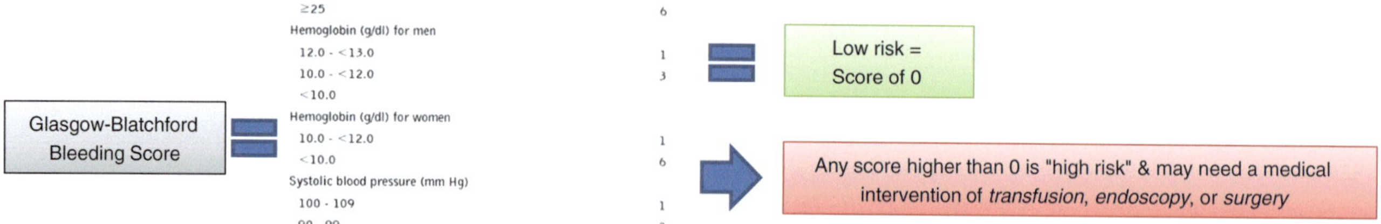

Criteria on admission	Score
Blood urea (mmol/l)	
6.5 - <8.0	2
8.0 - <10.0	3
10.0 - <25.0	4
≥25	6
Hemoglobin (g/dl) for men	
12.0 - <13.0	1
10.0 - <12.0	3
<10.0	
Hemoglobin (g/dl) for women	
10.0 - <12.0	1
<10.0	6
Systolic blood pressure (mm Hg)	
100 - 109	1
90 - 99	2
<90	3
Other markers	
Pulse ≥100 (per min)	1
Presentation with melena	1
Presentation with syncope	2
Hepatic disease	2
Cardiac failure	2

Introduction: Lower GI Bleed (LGIB)

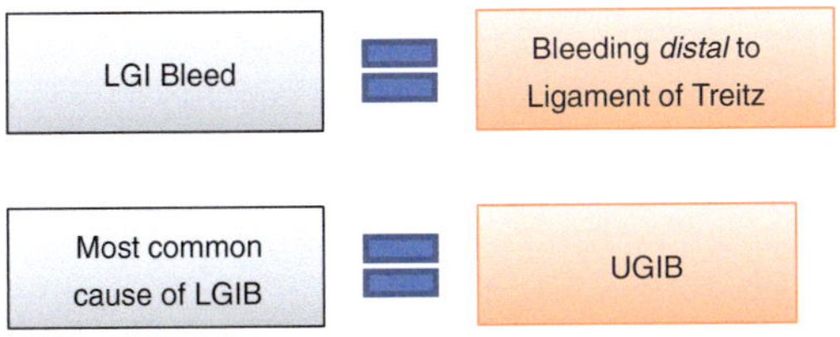

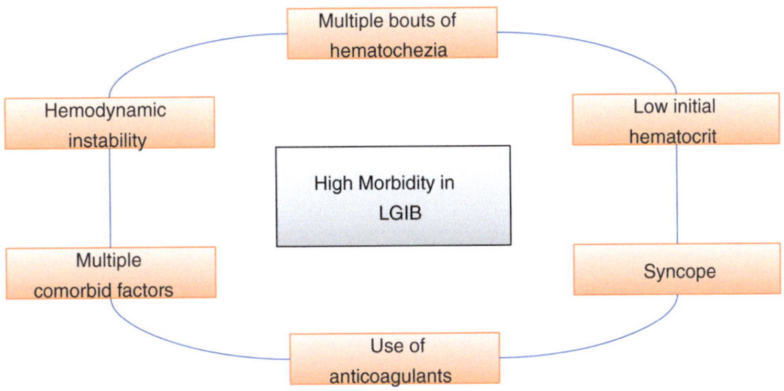

Some Causes of LGIB

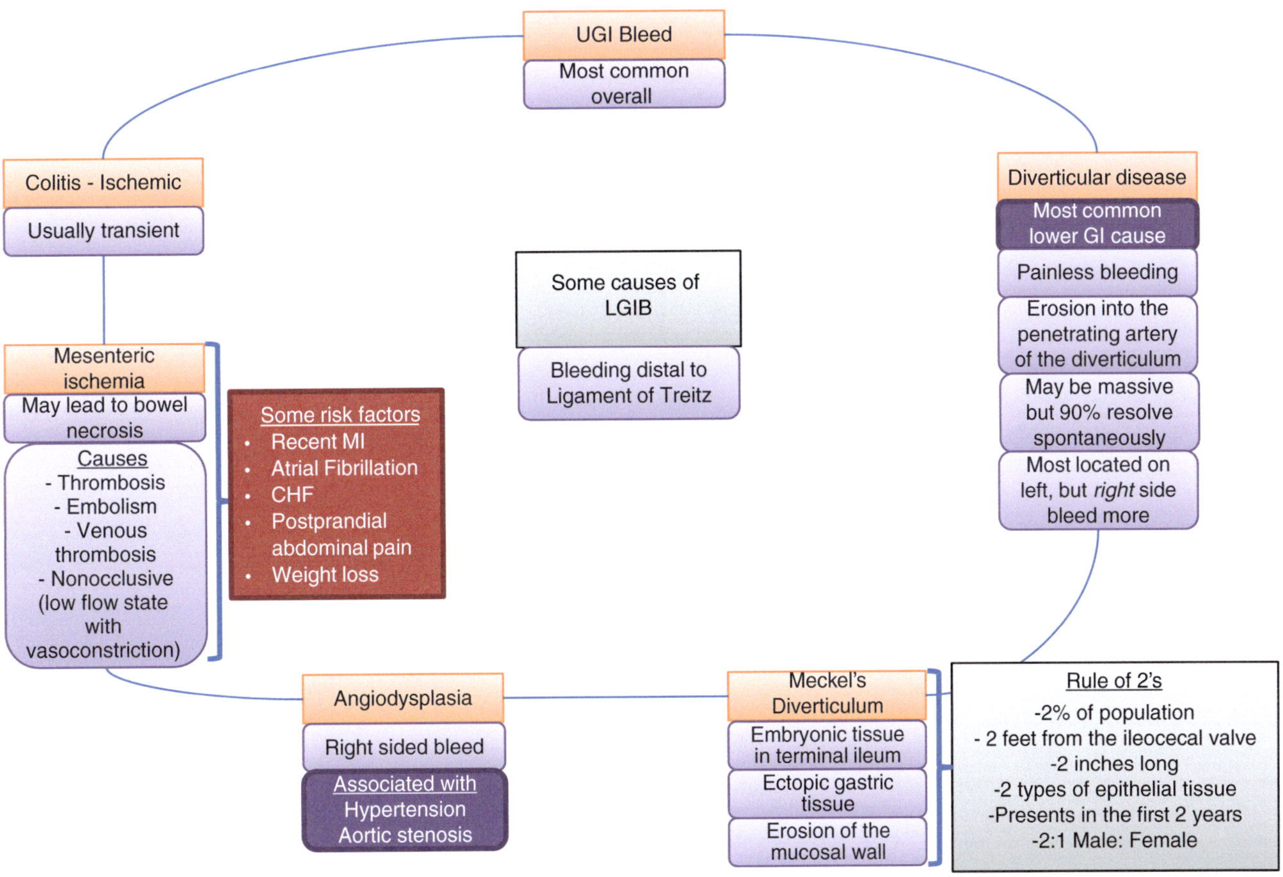

Other Causes of LGIB

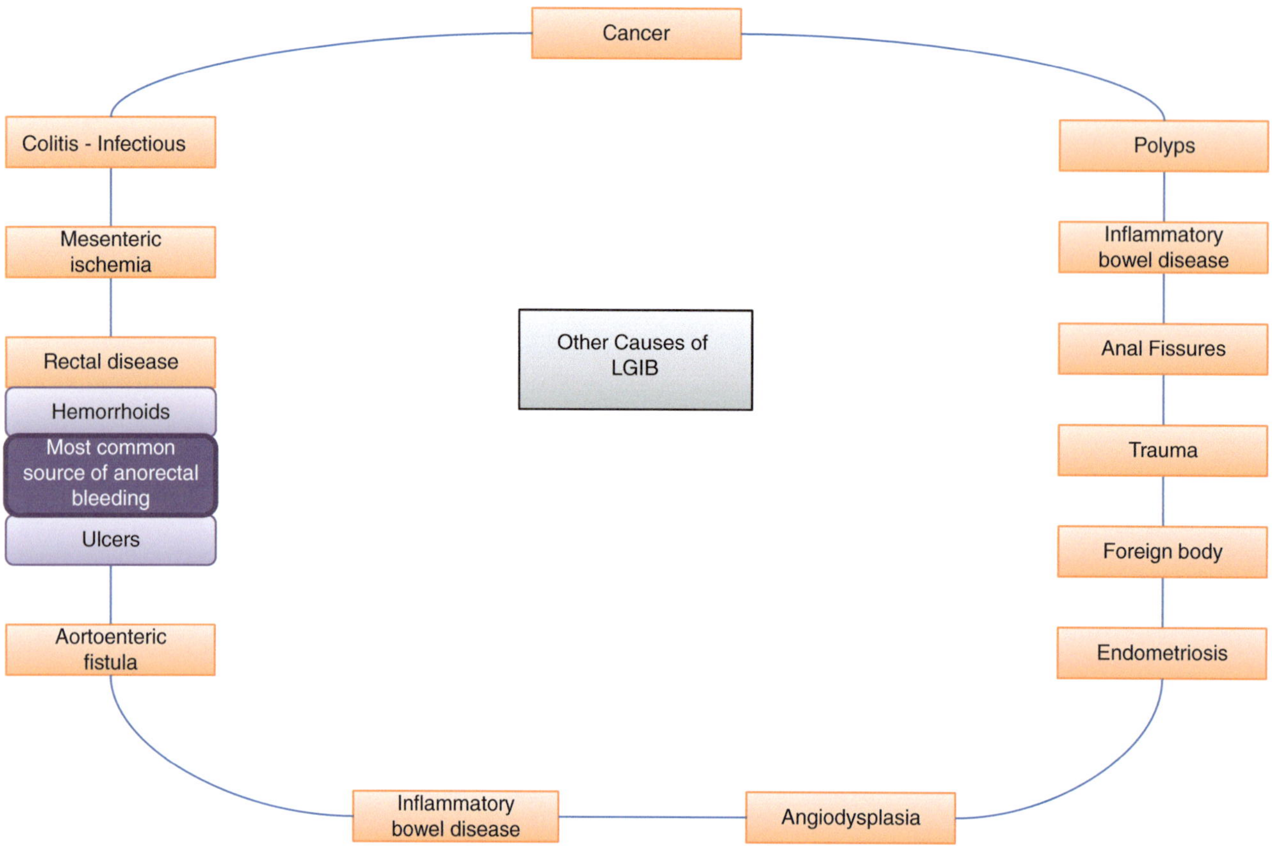

LGIB Diagnosis and Treatment

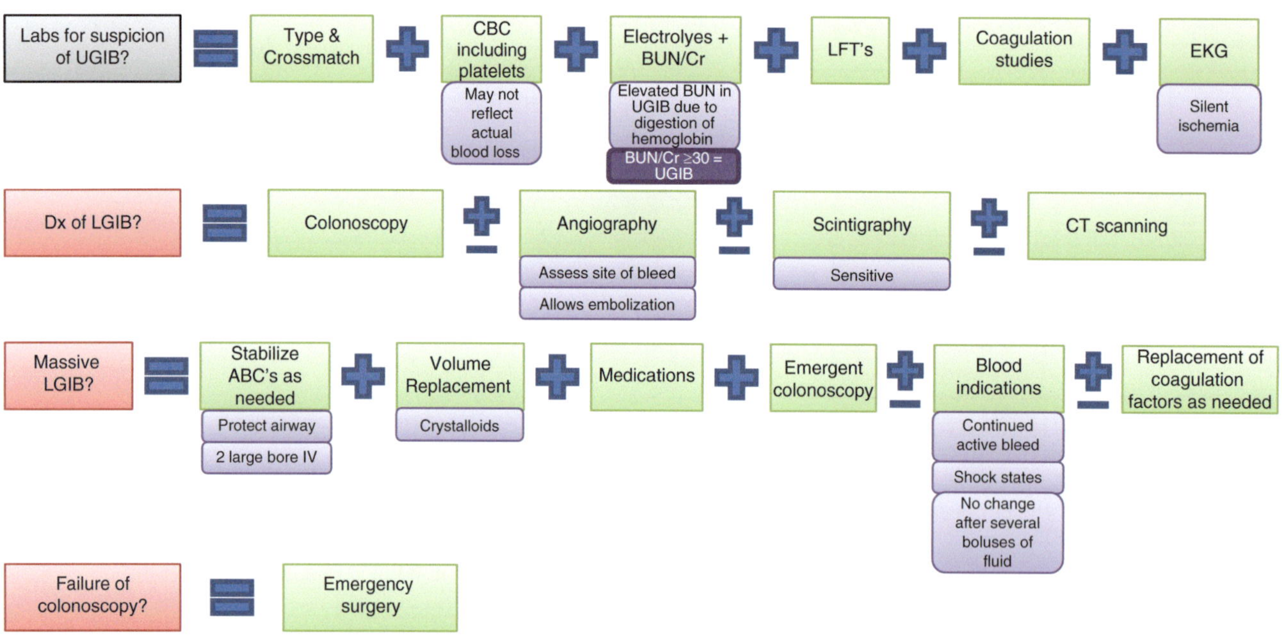

Disposition

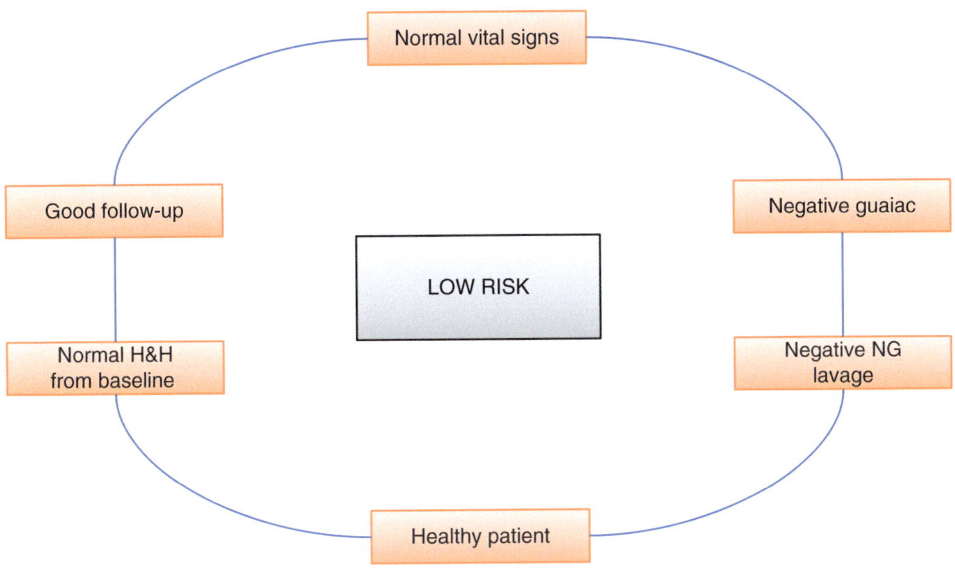

Liver and Gallbladder

Introduction: Liver

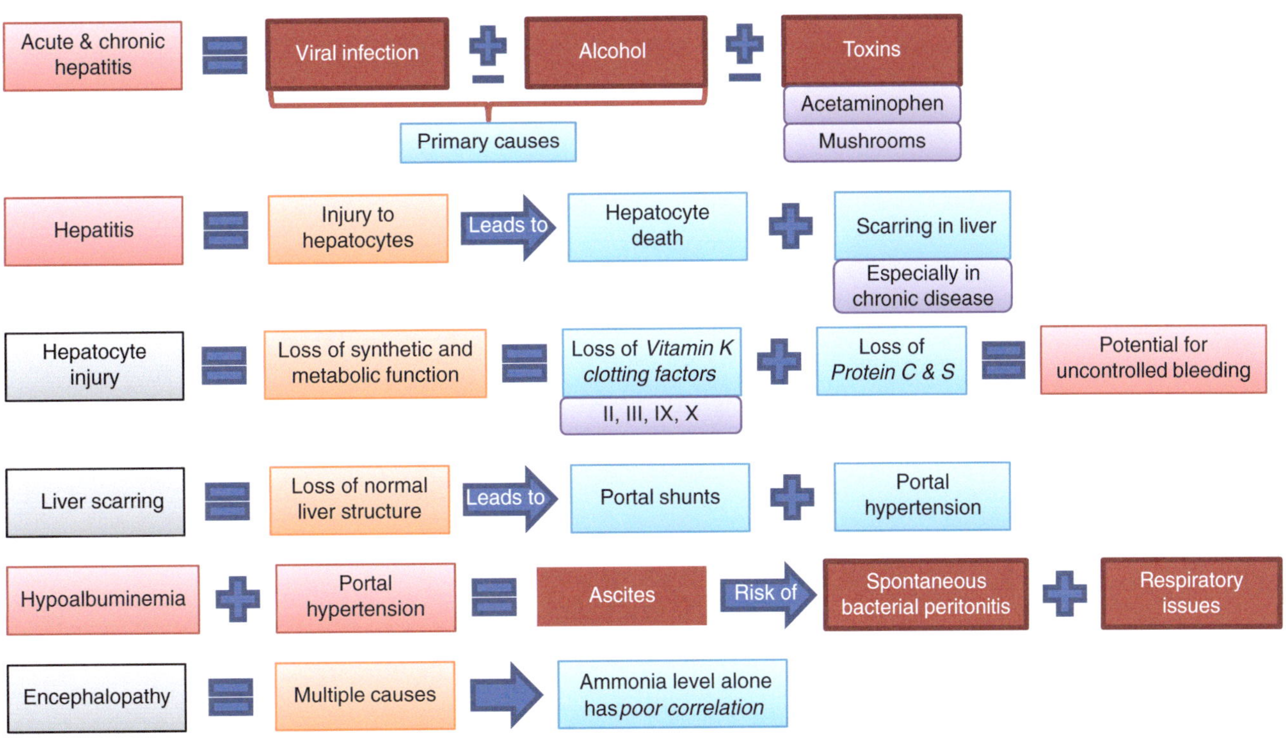

Bilirubin Evaluation

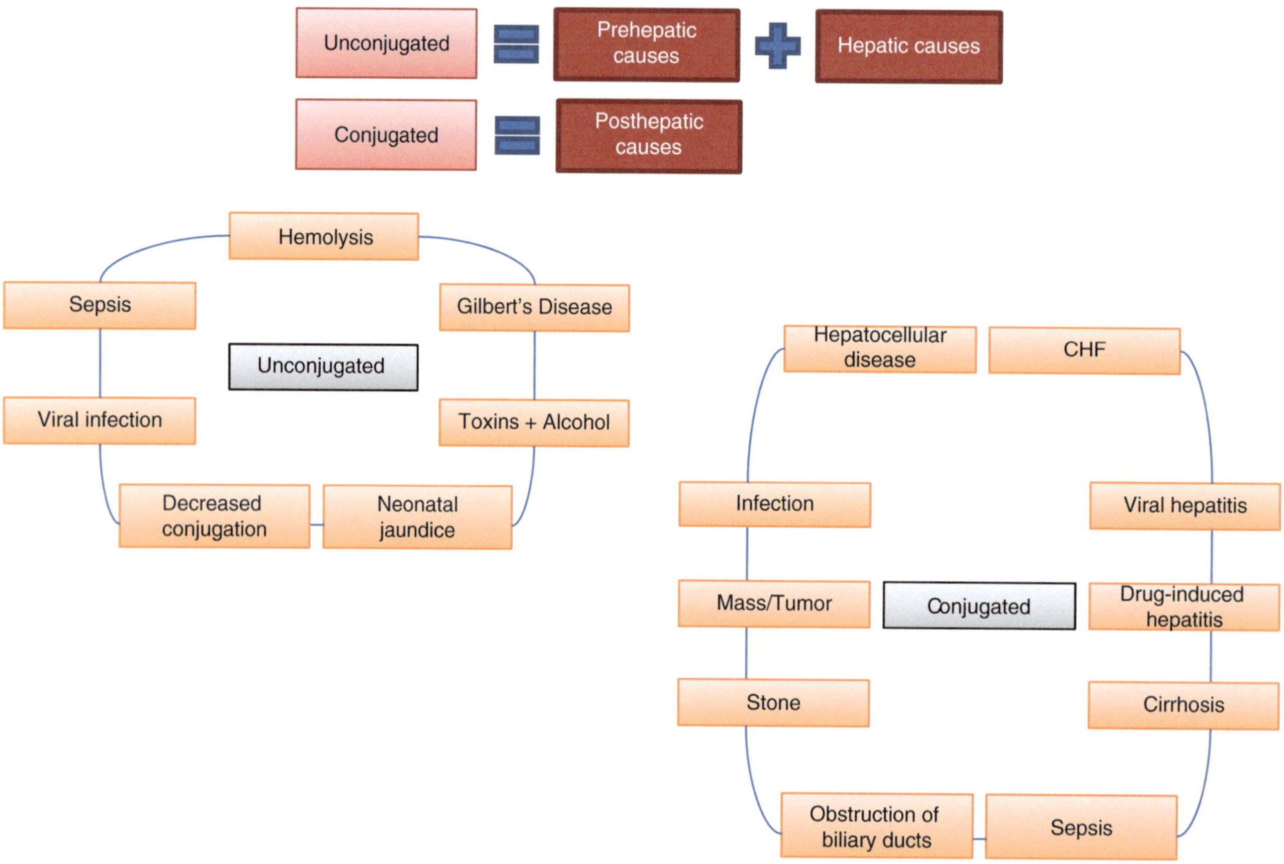

Neonatal Jaundice

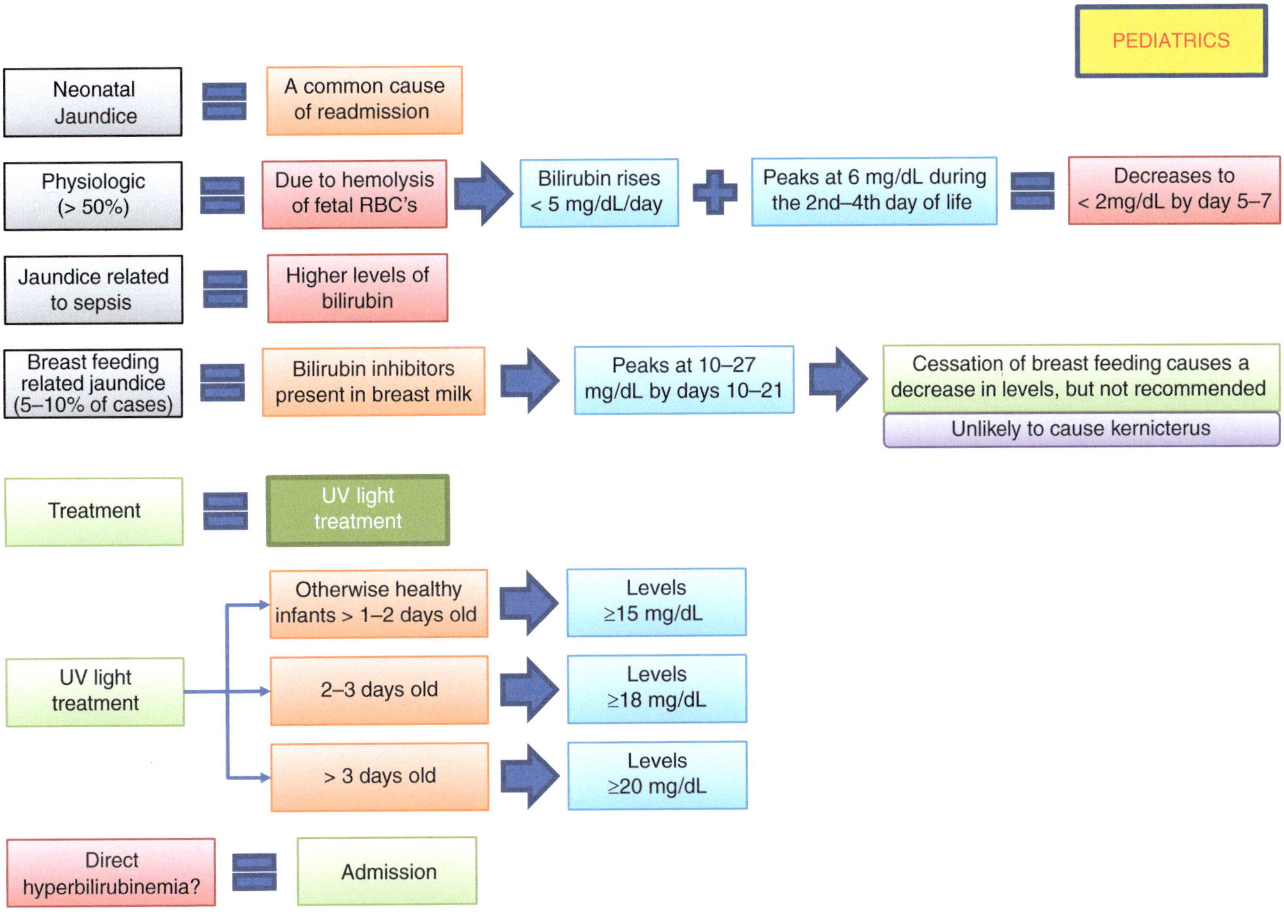

Hepatitis Symptoms and Signs

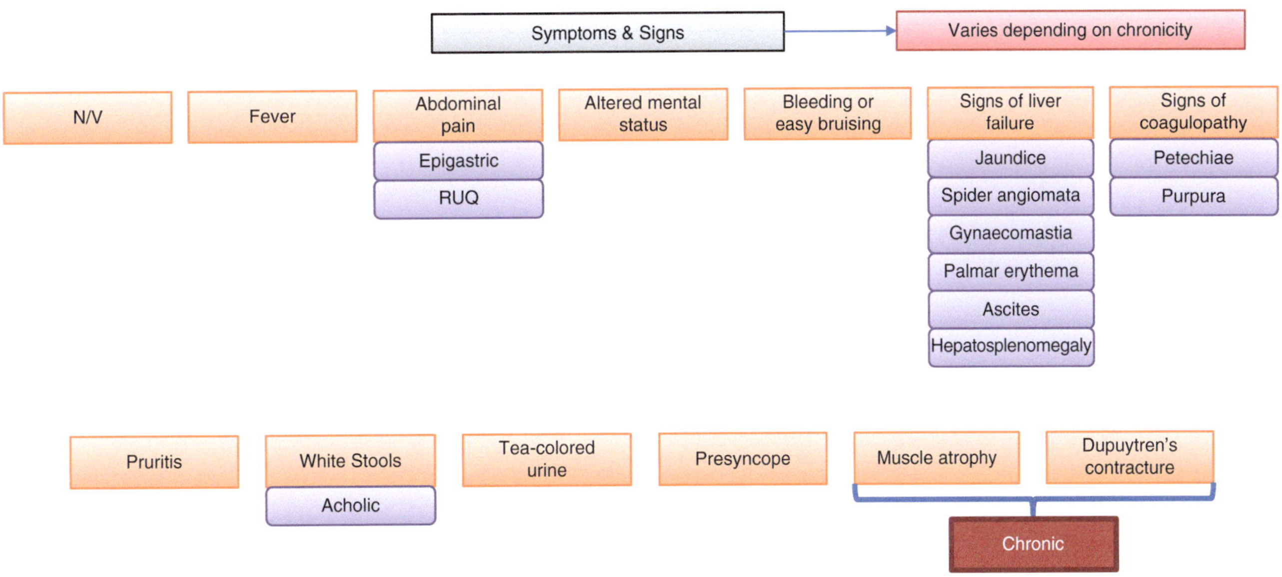

Laboratory Abnormalities in Hepatitis

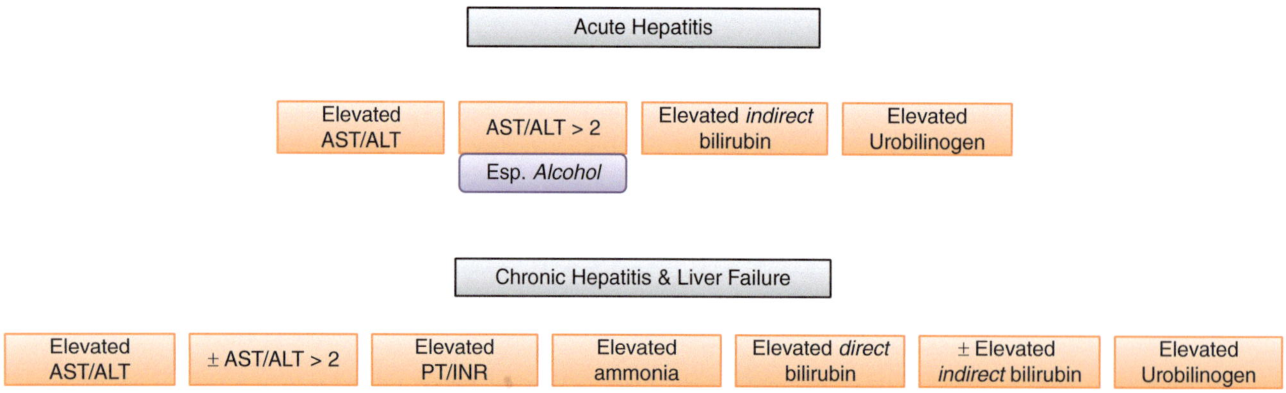

Indications for Hospitalization for Any Hepatitis

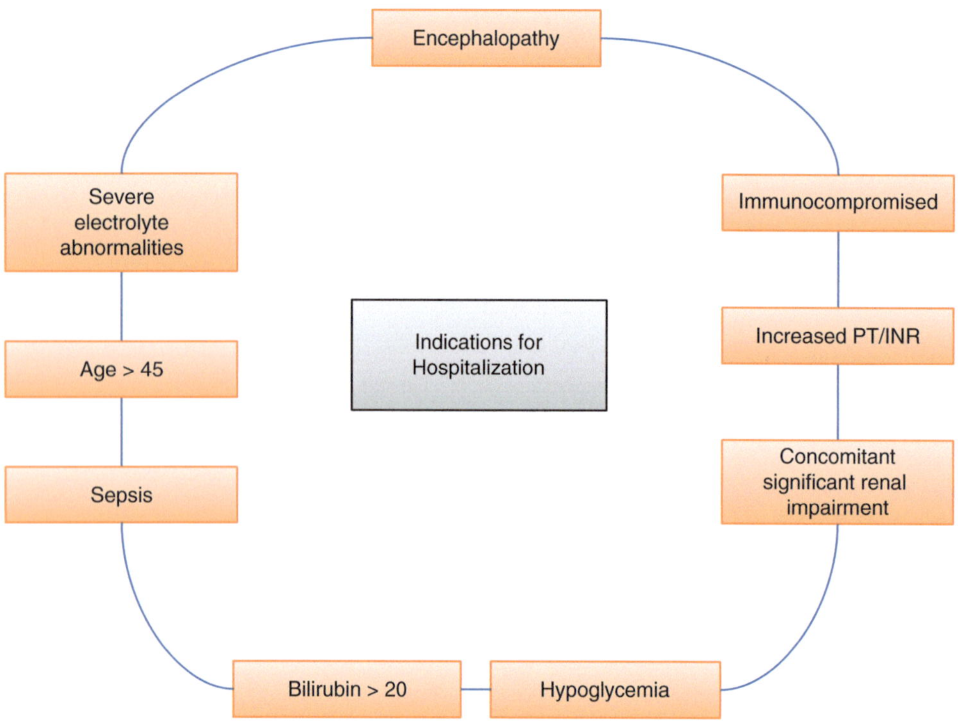

Hepatitis A

Hepatitis A = *Fecal-oral route* via contaminated water or food + Most common cause of *conjugated hyperbilirubinemia* in children + *No* chronic carrier state

Hepatitis A = Incubation of 15–50 days

Hepatitis A symptoms & signs = Nausea/Vomiting & Weakness → Dark urine → Jaundice + Light stools

Prophylaxis = Hepatitis A vaccine

Treatment = Immune globulin within *2 weeks of exposure*

Prognosis? = Majority are *self-limiting*

Hepatitis B

Hepatitis B = DNA virus + Transmission via blood, sexual exposure, & parenteral exposure

Hepatitis B complications = Cirrhosis + Liver cancer + 5-10% chronic carrier state → Hepatitis D co-infection increases risks of complications

Hepatitis B = Incubation of 1–6 months → Pts may be infectious for 5–15 weeks after Sx onset

Markers = HBsAg (+) early + HBsAb (+) after clearance of HbsAg; Best marker for immunity + HBeAg Marker for high infectivity; Risk of contracting HBV after exposure high if source is HbeAg(+) + HBcAb Appears *after* HbsAg; Best marker for *prior* infection

Treatment – Unvaccinated = HB immune globulin + Vaccination (0, 1, 6 months) → Repeat series if nonresponder

Risk of contracting HBV after exposure if **not** successfully vaccinated = 6-30%

Treatment – Vaccinated = NO TREATMENT if HbsAb positive → If (-) → HB immune globulin (Effective within 1 week of exposure) + Vaccination (0, 1, 6 months)

There are non-converters to the vaccine after vaccination!

Hepatitis C

Hepatitis C = RNA virus + Transmission via contaminated blood or blood products (Sexual transmission is *rare*) + Most common cause of viral infection with blood transfusion

Hepatitis C complications = 50% chronic disease + Cirrhosis + Hepatocellular carcinoma

Hepatitis C = Usually aymptomatic acutely

Hepatitis C = Higher incidence in pts with HIV

Hepatitis C = After exposure conversion rate is 2 % → No effective post-exposure prophylaxis

Hepatitis C = No vaccine available

Hepatitis D

Hepatitis D = Requires *Hepatitis B surface antigen* for co-infection + Most commonly from *injection drug use*

Hepatitis D complications = Rapidly progressive liver failure = High short term mortality

Hepatitis E and G

Hepatitis E = Fecal-oral transmission + Can occur in pregnancy + Higher incidence in Russia, Asia & Africa

Hepatitis G = Via *blood transfusions & sexual exposure*

Toxic Hepatitis

Toxic Hepatitis = Acetaminophen (Most common) + *Multiple* other prescription medications + Mushrooms (Amanita) + Alcohol

Acetaminophen overdose? = N-acetylcysteine

INH overdose? = Treat with B6

Severe hepatic necrosis with AST/ALT > 1000? → Consider: Acetaminophen OR Mushrooms OR Carbon tetrachloride

Hepatic Encephalopathy

Hepatic encephalopathy precipitants = Sedatives + Infection + Dehydration or volume loss + Electrolyte imbalances + GI bleeding

Ammonia level = Poor correlation

Early sign = Sleep inversion = Sleep during day, not night

Other signs = Asterixis ("Liver flap")

Pitfall? = Hypoglycemia

Treatment = Treat precipitants + Lactulose + Neomycin + Decreased dietary protein

Spontaneous Bacterial Peritonitis

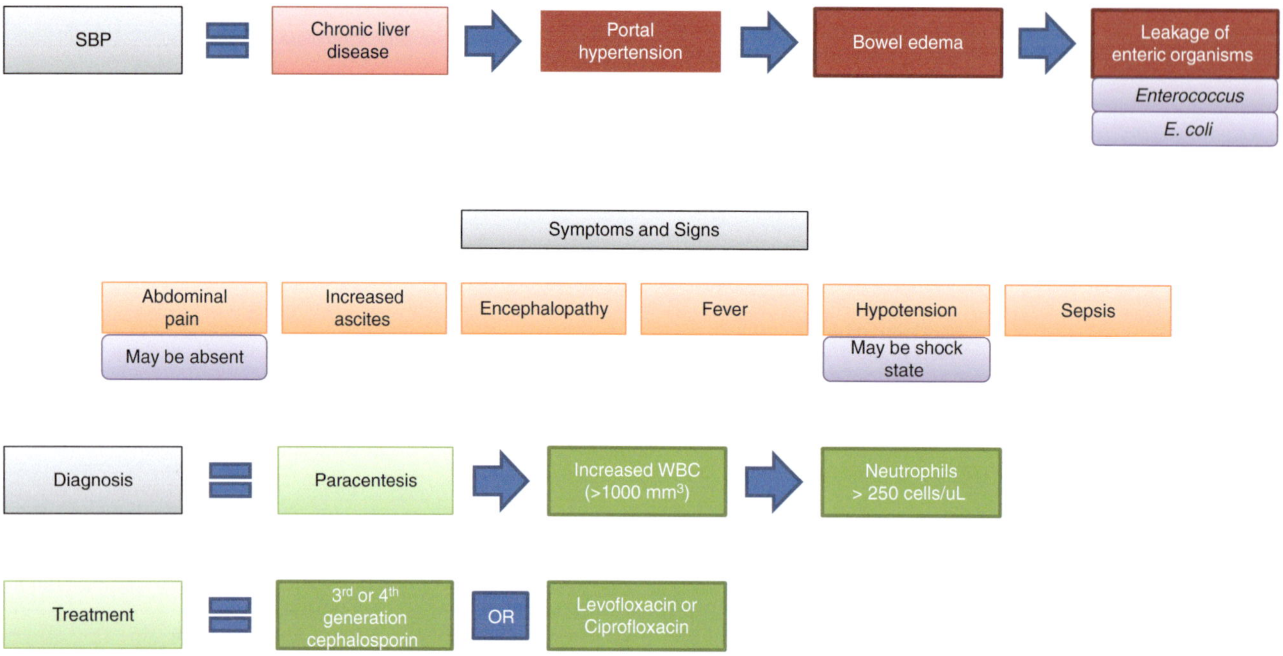

Introduction: Gallbladder

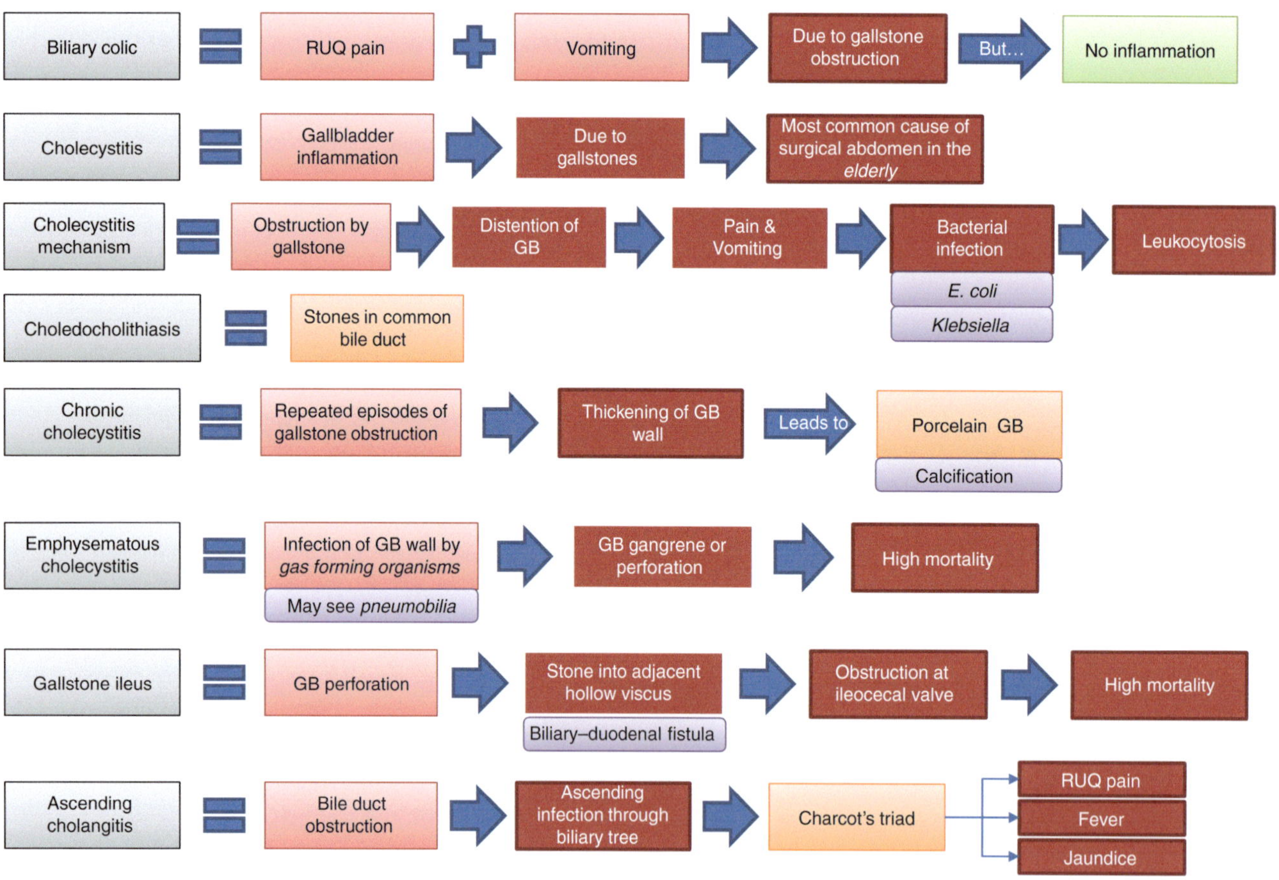

Acalculous Cholecystitis

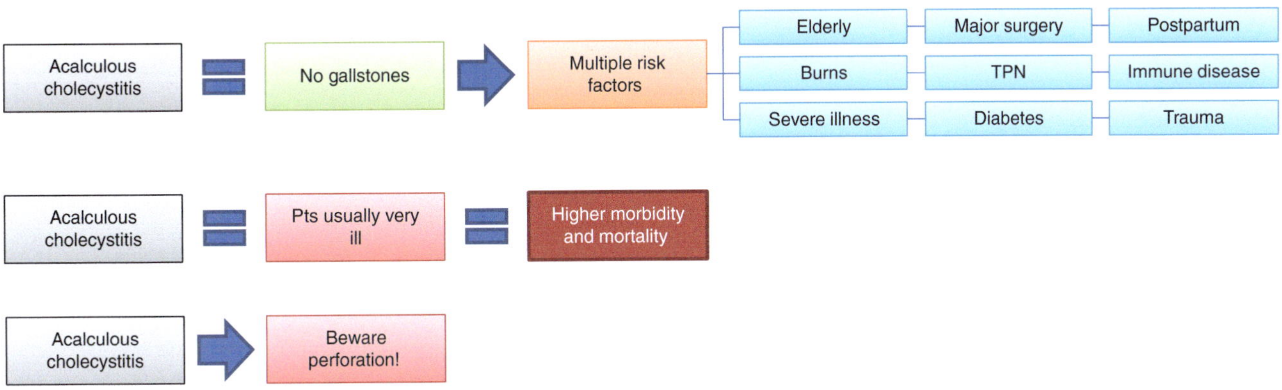

Ascending Cholangitis

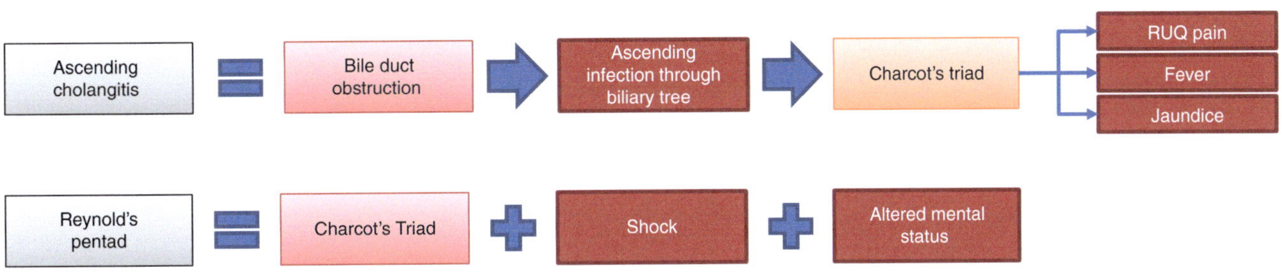

Pathophysiology

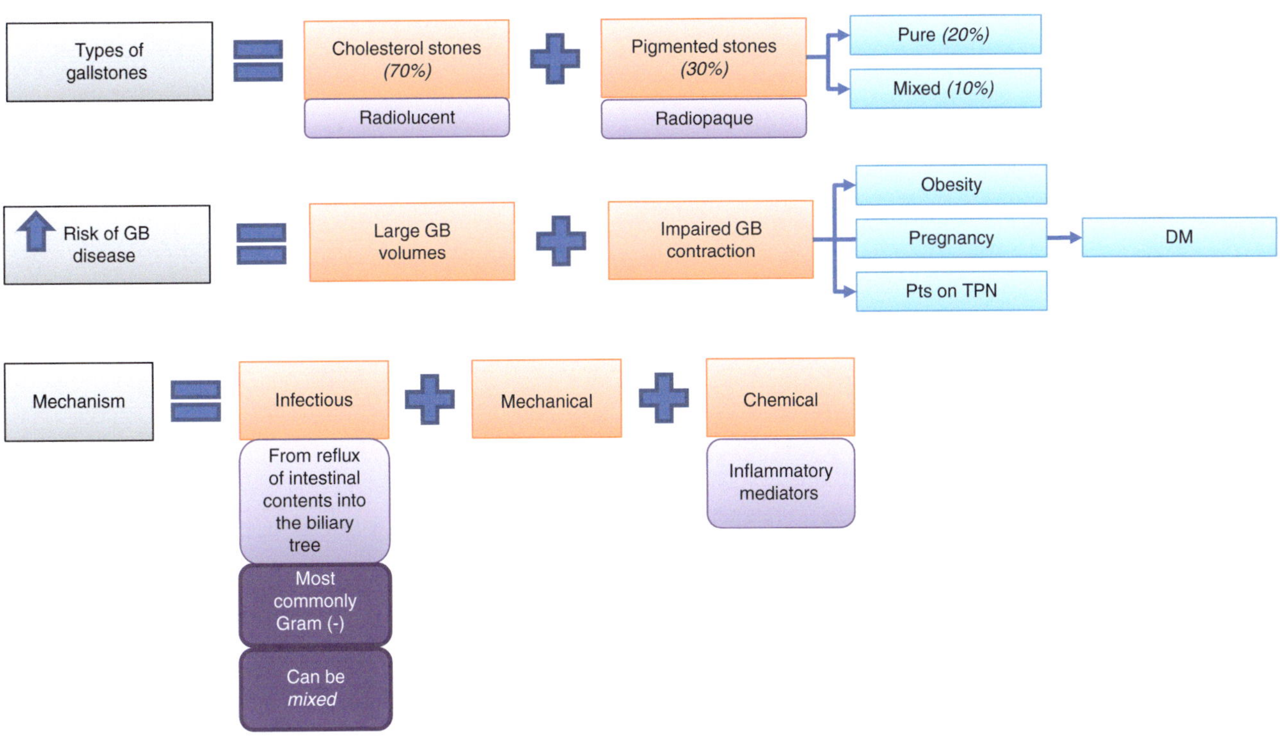

Symptoms and Signs

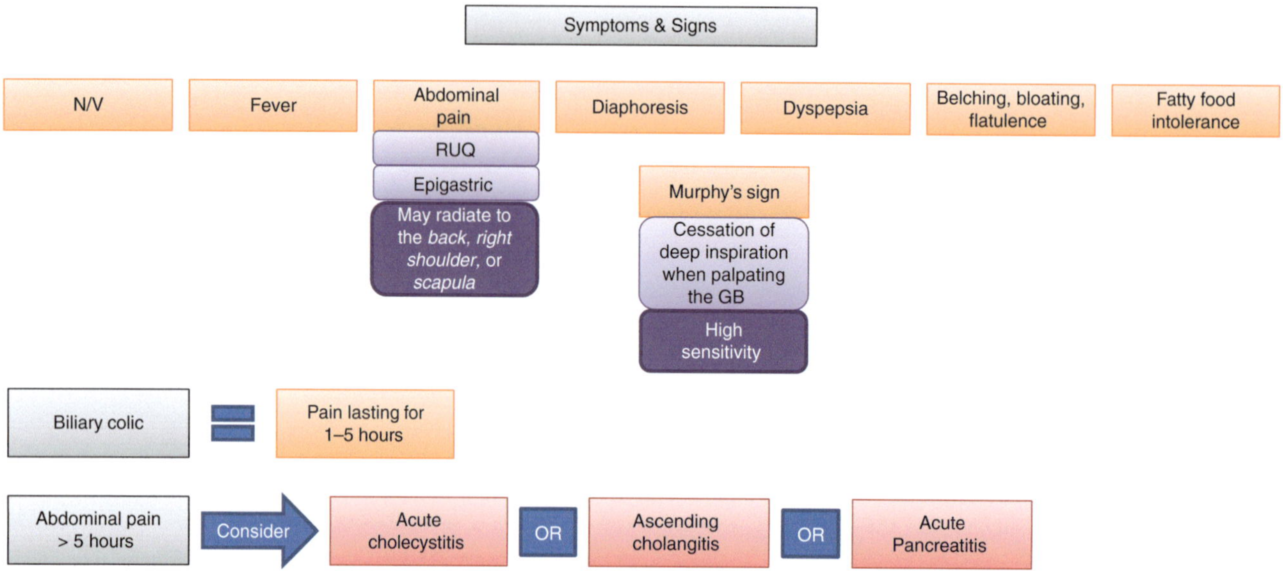

Diagnosis

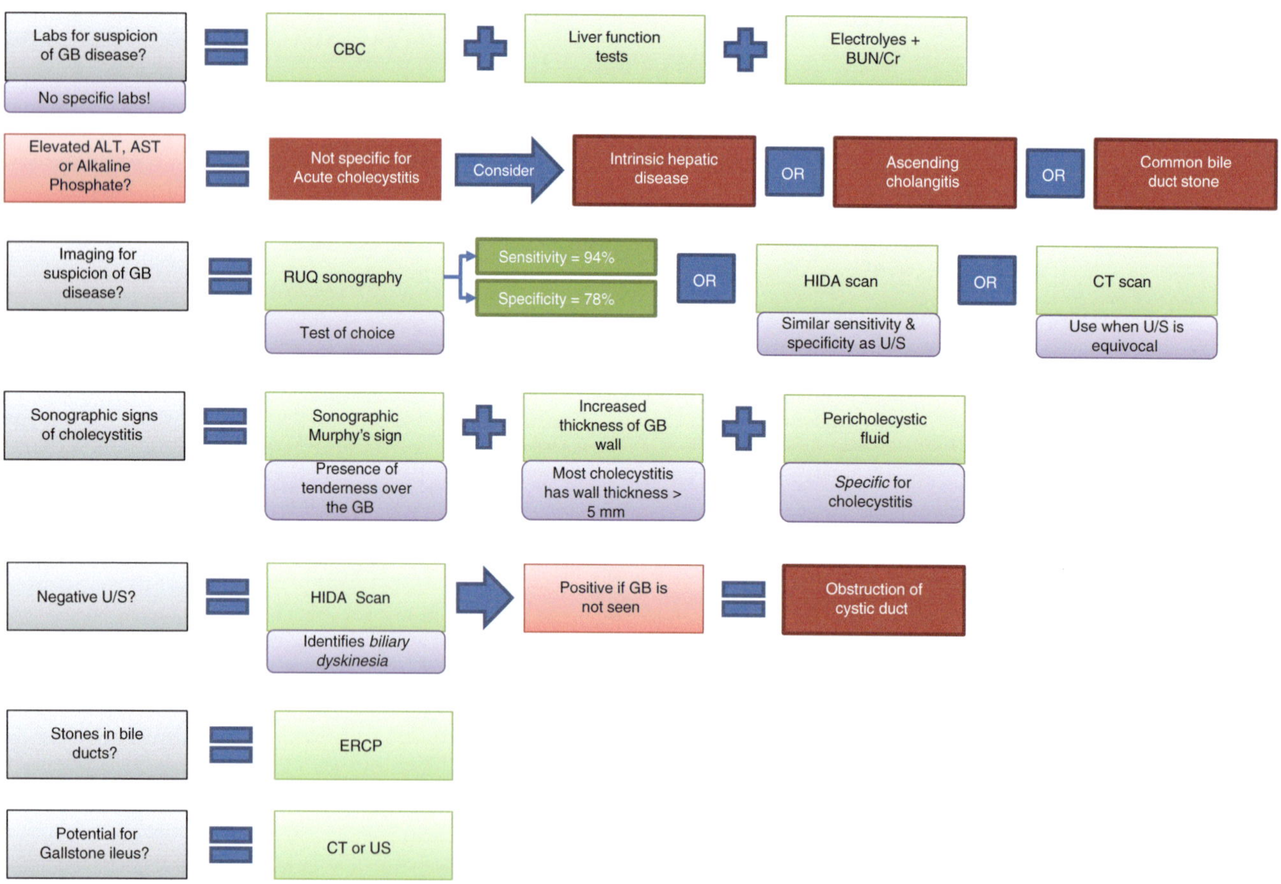

Treatment

Asymptomatic gallstones = No specific treatment → Refer to surgeon

Biliary colic? = Symptomatic treatment

Acute Cholecystitis? = Admission + Antibiotics + Symptomatic treatment + Surgical consultation

Ascending cholangitis? = Admission + Broad spectrum antibiotics + Surgical *or* Endoscopic GB decompression

Pancreatitis

Introduction and Some Causes of Pancreatitis

Pancreatitis
- Inflammation of the pancreas
- May involve other surrounding areas

Causes:

- Gallstones
  - Most common
- Alcohol
  - Acute
  - Chronic
  - 2nd most common
- Drugs and Medications
- Posterior penetrating peptic ulcer
- Hypertriglyceridemia
- Hyperparathyroidism
- Ischemia
- Trauma
  - Penetrating
- Hypercalcemia
- Toxins
  - Organophosphate poisoning
  - Scorpion venom
- Iatrogenic
  - ERCP
  - Post-op
- Cancer
- Autoimmune disease
- Infection
  - Bacterial
  - Viral
  - Parasites

Pancreatitis = Wide range in disease severity e.g., → Mild → Severe pancreatic necrosis → Multiorgan failure

Complications of Pancreatitis

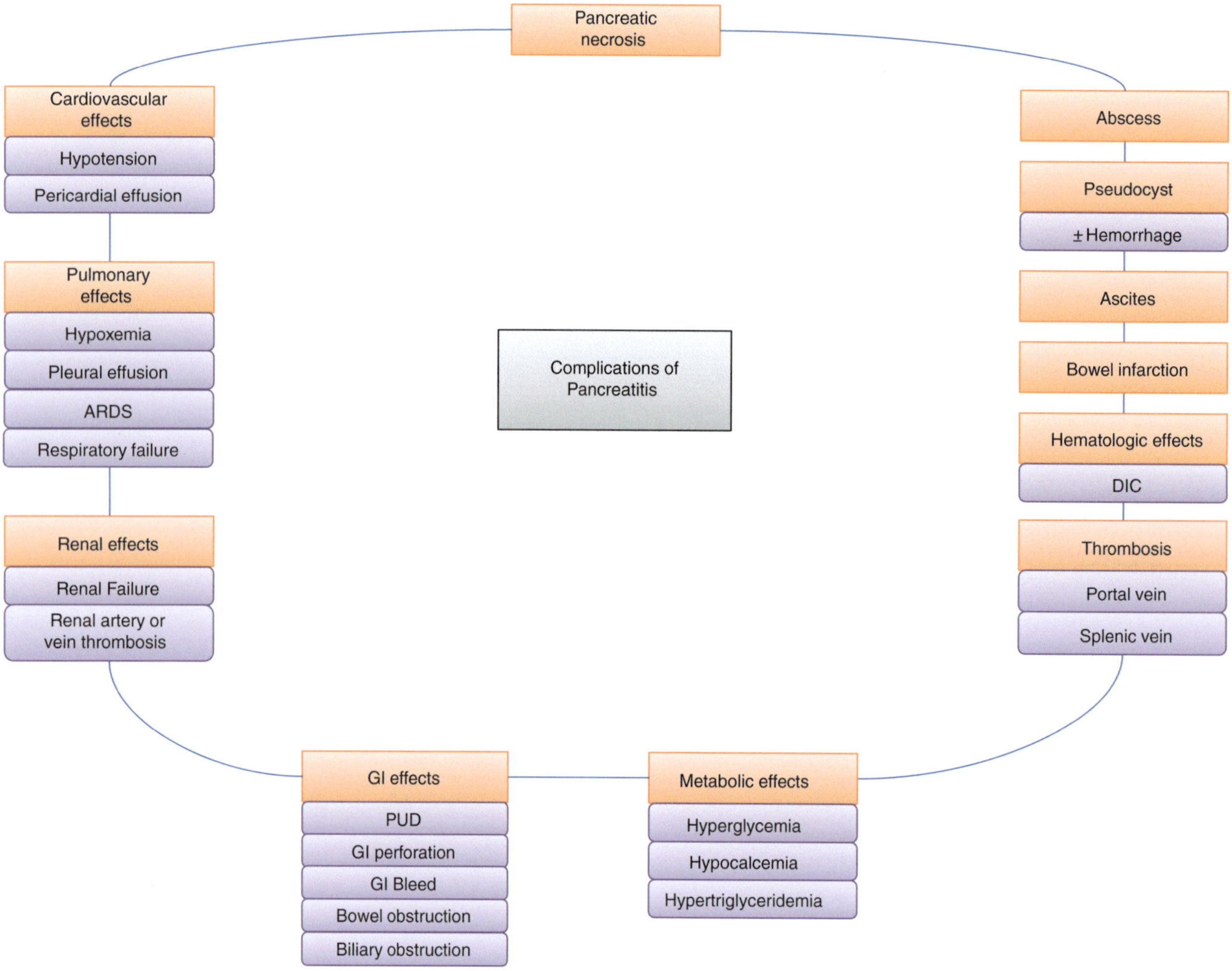

Symptoms and Signs

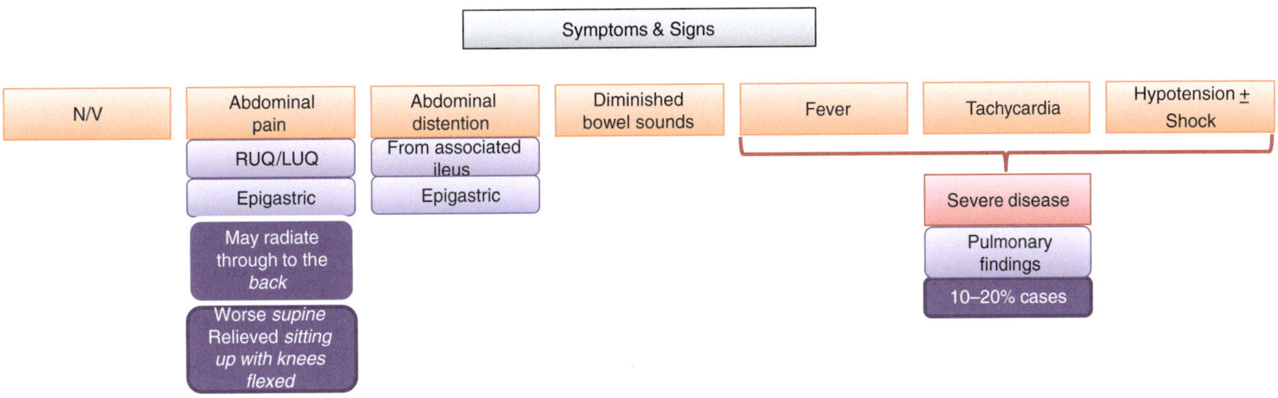

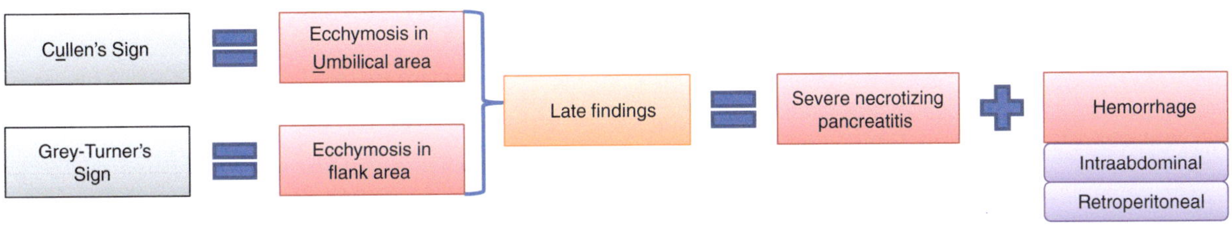

Diagnosis

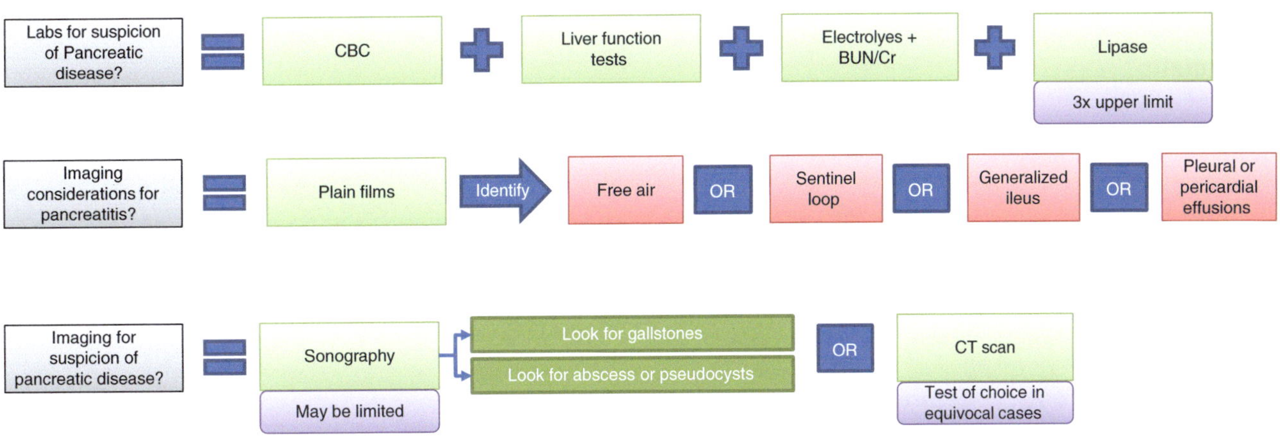

Ranson's Criteria: At Admission and 48 h

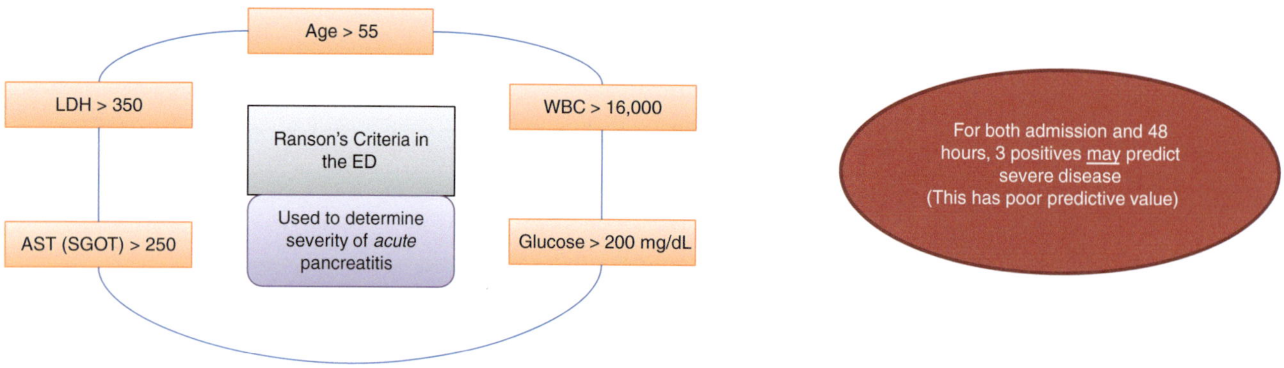

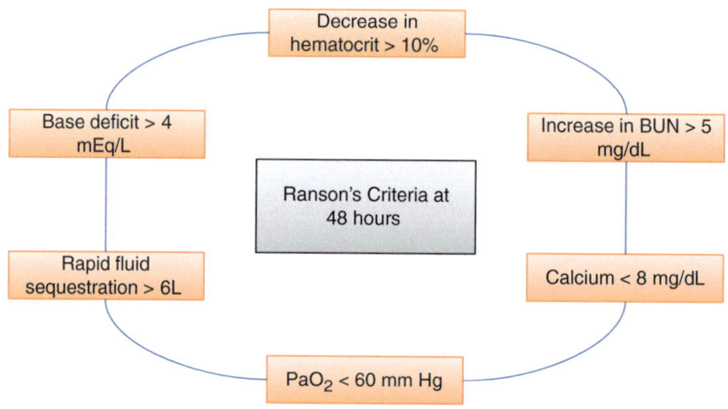

Treatment

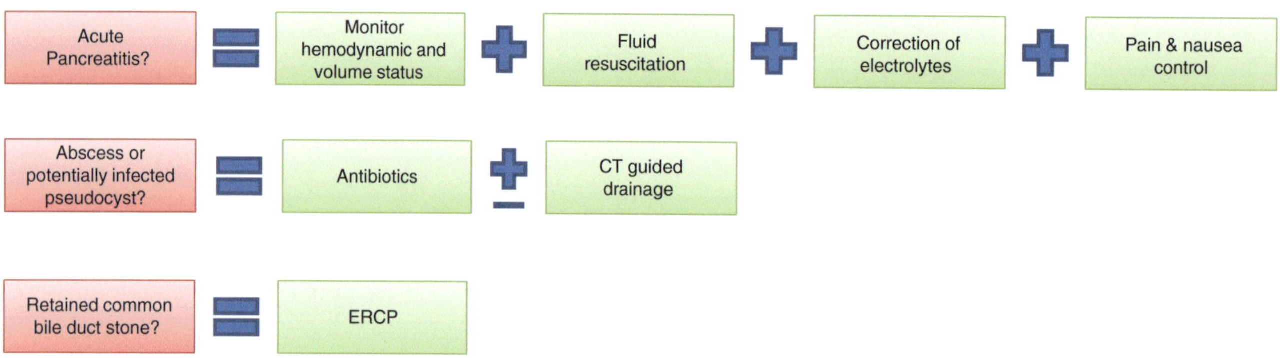

Ileus

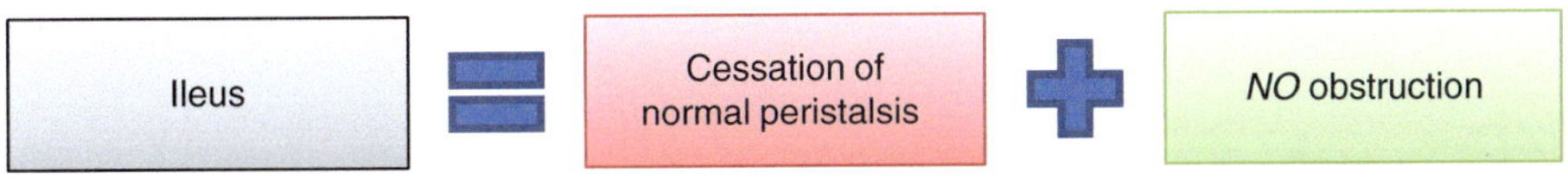
Ileus
Cessation of normal peristalsis
NO obstruction

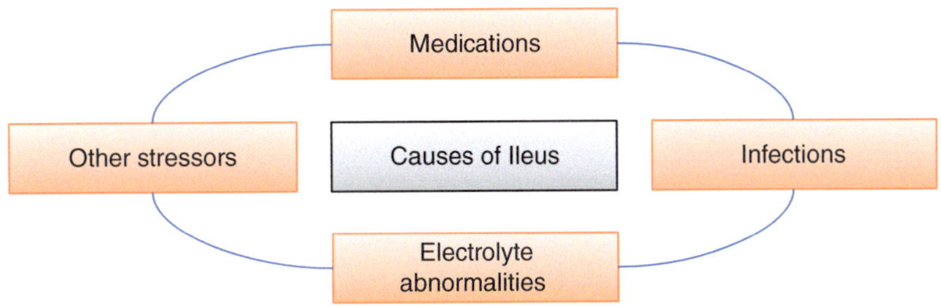
Medications
Other stressors
Causes of Ileus
Infections
Electrolyte abnormalities

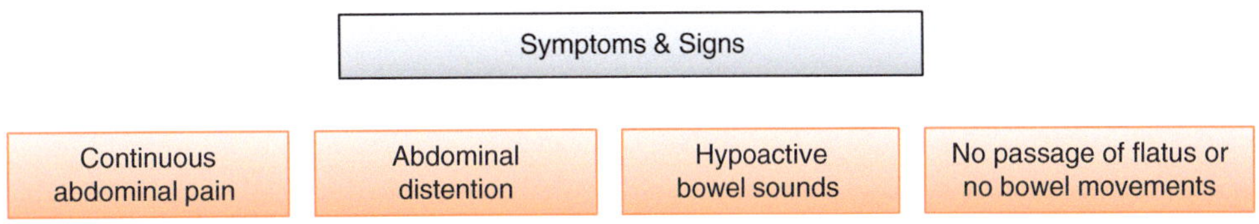
Symptoms & Signs
Continuous abdominal pain
Abdominal distention
Hypoactive bowel sounds
No passage of flatus or no bowel movements

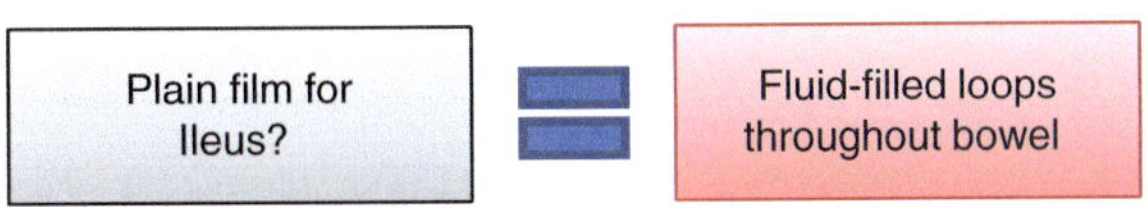
Plain film for Ileus?
Fluid-filled loops throughout bowel

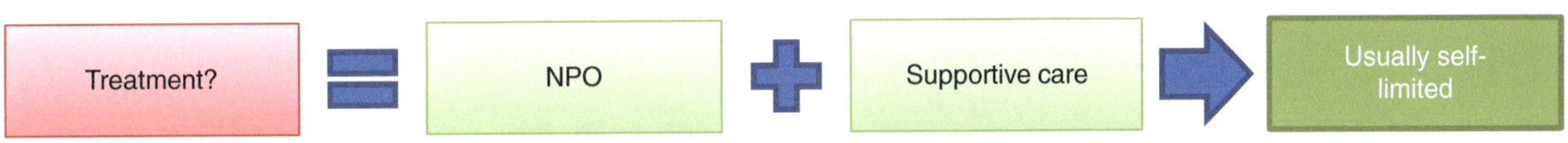
Treatment?
NPO
Supportive care
Usually self-limited

Bowel Obstruction

Introduction and Causes

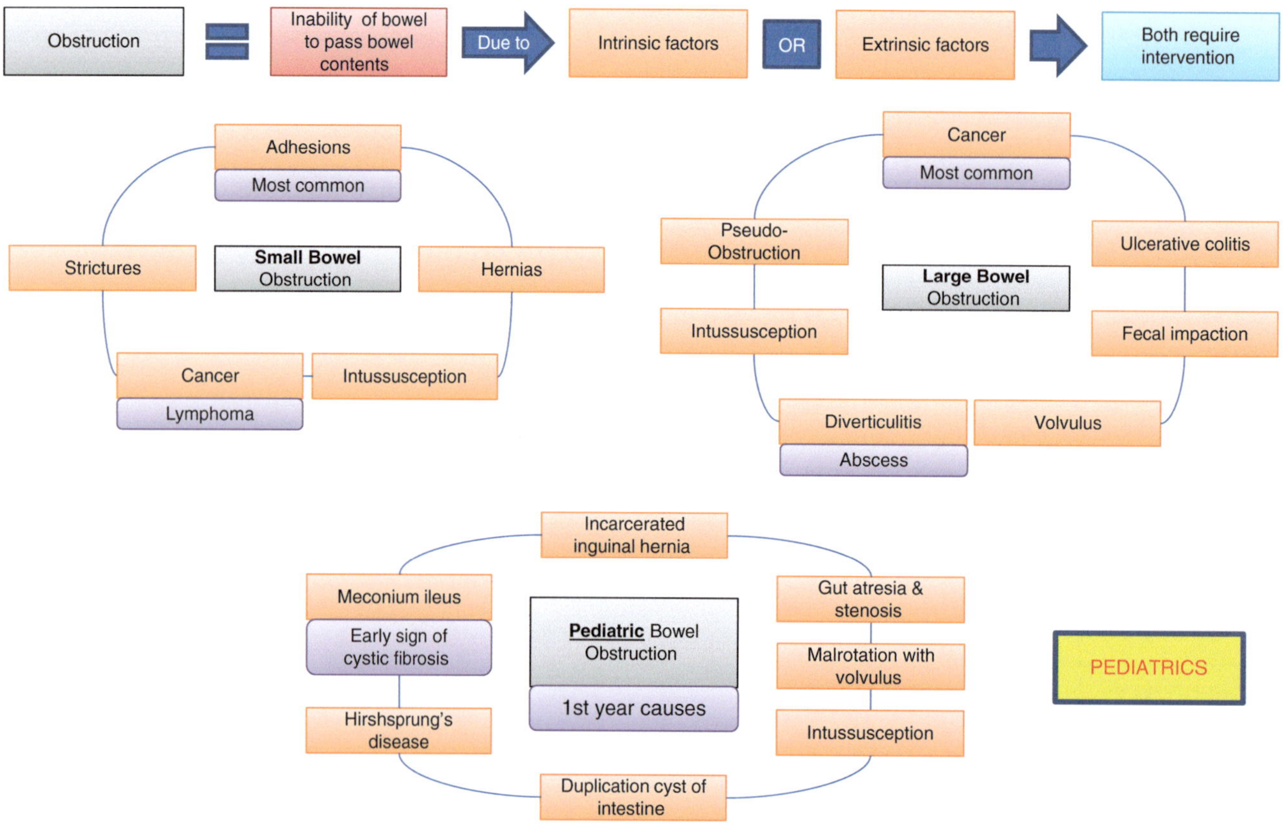

Bowel Obstruction Pathophysiology

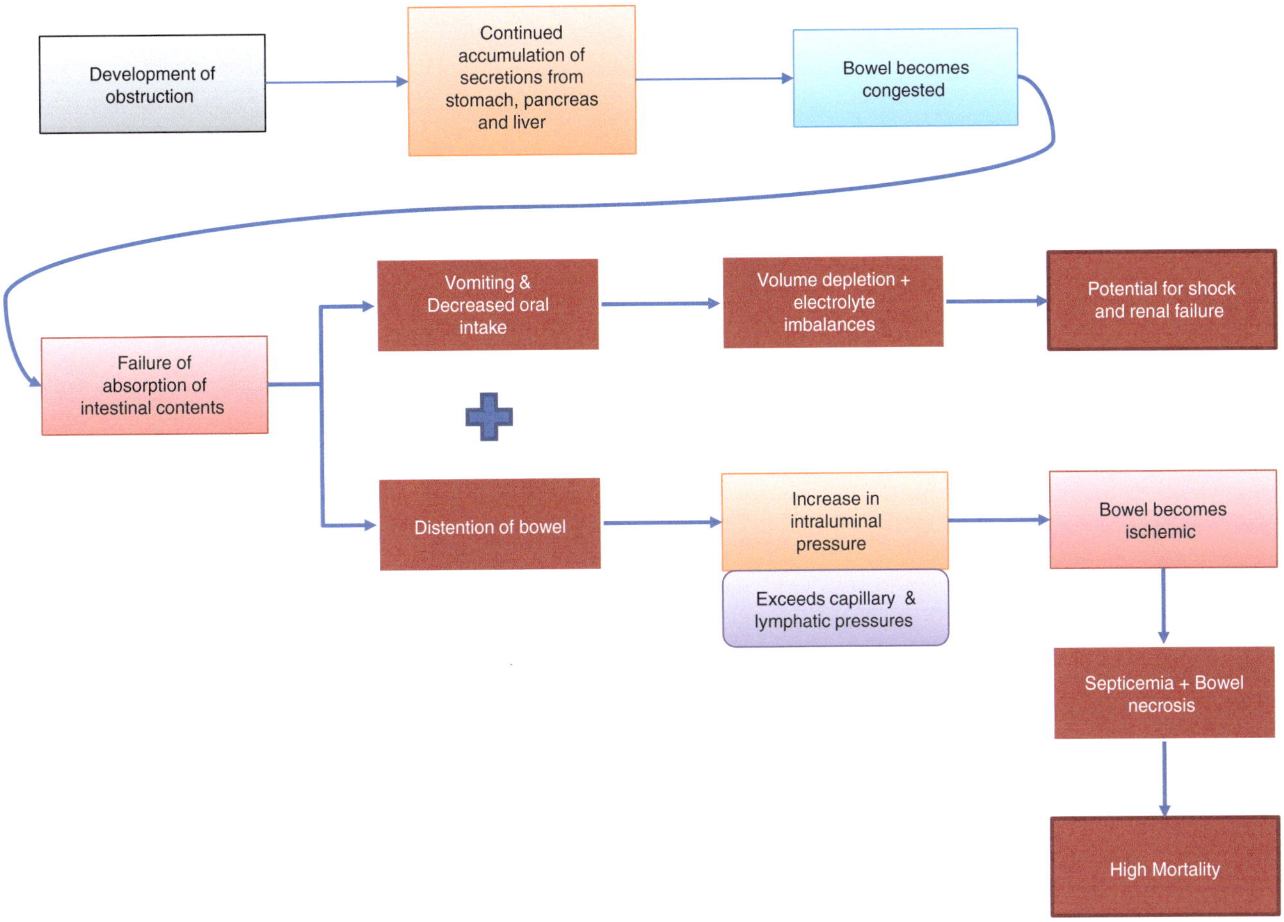

Symptoms and Signs

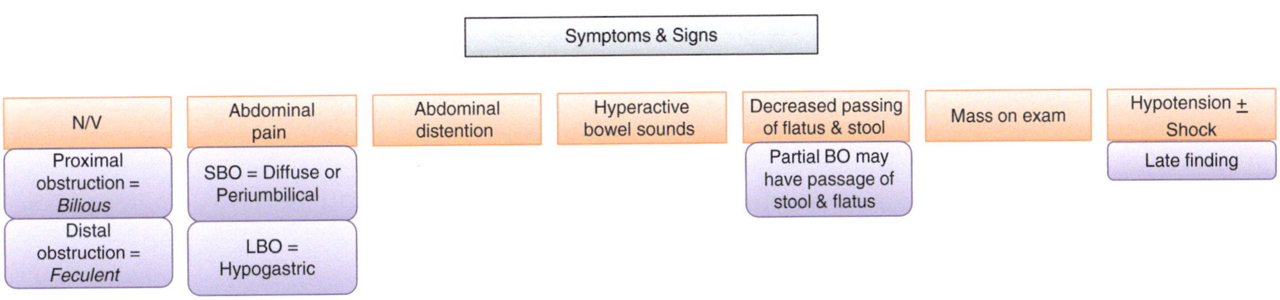

Diagnosis

Center bottom image (Reprinted from Pelaez CA, Agarwal N. The surgical abdomen. In: Pitchumoni CS, Dharmarajan TS, editors. Geriatric gastroenterology. New York: Springer Science; 2012. 607–13. With permission from Springer Science + Business Media)

Labs for suspicion of Bowel Obstruction? = CBC + Electrolytes + BUN/Cr + Others depending on DDx

No specific labs!

SBO X-ray Appearance? = Step Ladder or "String of pearls" → Plicae circulares are seen → Traverse the *entire* width of the bowel

LBO X-ray Appearance? = Distended colon → Haustra are seen → *DO NOT* traverse the entire width of the bowel

CT is diagnostic

"Coffee Bean" appearance on plain film? = Closed loop bowel obstruction = *Competent* ileocecal valve = High risk of perforation

Diagnostic method of choice? = CT scan

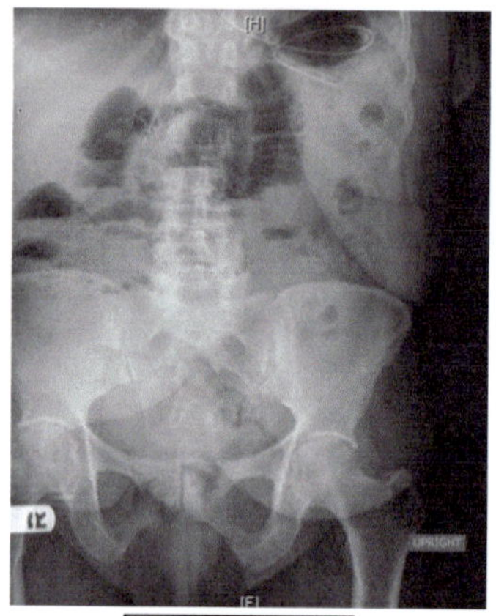

SBO

Treatment

Bowel obstruction? = Monitor hemodynamic and volume status + Fluid resuscitation + Correction of electrolytes + Pain & nausea control

Consider NG tube placement

True mechanical obstruction? = Surgery + Prophylactic broad spectrum antibiotics

Intussusception

(**a**) Top right image (Reprinted from Yoo S-Y. Non-neonatal gastrointestinal diseases. In: Kim I-O, editor. Radiology illustrated: pediatric radiology. Heidelberg: Springer Verlag; 2014. p. 629–63. With permission from Springer Verlag).
(**b**) Bottom right image (Reprinted from Gilger MA, Nazer HM. Gastrointestinal bleeding. In: Elzouki AY, Harfi HA, Nazer HM, Stapleton FB, Oh W, Whitley RJ, editors. Textbook of clinical pediatrics. Heidelberg: Springer Verlag; 2012. p. 1937–49. With permission from Springer Verlag)

Intussusception = Most common cause of surgical abdomen & SBO from ***3 months to 6 years***

Intussusception → Rare → < 3 months + Uncommon > 3 years

Intussusception = Increased risk with ***Cystic fibrosis, Henoch-Scholein Purpura, Meckel's diverticulum & Polyps***

Intussusception = "Sausage shaped" mass in right side of abdomen → Ileocecal valve is most common

Classic plain film findings = Crescent sign + Target sign + Bowel obstruction + Absent liver edge

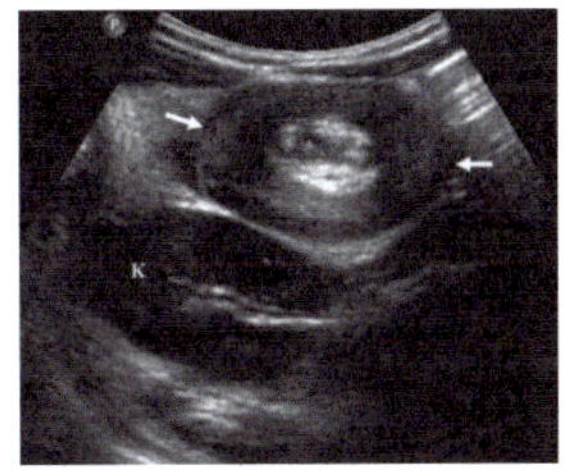

Ultrasound

Symptoms & Signs

- N/V
- Abdominal pain
  - Intermittent
  - Child appears well between paroxysms of pain
- Heme(+)stools
  - Currant jelly stool is *late* finding

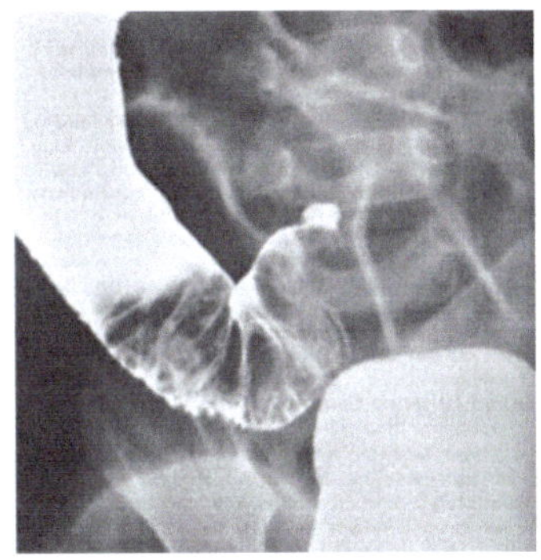

Coiled Spring sign

Diagnosis

Labs for suspicion of Intussusception? = CBC + Electrolyes + BUN/Cr + Others depending on DDx

No specific labs!

Imaging modalities? = Plain films + Ultrasound + Barium Enema

Appearance on Barium enema? = "Coiled spring" sign

Treatment

Intussusception? = Air contrast enema + Fluid resuscitation + Correction of electrolytes + Pain & nausea control

Consider NG tube placement

No relief with enema? = Surgery

Pyloric Stenosis

Image just right of center (Reprinted from Yoo S-Y. Non-neonatal gastrointestinal diseases. In: Kim I-O, editors. Radiology illustrated: pediatric radiology. Heidelberg: Springer Verlag; 2014. p. 629–63 (With permission from Springer Verlag)

PEDIATRICS

Pyloric stenosis = 3rd week to 3rd month of life → Most common cause of surgically correctable cause of vomiting in newborns

Pyloric stenosis = Increased incidence with ***1st born males*** + High incidence ***in families***

Pyloric stenosis = "Olive-shaped" mass in right upper quadrant

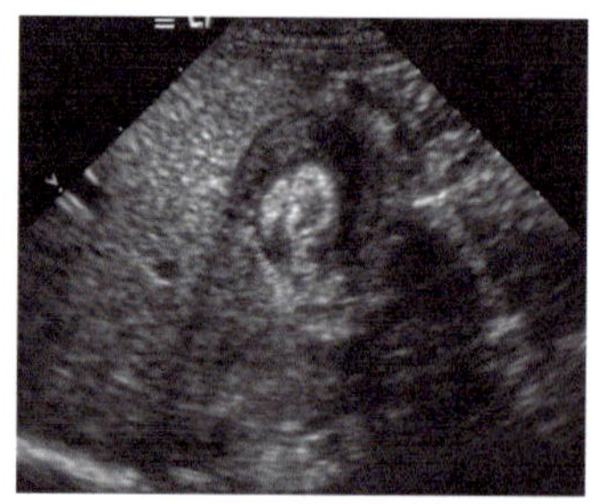

Symptoms & Signs

- N/V
  - *Non-bilious*
- Abdominal pain
  - Intermittent
  - Child appears well between paroxysms of pain
- Dehydration
  - Classic hypochloremic metabolic alkalosis
- Heme(+) stools
  - Currant jelly stool is late finding

Diagnosis

Labs for suspicion of Pyloric Stenosis? = CBC + Electrolyes + BUN/Cr + Others depending on DDx

No specific labs!

Electrolyes + BUN/Cr: Will see hypochloremic metabolic alkalosis

Imaging for Pyloric Stenosis? = Ultrasound OR Upper GI Series

Appearance on ultrasound? = "Target sign" (hypertrophied hypoechoic muscle surrounding echogenic mucosa) + Elongated pylorus with thickened muscle + "Cervix sign" + Exaggerated peristalsis & failure of the pylorus to open

Appearance on Upper GI series? = "String sign"

Treatment

Pyloric stenosis? = Monitor hemodynamic and volume status + Fluid resuscitation + Correction of electrolytes + Pain & nausea control

Pyloric stenosis? = Surgery

Hirschsprung's Disease

PEDIATRICS

Hirshsprung's Disease = Congenital megacolon → Usually the 1st month

Hirschsprung's Disease = Newborn: Failure to pass meconium + Children: Chronic constipation

Hirschsprung's Disease → Complication → Enterocolitis → Potentially fatal

Volvulus

Introduction

Bottom left image (Reprinted from Pelaez CA, Agarwal N. The surgical abdomen. In: Pitchumoni CS, Dharmarajan TS, editors. Geriatric gastroenterology. New York: Springer Science; 2012. p. 607–13. With permission from Springer Science + Business Media)
Bottom right image (Reprinted from Hellinger MD, Steinhagen RM. Colonic volvulus. In: Wolff BG, Fleshman JW, Beck DE, Pemberton JH, Wexner SD, Church JM, Garcia-Aguilar J, Roberts PL, Saclarides TJ, Stamos MJ, editors. The ASCRS textbook of colon and rectal surgery. New York: Springer Science; 2007. p. 286–98. With permission from Springer Science + Business Media)

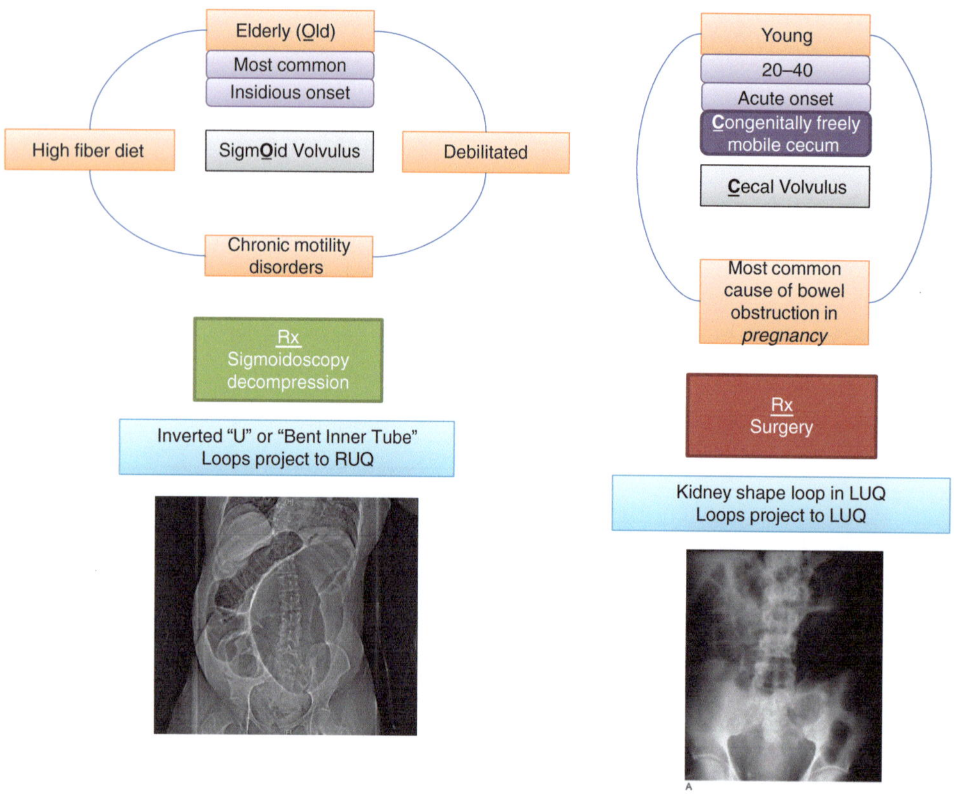

Malrotation with Volvulus

PEDIATRICS

Malrotation with Volvulus = Occurs in early infancy → Usually the 1st month

Malrotation with Volvulus = Abnormal rotation & fixation of midgut

Malrotation with Volvulus = Early diagnosis is important → Prevents → Midgut gangrene

Symptoms & Signs

- N/V
  - *Bilious*
  - Sudden onset
- Abdominal pain
- Abdominal distention
  - Rigid
- Heme(+) stools
- Shock (potential)

For ALL types of volvulus!

Diagnosis

Labs for suspicion of Malrotation? = CBC + Electrolyes + BUN/Cr + Others depending on DDx

No specific labs!

Appearance on Imaging? = "Double bubble sign" → Air-fluid levels in stomach & in distended duodenum

Treatment

Malrotation with Volvulus? = Monitor hemodynamic and volume status + Fluid resuscitation + Correction of electrolytes + Pain & nausea control (Consider NG tube placement)

Malrotation with Volvulus? = Surgery + Prophylactic broad spectrum antibiotics

Other Volvulus? = Surgical consultation + Prophylactic broad spectrum antibiotics

Hernias

Introduction

Hernia = Protrusion of a viscus from its surrounding tissue walls

Reducible hernia = Hernia is *soft* & *easy* to replace back through the defect

Incarcerated hernia = Hernia is *firm* & often *painful*. *Unable* to be replaced back through the defect

Strangulated hernia = Irreducible painful hernia developing as a result of incarceration (May have overlying skin changes) = Impairment of blood flow = Potential *obstruction& toxicity* = Acute surgical emergency (Do not reduce!)

Inguinal Hernias

Inguinal Hernia = Most common type of hernia for *males & females* → 2/3 are *Indirect*

Indirect Inguinal Hernia = Herniates through the *inguinal canal* → Extends into the scrotal sac (Common in boys)

Direct Inguinal Hernia = Herniates through the *abdominal wall* → Palpable at the inguinal ligament (Common in older men)

Pantaloon Hernia = Direct and Indirect at the *same time*

Ventral Hernias

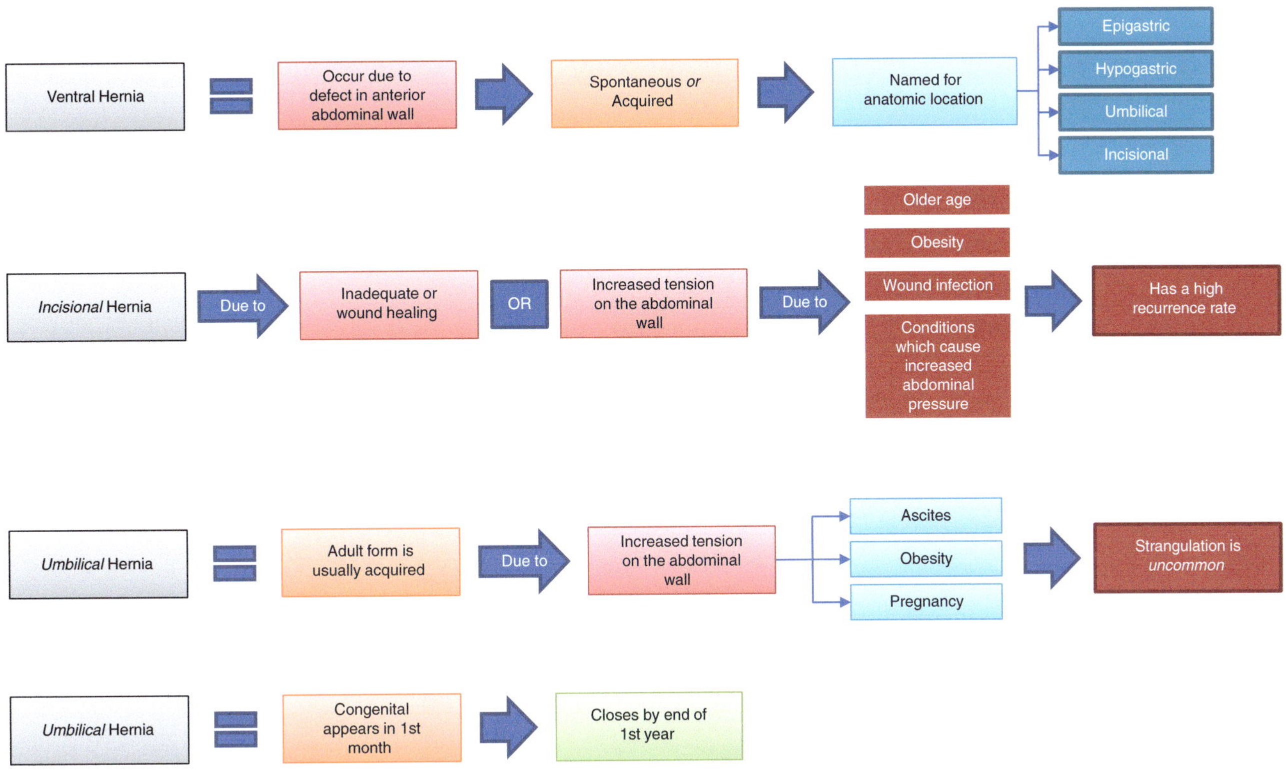

Other Hernias

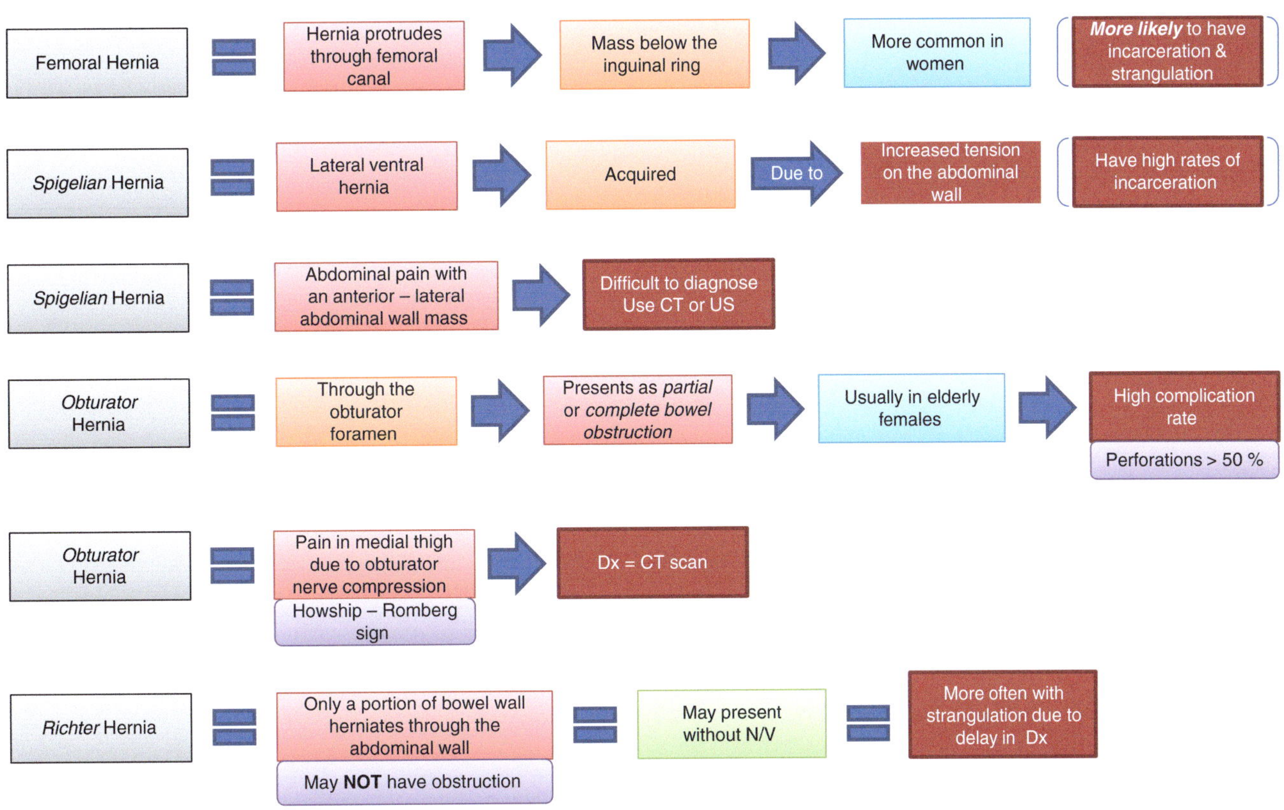

Diagnosis

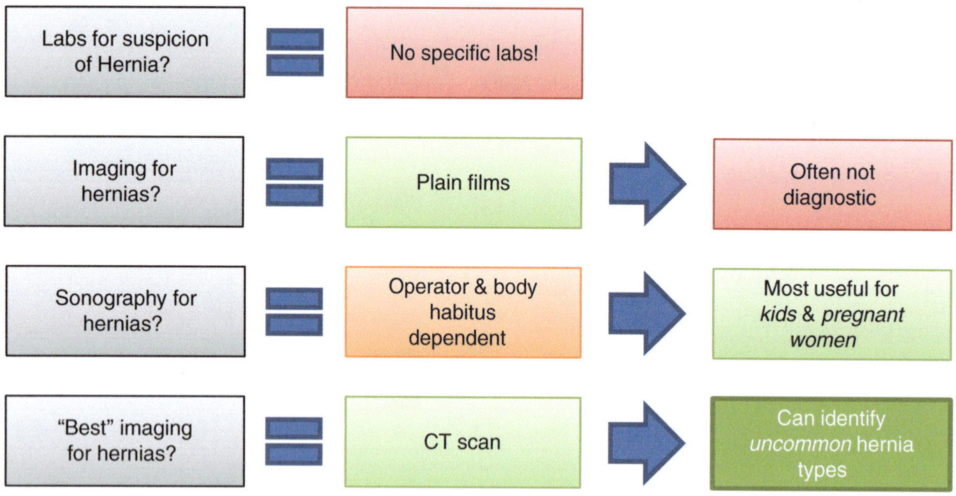

Treatment

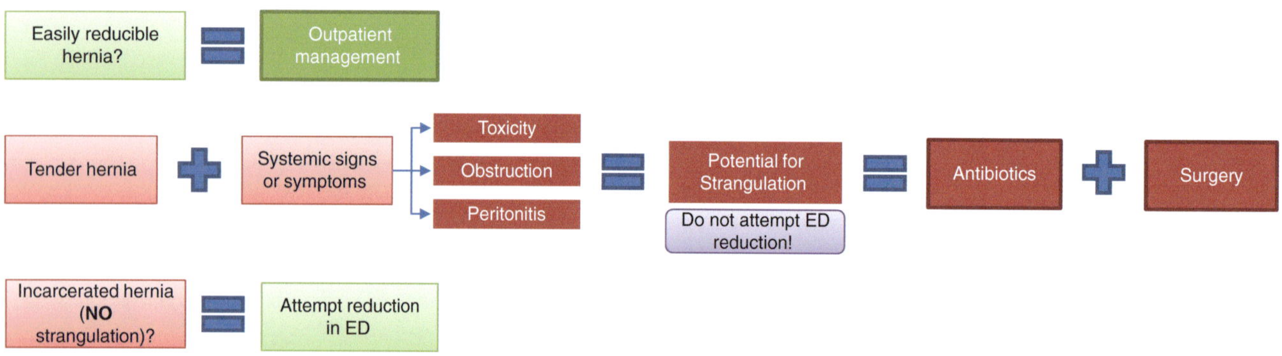

Bowel Perforation

Introduction

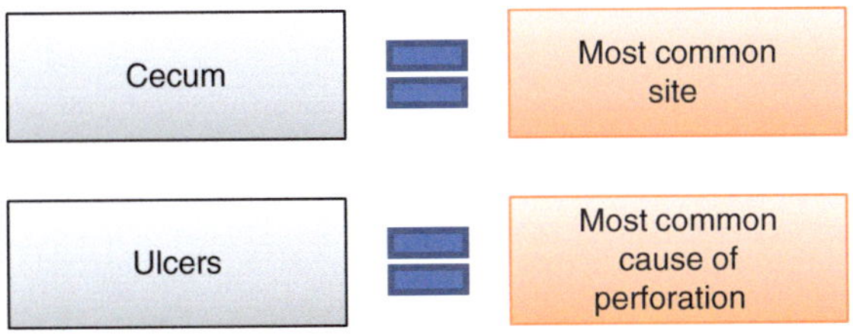

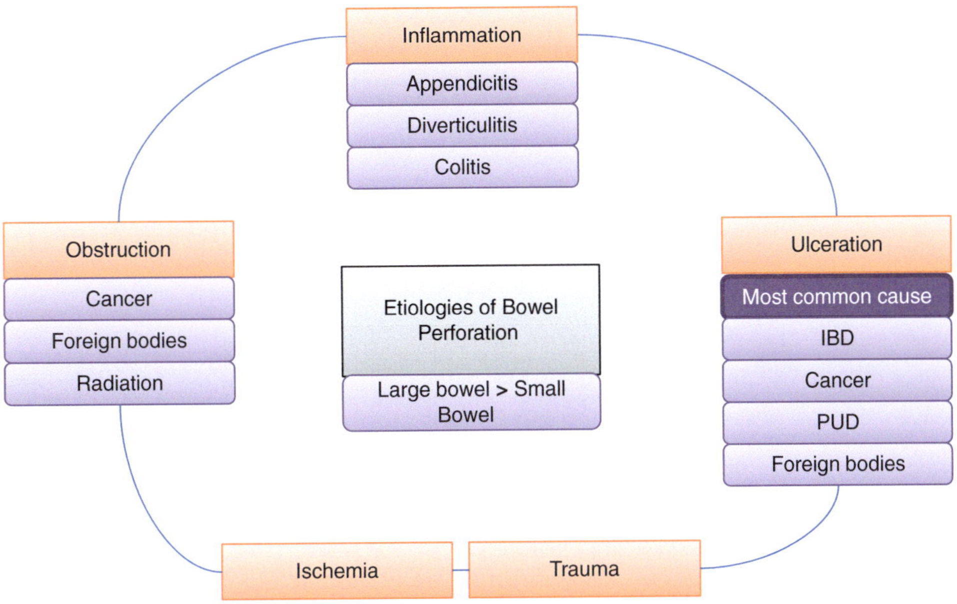

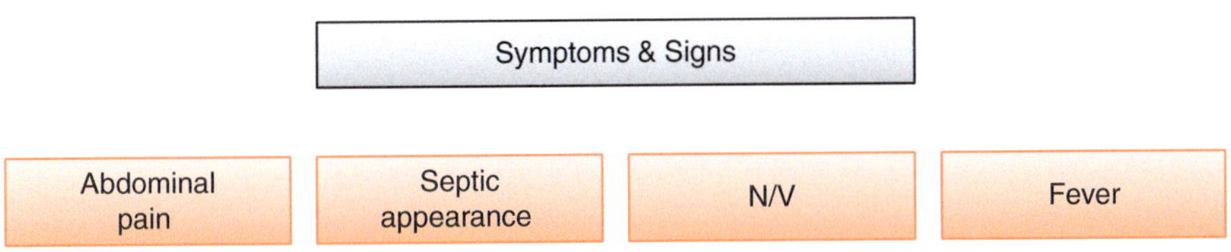

Diagnosis

Labs for suspicion of Bowel Perforation? (No specific labs!) = CBC + Electrolyes + BUN/Cr + Others depending on DDx

Imaging for Bowel perforation? = Plain films may miss small amounts of air + Plain films may miss retroperitoneal air = Get upright CXR!

Diagnostic method of choice? = CT scan

Treatment

Bowel perforation? = Monitor hemodynamic and volume status + Fluid resuscitation + Antibiotics + Surgery

True bowel perforation? = Surgery + Prophylactic broad spectrum antibiotics

Acute Appendicitis

Introduction

Appendicitis = Obstruction by fecalith of the vermiform appendix

Other causes of Appendicitis = Parasites OR Tumor OR Lymphatic tissue OR Gallstones

Appendicitis = Blockage of appendiceal lumen → Continued secretion from luminal mucosa → Increased luminal pressure → Vascular insufficiency → Inflammation with potential perforation

Appendicitis = <u>Visceral pain</u> Vague pain → <u>Parietal pain</u> Localizes to RLQ

Appendicitis = 33% have atypical presentations → But… → Most common is still RLQ

Appendicitis Confounders

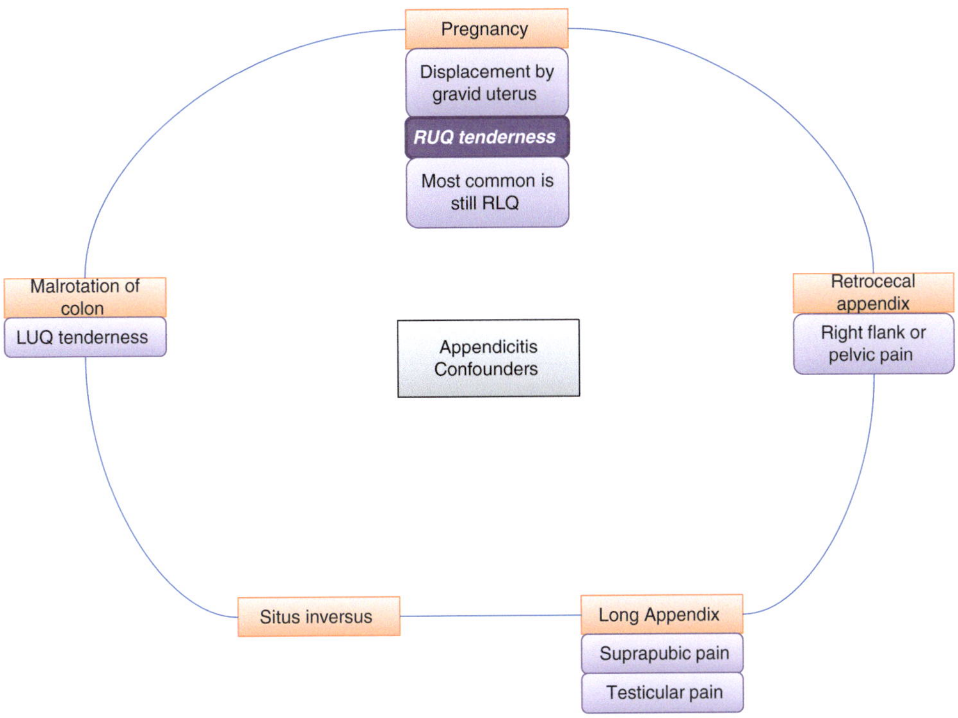

Symptoms and Signs

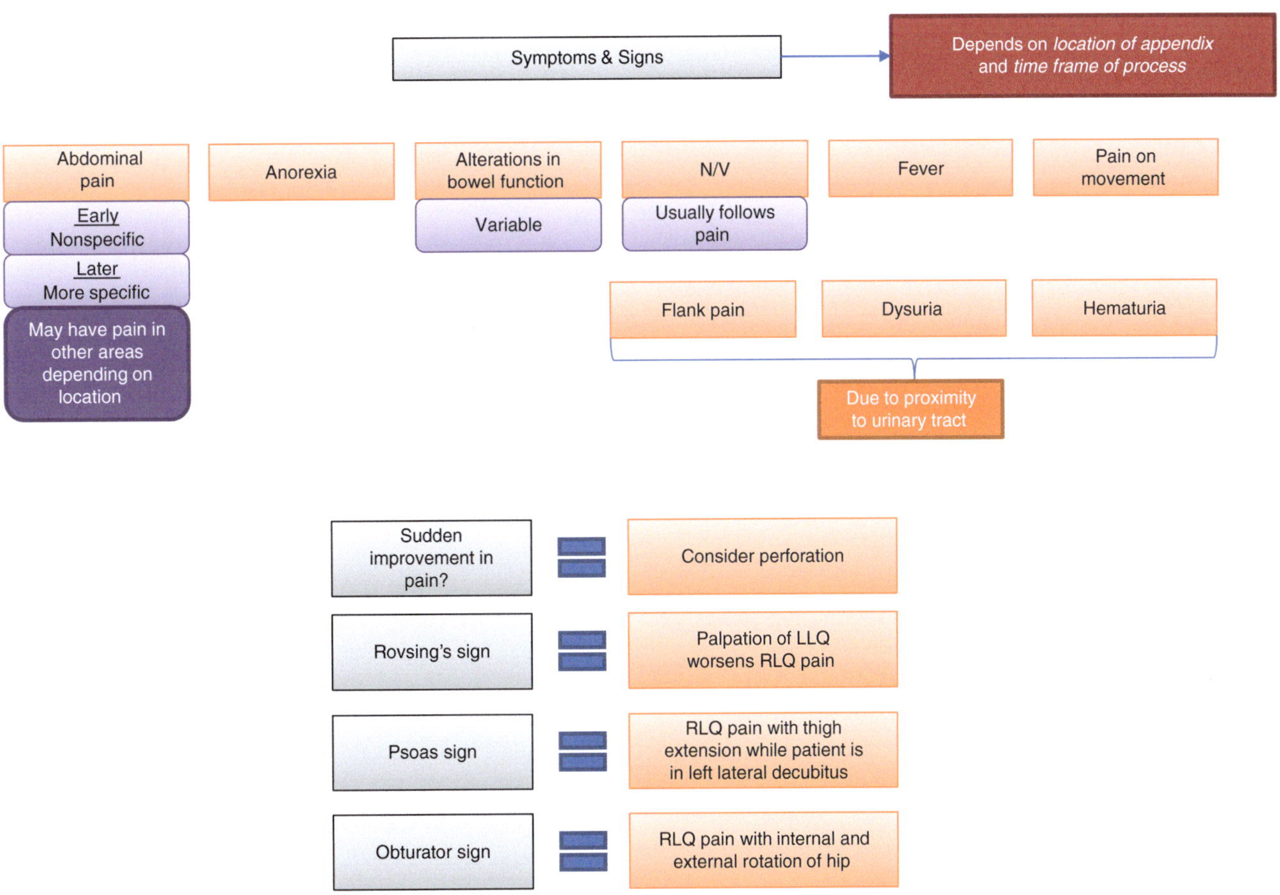

Diagnosis

Labs for suspicion of Appendicitis? (No specific labs!) = CBC (May not be helpful) + Electrolytes+ BUN/Cr + U/A (with pregnancy) ± CRP/ESR

Imaging for Appendicitis? = Ultrasound OR CT

Appearance on ultrasound? = Thickened noncompressible appendix > 6mm in diameter

CT for appendicitis? = Use when Dx is not clear

Appendicitis pitfall? = Mistaking pyuria for UTI

Treatment

Appendicitis? = Monitor hemodynamic and volume status + Fluid resuscitation + Pain & nausea control

Appendicitis? = Prophylactic broad spectrum antibiotics + Surgery

Acute Diverticulitis

Introduction: Diverticulitis

Diverticula = Outpouchings through the colonic wall near where vasa recta penetrate bowel wall (Involve only mucosal & submucosal layers) Due to Weakening of colonic wall + Increased intraluminal pressure (*Sigmoid* = highest pressures)

Diverticulitis = Erosion of diverticular wall Due to Thickened fecal material → Inflammation & microperforation (Free perforation is *rare*)

In the U.S. Diverticulitis = *Left* sided colonic process (Sigmoid) ≠ In Asia Diverticulitis = *Right* sided colonic process

Common bacterial agents = Gram (-) rods *E. coli* + *Clostridium* + *Peptostreptococci* + *Bacteriodes* + *Fusobacterium*

Risk Factors for Diverticulitis

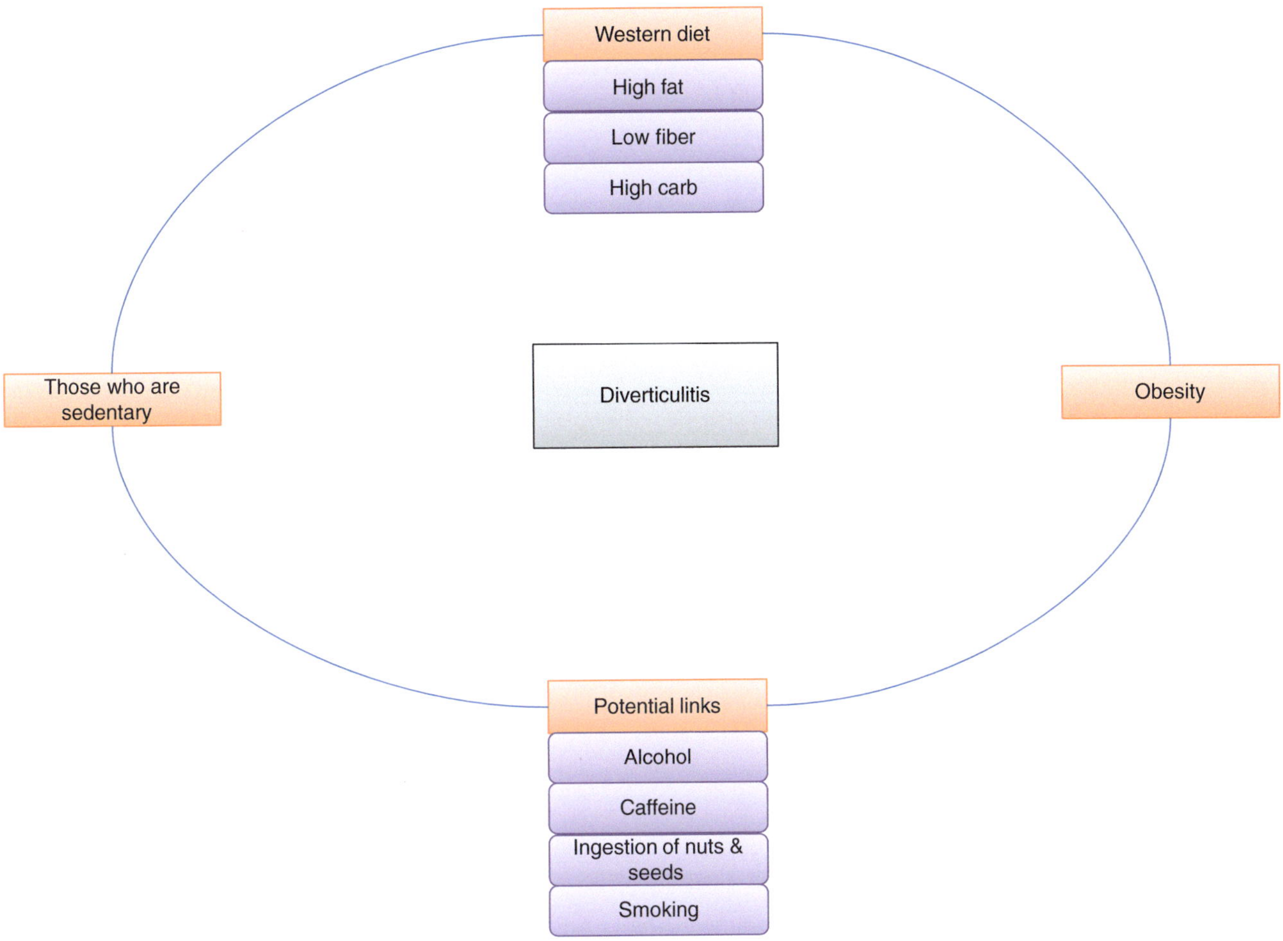

Symptoms and Signs

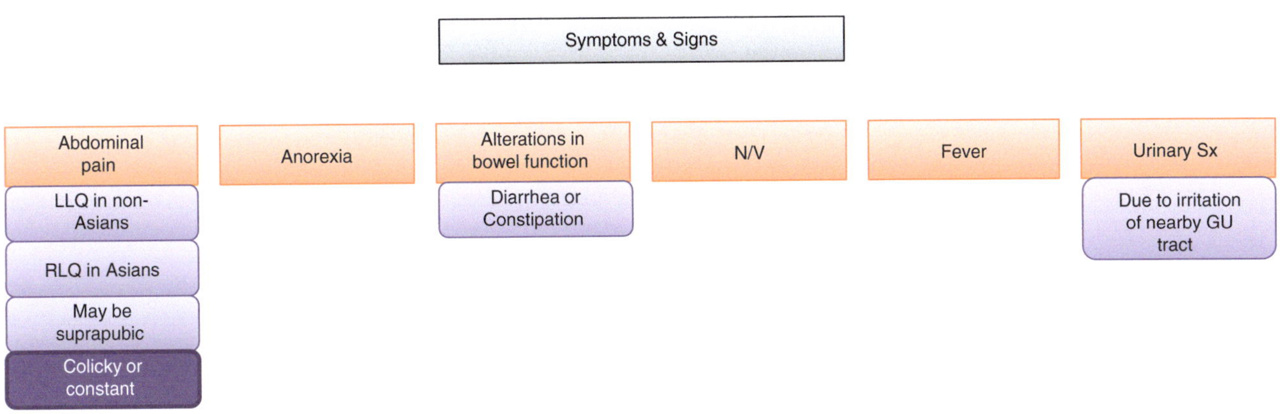

Diagnosis

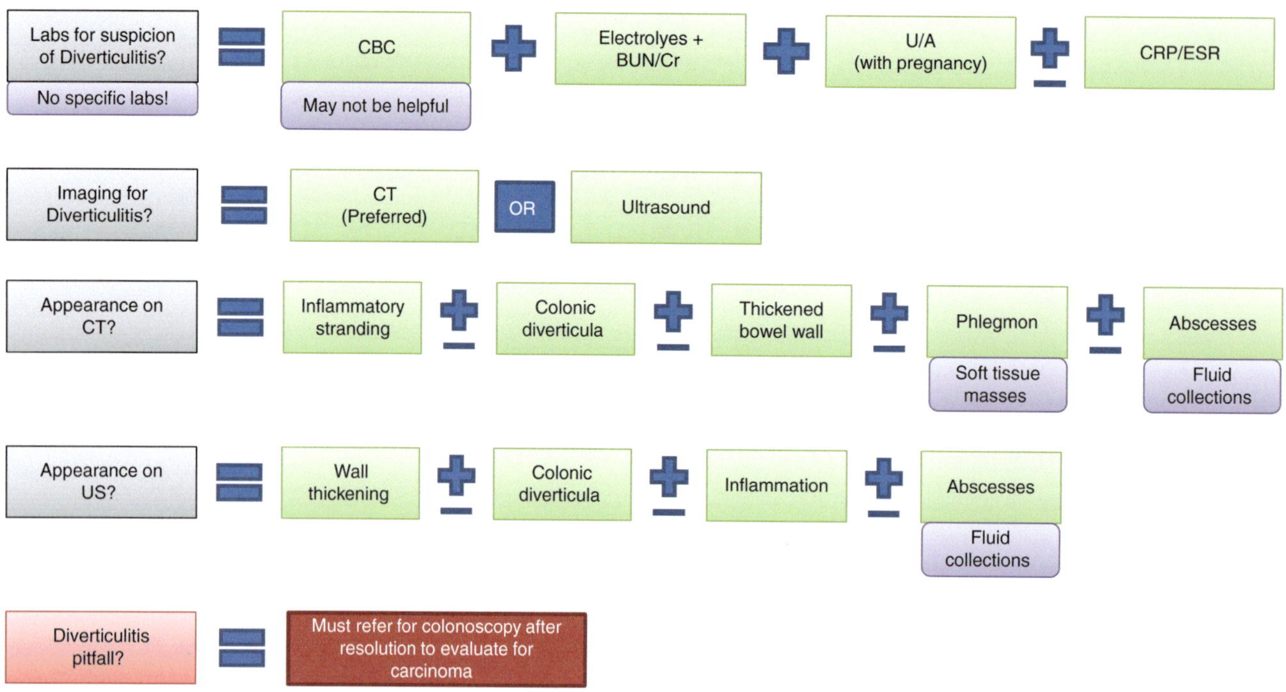

Treatment

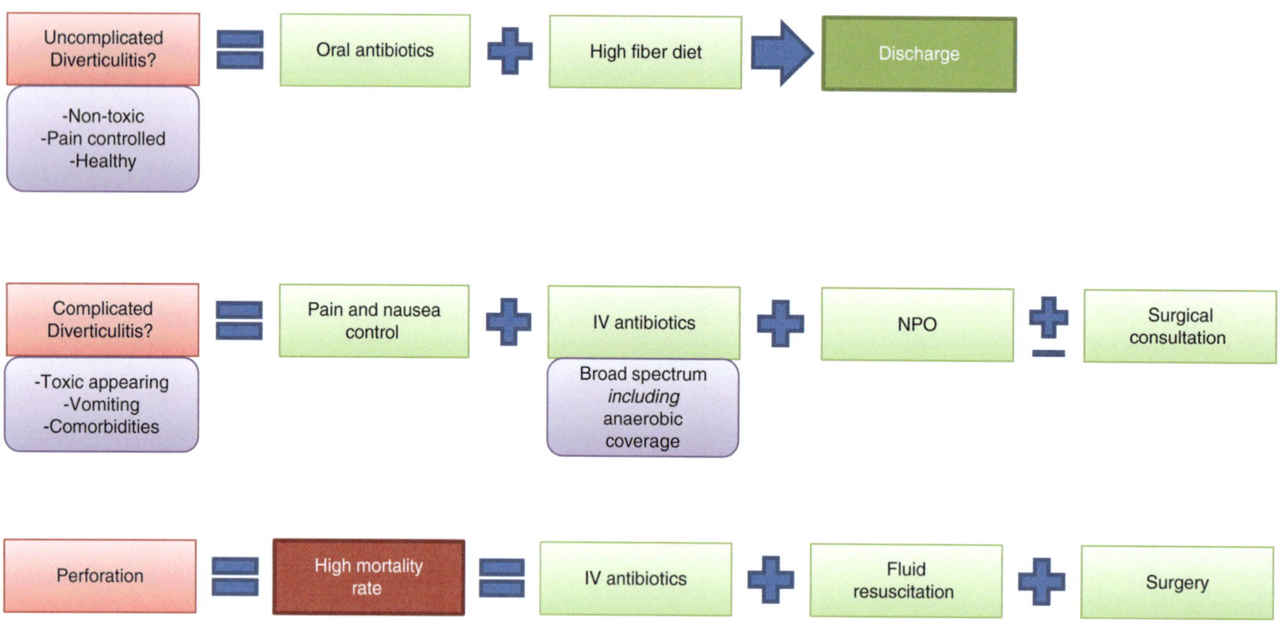

Mesenteric Ischemia

Introduction

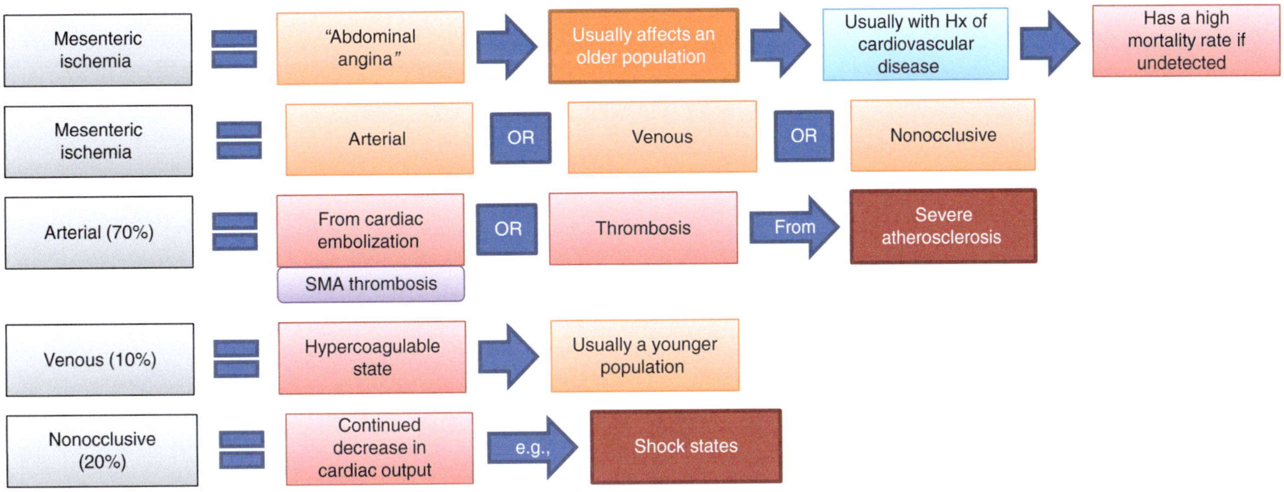

Risk Factors for Mesenteric Ischemia

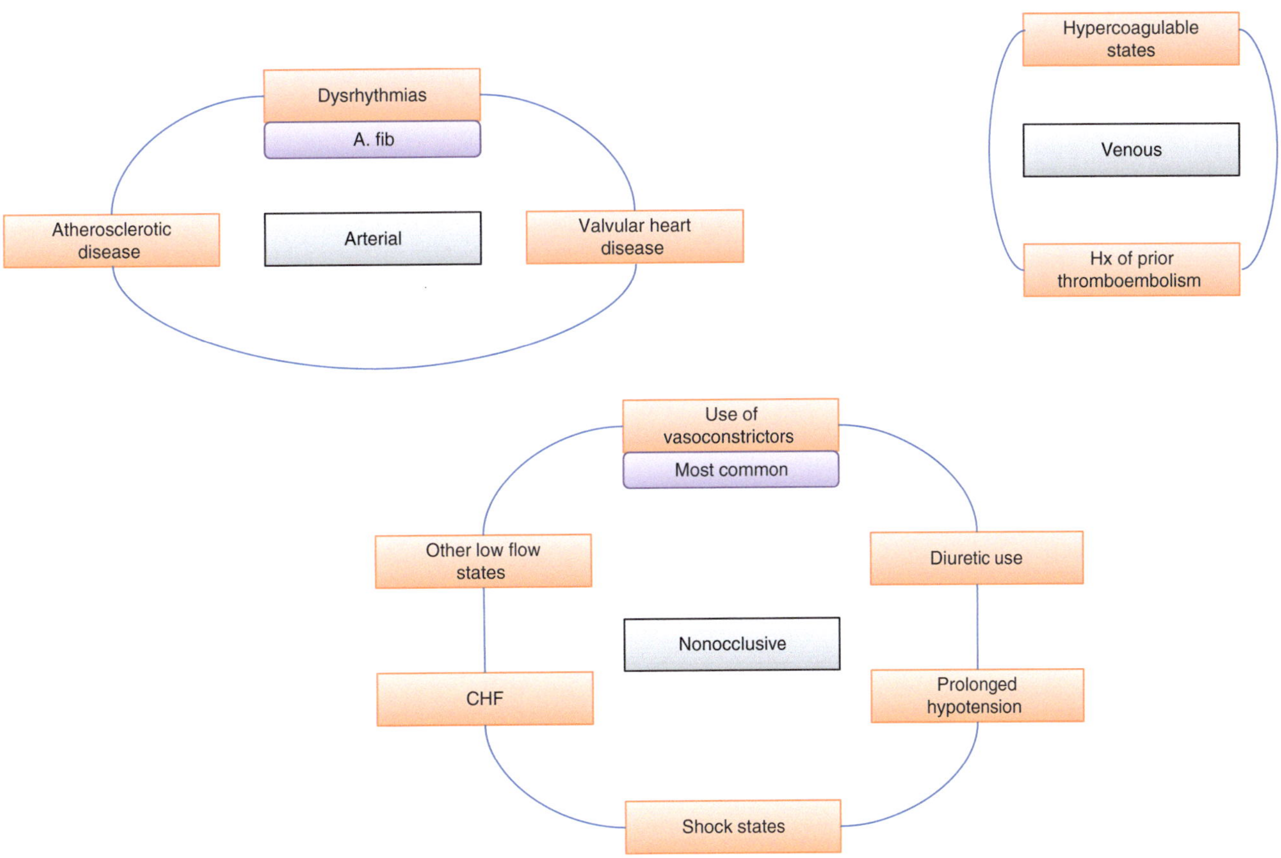

Symptoms and Signs

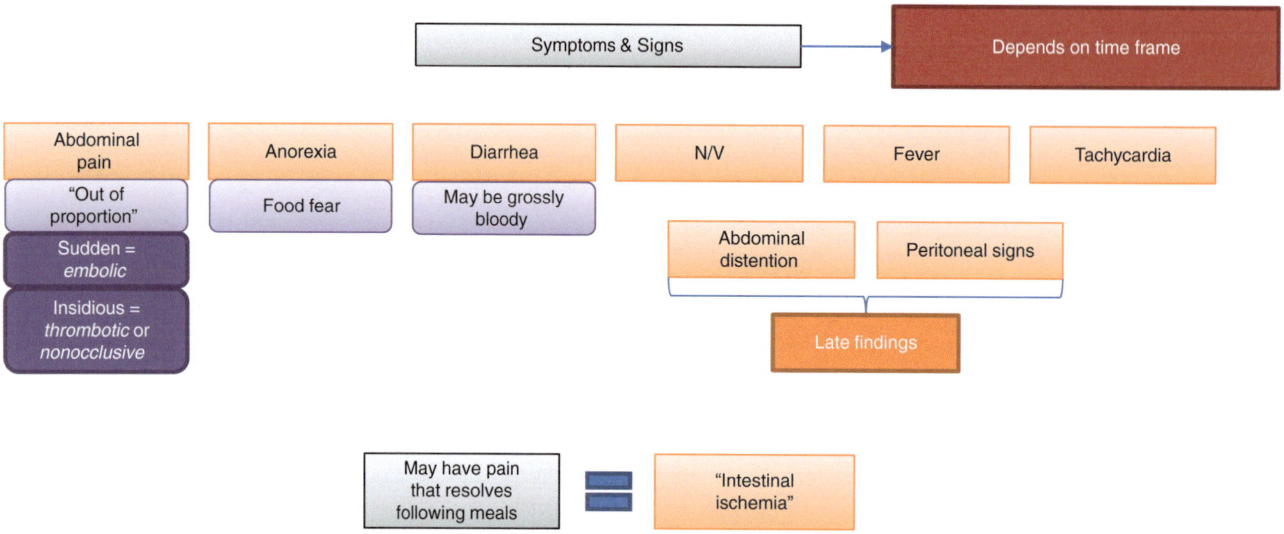

Diagnosis

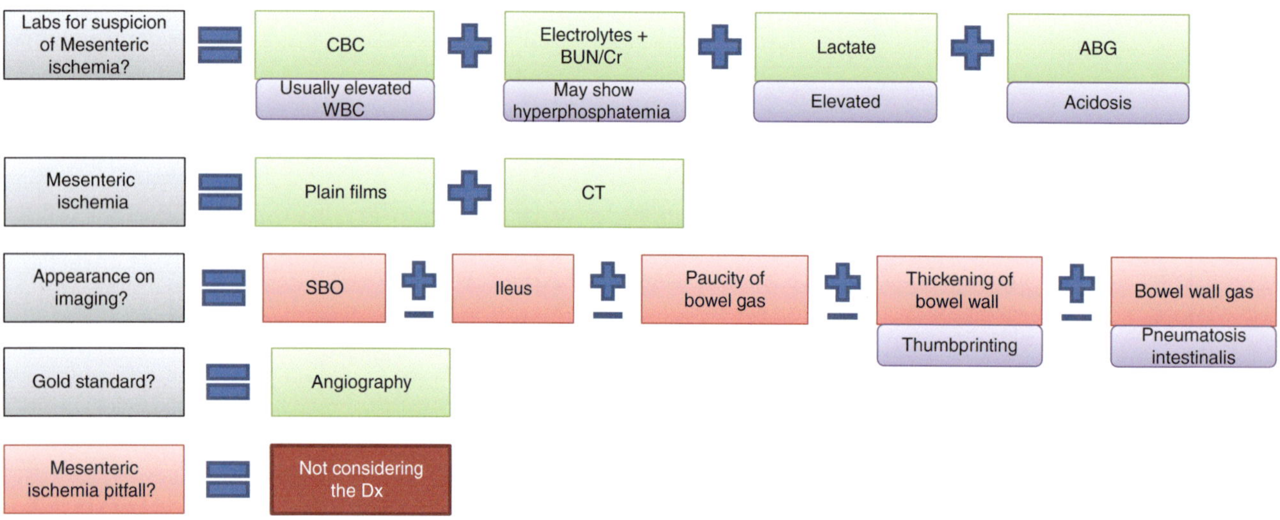

Treatment

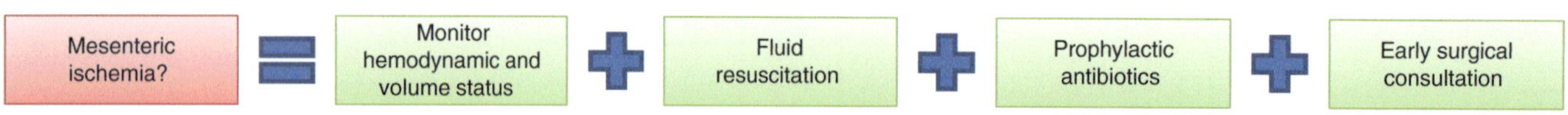

Crohn's Disease

Introduction

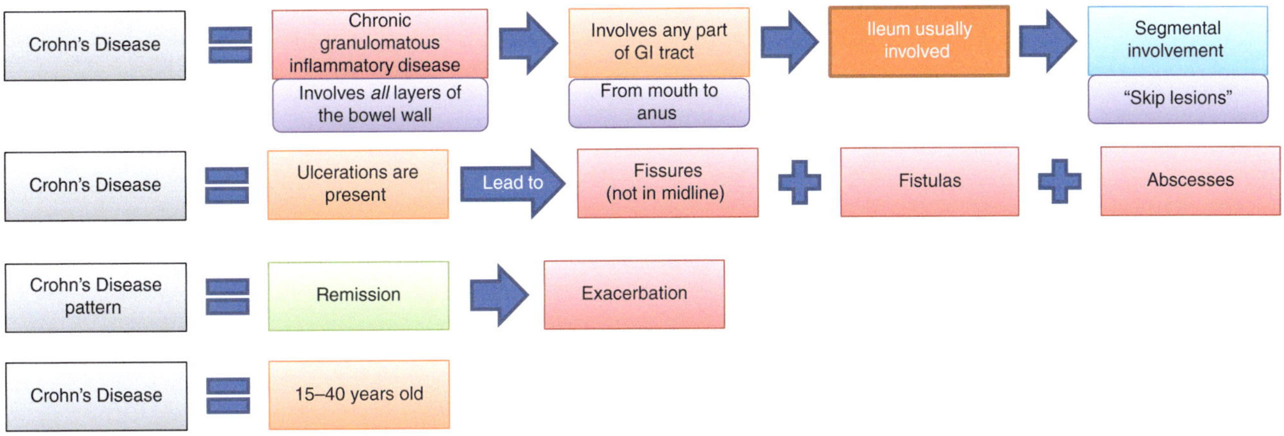

Symptoms and Signs

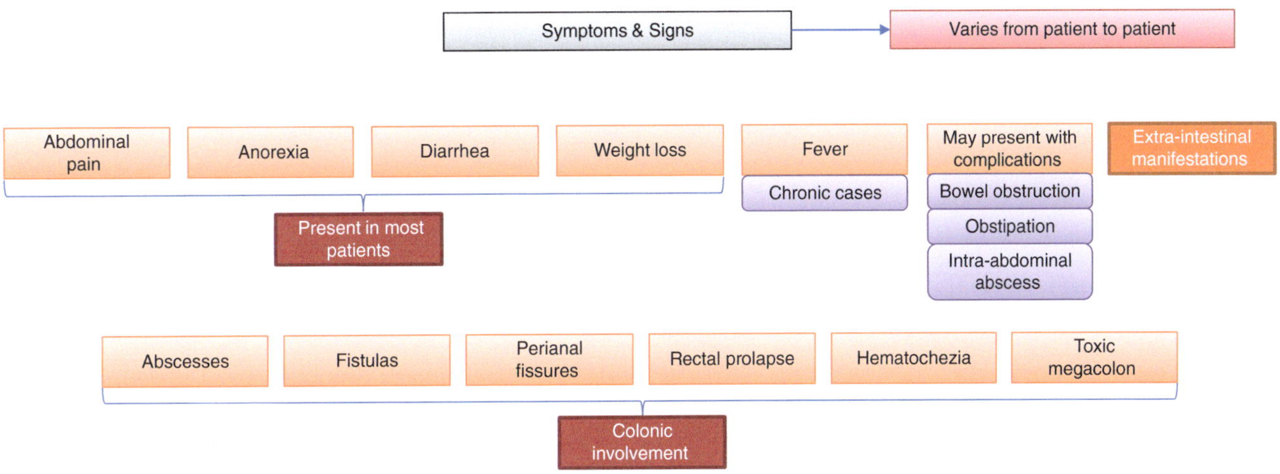

Extraintestinal Manifestations

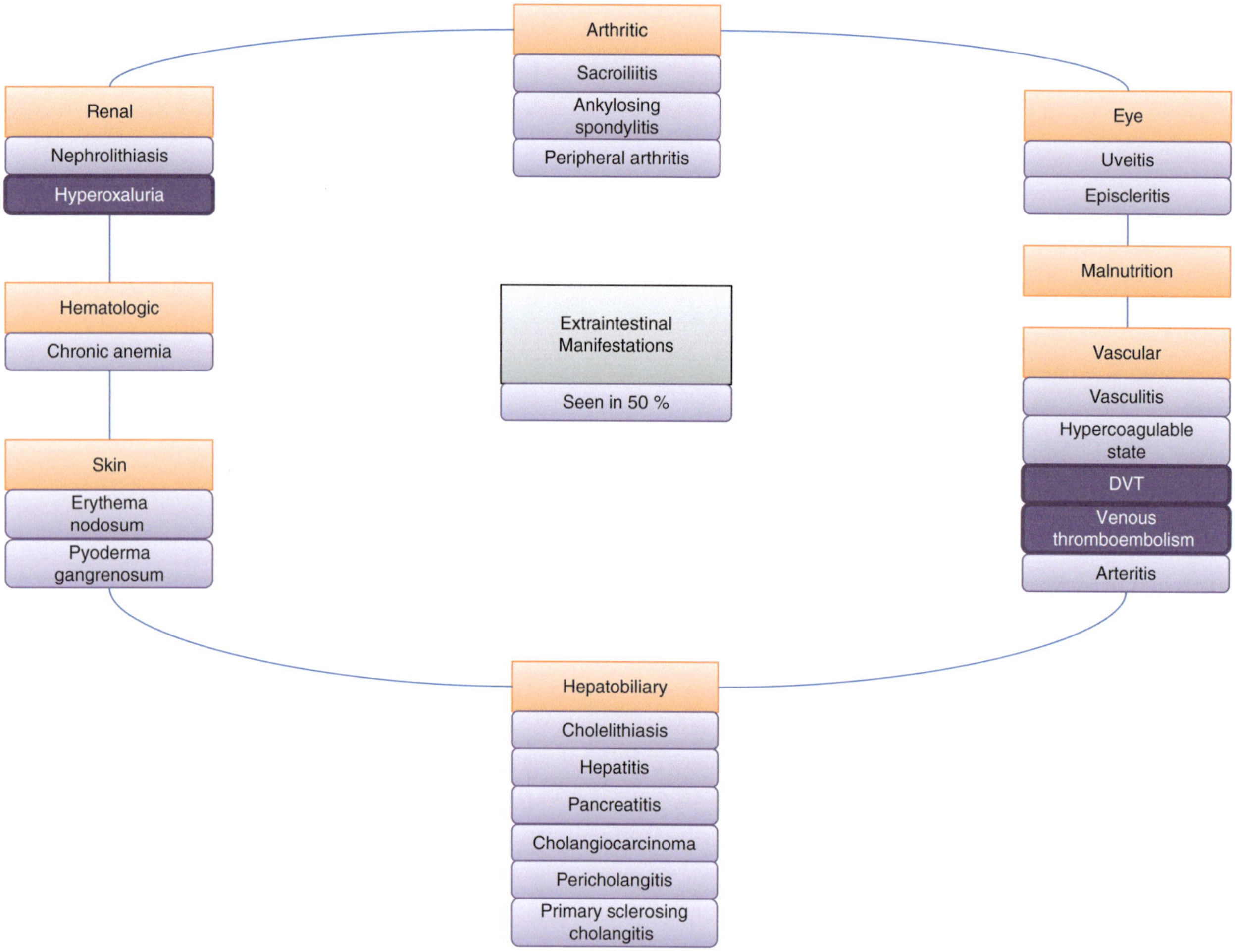

Diagnosis

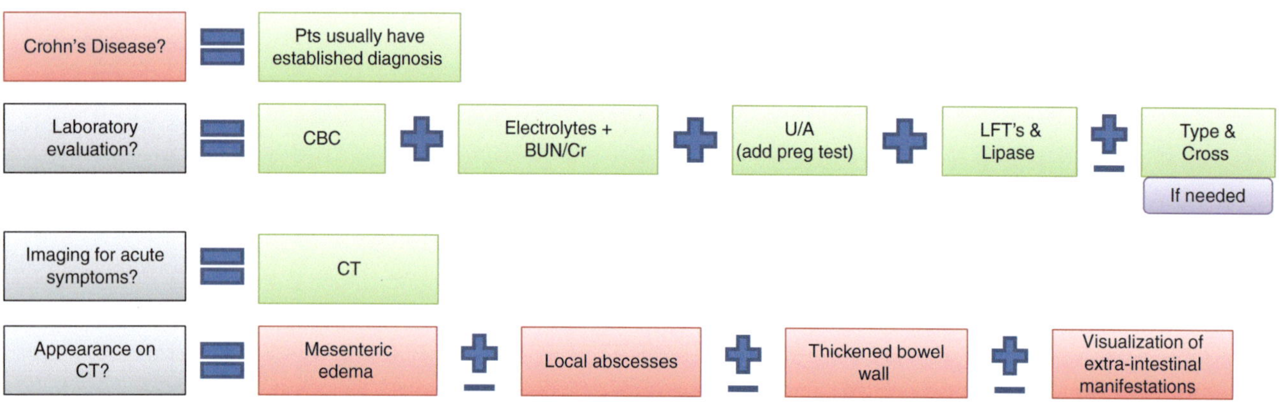

Treatment

Crohn's Disease? = Identify & treat complications

Crohn's disease? = Symptom relief + Prevention of complications + Nutritional maintenance

Mild to moderate Crohn's disease? = Sulfasalazine

Acute exacerbation of Crohn's disease? = Glucocorticoids

Antibiotics in Crohn's disease = Can help induce remission
Ciprofloxacin

Perianal complications & Fistulas = Metronidazole

Pitfall = Must screen for malignancy

Ulcerative Colitis

Introduction

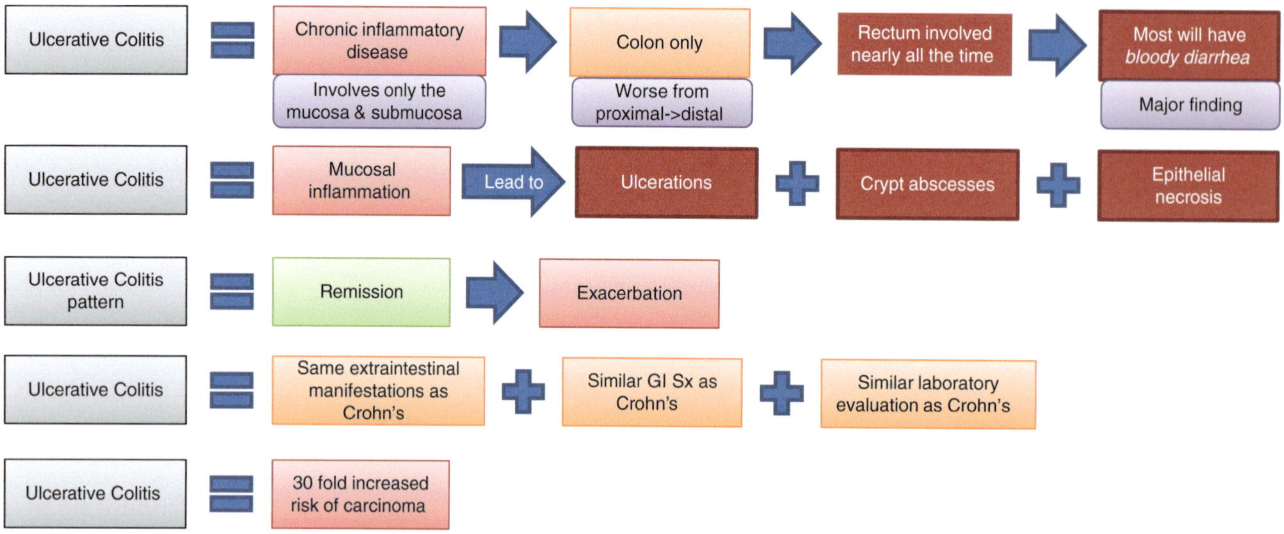

Toxic Megacolon

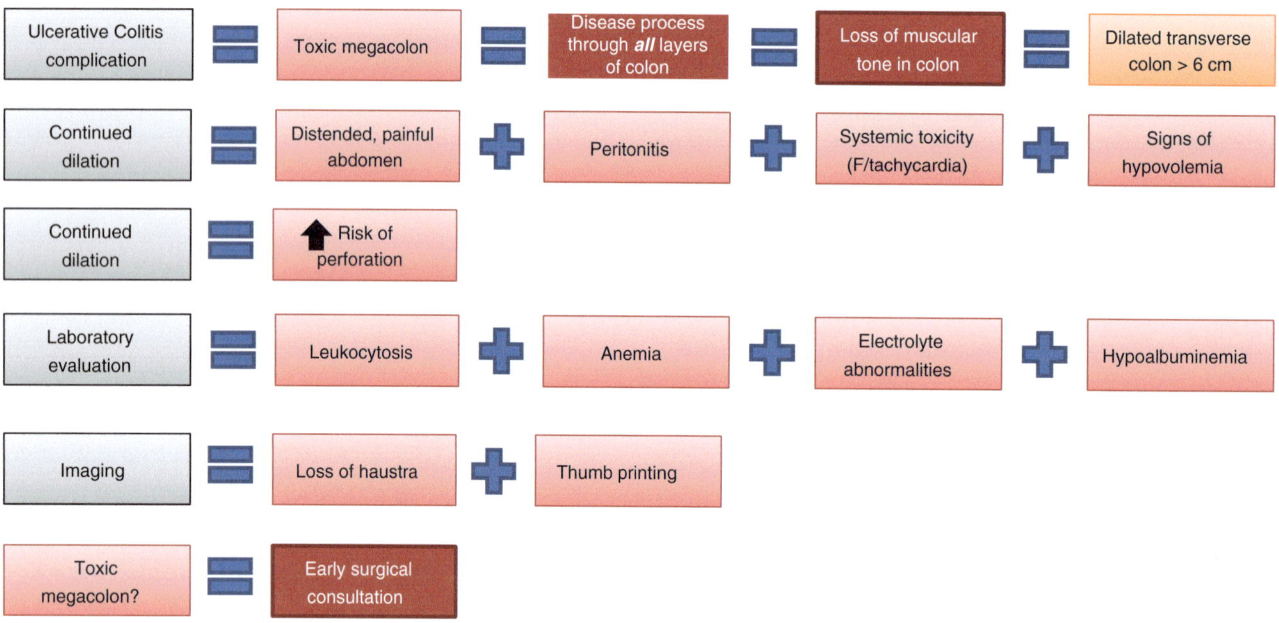

Irritable Bowel Syndrome

Irritable bowel syndrome = Altered gut motility + Altered gut sensation + Alterations in rectal evacuation

Irritable bowel syndrome = Abdominal pain + Bloating + Constipation OR Diarrhea

Irritable bowel syndrome = Usually concomitant psychiatric conditions

Diagnosis and Treatment

Diagnosis = Abdominal pain for 3 days/month in the last 3 months + Improvement with defecation + Change in frequency of bowel movements OR Change in appearance of stools

Treatment = Antispasmodics ± Laxatives OR Antidiarrheals (Depending on complaints)

Miscellaneous Anorectal Emergencies

Hemorrhoids

Hemorrhoids = *Engorgement, prolapse*, or *thrombosis* of hemorrhoidal veins

Internal hemorrhoids = Proximal to the dentate line → Found at → 2, 5, & 9 o'clock (When patient viewed prone) → Not easily palpable (Usually non-tender; Painless, self-limited bleeding) + Best seen with anoscope

External hemorrhoids = Distal to the dentate line = Seen on external examination = Tender to palpation if thrombosed

Treatment = Warm water sitz baths + Analgesia + Stool softeners + High fiber diet ± Topical steroids

Thrombosed hemorrhoid? = Clot excision

Pitfalls of excision (Don't excise) = Coagulopathy + Immune compromised + Pregnancy + Portal hypertension + Children

Surgical consultation? = Very large hemorrhoid + Incarcerated hemorrhoid + Strangulated hemorrhoid + Intractable pain + Continued bleeding

Risk Factors for Hemorrhoids

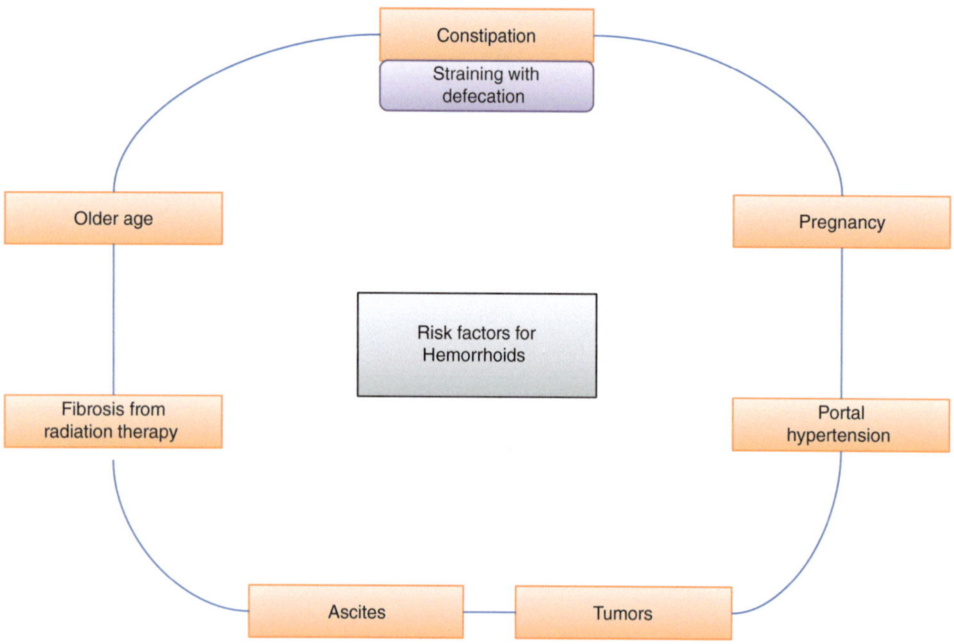

Anal Fissures

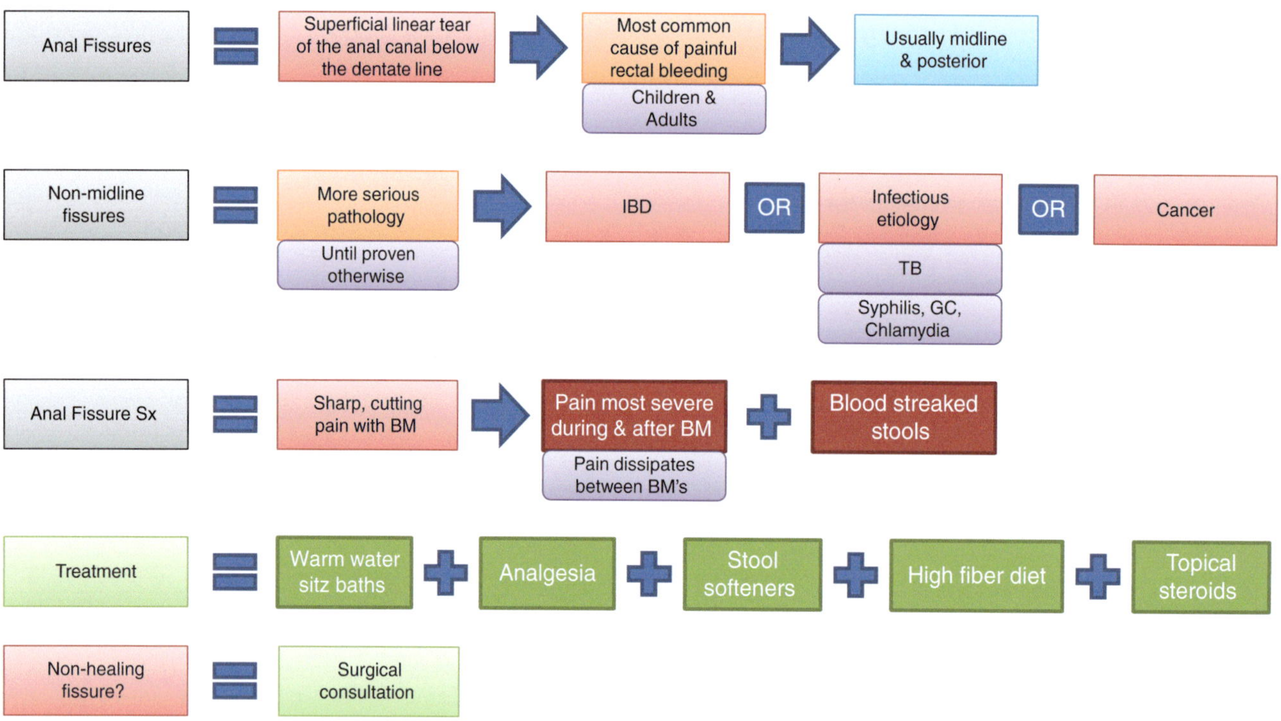

Anorectal Abscesses

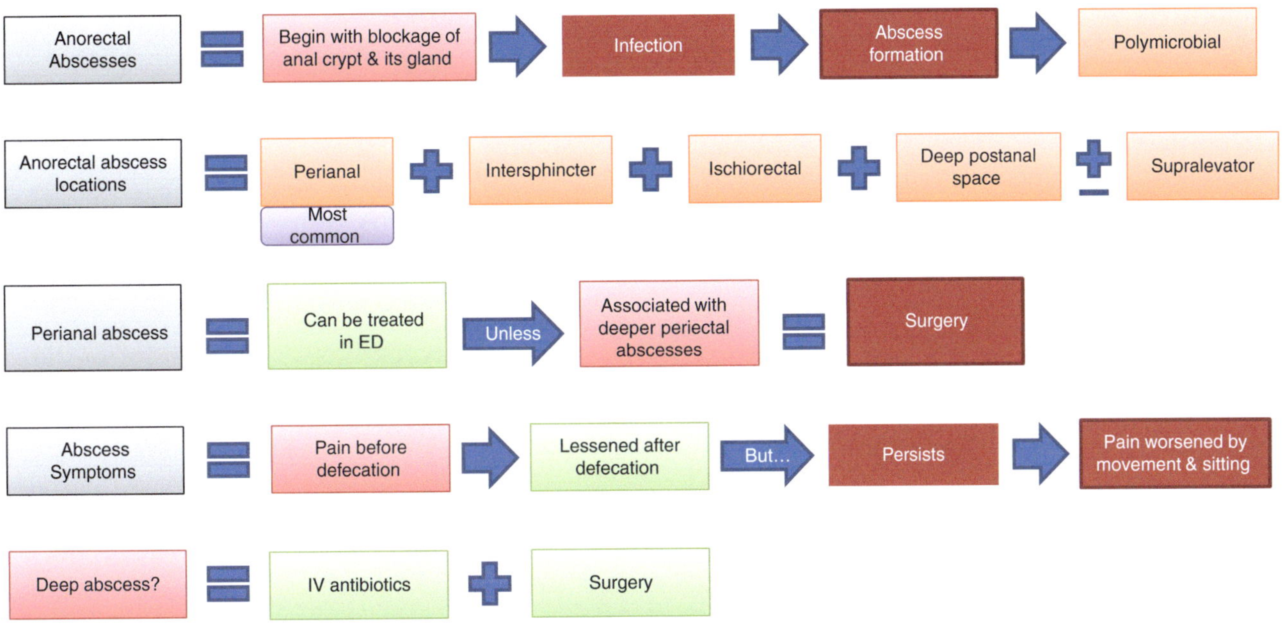

Rectal Prolapse

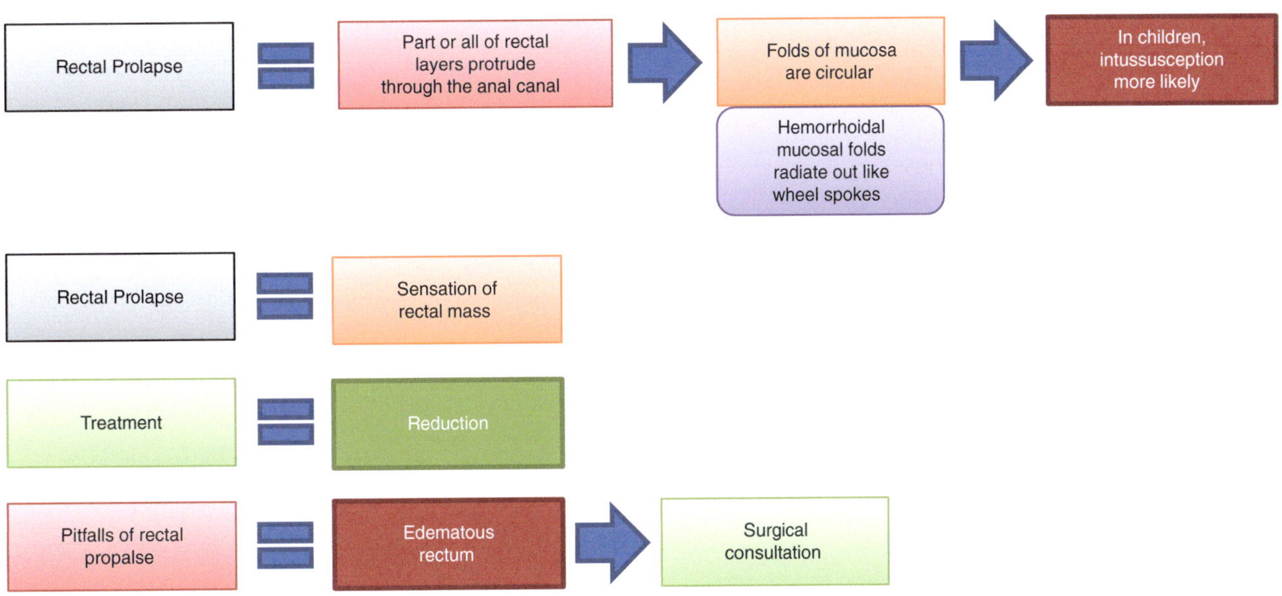

Nephrology and Urology

Bobby Desai

Contents

Acute Renal Failure ... 262
Rhabdomyolysis ... 274
Chronic Renal Failure ... 277
Hemodialysis ... 283
Urinary Tract Infections ... 288
Hematuria ... 292
Kidney Stones ... 293
Renal Transplant ... 295
Male Genital Emergencies ... 295
Sexually Transmitted Diseases ... 301

B. Desai, MD, MEd
Department of Emergency Medicine, University of Florida,
Gainesville, FL, USA
e-mail: bdesai@ufl.edu

B. Desai, B.R. Allen (eds.), *Nailing the Written Emergency Medicine Board Examination*,
DOI 10.1007/978-3-319-30838-8_4

Acute Renal Failure

Introduction

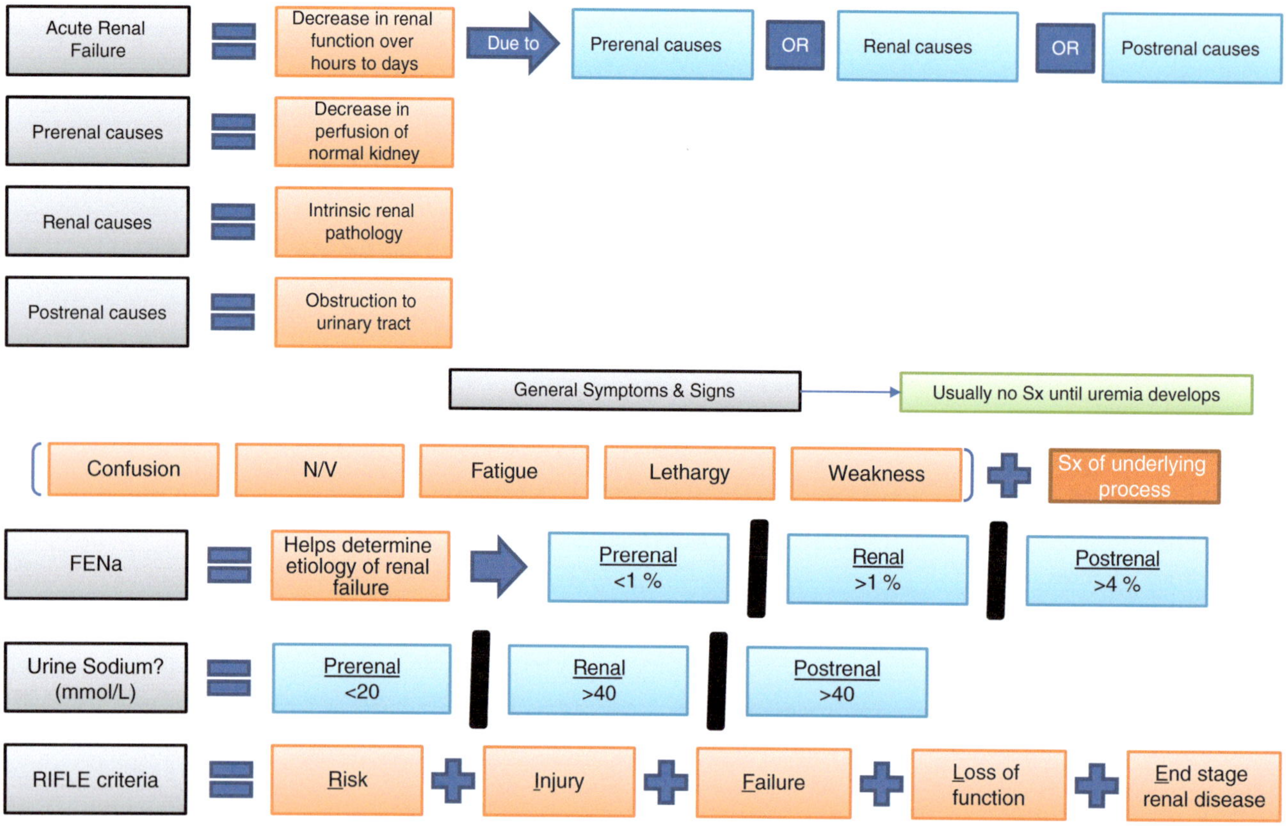

RIFLE Criteria

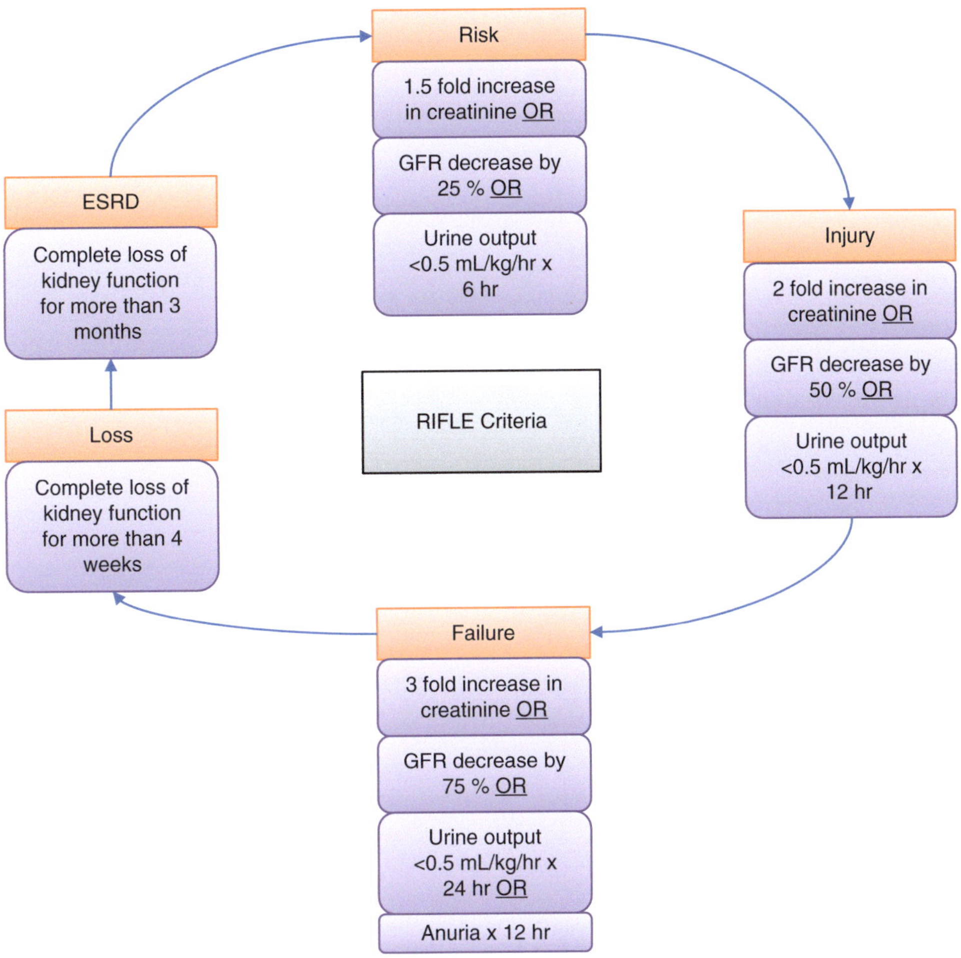

Common Causes of Acute Renal Failure in Children

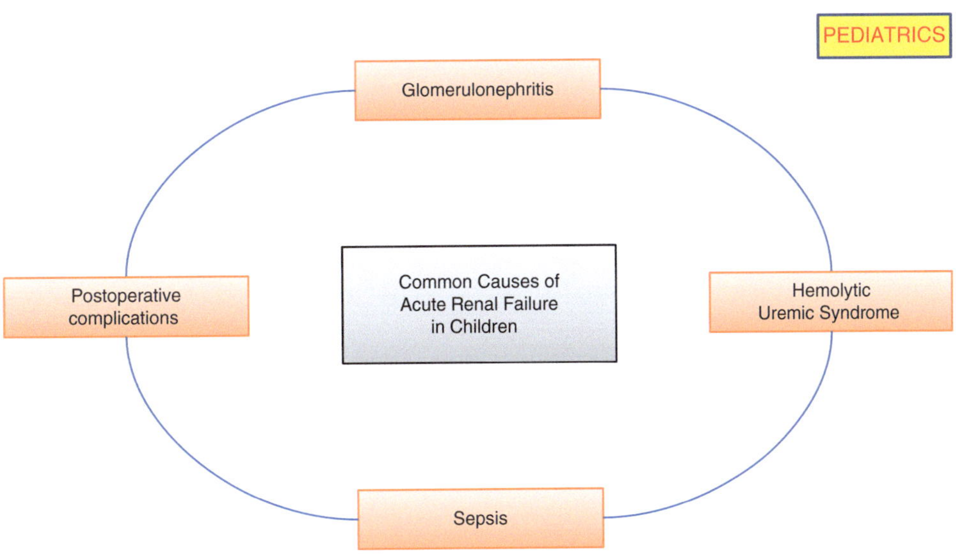

Prerenal Failure

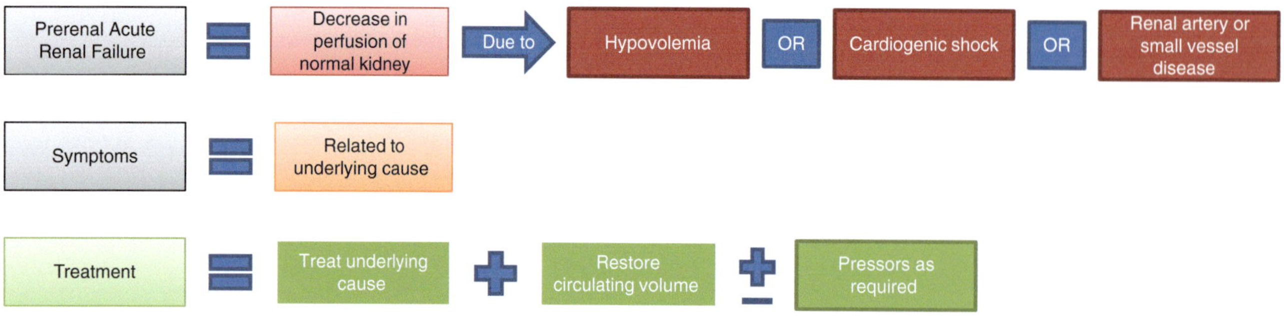

Causes of Prerenal Failure

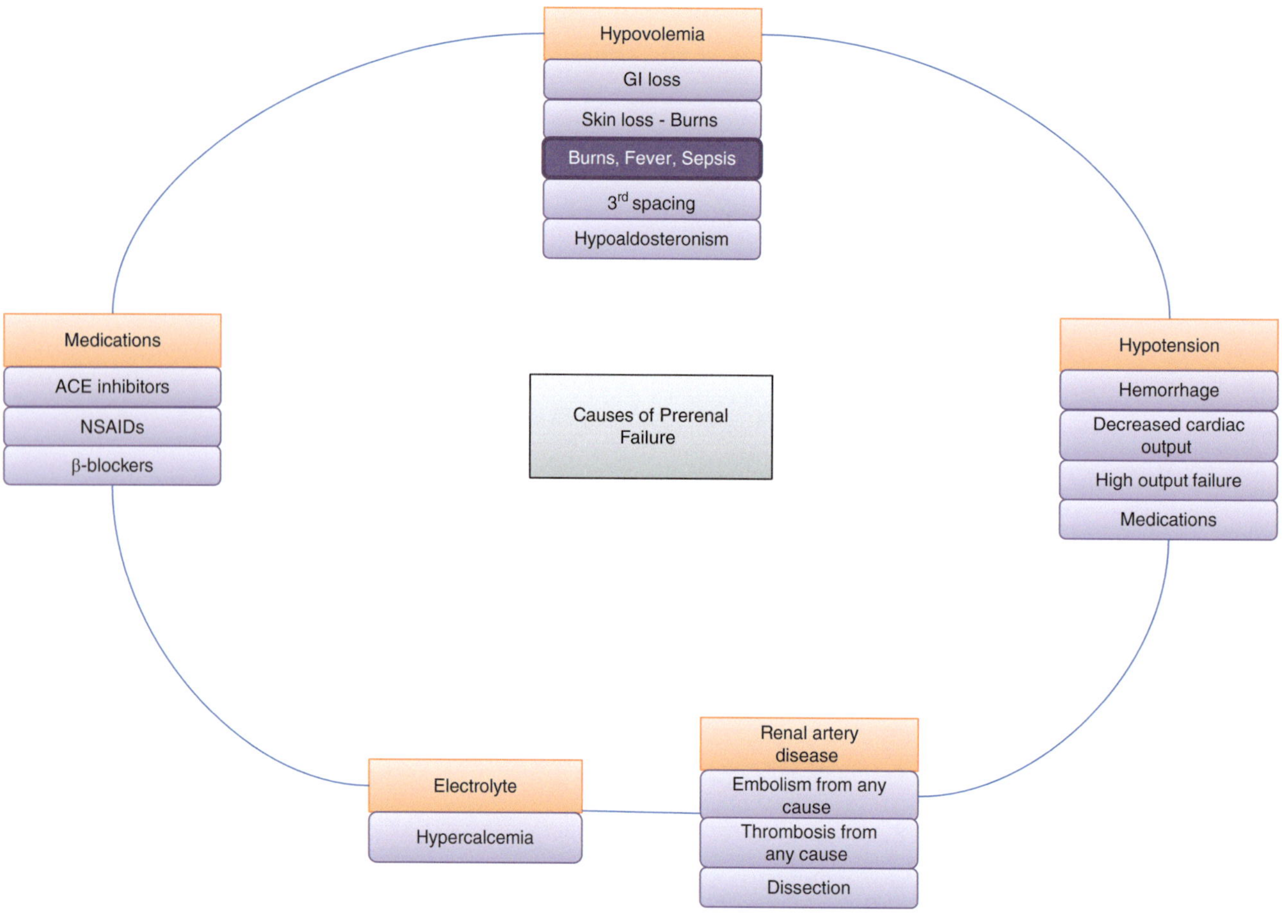

Intrinsic Renal Failure

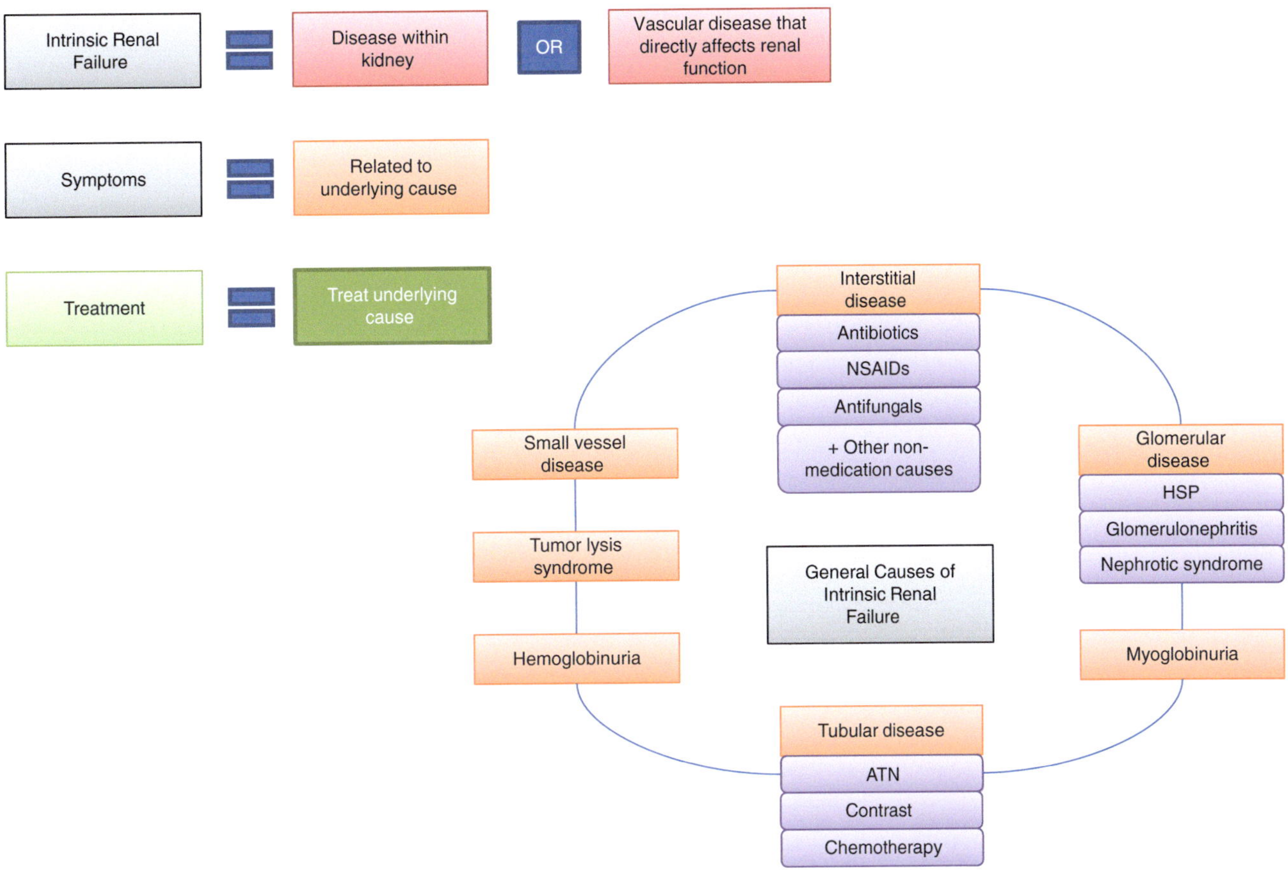

Some Causes of Interstitial Disease

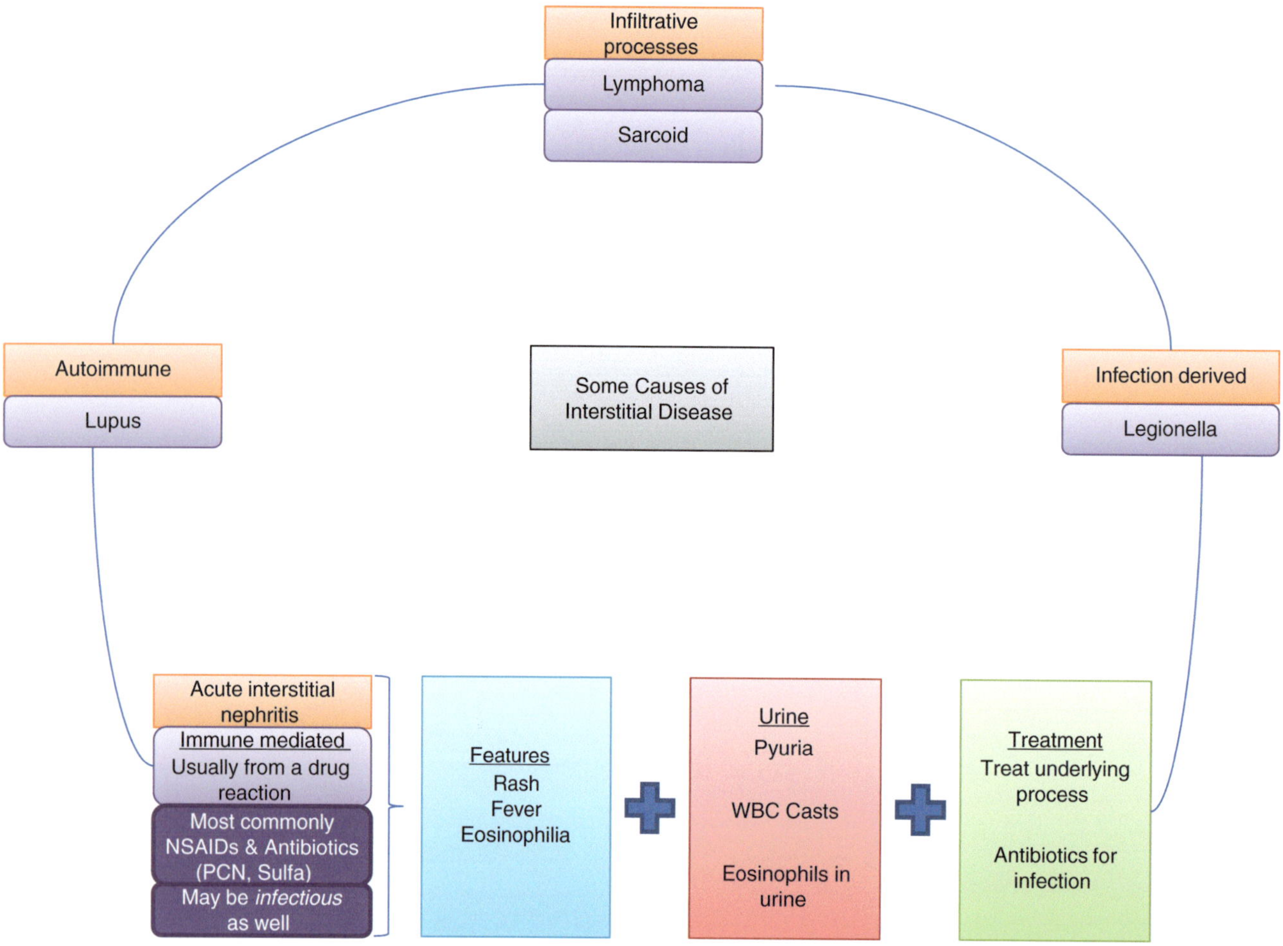

Some Causes of Glomerular Disease

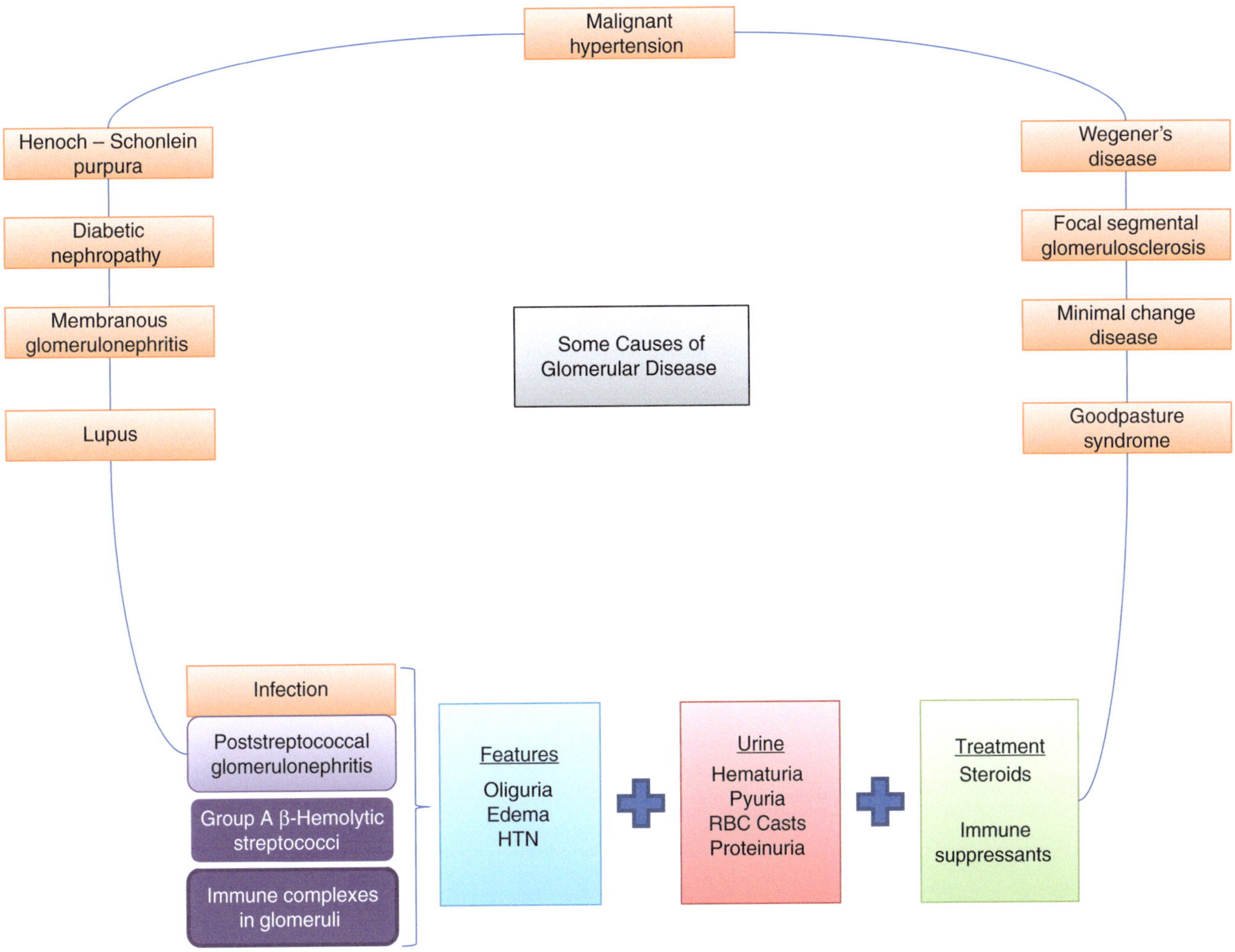

Some Causes of Tubular Disease

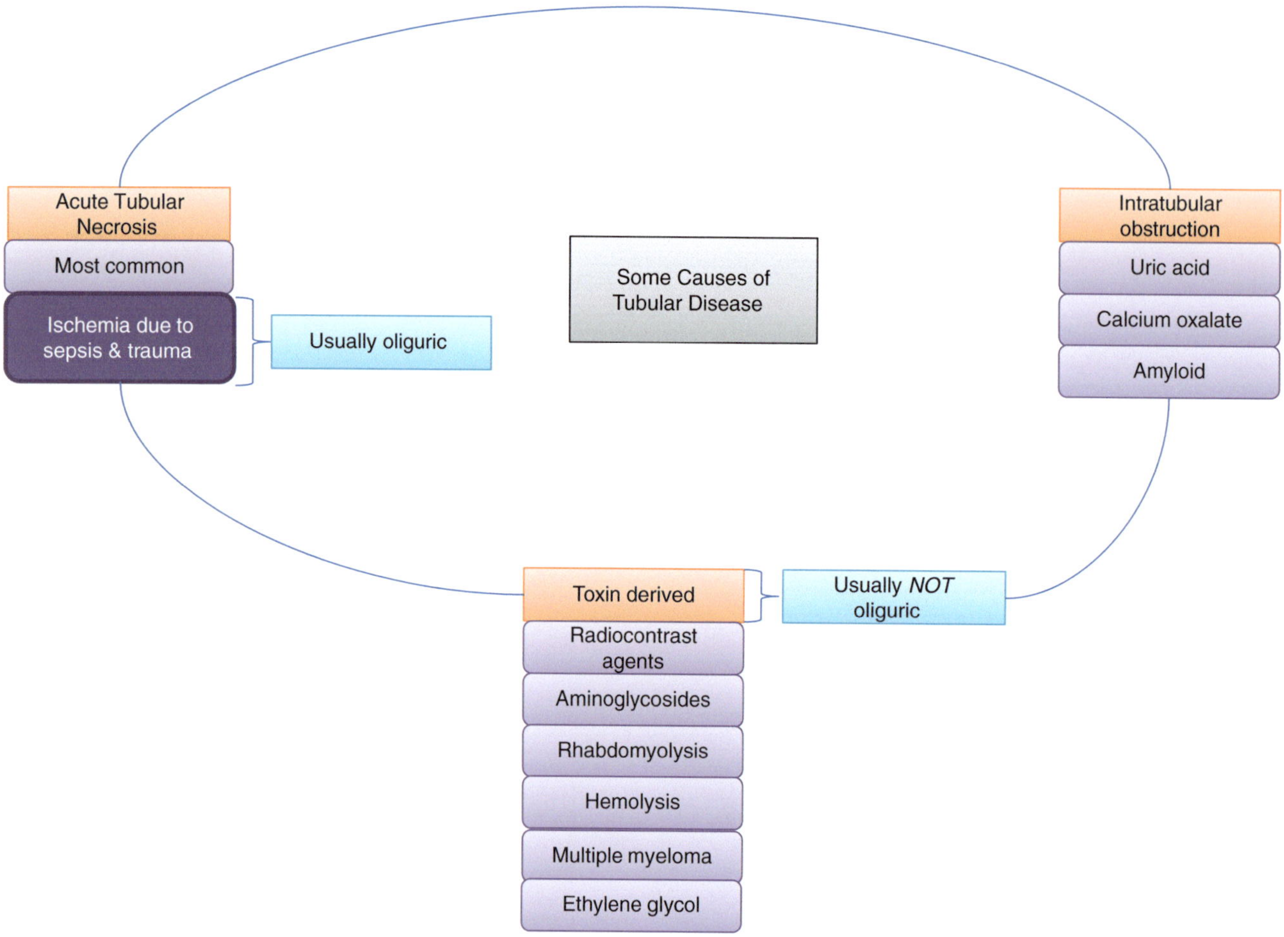

Risk for Radiocontrast-Induced Nephropathy

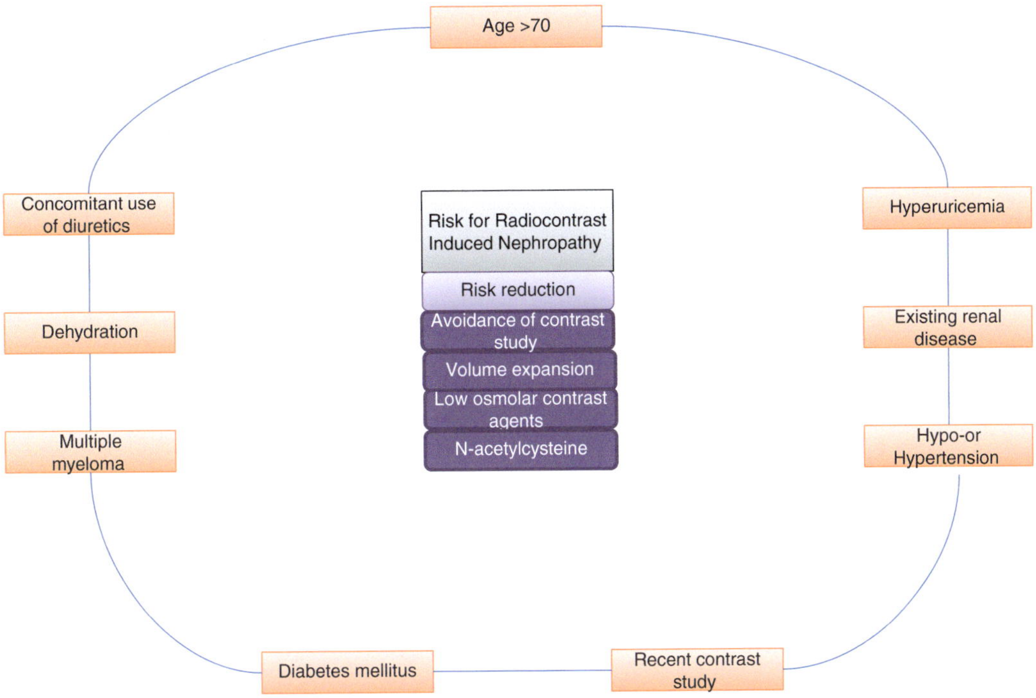

Vascular or Related Disease

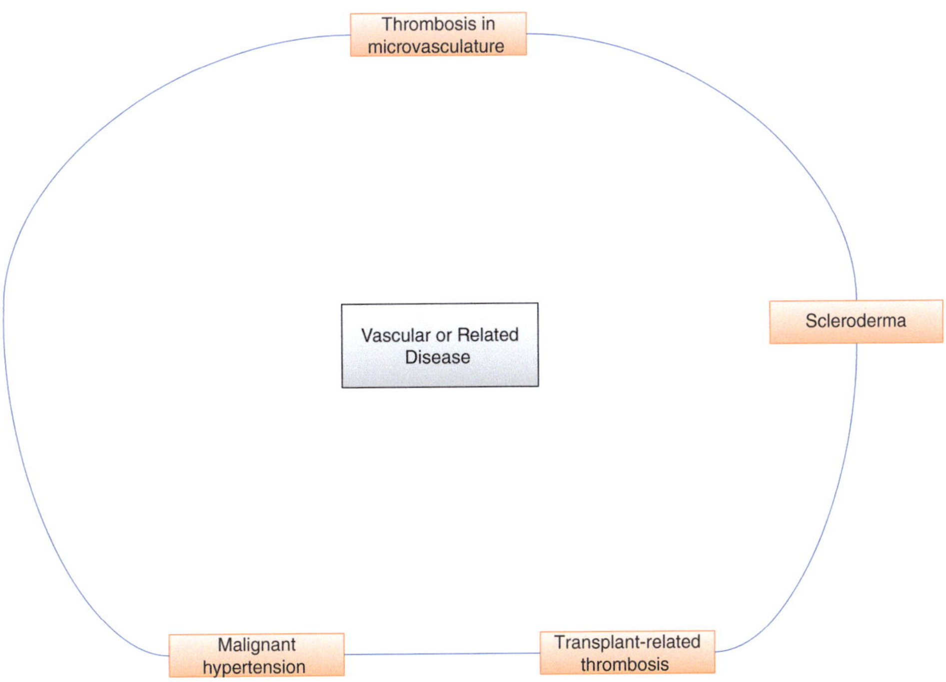

Causes of Microthrombosis

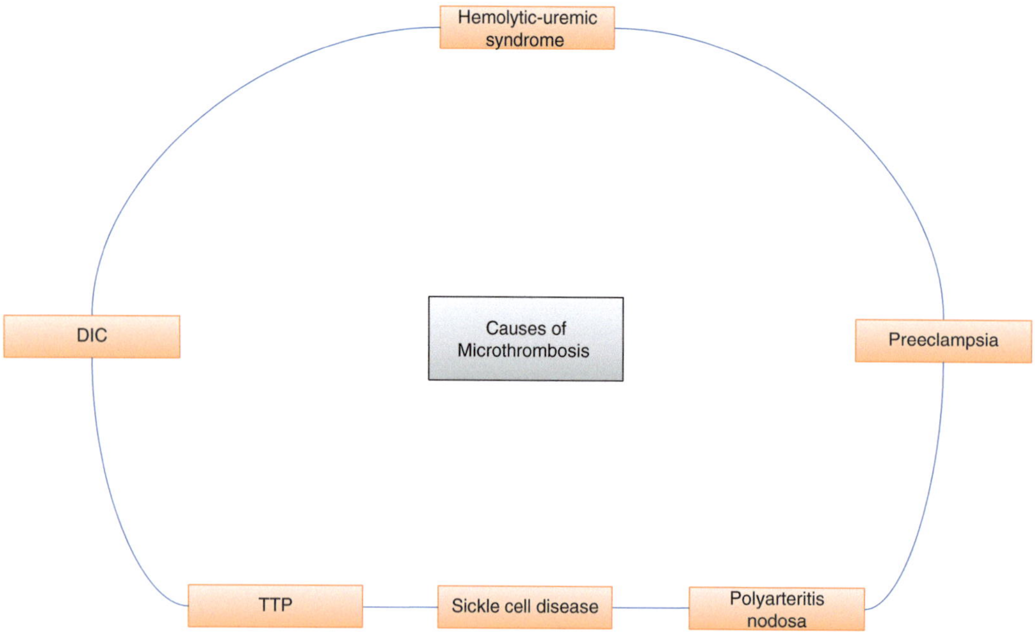

Postrenal Failure

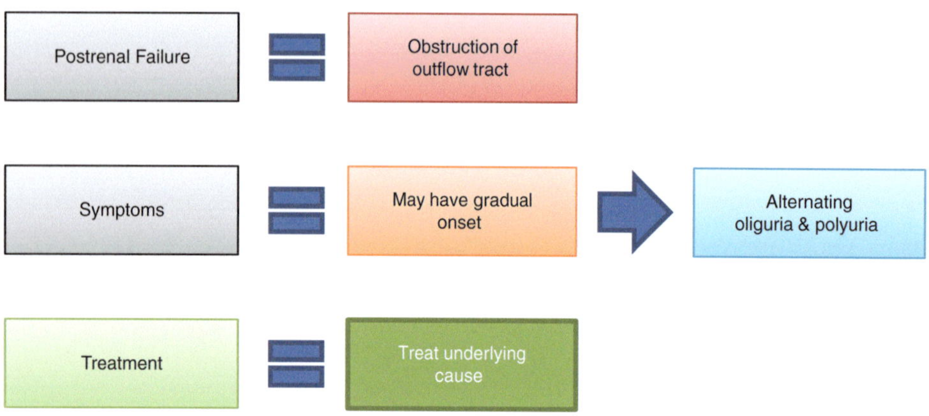

General Causes of Postrenal Failure

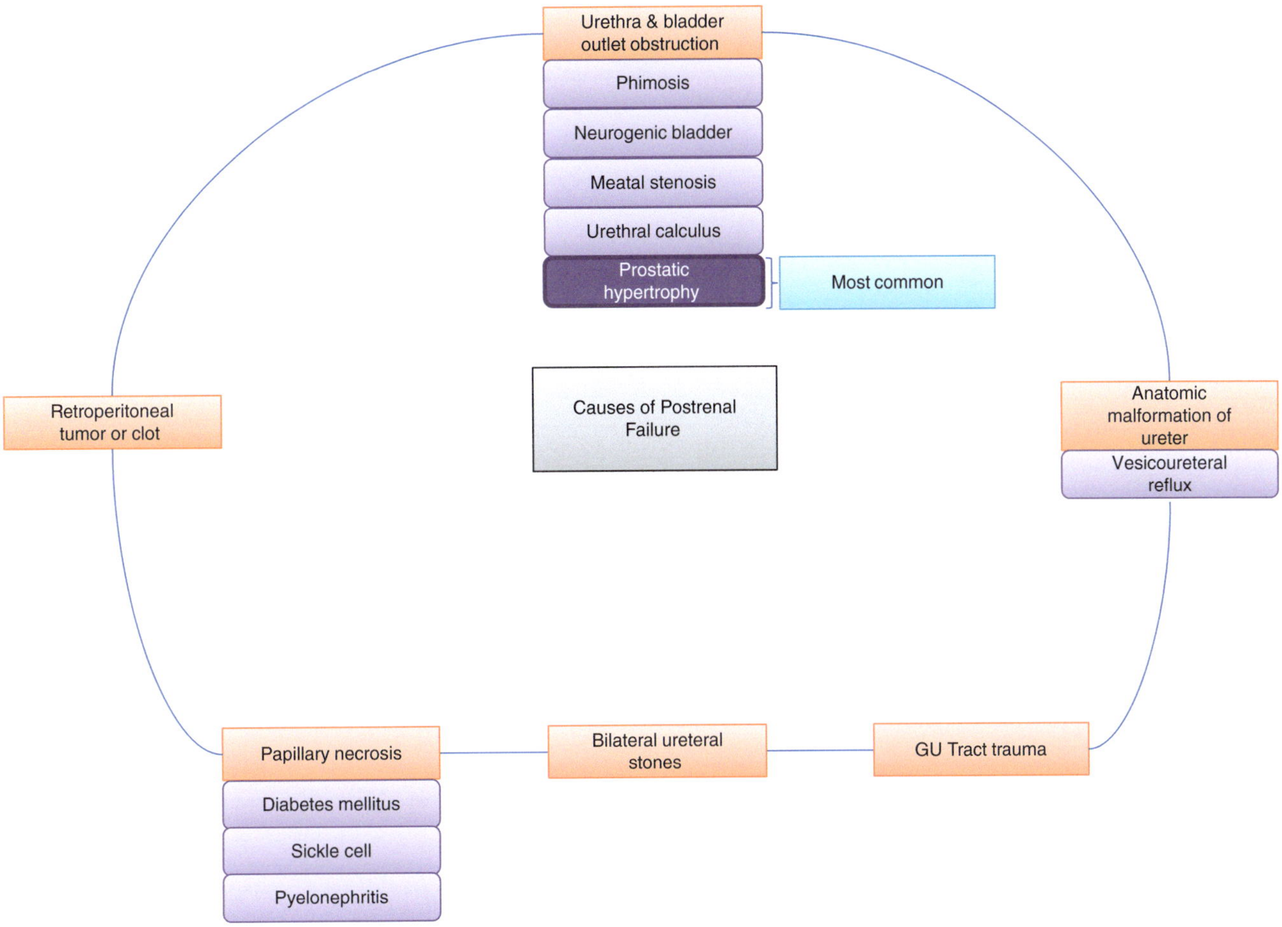

Some Laboratory Investigations for Renal Failure

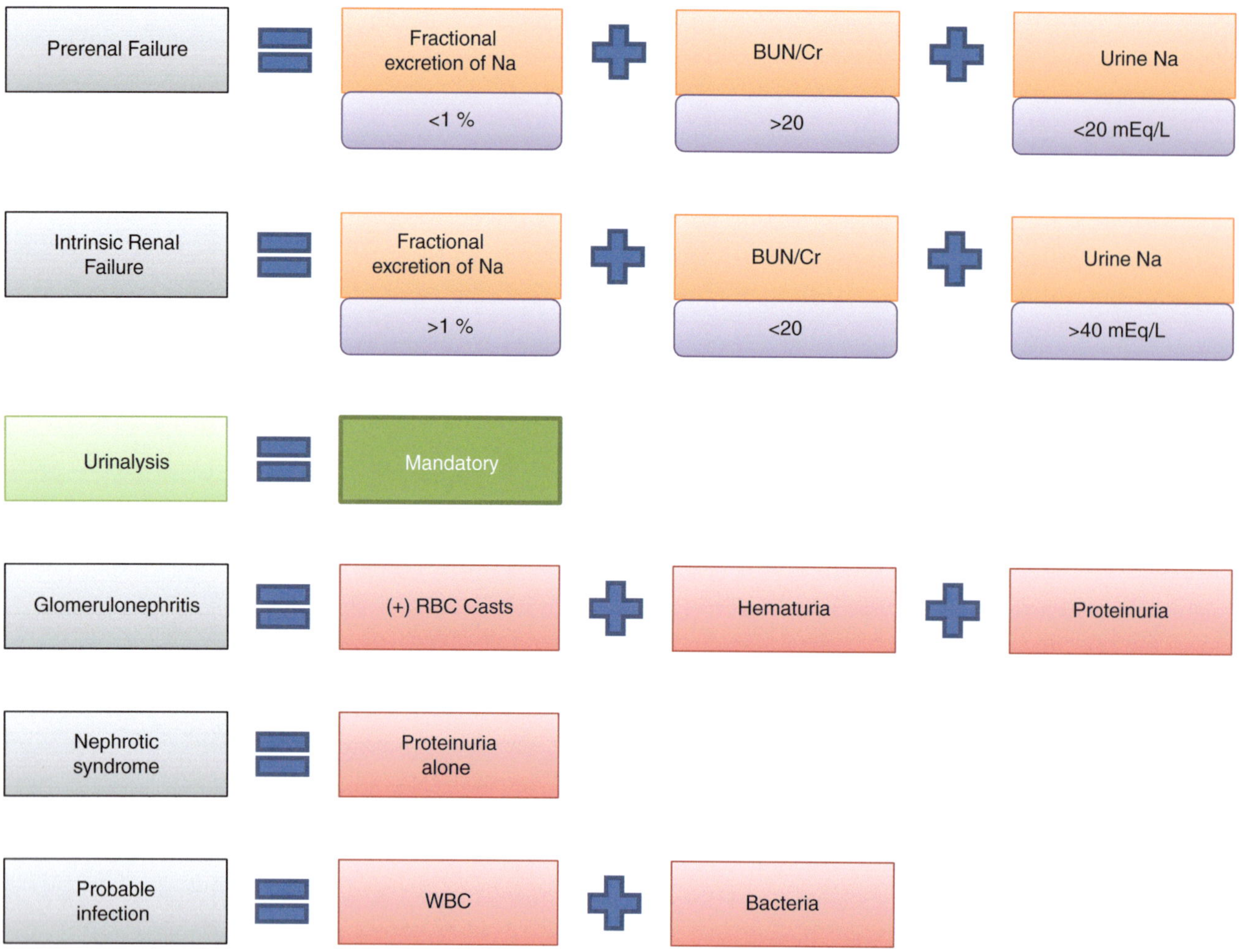

Macroscopic Urine

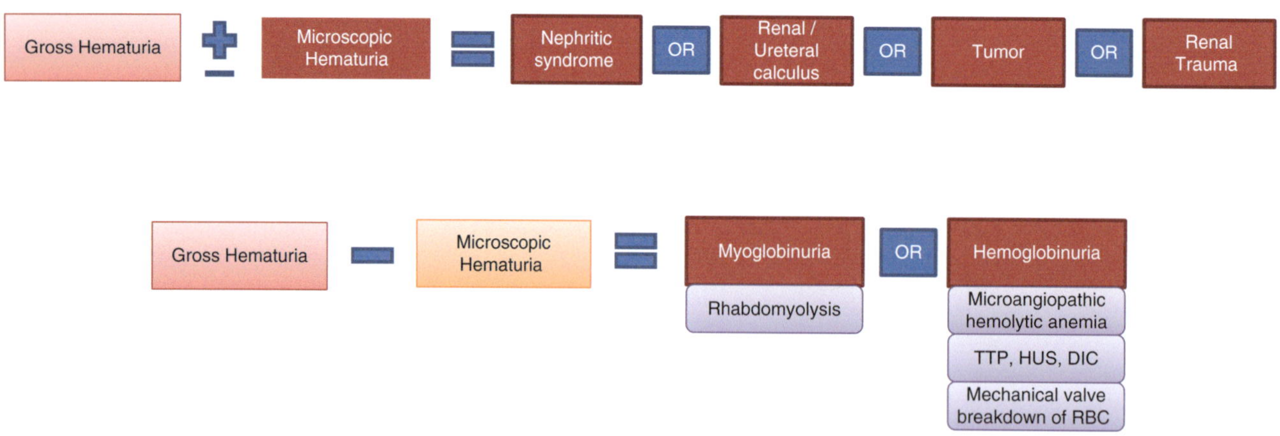

Urinalysis

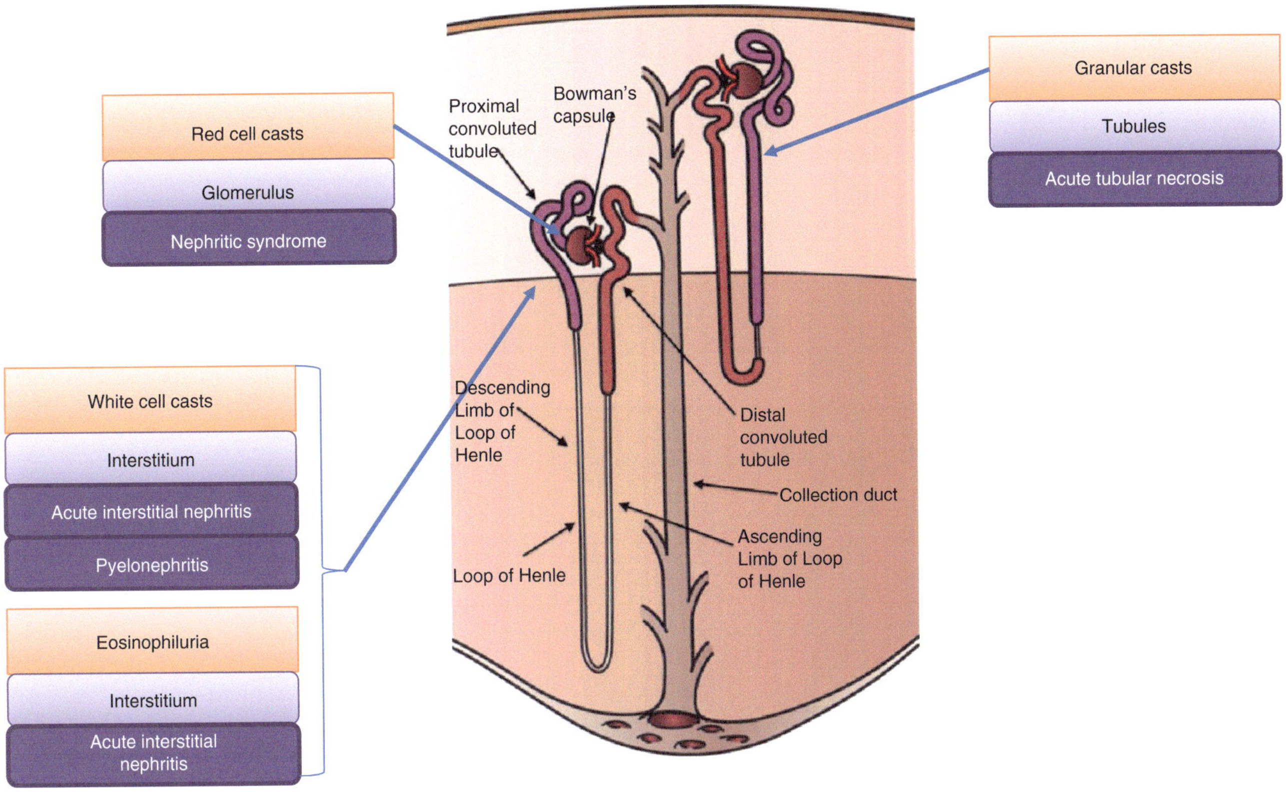

Center image (Adapted from Kidney Nephron: https://commons.wikimedia.org/wiki/File:Kidney_Nephron.png. Artwork by Holly Fischer with permission from Creative Commons License: https://creativecommons.org/licenses/by/3.0/deed.en)

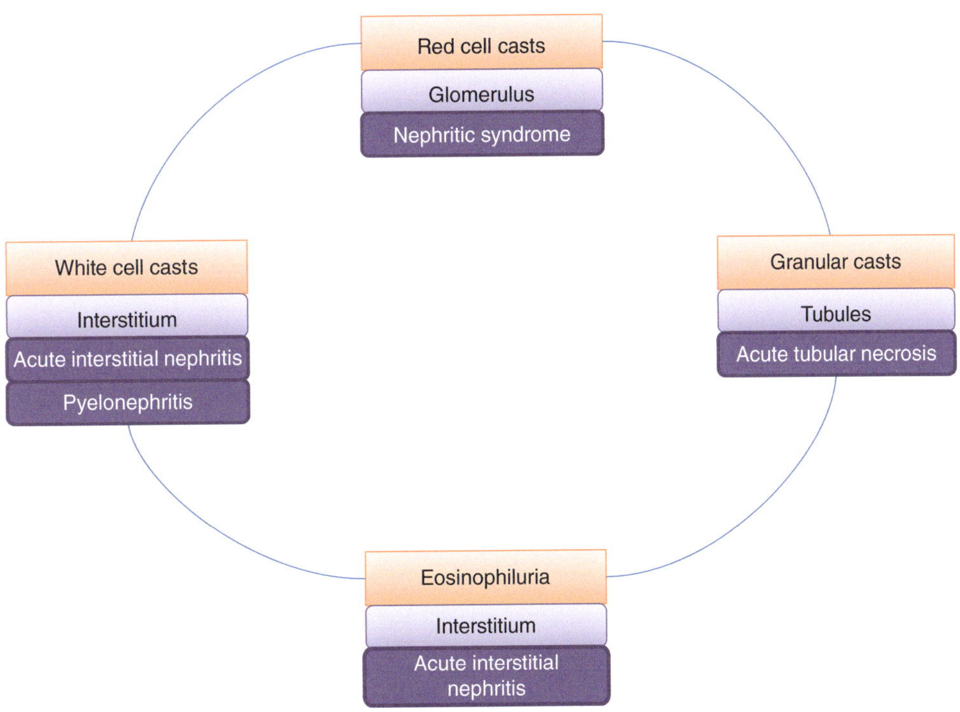

Rhabdomyolysis

Introduction

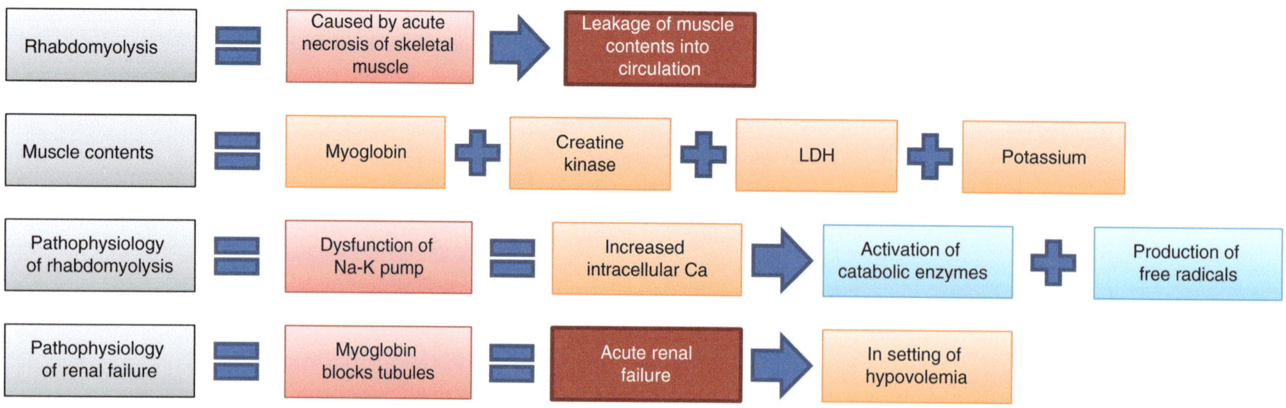

Causes of Rhabdomyolysis

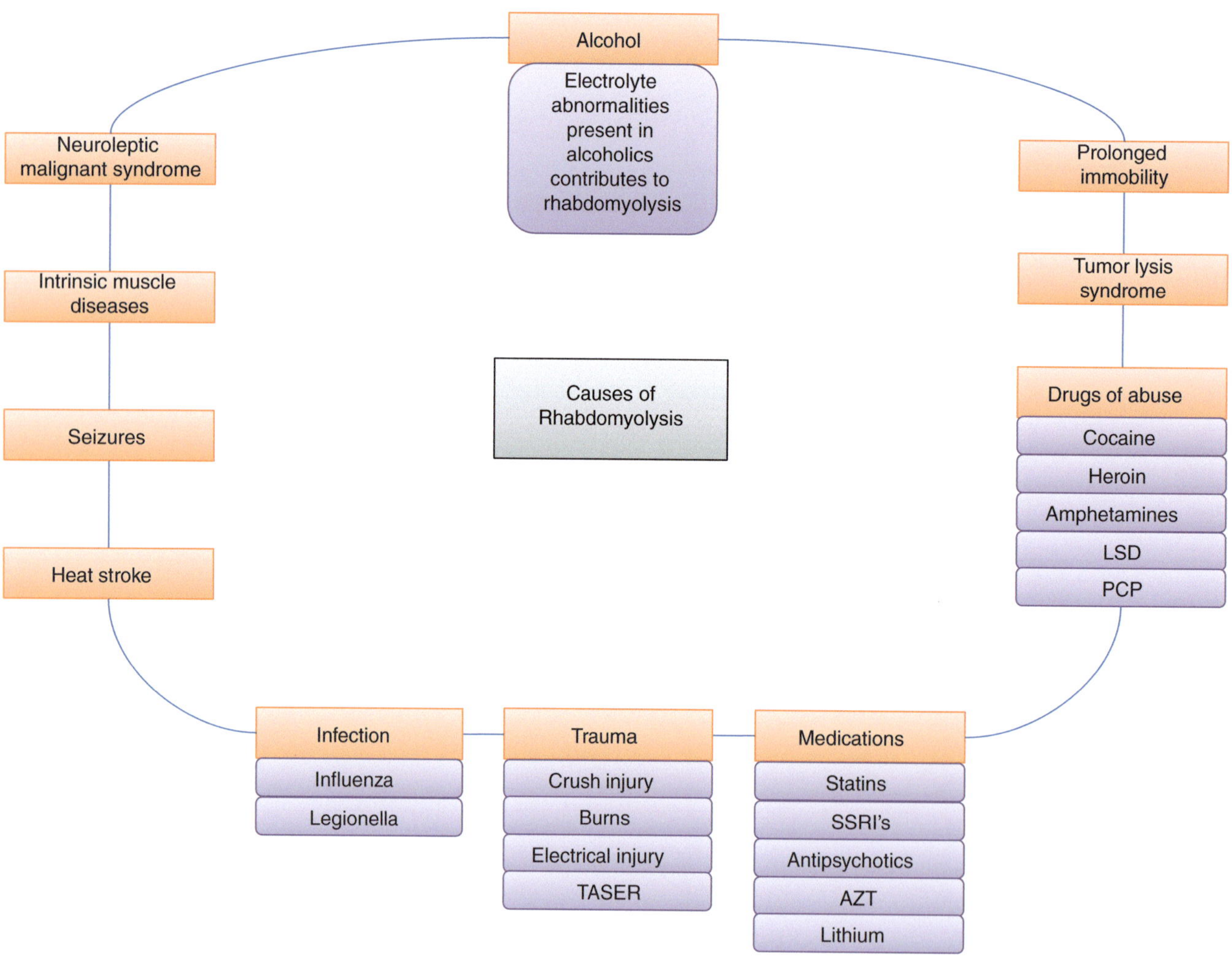

Clinical Features of Rhabdomyolysis

Symptoms & Signs

- **Acute**: Diffuse stiffness, Diffuse weakness, Myalgias, Malaise, Dark cola colored urine, ±Fever
- **More advanced stage**: N/V, Tachycardia, Abdominal pain, AMS

Diagnosis of Rhabdomyolysis

- **Creatine kinase** = 5 fold or greater increase in CK − Without heart or brain injury (CK rises 2-12 hours, peaks 24-72 hours)
- **Ongoing muscle necrosis** = Failure of CK to decrease over time
- **Other marker** = Acute rise in creatinine
- **Urine** = (+) dip for heme − RBC on microscopy
- **Other labs** = Serum electrolytes with BUN/Cr + Calcium + Phosphorus + Uric acid + Baseline CBC
- **Consider** = PT/PTT + Fibrinogen + Fibrin split products → Due to potential DIC as a complication

Complications of Rhabdomyolysis

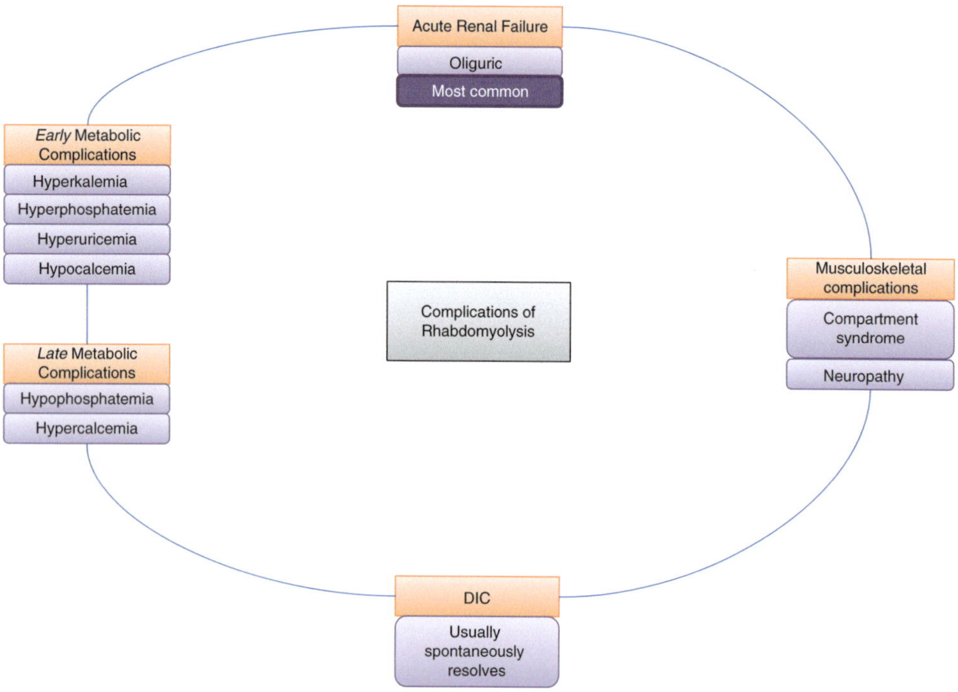

Treatment of Rhabdomyolysis

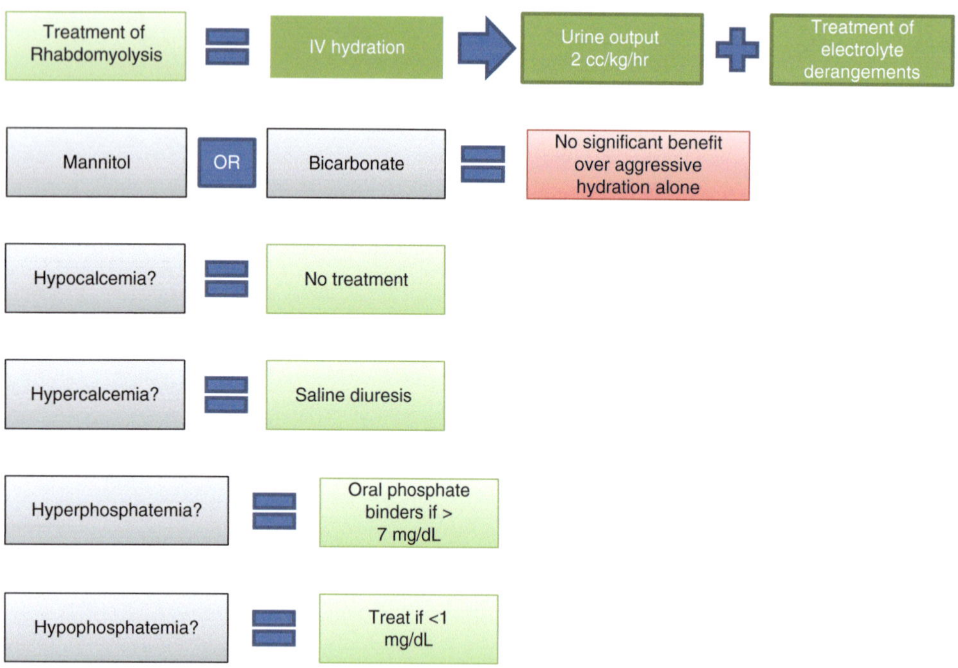

Chronic Renal Failure

Chronic Renal Failure and End-Stage Renal Disease (ESRD)

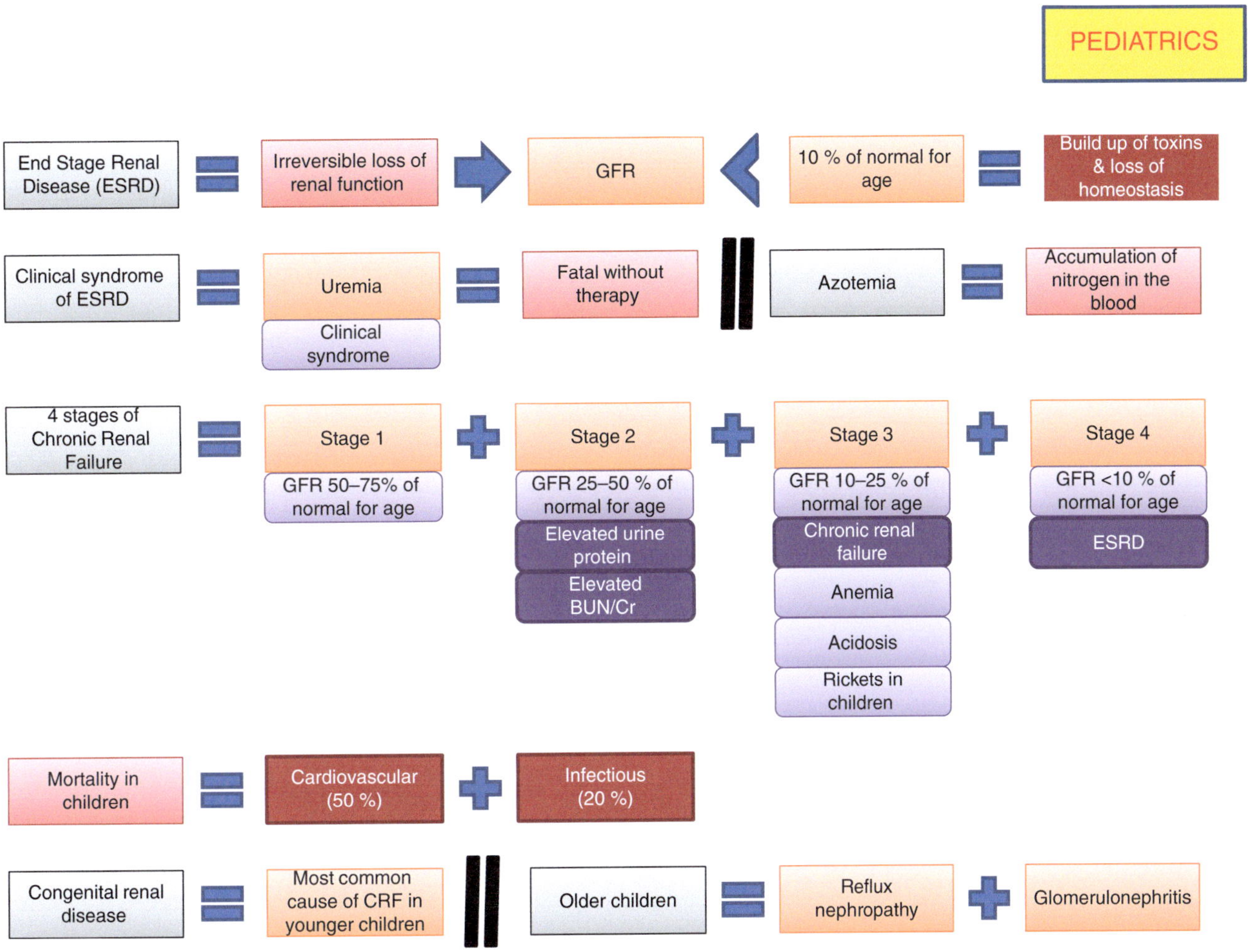

Nephrotic Syndrome

PEDIATRICS

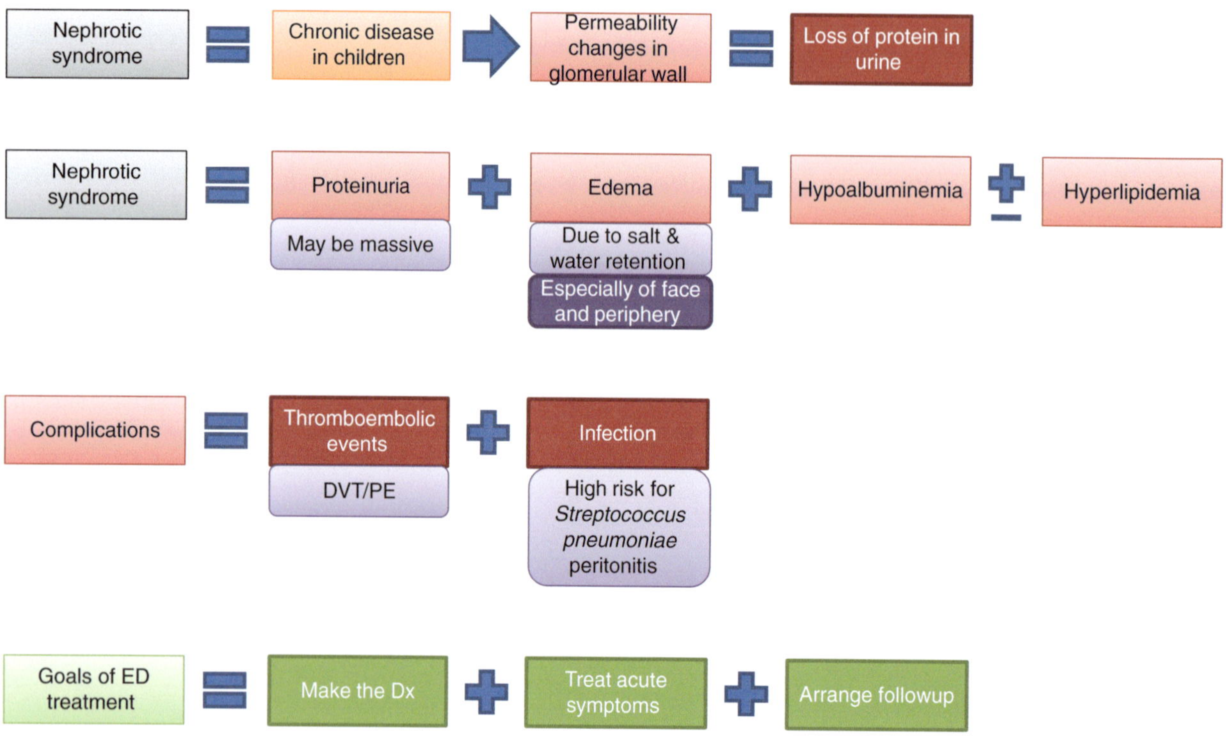

Causes of Nephrotic Syndrome

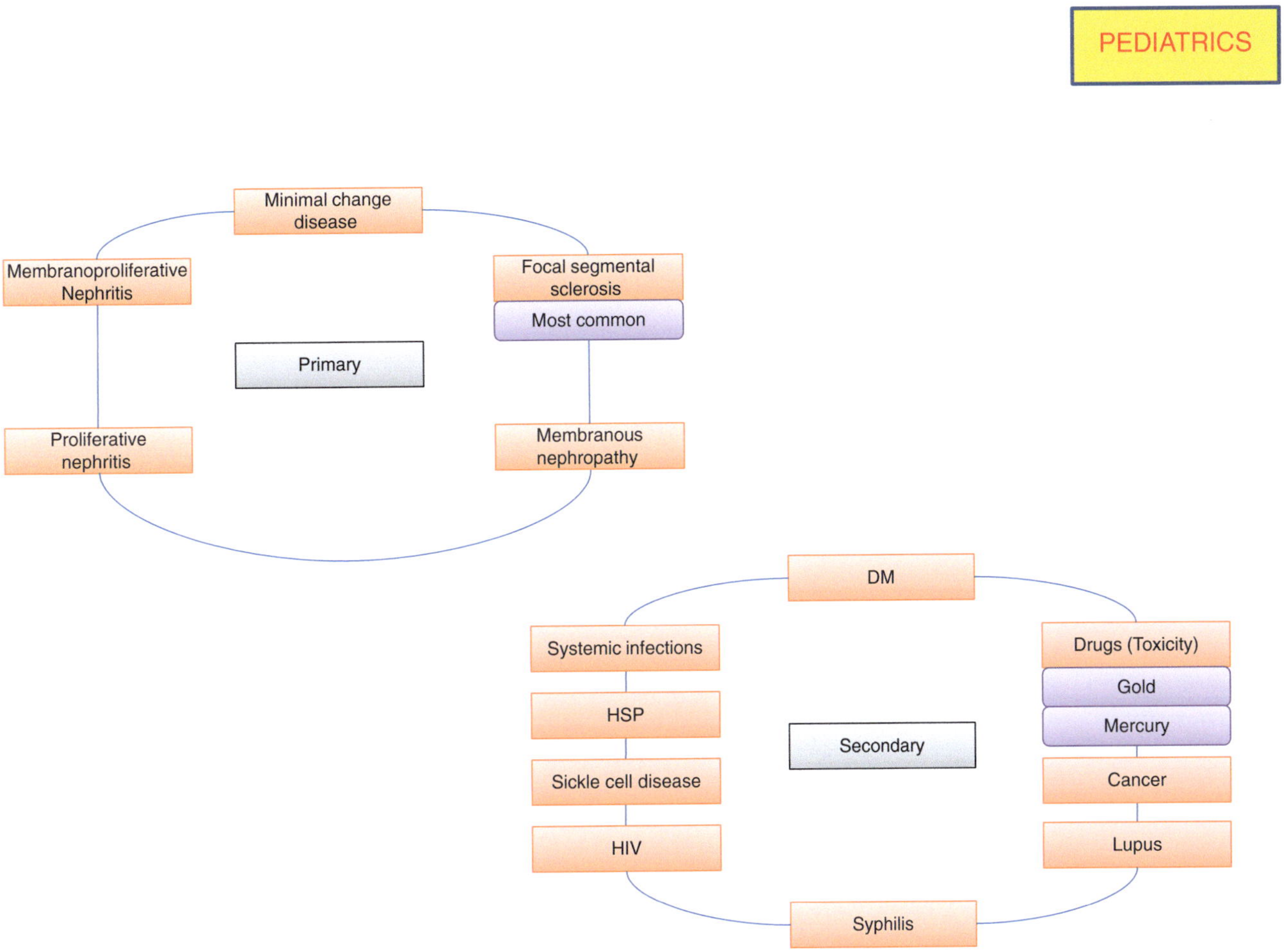

Renal Tubular Acidosis

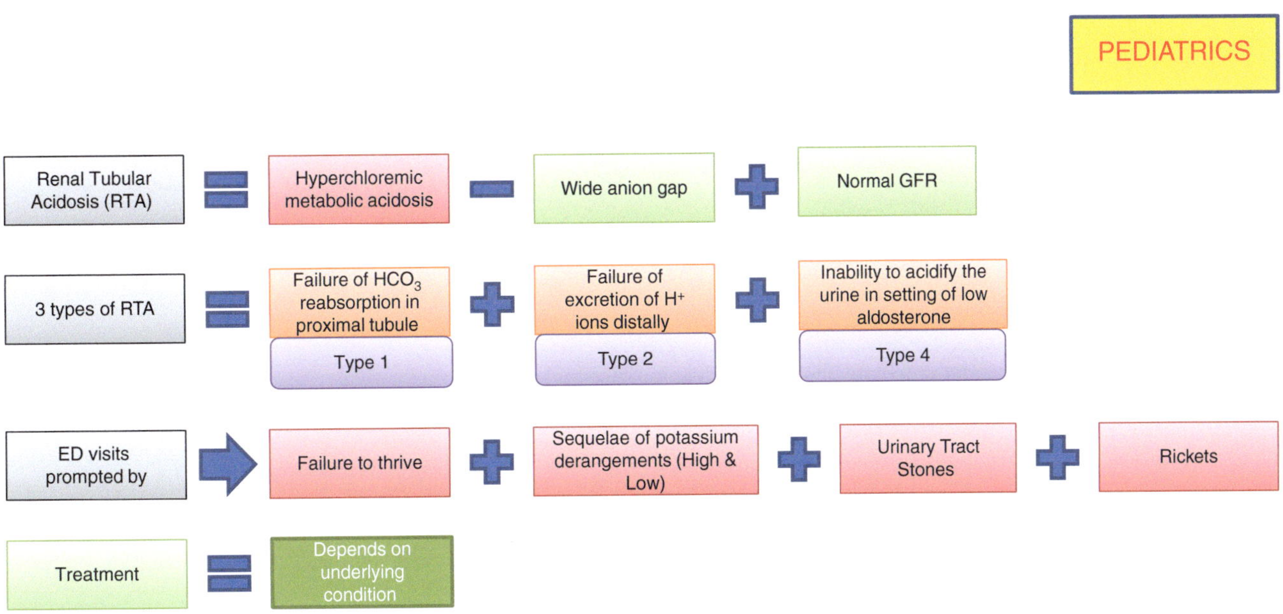

Polycystic Kidney Disease

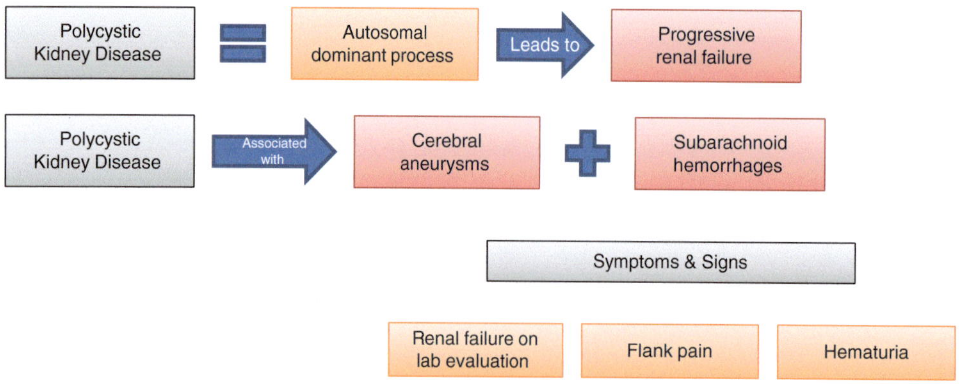

Cardiovascular Complications of Uremia

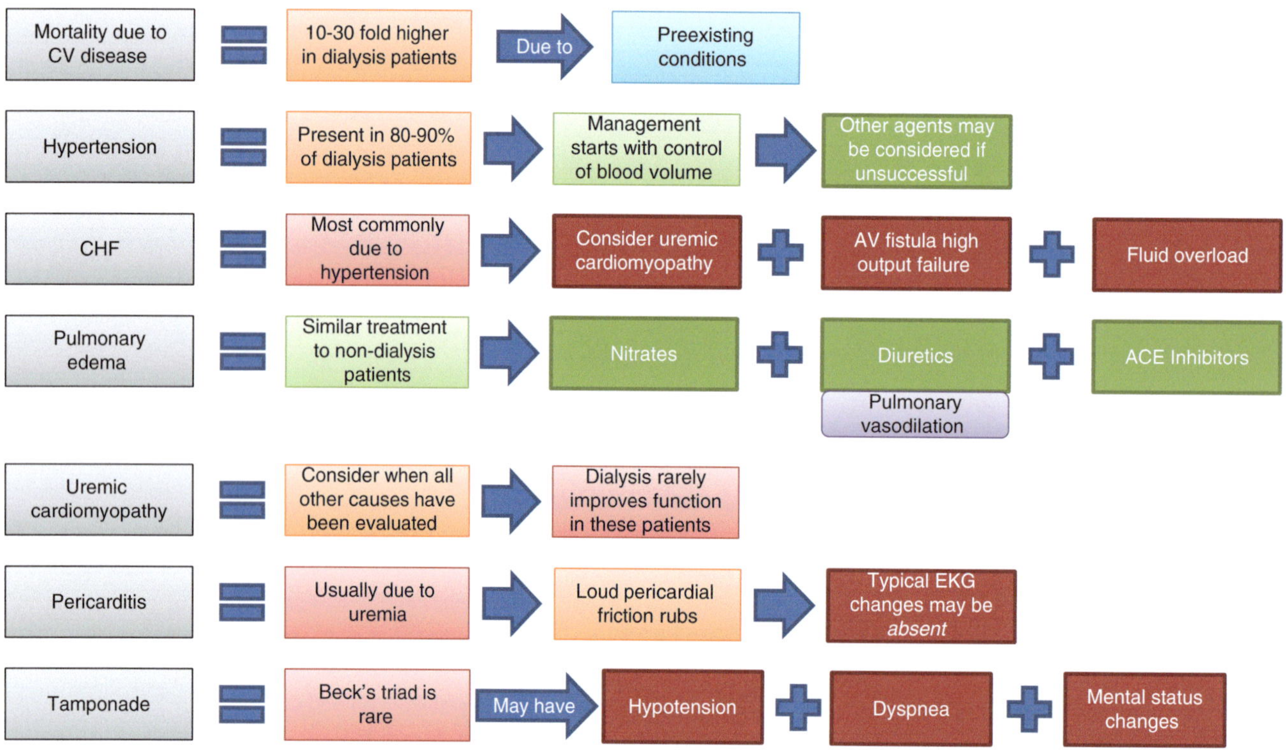

Neurologic Complications of Uremia

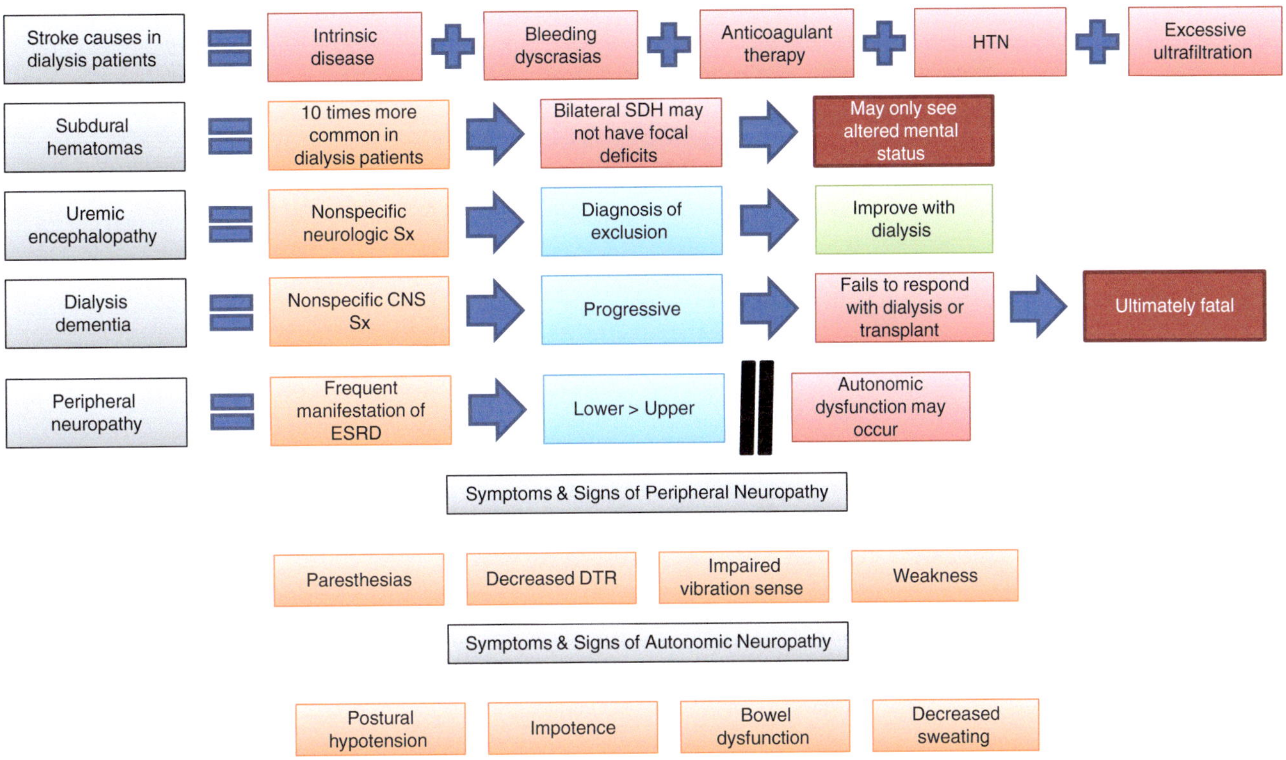

Hematologic Complications of Uremia

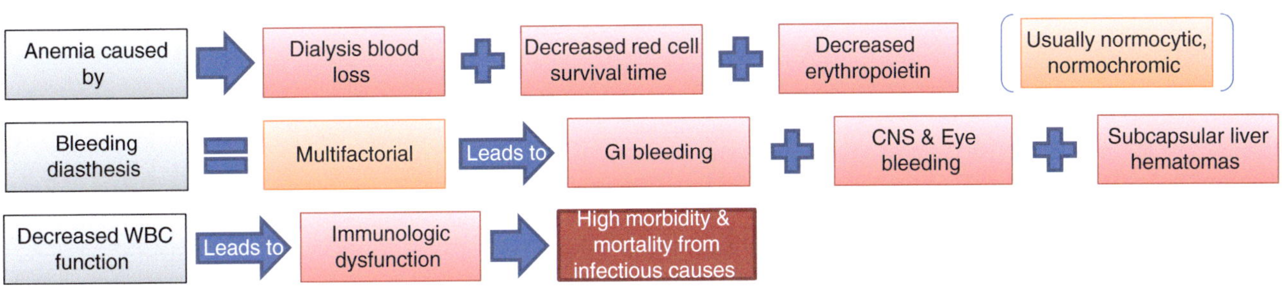

Gastrointestinal Complications of Uremia

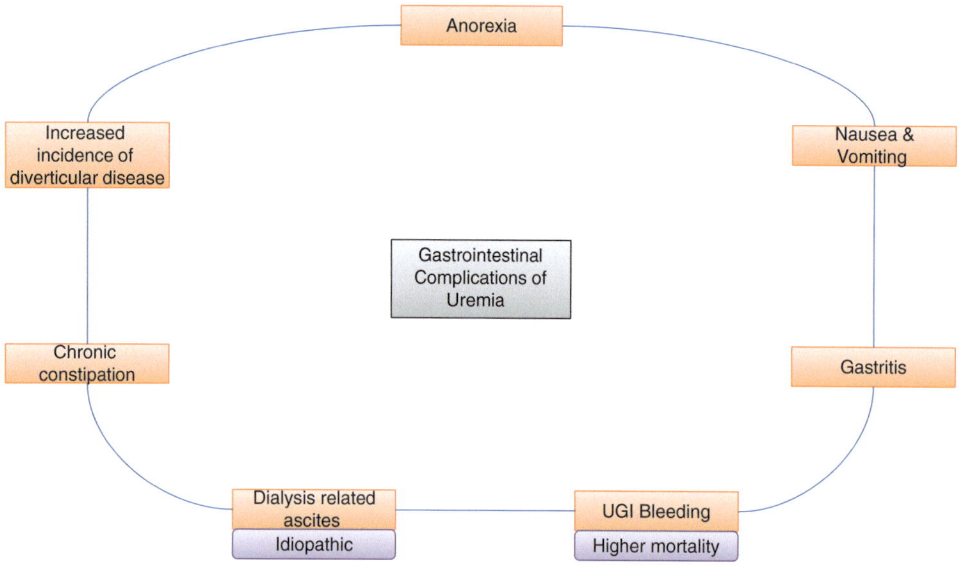

Electrolyte Complications of ESRD

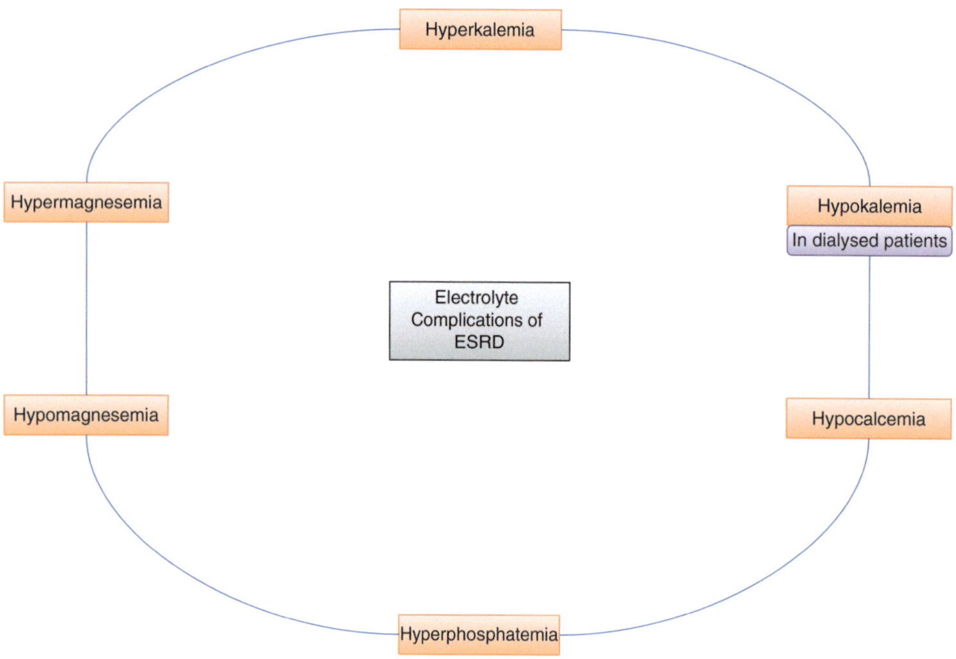

Hemodialysis

Indications for Emergency Dialysis

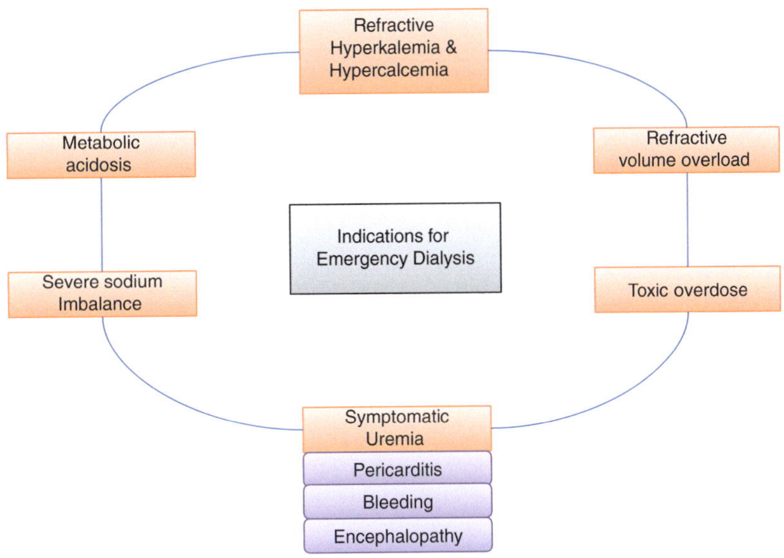

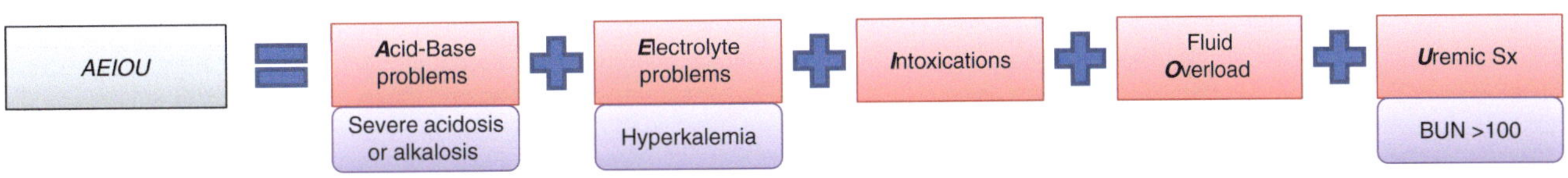

Complications of Hemodialysis

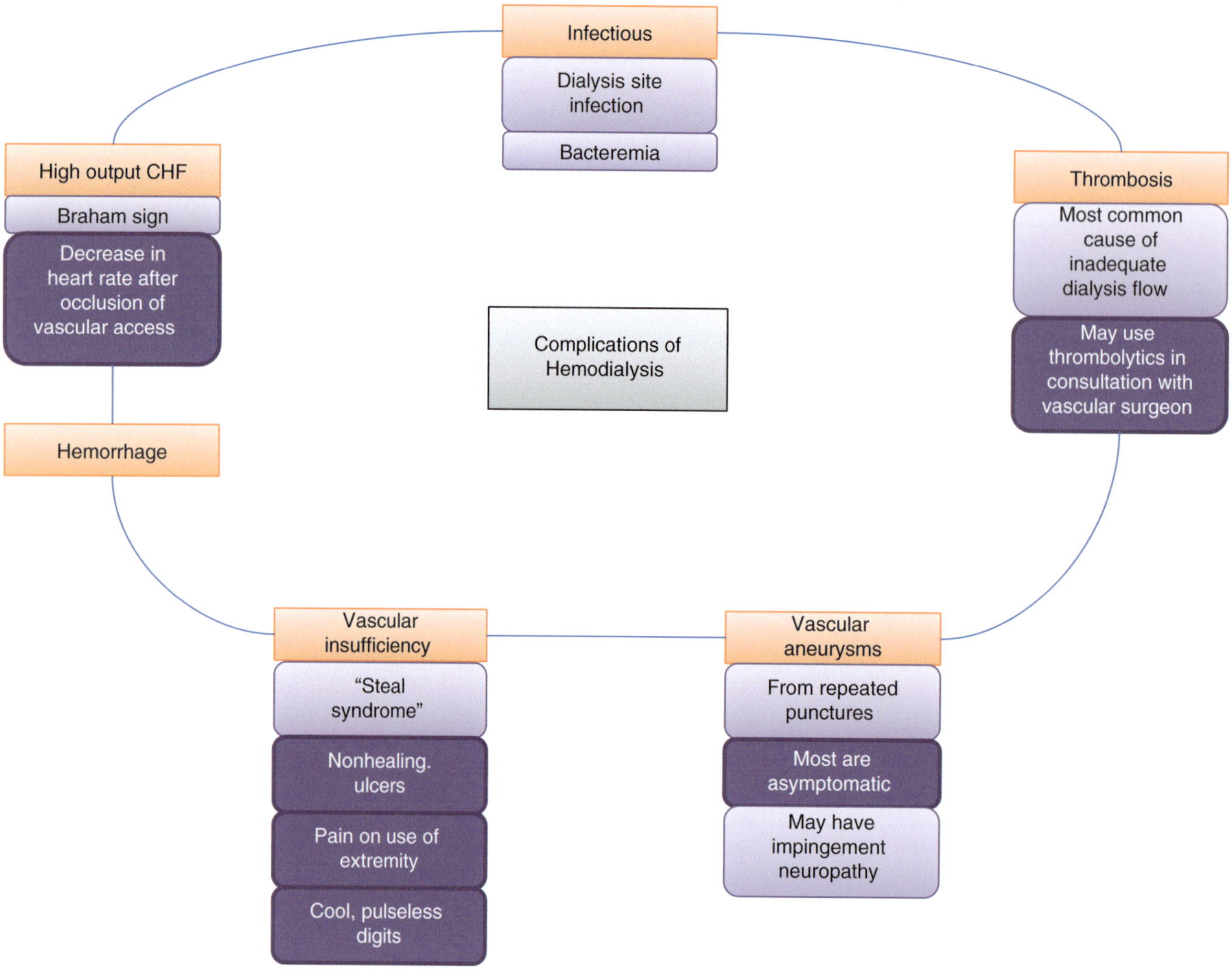

Infectious Complications of Hemodialysis

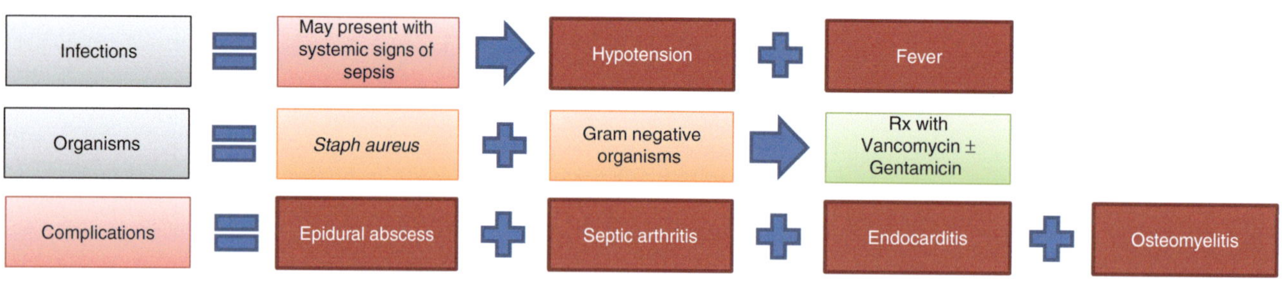

Hemorrhagic Complications of Hemodialysis

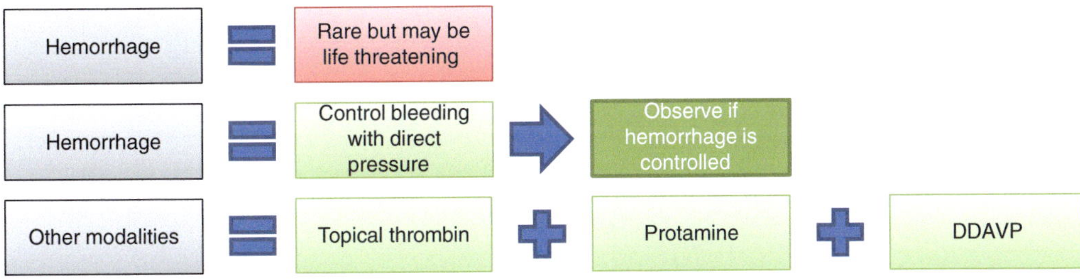

Hypotension During Hemodialysis (HD)

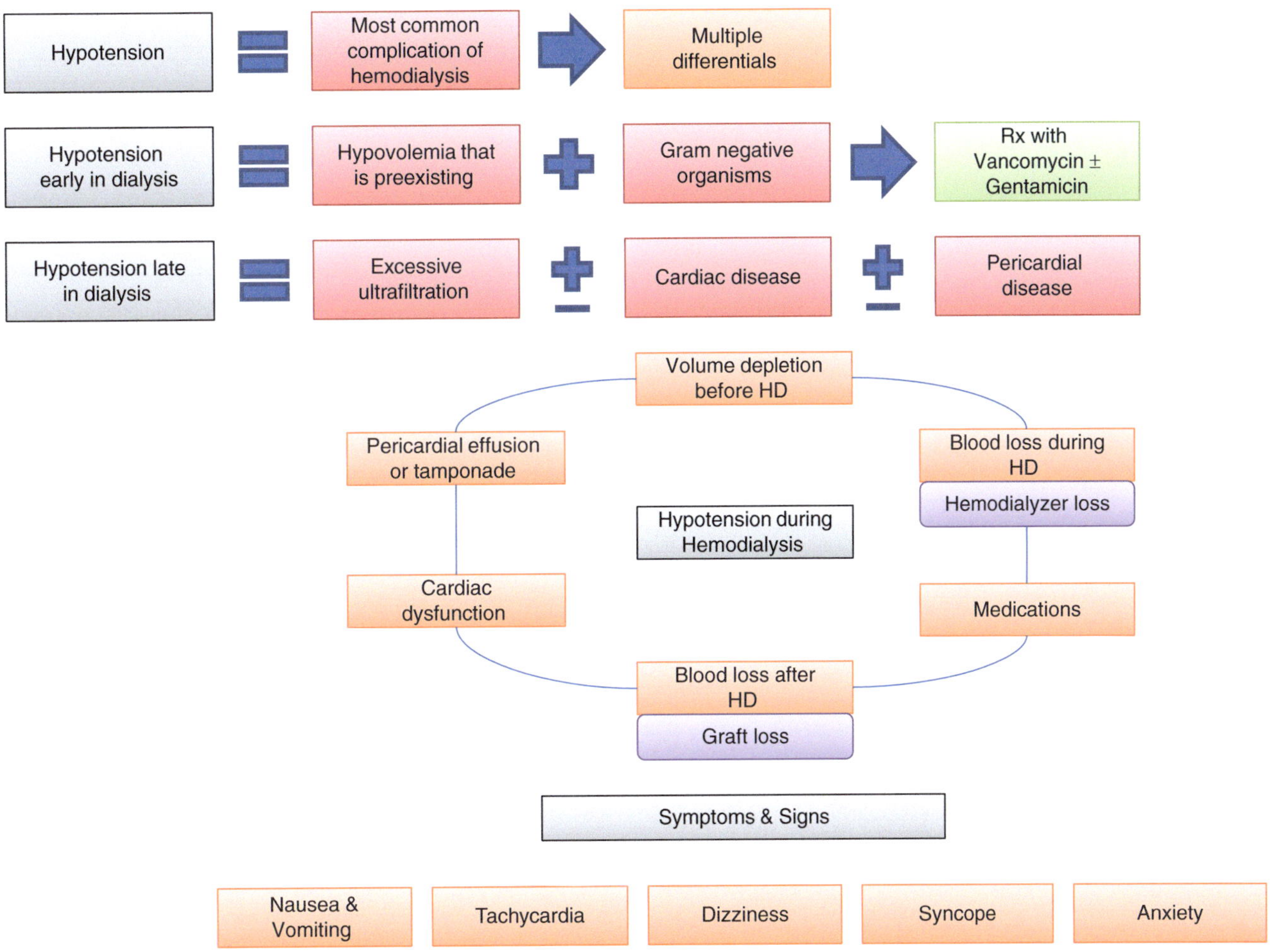

Dialysis Disequilibrium

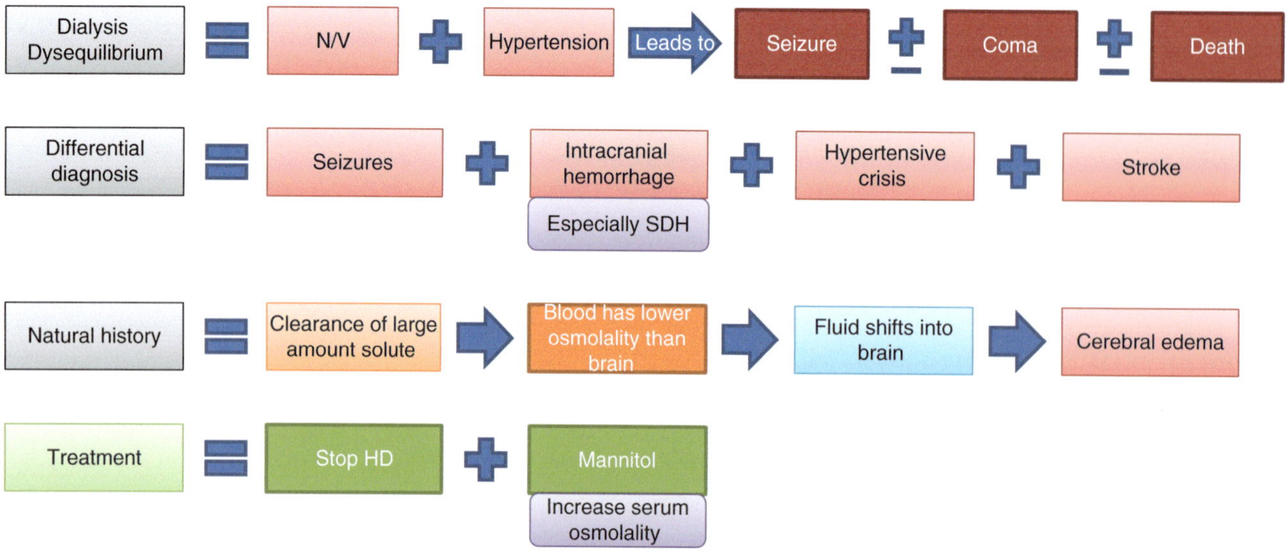

Altered Mental Status in Hemodialysis Patients

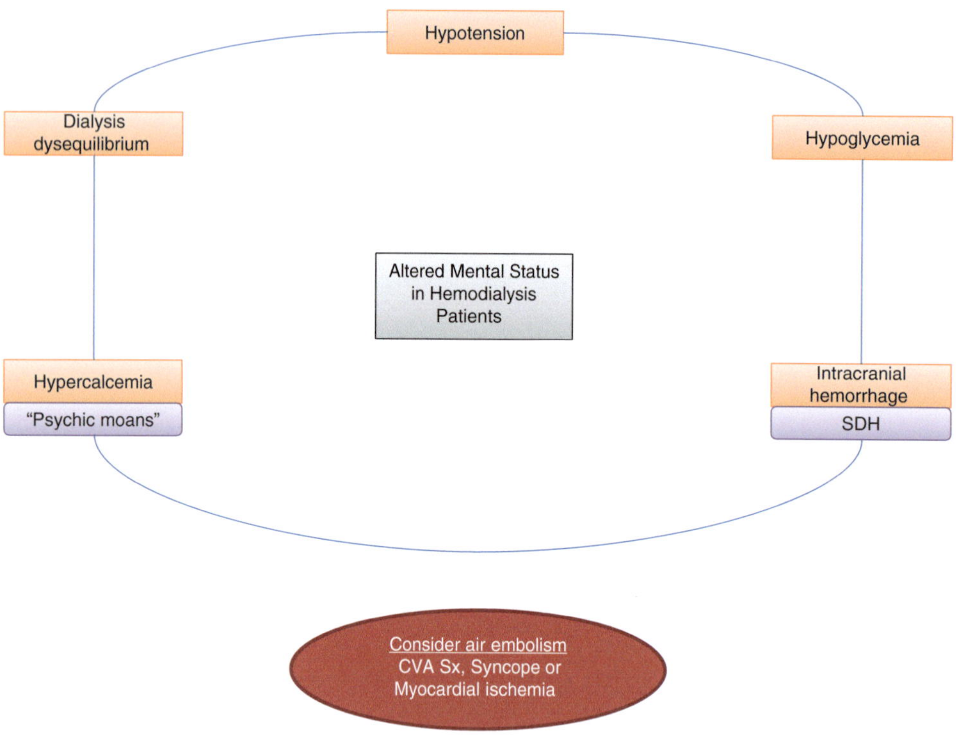

Peritoneal Dialysis

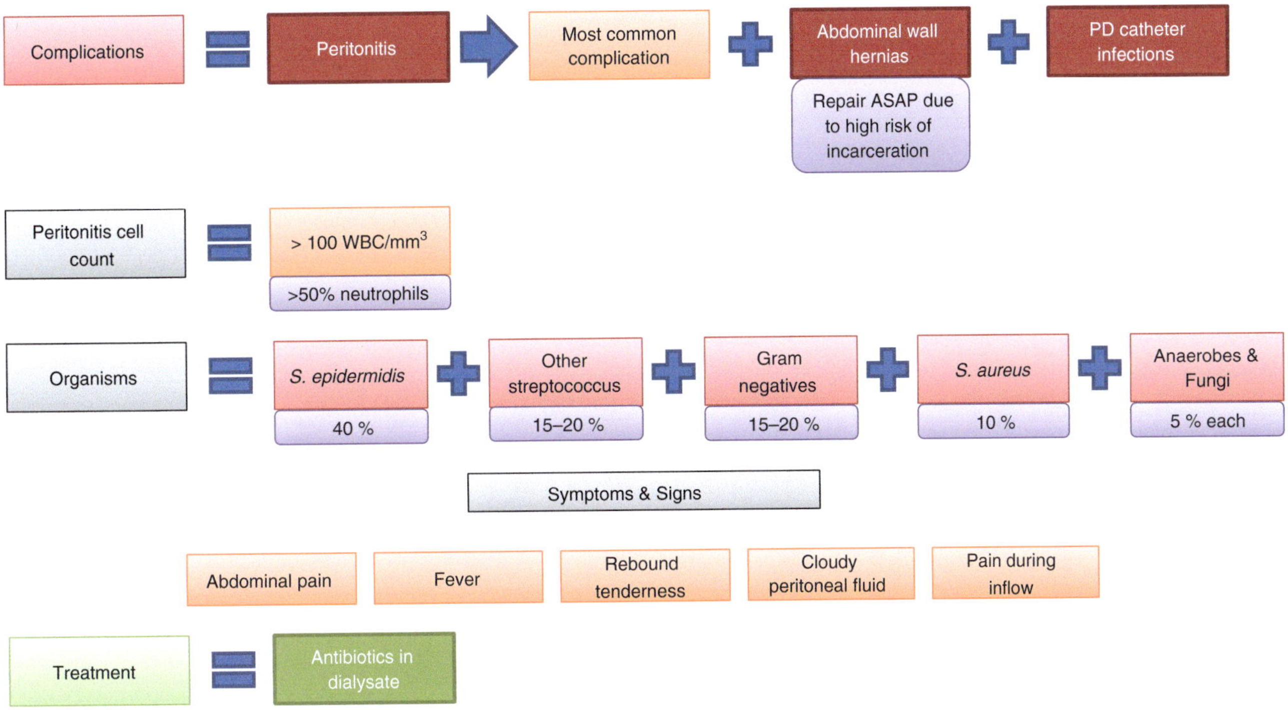

Urinary Tract Infections

UTI

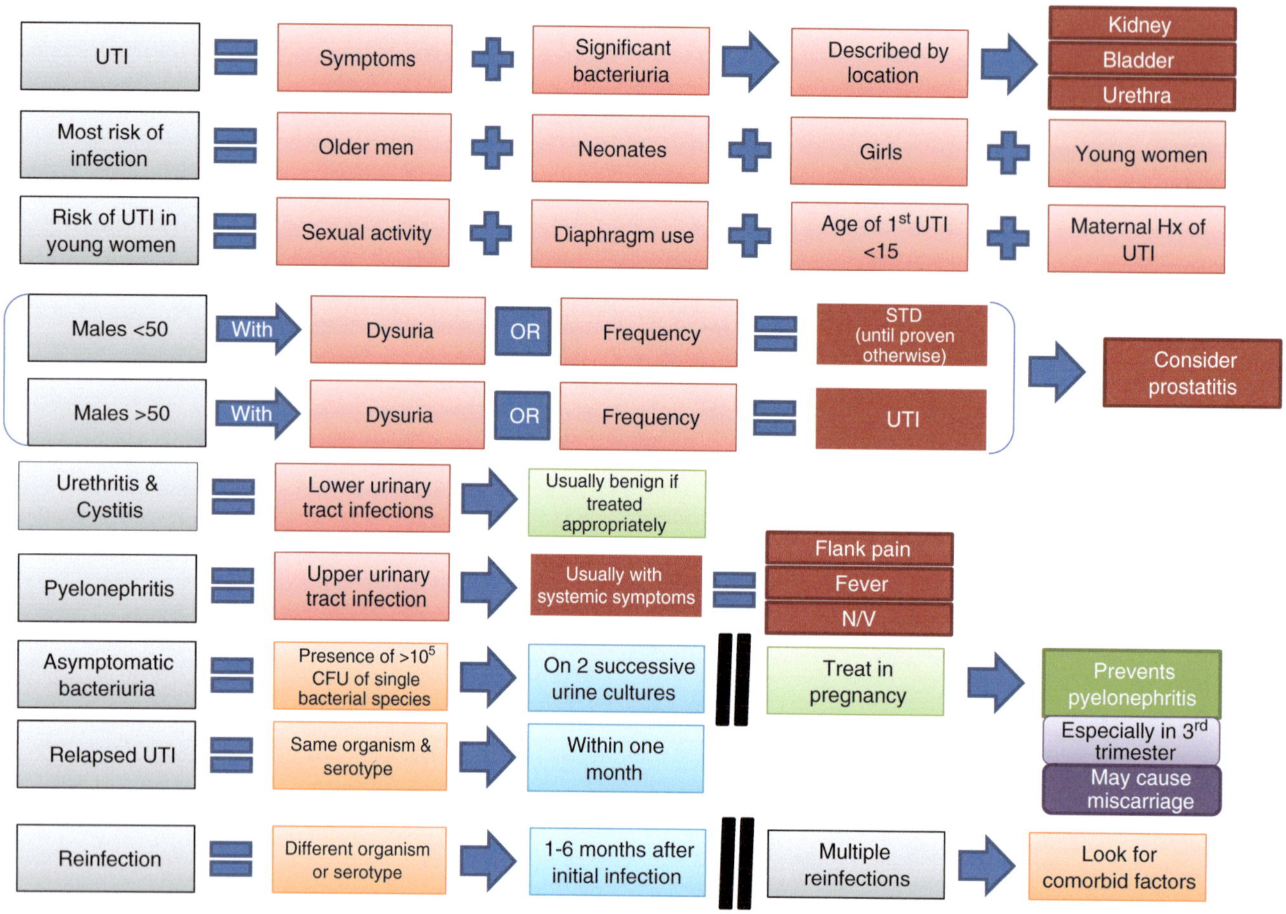

Complicated Versus Uncomplicated UTI

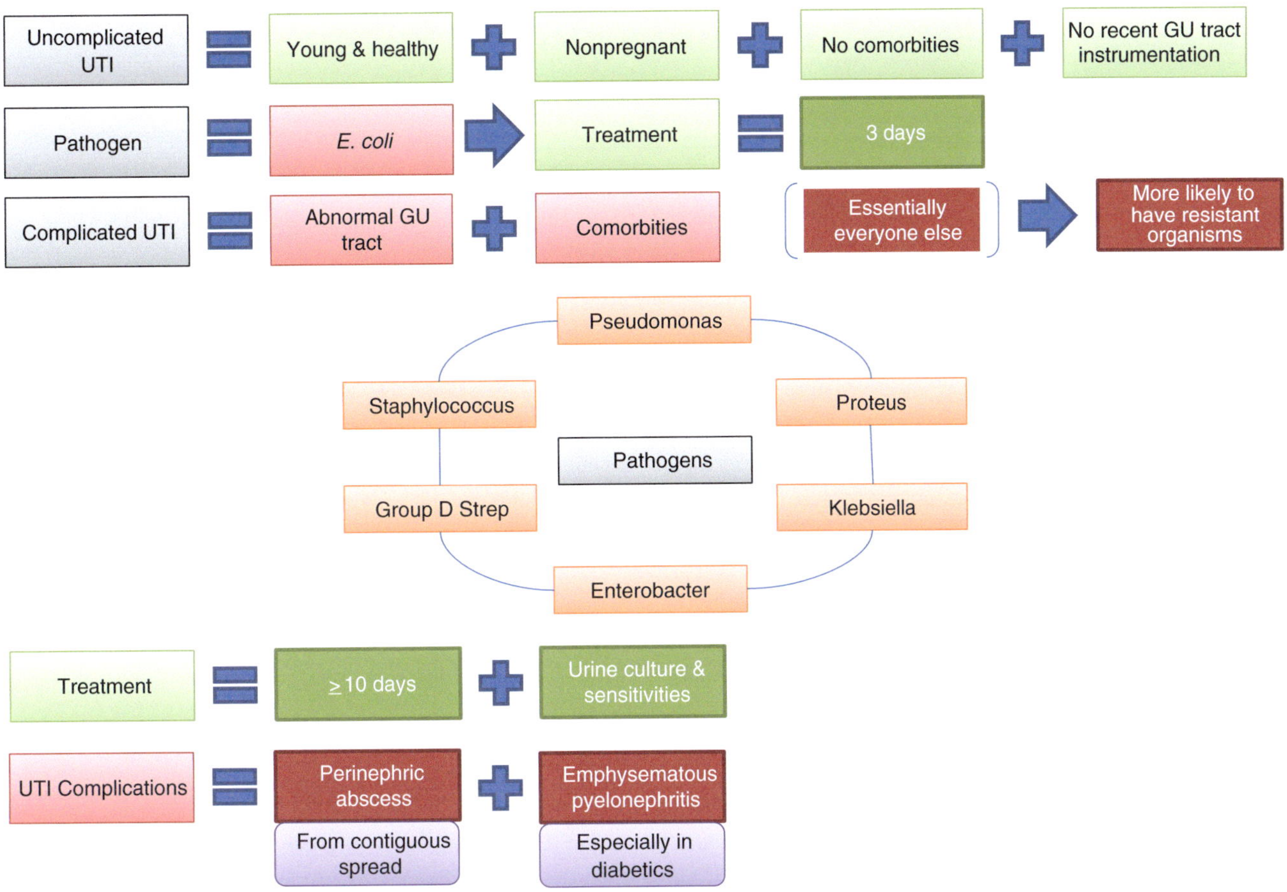

Clinical Features of UTI

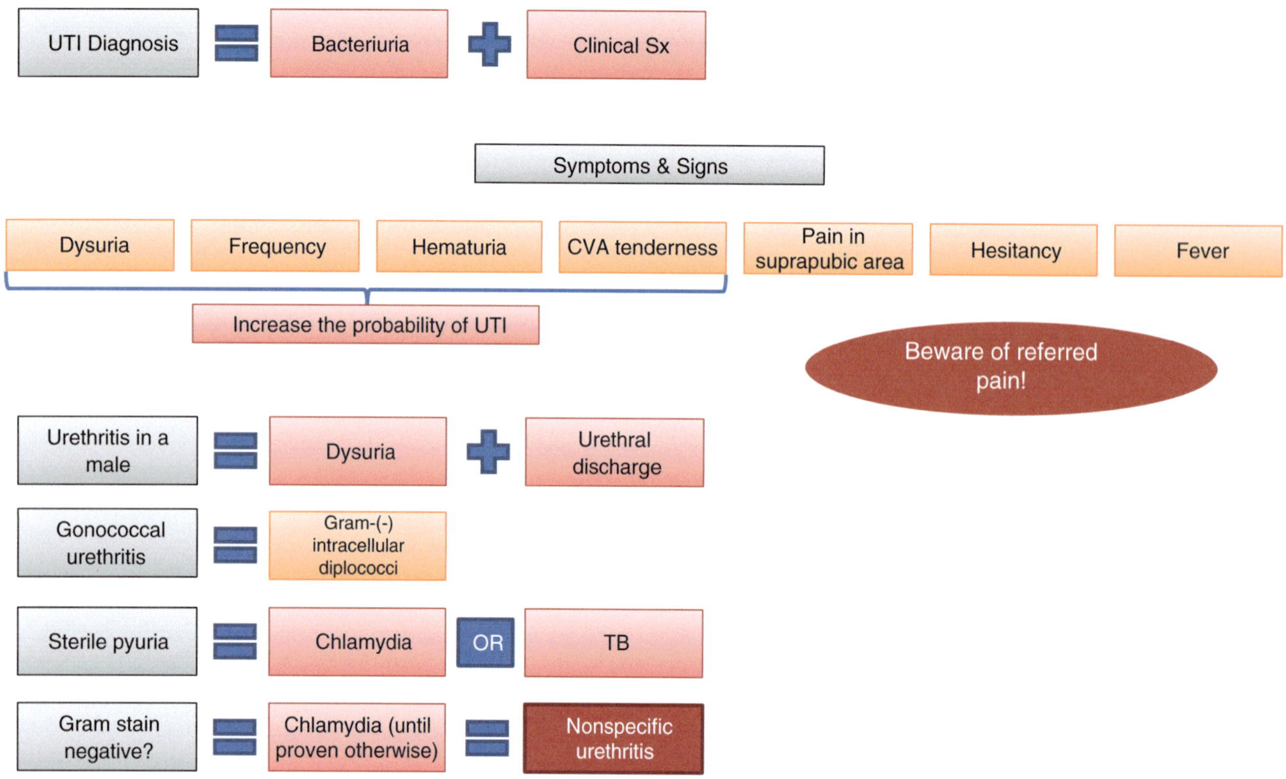

UTI Diagnosis

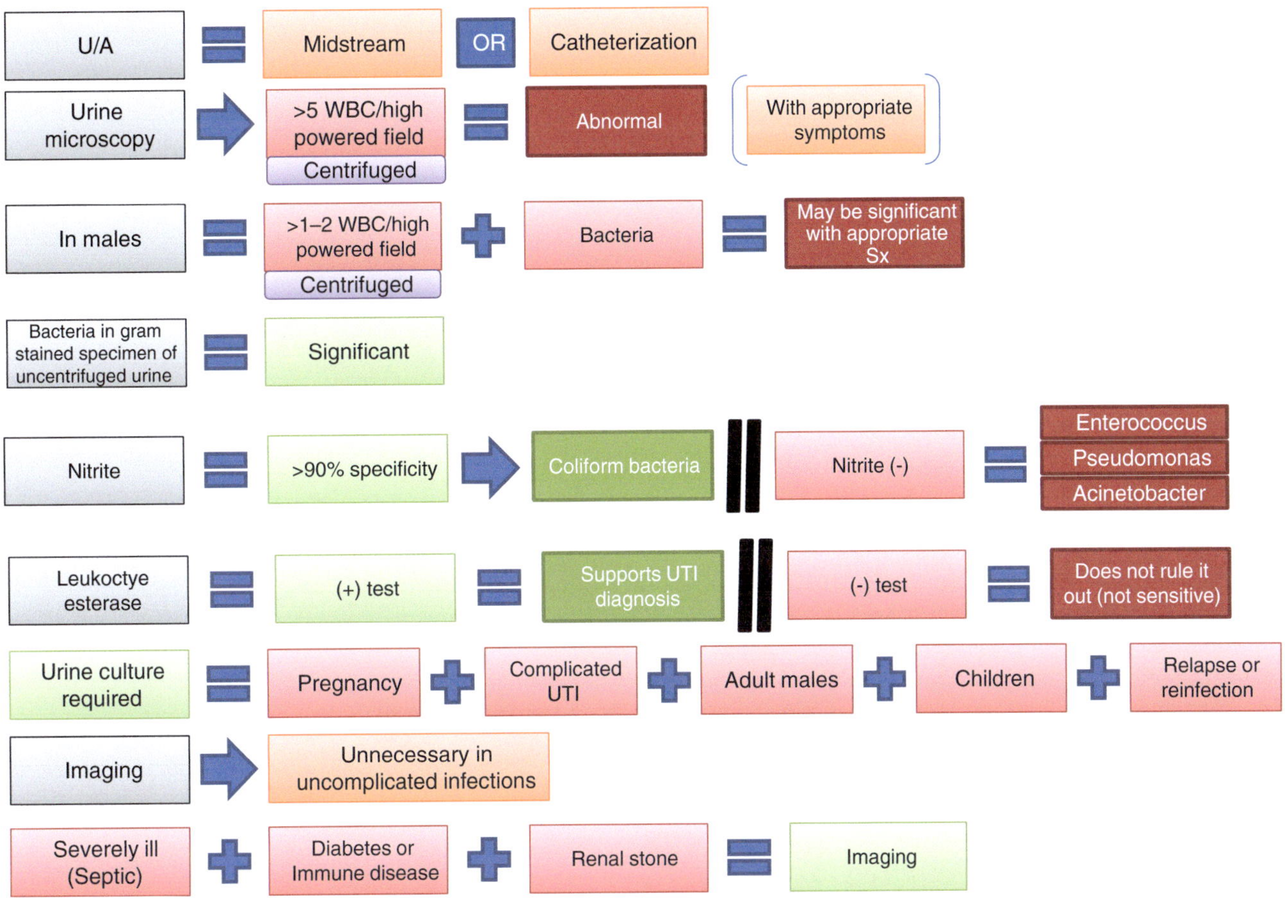

Hematuria

Most Common Causes of Hematuria

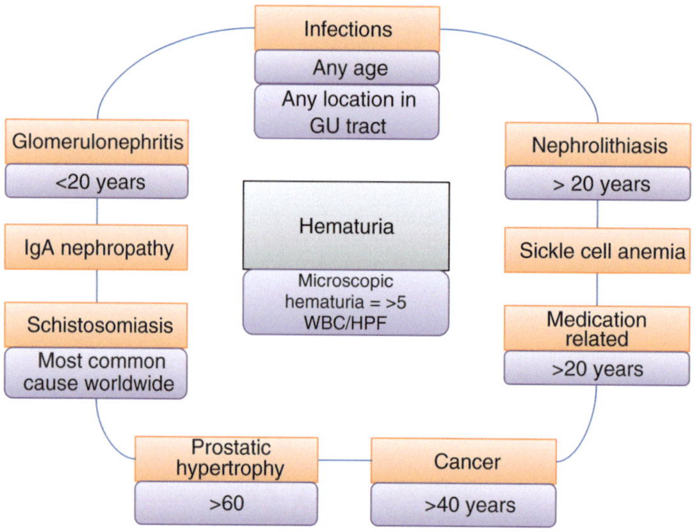

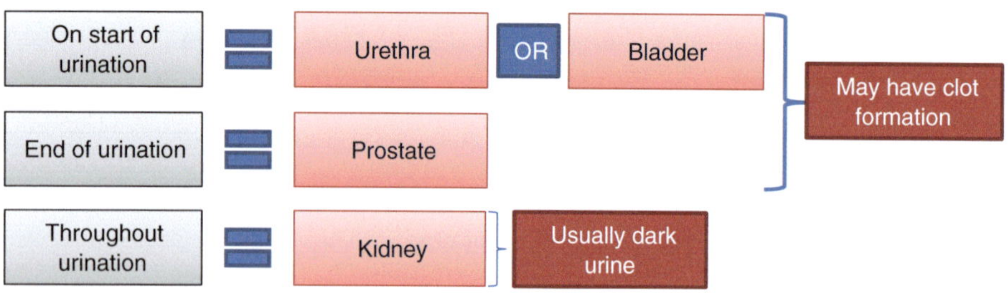

Kidney Stones

Kidney Stones Diagnosis and Treatment

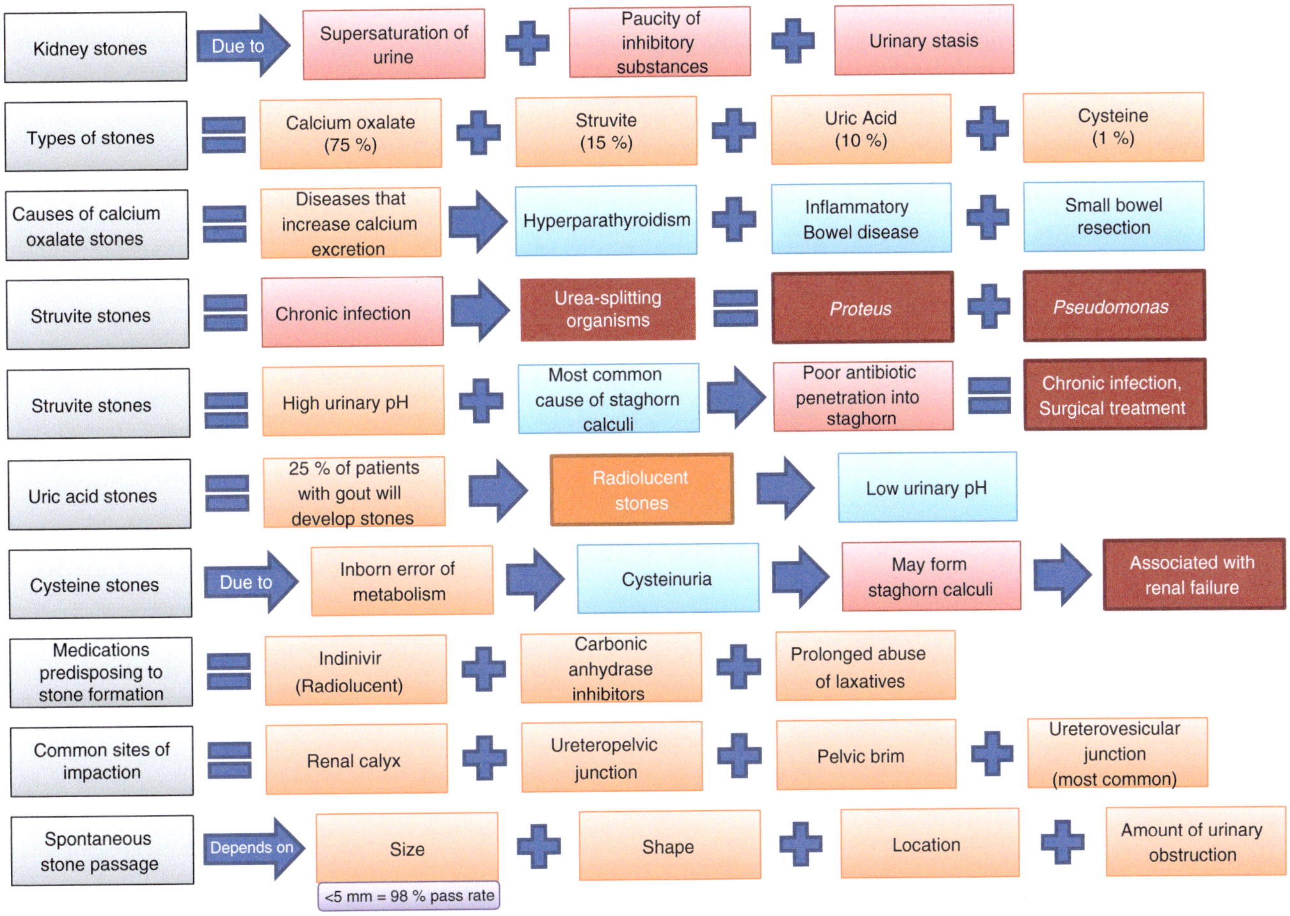

Diagnosis and Treatment

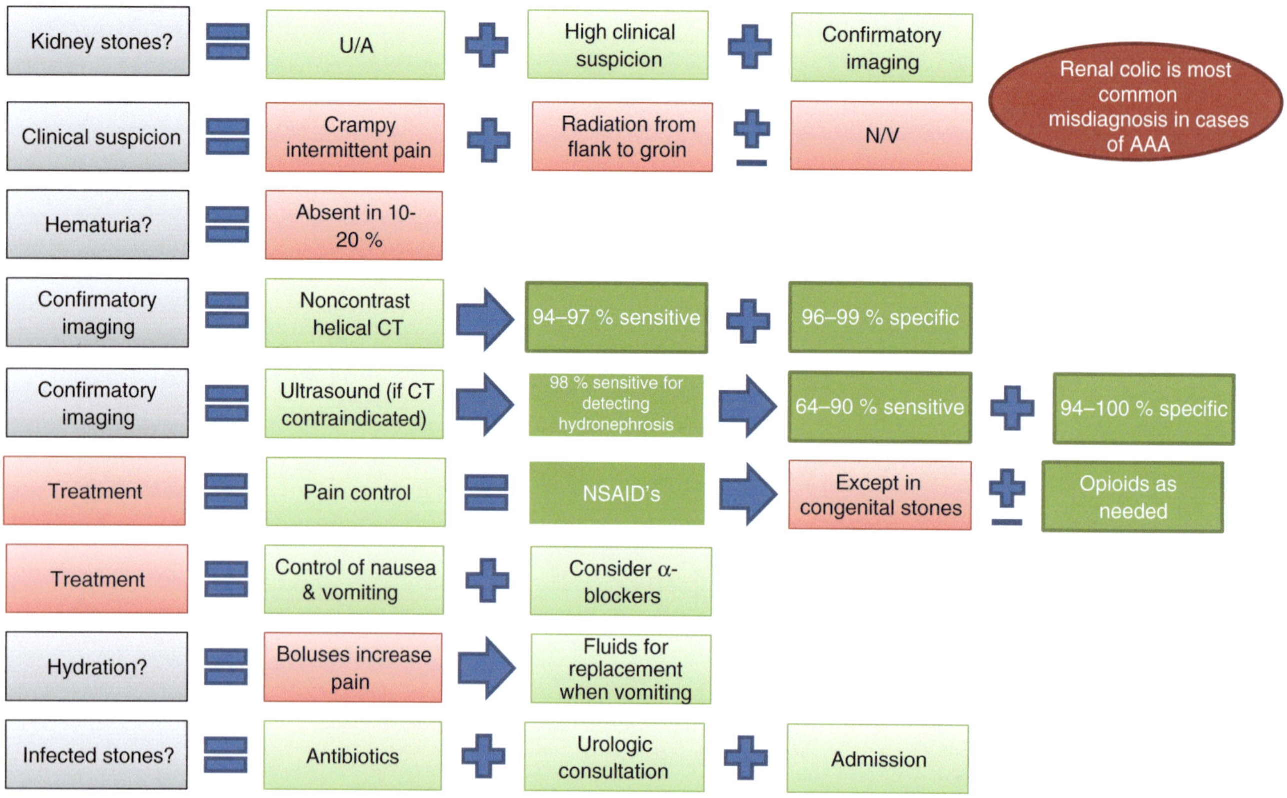

Stone Admission Criteria

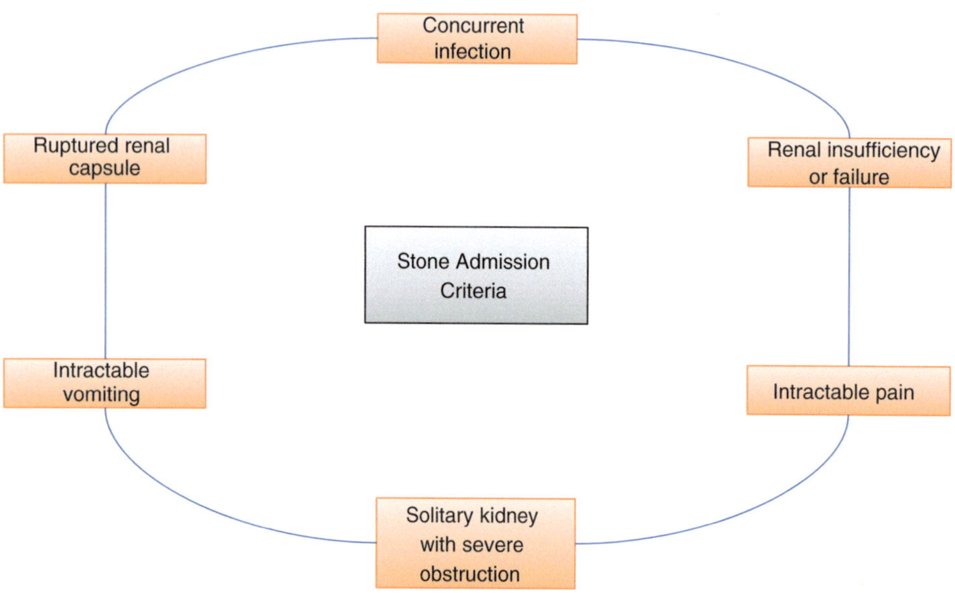

Renal Transplant

Renal Transplant = Most common solid organ transplant + Location = pelvis

Infection = Can be subtle

Rejection = Can be subtle → Minimal pain + May not have systemic signs

Antirejection meds = Cyclosporine → Is nephrotoxic

Male Genital Emergencies

Scrotal Disorders

Scrotal abscess = Usually from infected hair follicle → Simple I&D ± Antibiotics for complicated cases

Fournier's gangrene = Polymicrobial necrotizing fasciitis → Affects → Genital area ± Perianal area ± Perineal area

Fournier's gangrene = Starts as simple abscess or cellulitis → Spreads (immunosuppressed) → Microthrombi of subcutaneous vessels → Gangrene of overlying skin

↑ Risk of Fournier's = Diabetics + Alcohol abusers + IV Drug Users

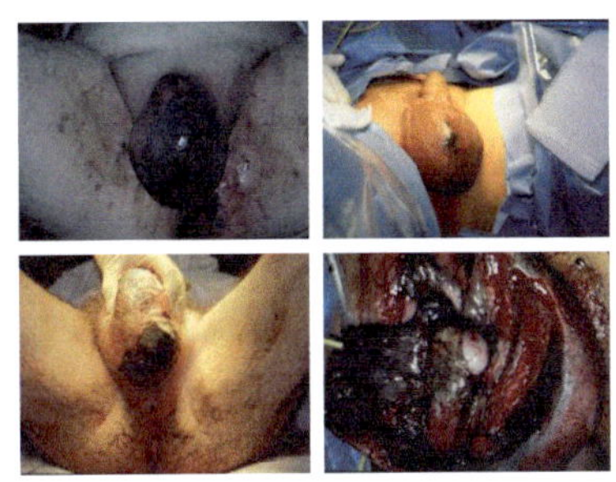

Symptoms & Signs

- Pain at involved area
- Swelling at involved area
- Ecchymosis
- Crepitus
- Fever
- Pain out of proportion to findings
- Pain extending beyond area of infection
- Foul odor

(Pain out of proportion to findings / Pain extending beyond area of infection → Immunocompromised)

Treatment = Prompt recognition + Fluid resuscitation + Polymicrobial antibiotics + Prompt surgical debridement

Center right image (Reprinted from Wessells H, Sorensen MD. Fournier's gangrene. In: Wessells H, editor. Urological emergencies: a practical approach. New York: Humana Press; 2013. p. 141–50. With permission from Springer Science + Business Media)

Glans Penis and Foreskin Disorders

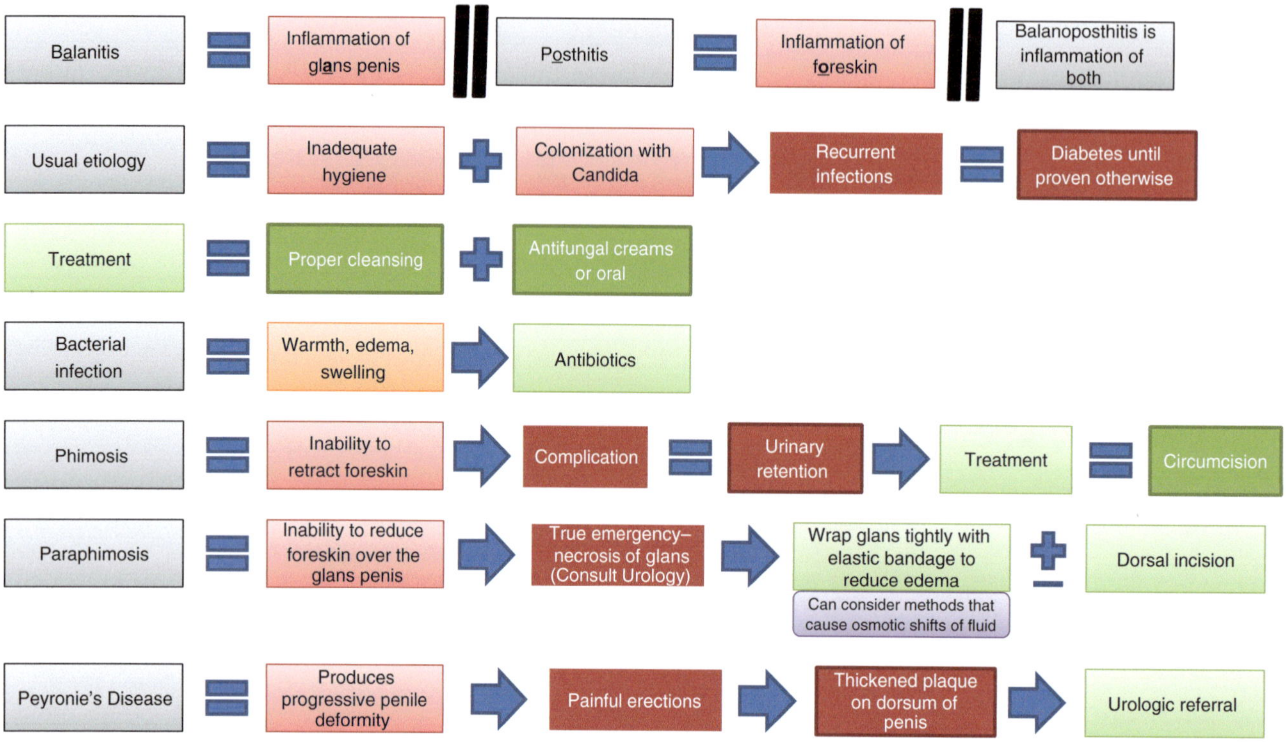

Traumatic Penis and Foreskin Disorders

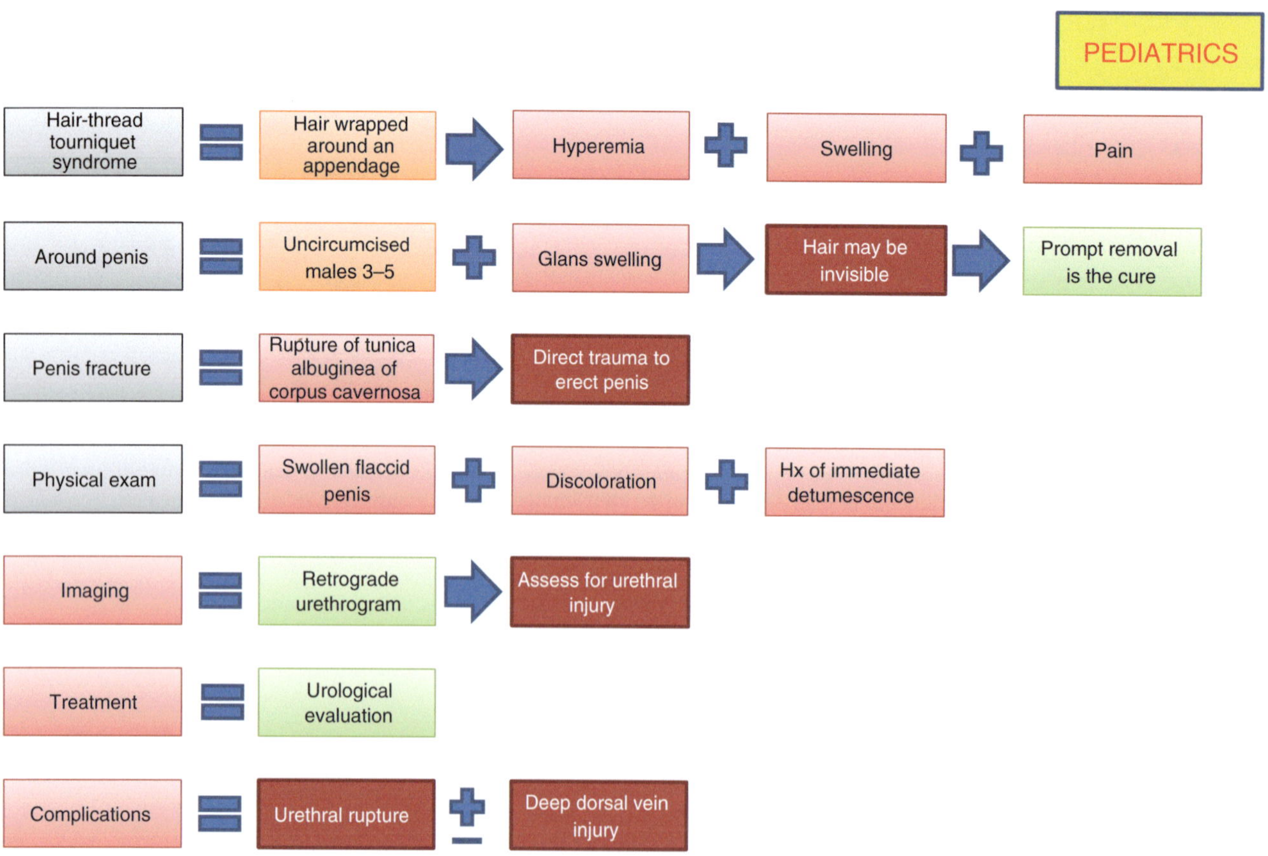

Priapism

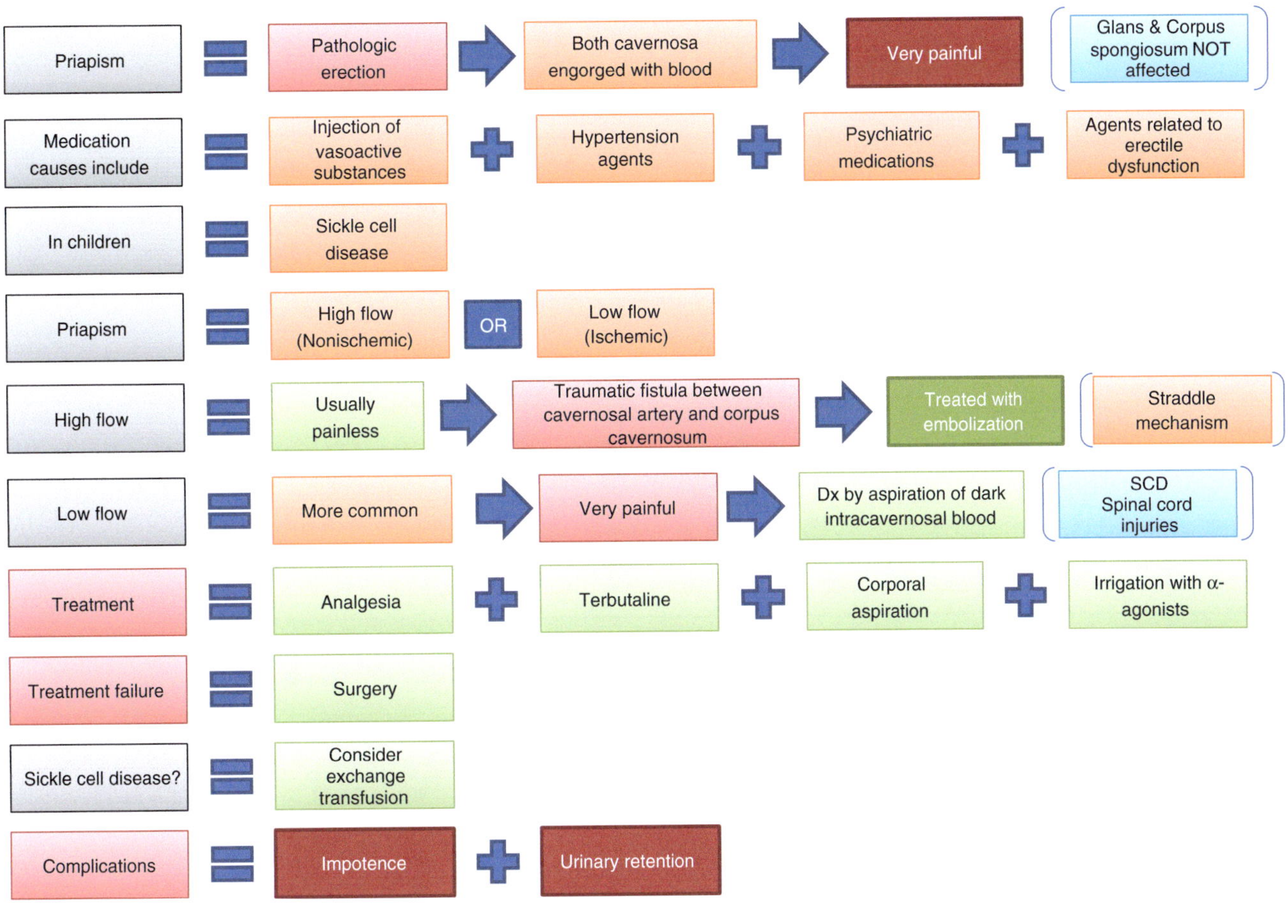
Priapism
Pathologic erection
Both cavernosa engorged with blood
Very painful
Glans & Corpus spongiosum NOT affected
Medication causes include
Injection of vasoactive substances
Hypertension agents
Psychiatric medications
Agents related to erectile dysfunction
In children
Sickle cell disease
Priapism
High flow (Nonischemic)
OR
Low flow (Ischemic)
High flow
Usually painless
Traumatic fistula between cavernosal artery and corpus cavernosum
Treated with embolization
Straddle mechanism
Low flow
More common
Very painful
Dx by aspiration of dark intracavernosal blood
SCD
Spinal cord injuries
Treatment
Analgesia
Terbutaline
Corporal aspiration
Irrigation with α-agonists
Treatment failure
Surgery
Sickle cell disease?
Consider exchange transfusion
Complications
Impotence
Urinary retention

Testicular Torsion

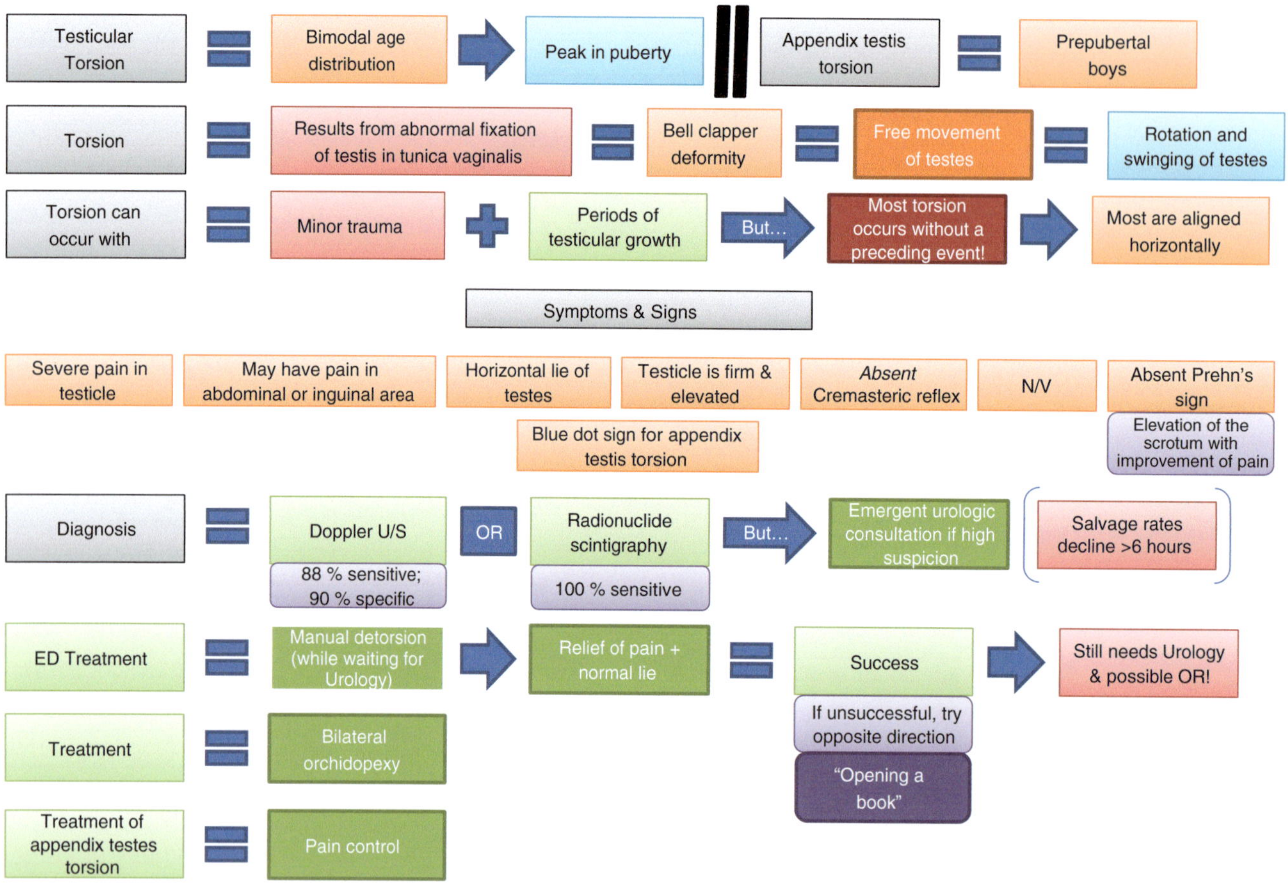

Epididymitis and Orchitis

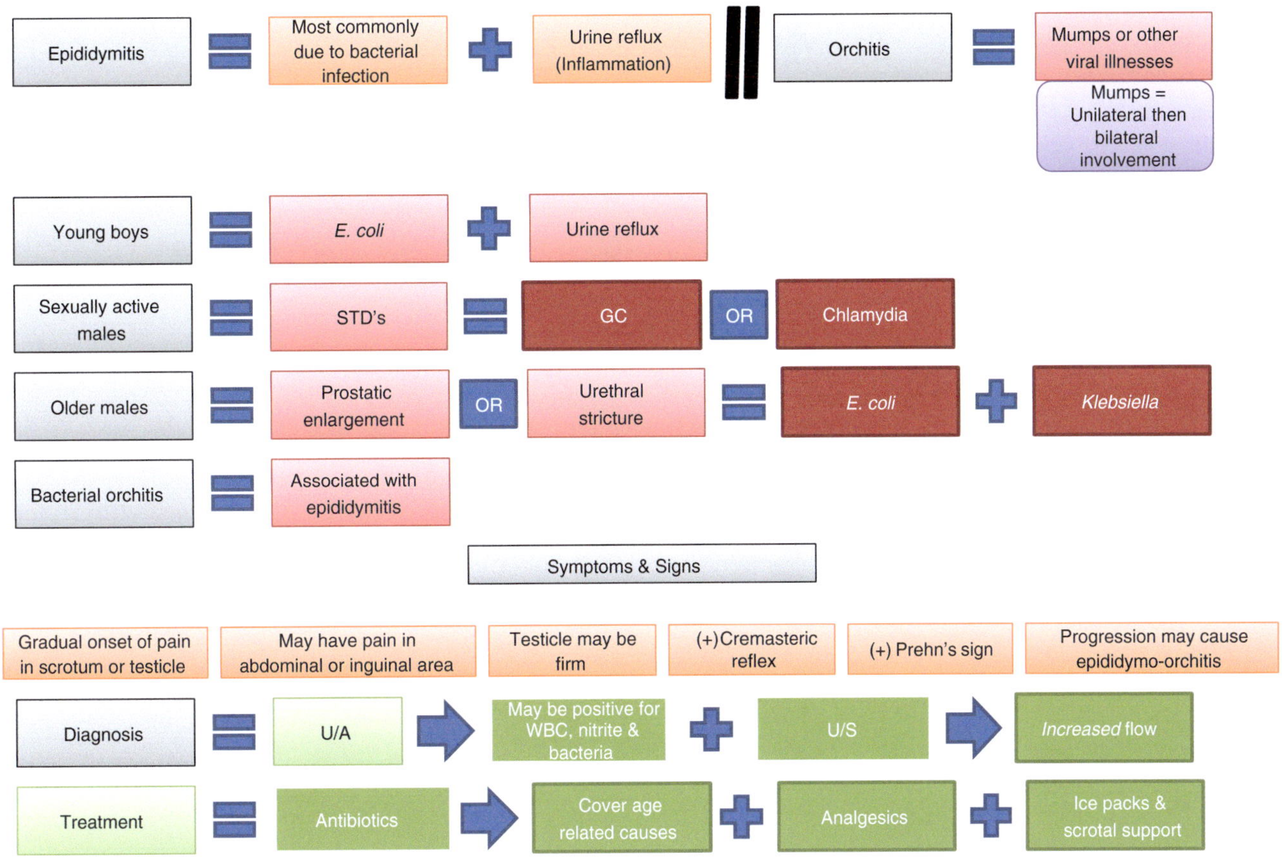

Prostatitis

Prostatitis = Same etiologies as epididymitis + Same age related considerations

Risk factors = Epididymitis or urethritis + Phimosis + Foley catheter + Rectal intercourse + Lower urinary tract obstruction

Causative agents = *E. coli* (most common) + *Klebsiella* + *Pseudomonas* + *Serratia* + *Staph*

Symptoms & Signs

Pain in perineum | Low back pain | Pain in genital area | Frequency | Dysuria | F/C | Difficulty in defecating | Urinary retention | Enlarged & tender prostate – "boggy"

Diagnosis = Evaluate for GC/Chlamydia + U/A

Treatment = Antibiotics (long term = 30 days) + Analgesics − Foley

Severe? = Suprapubic catheter (Especially for retention) + IV antibiotics

Urethritis

Urethritis = Purulent urethral discharge

GC = Whitish discharge + *Intracellular gram (-) diplococci*

Chlamydia = Watery or no discharge + *Negative* gram stain

Diagnosis = DNA probes + U/A

Treatment = Ceftriaxone 250 mg IM + Azithromycin 1 g po + Treat partners

Urinary Retention

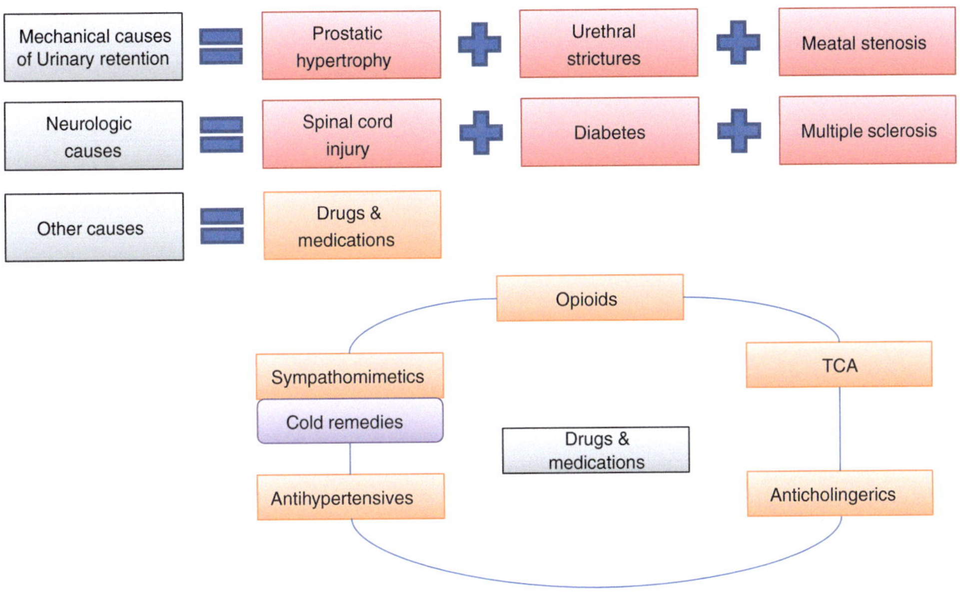

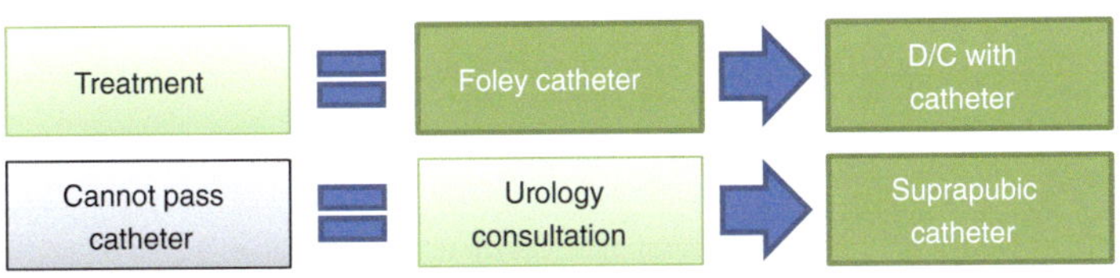

Sexually Transmitted Diseases

Ulcer-Forming Processes

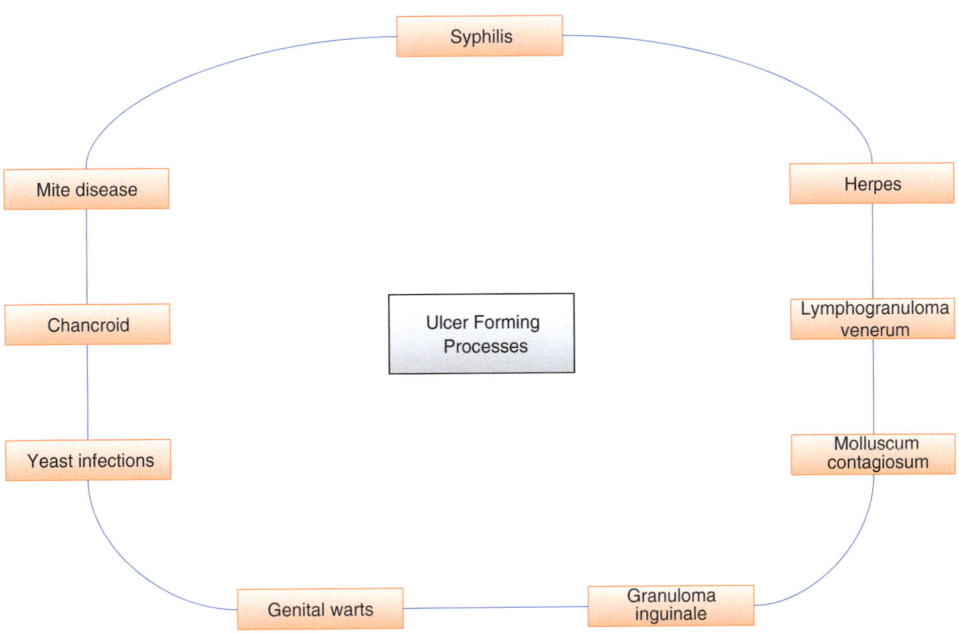

Non-ulcer-Forming Processes

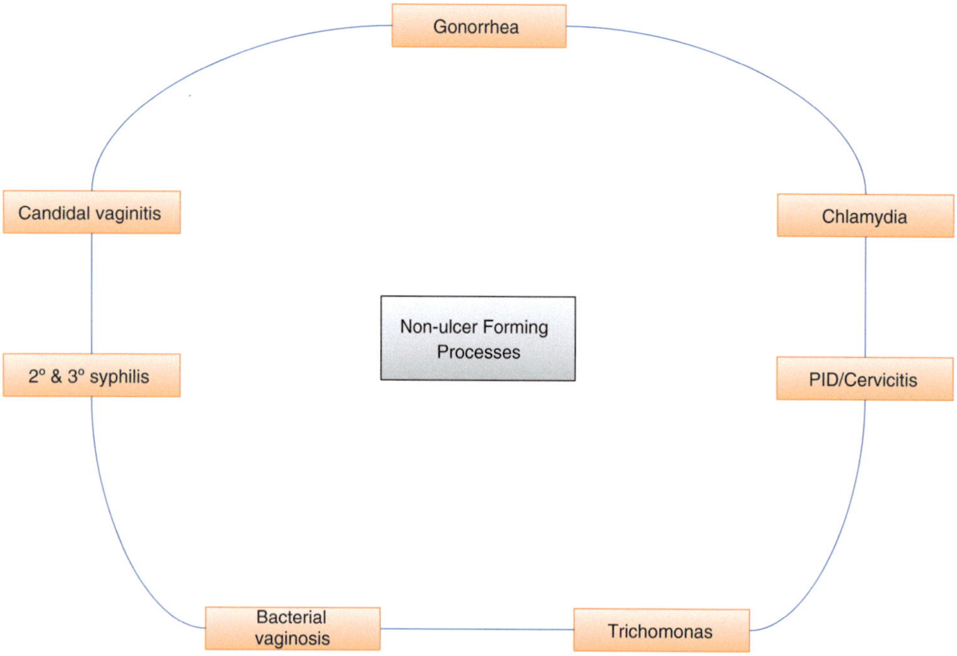

Chlamydia

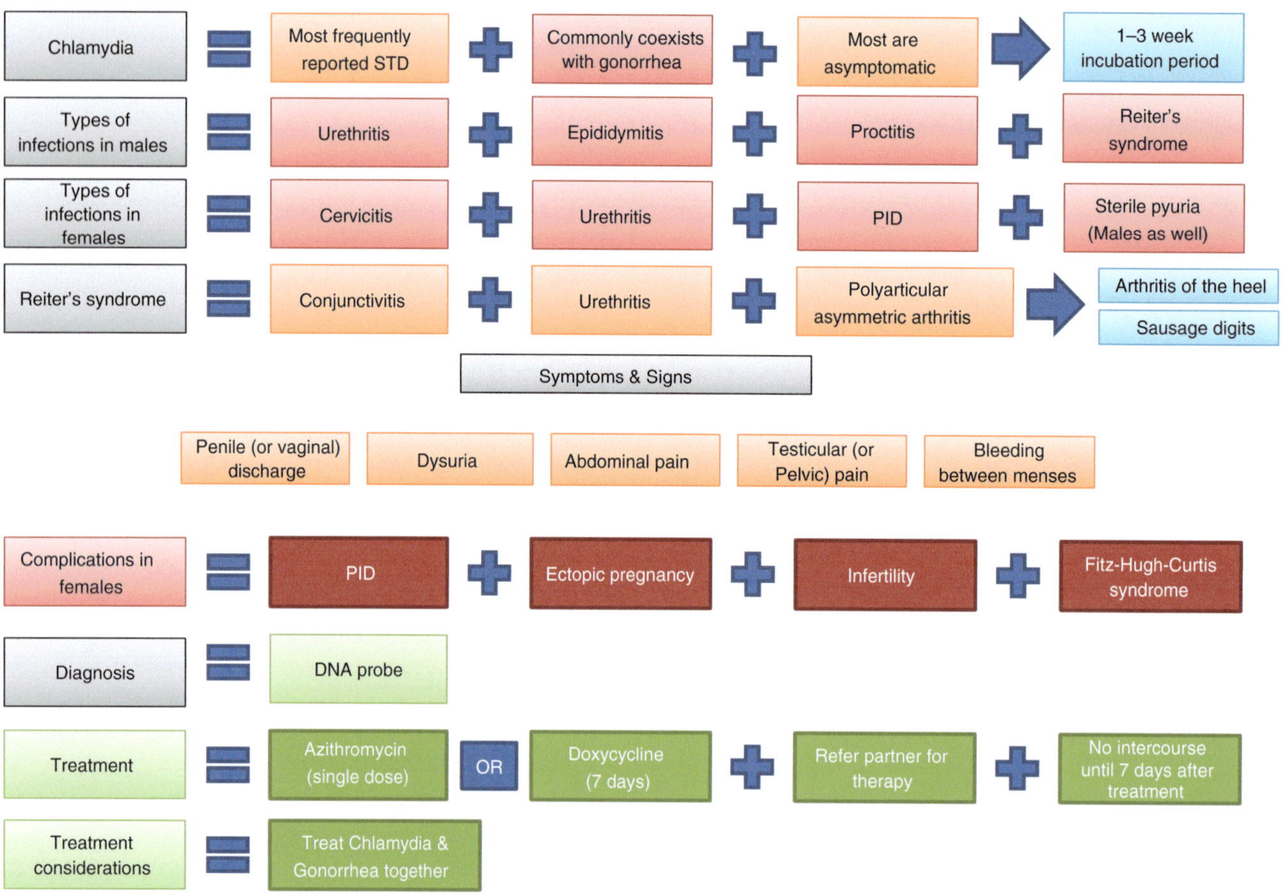

Gonorrhea

Gonorrhea = 2nd most frequently reported STD + Commonly coexists with chlamydia + Most are asymptomatic → 1–2 week incubation period

Types of infections in males = Urethritis + Epididymitis + Prostatitis + Proctitis

Types of infections in females = Cervicitis + Urethritis + PID (20% of untreated females get PID)

Symptoms & Signs

- In males: Penile discharge; Dysuria
- Mucopurulent anal discharge
- Testicular (or Pelvic) pain
- Bleeding between menses
- In females: Lower abdominal pain; Mucopurulent cervicitis
- GC conjunctivitis
- GC Pharyngitis
- Septic arthritis (most common cause <50 years)

Complications in females = PID + Ectopic pregnancy + Chronic pelvic pain

Disseminated Gonococcemia = Petechial rash on red base + Tenosynovitis + Fever & Malaise + Asymmetric arthralgias + Septic arthritis

Diagnosis = Gram stain of urethral swab + DNA amplification

Treatment = IM Ceftriaxone + (Doxycycline (7 days) OR Azithromycin 1 g dose) + Treatment of partner & no intercourse until 7 days after treatment

Treatment disseminated GC = IV antibiotics + Hospitalization + Evaluation for endocarditis + Evaluation for meningitis

Trichomoniasis

T.vaginalis = Protozoan infection + Infections mostly in women + High prevalence of coinfection with other STD → 3 days to 4 weeks incubation period

Symptoms & Signs

- Thin, malodorous watery discharge
- Vulvar irritation
- Dysuria
- Frequency
- Dyspareunia
- Lower abdominal pain
- Inflamed vaginal mucosa
- Punctate cervical hemorrhages
- Males: May be asymptomatic in men; Urethritis

Diagnosis = Motile organisms on microscopy

Treatment = Metronidazole + Refer partner for therapy + No intercourse until 7 days after treatment

Syphilis

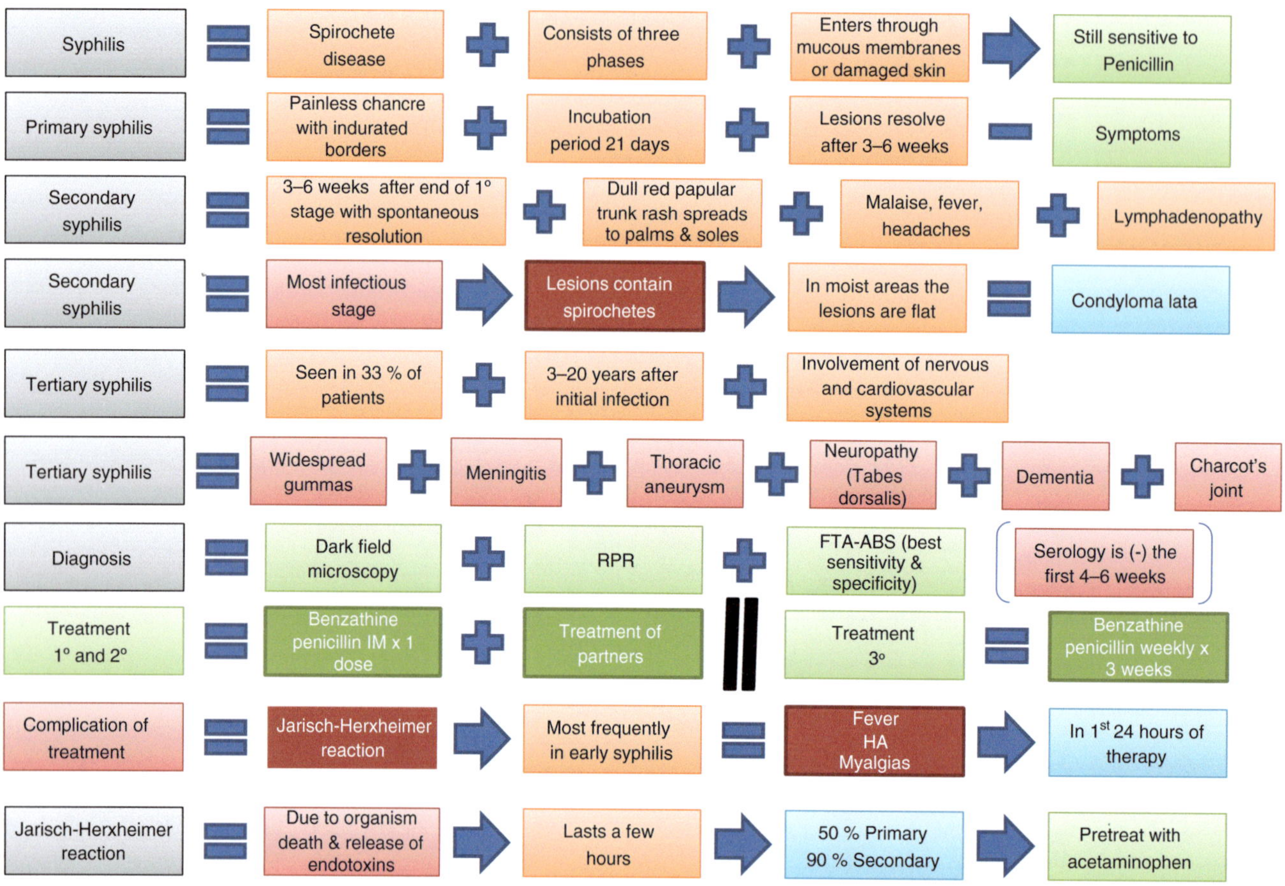
Syphilis = Spirochete disease + Consists of three phases + Enters through mucous membranes or damaged skin → Still sensitive to Penicillin
Primary syphilis = Painless chancre with indurated borders + Incubation period 21 days + Lesions resolve after 3–6 weeks − Symptoms
Secondary syphilis = 3–6 weeks after end of 1° stage with spontaneous resolution + Dull red papular trunk rash spreads to palms & soles + Malaise, fever, headaches + Lymphadenopathy
Secondary syphilis = Most infectious stage → Lesions contain spirochetes → In moist areas the lesions are flat = Condyloma lata
Tertiary syphilis = Seen in 33 % of patients + 3–20 years after initial infection + Involvement of nervous and cardiovascular systems
Tertiary syphilis = Widespread gummas + Meningitis + Thoracic aneurysm + Neuropathy (Tabes dorsalis) + Dementia + Charcot's joint
Diagnosis = Dark field microscopy + RPR + FTA-ABS (best sensitivity & specificity) (Serology is (-) the first 4–6 weeks)
Treatment 1° and 2° = Benzathine penicillin IM x 1 dose + Treatment of partners
Treatment 3° = Benzathine penicillin weekly x 3 weeks
Complication of treatment = Jarisch-Herxheimer reaction → Most frequently in early syphilis = Fever HA Myalgias → In 1st 24 hours of therapy
Jarisch-Herxheimer reaction = Due to organism death & release of endotoxins → Lasts a few hours → 50 % Primary 90 % Secondary → Pretreat with acetaminophen

Herpes Simplex

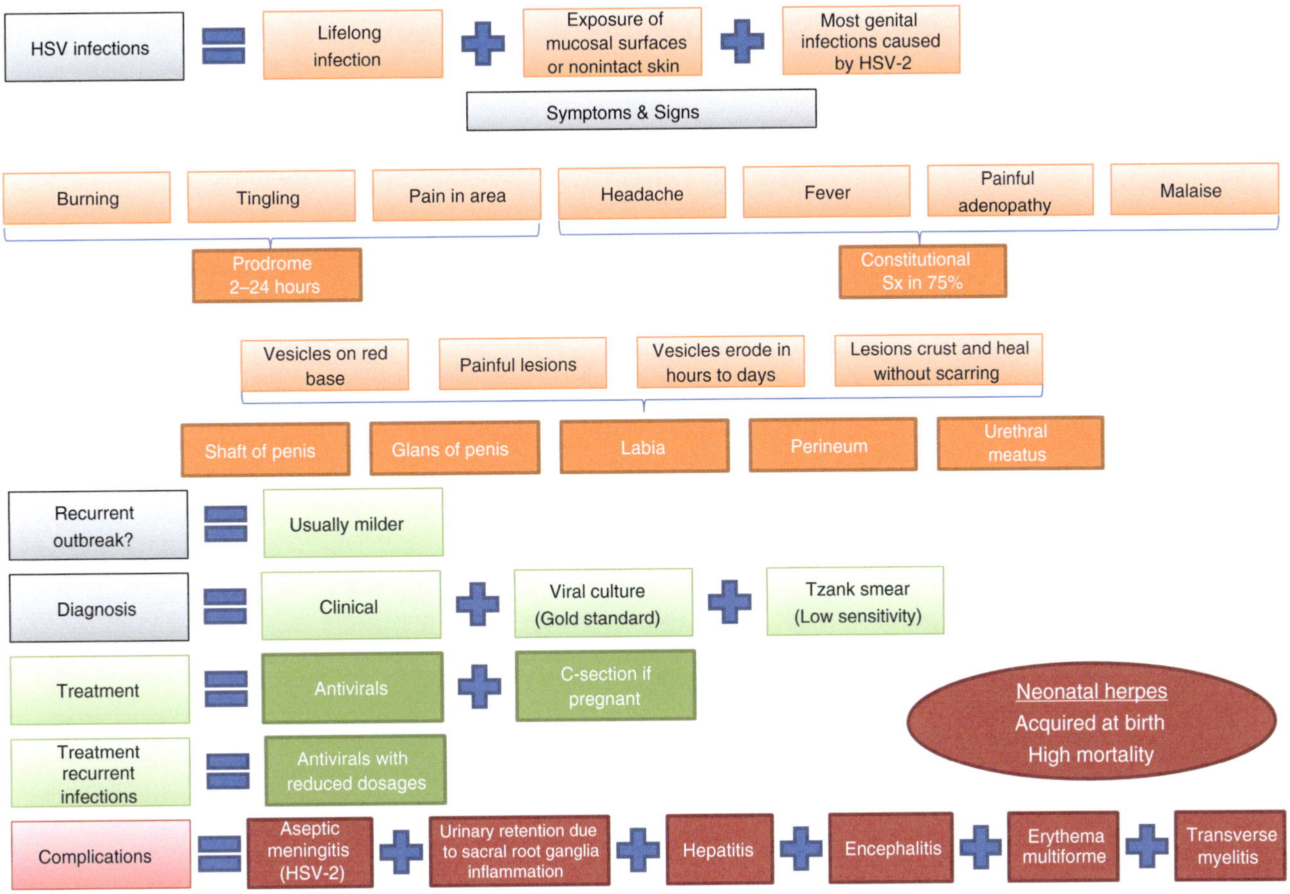

Chancroid

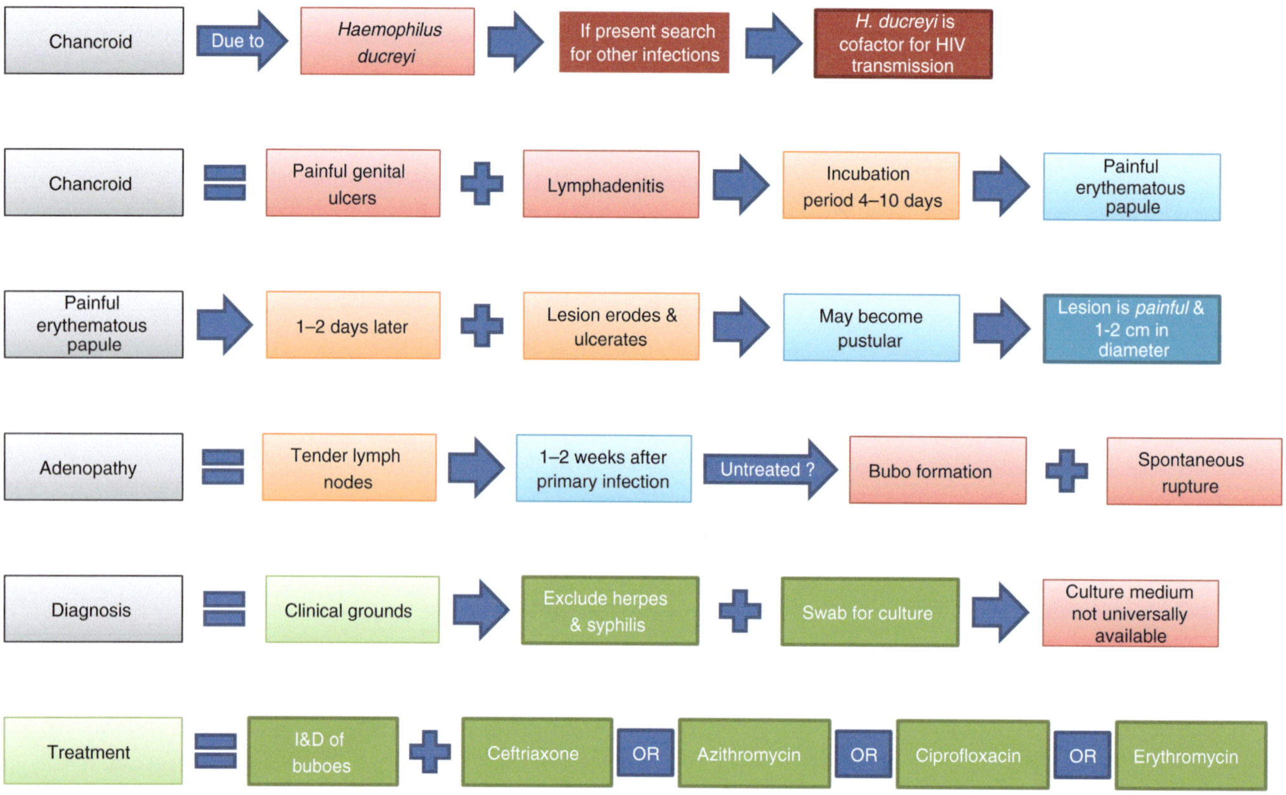

Lymphogranuloma Venereum (LGV)

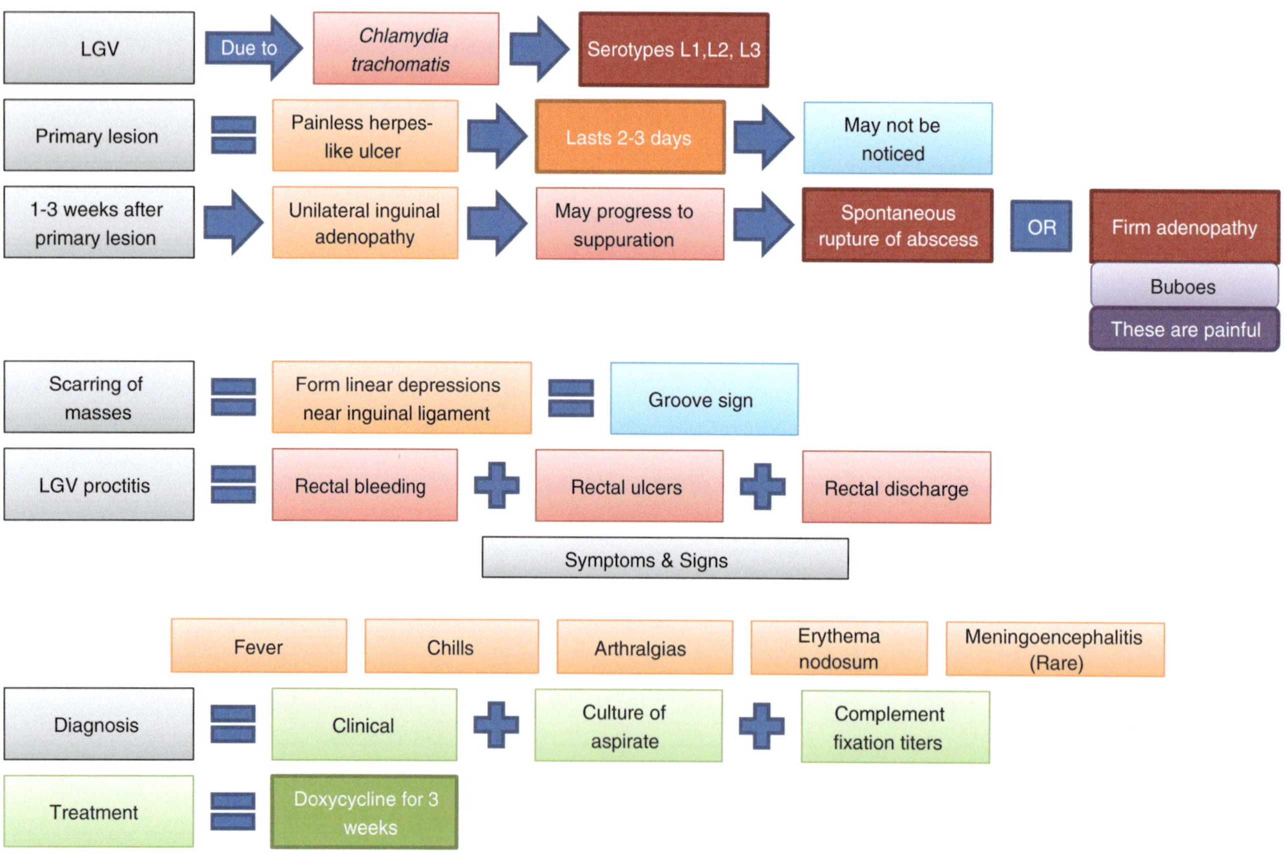

Granuloma Inguinale

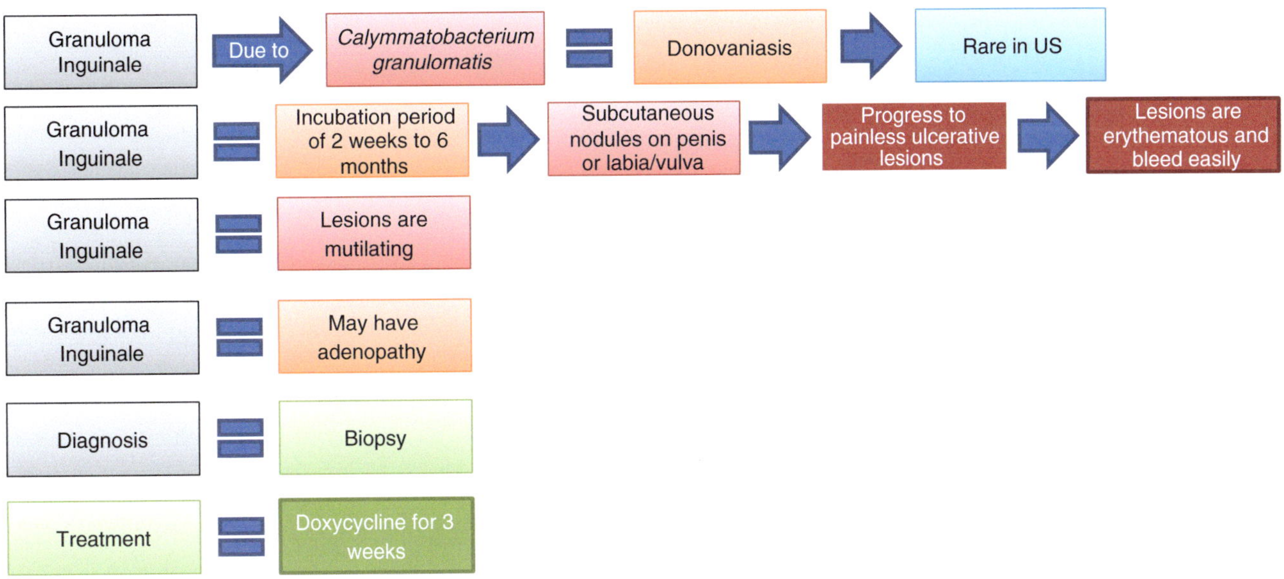

Lesions

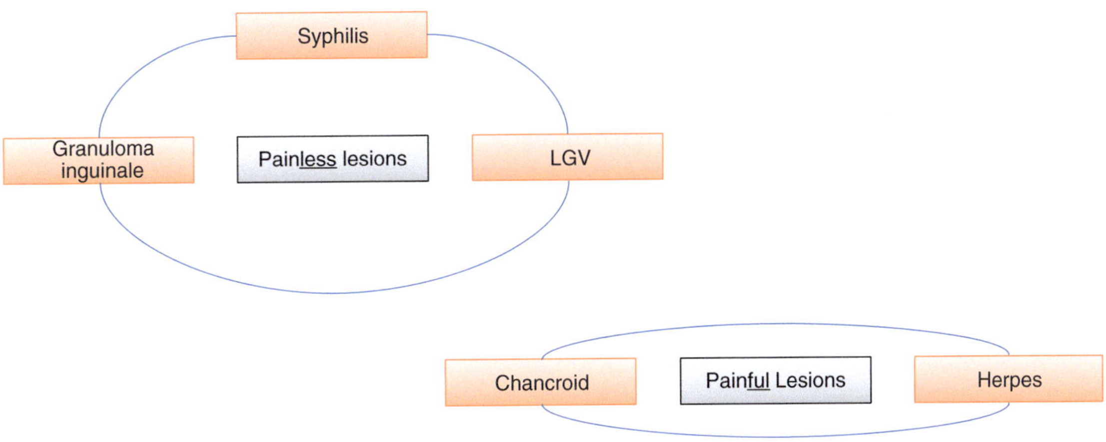

Genital Warts

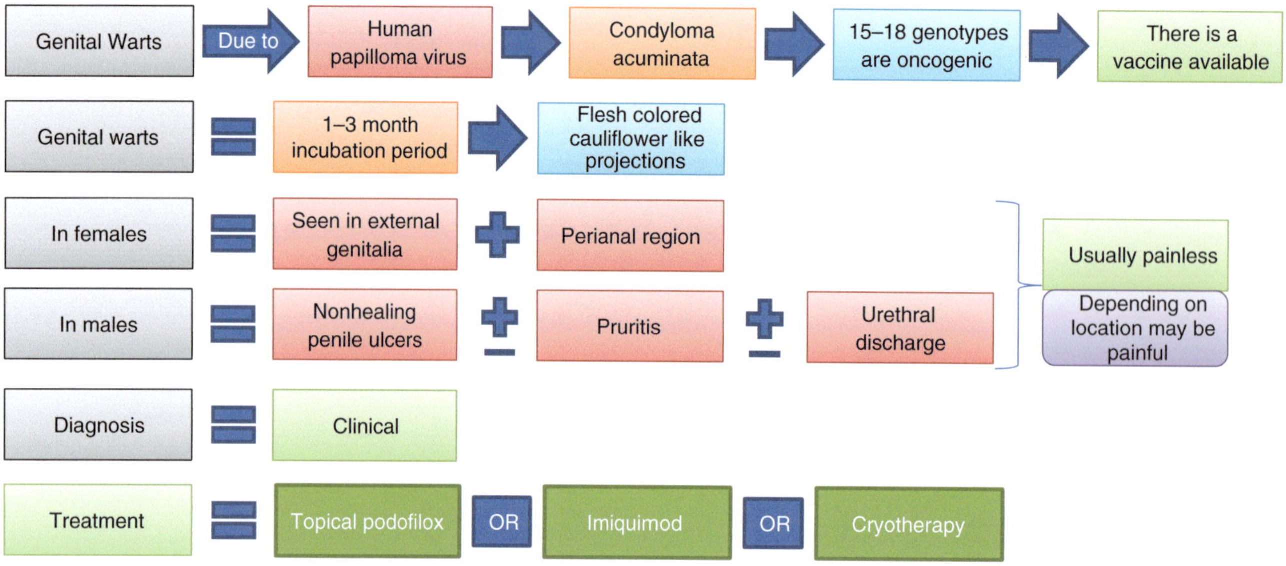

Hematologic and Oncologic Emergencies

Bobby Desai

Contents

Anemia 310
Transfusion Therapy 314
Complications of Transfusion Therapy 317
Dyshemoglobinemias 321
Hemostasis Tests 323
Sickle Cell Anemia 325
Hereditary Hemolytic Anemias 329
Specific Labs for Hemolytic Anemia 330
Platelet Disorders 333
Hemophilia 338
Von Willebrand's Disease 339
Anticoagulants 339
Absolute and Relative Contraindications to Thrombolysis 342
Complications of Malignancy 343

B. Desai, MD, MEd
Department of Emergency Medicine, University of Florida,
Gainesville, FL, USA
e-mail: bdesai@ufl.edu

B. Desai, B.R. Allen (eds.), *Nailing the Written Emergency Medicine Board Examination*,
DOI 10.1007/978-3-319-30838-8_5

Anemia

Introduction

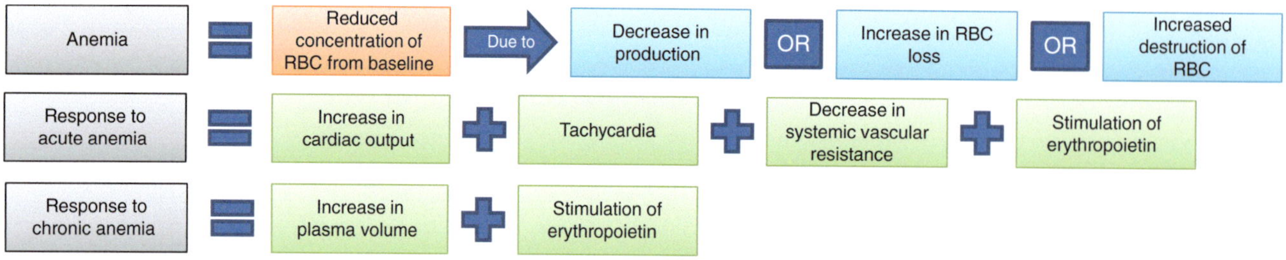

Causes of Anemia

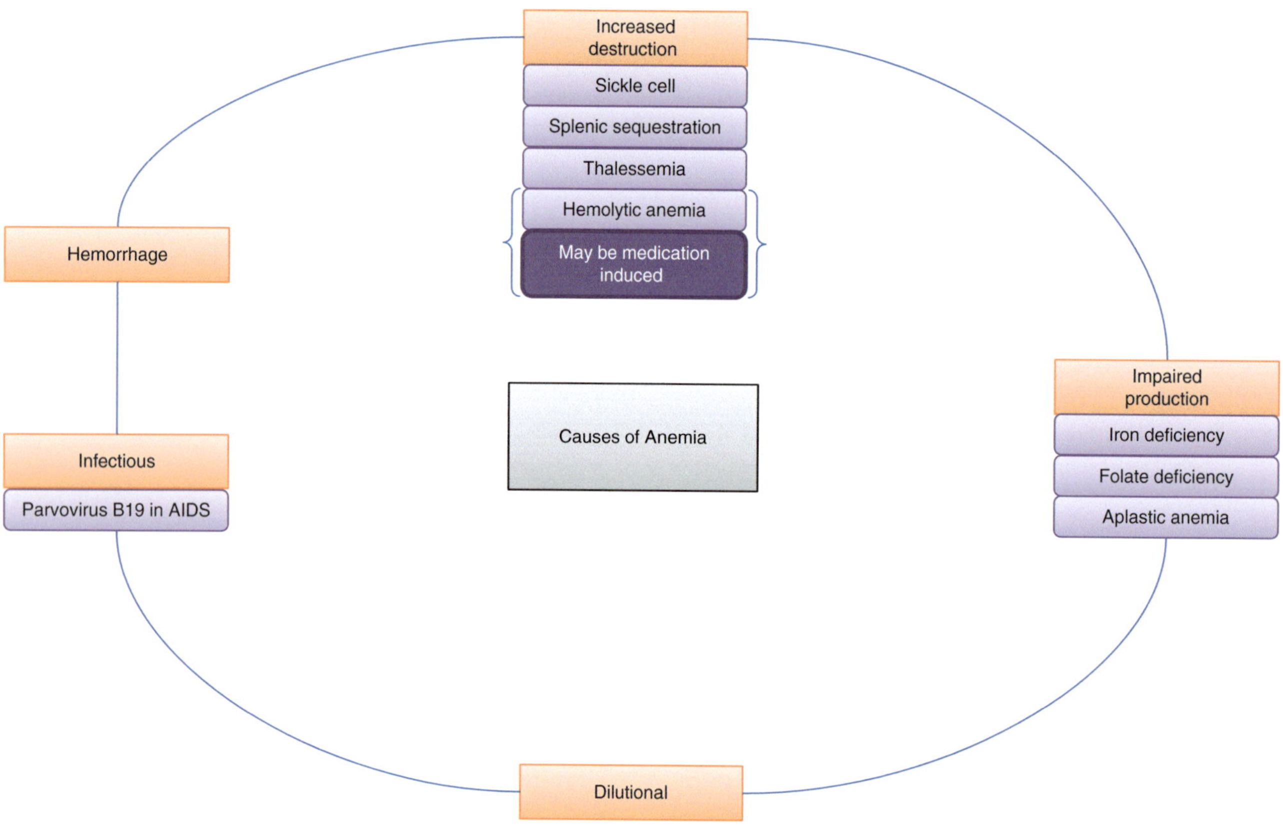

Symptoms and Signs

Symptoms & Signs → Depend on → Rate of development + Age and condition of patient + Comorbidities + Extent of anemia

Most symptoms & signs = Hemoglobin of ≤7 g/dL

Symptoms & Signs

Chronic anemia:
- Fatigue
- Weakness
- Orthostasis
- Lethargy
- Dyspnea on exertion
- Palpitations ± Chest pain
- Tachycardia
- Pallor of skin & mucosal surfaces
- Wide pulse pressure
- Systolic ejection murmur
- Hepatosplenomegaly
- Jaundice

Hepatosplenomegaly, Jaundice → Hemolytic anemia

Acute anemia:
- Hypotension
- Resting dyspnea
- Palpitations ± Chest pain
- Diaphoresis
- Altered mental status

Specific Labs for Anemia

Anemia	=	Decreased Hemoglobin & Hematocrit	+	Decreased RBCs		
Consideration of anemia	=	Look for GI or GU bleeding	+	CBC	+	Reticulocyte count + Consider sending peripheral smear
MCV	=	Mean corpuscular volume	=	Red blood cell size		
RDW	=	Red cell distribution	=	Size variability of RBC's		
Reticulocyte count	=	RBC production				
Best indicator for iron deficiency anemia	=	Serum ferritin				
Direct Coomb's Test	=	Demonstrates presence of antibodies ***on RBC's***	=	(+) in Hemolytic anemia	+	Transfusion reactions
Indirect Coomb's Test	=	Demonstrates presence of antibodies ***in serum***	=	Tested before transfusion		

Classification of Anemia

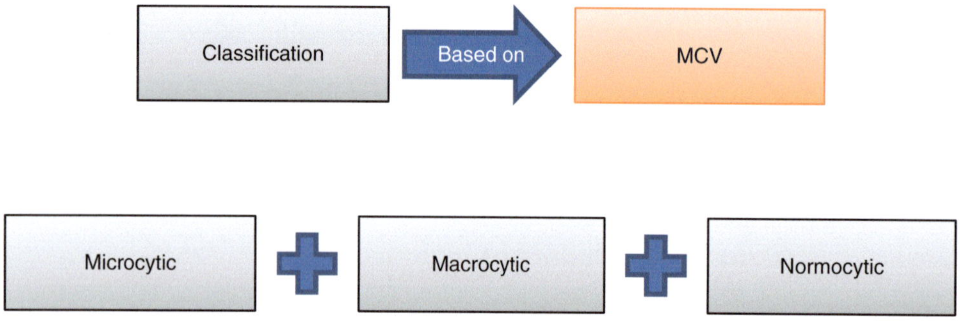

Low MCV (Microcytic)

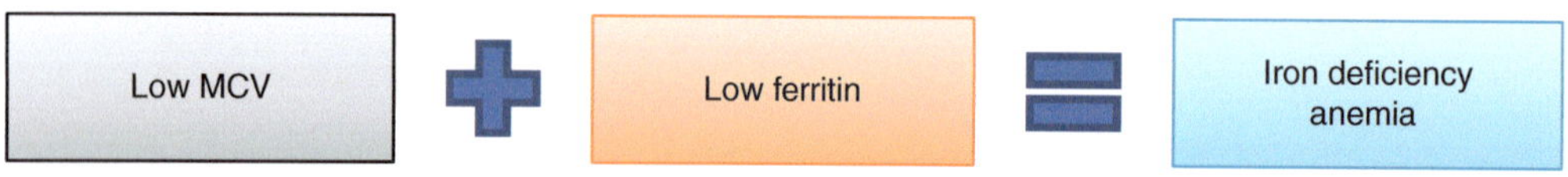

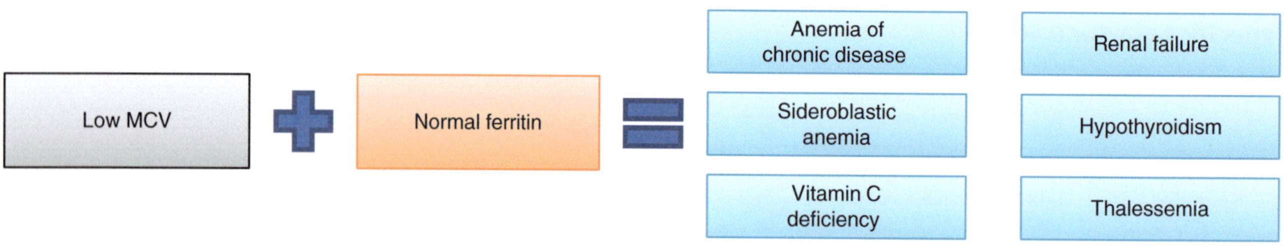

High MCV (Macrocytic)

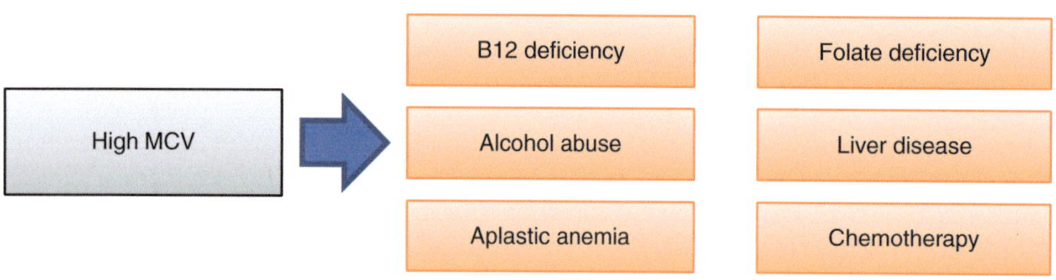

Normal MCV (Normocytic)

Normal MCV + Normal reticulocyte count = Anemia of chronic disease / Renal failure / Iron deficiency / B12 deficiency / Folate deficiency

Normal MCV + High reticulocyte count + Positive Coomb's test = Autoimmune related

Normal MCV + High reticulocyte count + Negative Coomb's test = Sickle cell disease / Hereditary spherocytosis / G6PD deficiency / Microangiopathic hemolysis

Treatment

Treatment = Depends on etiology of anemia

Significant blood loss OR Limited cardiac reserve OR Evidence of hypoxia OR Cardiac ischemia OR Hemodynamic instability = Type & cross-matched RBC

Iron deficiency anemia = Elemental iron

B12 or Folate deficiency anemia = IM Cyanocobalamin OR PO Folate

Sideroblastic anemia = Evaluate for reversible causes → Supportive care

Aplastic anemia = Transfusion + Supportive care

Anemia of chronic disease = Transfusion as needed + Supportive care

Transfusion Therapy

Packed Red Blood Cells (PRBC)

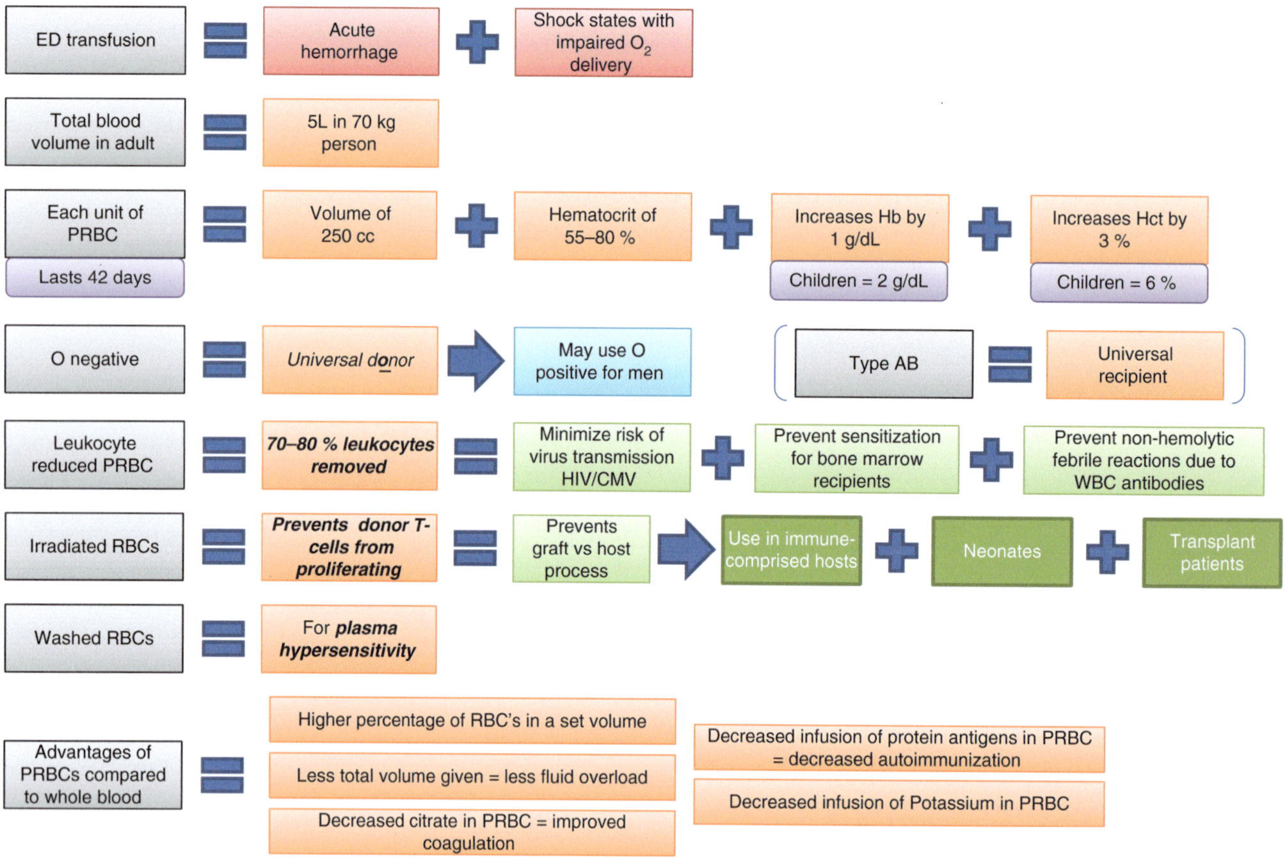

Massive Blood Transfusion

Bottom figure image (Reprinted from Allen B, Ganti L, Desai B. Trauma and ATLS. In: Allen B, Ganti L, Desai B, editors. Quick hits in emergency medicine. New York: Springer; 2013. p. 37–44. With permission from Springer Science + Business Media)

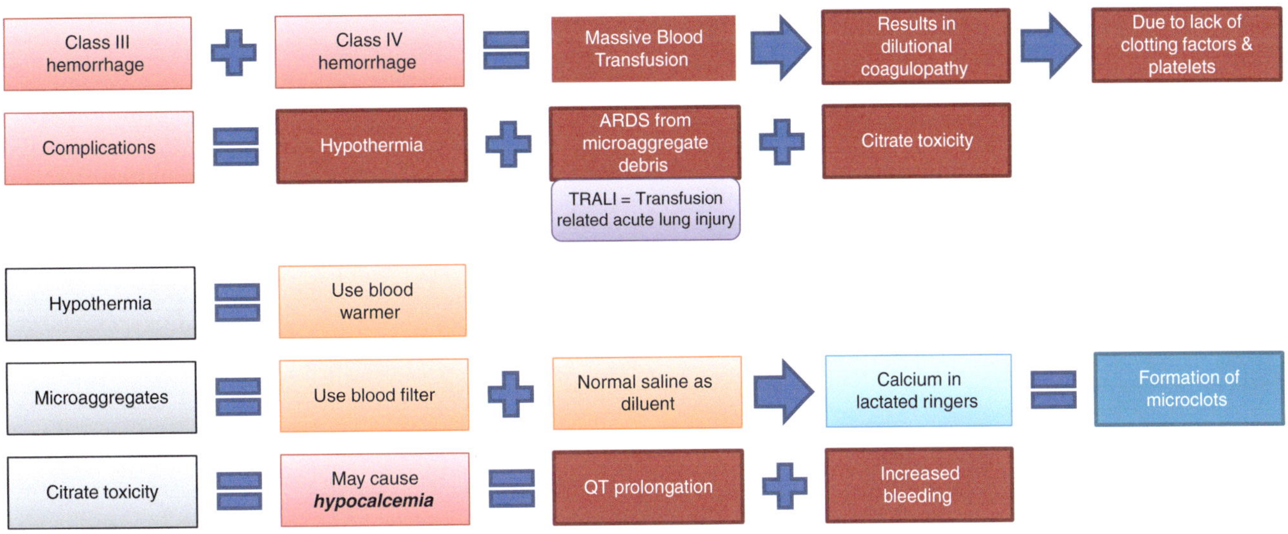

	Class I	Class II	Class III	Class IV
Blood Loss	< 750	750-1500	1500-2000	> 2000
% Blood Vol.	< 15%	15 – 30%	30 – 40%	> 40%
Pulse	< 100	**> 100**	> 120	> 140
Blood Pressure	Normal	Normal	**Decreased**	**Decreased**
Pulse Pressure	Normal	**Decreased**	**Decreased**	**Decreased**
Resp. Rate	14 – 20	**20 – 30**	**30 – 40**	**> 40**
UOP	> 30	**20 – 30**	**5 – 15**	**negligible**
Mental Status	sl. Anxious	mildly anx	**confused**	**lethargic**
Fluid	crystalloid	crystalloid	**blood**	**blood**

Platelet Transfusion

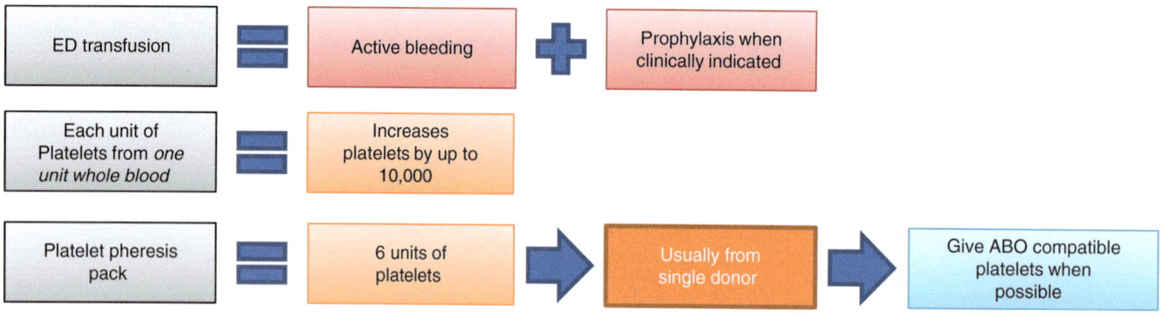

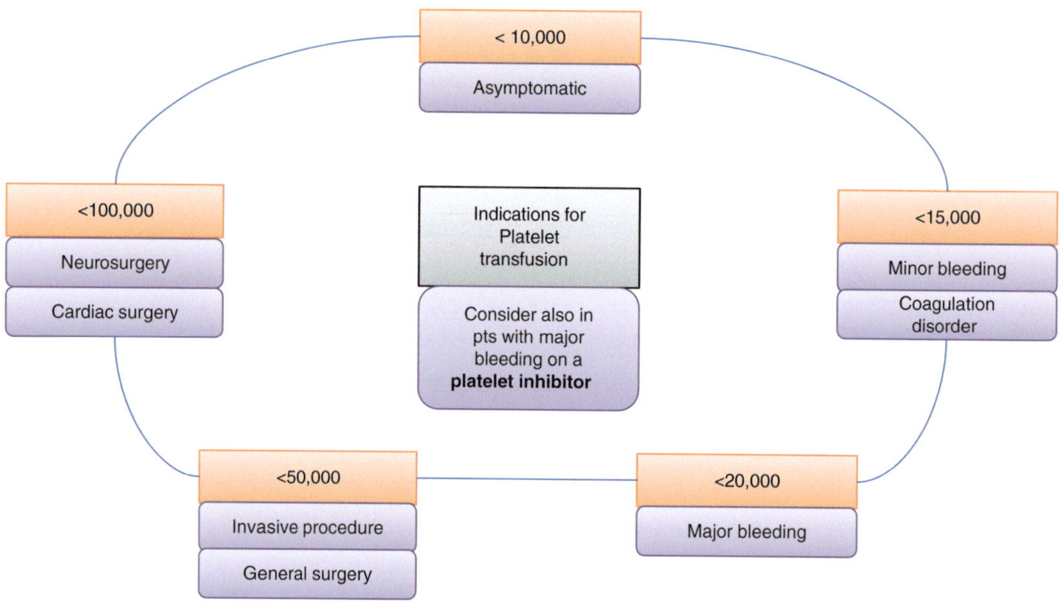

Fresh Frozen Plasma

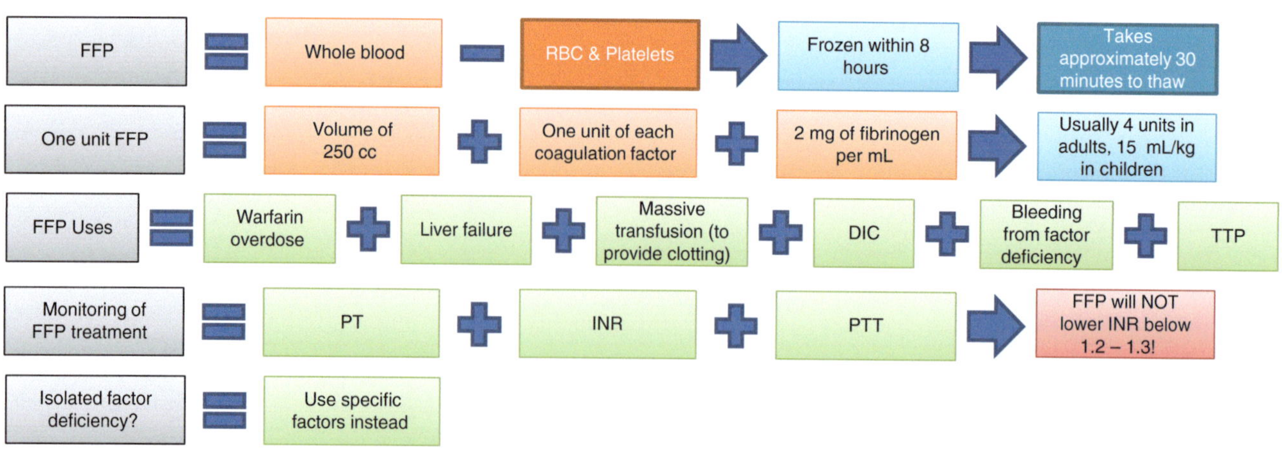

Cryoprecipitate

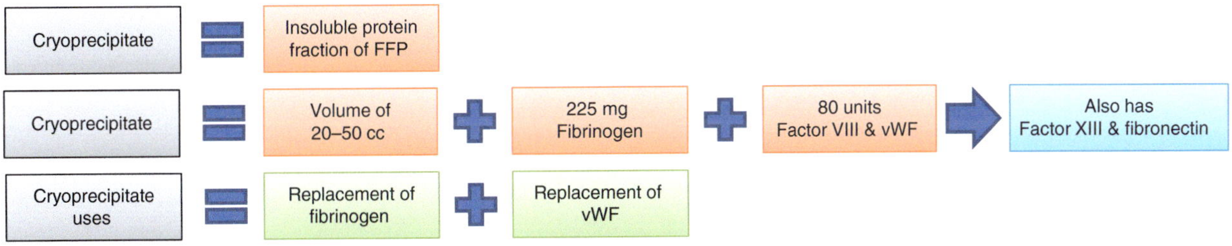

Complications of Transfusion Therapy

Acute Hemolytic Transfusion Reaction

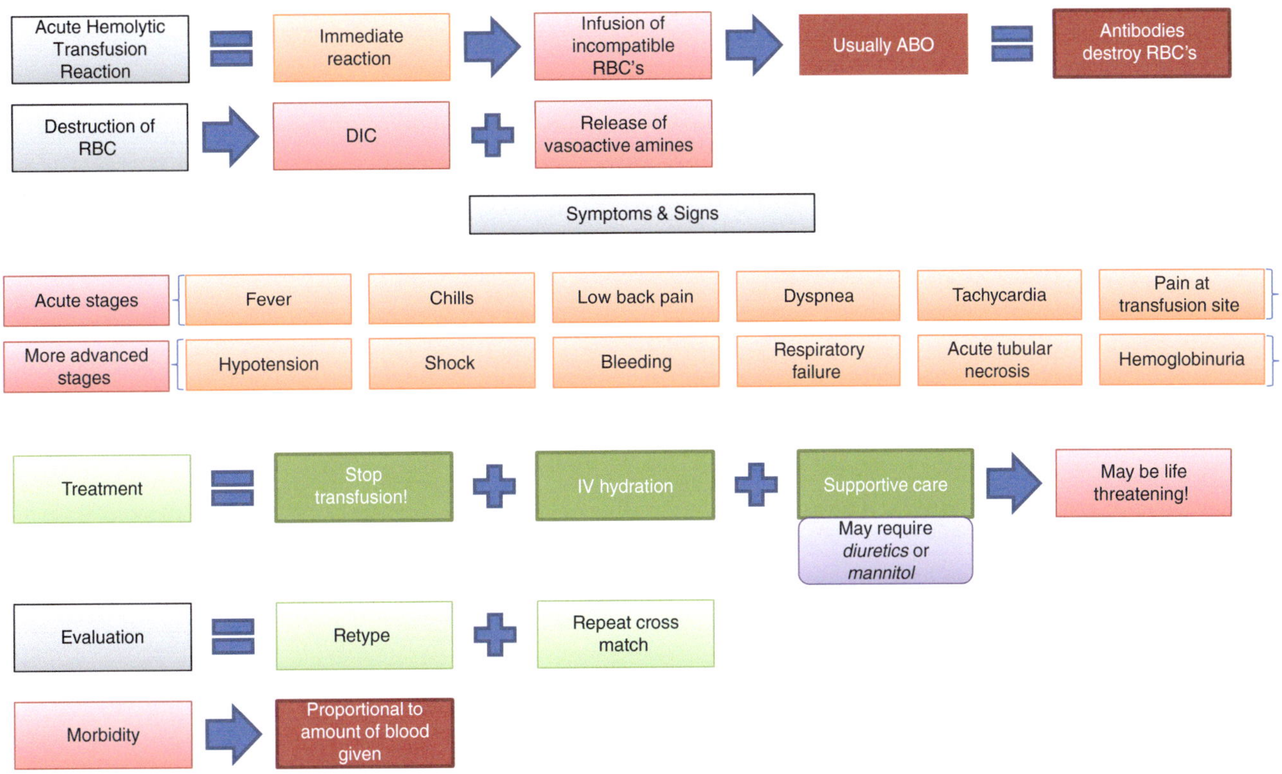

Laboratory Investigation for Acute Hemolytic Transfusion Reaction

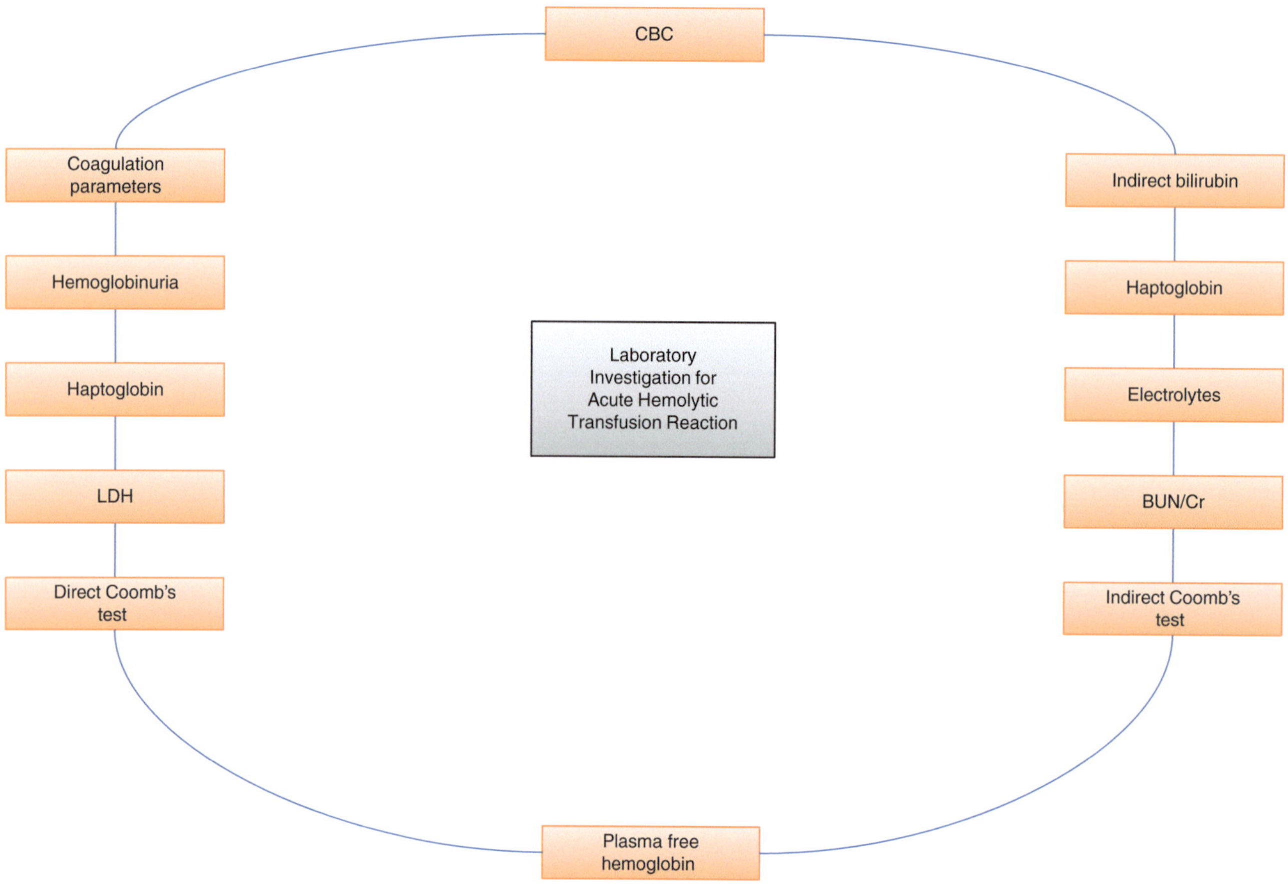

Febrile Nonhemolytic Reaction

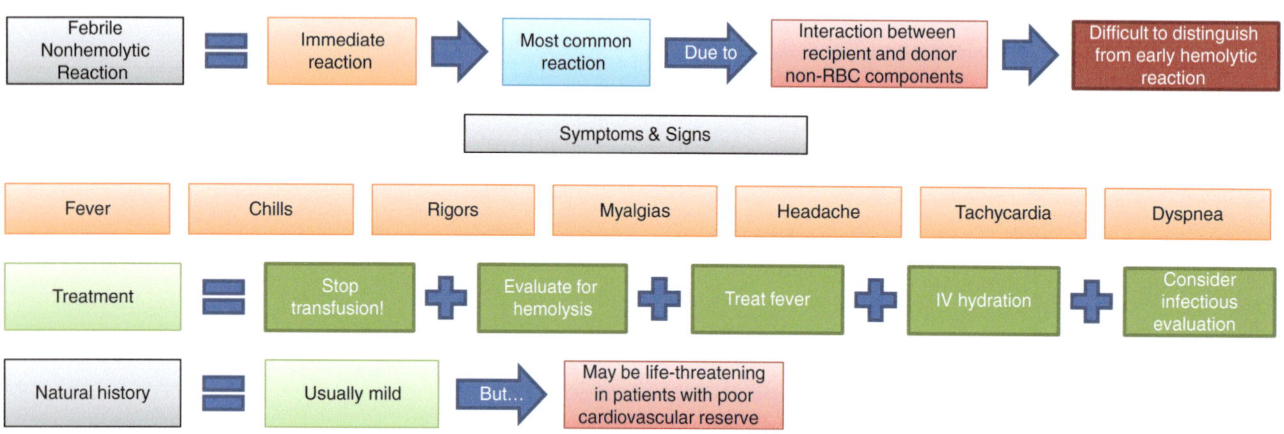

Delayed Transfusion Reaction

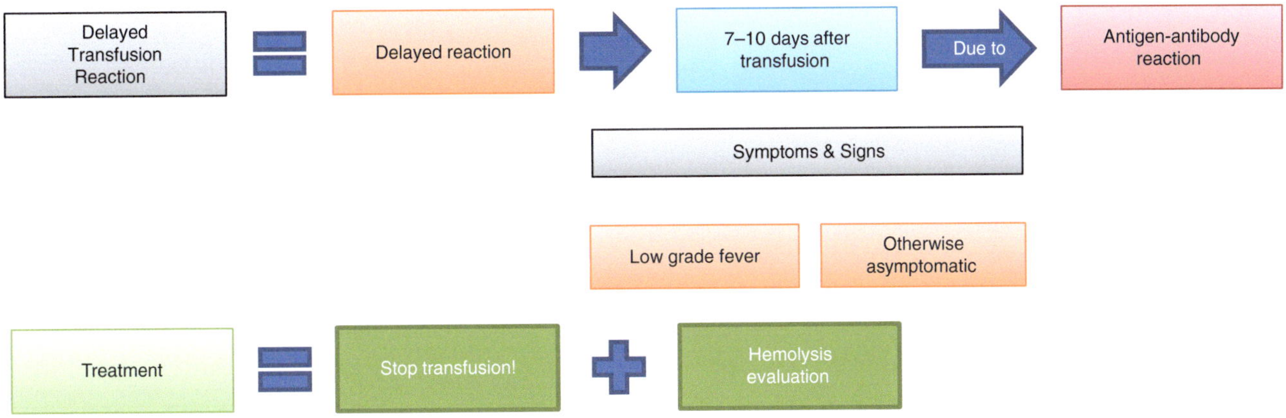

Allergic Transfusion Reaction

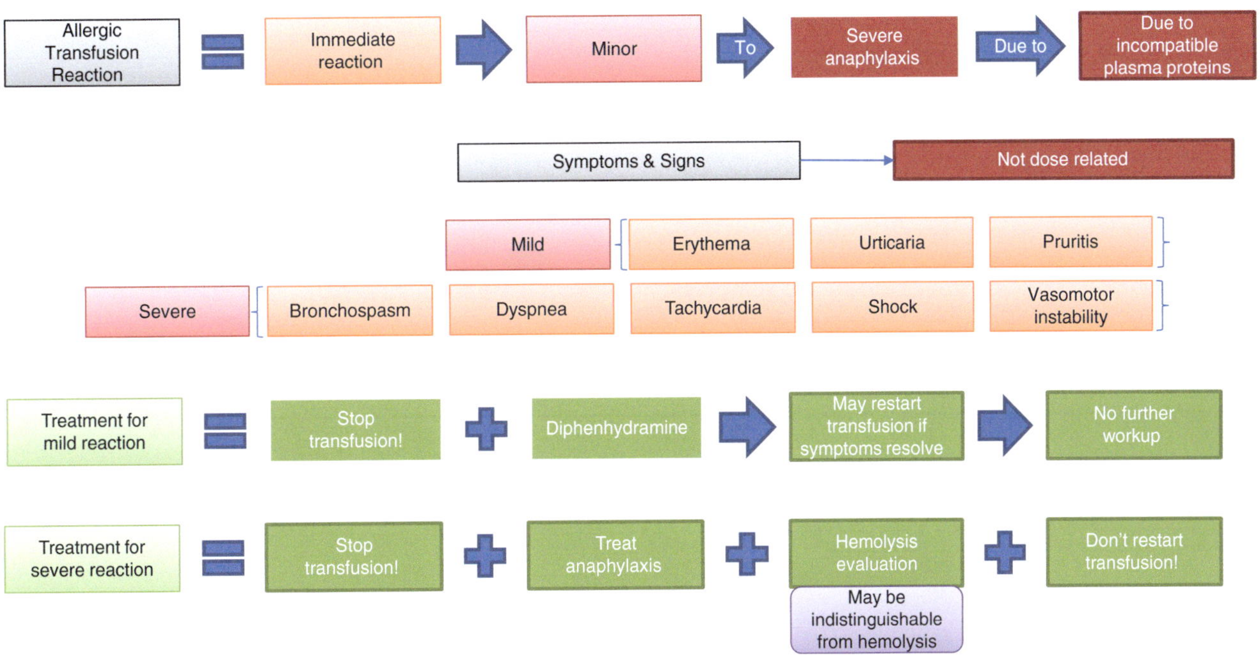

Infectious Complications of Transfusion

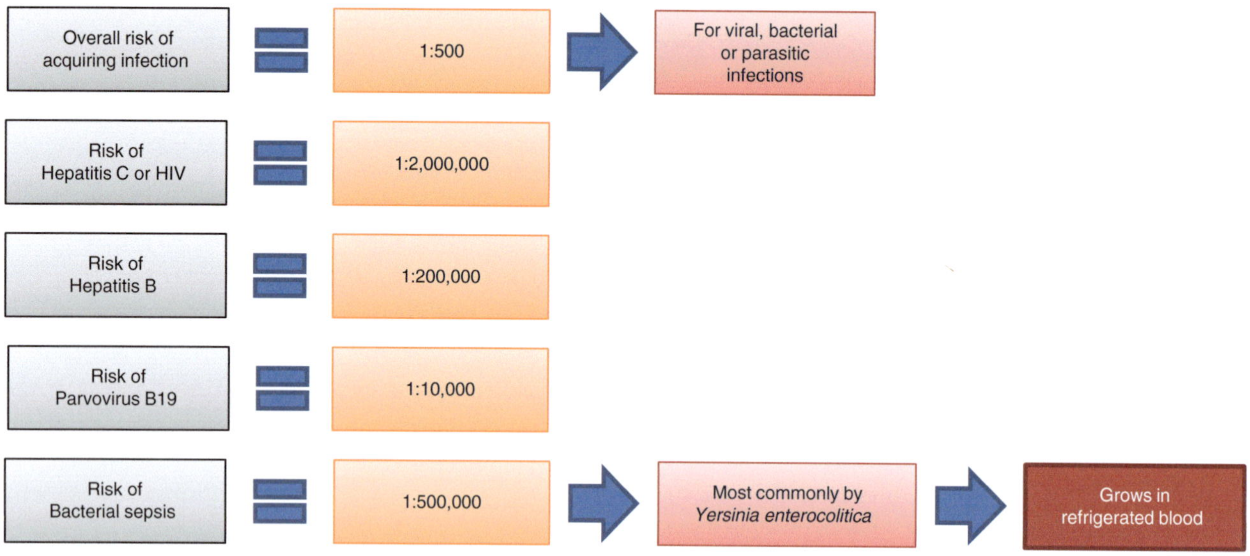

Other Complications of Transfusion

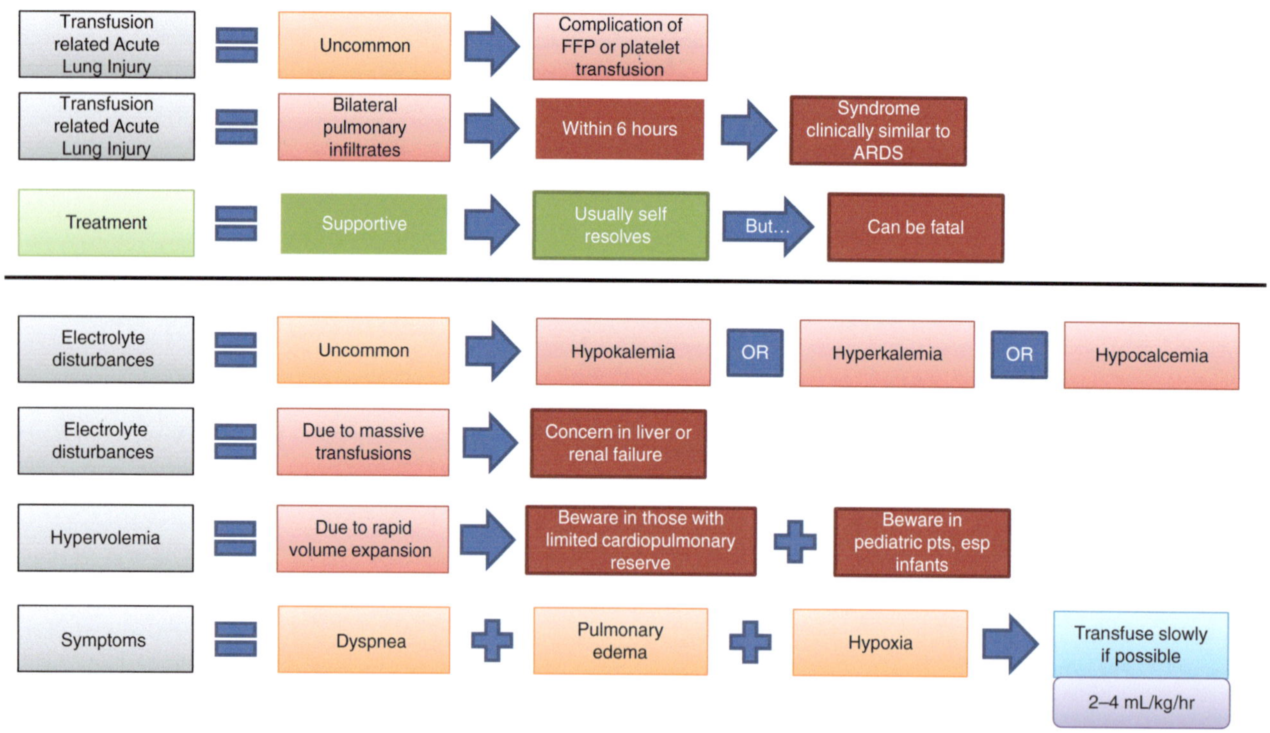

Dyshemoglobinemias

Introduction: Methemoglobin (MHb)

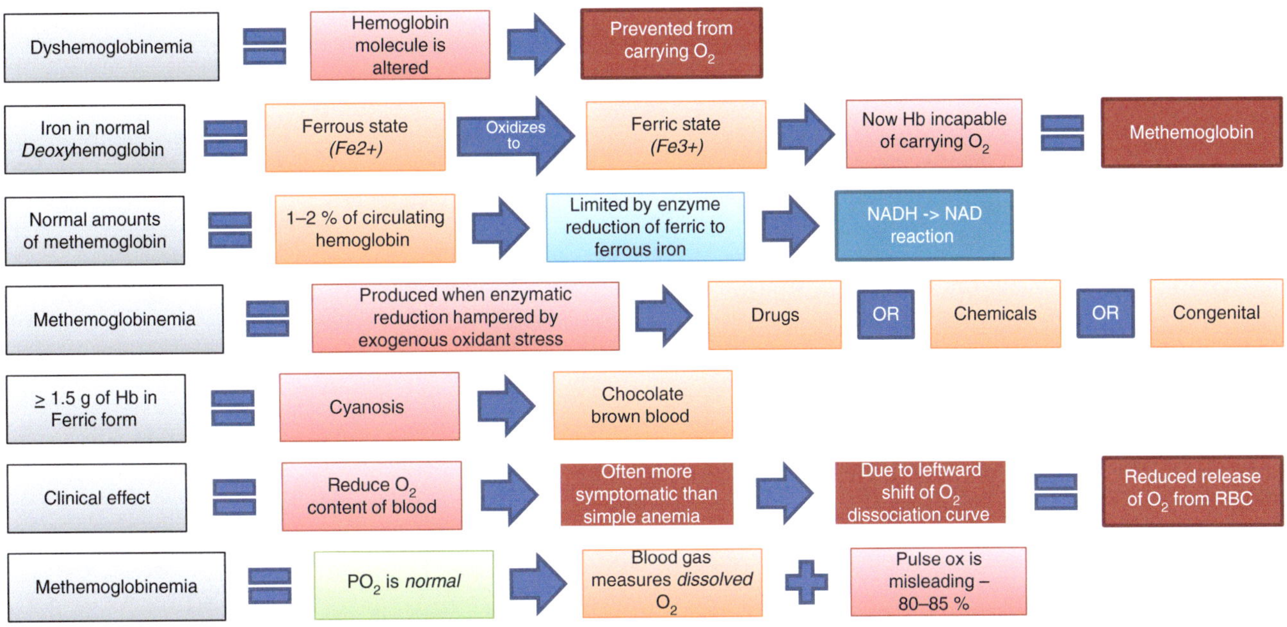

Drugs Causing Methemoglobinemia

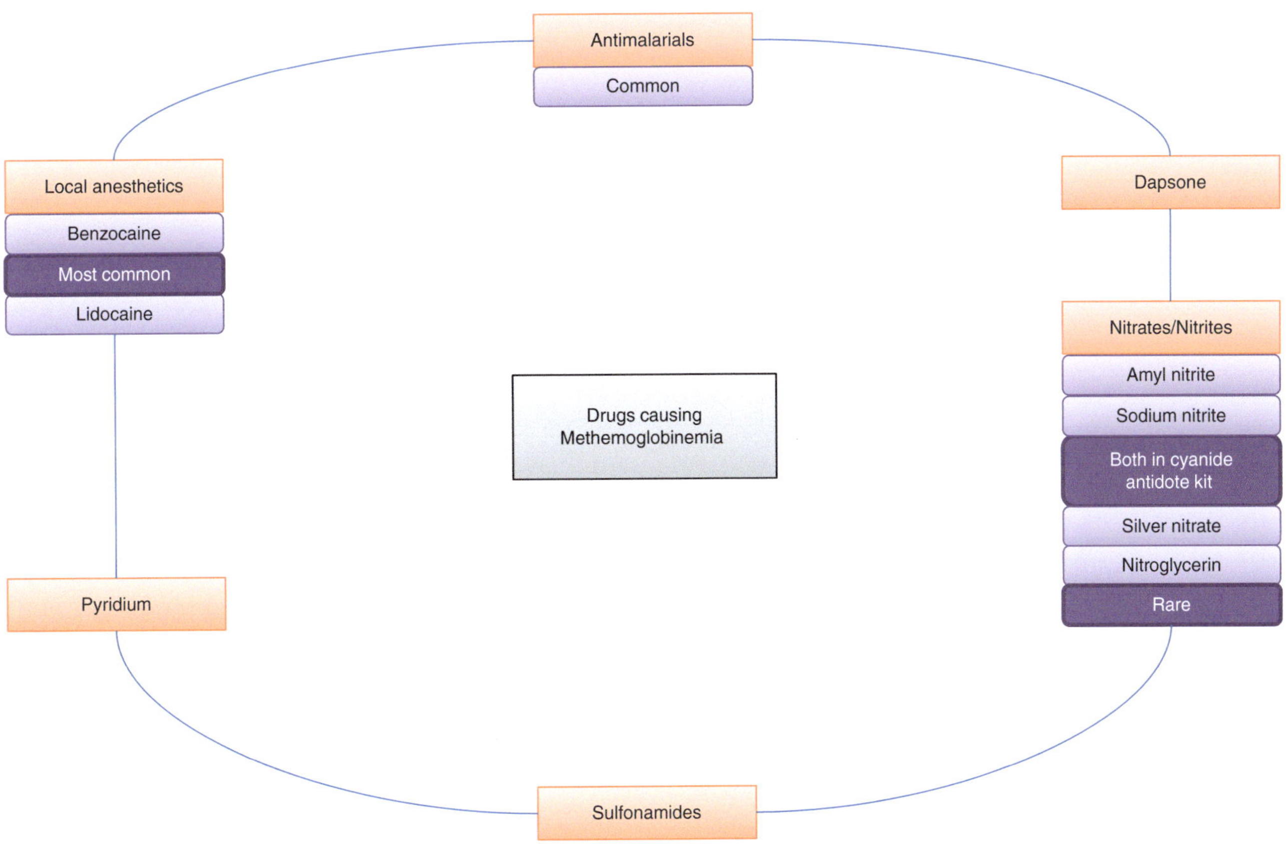

Types of Methemoglobinemia

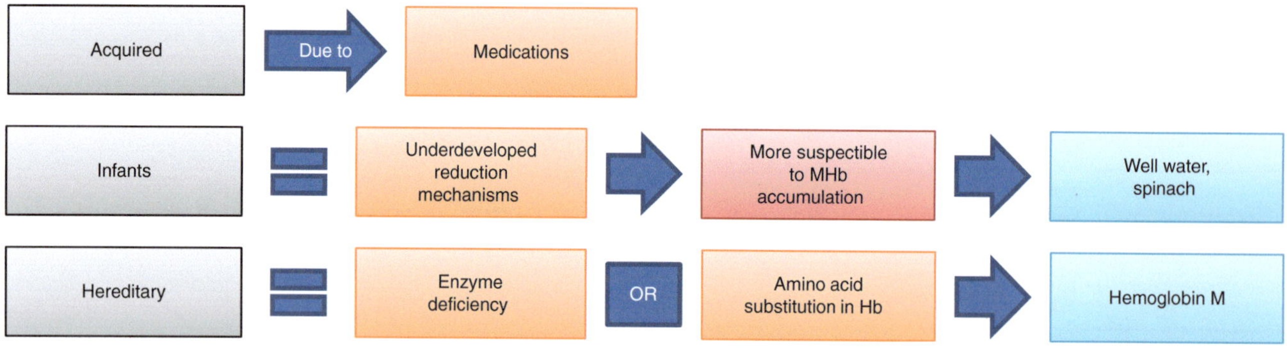

Clinical Features

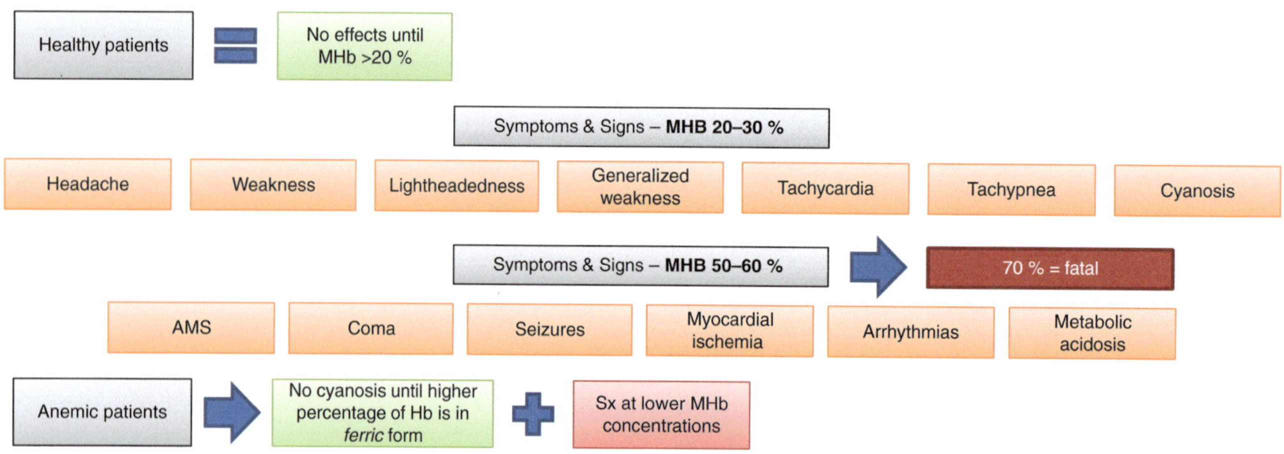

Treatment

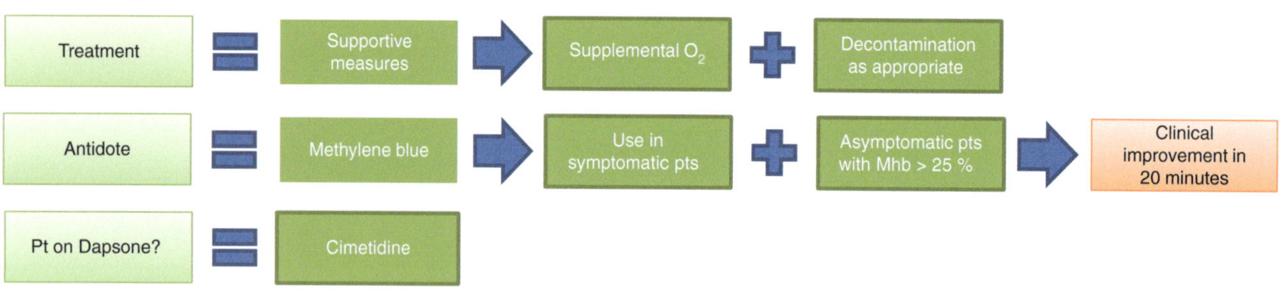

Hemostasis Tests

Bleeding Time

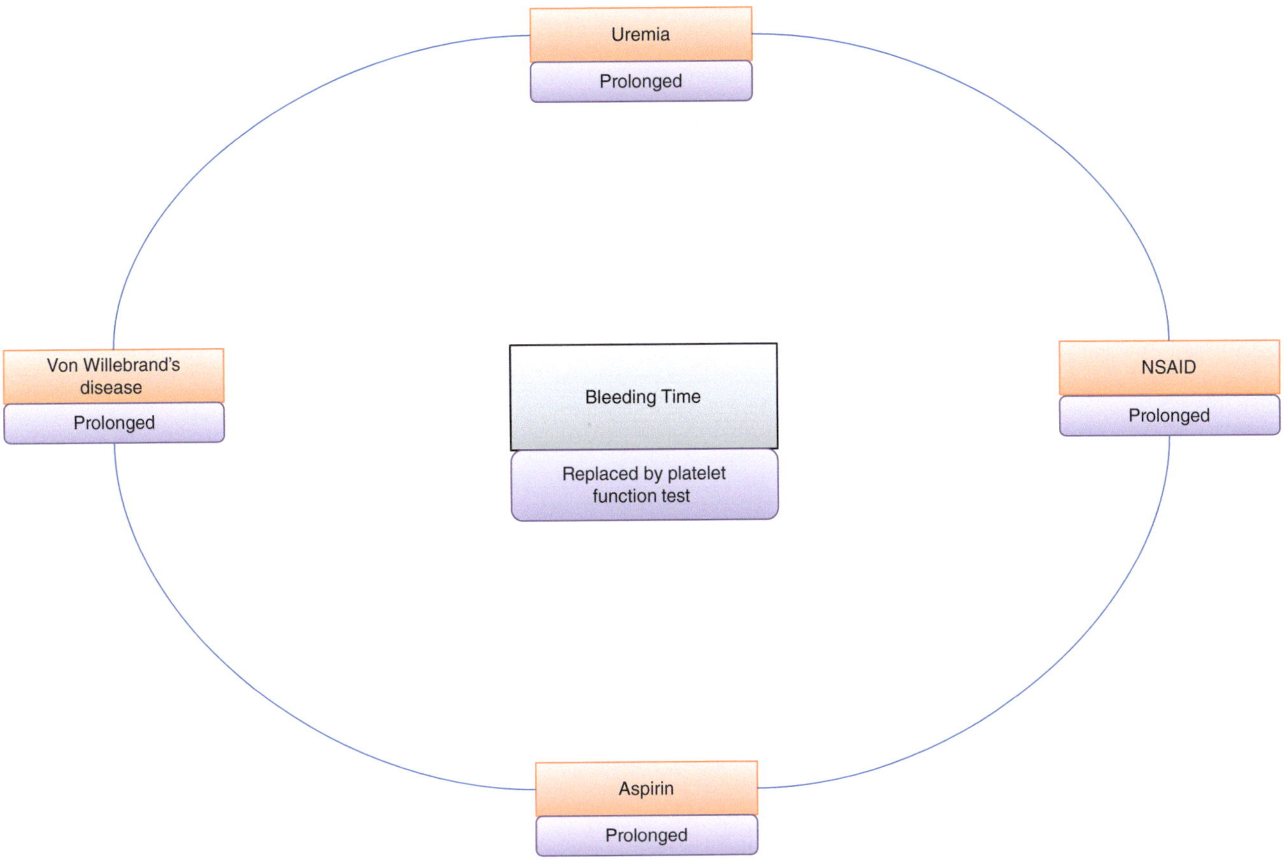

Prothrombin Time

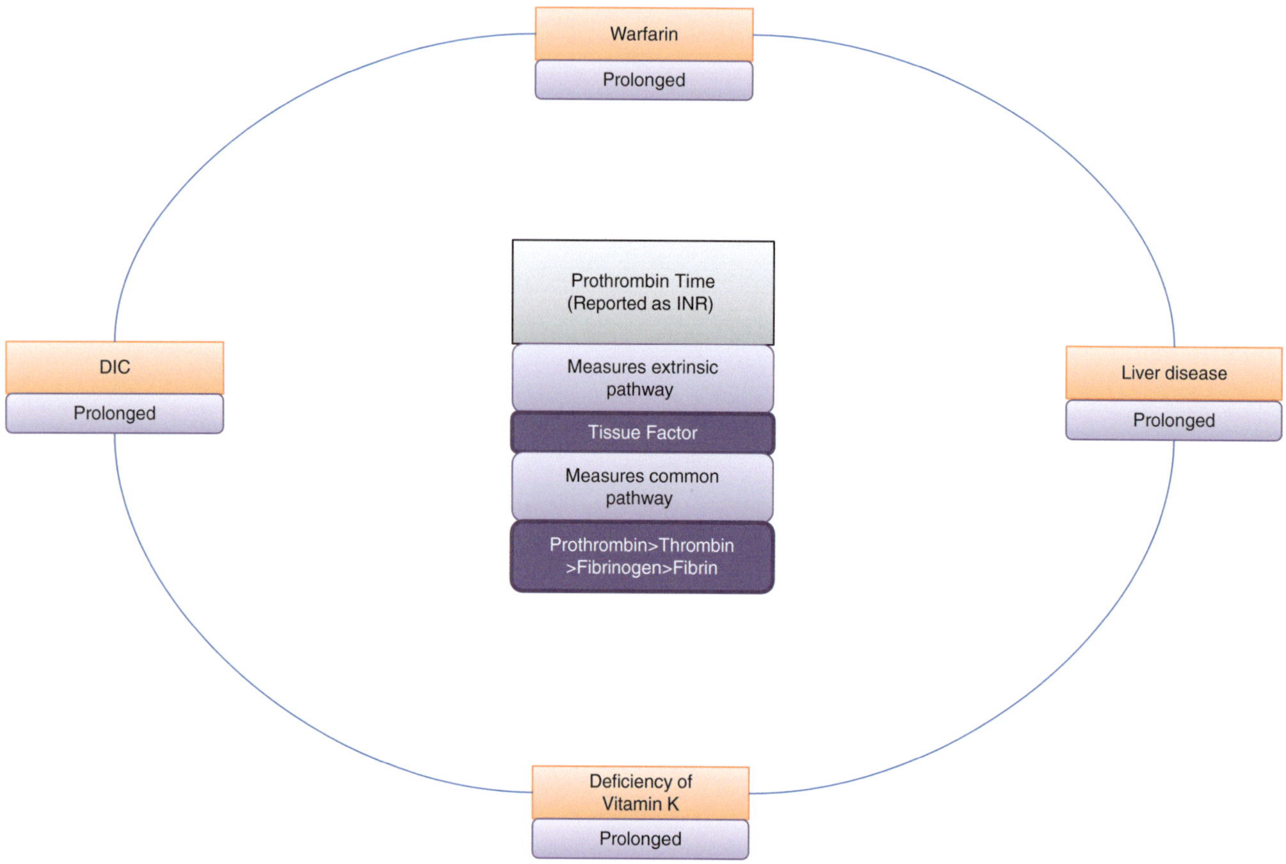

Activated Partial Thromboplastin Time

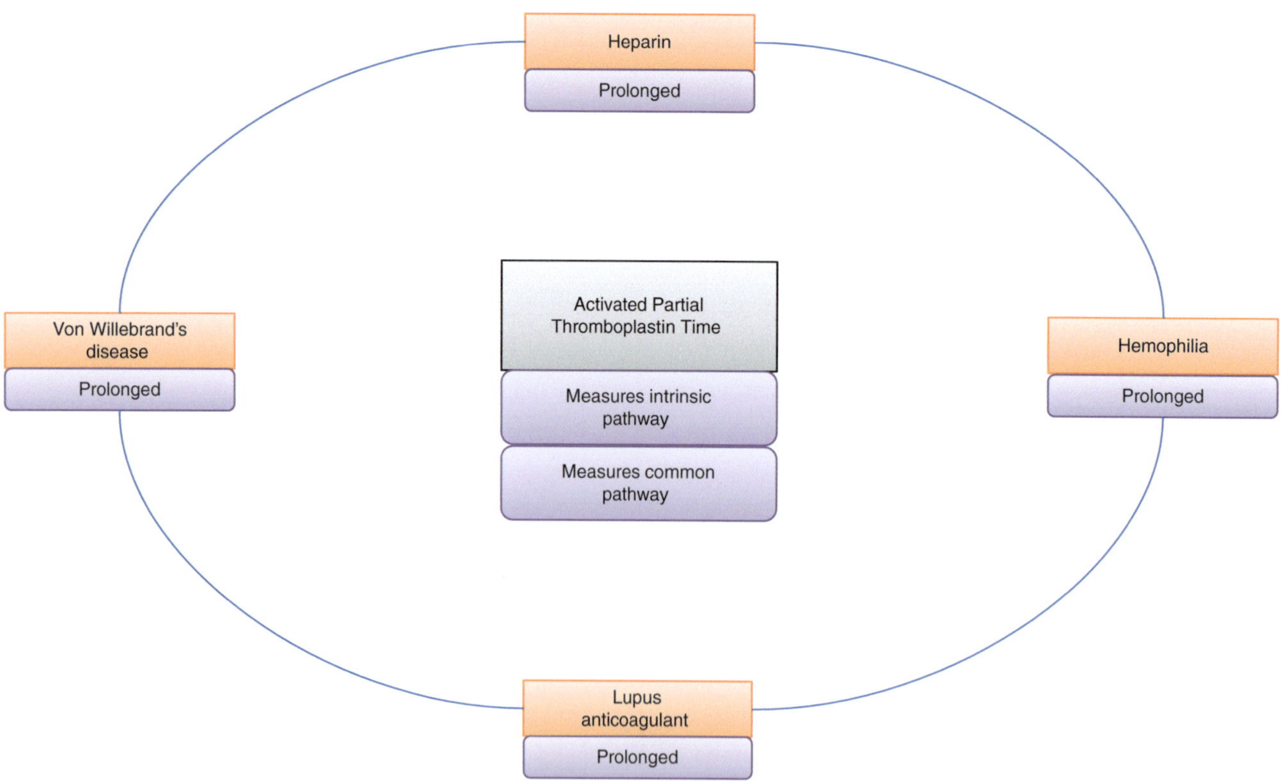

Sickle Cell Anemia

Introduction

Sickle cell disease = Genetically based → Due to abnormal Hb molecule → Hemoglobin S → Under certain conditions causes RBC sickling

Sickled cells → Cannot pass through microcirculation → Leads to → Ischemia + Infarction

Sickled cells → Higher rate of hemolysis than normal RBC → Chronic hereditary hemolytic anemia → May be icteric

Sickle cell *Trait* = Usually asymptomatic → May have → Vaso-occlusive crisis under *extreme conditions* + Spontaneous bleeding

Sickle cell Anemia = Have a reticulocytosis → 10–15 %

Sickle cell Anemia = Higher risk of infection with encapsulated organisms (*Strep pneumoniae*, *Neisseria*) → Due to → Autosplenectomy

Minimal laboratory investigation = CBC + Reticulocyte count + CXR + Urine

Sickle Cell Tidbits

PEDIATRICS

Early sign of sickle cell in children = Dactylitis = Hand-foot syndrome = Marrow infarction in bones of hands & feet

Hip pain in sickle cell disease = Consider *avascular necrosis* of femoral head = 30 % of patients will have this

Priapism = 30 % of patients will have this → Same treatment → But… → May consider exchange transfusion for severe cases

SCD = May have loud systolic ejection murmur

SCD = May have chronic poor healing leg ulcers around the malleoli

Vaso-occlusive Crisis

Vaso-occlusive Crisis = Obstruction of microvasculature → Due to → Sludging of sickled cells

Vaso-occlusive Crisis → Increased viscosity of blood → Leads to → Ischemia + Infarction

Precipitants or stressors = Infection + Dehydration + Cold weather + Changes in altitude

Manifestations = Joint pain + Bone pain + Muscle pain

Musculoskeletal pain = Most common presentation → Back ± Arms ± Legs

Abdominal pain = 2nd most common presentation → Diffuse + Poorly localized → Cholelithiasis is common

Papillary necrosis of kidney = Microscopic or gross hematuria + Flank pain → Treat with hydration + Monitoring of Hb levels

Treatment = Hydration + Analgesia ± (Hydroxyurea + Folate)

Elevated WBC + Evidence of infection? = Antibiotics

Acute Chest Syndrome

Acute Chest Syndrome = New infiltrate on CXR involving 1 complete lung segment (usually lower lobes) + Fever + Chest pain + Cough or wheeze + Tachypnea

Acute Chest Syndrome → Leading cause of death + 2nd most common cause of hospitalization → Most common in 2–4 years

Acute Chest Syndrome Etiologies = Infection + Rib infarction + Fat emboli + Iatrogenic – over hydration leading to pulmonary edema

Infectious organisms = *Chlamydia pneumoniae* + *Mycoplasma pneumoniae* + *Streptococcus pneumoniae* + *Staph aureus* + *Hemophilus influenzae*

Acute Chest Syndrome = May be a combination of factors → May occur during hospitalization

Treatment = O_2 + Antibiotics (Don't forget a *macrolide*) + Pain control + Hydration + Broncho-dilators ± Exchange transfusions

Aplastic Crisis

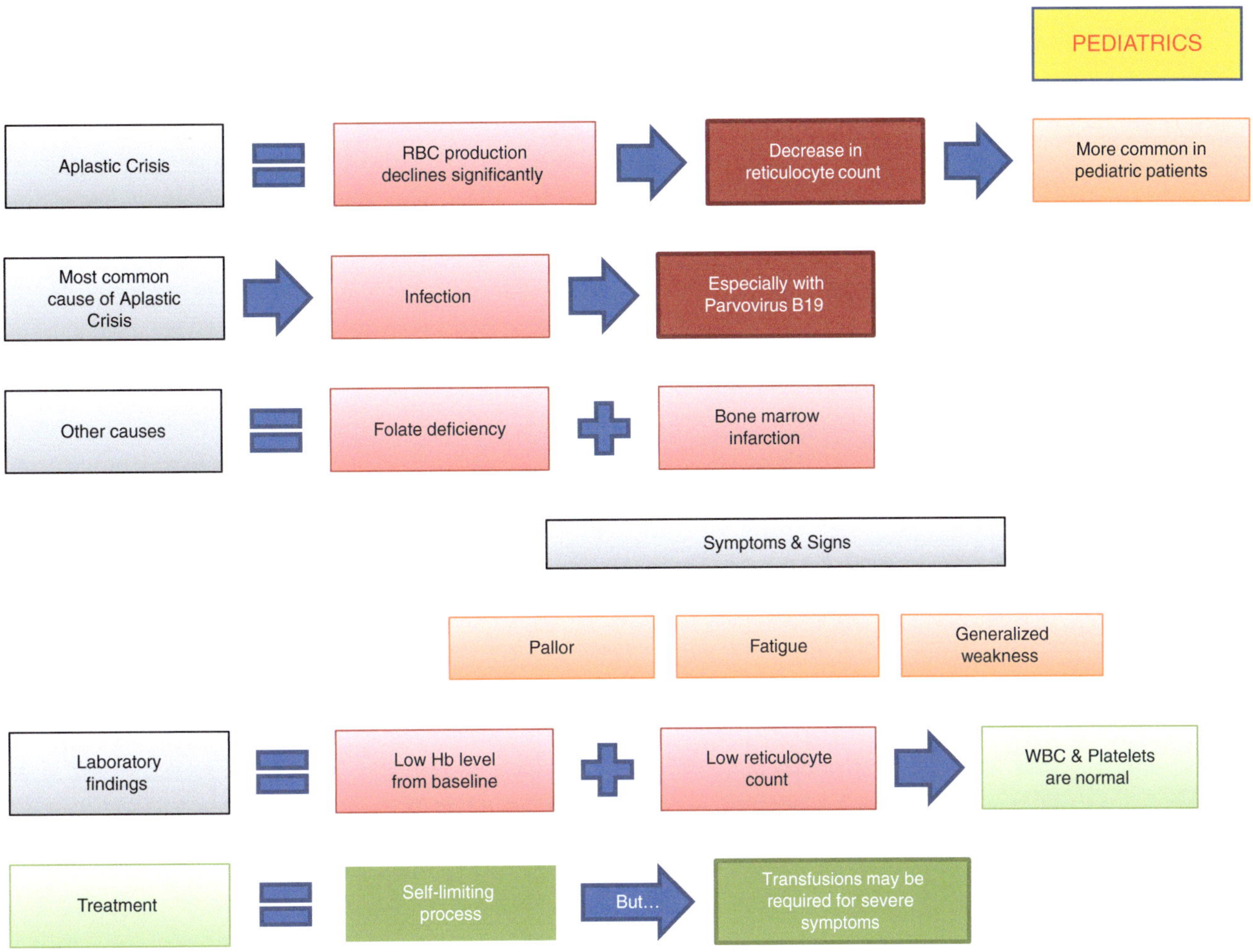

Splenic Sequestration

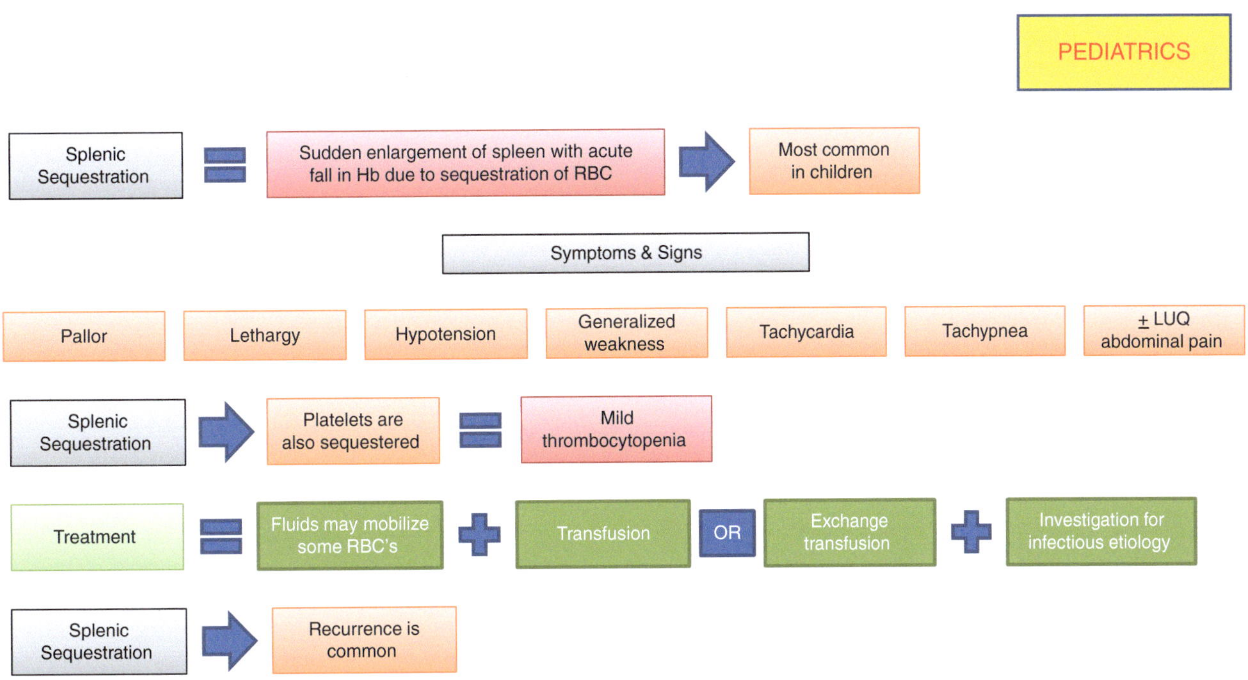

Neurologic Complications of SCD

Neurologic sequelae = Ischemic & Hemorrhagic stroke + TIA + Seizures + Paresthesias

Strokes = Ischemic in children + Hemorrhagic in adults

Cerebral aneurysms → More common in SCD

Treatment = Exchange transfusion

Neurologic sequelae → Recurrence is common

Infectious Complications of SCD

Sickle cell disease = Functionally asplenic = High risk of infection from encapsulated organisms = *Streptococcus pneumoniae* + *Hemophilus influenzae*

Pneumonia = *Chlyamdia pneumoniae* + *Mycoplasma pneumoniae* + *Streptococcus pneumoniae* + *Staph aureus* + *Hemophilus influenzae*

Osteomyelitis in SCD = *Salmonella typhimurum* + *Staph aureus* + *E. coli*

Fever OR Infectious symptoms = Early antibiotics

SCD → Need immunizations → Especially pneumococcal vaccine

Hereditary Hemolytic Anemias

G6PD Deficiency

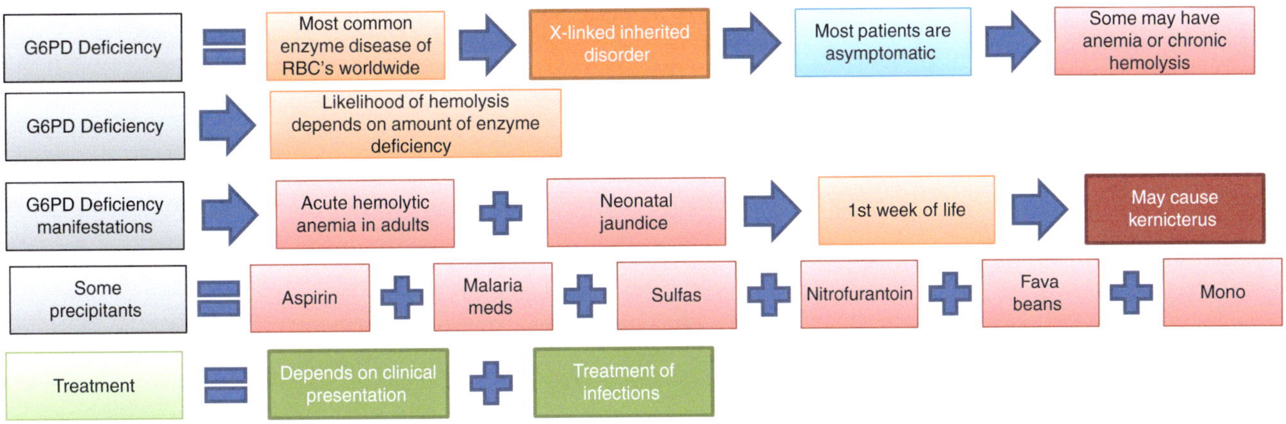

Hereditary Spherocytosis

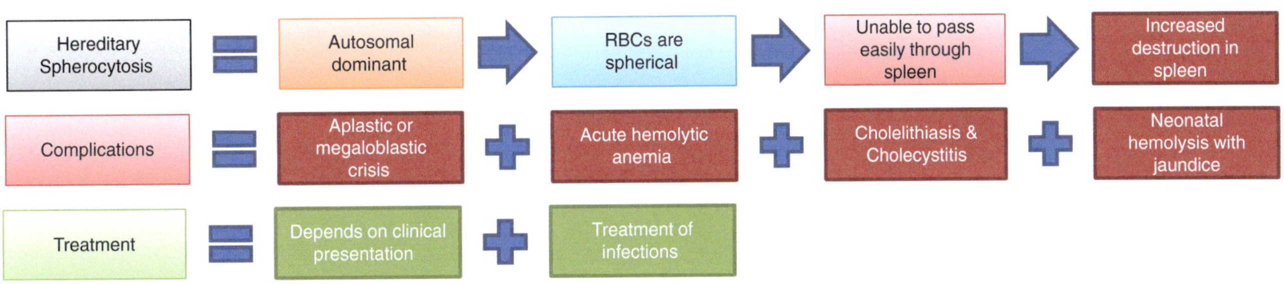

Specific Labs for Hemolytic Anemia

Acquired Hemolytic Anemia

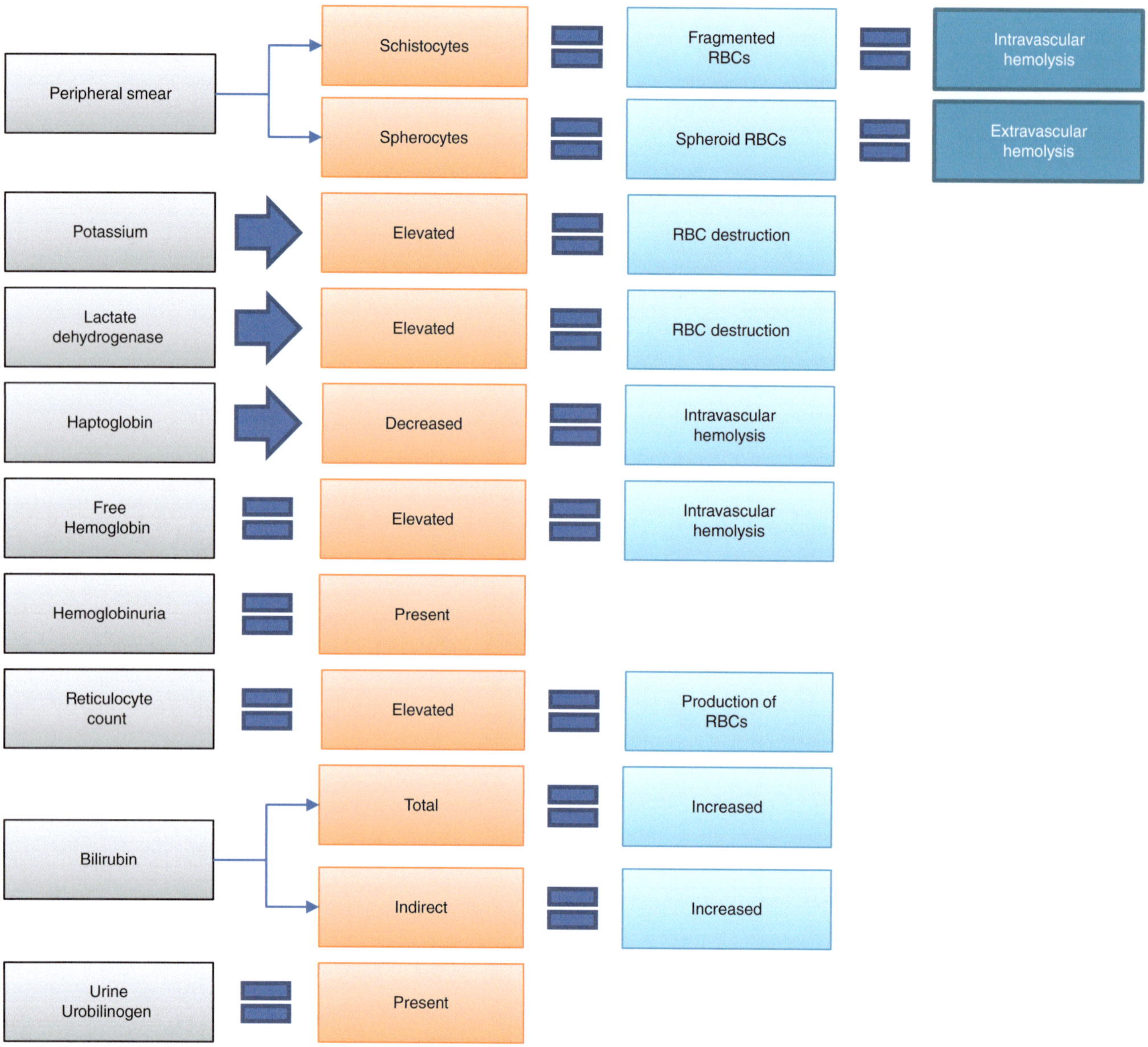

Microangiopathic Hemolytic Anemia (MAHA)

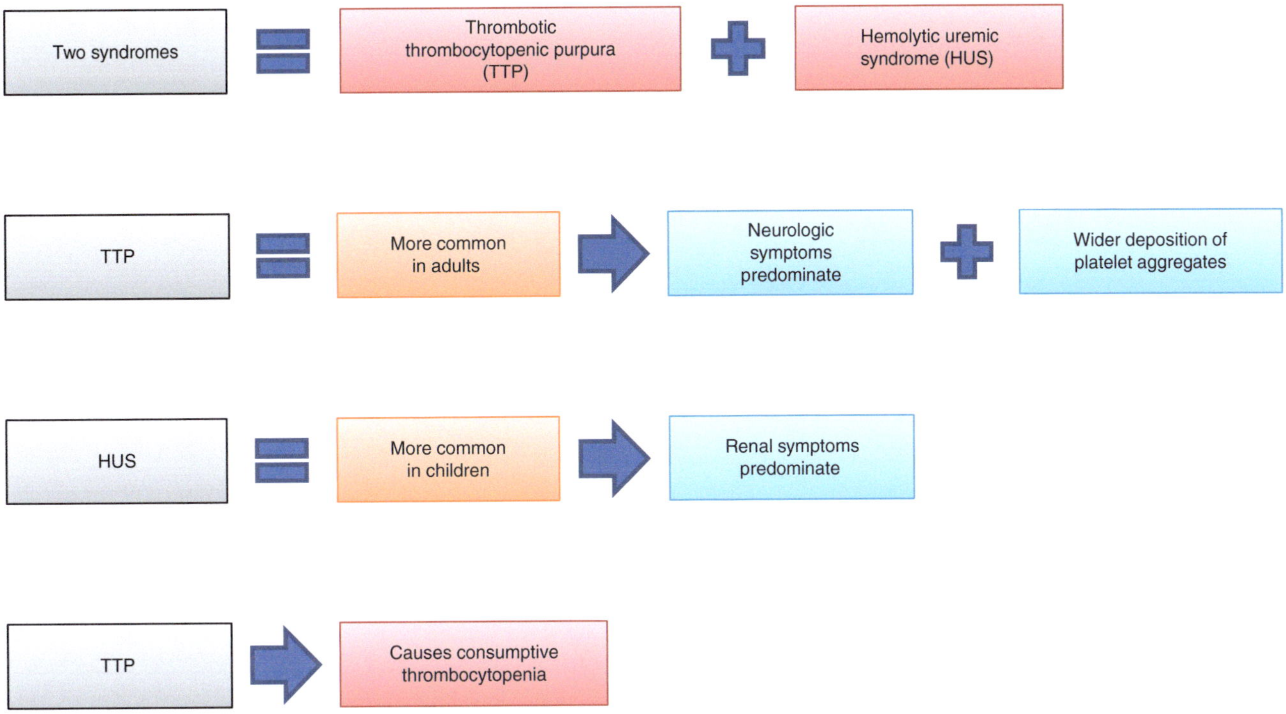

Thrombotic Thrombocytopenic Purpura (TTP)

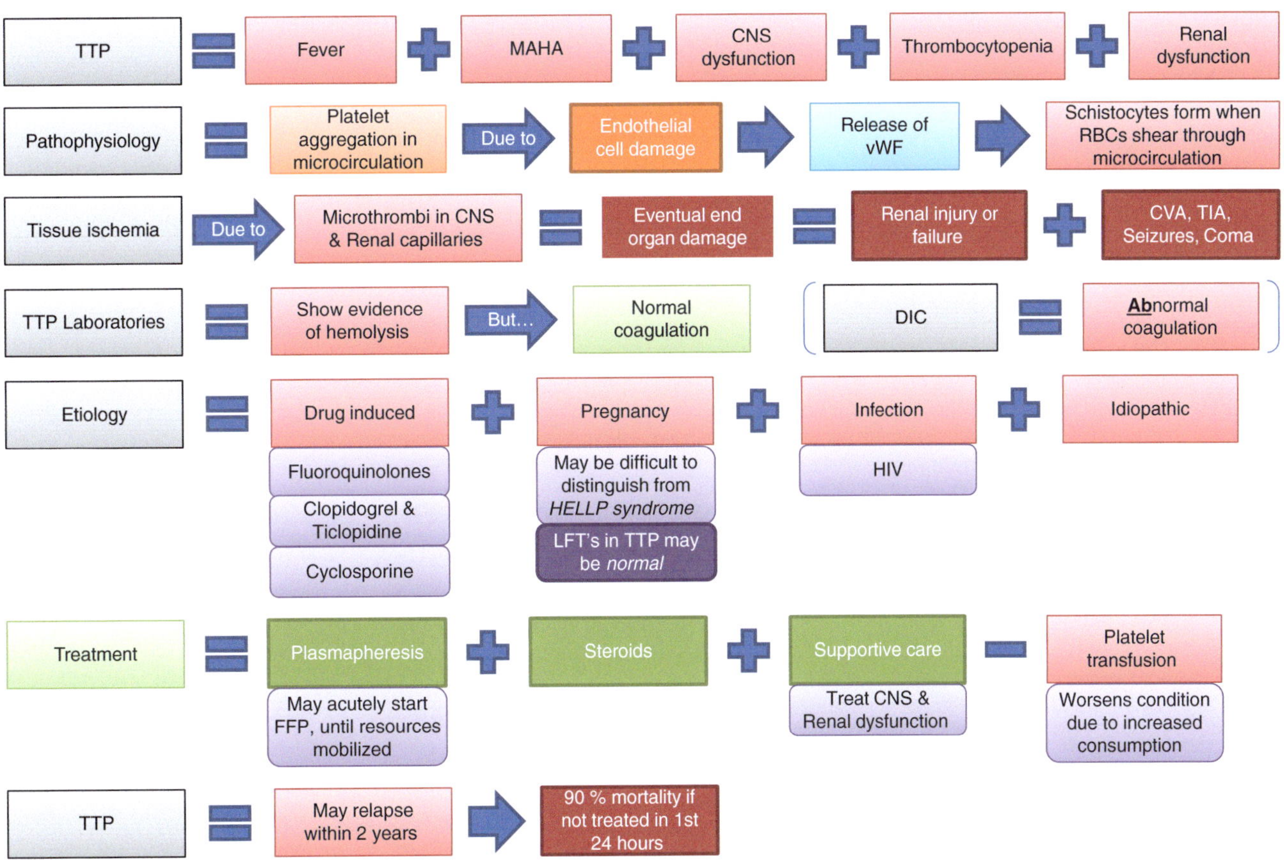

Hemolytic Uremic Syndrome (HUS)

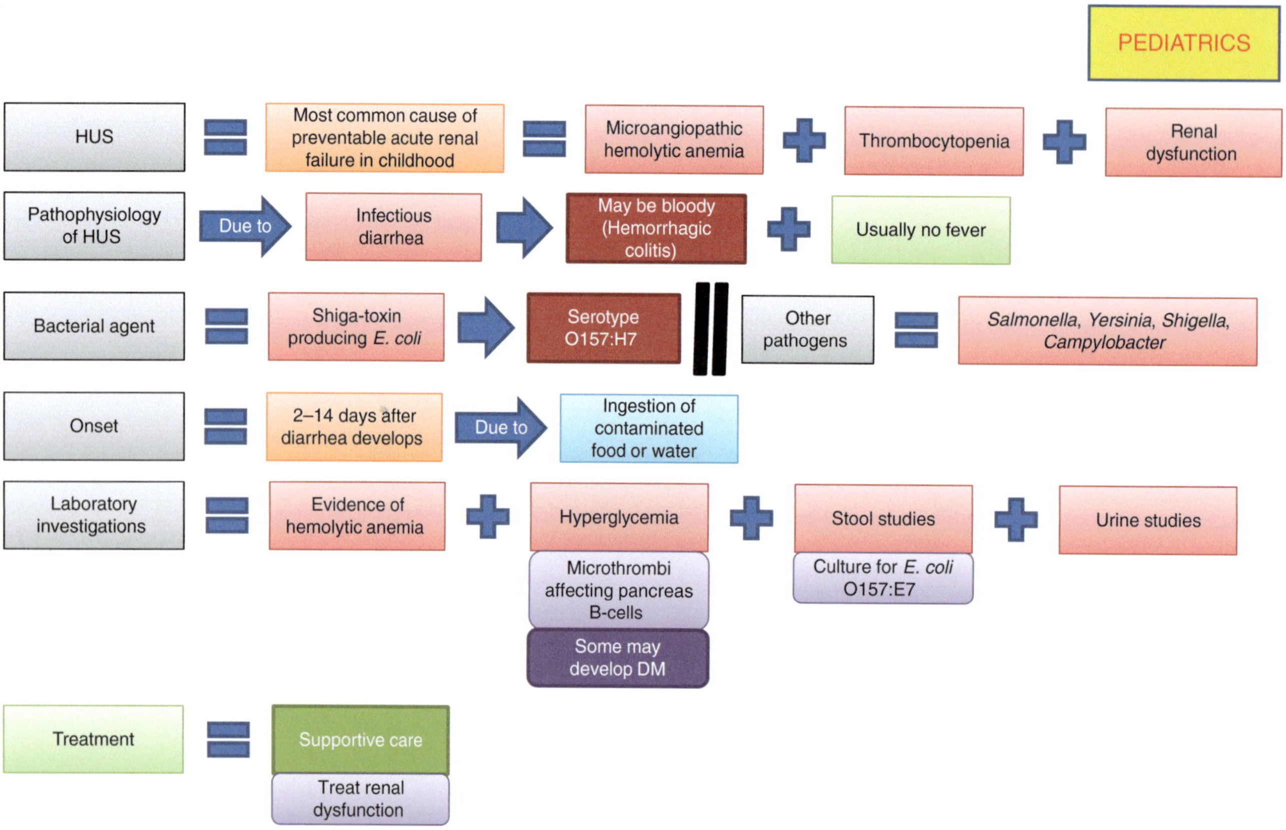

Platelet Disorders

Introduction

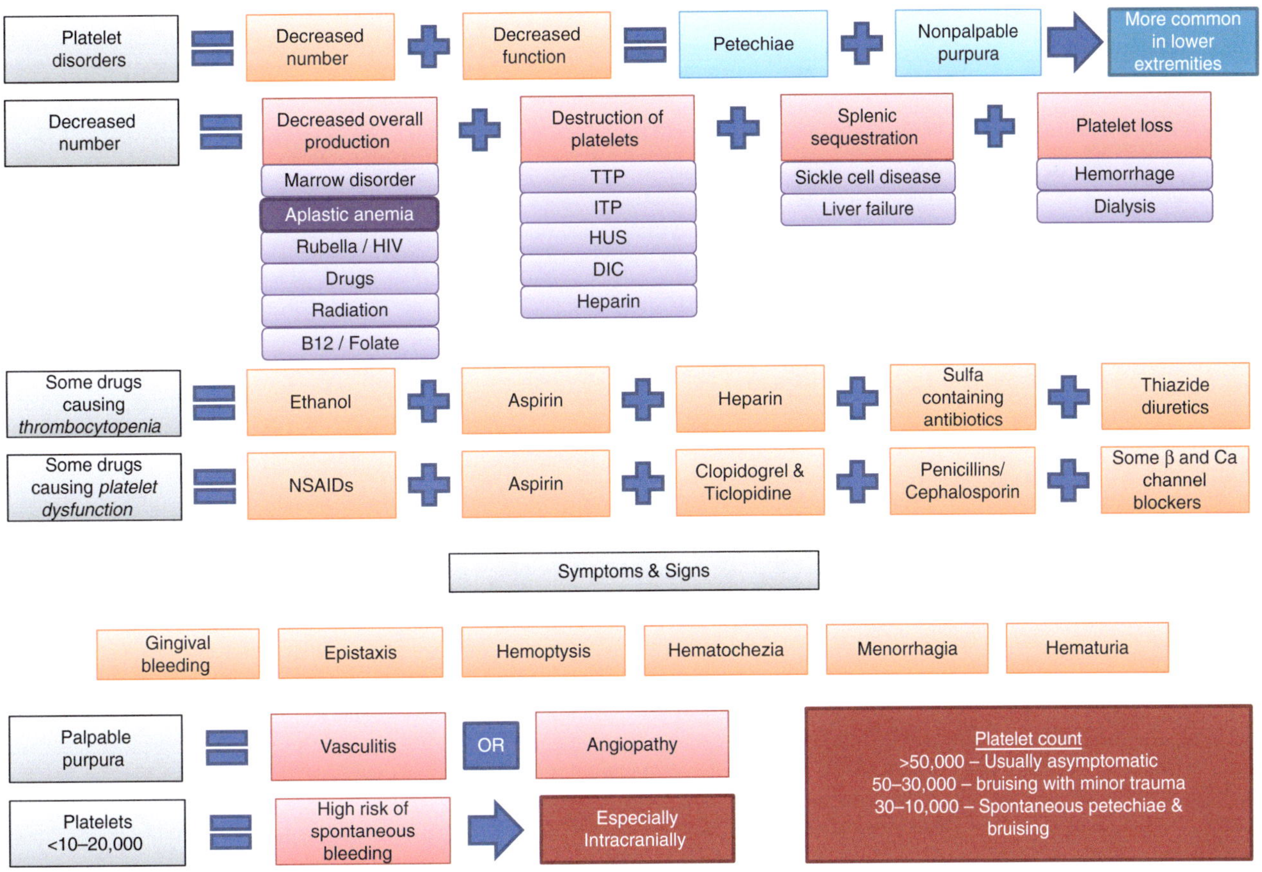

Idiopathic Thrombocytopenic Purpura (ITP)

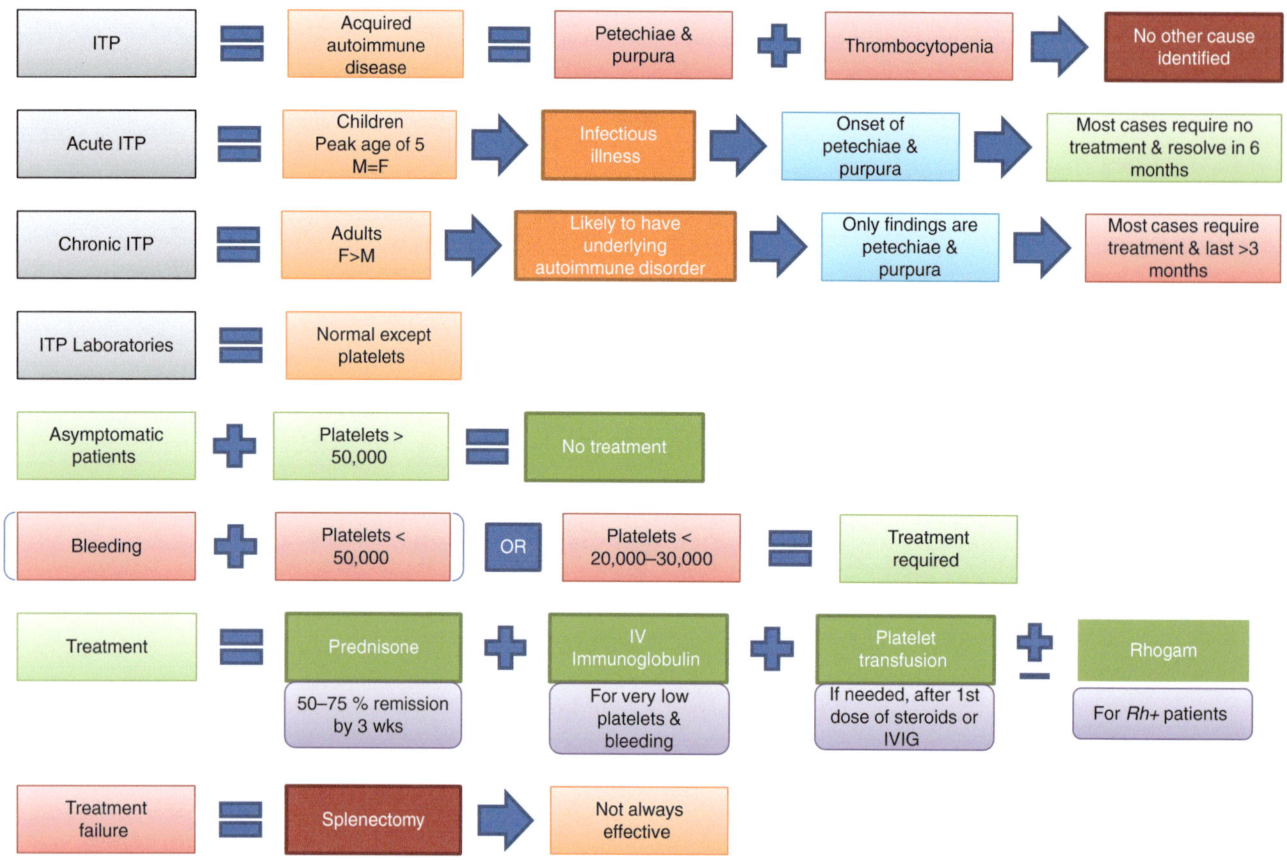

Etiologies of Disseminated Intravascular Coagulation (DIC)

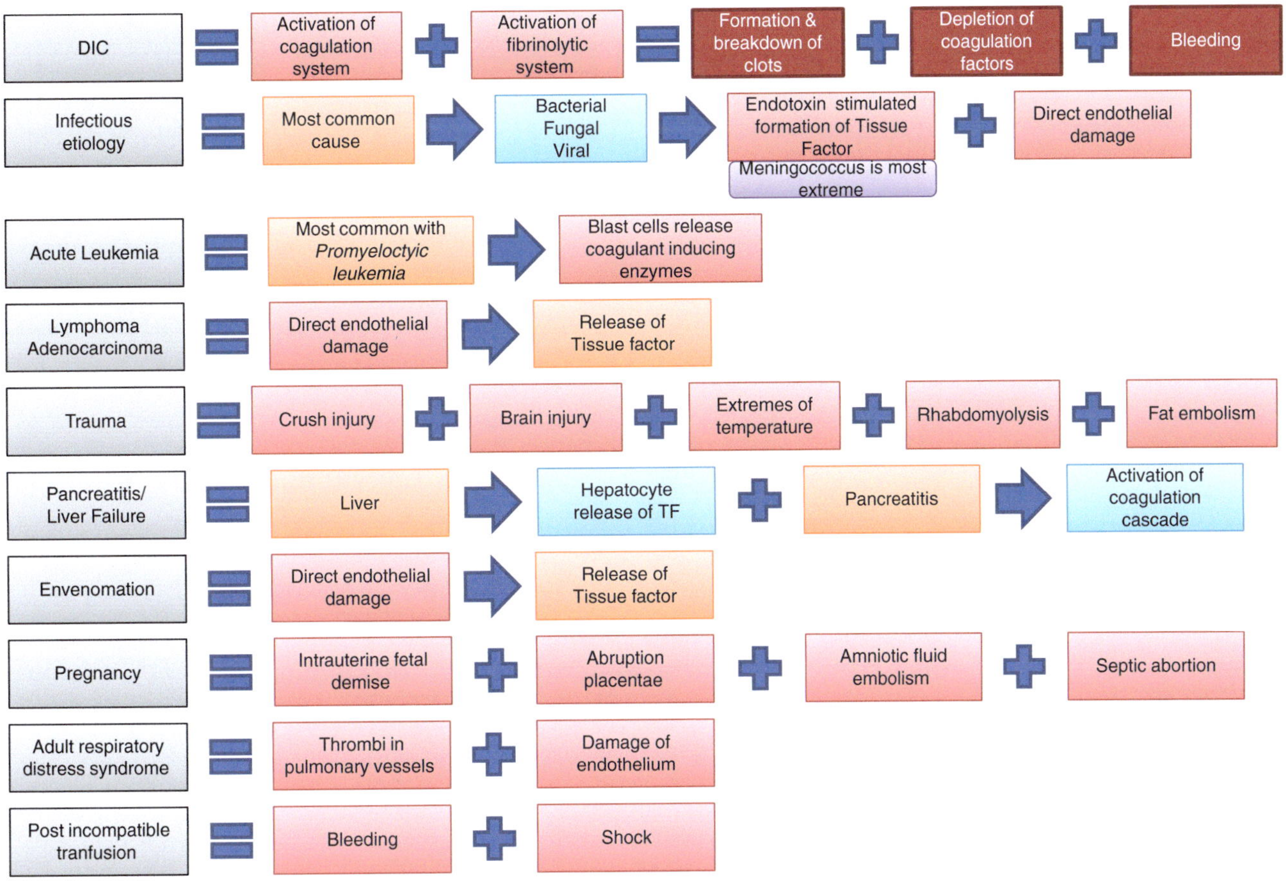

Disseminated Intravascular Coagulation (DIC)

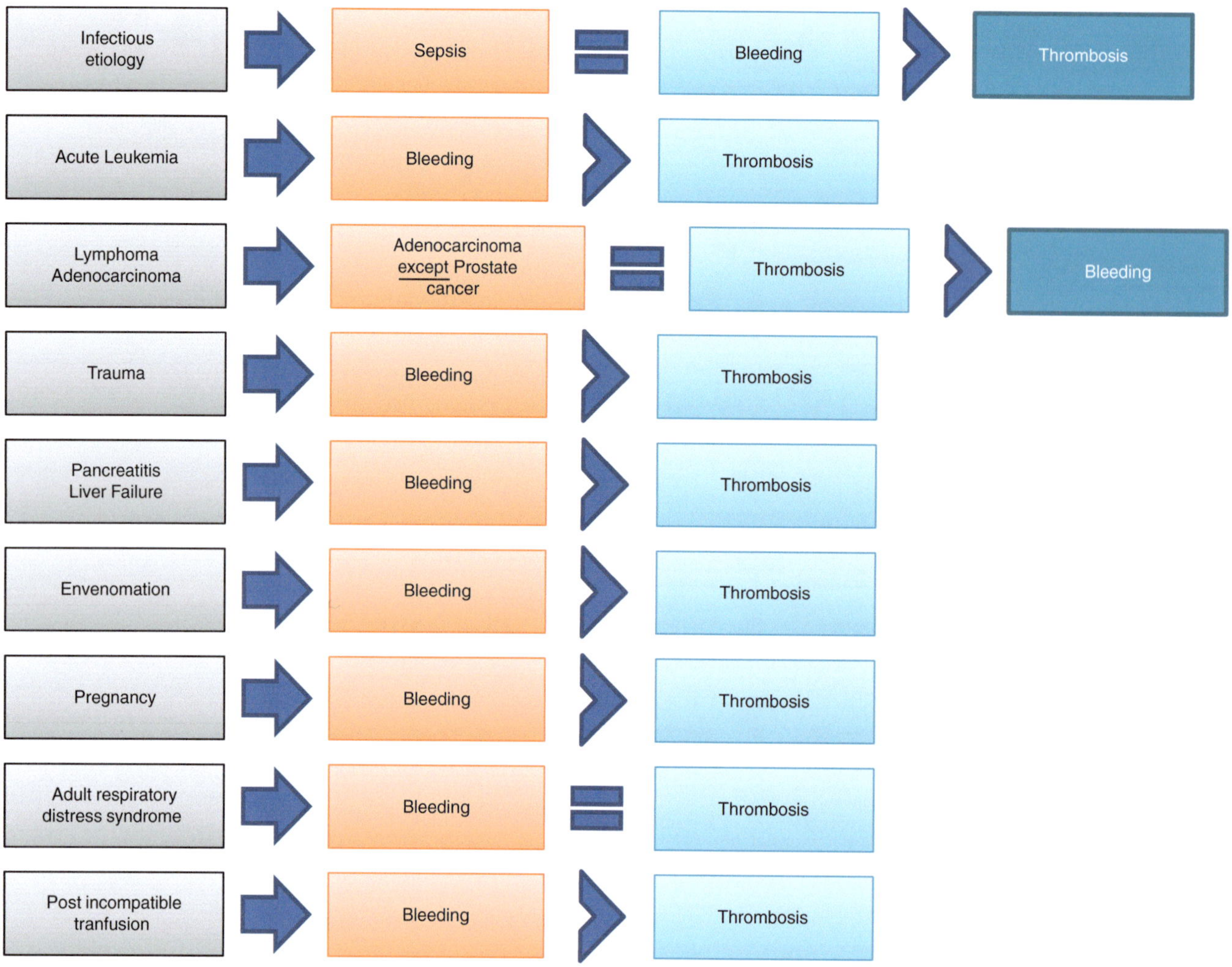

Clinical Features of DIC

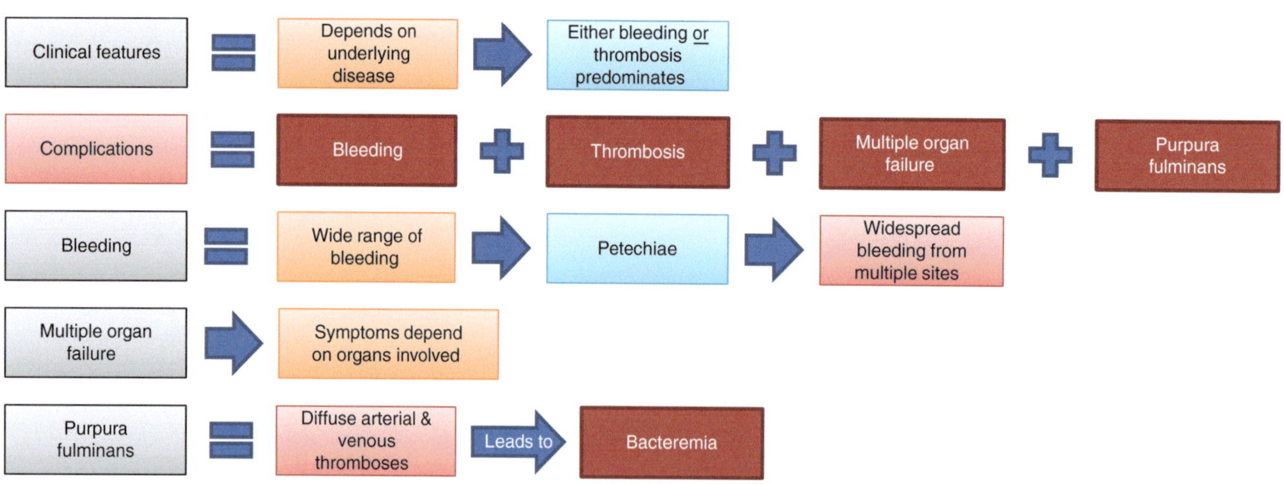

Laboratory Findings in DIC

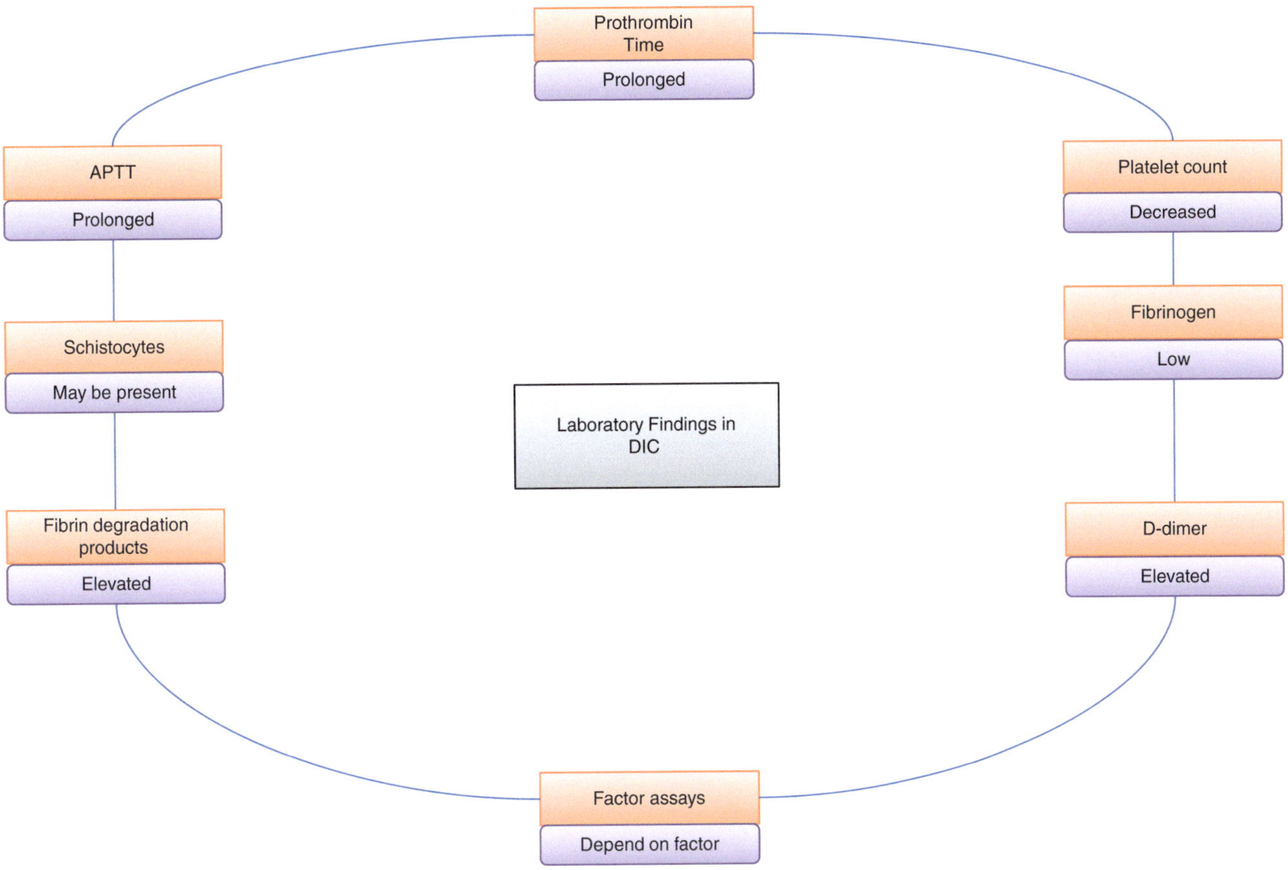

Treatment of DIC

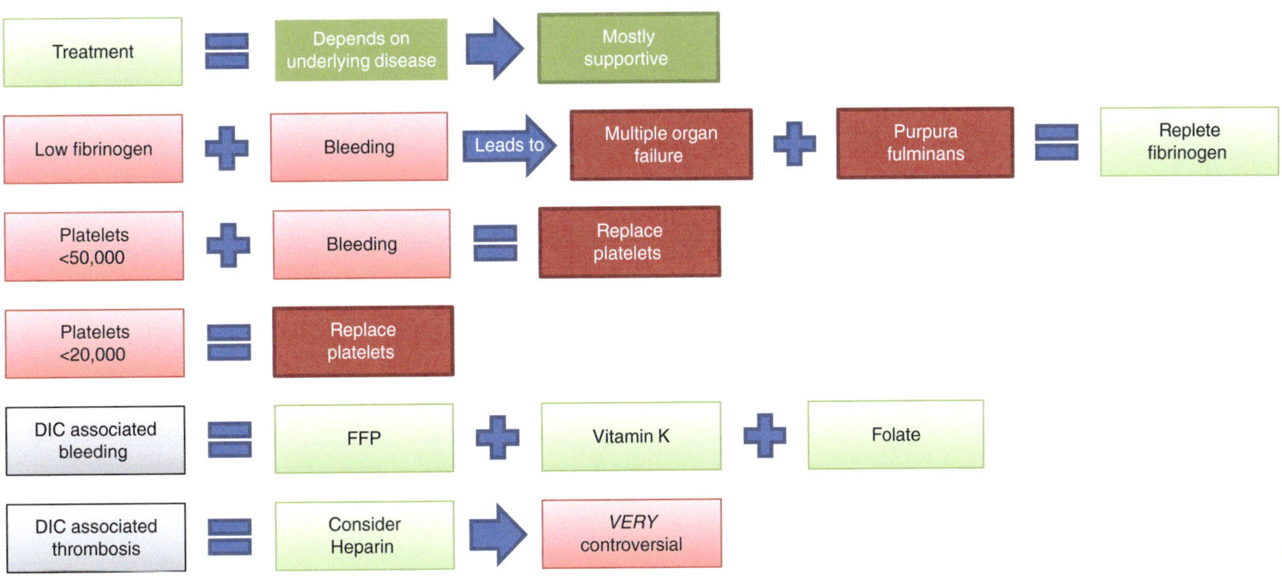

Hemophilia

Introduction

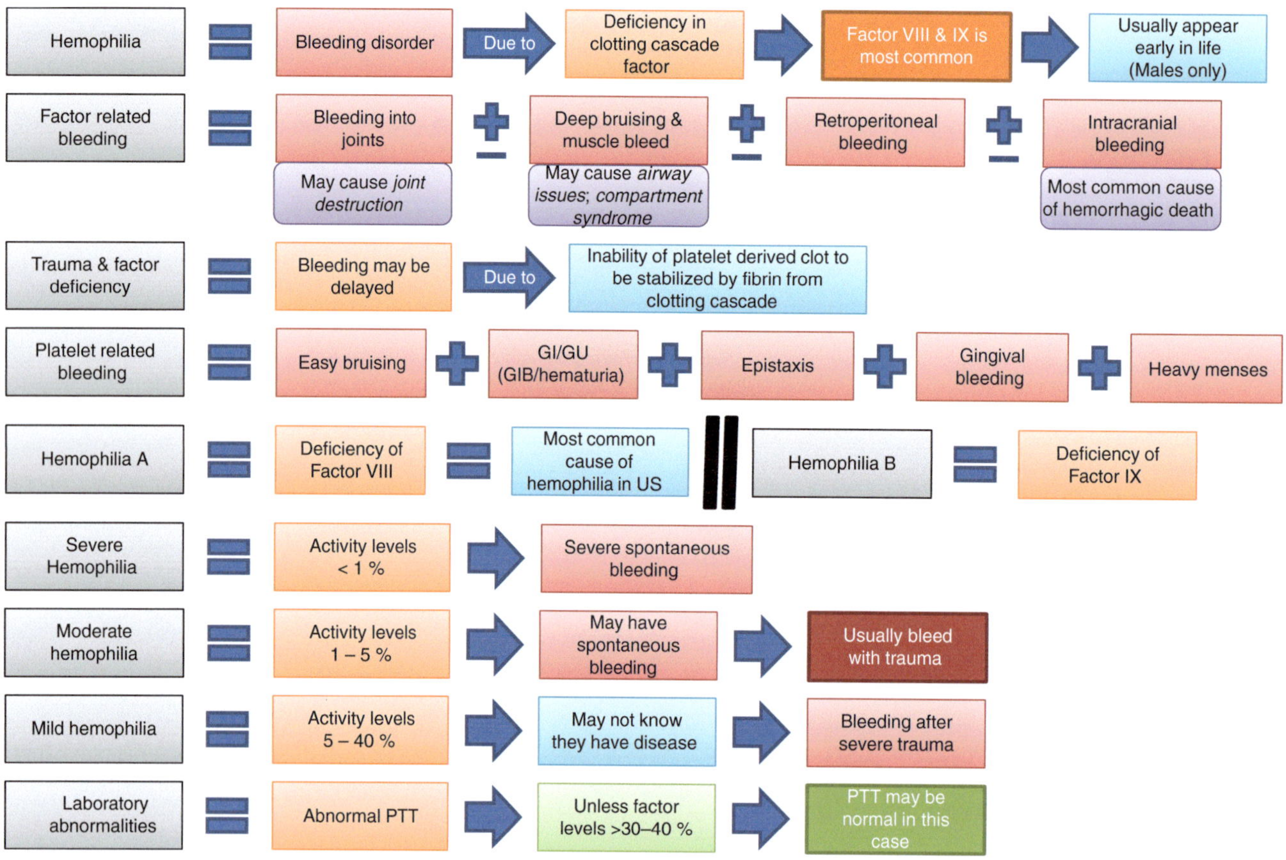

Treatment

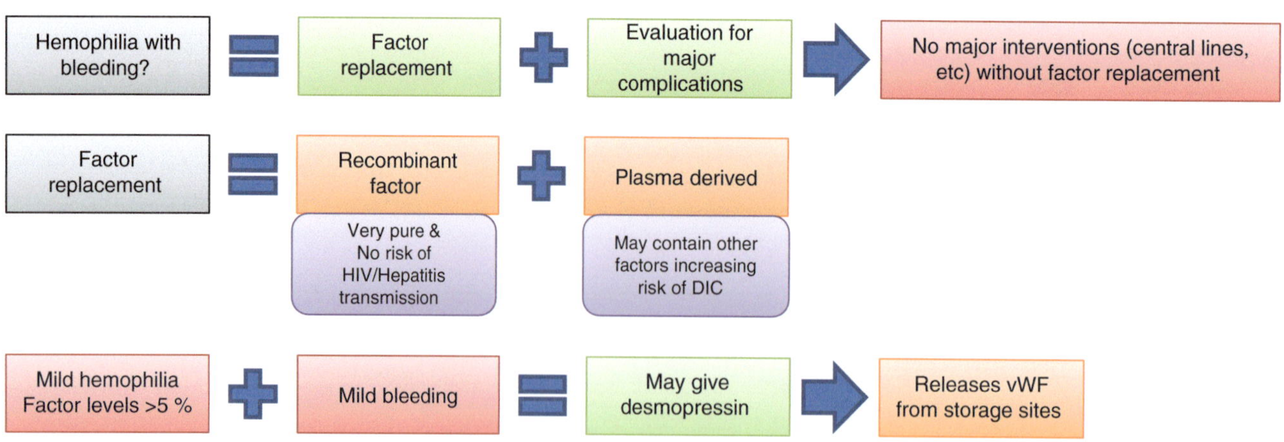

Von Willebrand's Disease

Introduction: VWD

- VWD = Most common congenital bleeding disorder → Due to → Deficiency in von Willebrand factor (VWF) → Made & stored in vascular endothelial cells
- Von Willebrand Factor = Cofactor for platelet adhesion + Carrier protein for factor VIII → Leads to platelet activation & adhesion to other platelets
- Clinical features = Easy bruising + GI/GU (GIB/hematuria) + Epistaxis + Gingival bleeding + Heavy menses
- Clinical features = NO Hemarthosis → Unless severe disease
- Diagnosis = Bleeding time (Prolonged) + PTT (Prolonged depending on severity) + vWF activity (Decreased)
- Treatment for Mild disease = Desmopressin
- Treatment for Moderate to severe disease = Cryoprecipitate OR Factor VIII products that have vWF

Anticoagulants

Introduction: Warfarin

- Warfarin = Blocks action of vitamin K → Disrupts synthesis of Vitamin K dependent factors = II, VII, IX, X (Also Proteins C&S) = Extrinsic pathway blocked (Has mild thrombotic effect through Protein C&S blockade)
- Warfarin dosing = Guided by INR → Therapeutic range usually from 2–3 → But… → Over anti-coagulation will raise PTT as well due to effect on common final pathway of coagulation
- Warfarin = Multiple interfering factors = Drugs or Medications + Albumin binding + Change in hepatic metabolism
- Warfarin = NOT in Pregnancy → Teratogenic
- Major Warfarin complications = Bleeding + Skin necrosis

Bleeding from Warfarin

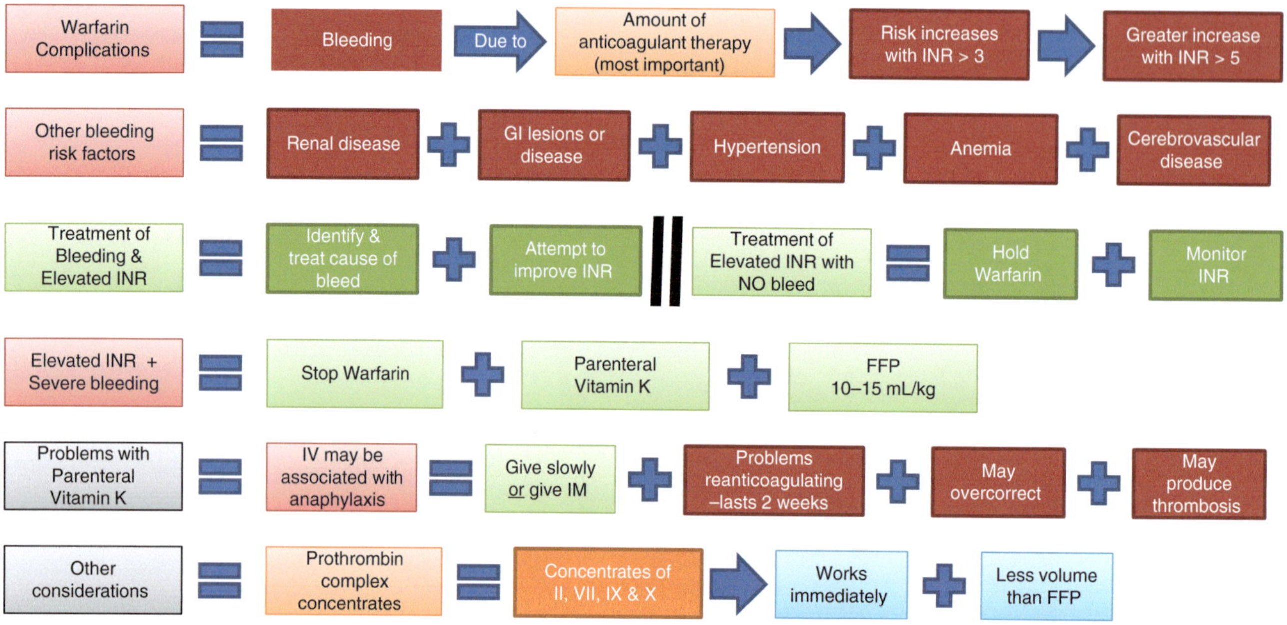

Skin Necrosis from Warfarin

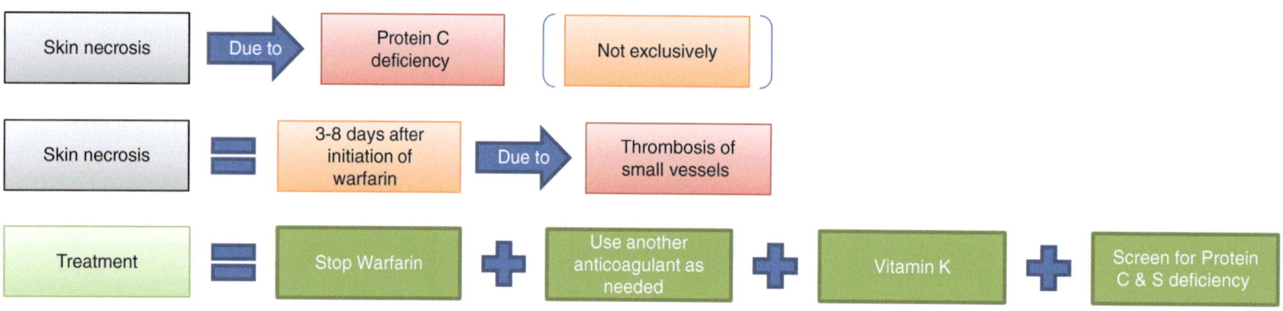

Introduction: Heparin

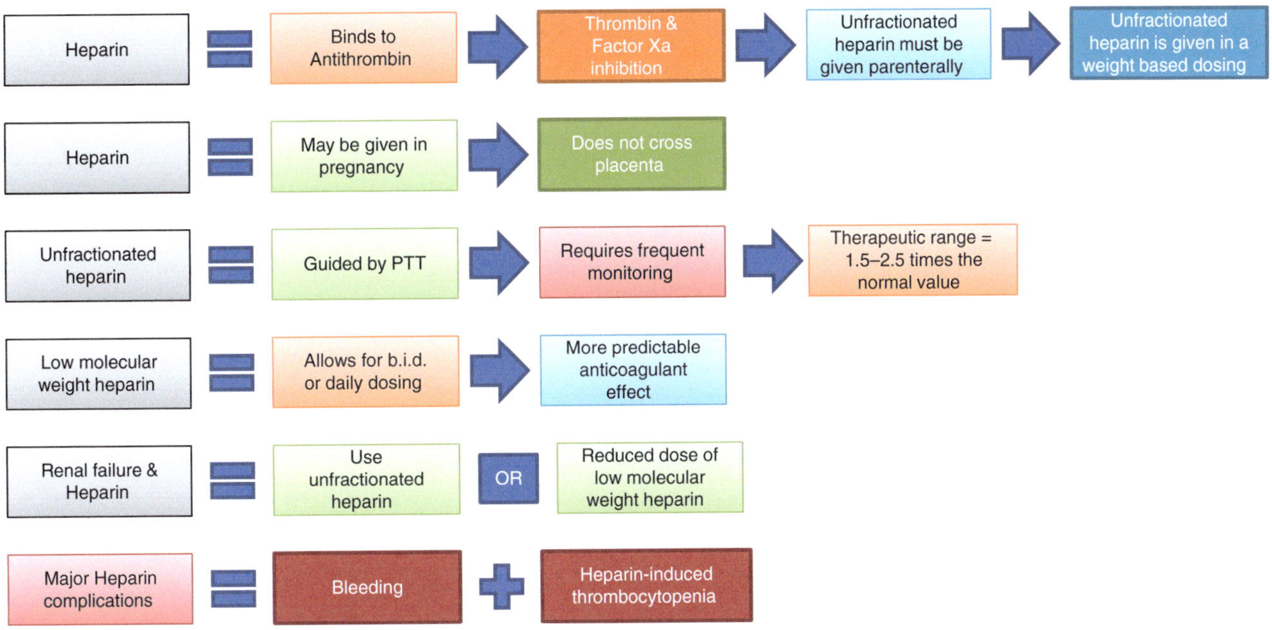

Bleeding from Heparin

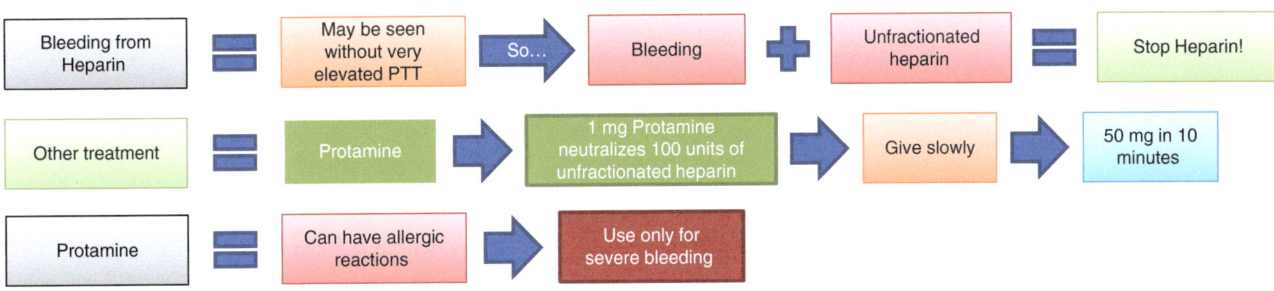

Heparin-Induced Thrombocytopenia (HIT)

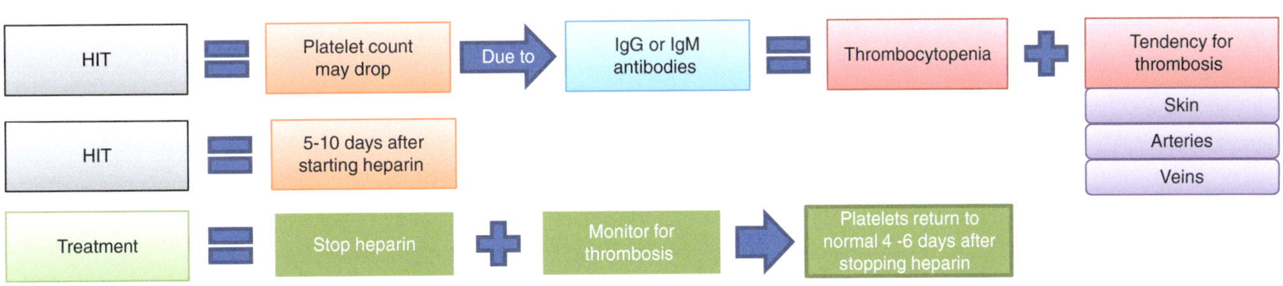

Absolute and Relative Contraindications to Thrombolysis

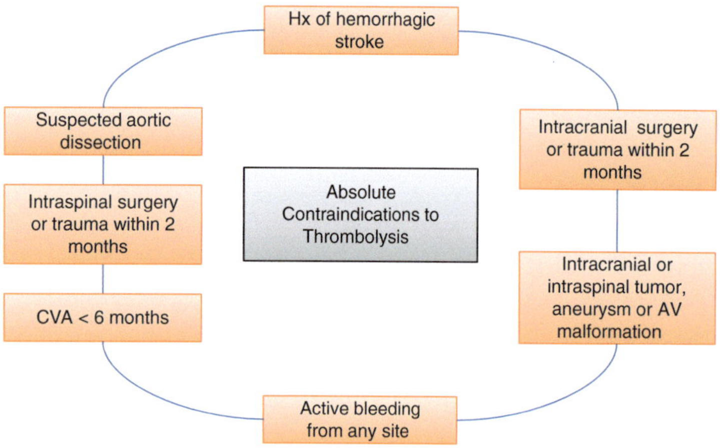

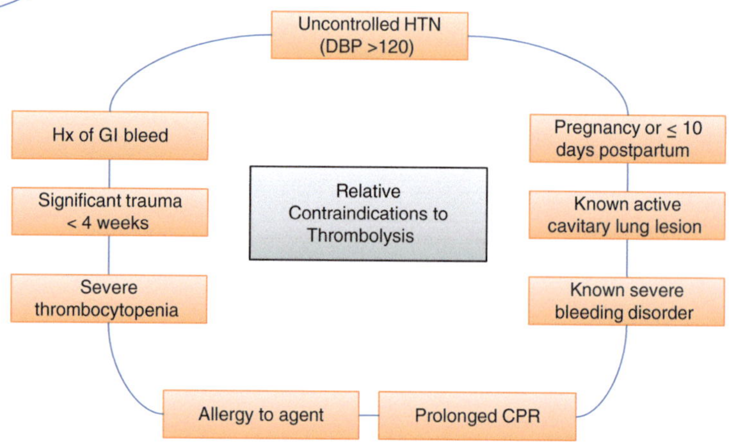

Complications of Malignancy

Introduction

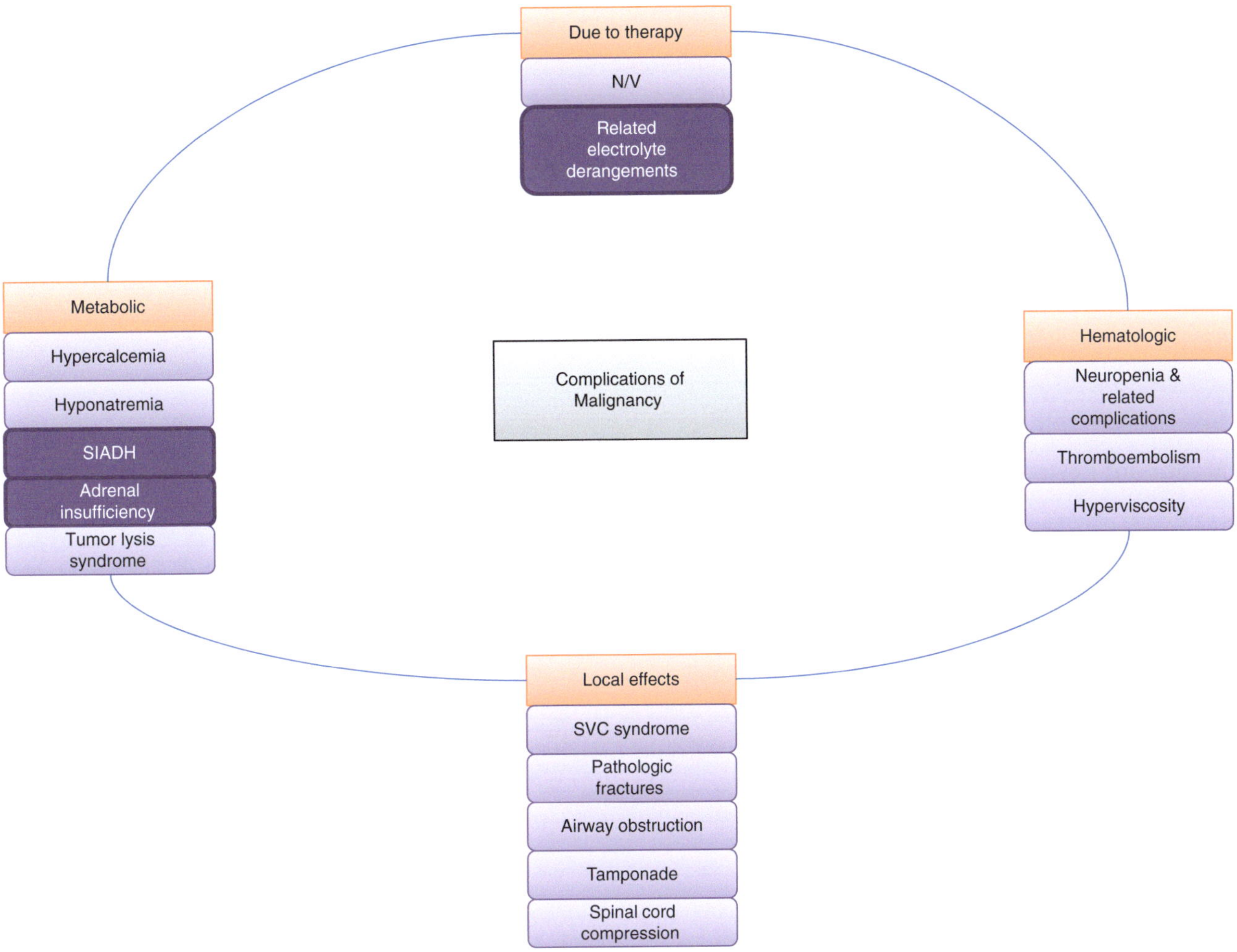

Malignant Airway Obstruction

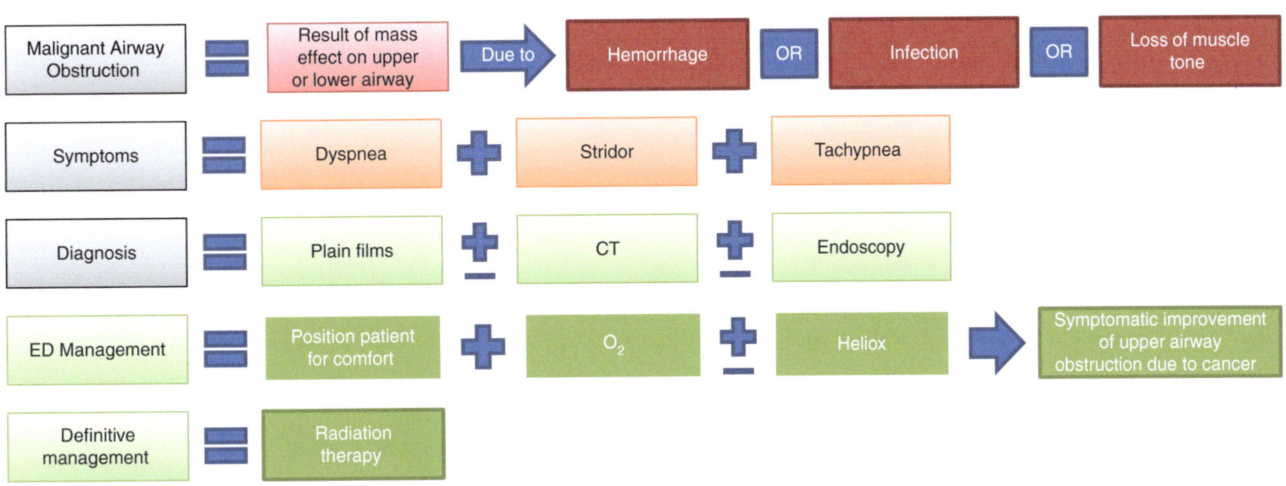

Pathologic Fractures from Bone Metastases

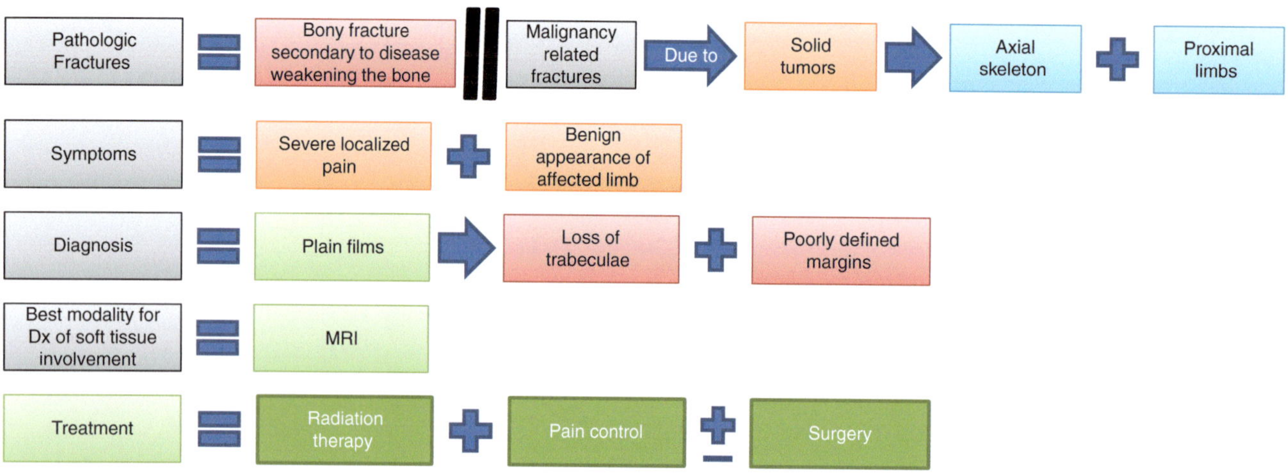

Malignant Pericardial Effusion and Tamponade

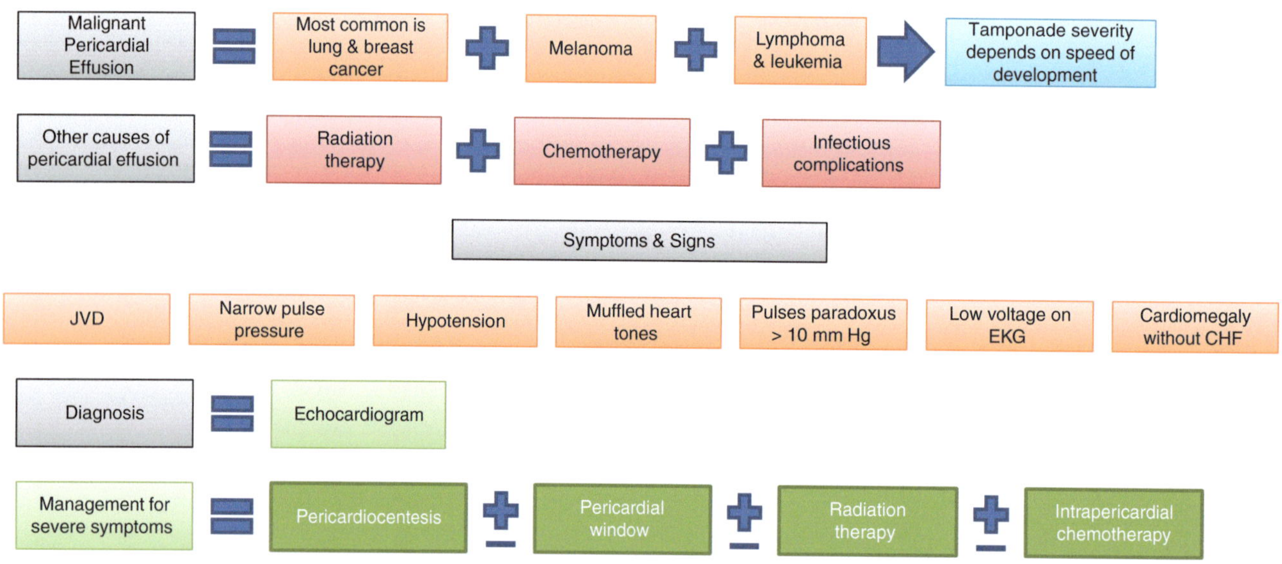

Malignant Spinal Cord Compression

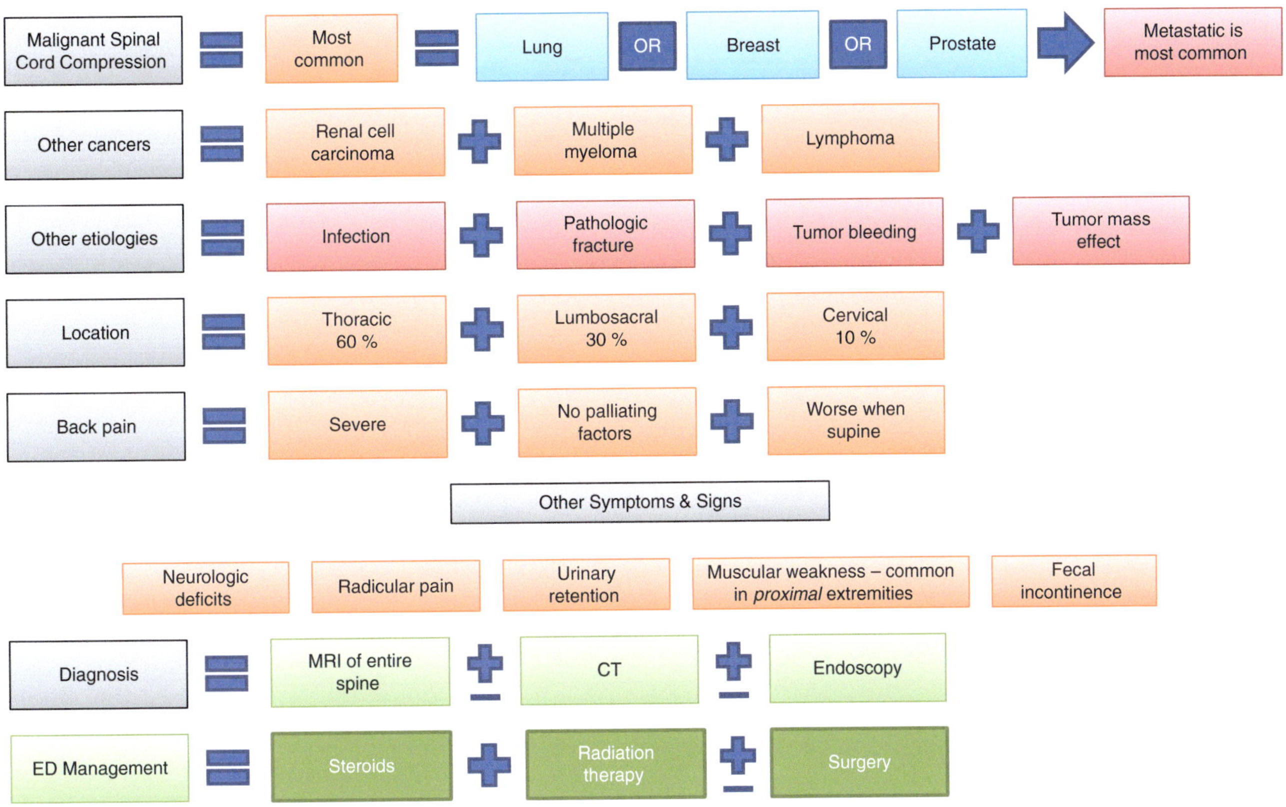

Superior Vena Cava Syndrome

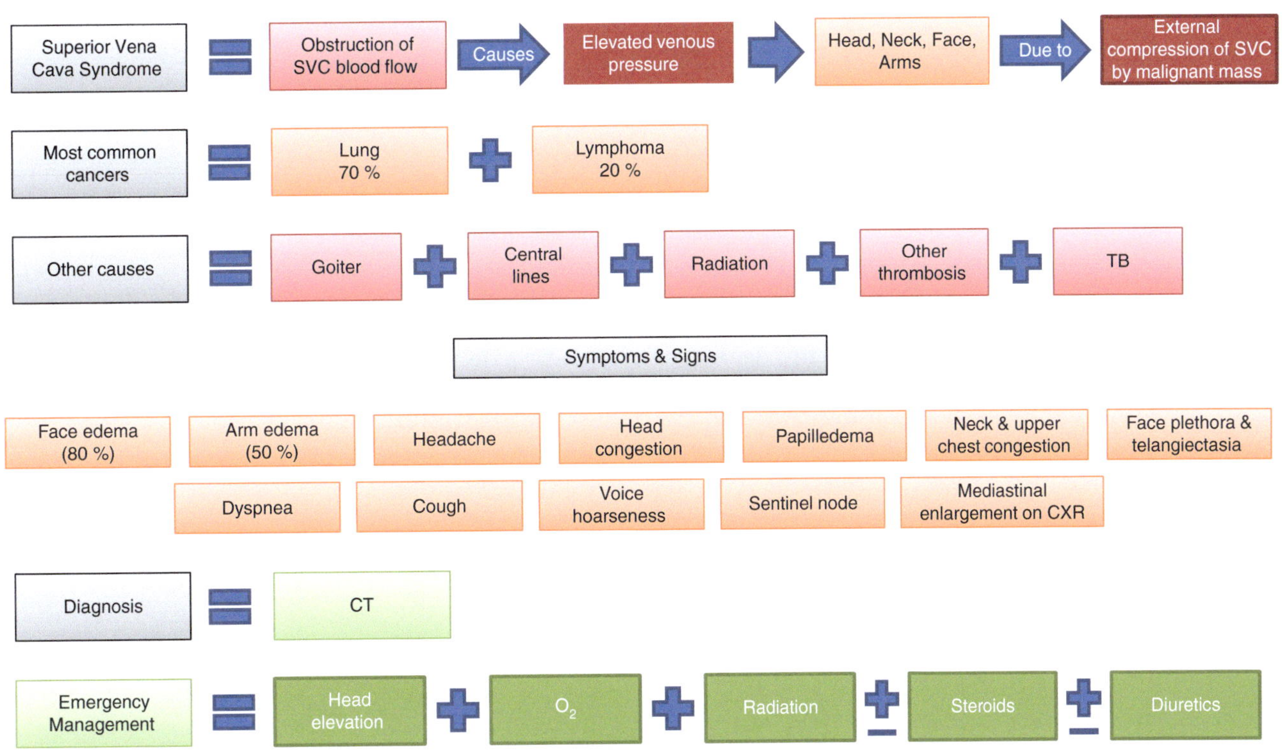

Hypercalcemia Due to Malignancy

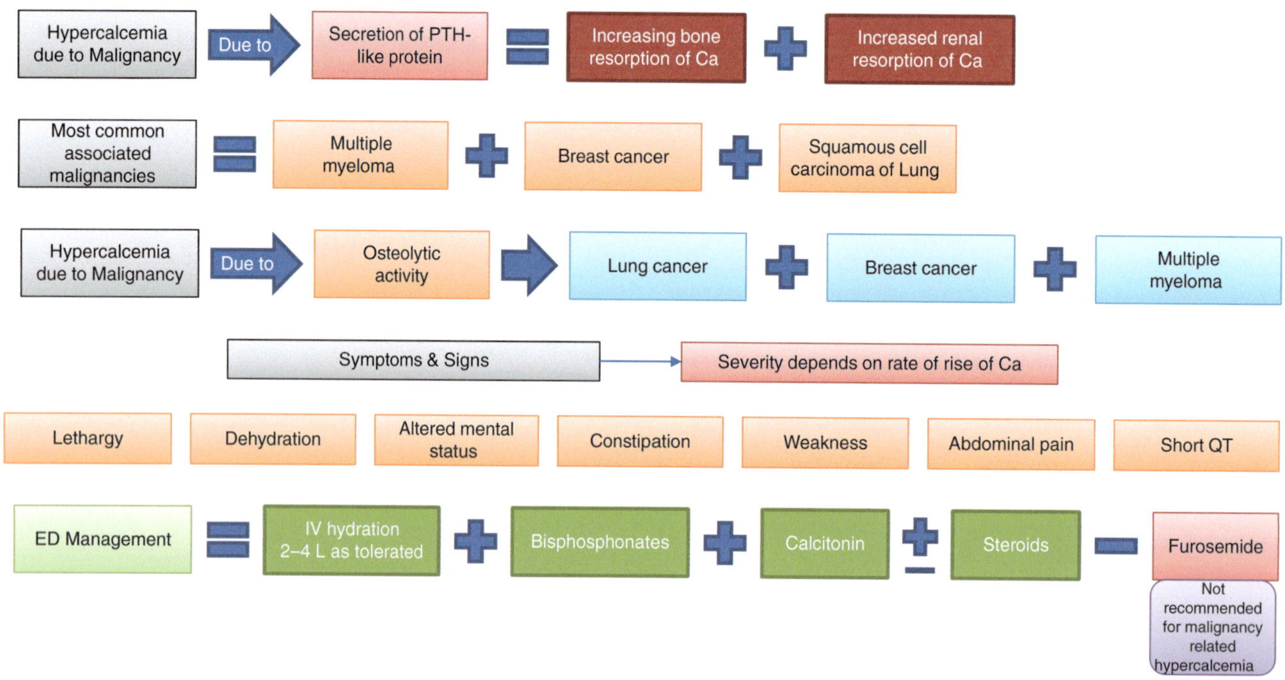

SIADH Due to Malignancy

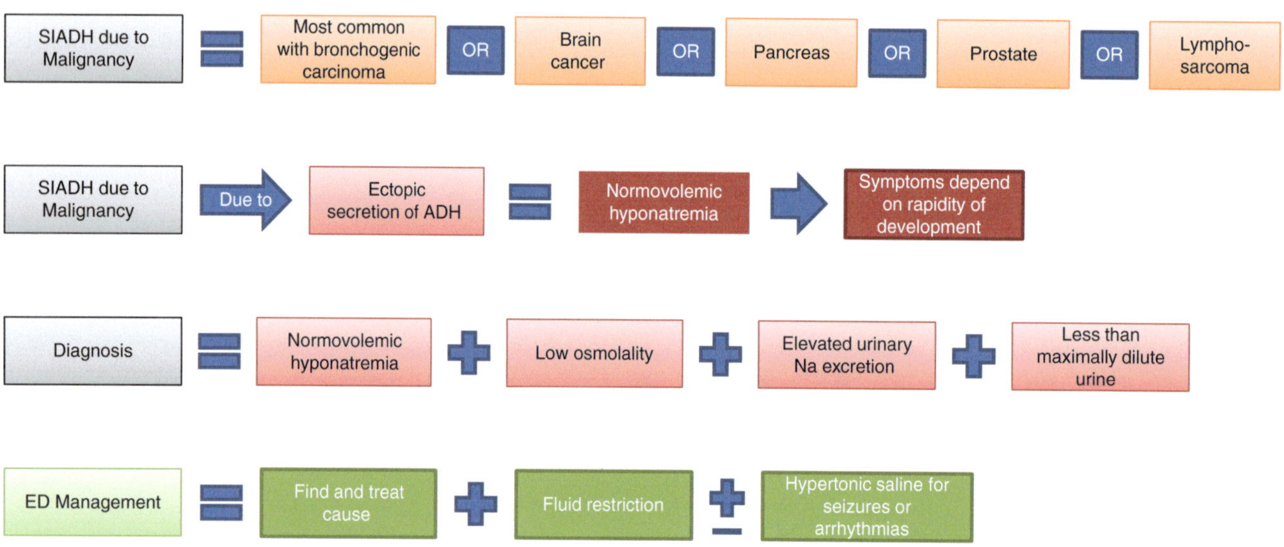

Adrenal Insufficiency Due to Malignancy

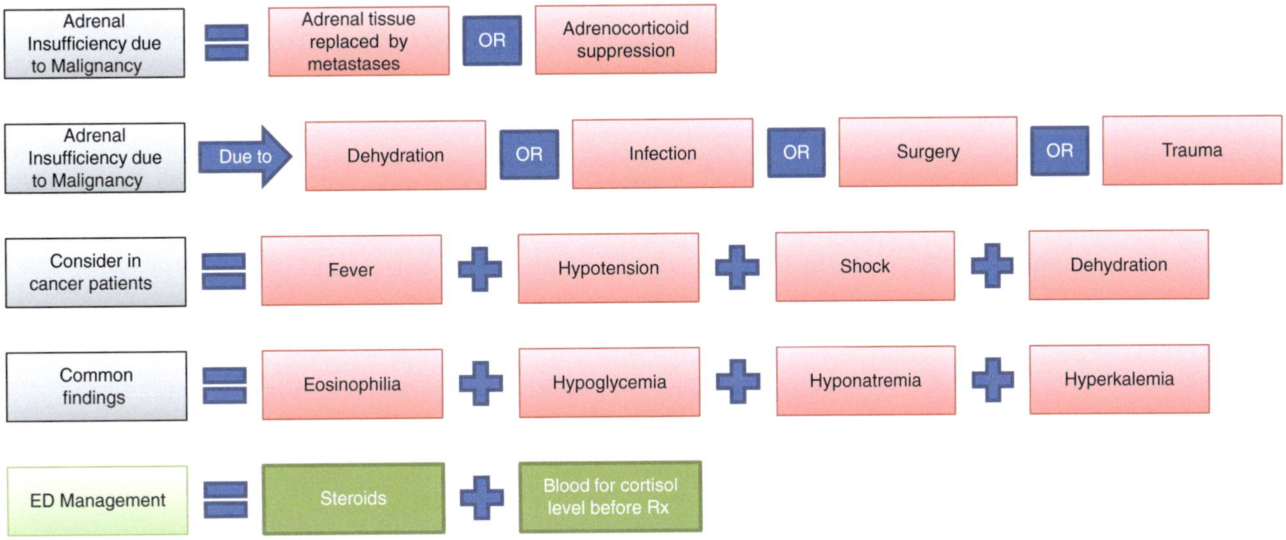

Tumor Lysis Syndrome

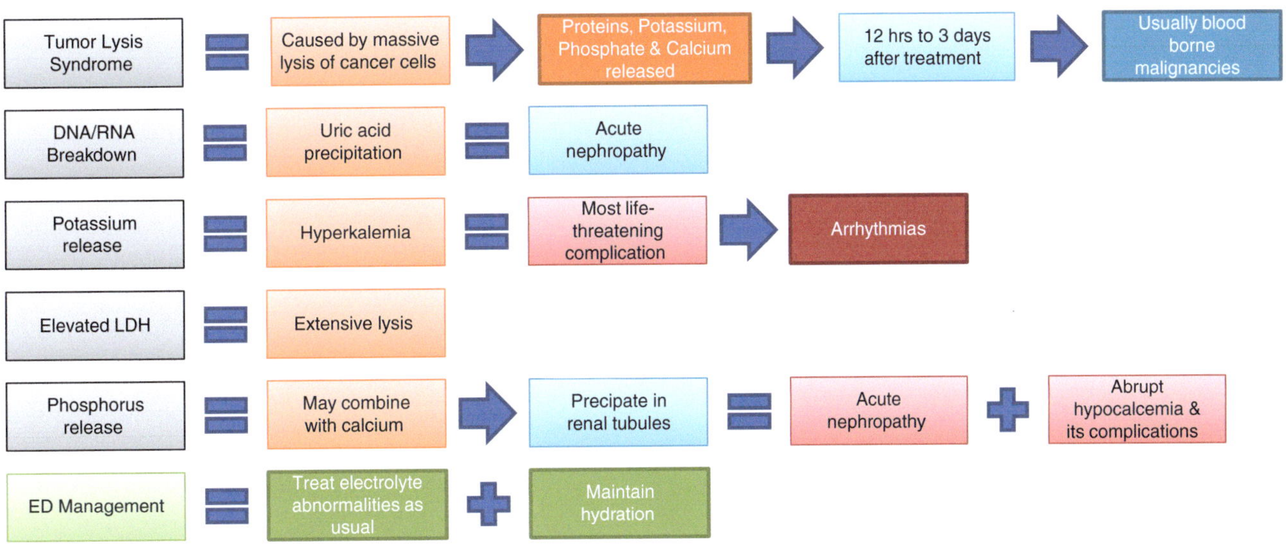

Febrile Neutropenia

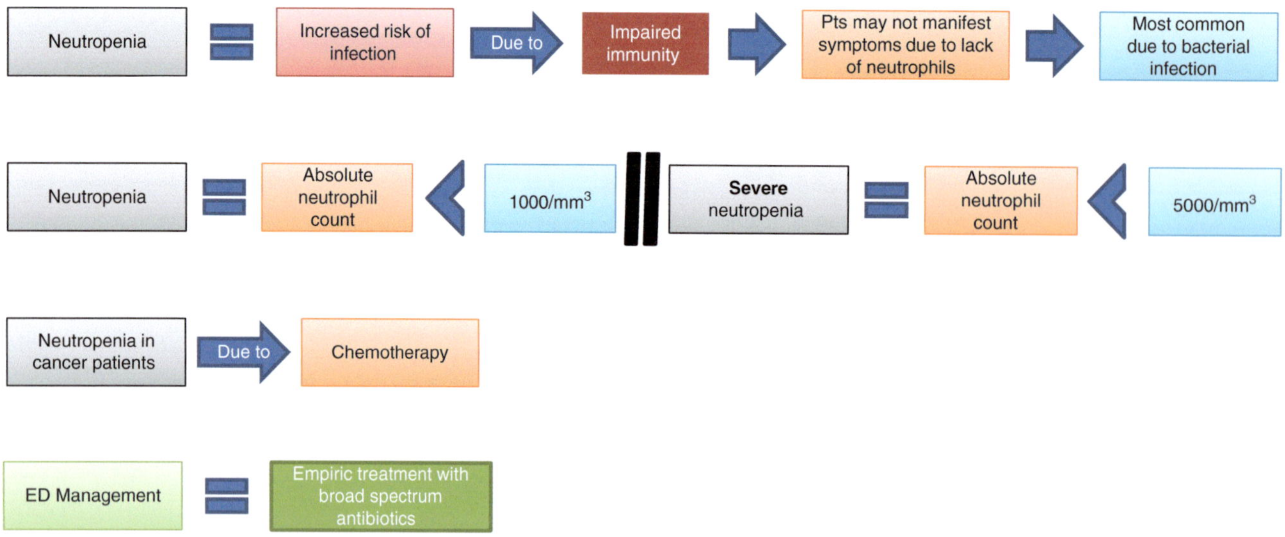

Hyperviscosity Syndrome Due to Malignancy

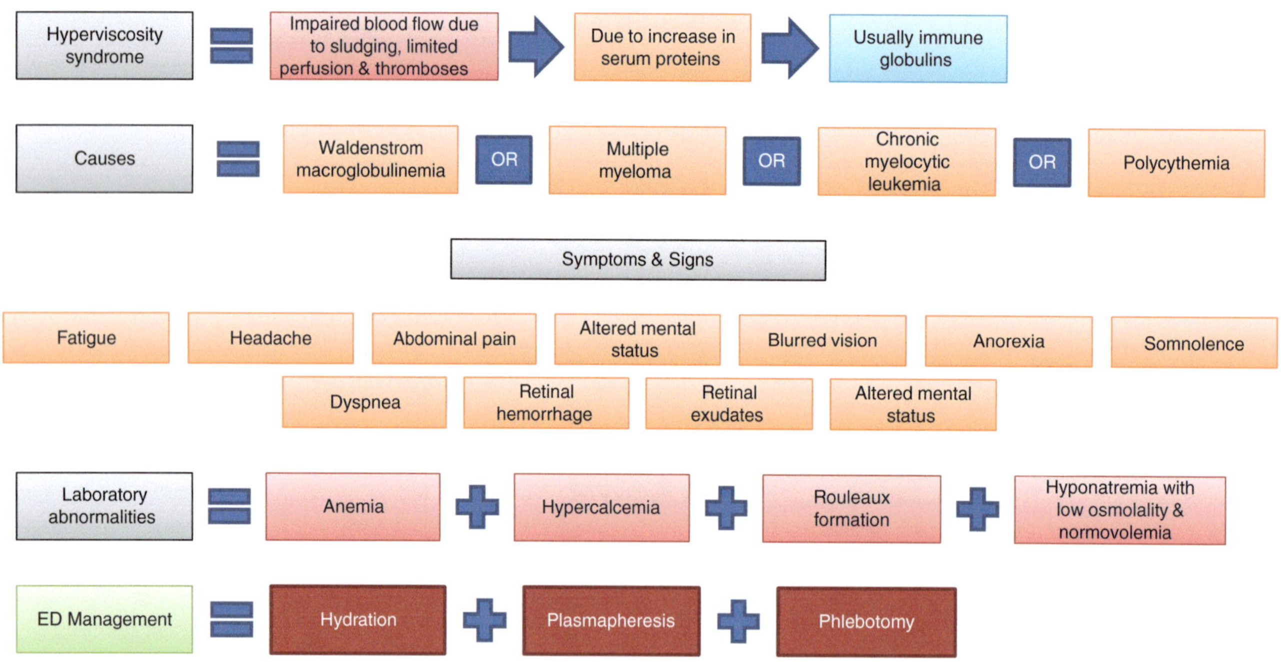

Disorders Affecting the Skin

Bobby Desai

Contents

Generalized Skin Rashes and Disorders 350
Allergic Processes 363
Skin Cancers 365
Infectious Diseases and Associated Skin Lesions 366
Viral Infections 372
Malaria 376
Pediatric Rashes 376
Miscellaneous Skin-Related Disorders 385

B. Desai, MD, MEd
Department of Emergency Medicine, University of Florida,
Gainesville, FL, USA
e-mail: bdesai@ufl.edu

B. Desai, B.R. Allen (eds.), *Nailing the Written Emergency Medicine Board Examination*,
DOI 10.1007/978-3-319-30838-8_6

Generalized Skin Rashes and Disorders

Erythema Multiforme

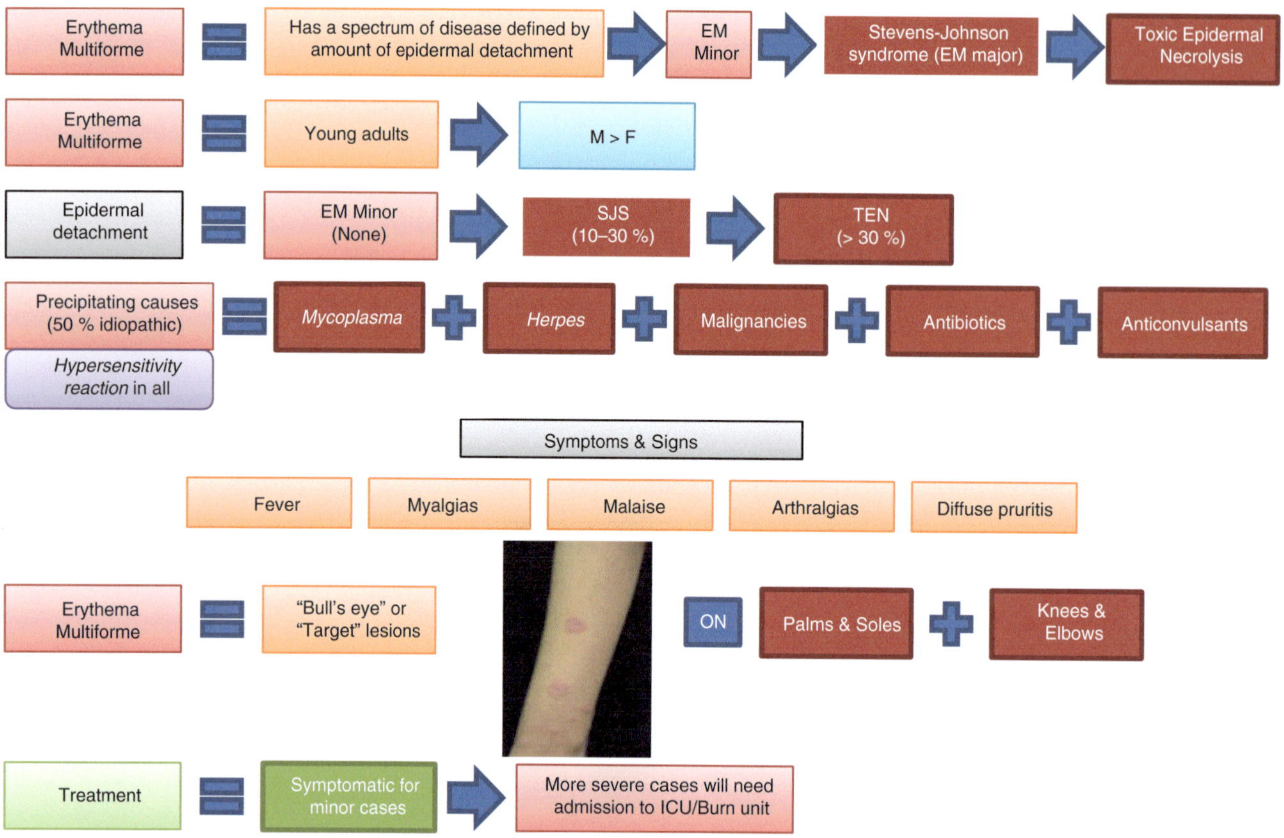

Bottom center image (Reprinted from Zaidi Z, Lanigan SW. Vasculitis, common erythemas, and lymphatic disorders. In: Zaidi Z, Lanigan SW, editors. Dermatology in clinical practice. London: Springer; 2010. p. 253–70. With permission from Springer Verlag)

Stevens-Johnson Syndrome (SJS) and Toxic Epidermal Necrolysis (TEN)

SJS = Severe bullous form of EM → Affects 10–30 % of body surface area + Has mucosal involvement → May be fatal

TEN = Affects > 30 % of body surface area

Precipitating causes (50 % idiopathic) = *Mycoplasma* + *Herpes* + Malignancies + Antibiotics + Anticonvulsants

Hypersensitivity reaction in all

Common medication precipitants = Sulfonamides PCN Tetracyclines + Thiazides + Barbiturates + Phenytoin

Symptoms & Signs

SJS { Bullous cutaneous lesions, Stomatitis, Conjunctivitis, Mucositis }

TEN { Hypotension, Shock, Tachycardia, Very large bullae, Severe mucositis }

Nikolsky's sign: Skin peels off with light pressure

Increased mortality = Older age + Dehydration + Secondary infection

Primary causes of death = Sepsis + Pneumonia

Disposition = ICU Admission

PEDIATRICS

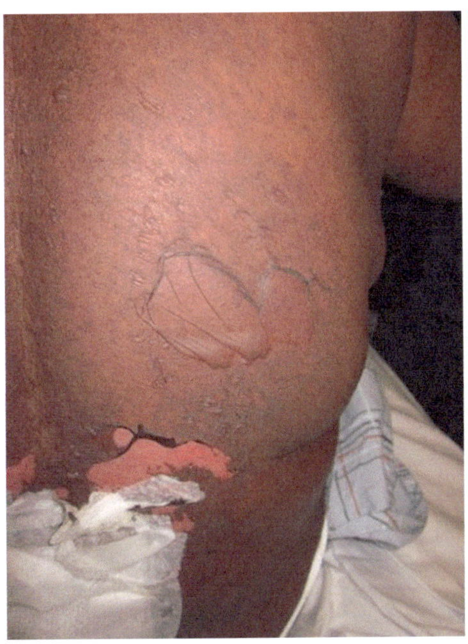

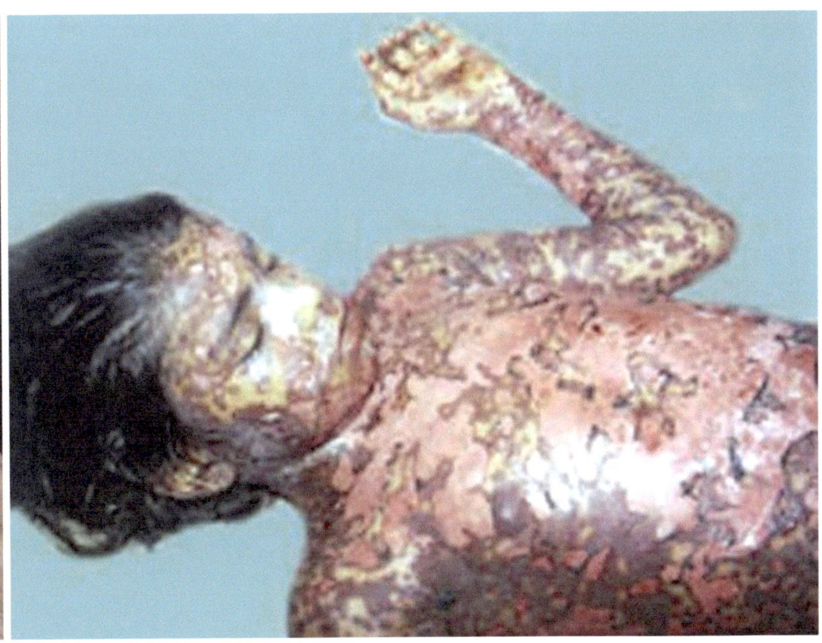

Right side image (Reprinted from Zaidi Z, Lanigan SW. Exanthems and Hypersensitivity Syndromes. In: Zaidi Z, Lanigan SW, editors. Dermatology in clinical practice. London: Springer; 2010. p. 271–80. With permission from Springer Verlag)

Staphylococcal Scalded Skin Syndrome (SSSS)

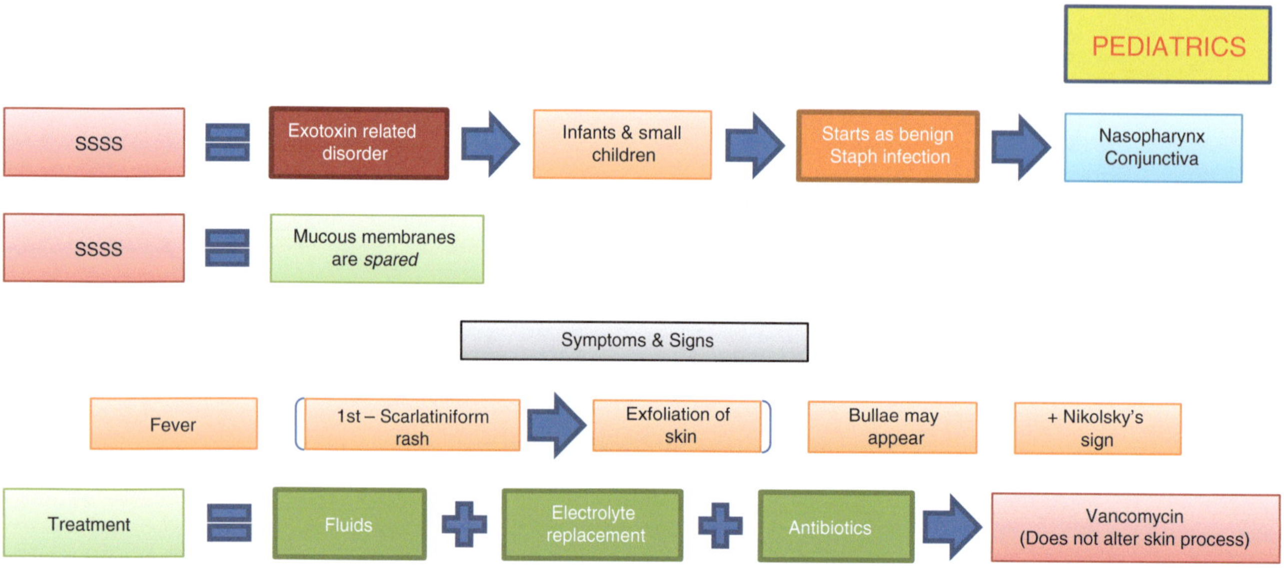

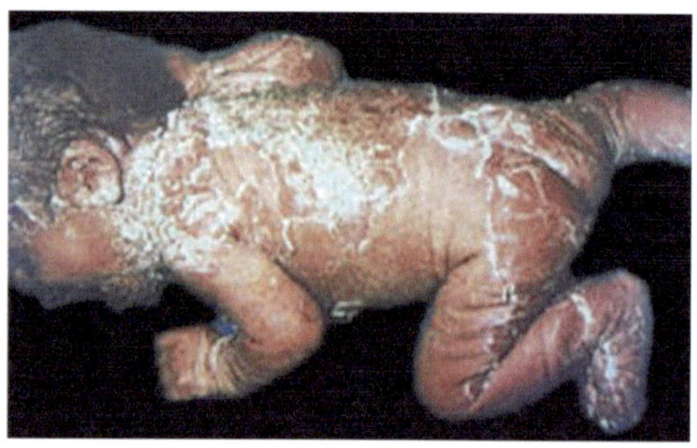

Bottom center image (Reprinted from Zaidi Z, Lanigan SW. Exanthems and hypersensitivity syndromes. In: Zaidi Z, Lanigan SW, editors. Dermatology in clinical practice. London: Springer; 2010. p. 271–80. With permission from Springer Verlag)

Pemphigus Vulgaris

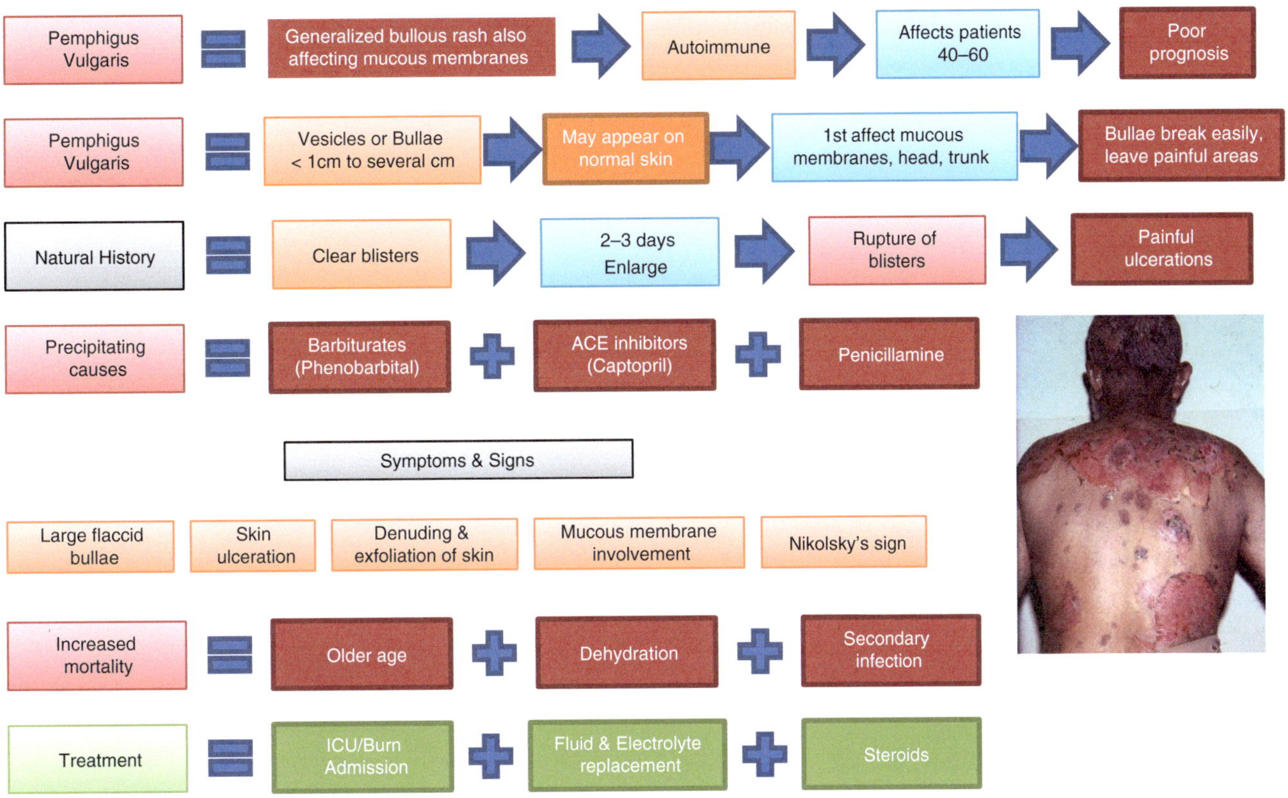

Right side image (Reprinted from Zaidi Z, Lanigan SW. Bullous disorders: autoimmune and childhood bullous dermatoses. In: Zaidi Z, Lanigan SW, editors. Dermatology in clinical practice. London: Springer; 2010. p. 233–52. With permission from Springer Verlag)

Bullous Pemphigoid

Bullous Pemphigoid = Benign chronic bullous rash → Autoimmune process (IgE) → Affects pts > 60 → F > M

Bullous Pemphigoid = Begins with urticaria → Formation of tense blisters → Blisters may exceed 10 cm → Leads to exfoliation

Bullous Pemphigoid = Minimal involvement of mucous membranes + *NO* Nikolsky sign

Precipitating causes = Medications (Sulfa) + Malignancy

Complications = Infection + Electrolyte loss

Treatment = Supportive → Much more benign course than pemphigus vulgaris

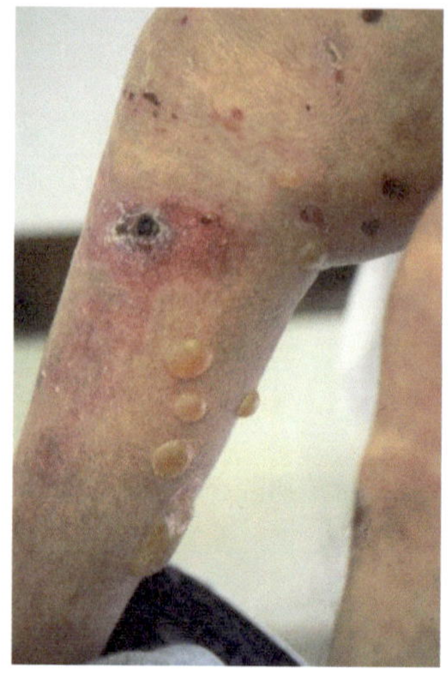

Right side image (Reprinted from Cashman MW, Doshi D, Krishnamurthy K. Vesiculobullous dermatoses. In: Buka B, Uliasz A, Krishnamurthy K, editors. Buka's emergencies in dermatology. New York: Springer; 2013. p. 147–73. With permission from Springer Science + Business Media)

Exfoliative Dermatitis (Erythroderma)

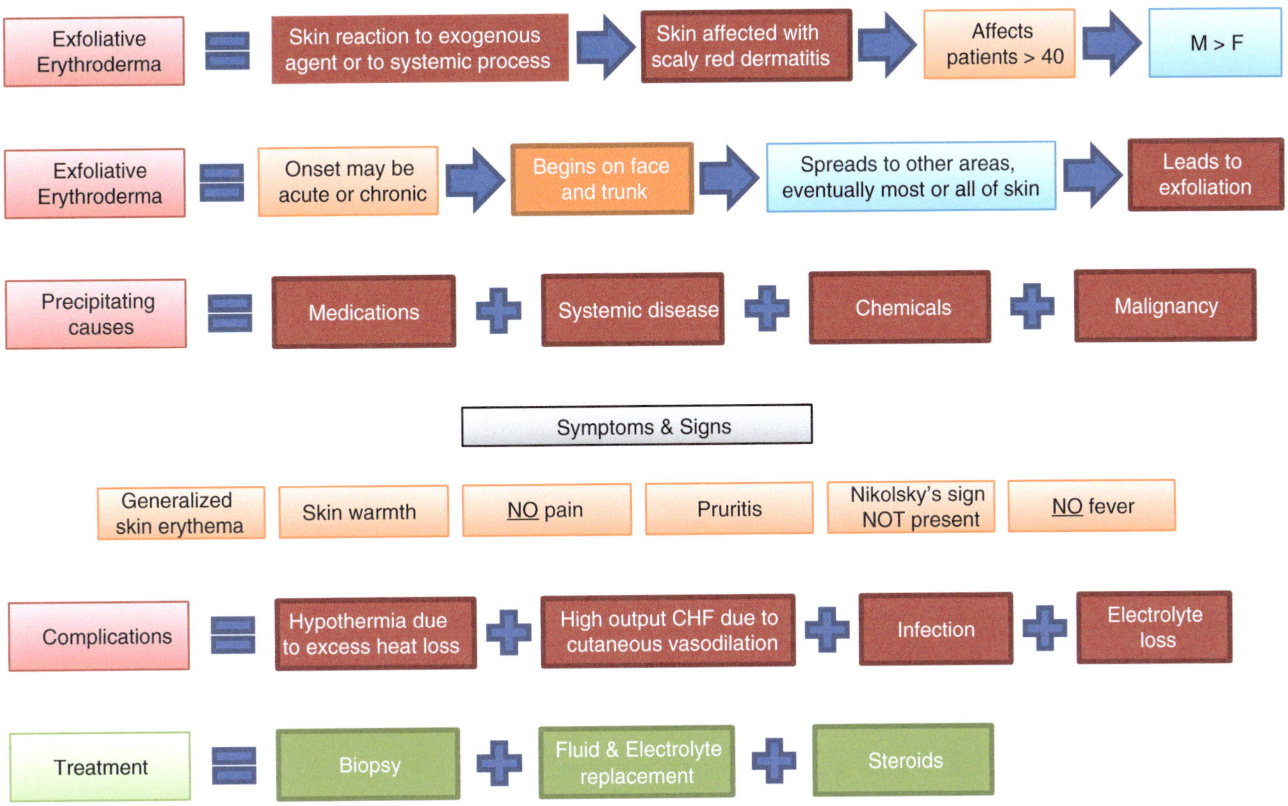

Drug Rash or Eruption

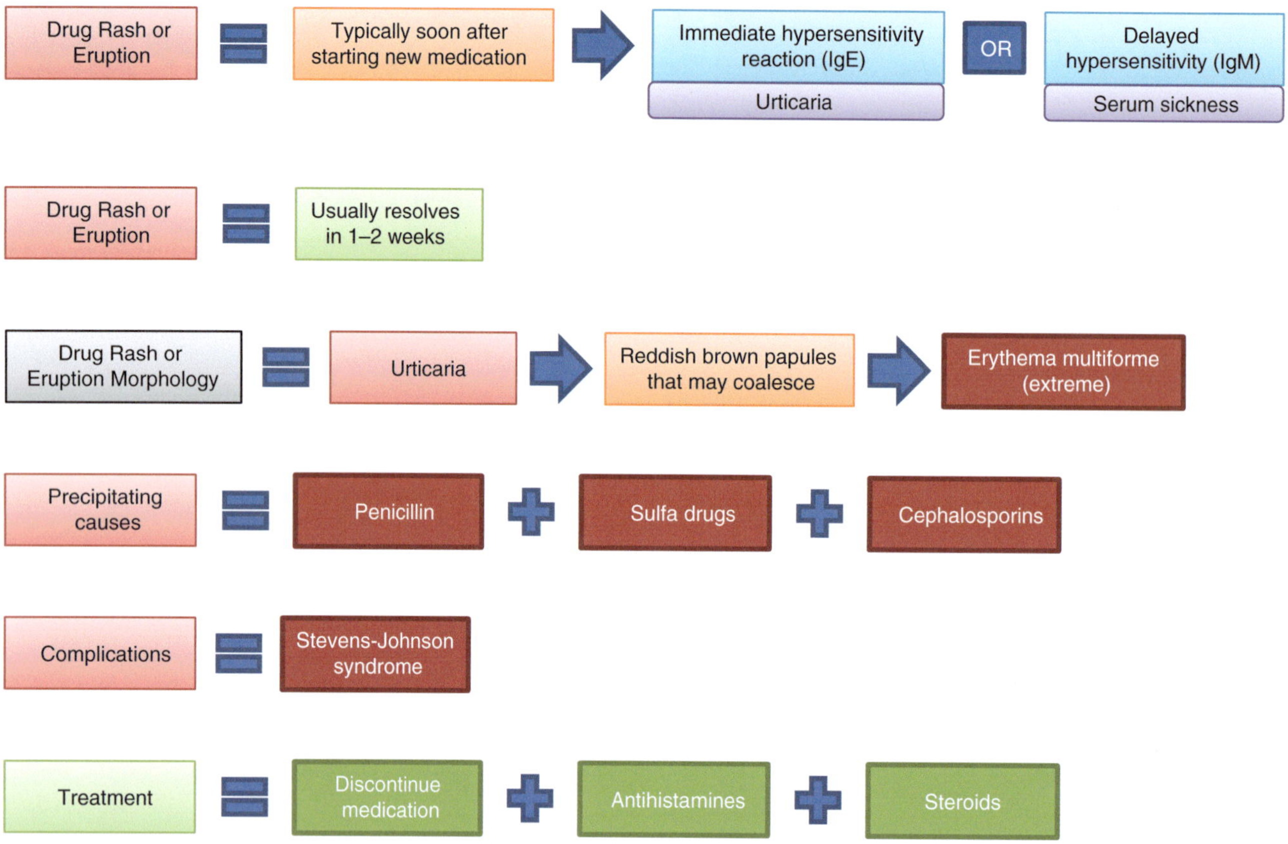

Erythema Nodosum

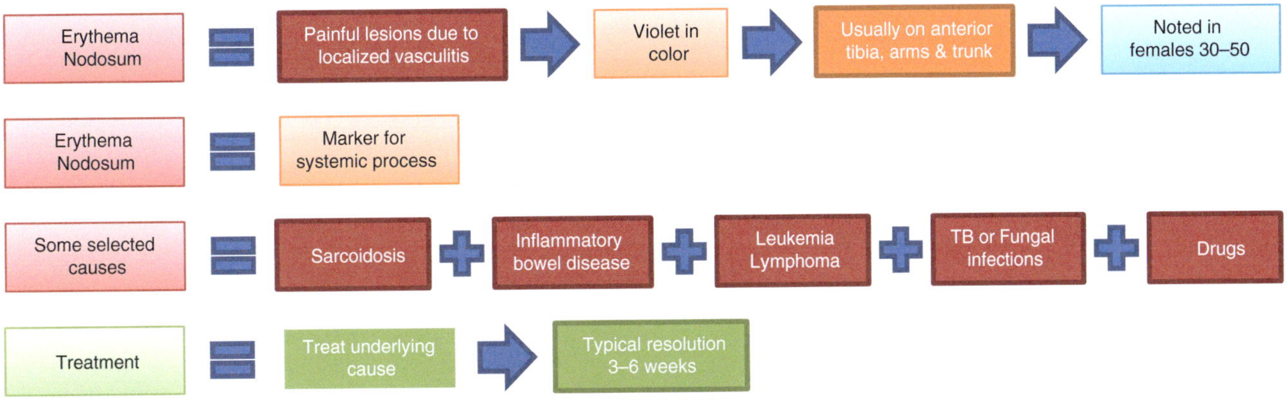

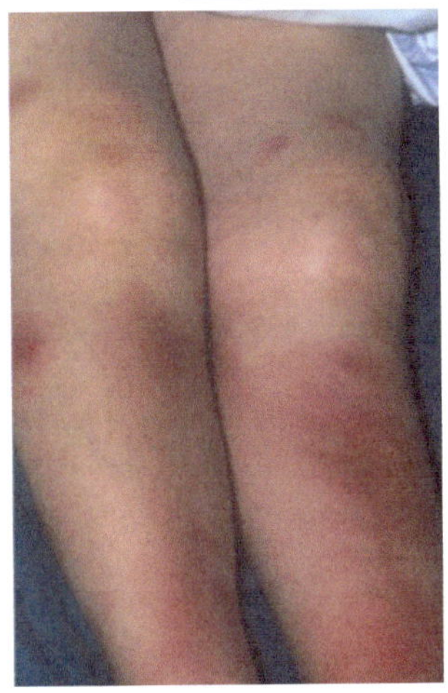

Bottom center image (Reprinted from Vázquez-Roque MI, De Jesús-Monge WE. Cutaneous manifestations of gastrointestinal diseases. In: Sánchez NP, editors. Atlas of dermatology in internal medicine. New York: Springer; 2012. p. 41–51. With permission from Springer Science + Business Media)

Eczema

Eczema = Has association with multiple processes → Allergic rhinitis / Asthma / Nasal Polyps → Chronic & itchy / (+) Family hx / Worse in winter

Skin findings = Lichenification + Crusting + Redness + Excoriations + Pruritis + Fissures

Eczema in infants = Face, scalp & extremities → Crusting and blistering → Resolves by age 2

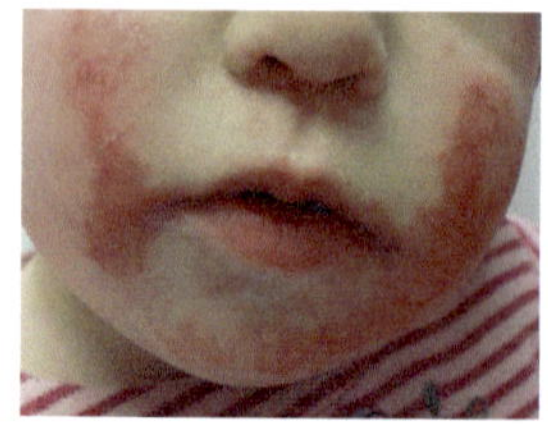

Eczema in adults = Antecubital & Popliteal fossa → Dryness and skin thickening

Complications = Eczema herpeticum → HSV infection with underlying eczema + Secondary infection

Treatment = Antipruritics + Steroids

Right center image (Reprinted from Silverberg NB. Eczematous diseases. In: Silverberg NB, editor. Atlas of pediatric cutaneous biodiversity: comparative dermatologic atlas of pediatric skin of all colors. New York: Springer; 2012. p. 69–88. With permission from Springer Science + Business Media)

Allergic Contact Dermatitis

Allergic Contact Dermatitis = Delayed hypersensitivity reaction → 48 hours to days after allergen contact

Causes = Poison Ivy, Oak or Sumac + Detergents + Nickel in metal jewelry

Symptoms & Signs

Erythema | Pruritis | Vesicles | Bullae | May be limited to area of contact

Treatment = Steroids

Psoriasis

Psoriasis = Red papules & plaques with silvery-white scale → Chronic Starts in 20's → Due to overproduction of keratinocytes

Psoriasis = May be accompanied by psoriatic arthritis

Symptoms & Signs

Auspitz sign → Removal of scale shows areas of bleeding

Pitting of nails

Treatment = Steroid creams + Tar + UV light + Methotrexate

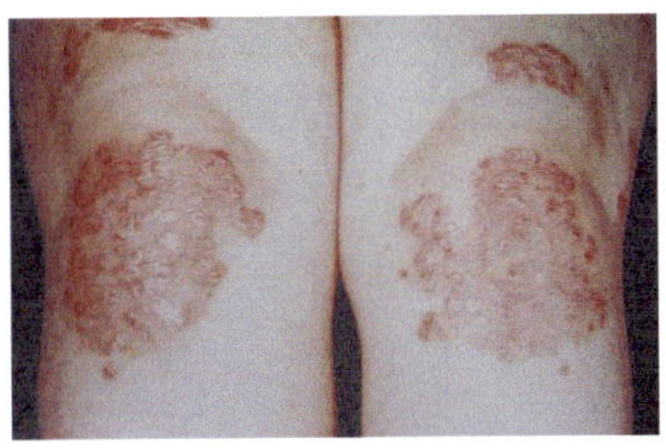

Bottom center image (Reprinted from Norman RA, Young, Jr. EM. Psoriasis. In: Norman RA, Young EM Jr, editors. Atlas of geriatric dermatology. London: Springer; 2014. p. 83–95. With permission from Springer Verlag)

Seborrheic Dermatitis

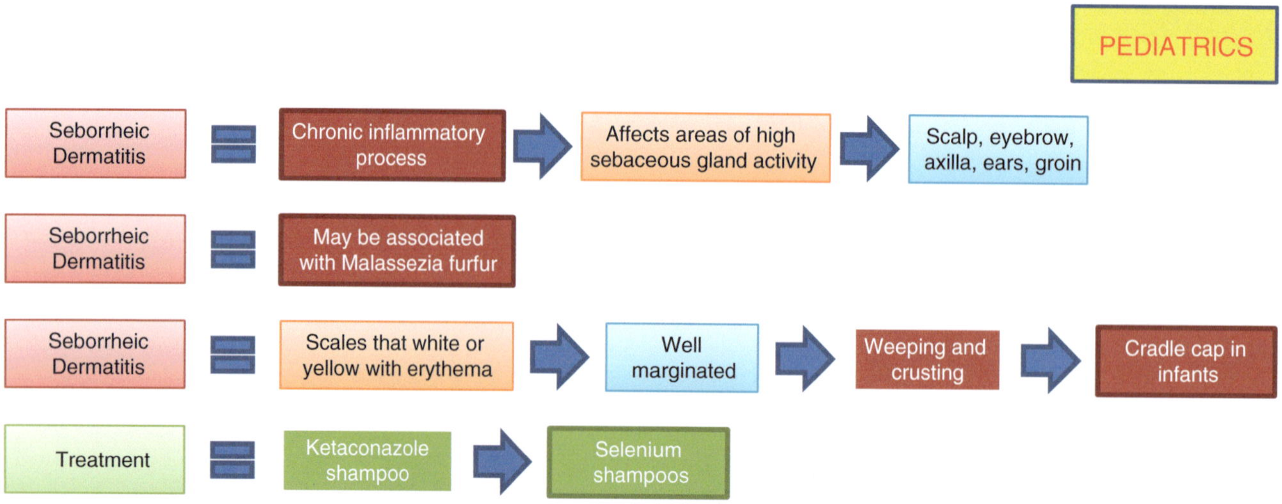

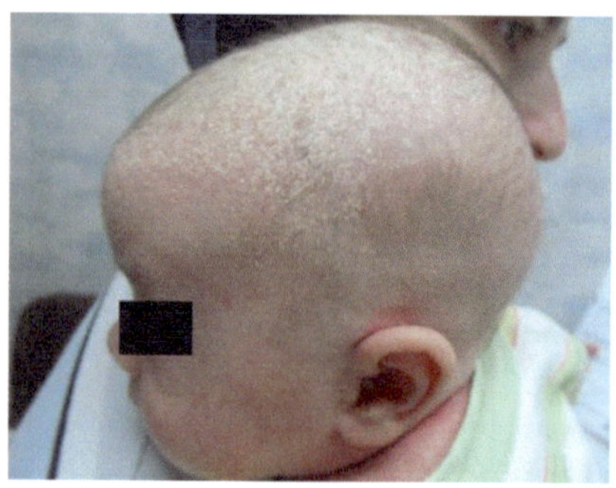

Bottom center image (Reprinted from Silverberg NB. Eczematous diseases. In: Silverberg NB, editor. Atlas of pediatric cutaneous biodiversity: comparative dermatologic atlas of pediatric skin of all colors. New York: Springer; 2012. p. 69–88. With permission from Springer Science + Business Media)

Pityriasis Rosea

PEDIATRICS

Pityriasis Rosea = Affects F > M 15–40 → Especially in spring & fall → Unknown etiology → Not contagious, resolves 1–2 months

PityriasisRosea = Starts with "herald patch" → Single salmon colored lesion with raised border → Seen on trunk → 1–5 cm large

Natural History = Herald patch → 1–2 weeks Pink maculopapular oval patches that follow ribs = Christmas tree pattern

Pityriasis Rosea mimics = Syphilis (*no* herald patch) + Drug reaction

Treatment = Symptomatic + Antihistamines for pruritis

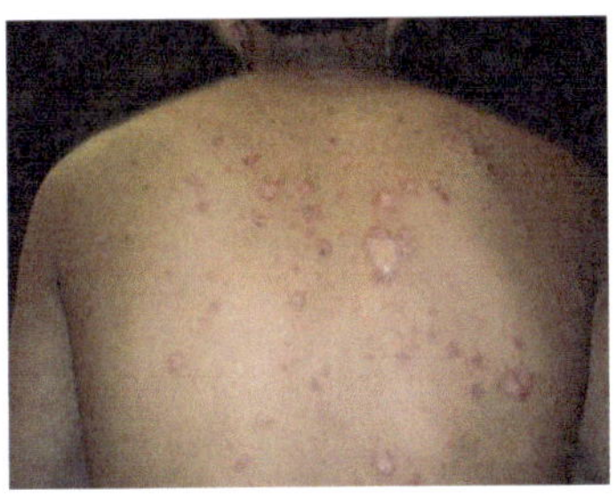

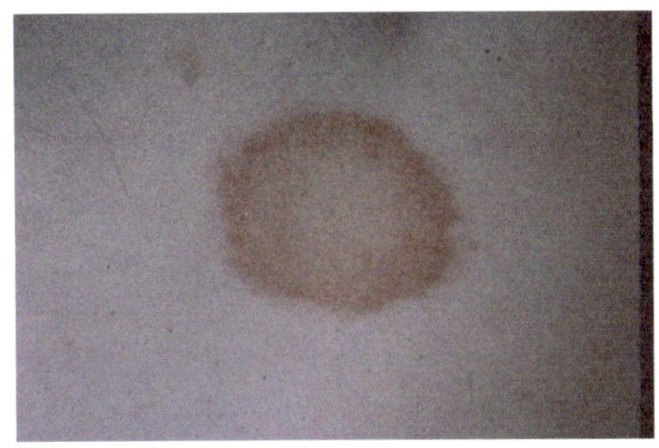

Left side image (Reprinted from Zaidi Z, Lanigan SW. Keratinizing and papulosquamous disorders. In: Zaidi Z, Lanigan SW, editors. Dermatology in clinical practice. London: Springer; 2010. p. 179–209. With permission from Springer Verlag)

Right side image (Reprinted from Silverberg NB. Papulosquamous disorders. In: Silverberg NB, editor. Atlas of pediatric cutaneous biodiversity: comparative dermatologic atlas of pediatric skin of all colors. New York: Springer; 2012. p. 53–60. With permission from Springer Science + Business Media)

Dermatophyte Infections

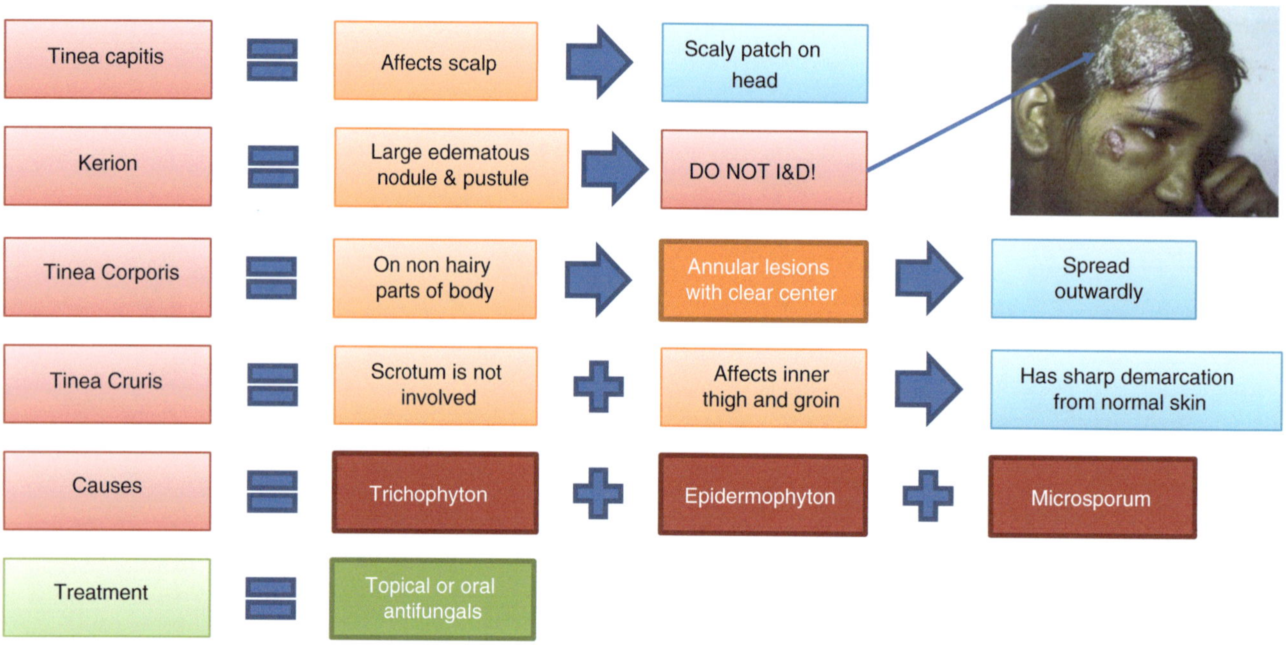

Right side image (Reprinted from Zaidi Z, Lanigan SW. Superficial fungal infections. In: Zaidi Z, Lanigan SW, editors. Dermatology in clinical practice. London: Springer; 2010. p. 73–99. With permission from Springer Verlag)

Tinea Versicolor

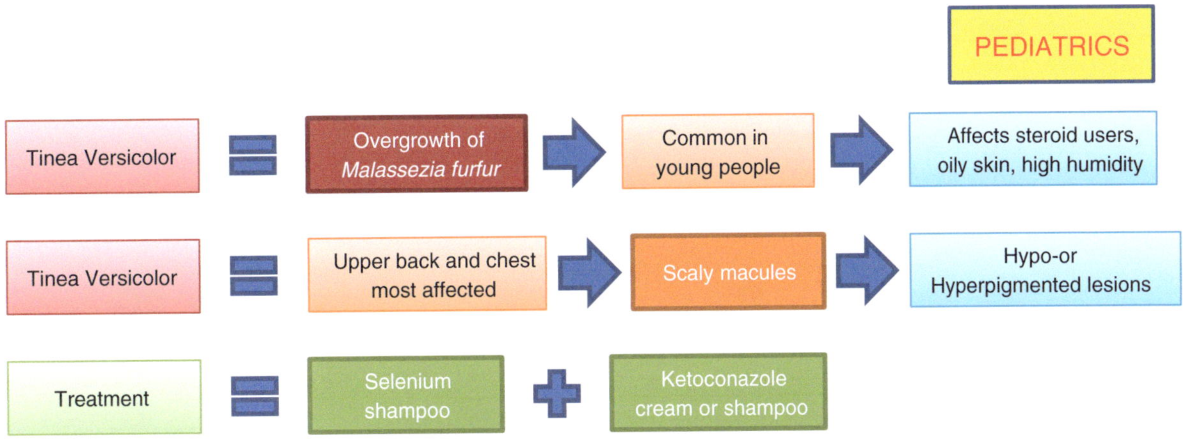

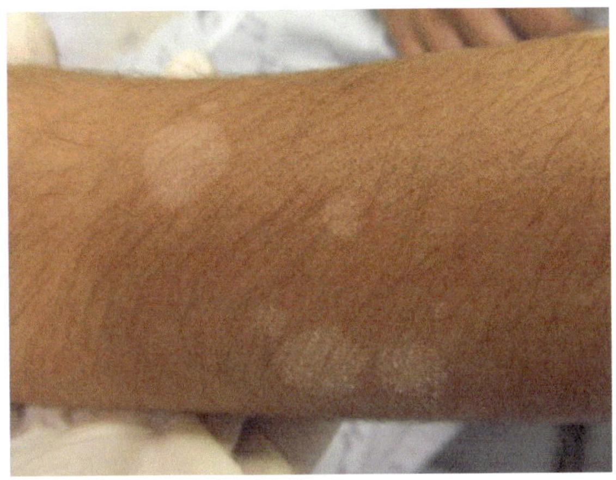

Bottom center image (Reprinted from Silverberg NB. Cutaneous infections. In: Silverberg NB, editor. Atlas of pediatric cutaneous biodiversity: comparative dermatologic atlas of pediatric skin of all colors. New York: Springer; 2012. p. 113–25. With permission from Springer Science + Business Media)

Allergic Processes

Urticaria

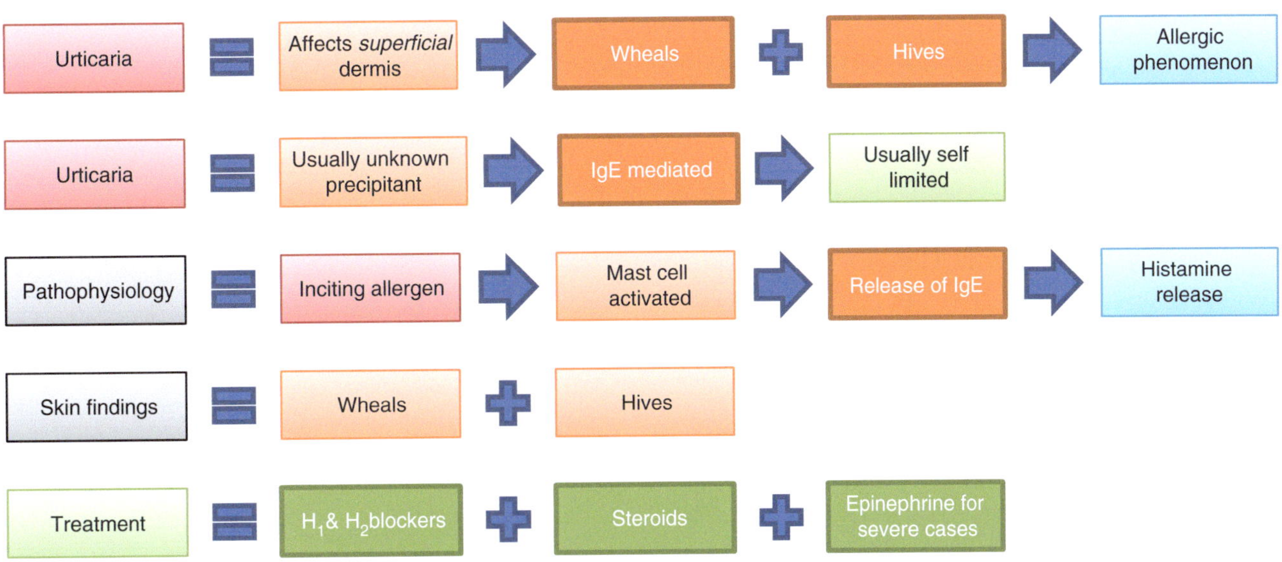

Angioedema

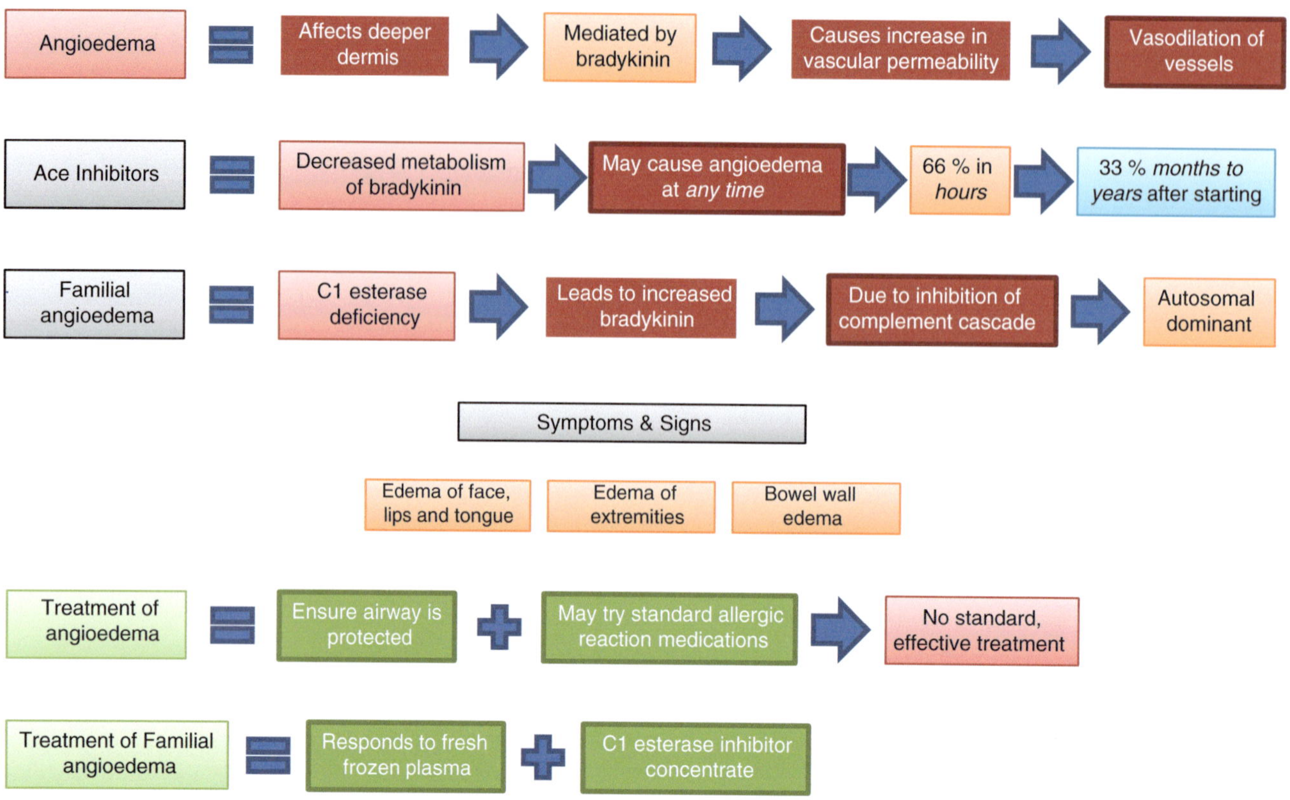
Angioedema
Affects deeper dermis
Mediated by bradykinin
Causes increase in vascular permeability
Vasodilation of vessels
Ace Inhibitors
Decreased metabolism of bradykinin
May cause angioedema at *any time*
66 % in *hours*
33 % *months to years* after starting
Familial angioedema
C1 esterase deficiency
Leads to increased bradykinin
Due to inhibition of complement cascade
Autosomal dominant
Symptoms & Signs
Edema of face, lips and tongue
Edema of extremities
Bowel wall edema
Treatment of angioedema
Ensure airway is protected
May try standard allergic reaction medications
No standard, effective treatment
Treatment of Familial angioedema
Responds to fresh frozen plasma
C1 esterase inhibitor concentrate

Skin Cancers

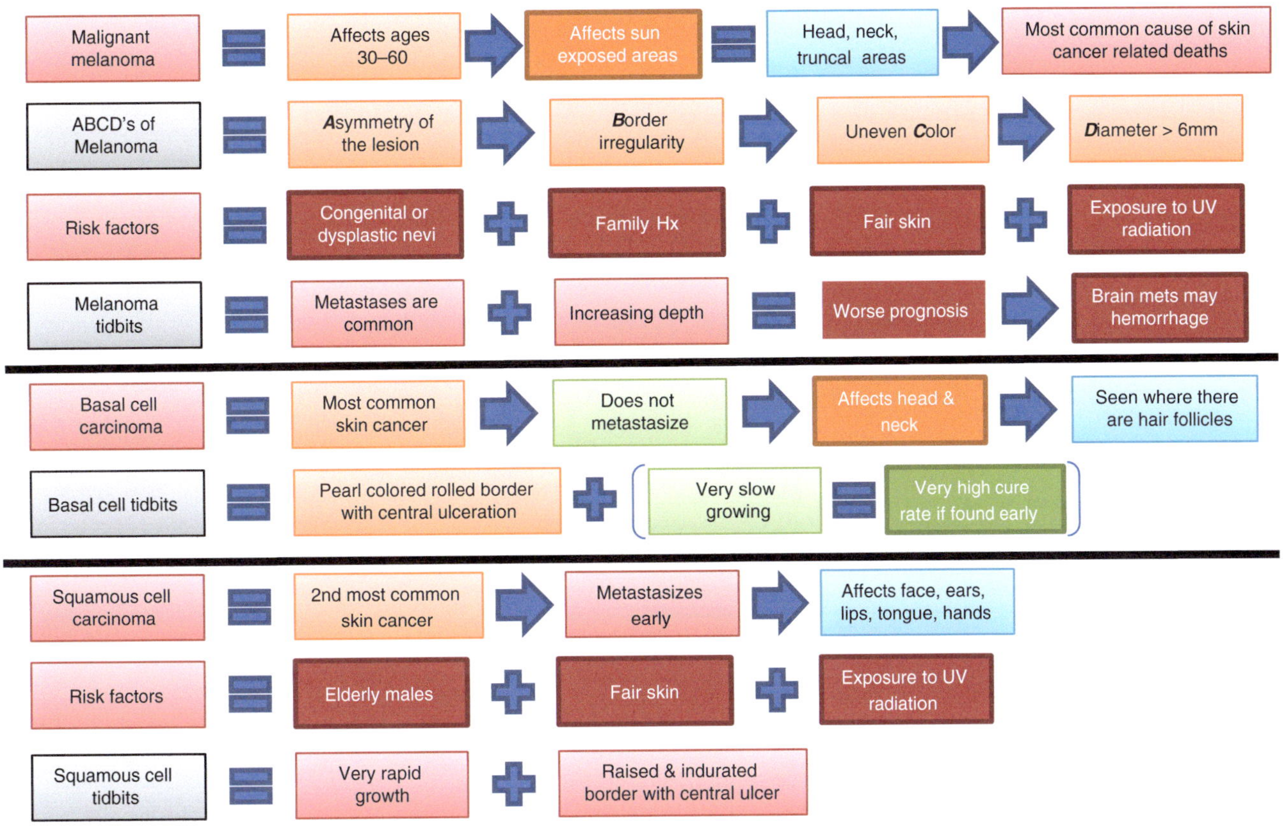

Infectious Diseases and Associated Skin Lesions

Meningococcemia

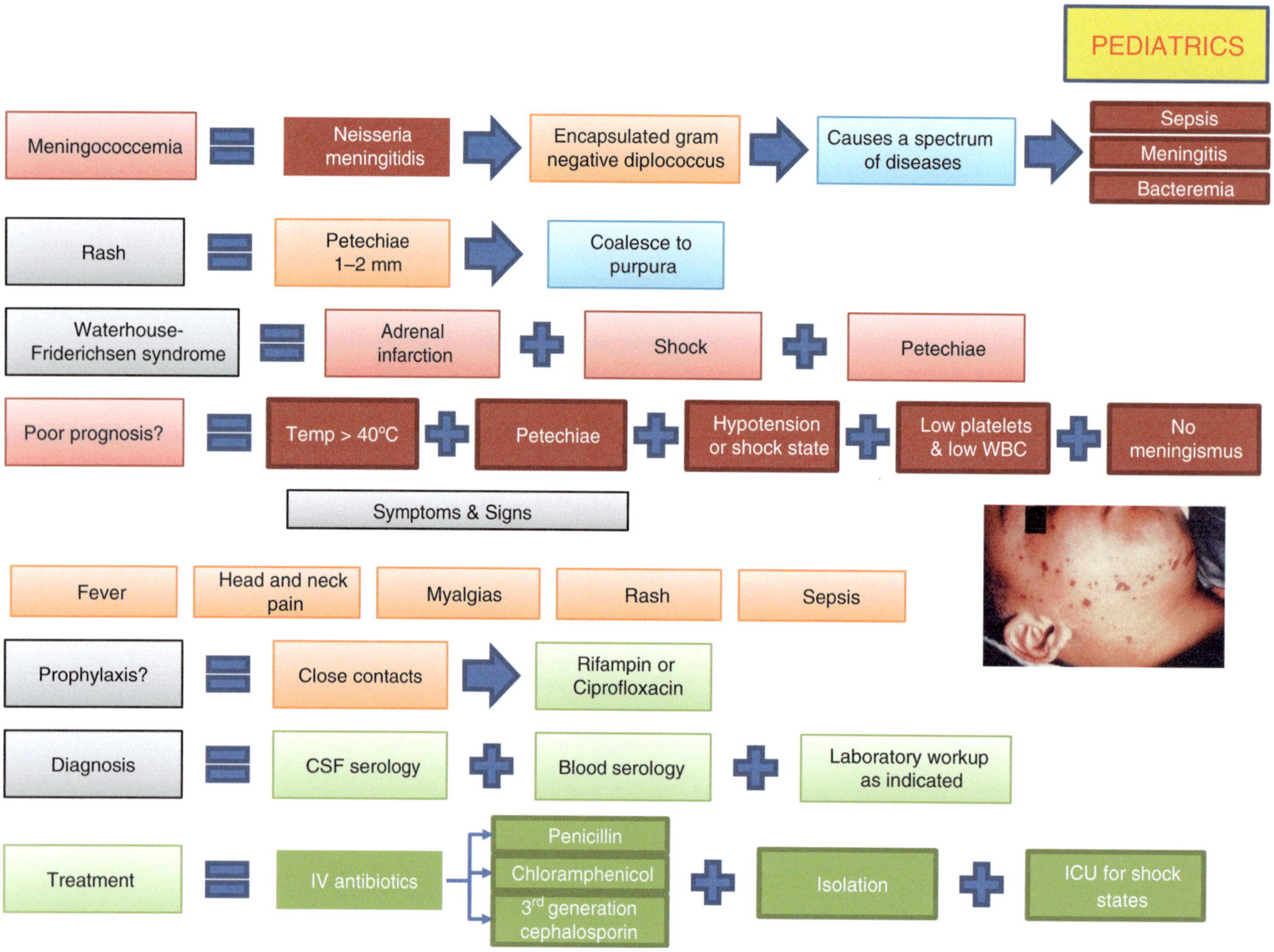

Right side image (Reprinted from Stamell E, Krishnamurthy K. Infectious emergencies in dermatology. In: Buka B, Uliasz A, Krishnamurthy K, editors. Buka's emergencies in dermatology. New York: Springer; 2013. p. 19–41. With permission from Springer Science+Business Media)

Gonococcemia and GC Arthritis

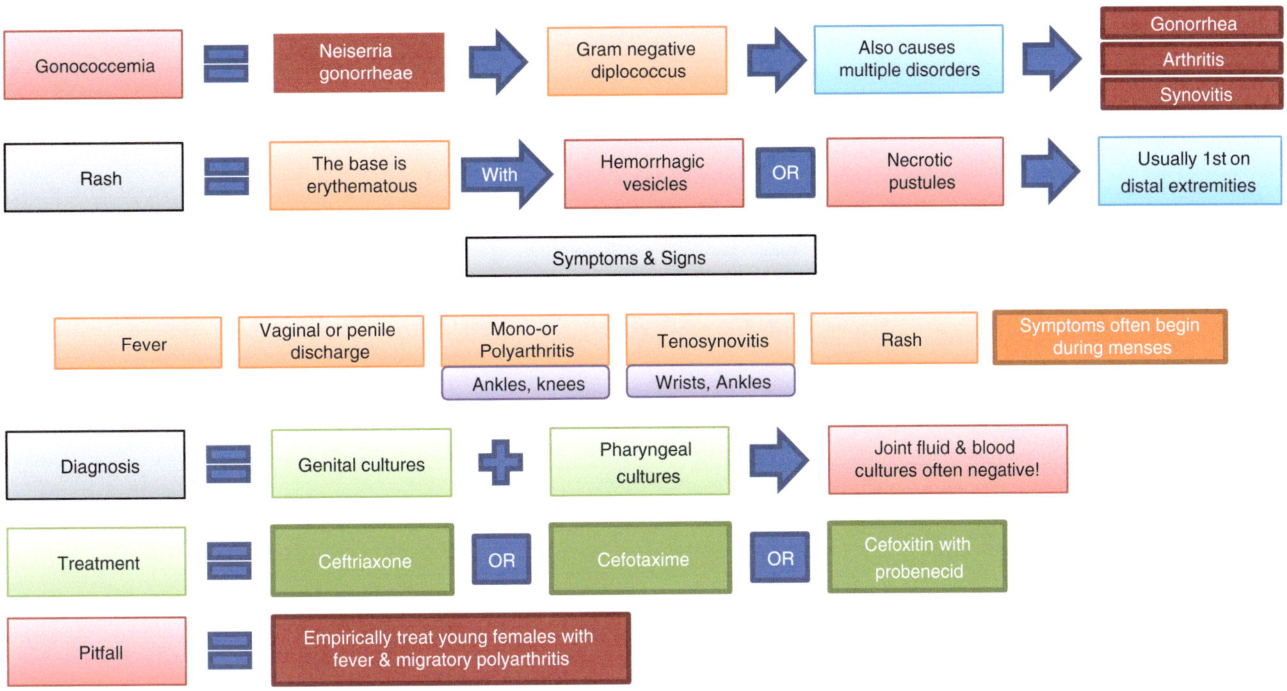

Lyme Disease

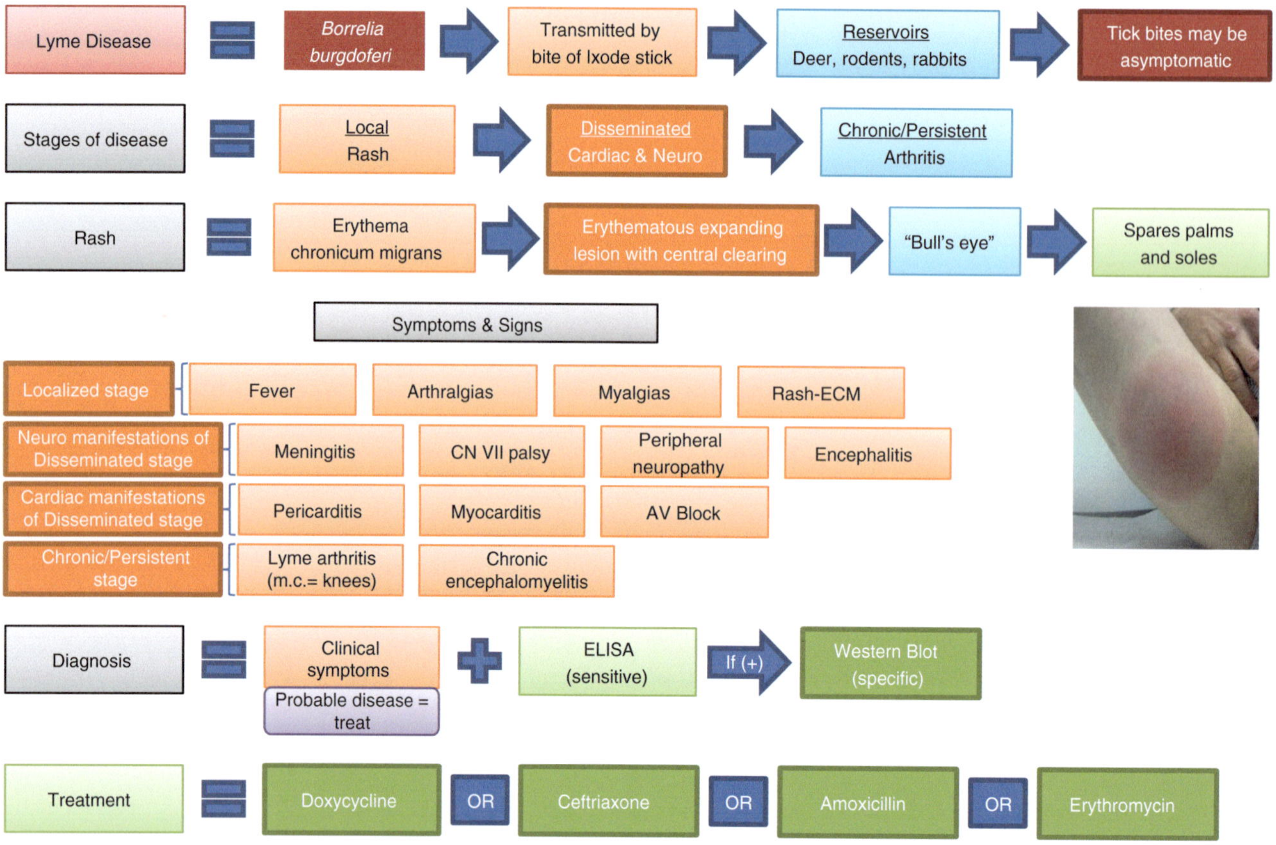

Right side image (Reprinted from Miró EM, Sánchez NP. Cutaneous manifestations of infectious diseases. In: Sánchez NP, editor. Atlas of dermatology in internal medicine. New York: Springer; 2012. p. 77–119. With permission from Springer Science + Business Media)

Leptospirosis

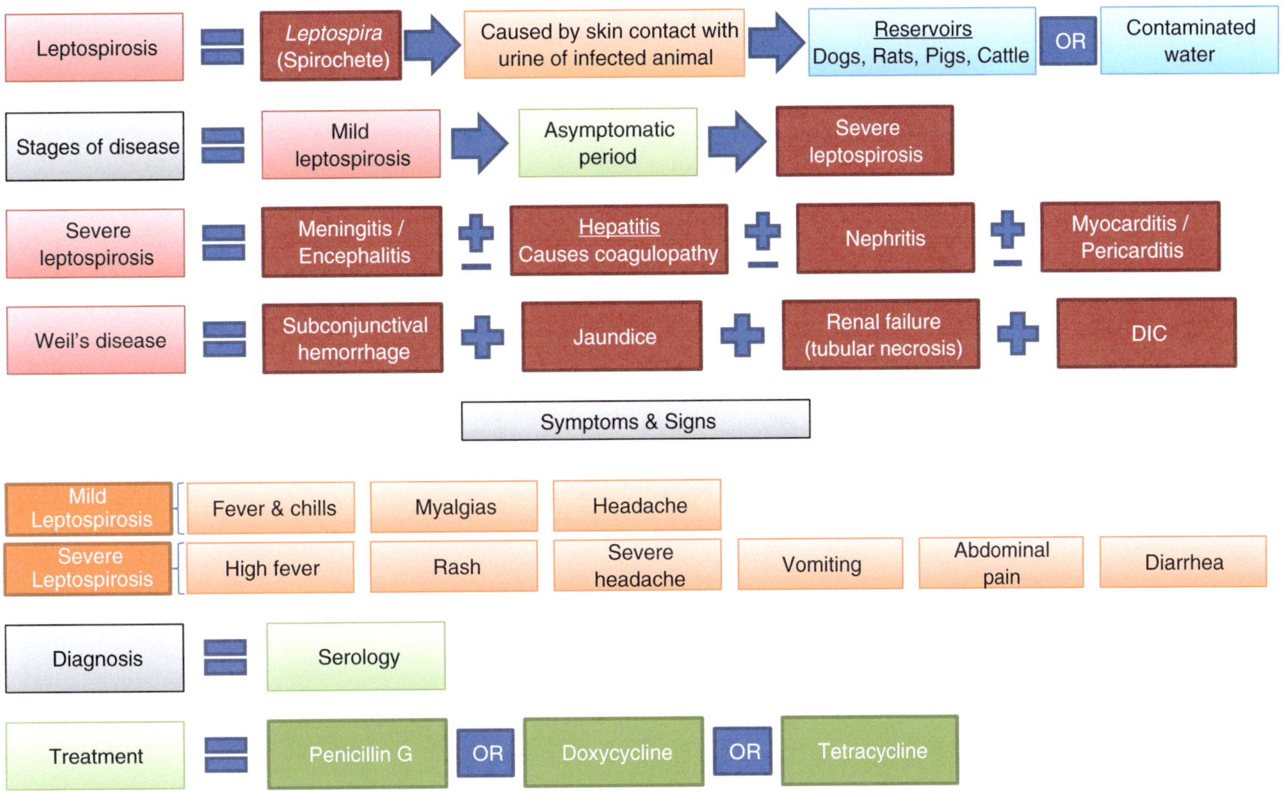

Rocky Mountain Spotted Fever (RMSF)

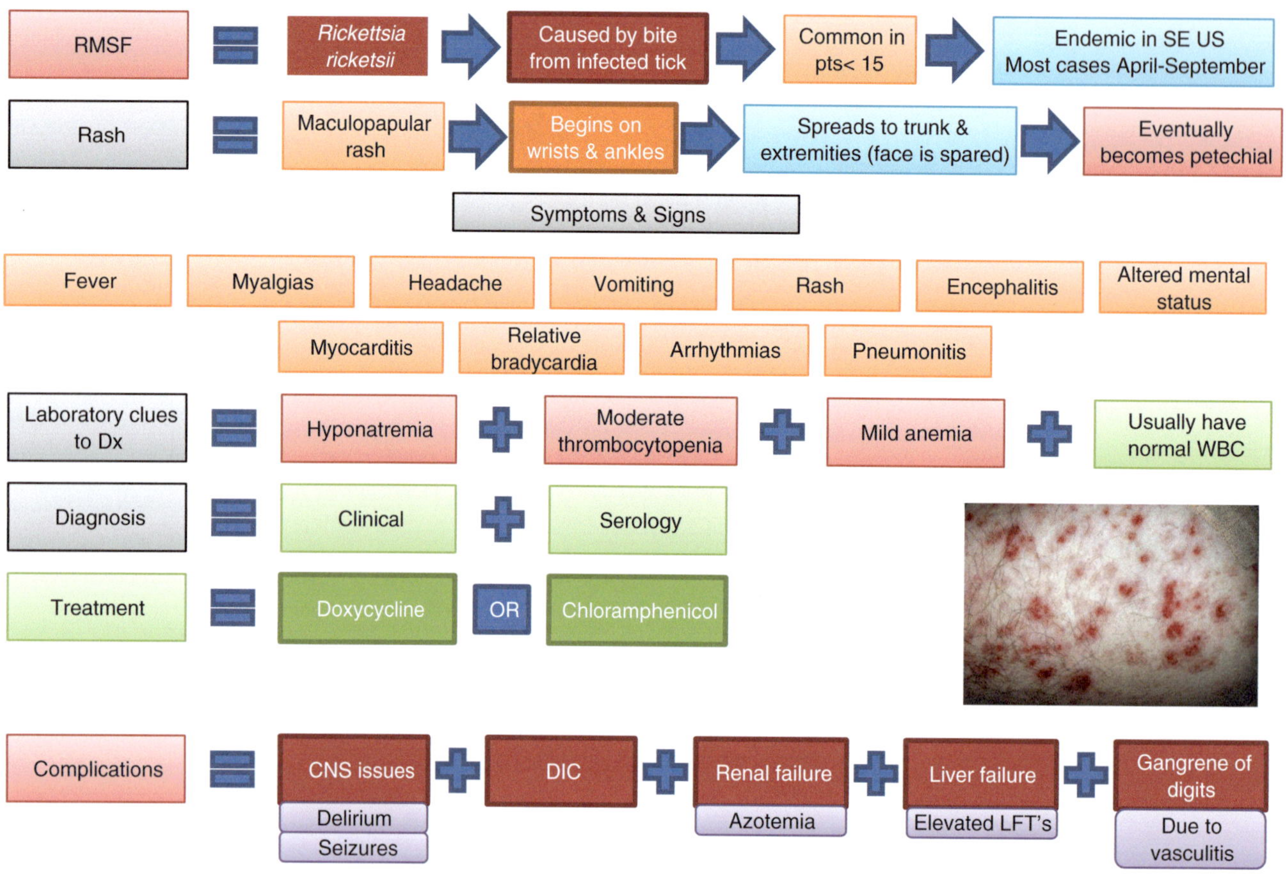

Bottom right image (Reprinted from Morgan MB, Smoller BR, Somach SC. Rocky mountain spotted fever and the rickettsioses. In: Morgan MB, Smoller BR, Somach SC, editors. Deadly dermatologic diseases: clinicopathologic atlas and text. New York: Springer; 2007. p. 125–8. With permission from Springer Science + Business Media)

Ehrlichiosis

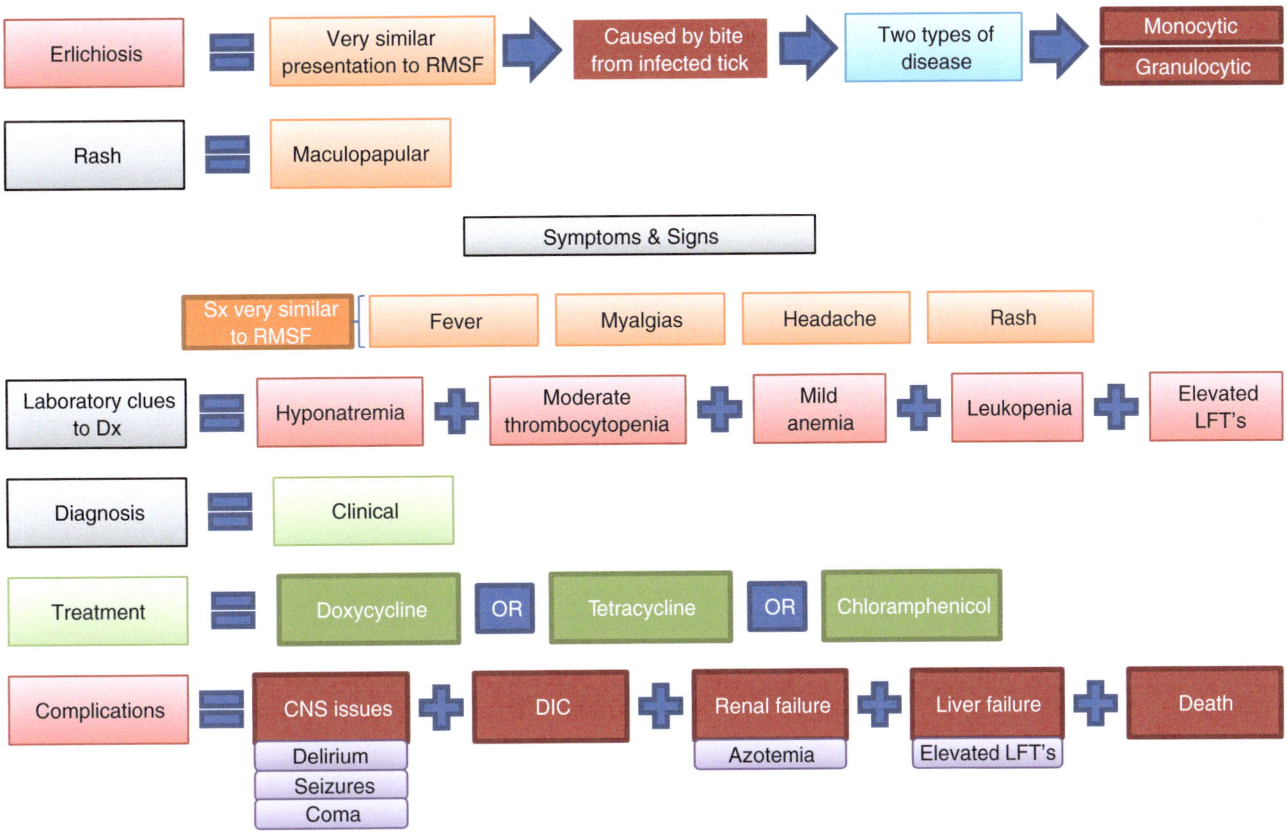

Babesiosis

Babesiosis = *Babesia* (protozoan parasite) → Caused by bite from infected tick → Endemic in NE US → 2nd most common blood parasite / Malaria #1

Symptoms & Signs

- Fever
- Chills
- Fatigue
- Malaise
- Diarrhea
- Signs of hemolytic anemia
- Signs of ARDS (Severe cases)
- Hepatomegaly
- Splenomegaly
- Jaundice

Diagnosis = Serology + Blood smear with intra-RBC parasites → Protozoa in blood smear → "Maltese cross"

Treatment = Clindamycin + Quinine OR Azithromycin + Atovaquone

Usually mild unless = Asplenic + Immune compromised + Elderly

Viral Infections

TORCHES

PEDIATRICS

TO	Toxoplasmosis
R	Rubella
C	CMV
H	Herpes/HIV
E	Epstein-Barr Virus
S	Syphilis

These organisms are associated with congenital transmission

Cytomegalovirus (CMV)

PEDIATRICS

CMV = Most common of the TORCHES → Member of Herpes virus family → 3 disease processes → Congenital / Acquired / Immunocompromised

Congenital = Chorioretinitis + Liver & spleen enlargement (± Jaundice) + Deafness + Rash

Acquired = Usually benign → Flu-like illness OR Mono-like illness

CMV effects on immunocompromised pts? = Nephritis + Pneumonitis + Retinitis + Colitis

Immune compromised + CMV = High mortality

Diagnosis = ELISA + Atypical lymphocytes on peripheral smear

Treatment = Ganciclovir + Foscarnet

Epstein-Barr Virus (EBV)

PEDIATRICS

EBV = Infectious mononucleosis → Member of Herpes virus family → Common in adolescents → May be asymptomatic in younger children

Symptoms & Signs

Fever | Exudative pharyngitis | Splenomegaly | Lymphadenopathy

Diagnosis = Monospot + Serology + Atypical lymphoctyes on peripheral smear

Complications = Splenic rupture + Thrombocytopenia + Macular rash if given Amoxicillin → May be diagnostic

Treatment = Rest + Supportive care → Instructions for no contact sports

Herpes Zoster (HZV)

Herpes Zoster = Varicella virus → Member of herpes virus family → Located in dorsal root ganglion-Zoster is a *reactivation* process → Dermatomal distribution of painful vesicles

Complications = Meningitis + Pneumonia + Disseminated VZV + Post-herpetic neuralgia

Treatment = Valacyclovir OR Acyclovir + Steroids

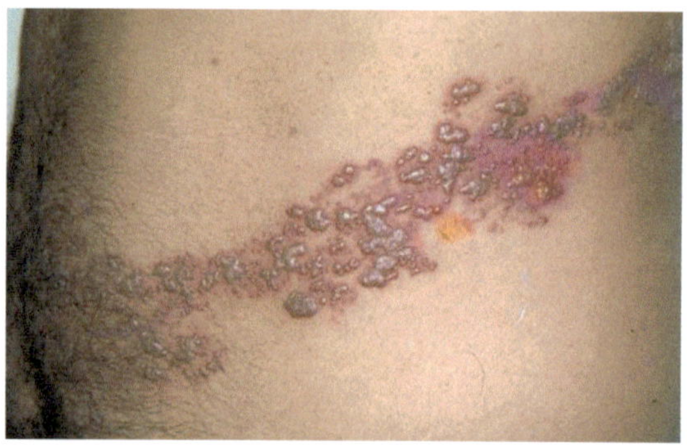

Bottom center image (Reprinted from Zaidi Z, Lanigan SW. Viral infections. In: Zaidi Z, Lanigan SW, editors. Dermatology in clinical practice. London: Springer; 2010. p. 101–23. With permission from Springer Verlag)

Complications of AIDS

Pulmonary = *Pneumocystis* = Most frequent infection → Hypoxemia with bilateral infiltrates → TMP/SMX & Steroids

Meningitis = *Cryptococcal* meningitis = Most common CNS fungal infection → Dx with CSF studies → Amphotericin B

Encephalitis = Toxoplasmosis = Most common cause of encephalitis → Dx = CT with ring enhancing lesions → Pyrimethamine & Sulfadiazine

Kaposi's Sarcoma (KS) = 2nd most common AIDS manifestation → Seen in homosexual males → No significant morbidity

KS Skin Findings = Painless macular purple areas → Nonpruritic → These may coalesce & bleed OR Raised strawberry like plaques

Extracutaneous findings = GI tract, especially liver & spleen + Lungs + Central nervous system

Percutaneous exposure = Transmission rate 0.3 % → Post exposure prophylaxis recommended for significant exposure

Increased Risk = Deep injury + Source with high viral load + Contamination due to hollow bore needle

Post exposure prophylaxis = Start meds within 1–2 hours, continue for 4 weeks → Multiple drugs are standard → Reverse transcriptase inhibitors + Protease inhibitors

Molluscum Contagiosum

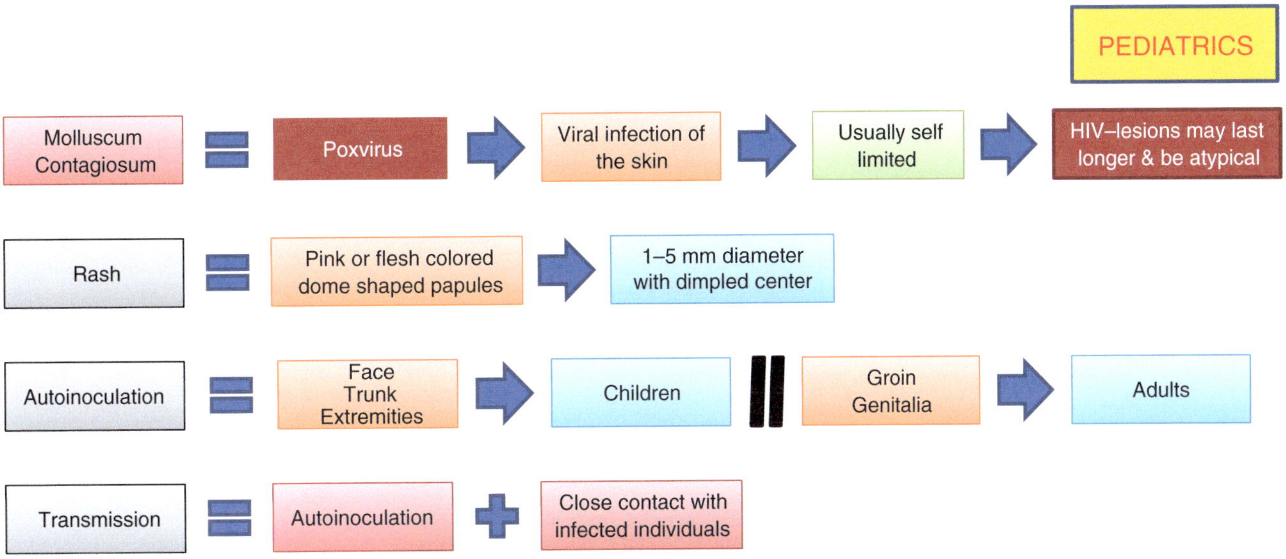

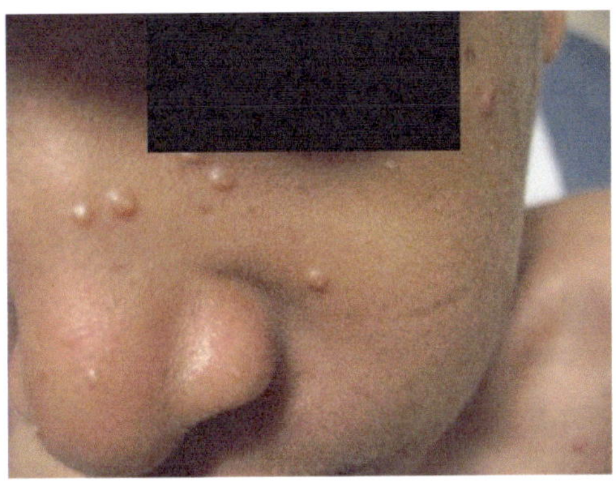

Bottom center image (Reprinted from Silverberg NB. Cutaneous infections. In: Silverberg NB, editor. Atlas of pediatric cutaneous biodiversity: comparative dermatologic atlas of pediatric skin of all colors. New York: Springer; 2012. p. 113–25. With permission from Springer Science + Business Media)

Malaria

Malaria = Intra-RBC parasite → Transmitted via infected female Anopheles mosquito → Prevalent in Asia, Latin America & Sub-Saharan Africa

Organisms = Plasmodium falciparum + Plasmodium ovale + Plasmodium vivax + Plasmodium malariae

Plasmodium falciparum = Most severe → Due to → Causes more complications + Widespread medication resistance + High likelihood of parasitemia

Symptoms & Signs

Fever & Chills | Splenomegaly | Headache | Malaise | Joint pain | N/V | "Blackwater fever"

Cerebral malaria: AMS | Seizures | Abnormal posturing | Opisthotonus

"Blackwater fever": Massive hemolysis

Classic Paroxysm = Coldness → Shivering → Fever

Diagnosis = Thick and thin blood smears

Treatment = Depends on organism and resistance pattern

Pediatric Rashes

Erythema Infectiosum

PEDIATRICS

Erythema Infectiosum = Parvovirus B19 → Fifth Disease

Rash = Bright red face & cheeks → Spares eyelids & chin + "Lace-like" red papules → Limbs & Trunk

Symptoms & Signs

Fever | Headache | Myalgias | URI/Flu Sx | Diarrhea → Rash follows these Sx

Treatment = NSAID's

Complications = Arthritis + Aplastic crisis (Sickle cell) + Fetal anemia if acquired in pregnancy

Rubella

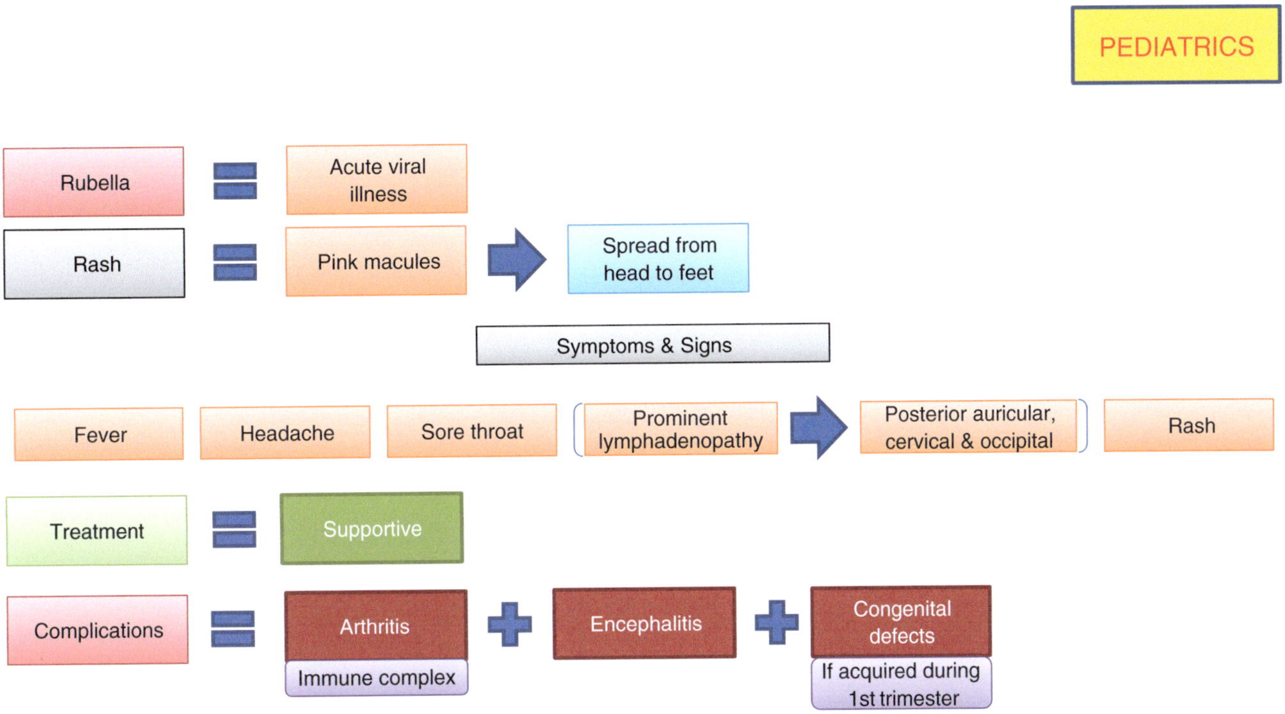
PEDIATRICS
Rubella
Acute viral illness
Rash
Pink macules
Spread from head to feet
Symptoms & Signs
Fever
Headache
Sore throat
Prominent lymphadenopathy
Posterior auricular, cervical & occipital
Rash
Treatment
Supportive
Complications
Arthritis
Immune complex
Encephalitis
Congenital defects
If acquired during 1st trimester

Measles (Rubeola)

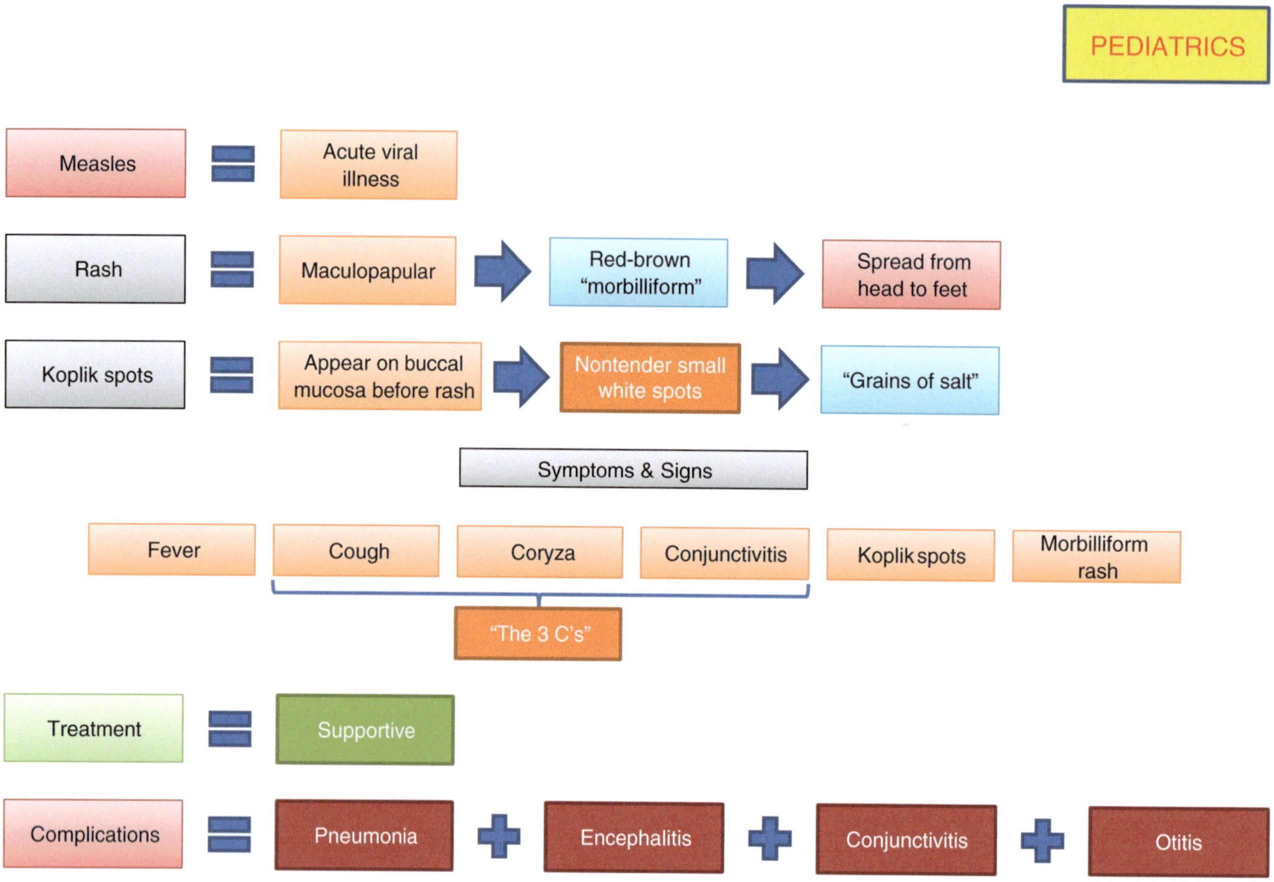

Roseola Infantum

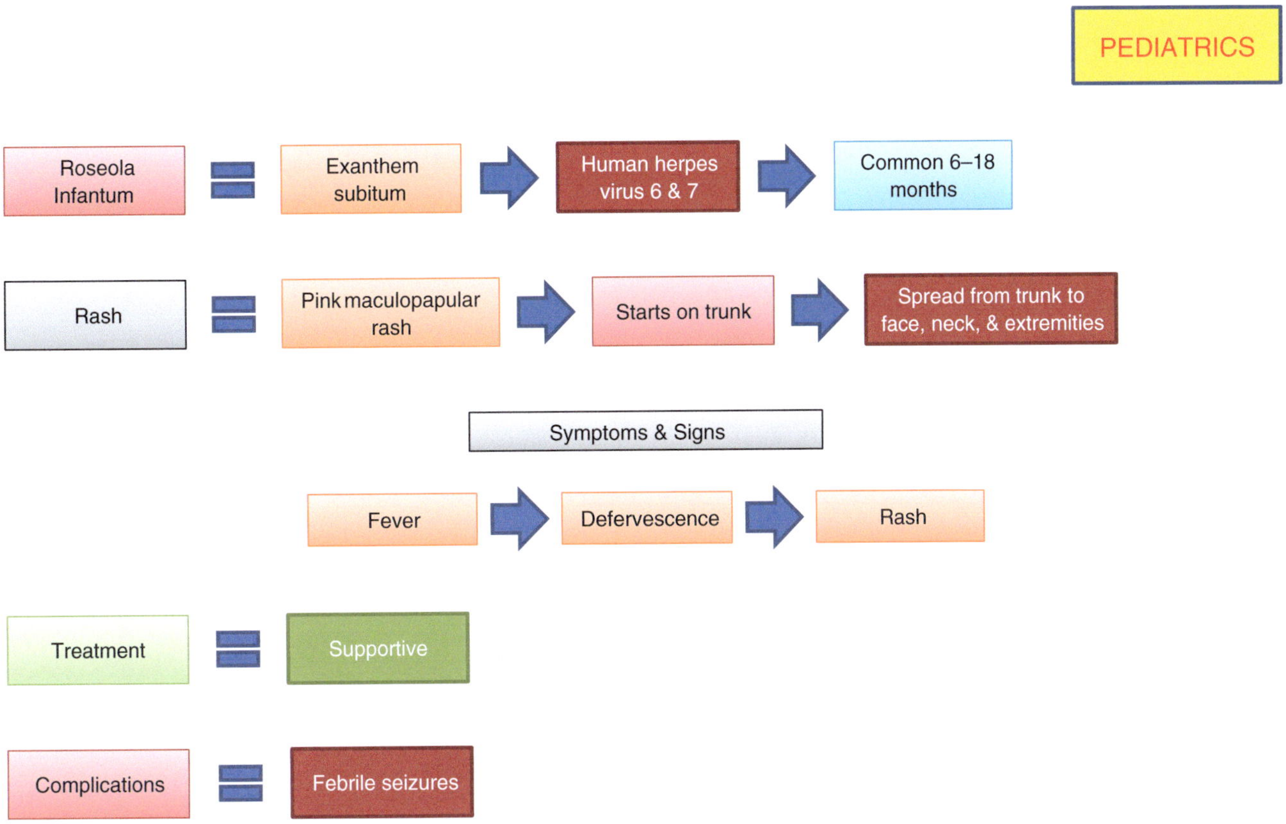

Varicella (Chicken Pox)

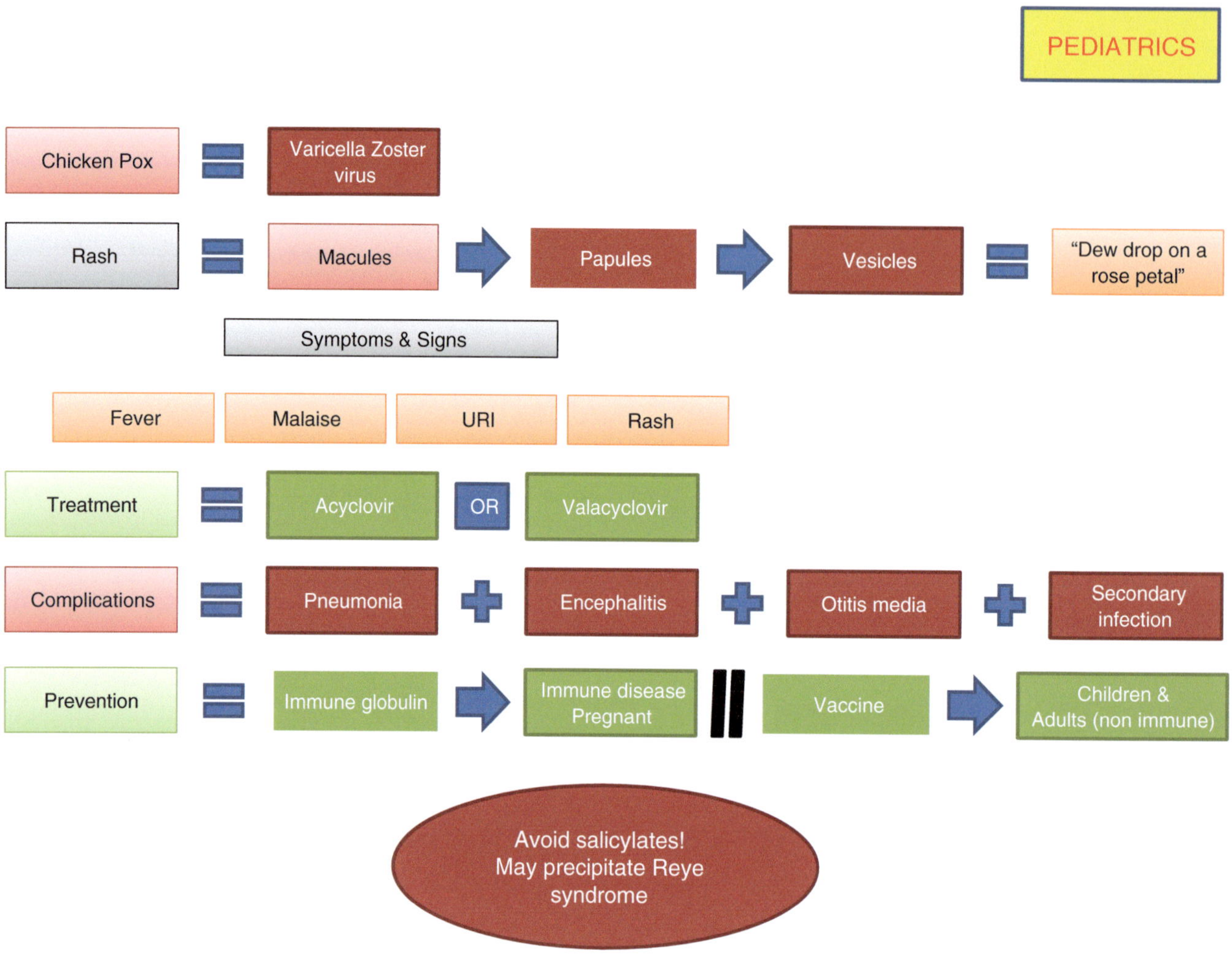

Hand-Foot-Mouth Disease

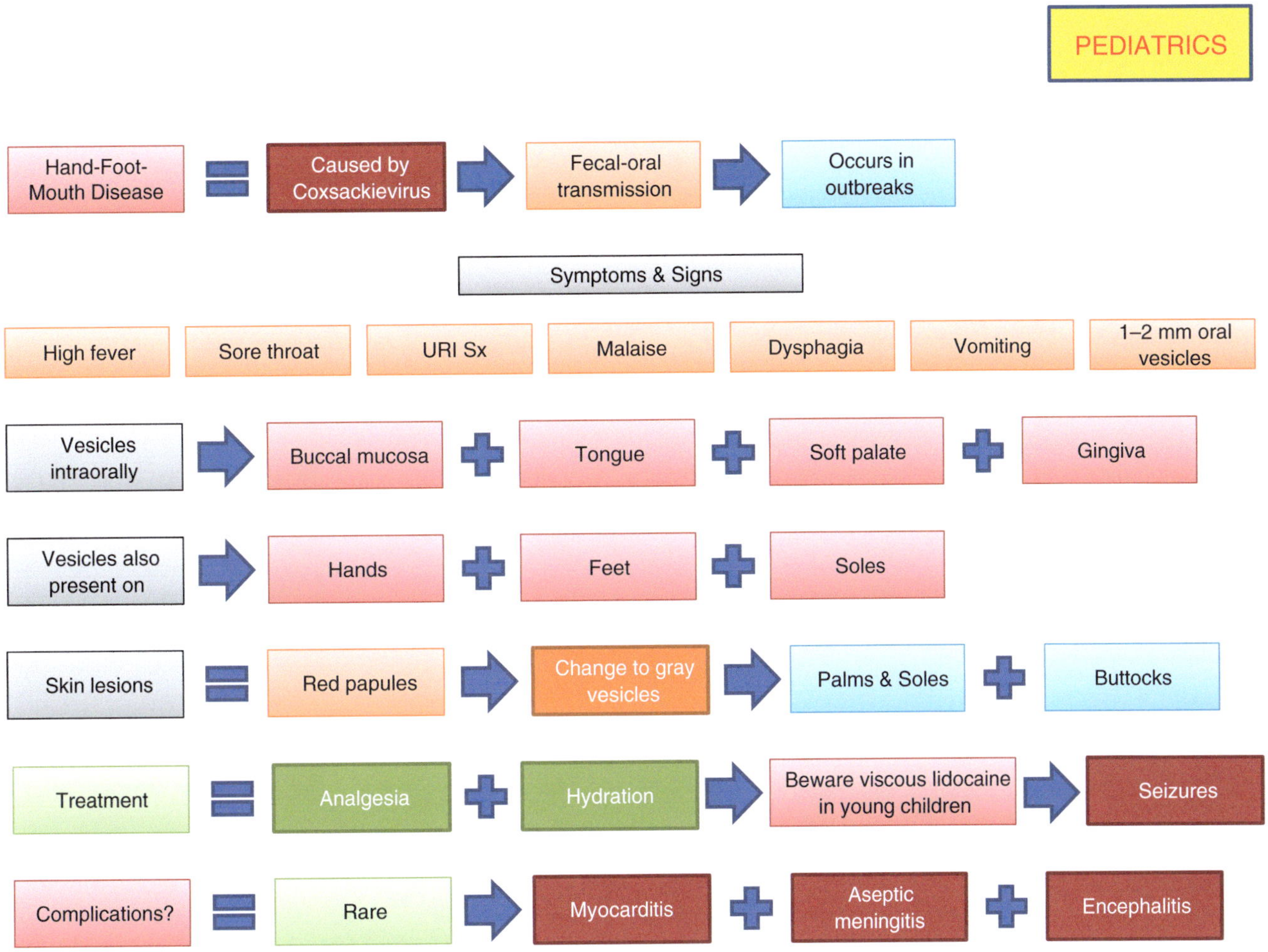

Henoch-Schonlein Purpura (HSP)

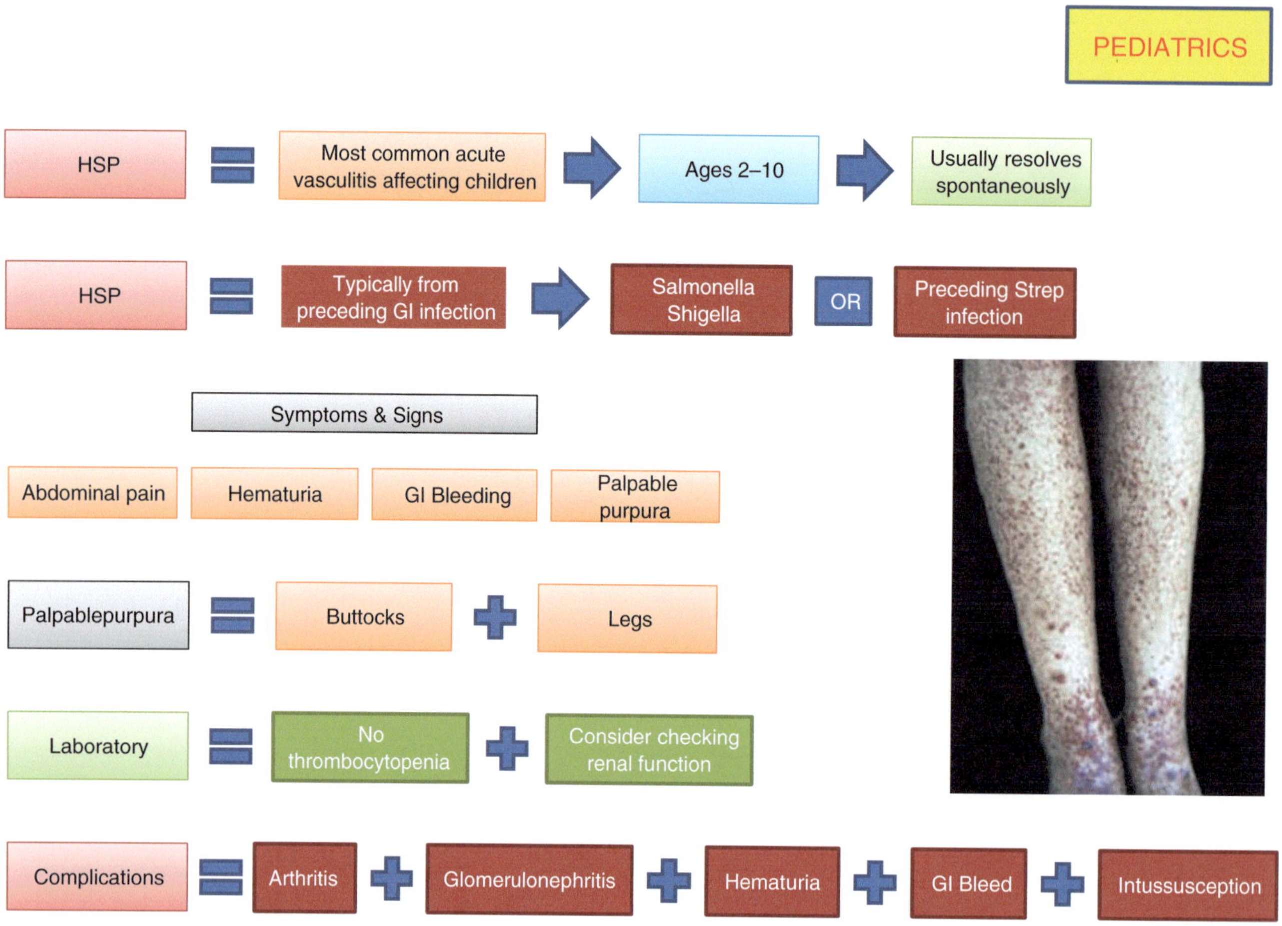

Right side image (Reprinted from Zaidi Z, Lanigan SW. Vasculitis, common erythemas, and lymphatic disorders. In: Zaidi Z, Lanigan SW, editors. Dermatology in clinical practice. London: Springer; 2010. p. 253–70. With permission from Springer Verlag

Kawasaki's Disease

PEDIATRICS

Kawasaki's Disease = Mucocutaneous lymph node syndrome → Ages 2–5 → Typically in males & of Asian descent → Self-limited vasculitis; Predilection for coronary arteries

Criteria for Diagnosis = Fever >5 days PLUS 4

- Eyes: Bilateral conjunctival injection
- Oral: Strawberry tongue; Lip fissures & cracking
- Skin: Erythematous rash starting on palms & soles; Swelling or desquamation of fingers & toes
- Nodes: Enlarged (≥15 mm) cervical lymph nodes

Laboratory = Increased WBC + Elevated ESR + Increased platelets

Treatment = Aspirin + IV immunoglobulin

Complication = Coronary artery aneurysm

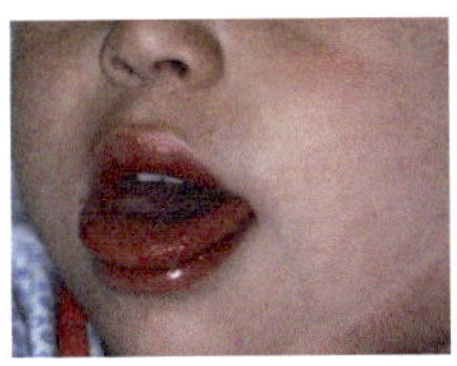
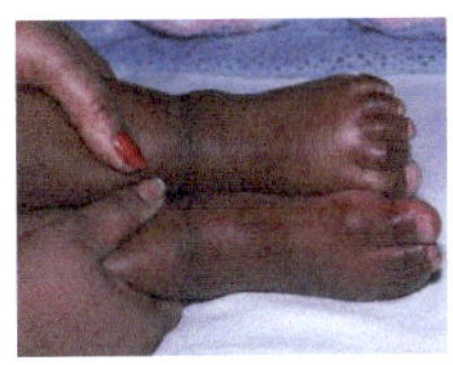
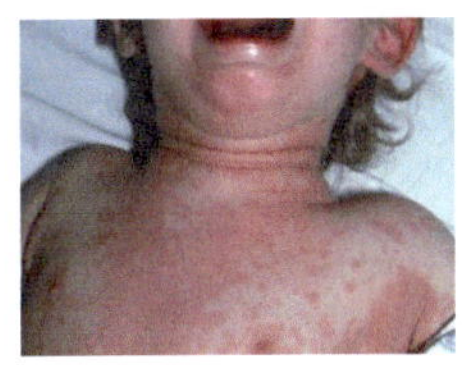

Scarlet Fever

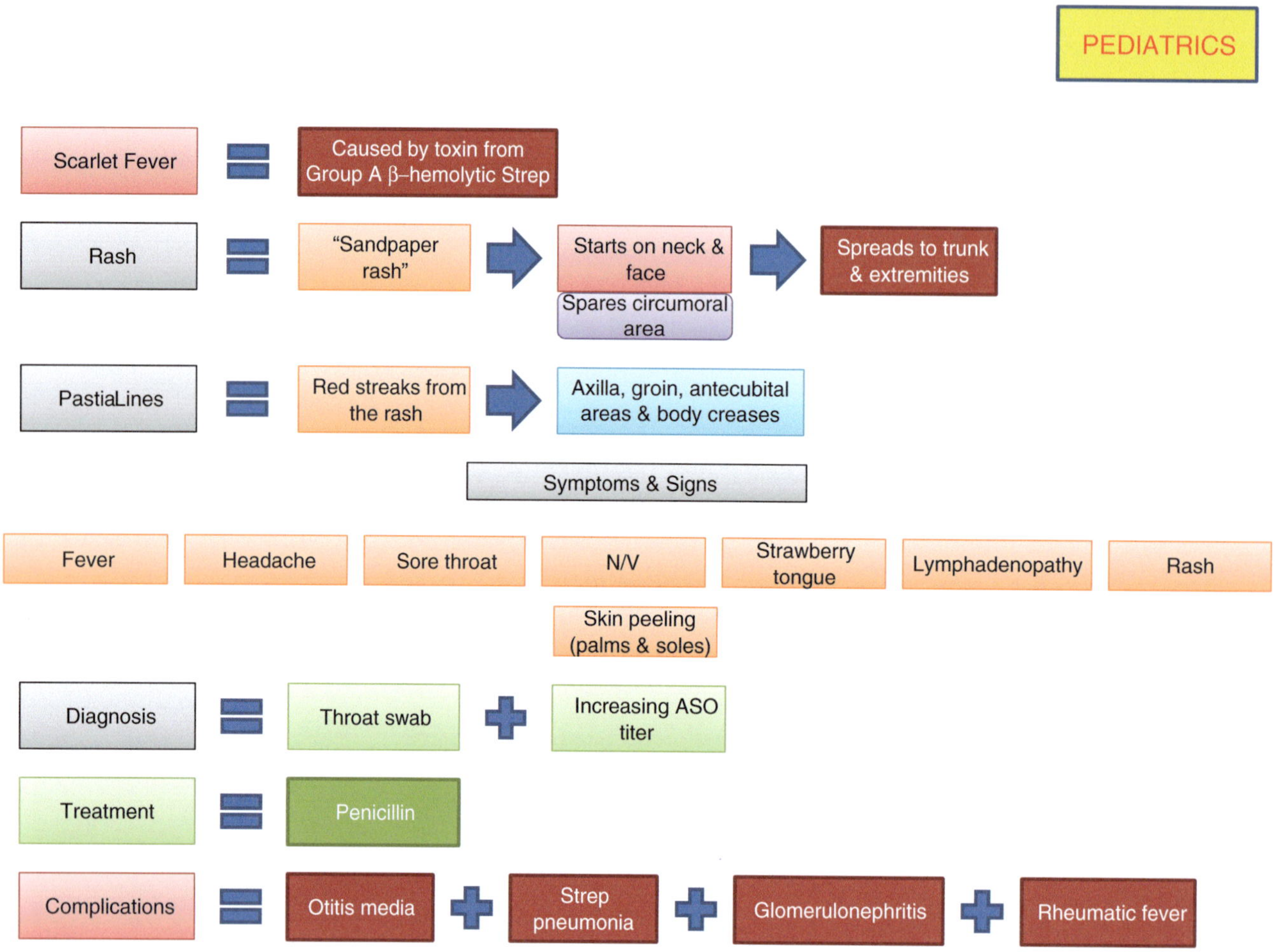

Miscellaneous Skin-Related Disorders

Venous Stasis Ulcers

Venous Stasis Ulcers = Result from chronic venous insufficiency → Caused by episodes of phlebitis or varicose veins → Poor venous return from LE leading to edema & stasis dermatitis

Risk Factors = Older age + Female + Pregnancy + Prolonged standing + Genetic + Tall person

Tidbits = Medial distal legs & pretibial areas most affected for dermatitis
Ulcers – medial & lateral malleolus
|| Honey crusted lesions or pustules? = Secondary infection → Cellulitis or lymphangitis

Symptoms & Signs

- Dependent edema
- Erythema
- Hyperpigmentation Orange/Brown
- Ulceration in severe cases
- Pruritis

Diagnosis = Clinical

Treatment = Leg elevation + Support stockings + Anitbiotics for infection

Pilonidal and Sebaceous Cysts and Abscess

Pilonidal Cysts = Located along the gluteal fold → These sinuses are lined with squamous epithelium & hair → Sinuses can get blocked & lead to bacterial infection

Organisms = Skin flora → *Staphylococcus* spp
Most common

Sebaceous cysts = Occur diffusely → Blockage of sebaceous gland duct may lead to bacterial infection

Symptoms & Signs

- Tender, swollen nodule along gluteal fold
  - For pilonidal
  - Sebaceous may be located anywhere
- Nodule is fluctuant
- May have surrounding erythema

Diagnosis = Clinical

Treatment = Incision & drainage + Packing → Antibiotics generally not needed

Pitfall = Not removing capsule of sebaceous cyst → May lead to recurrence

Decubitus Ulcers

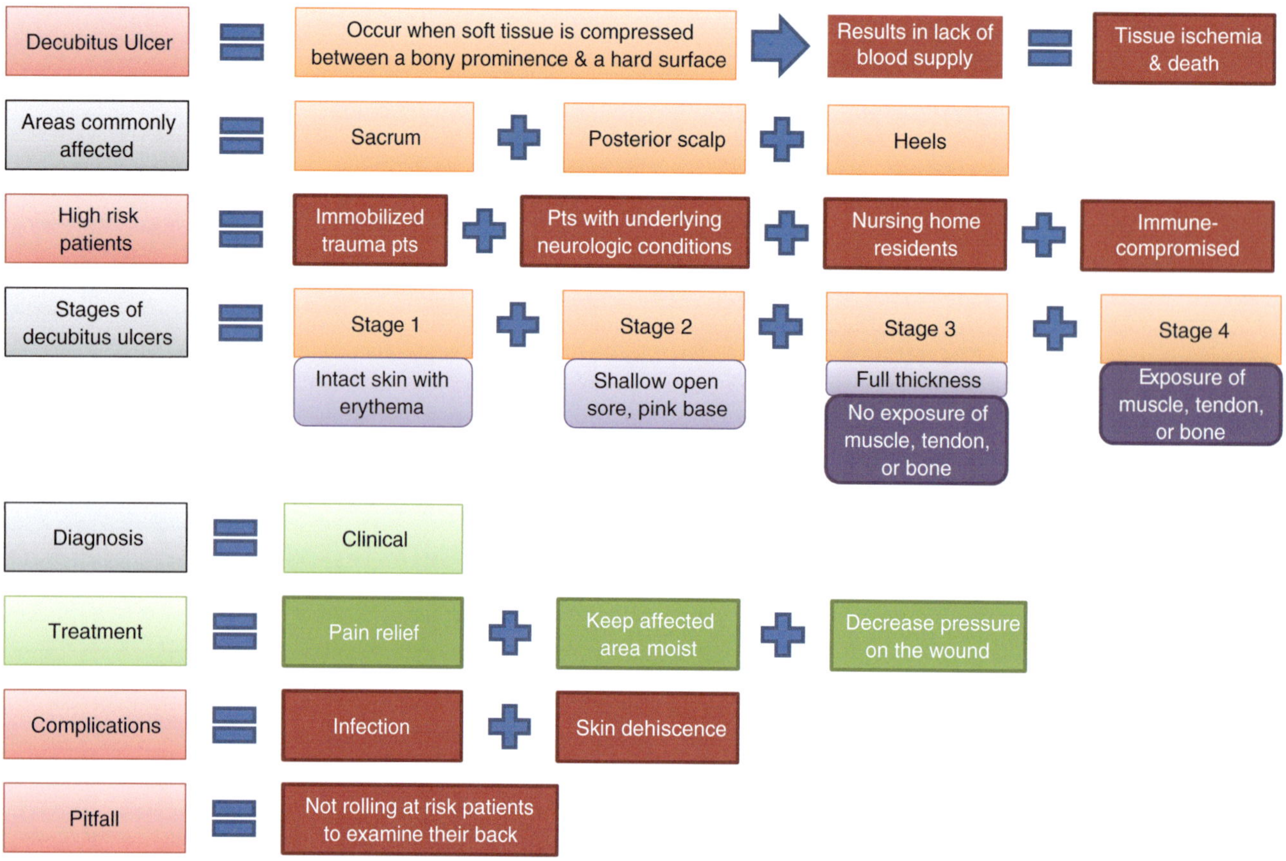

Lipoma

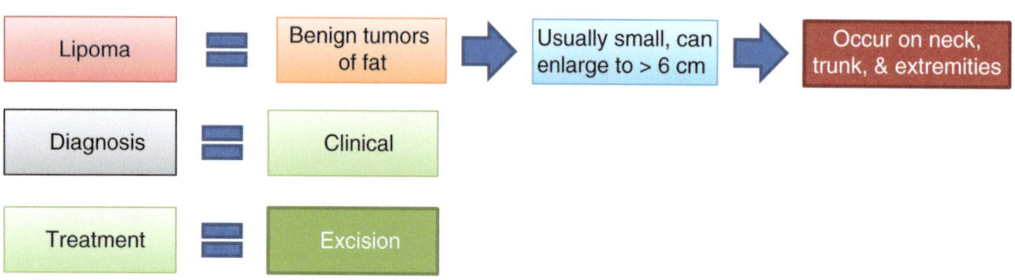

Hemangiomas

PEDIATRICS

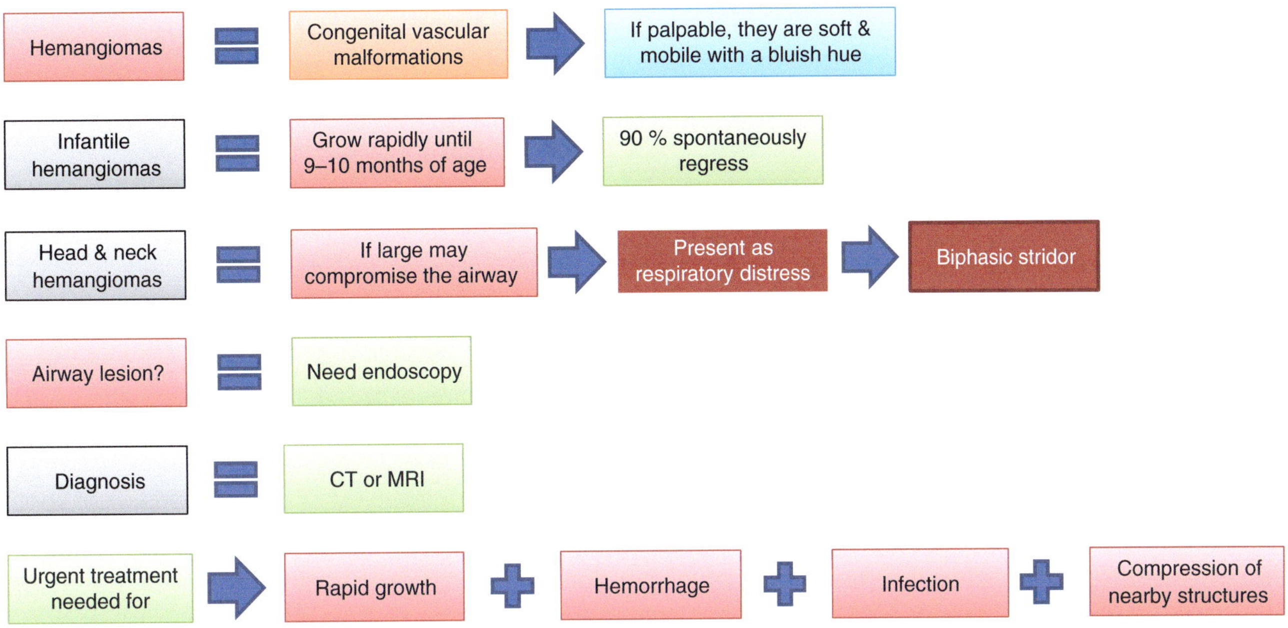

Lymphangiomas (Cystic Hygroma)

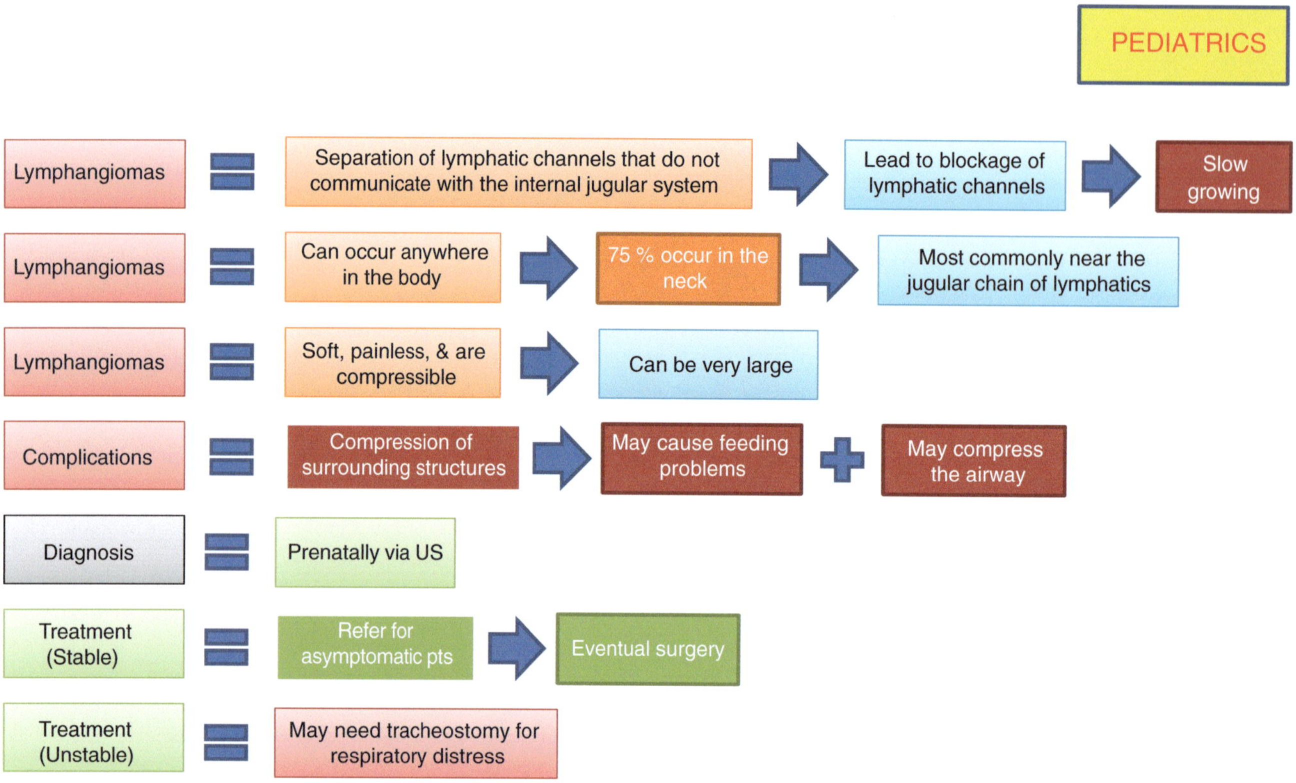

Endocrine/Metabolic/Electrolytes

Bobby Desai

Contents

Hypoglycemia ... 390
Diabetes Mellitus ... 393
Diabetic Ketoacidosis ... 395
Alcoholic Ketoacidosis ... 401
Hyperosmolar Hyperglycemic Nonketotic Syndrome ... 404
Thyroid Disorders ... 407
Hypothyroidism and Myxedema Coma ... 408
Hyperthyroidism and Thyroid Storm ... 415
Adrenal Insufficiency and Crisis ... 423
Pheochromocytoma ... 429
ADH-Related Diseases ... 430
Electrolytes and Acid-Base ... 437
The Osmolal Gap ... 466

B. Desai, MD, MEd
Department of Emergency Medicine, University of Florida,
Gainesville, FL, USA
e-mail: bdesai@ufl.edu

B. Desai, B.R. Allen (eds.), *Nailing the Written Emergency Medicine Board Examination*,
DOI 10.1007/978-3-319-30838-8_7

Hypoglycemia

Agents for Glucose Control

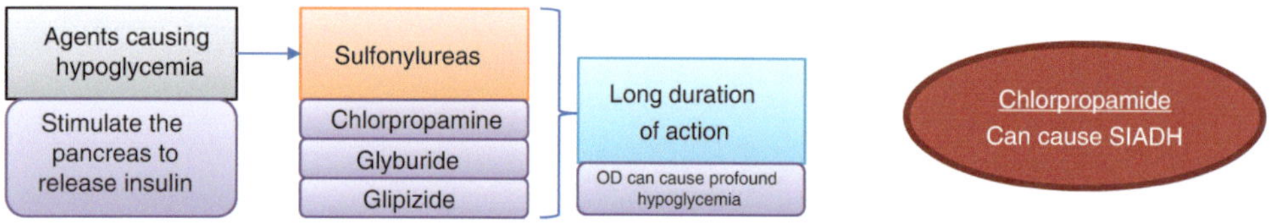

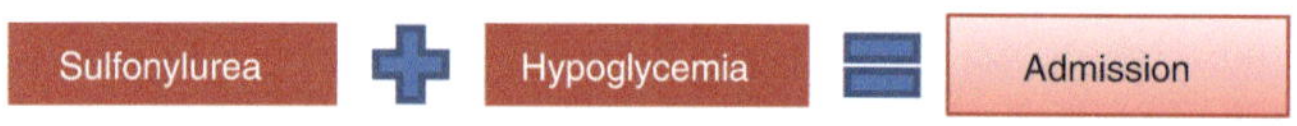

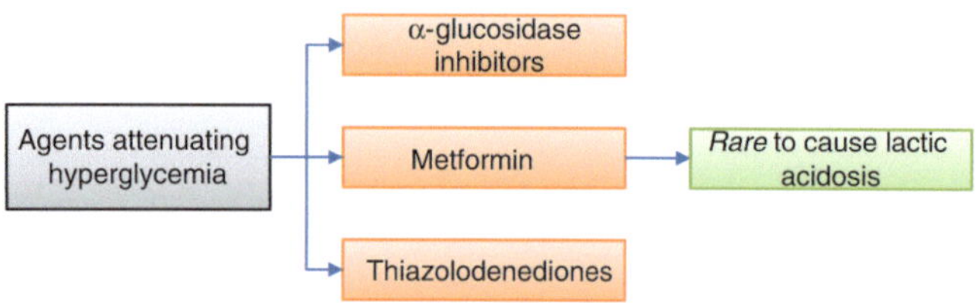

Hypoglycemia

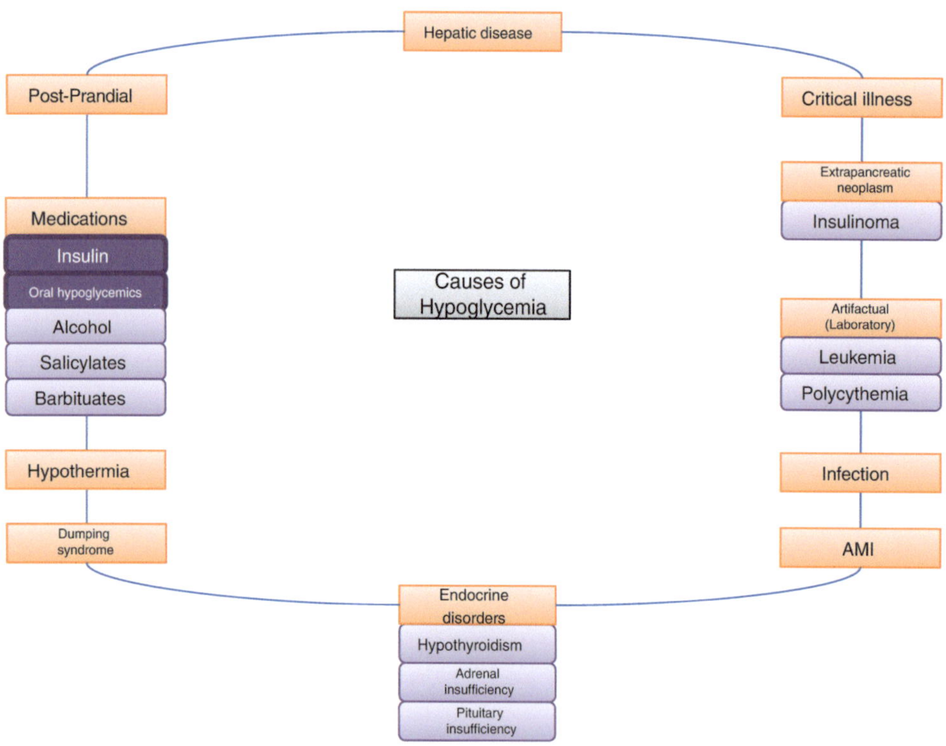

Hypoglycemia: Clinical Features

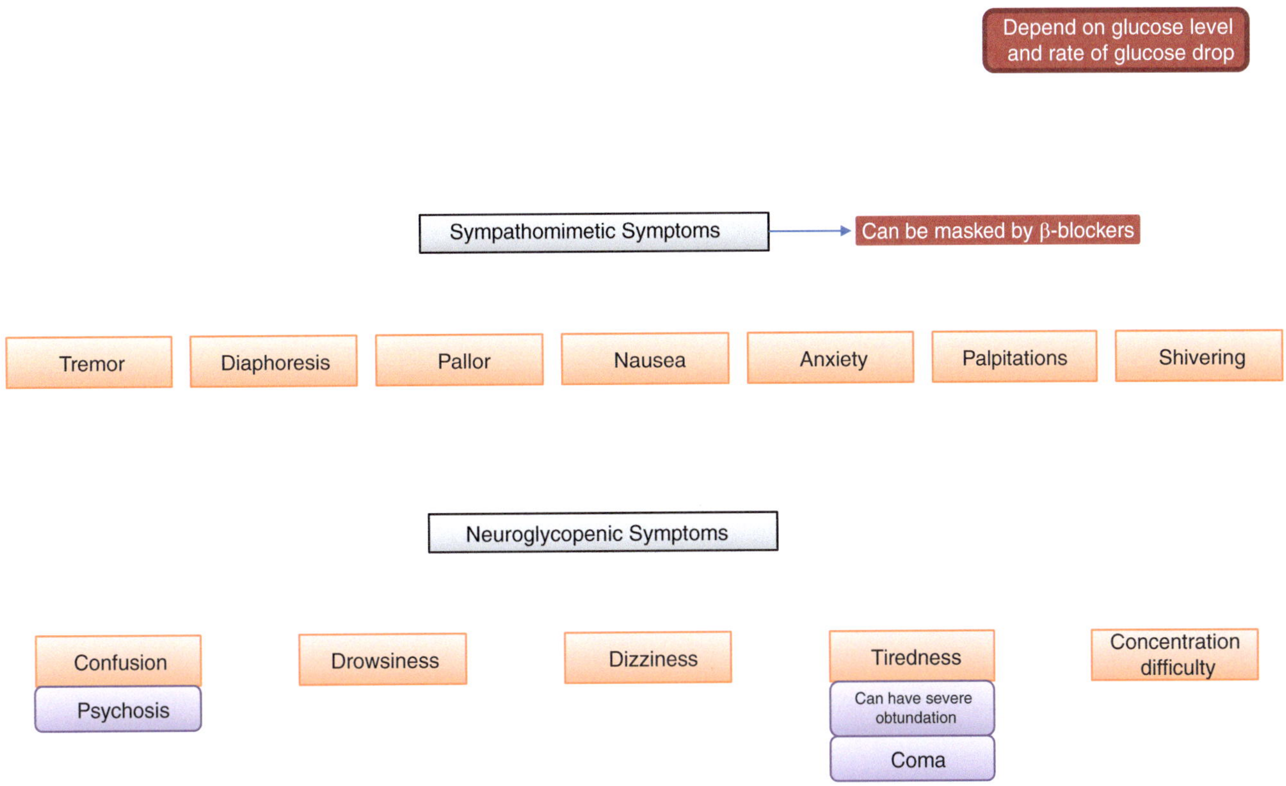

Tidbits of Hypoglycemia

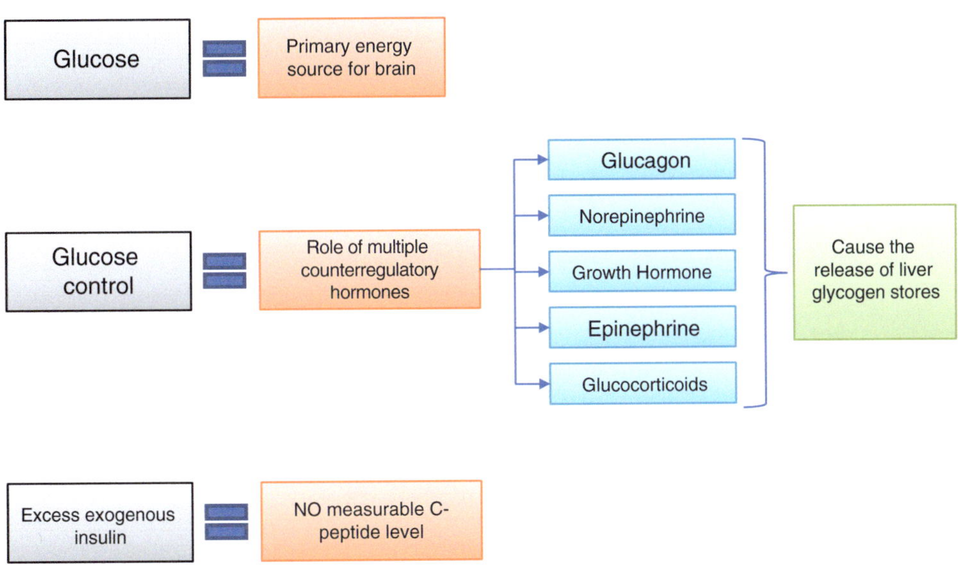

Hypoglycemia Differential Diagnosis

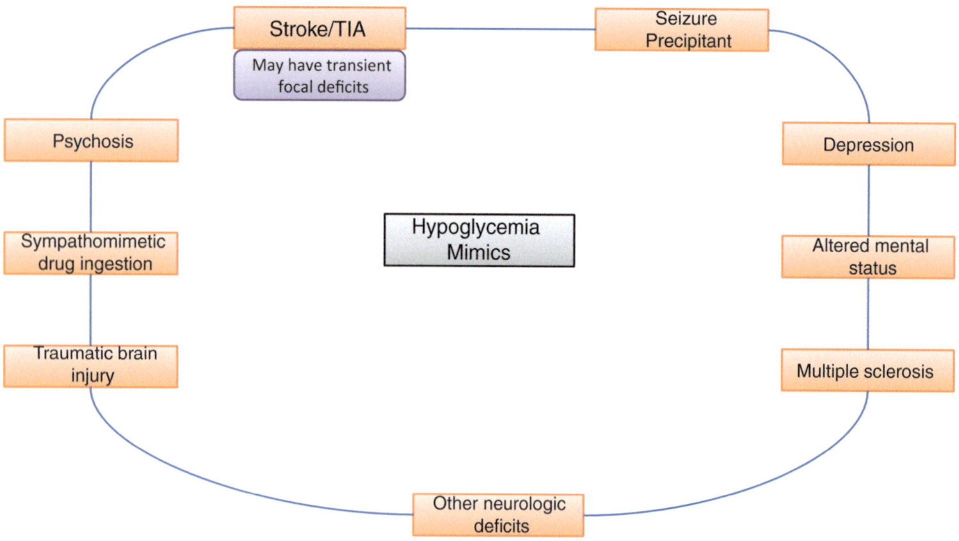

Treatment of Hypoglycemia

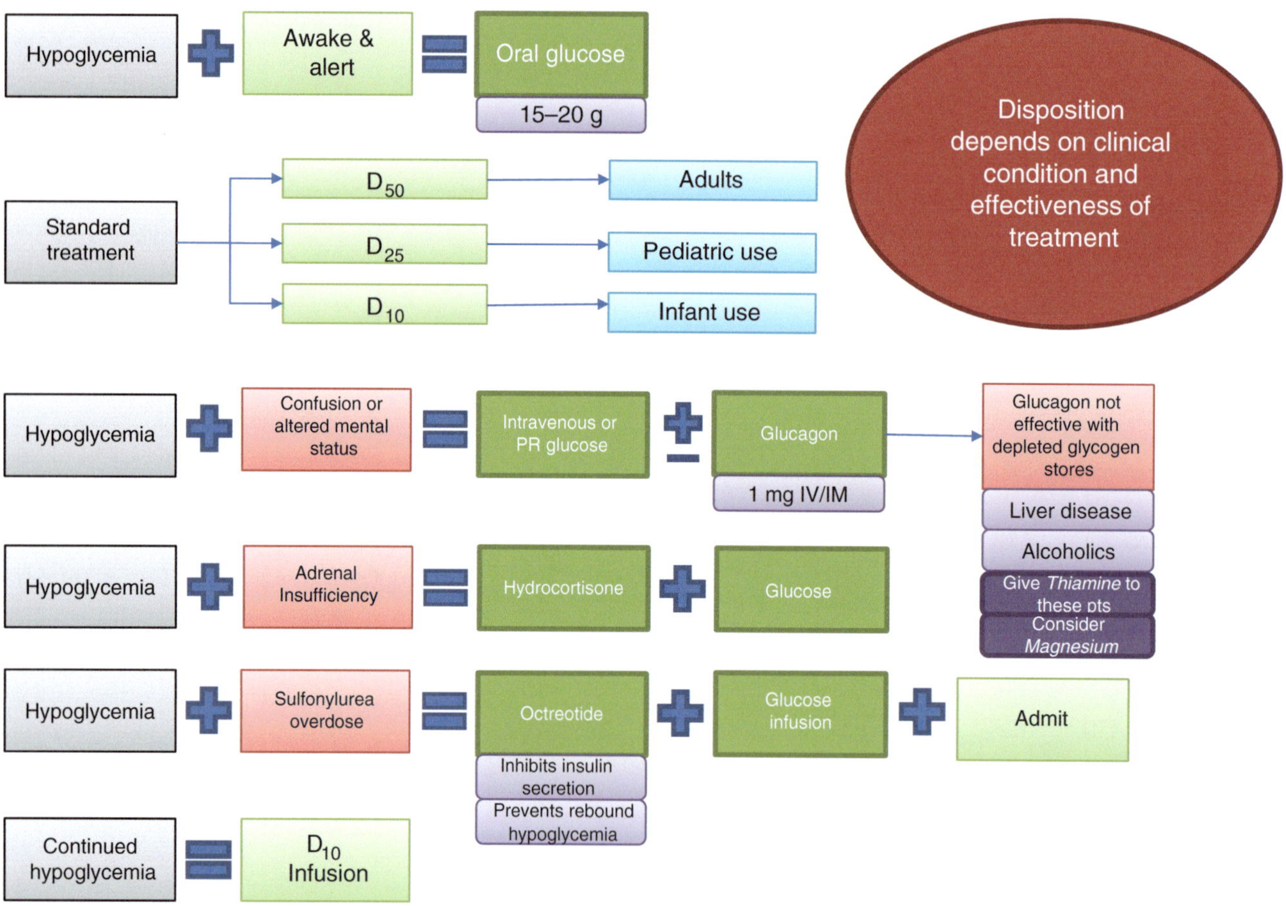

Diabetes Mellitus

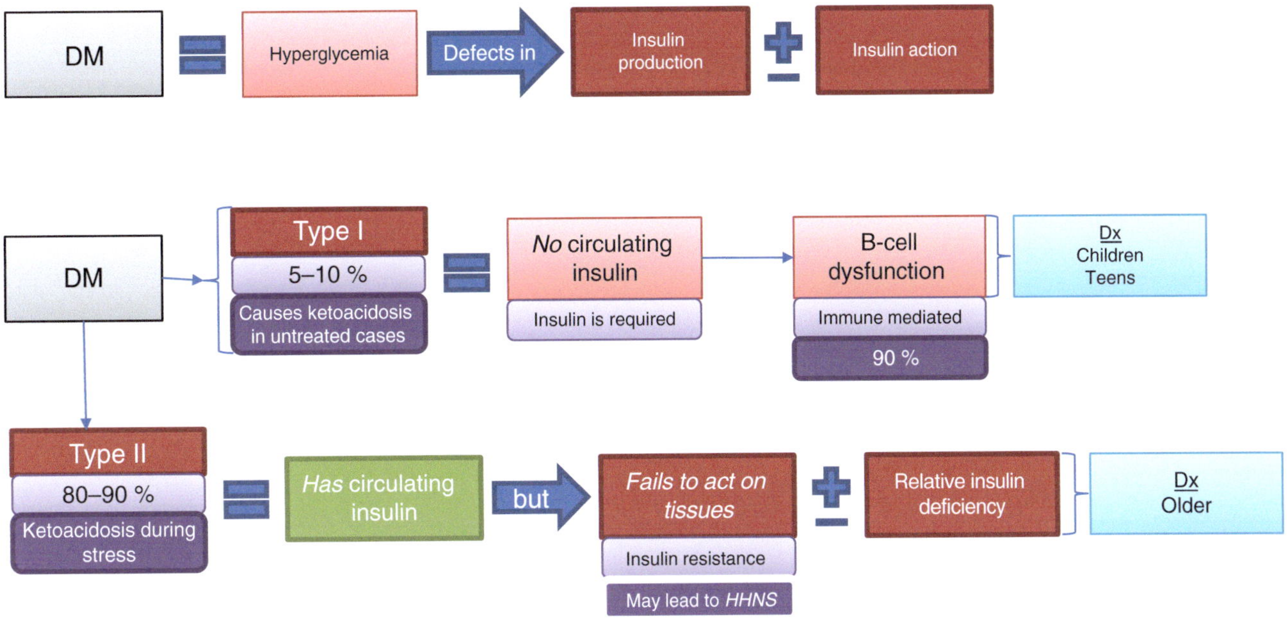

Tidbits About Hormones

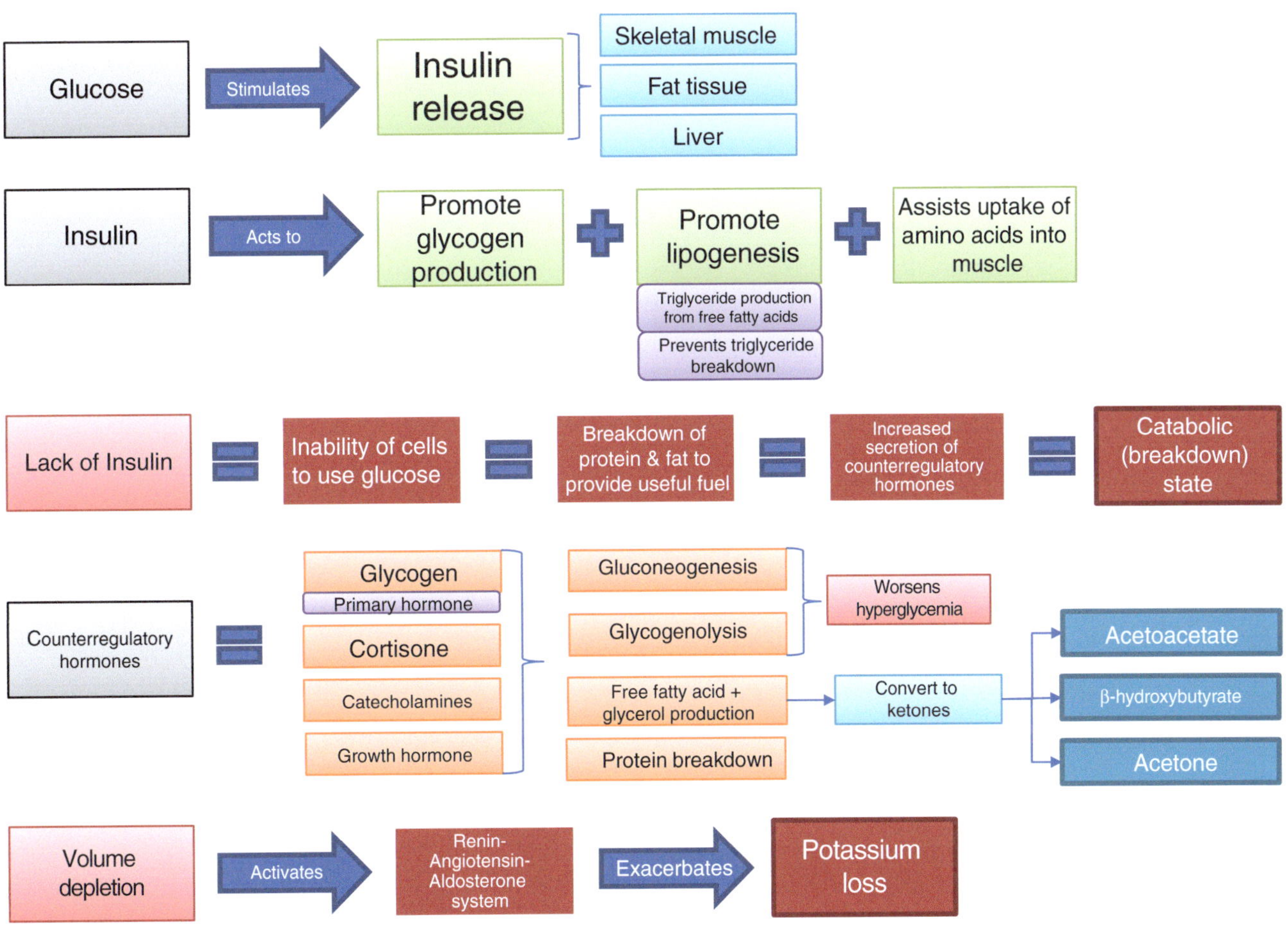

Types of Insulin

	Rapid	Short	Intermediate	Long
Time of Onset	6 – 15 min	15 – 60 min	1–4 hrs	90 min
Time to Peak	1–2 hrs	2–4 hrs	6–9 hrs	No peak
Duration of effect	3–6 hrs	6–8 hrs	6–24 hrs	24 hrs

Insulin Administration

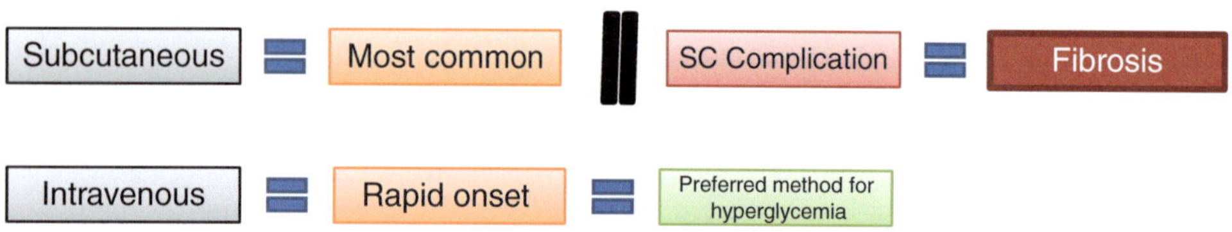

Insulin Pump

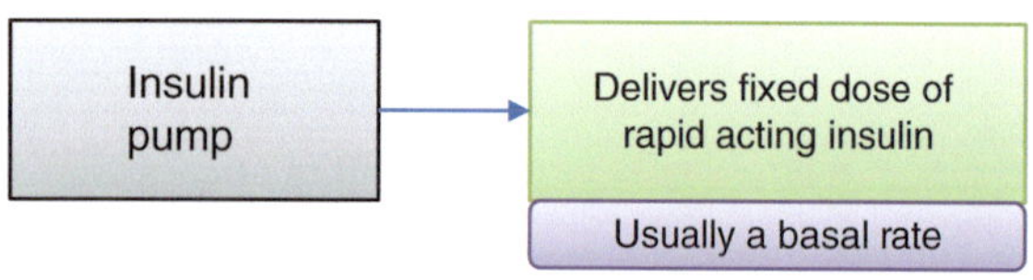

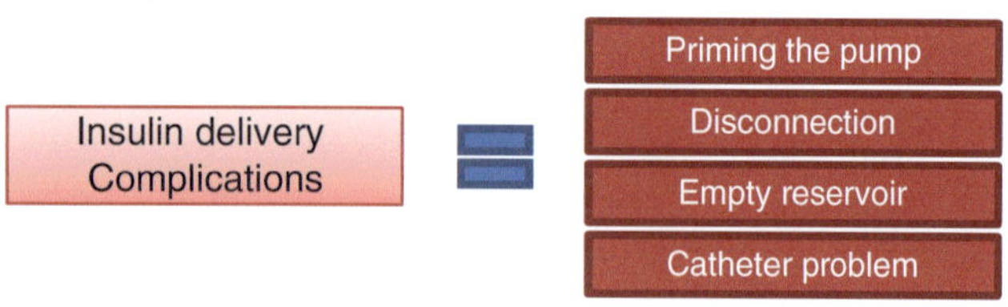

Diabetic Ketoacidosis

Some Causes of Diabetic Ketoacidosis

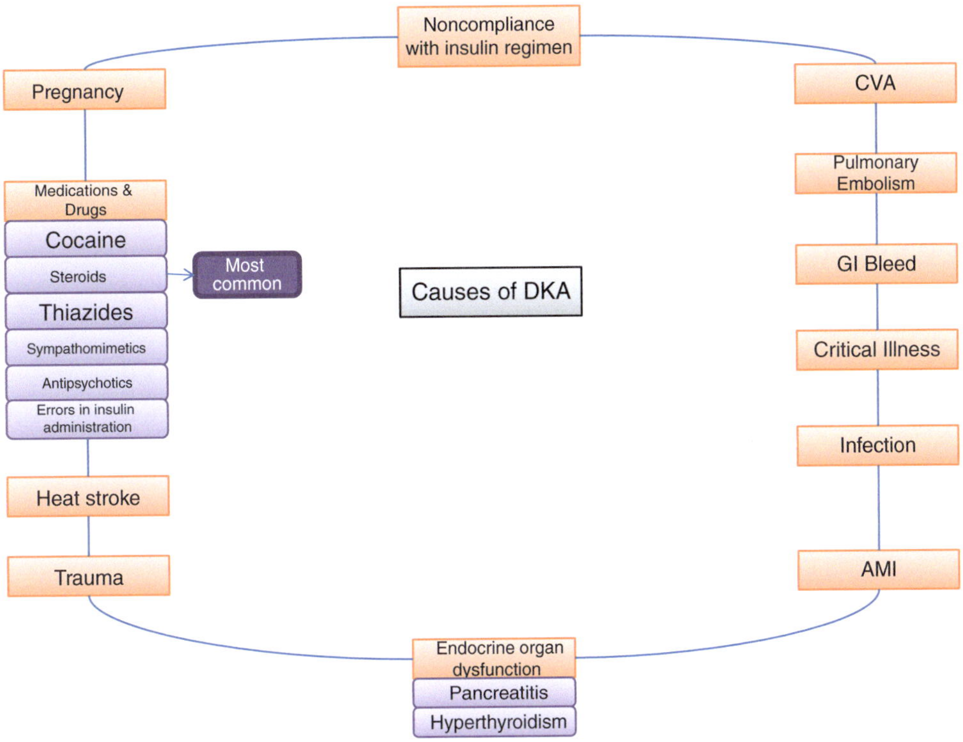

Diabetic Ketoacidosis

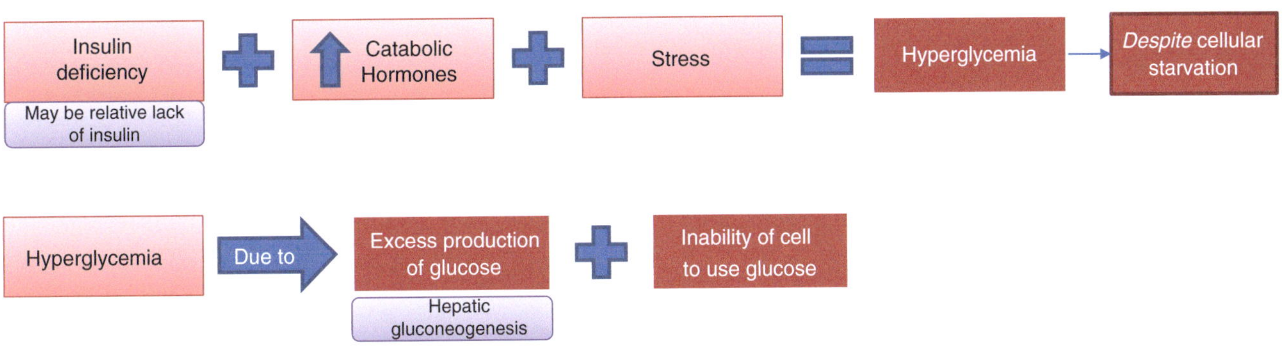

Effects of Hyperglycemia

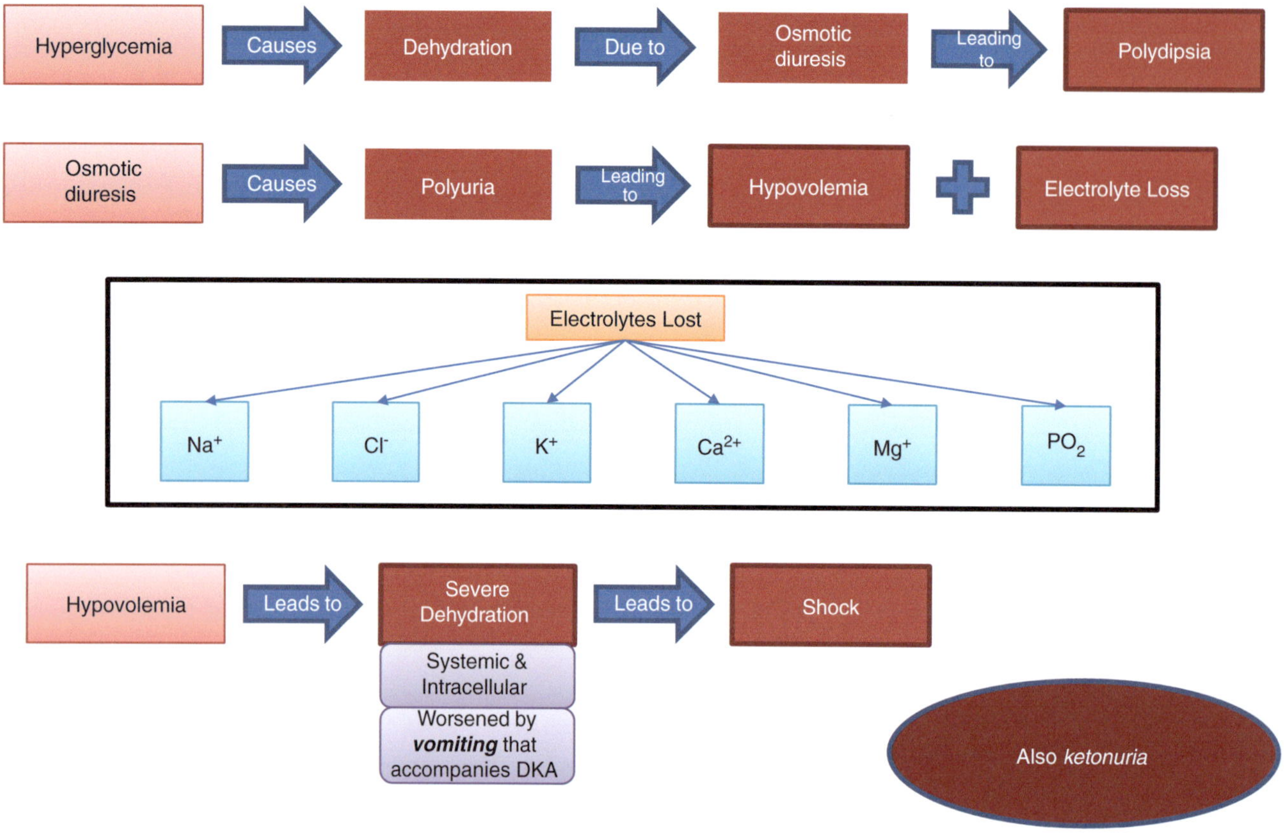

Systemic Effects of Hyperglycemia

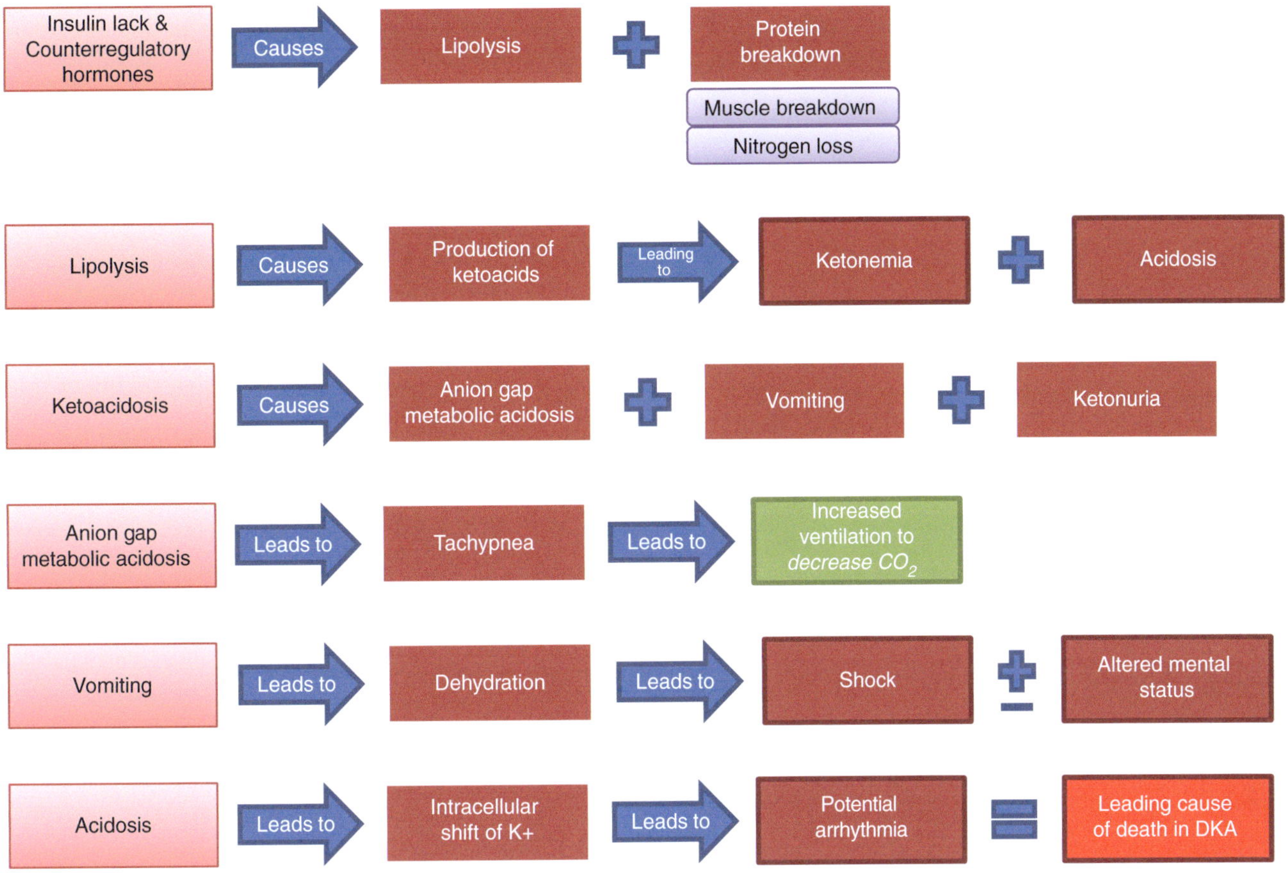

DKA: Clinical Features

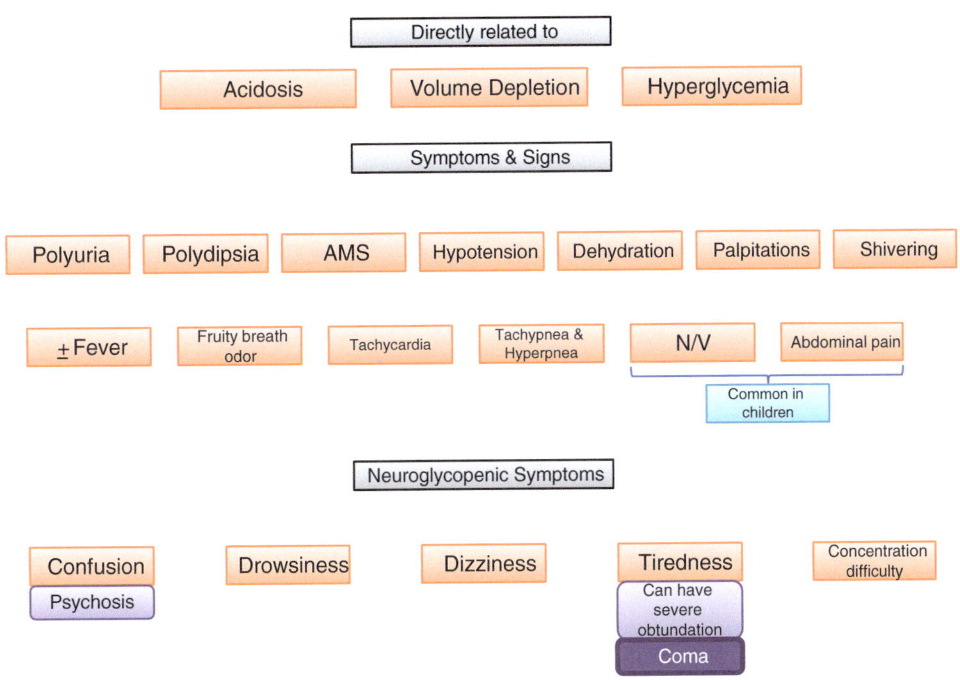

Diagnosis: DKA

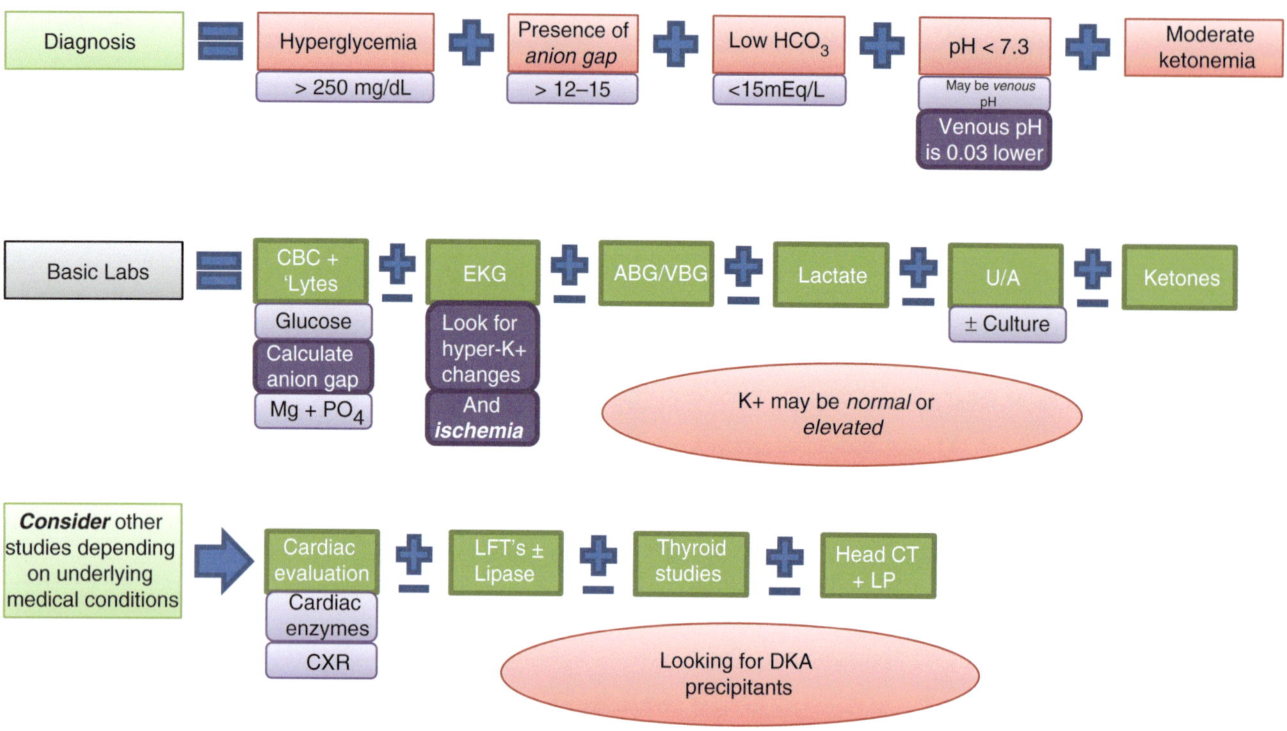

DKA Precipitants

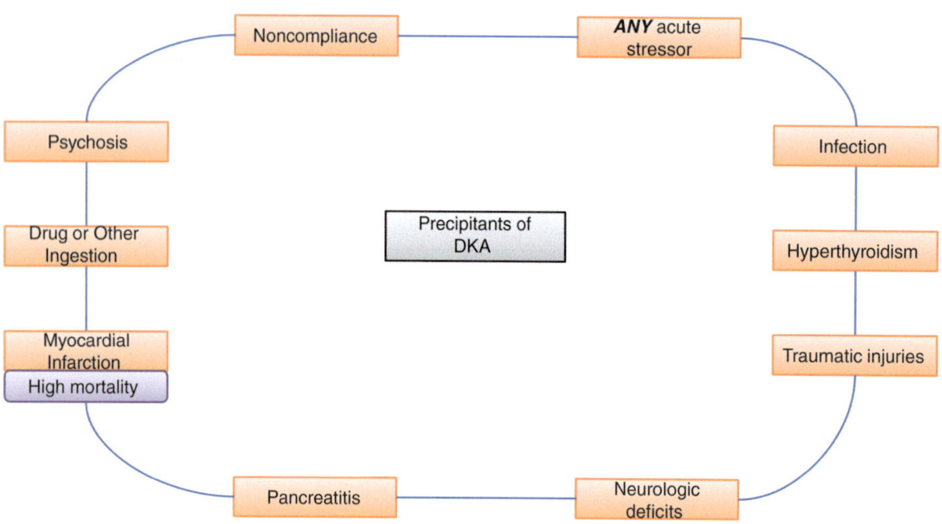

DKA Differential Diagnosis

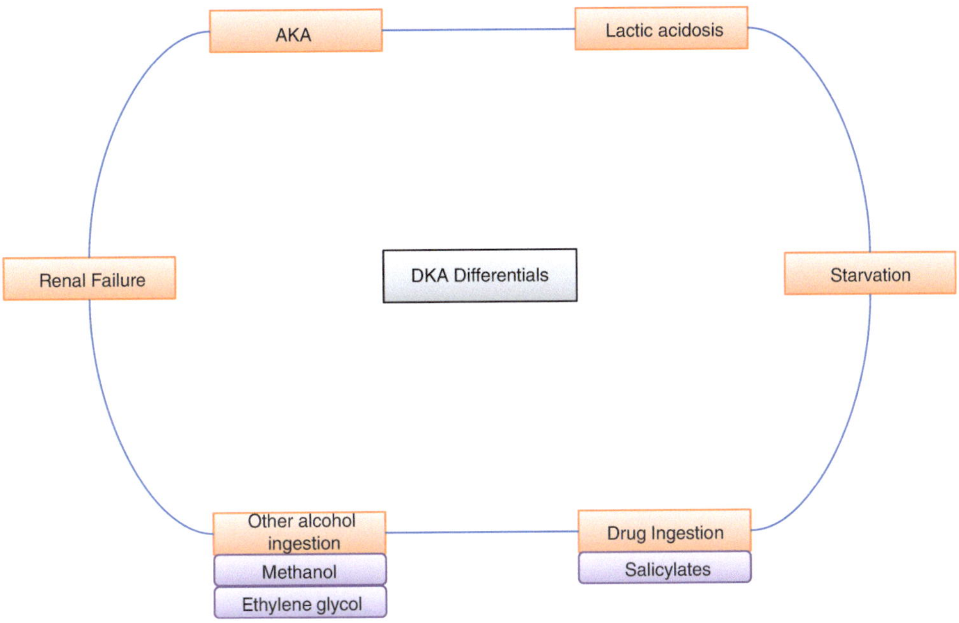

DKA Treatment

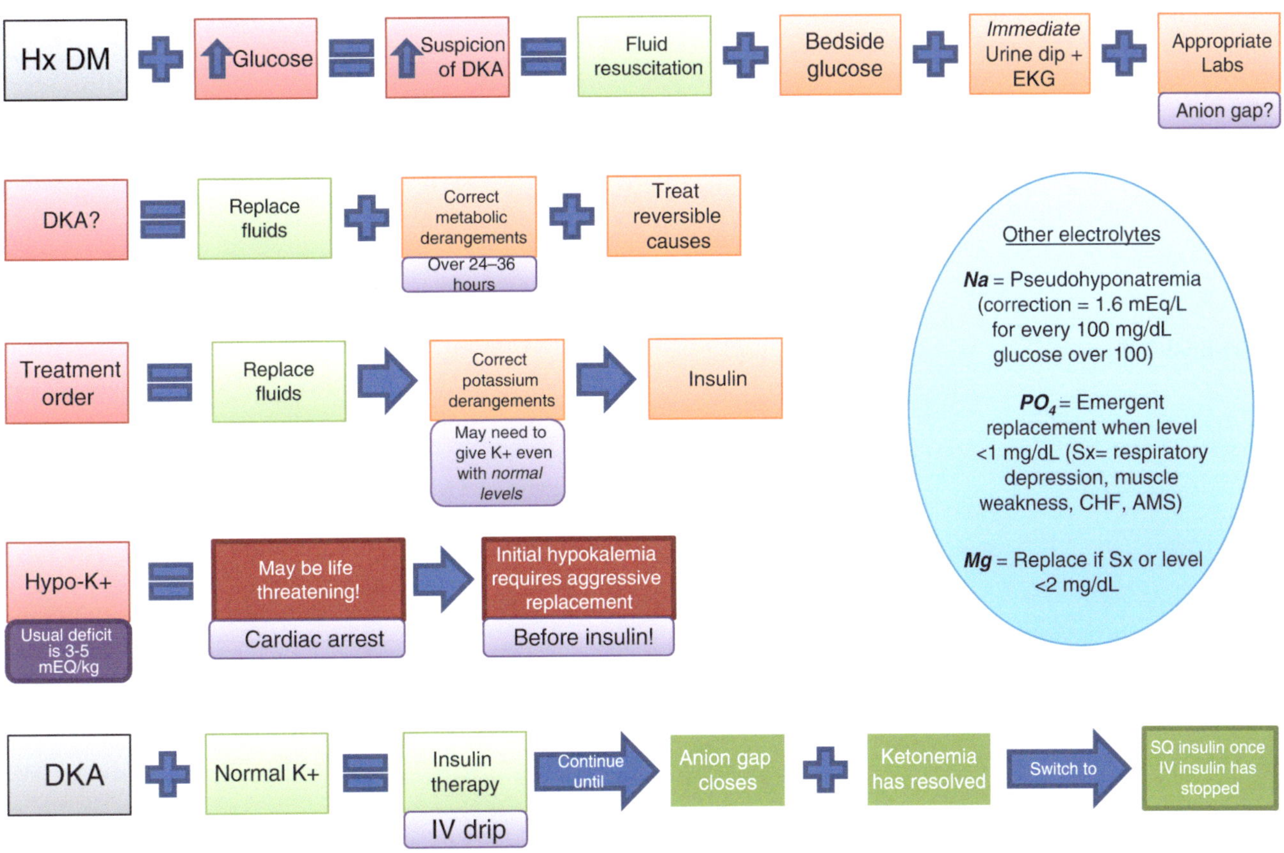

Bicarbonate in DKA

HCO_3 = Rarely indicated!

Potential complications = Cerebral edema (Especially in *children*) + Electrolyte problems (Hypo-K+; Hypo-PO_4) + Sodium overload + Impaired oxygen–hemoglobin dissociation (Curve shifts to *left*) + Paradoxical CSF acidosis (Also worsening *intracellular* acidosis)

DKA Complications

↑ Mortality = ↓ HCO_3 + ↑ Serum osmolarity + ↑ Glucose + ↑ BUN

Precipitating factors with highest mortality = MI + Infection

Over-aggressive fluids? = Acute Respiratory Distress Syndrome

Cerebral edema (High mortality) = Young persons + New-onset DM

Cerebral edema → May be due to → Over-hydration ± Osmotic changes ± Hypoxemia

Cerebral Edema

Symptoms/Signs

Bradycardia | Headache | Drowsiness or Obtundation | Incontinence | Pupillary changes | Seizures | Hypo-or Hyperthermia

Treatment (High mortality) = Intubation + Fluid restriction + Mannitol

Disposition

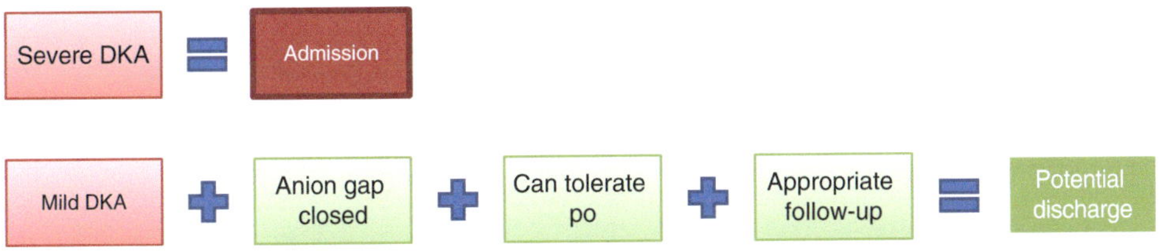

Alcoholic Ketoacidosis

Introduction

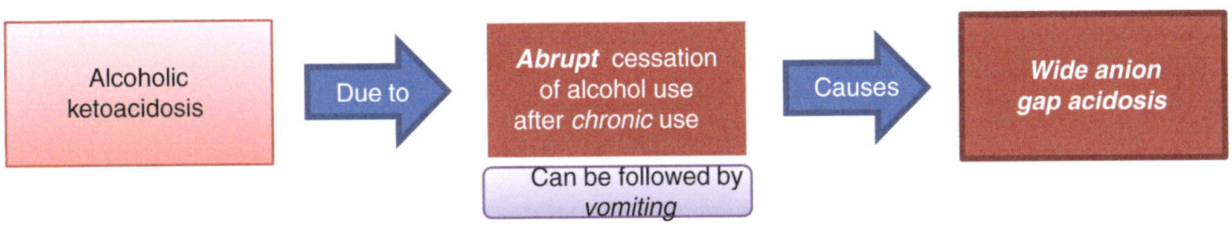

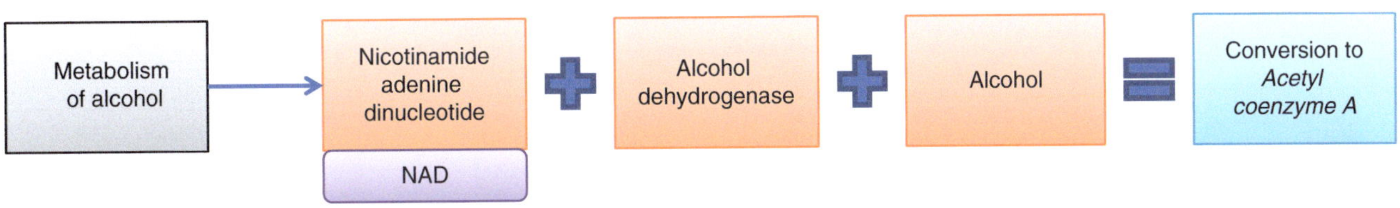

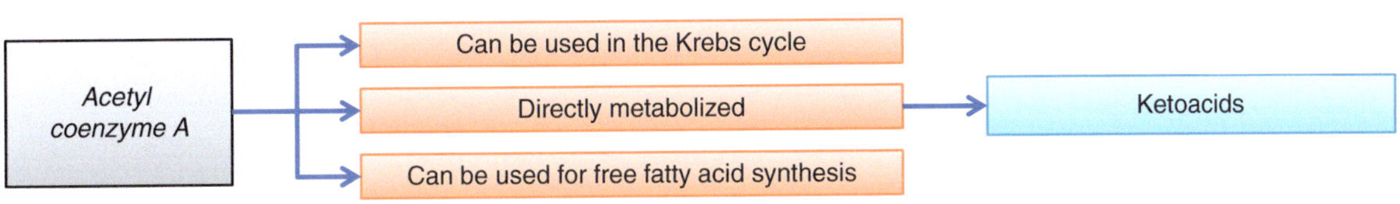

Pathophysiology

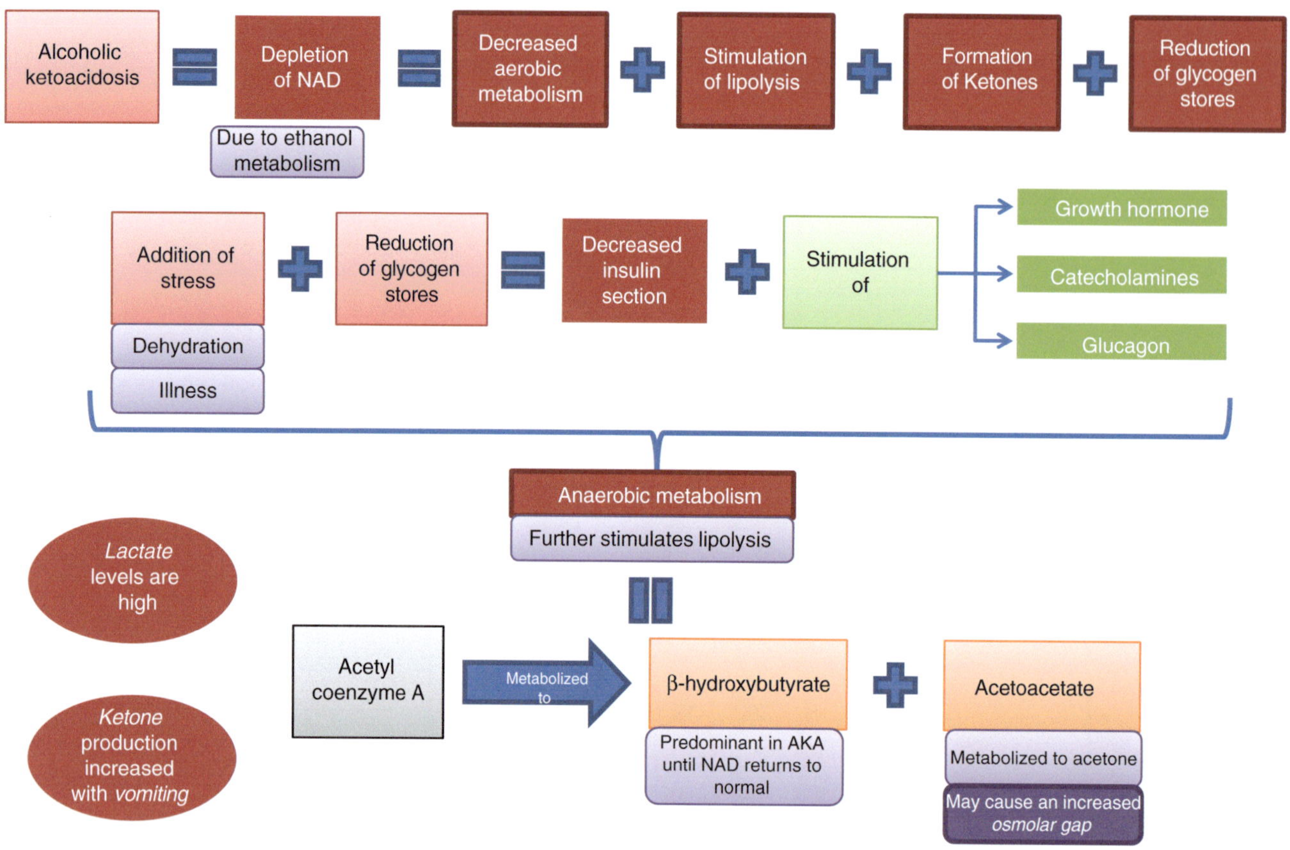

Alcoholic Ketoacidosis: Clinical Features

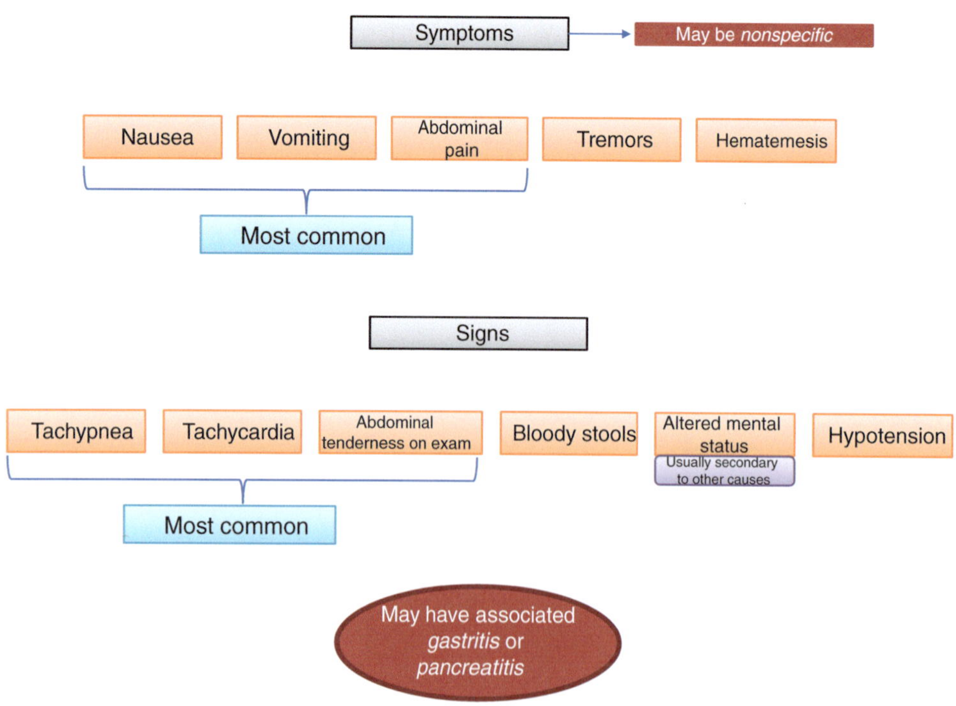

Diagnosis

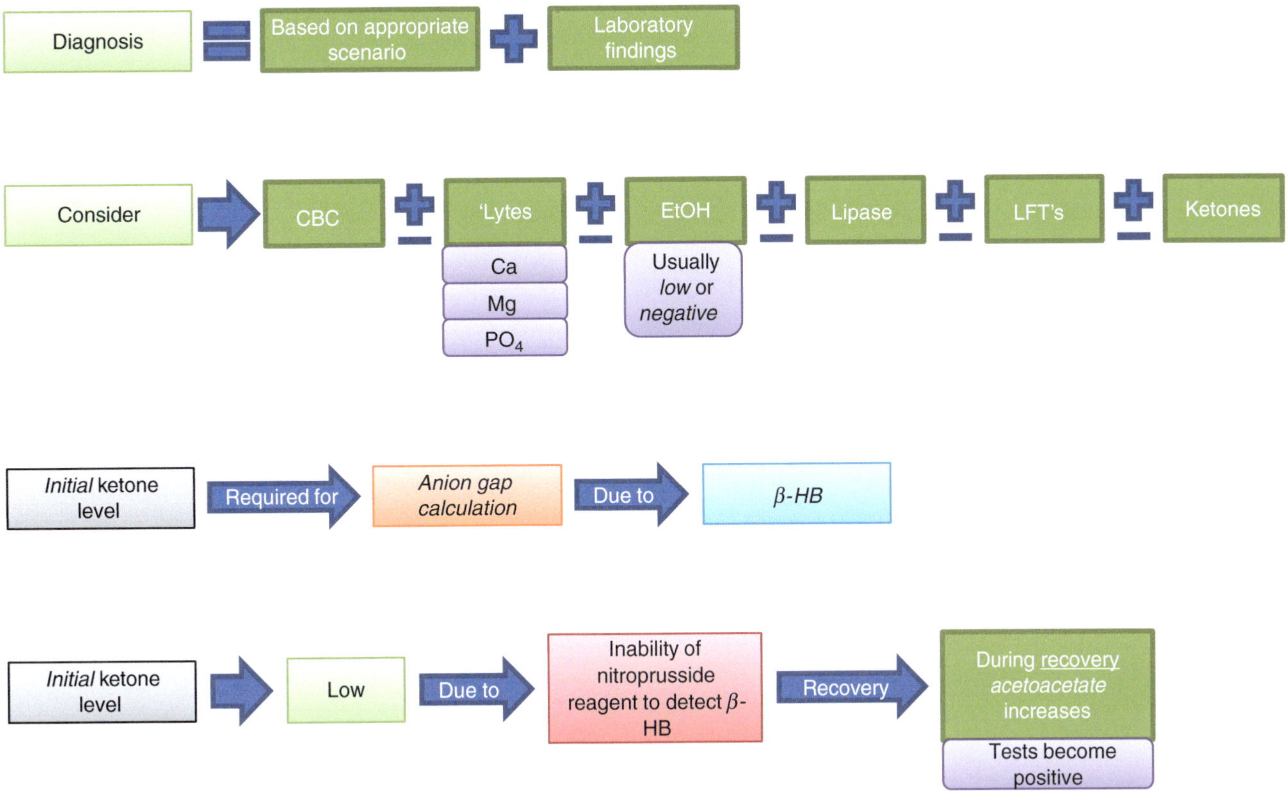

Treatment

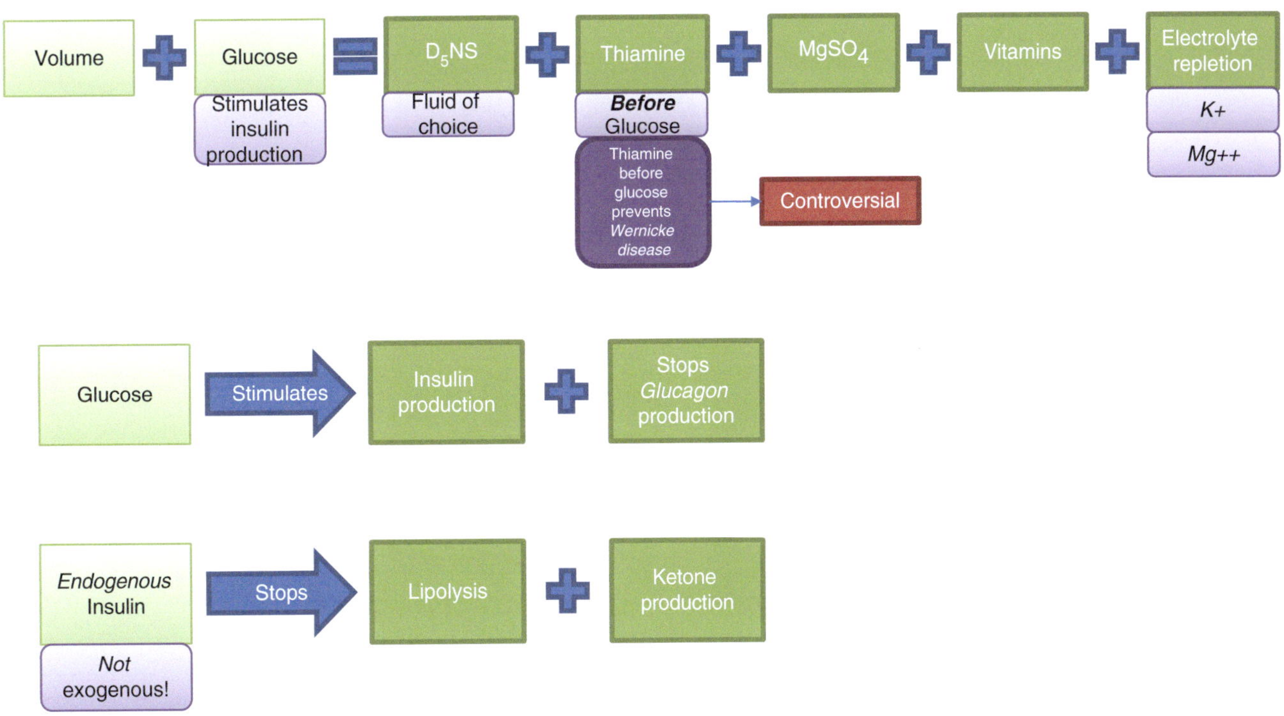

Disposition

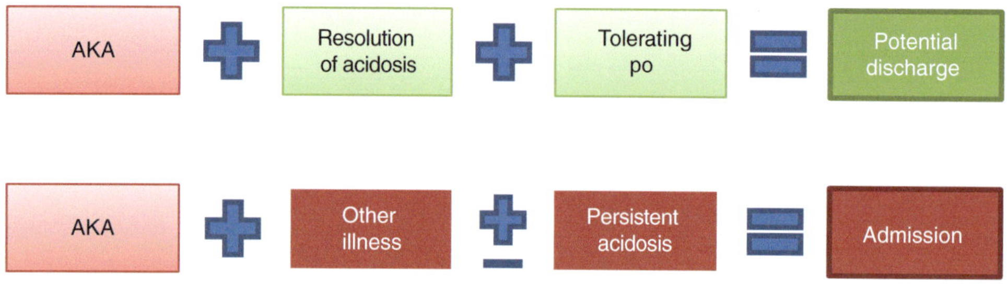

Hyperosmolar Hyperglycemic Nonketotic Syndrome

Introduction

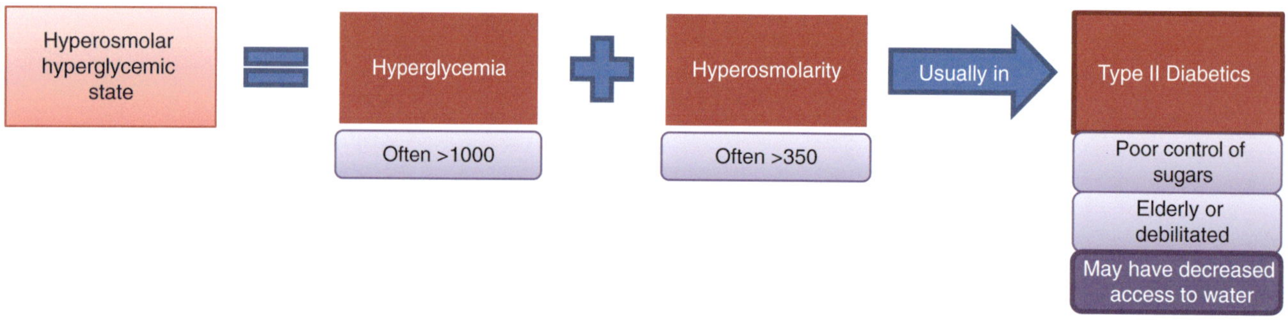

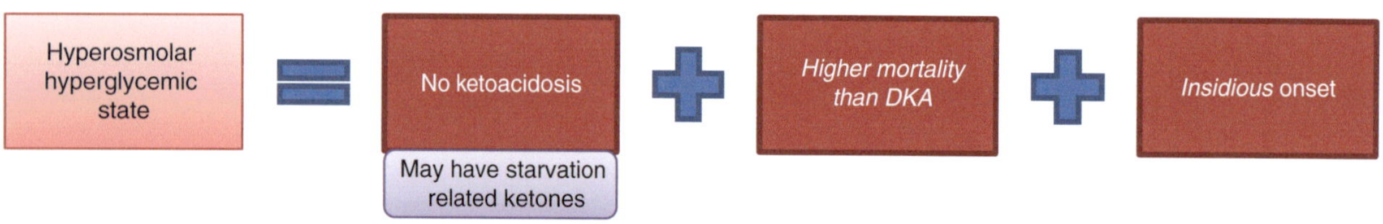

Pathophysiology

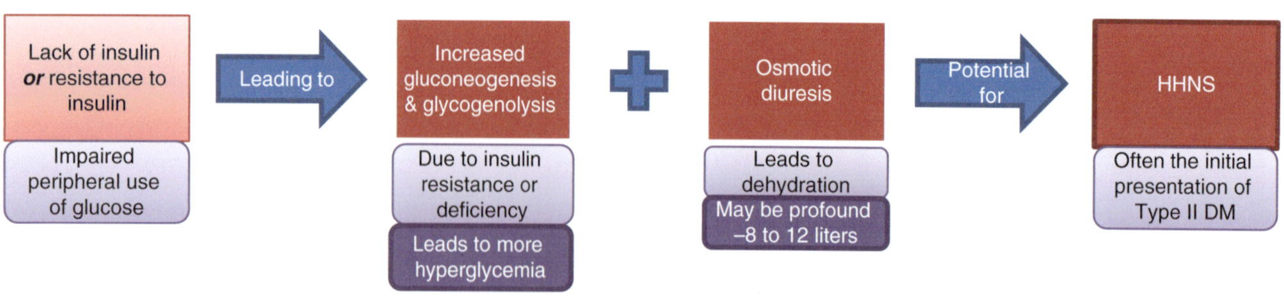

HHNS: Clinical Features

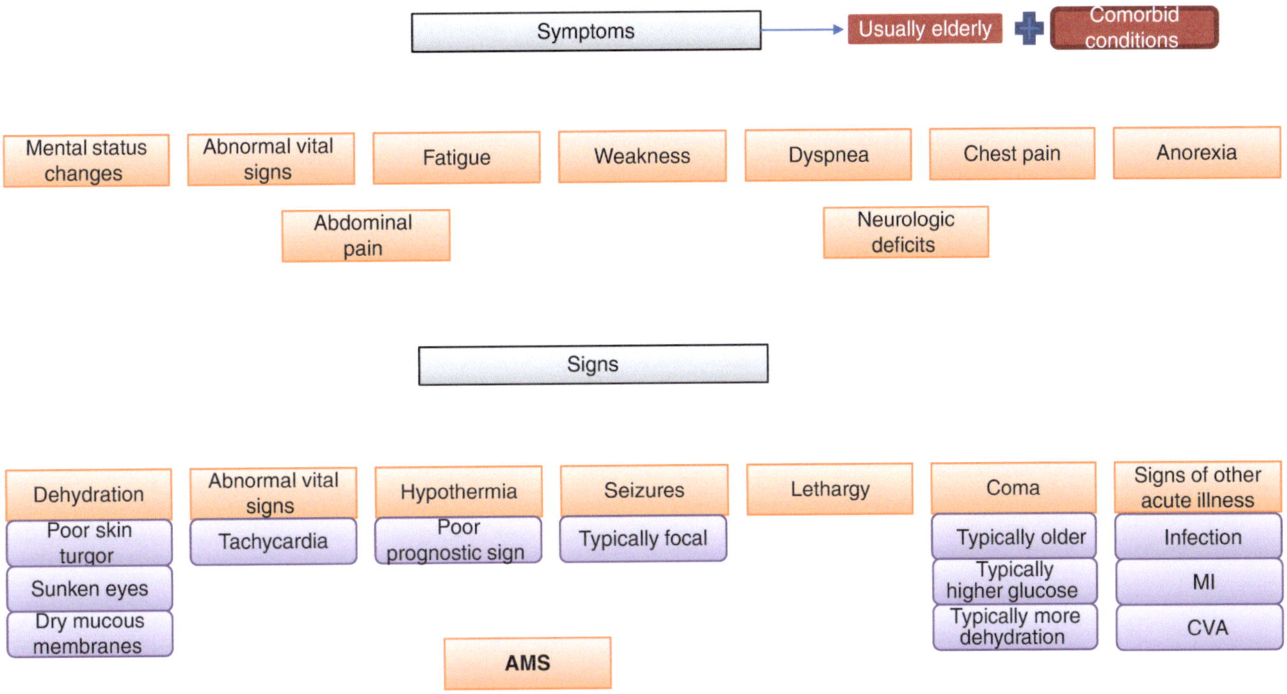

Precipitating Factors for HHNS

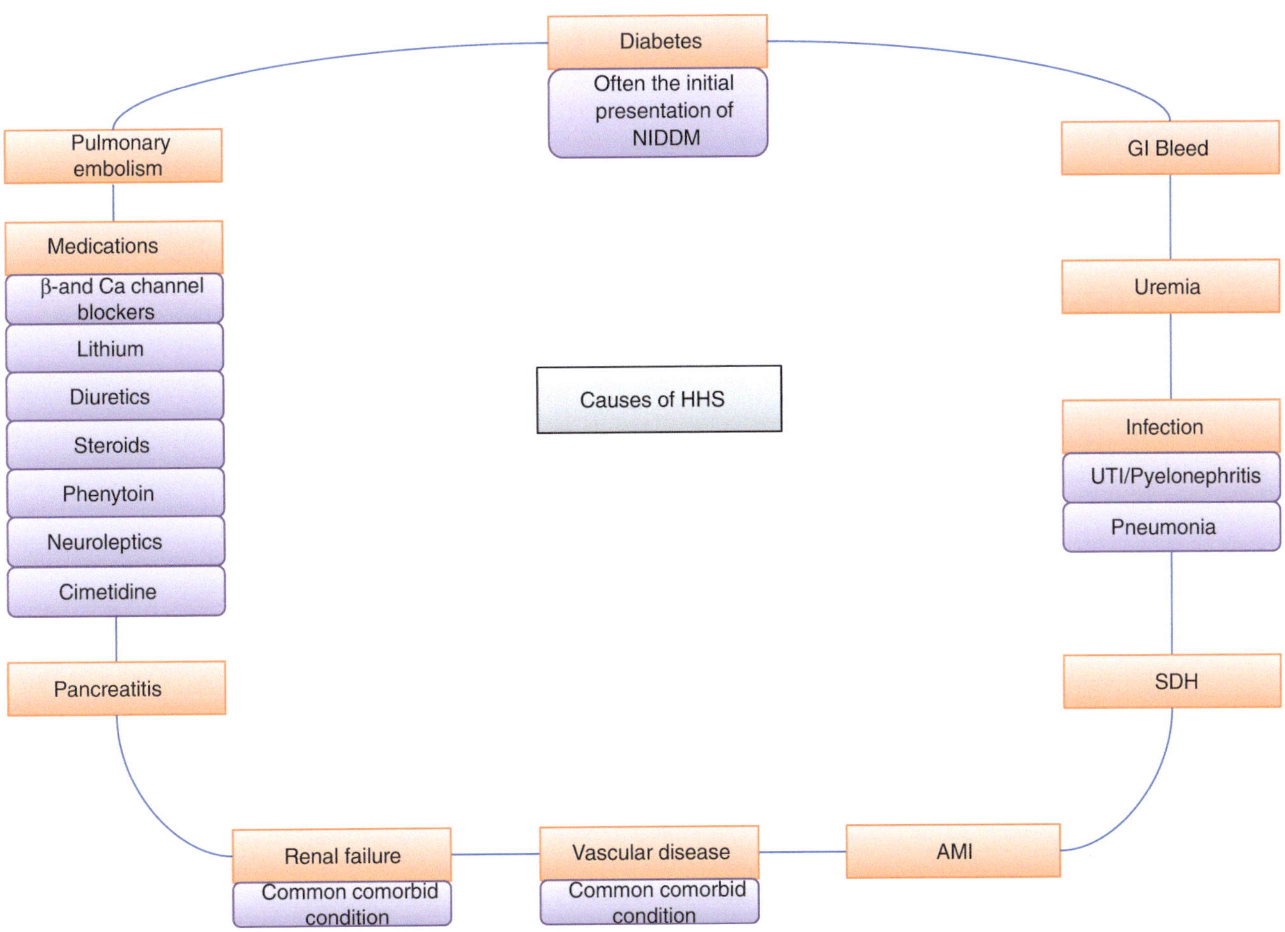

Diagnosis

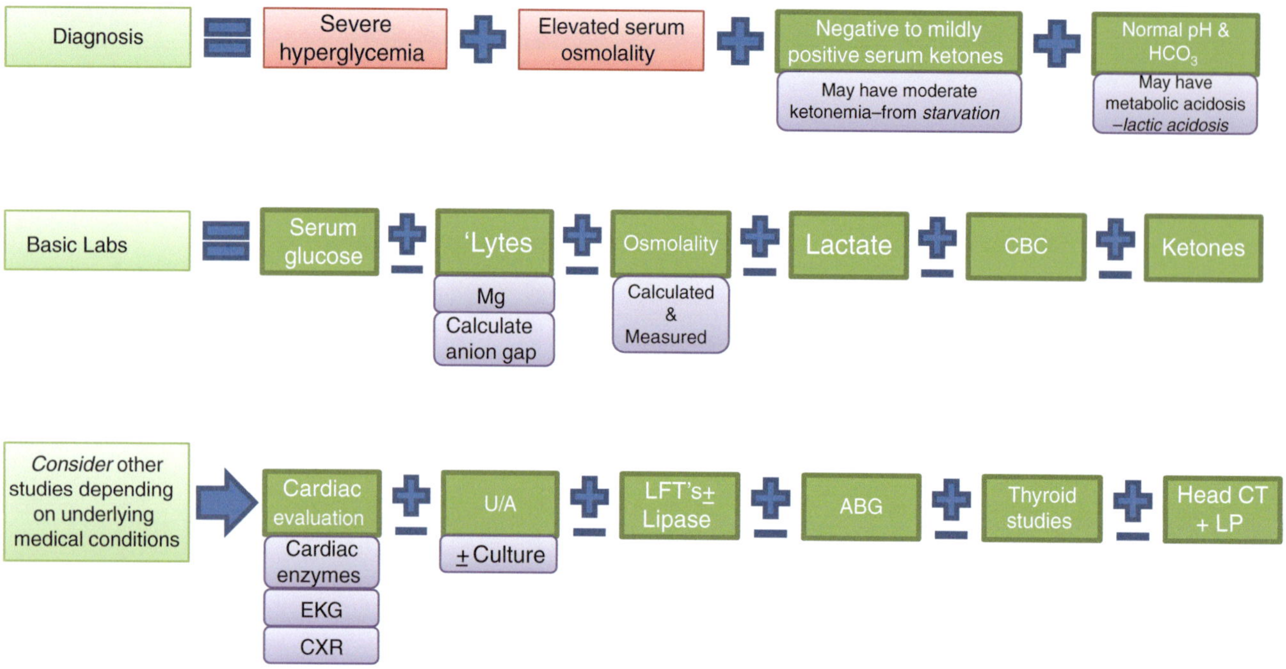

Treatment

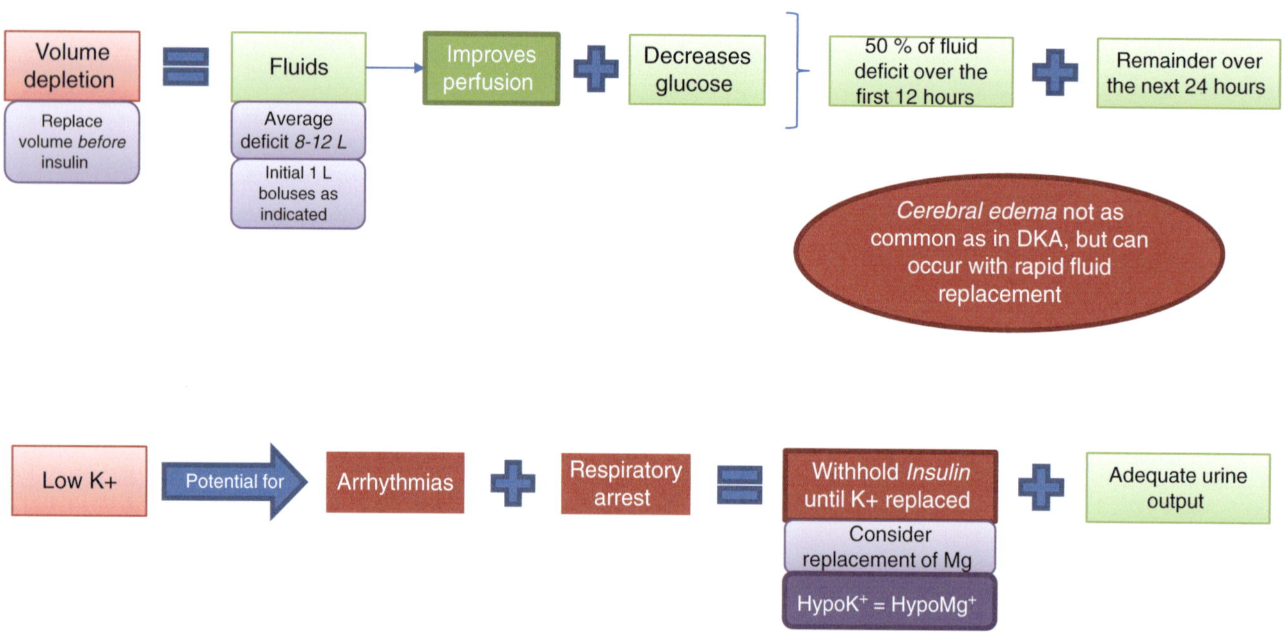

Disposition

Thyroid Disorders

Thyroid Hormones

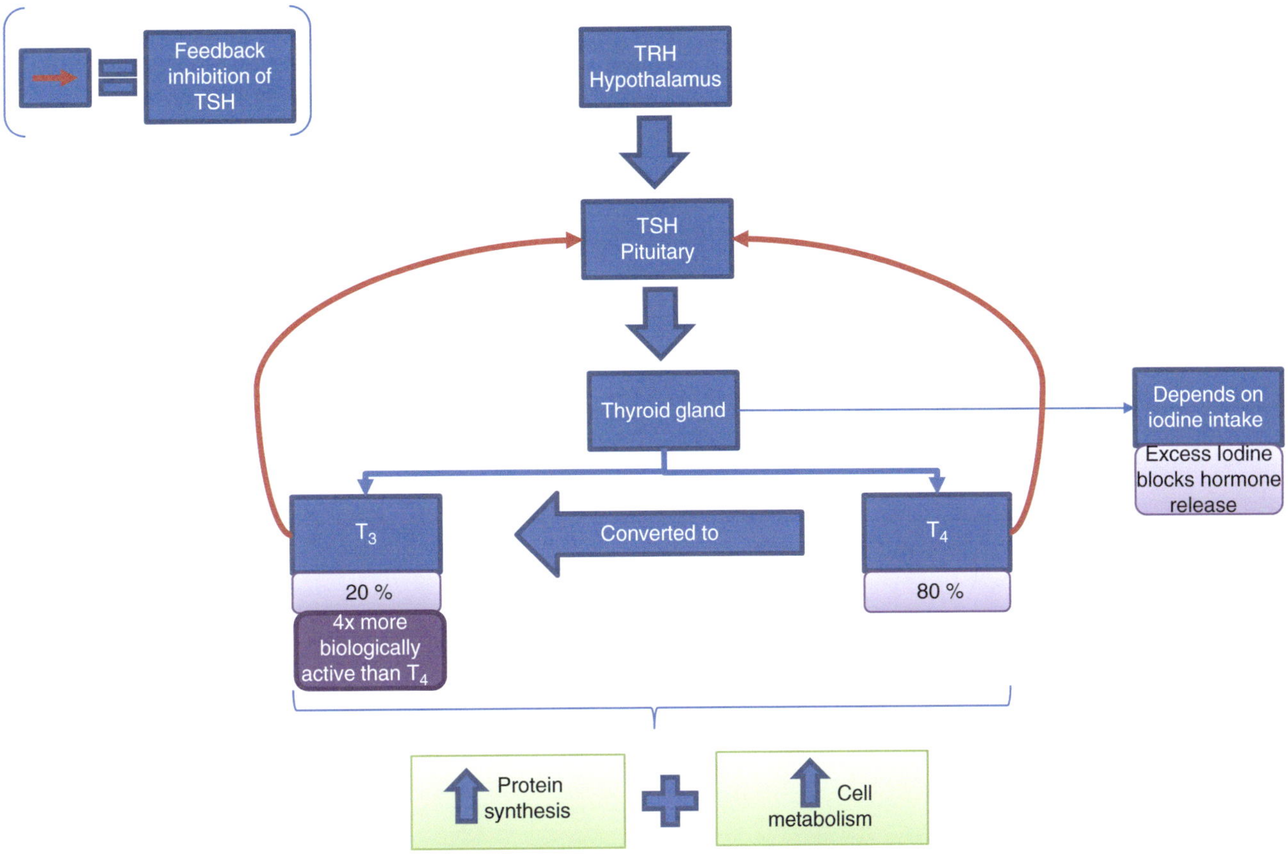

Hypothyroidism and Myxedema Coma

Introduction: Hypothyroidism

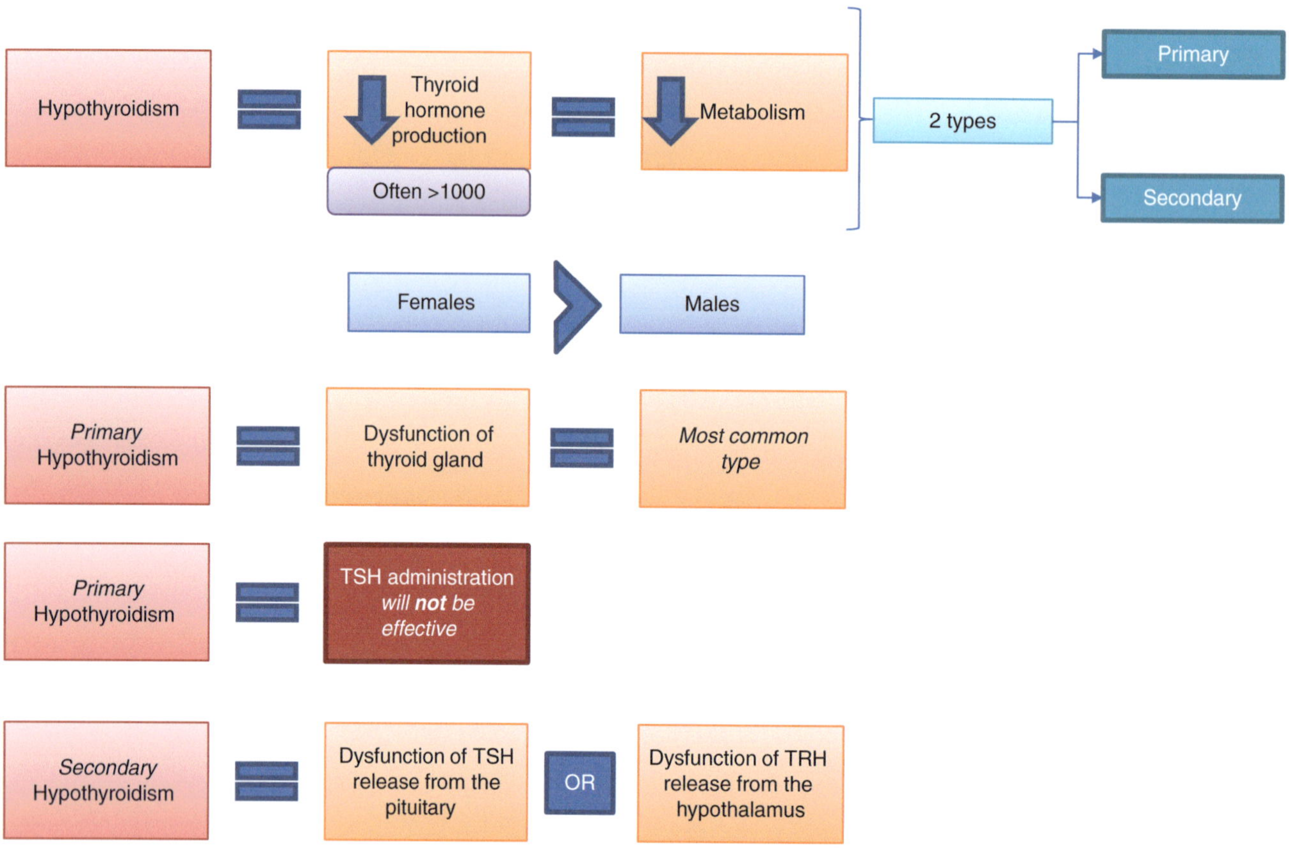

Some Causes of Hypothyroidism

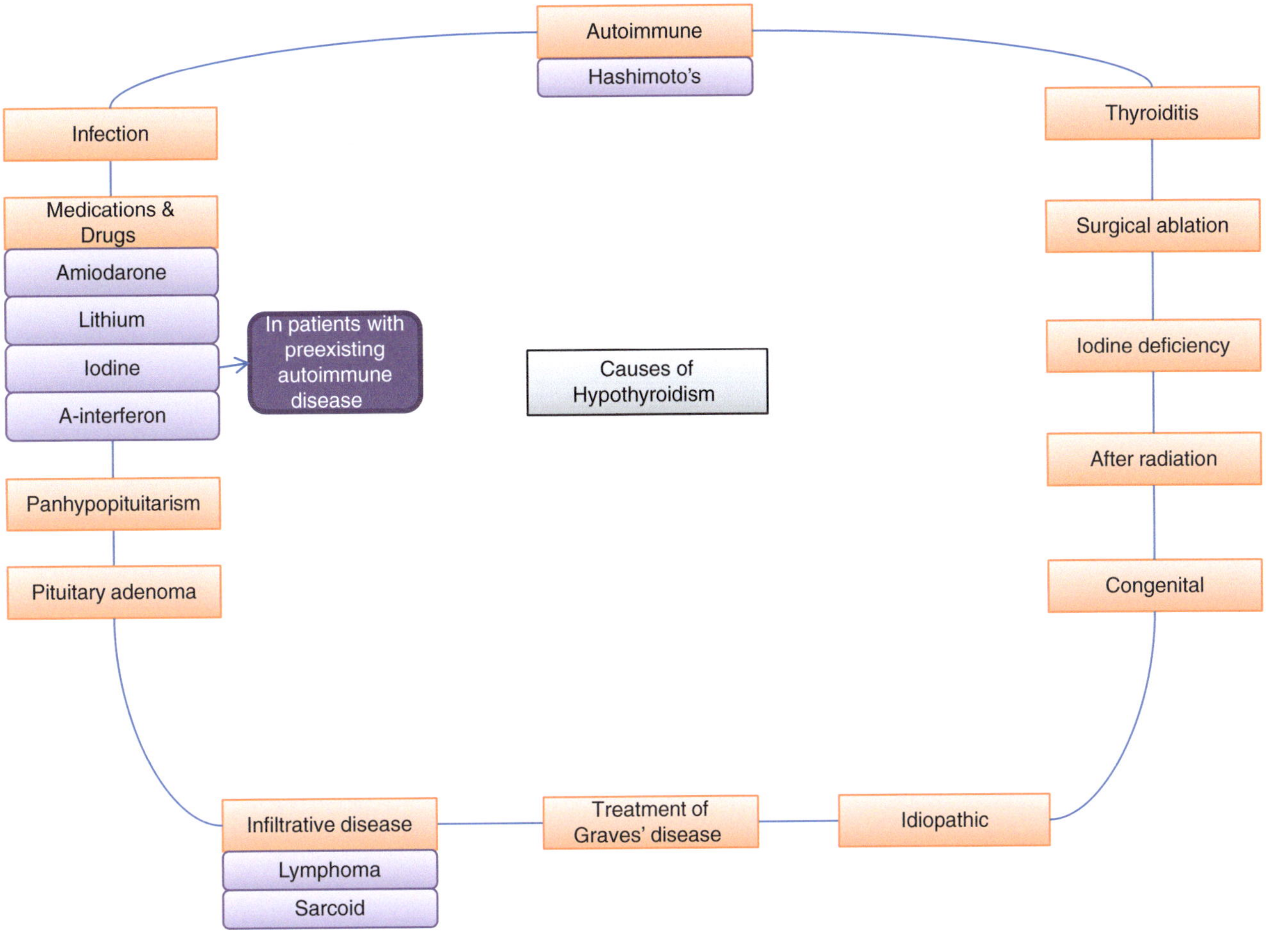

Hypothyroidism: Clinical Features

Symptoms

- Thinning or loss of hair
- Depression
- Weakness & Fatigue
- Muscle and joint pain
- Weight gain
- Shortness of breath
- Constipation
- Irregular menstrual cycles
  - Dysfunctional uterine bleeding
- Cold intolerance
  - Due to *decreased metabolic rate*
  - And…decreased shivering

Signs

- Puffiness around orbits
- Pallor
- Hoarseness
- Macroglossia
- Bradycardia
- Hypoventilation
- Decreased or absent bowel sounds
- Hypothermia
  - Severe in Myxedema coma
- Edema
  - Non-pitting
  - Pretibial myxedema
  - May also be a rare sign of *hyperthyroidism*
- Delay in relaxation of reflexes
  - "Hung -up" reflexes
- Peripheral neuropathy
- Cool dry skin
- Hypoxemia
  - Myxedema coma

Severe Hypothyroidism: Specific Clinical Features

Cardiopulmonary

- Low EKG voltage
- Angina
- Bradycardia
- Distant heart sounds
- Pericardial & Pleural effusions
- Cardiomyopathy
- Hypoventilation

Dermatologic

- Dry skin
- Non-pitting edema
- Hair loss
- Macroglossia
- Facial swelling
- Periorbital edema
- Ptosis

Neuropsychiatric

- Delayed DTR's
- Dementia
- Paresthesias
- Psychosis
- Depression
- Confusion
- Ataxia

Myxedema Coma

Myxedema Coma = Preexisting hypothyroidism + Mental status changes (Or *coma*) + Hypothermia (<35.5°C) + Some type of ***stress***

Myxedema Coma = Occurs in elderly females + High mortality rate + Consider in winter months

Signs (Infection may be present despite these signs) = Bradycardia + Hypotension (May be in shock) + Hypoventilation + Hypothermia (Very common) + AMS or Coma

Poor prognostic factors for Myxedema Coma = The elderly + Persistent hypotension + Bradycardia

Precipitating Factors of Myxedema Coma

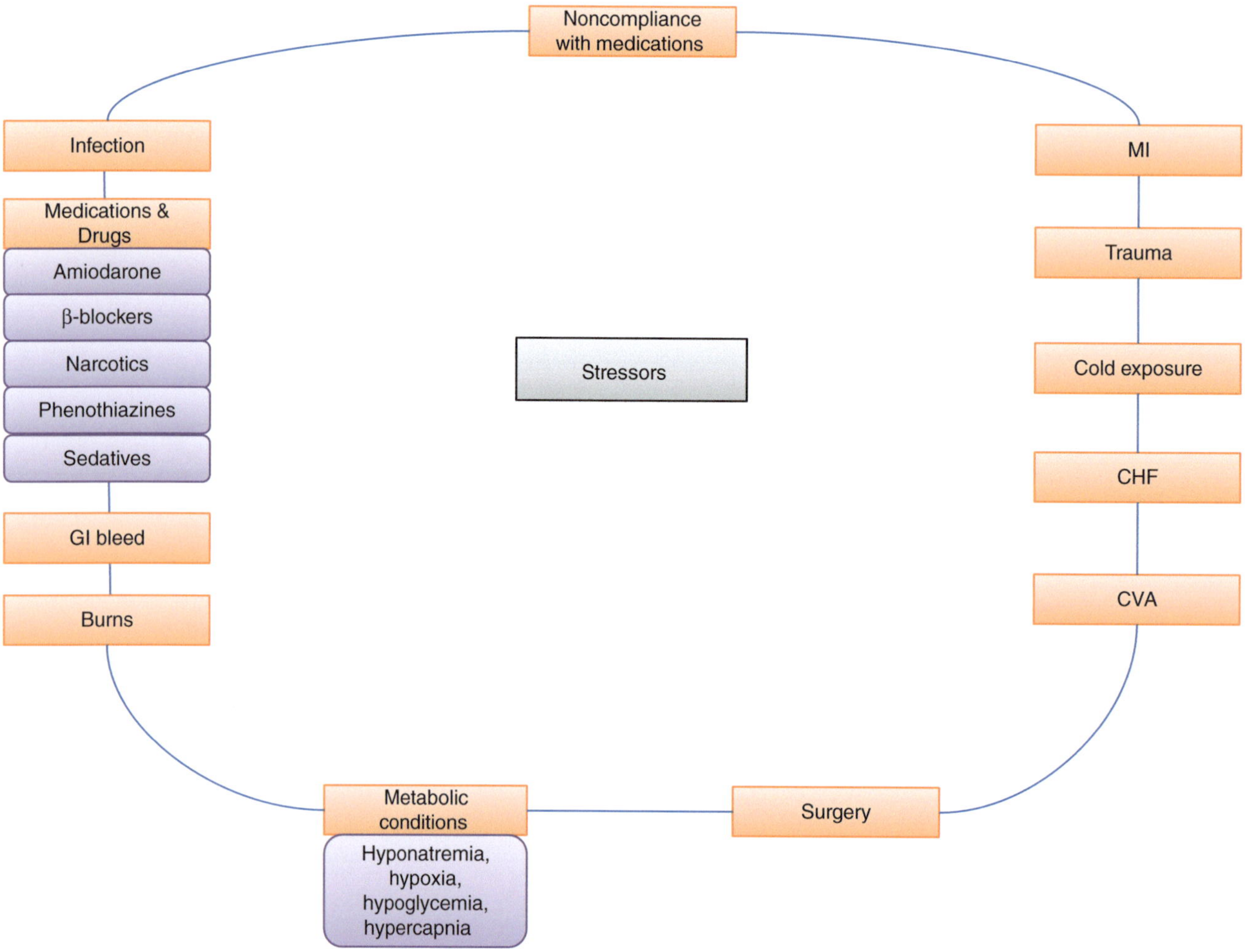

Differential Diagnosis of Myxedema Coma

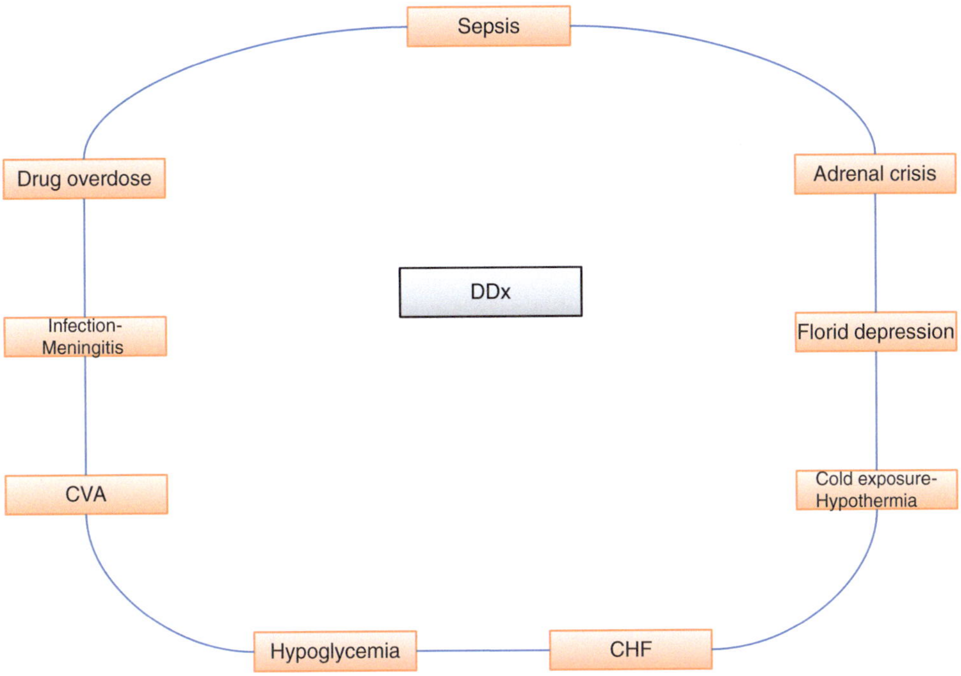

Myxedema Diagnosis

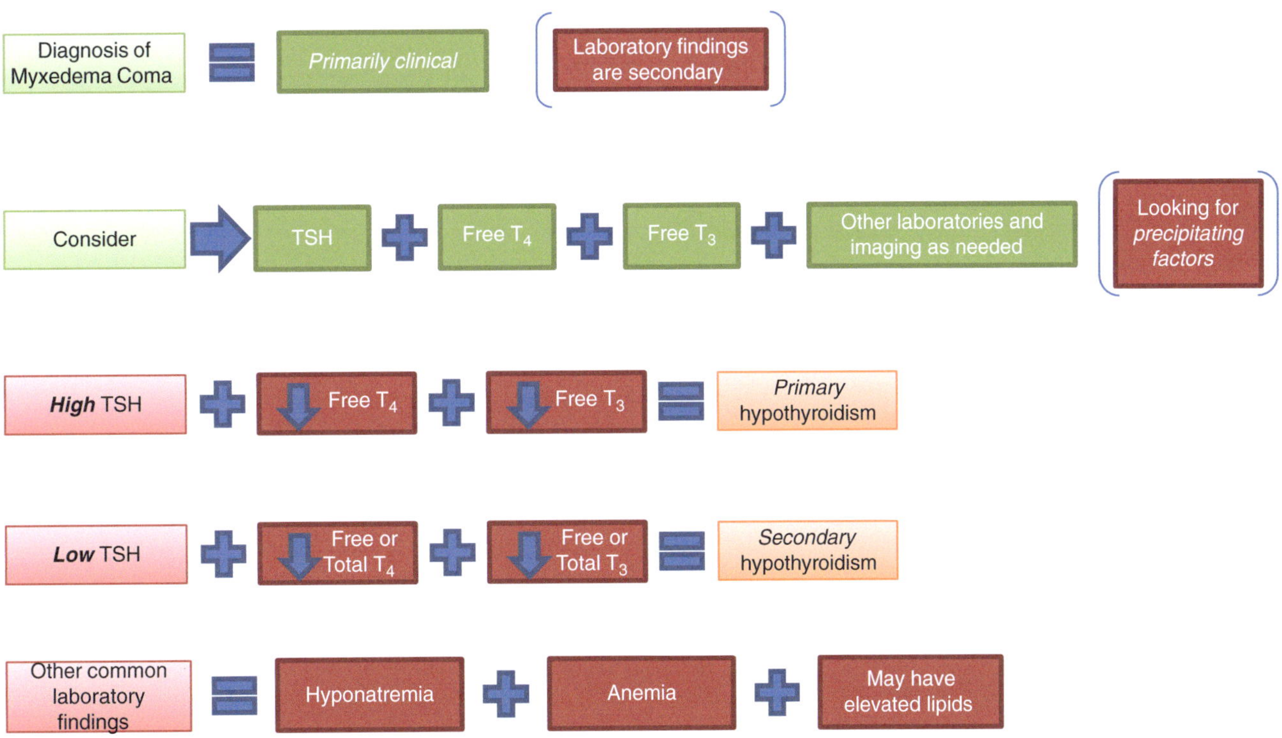

Treatment

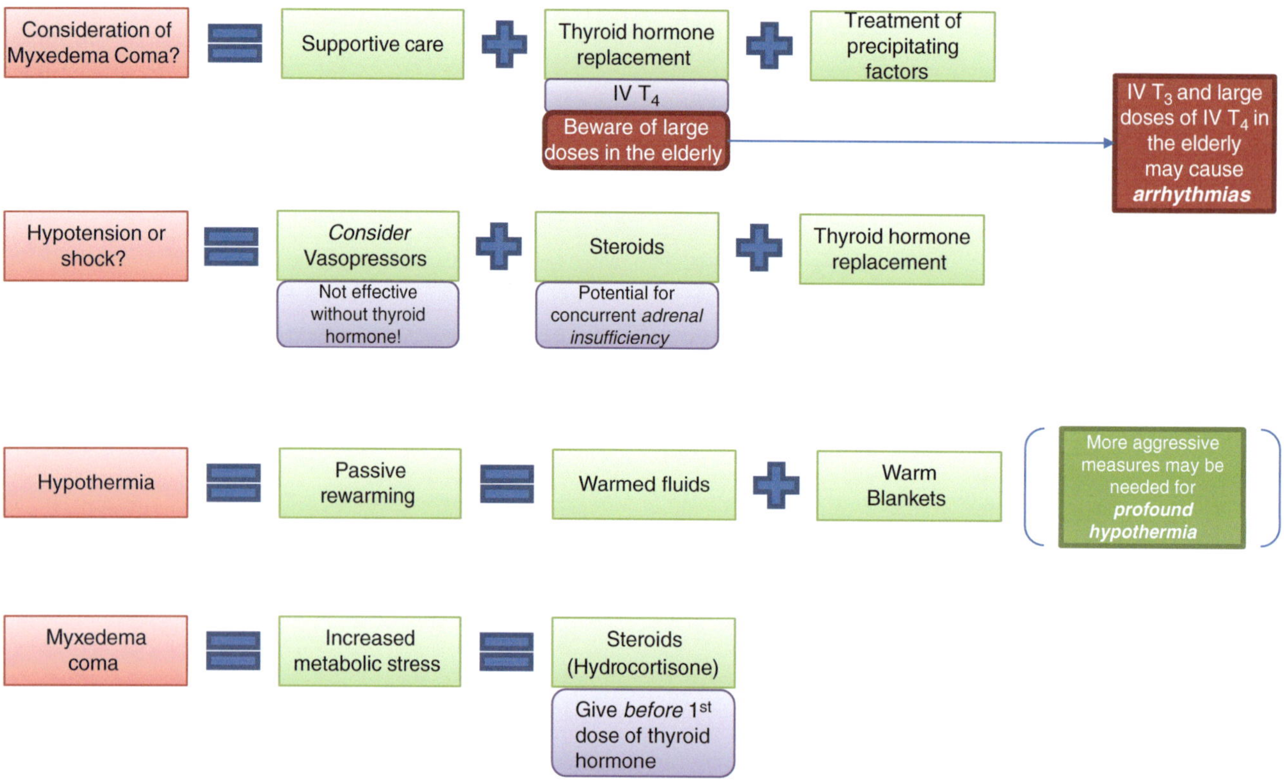

Disposition

Hyperthyroidism and Thyroid Storm

Introduction: Hyperthyroidism

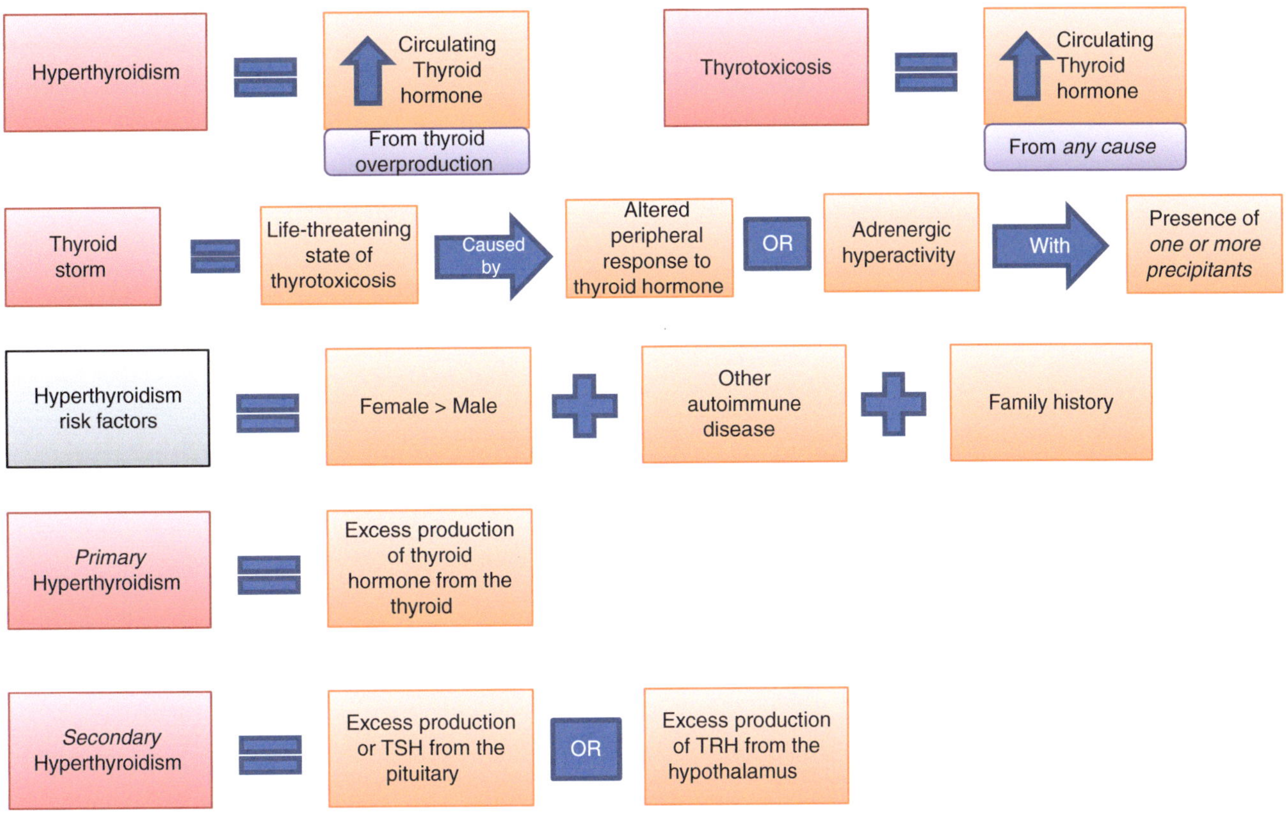

Causes of Primary Hyperthyroidism

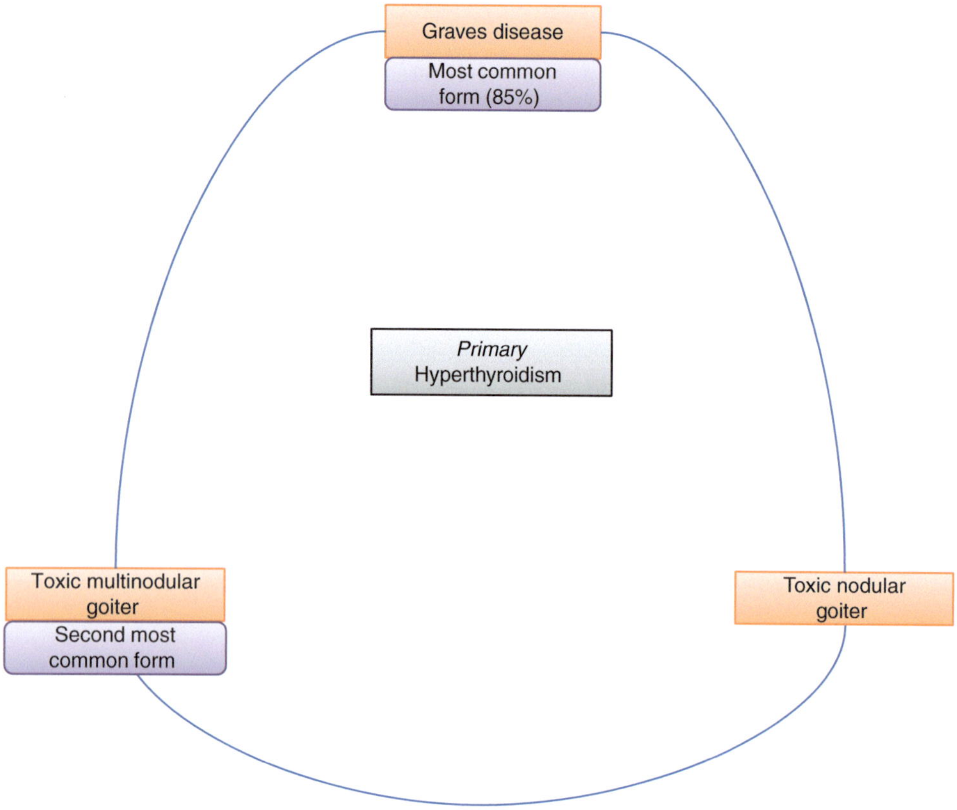

Graves' Disease

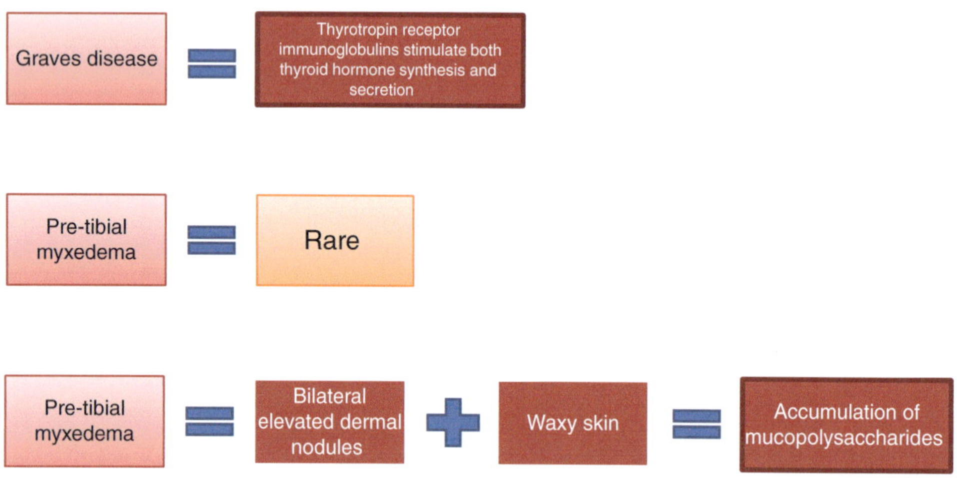

Causes of Hyperthyroidism

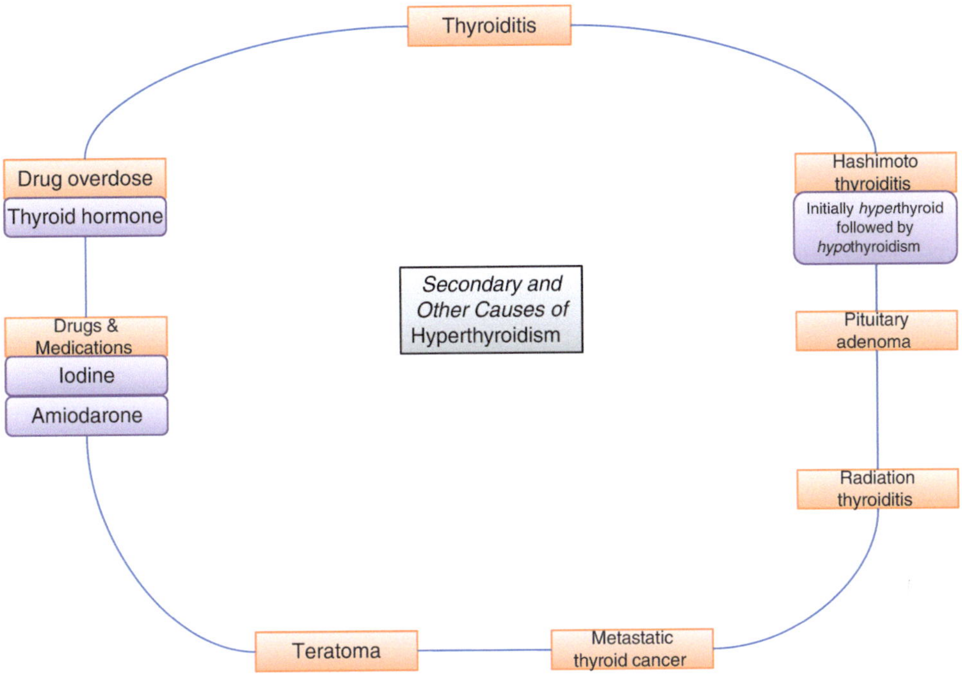

Hyperthyroidism: Clinical Features

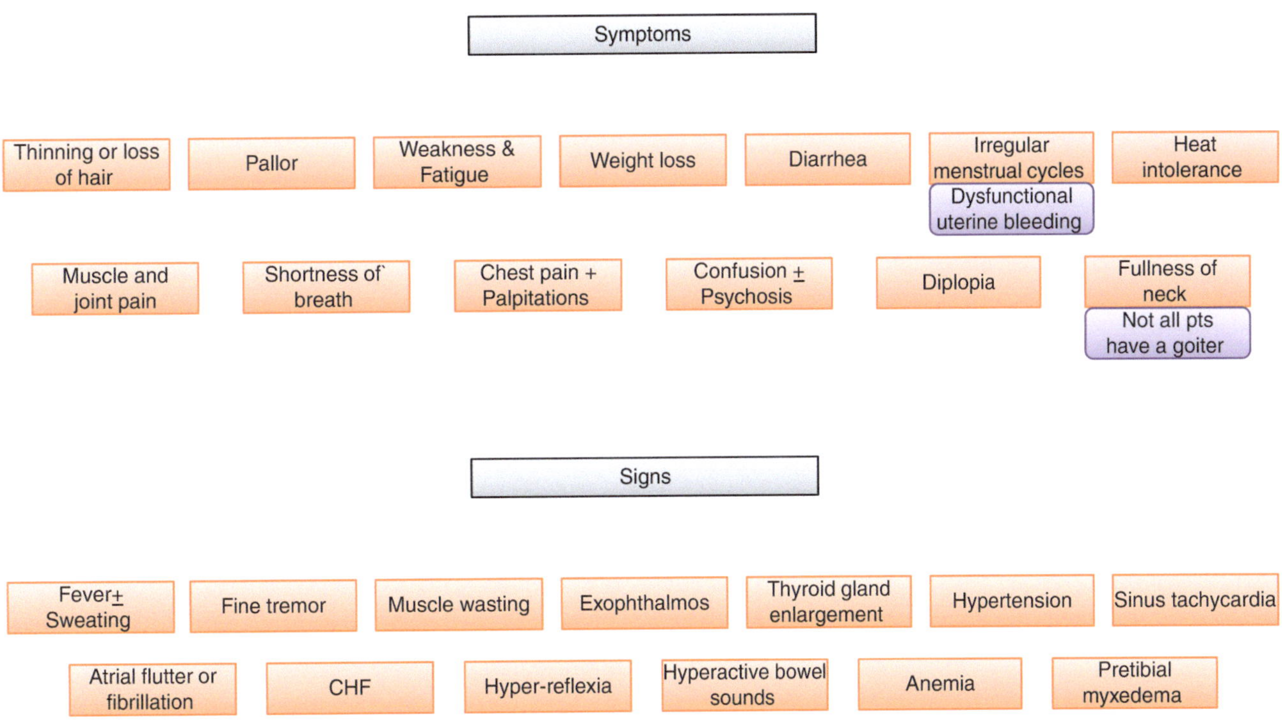

Thyroid Storm: Specific Clinical Features

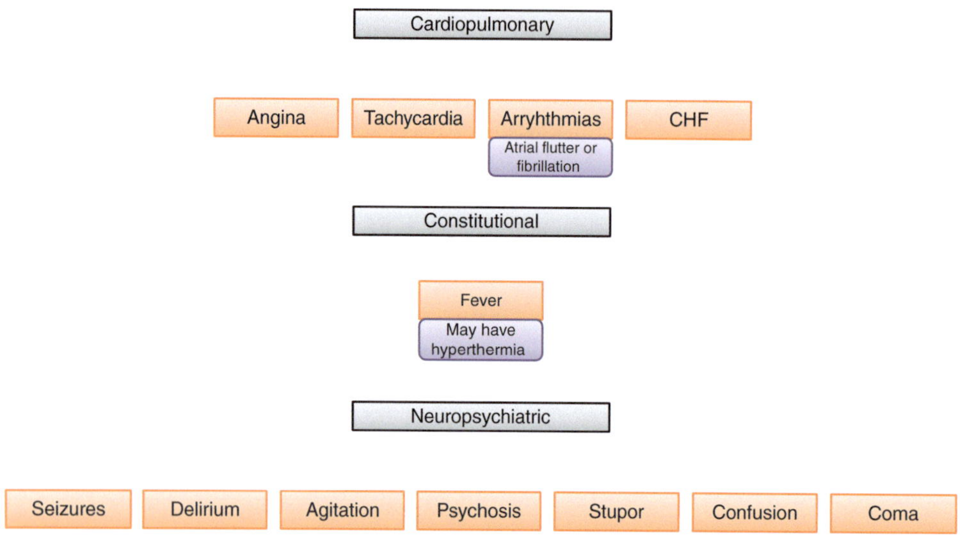

Precipitating Factors of Thyroid Storm

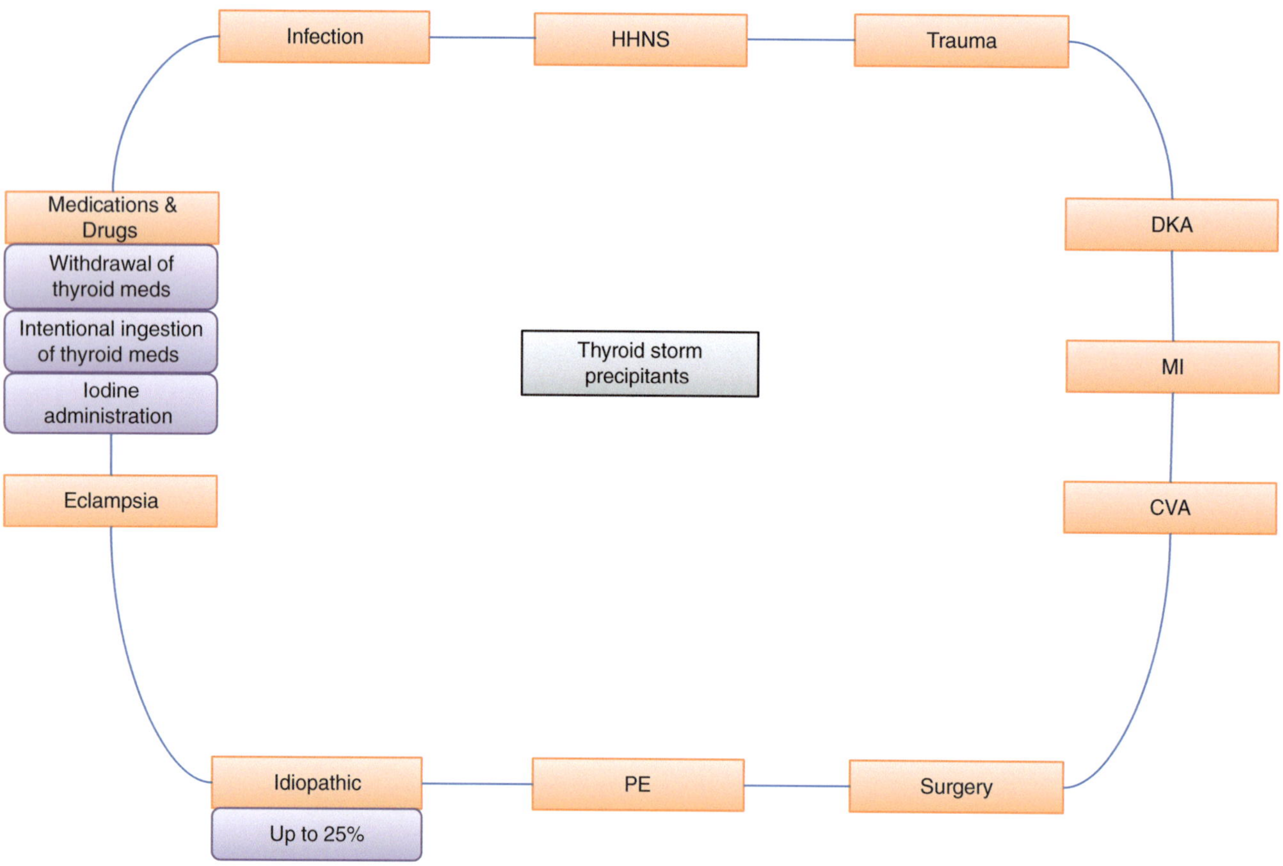

Differential Diagnosis of Thyroid Storm

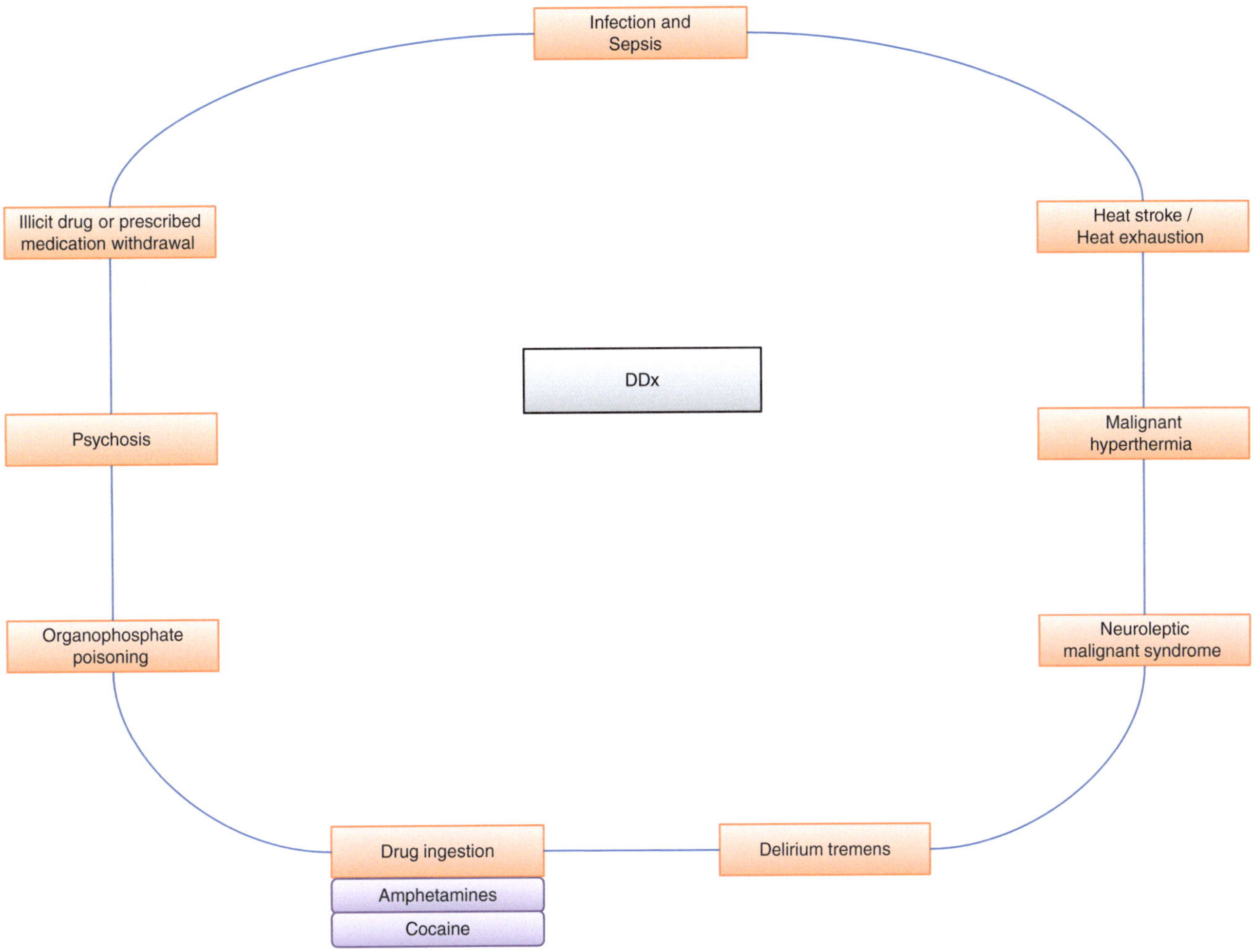

Thyroid Storm Diagnosis

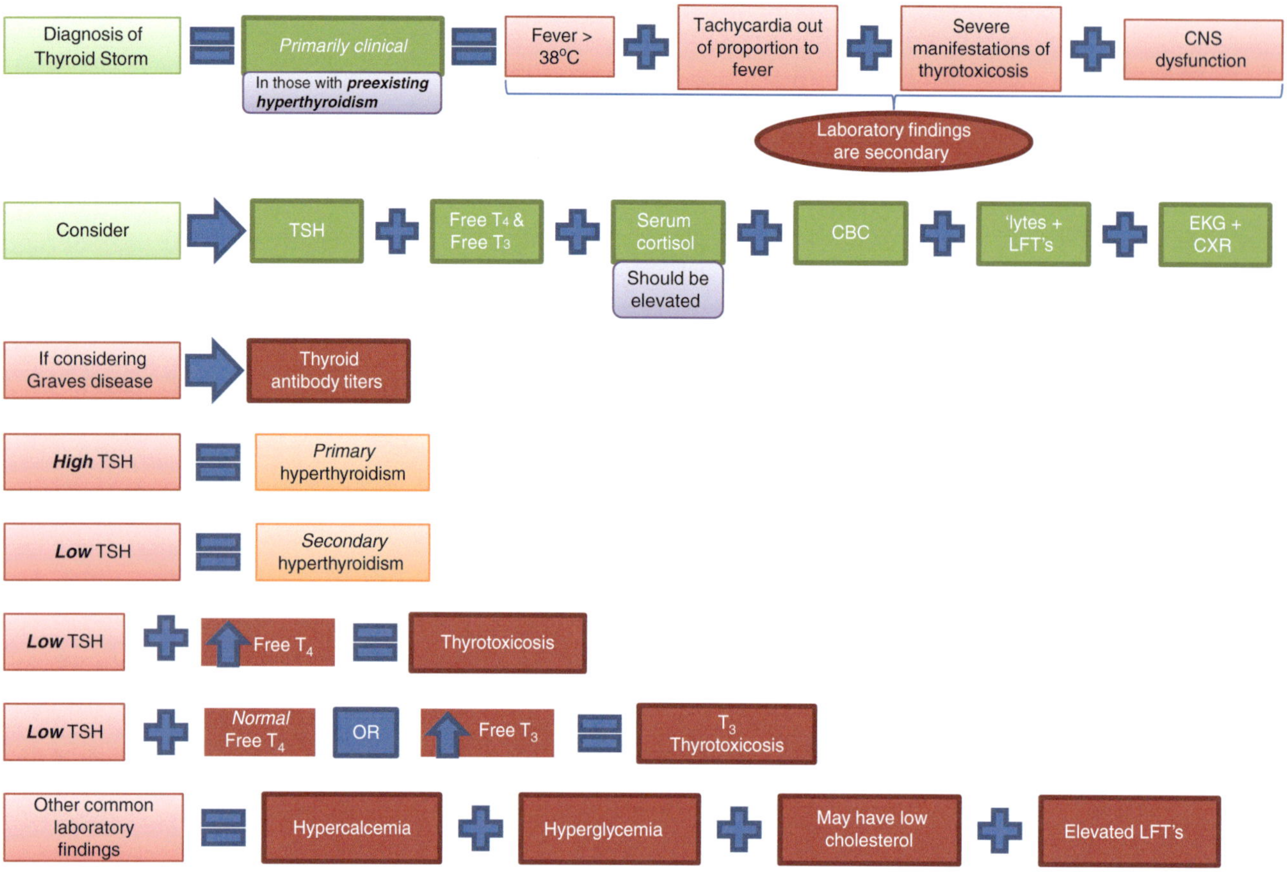

Treatment

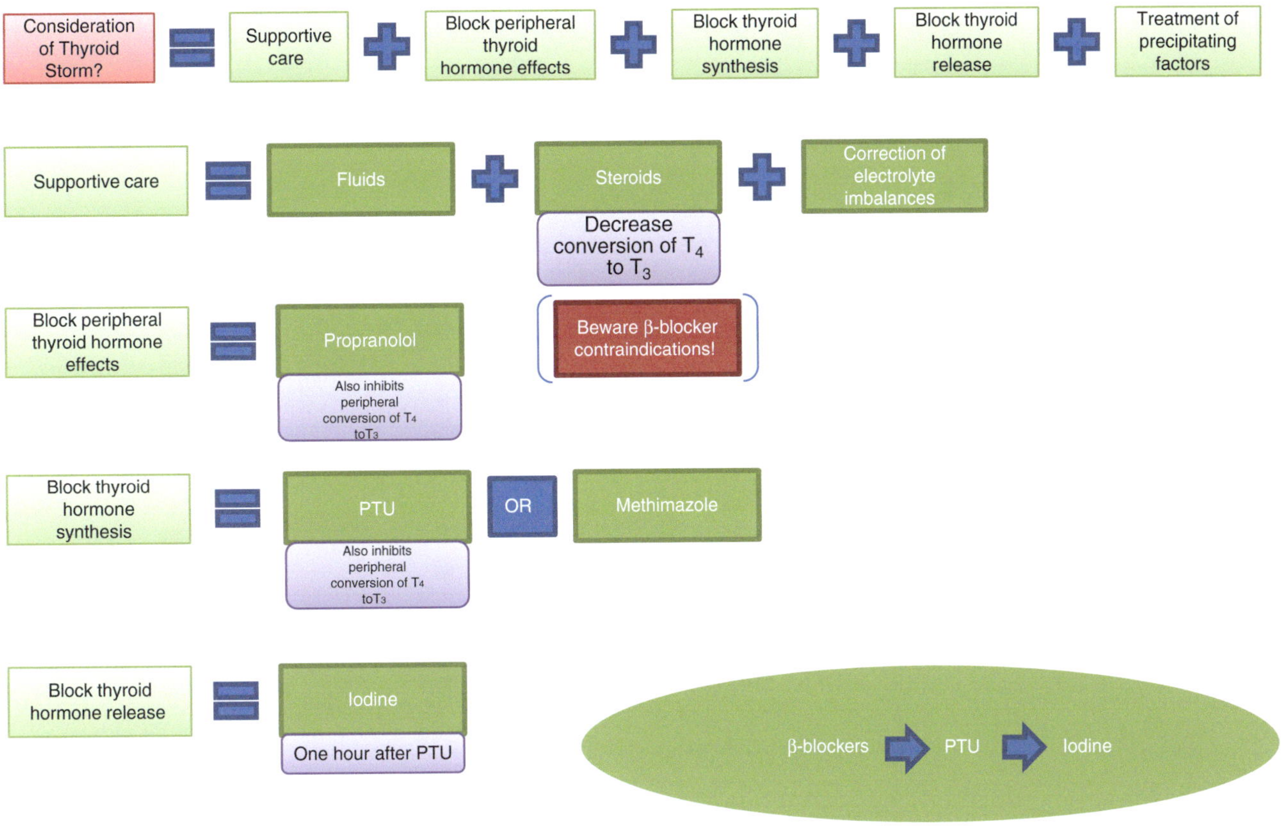

Disposition

Apathetic Thyrotoxicosis

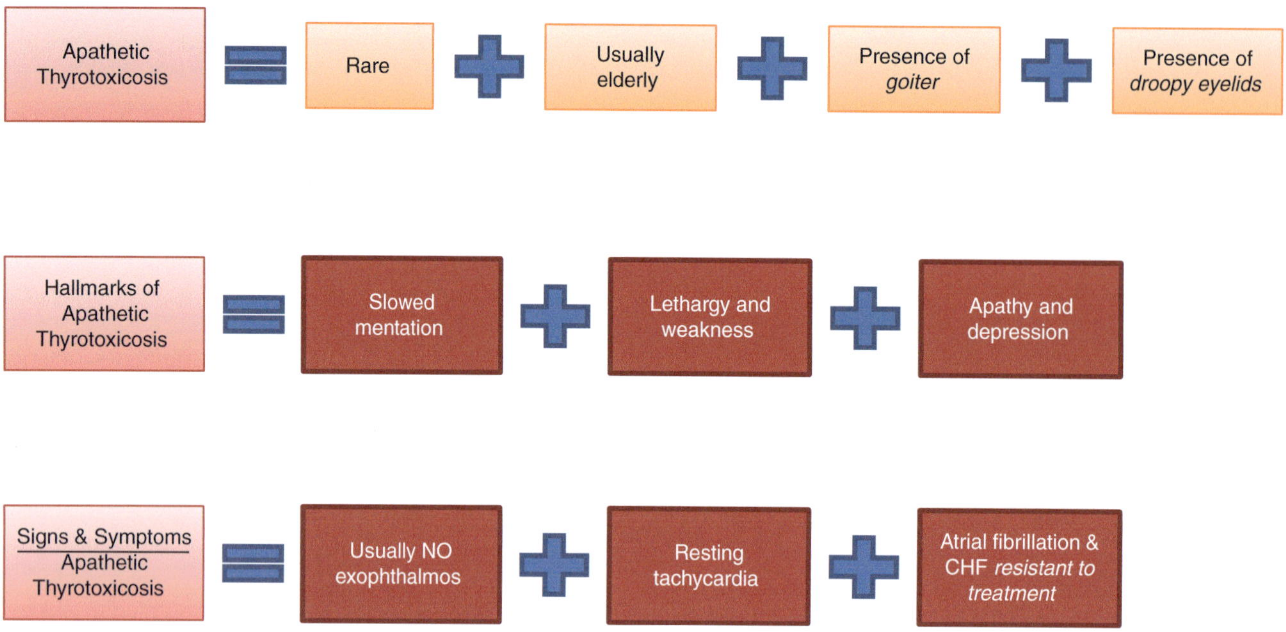

Adrenal Insufficiency and Crisis

Adrenal Hormones

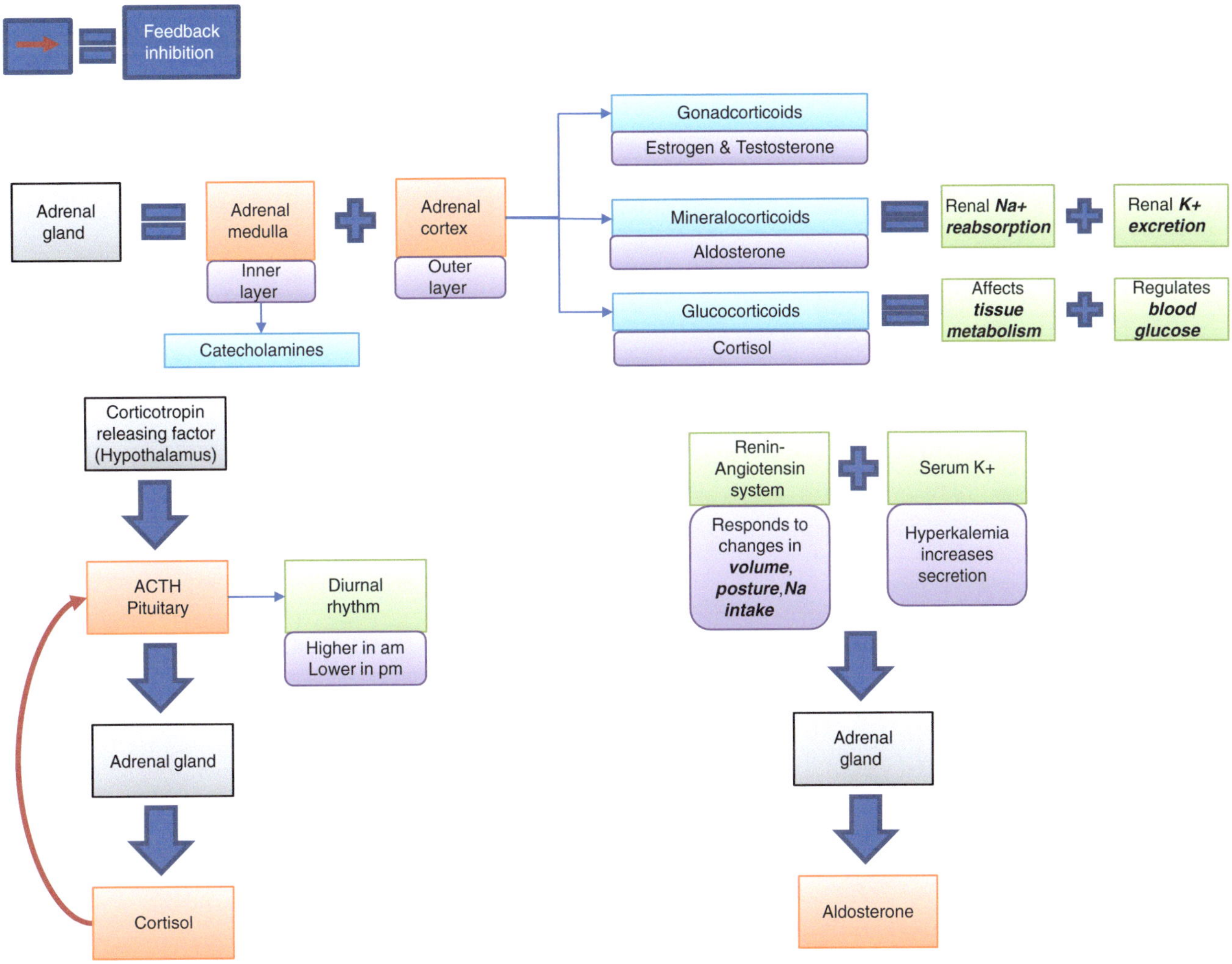

Introduction: Adrenal Insufficiency and Crisis

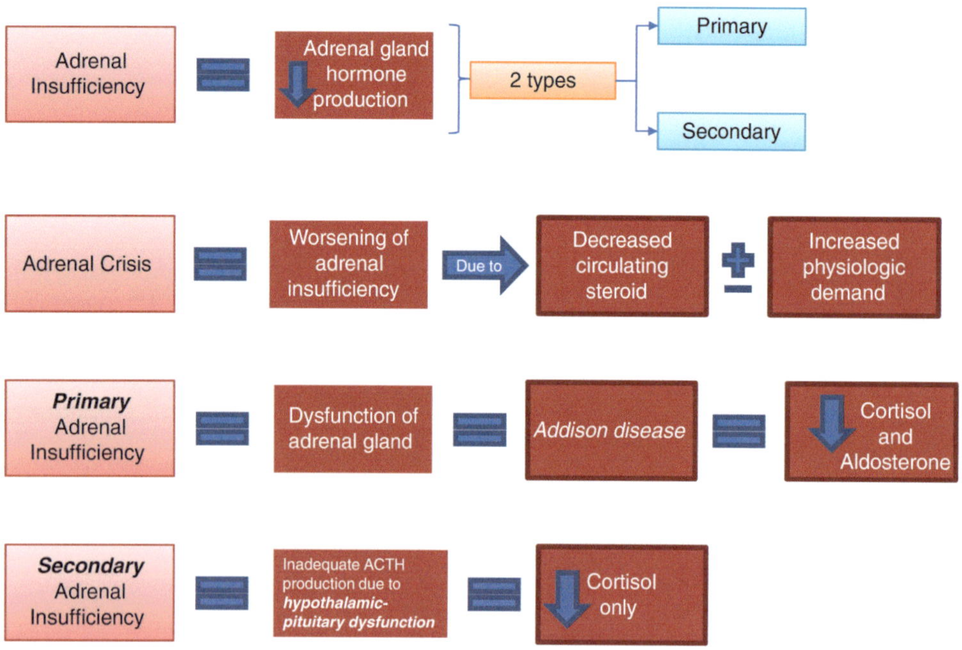

Some Causes of Primary Adrenal Insufficiency

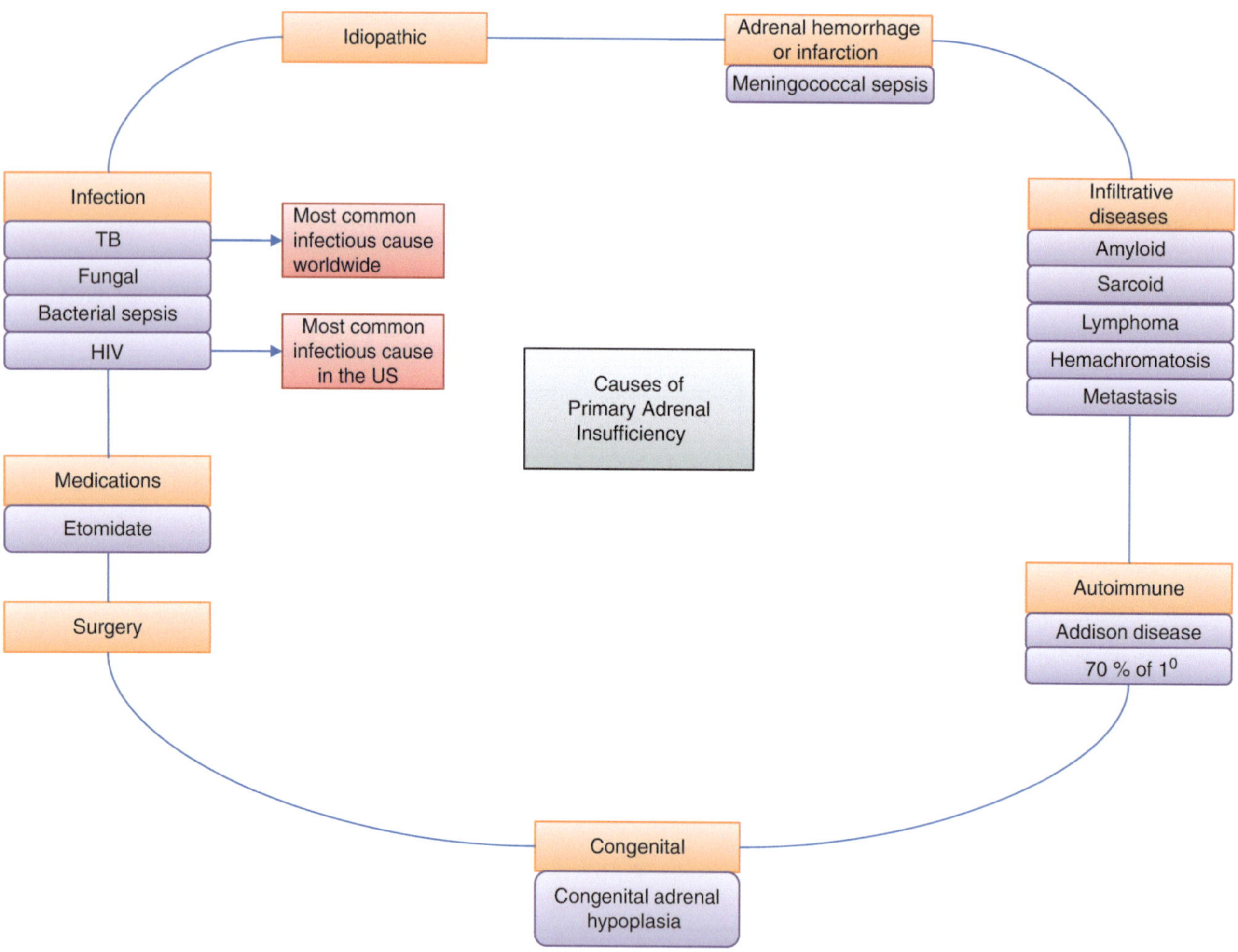

Some Causes of Secondary Adrenal Insufficiency

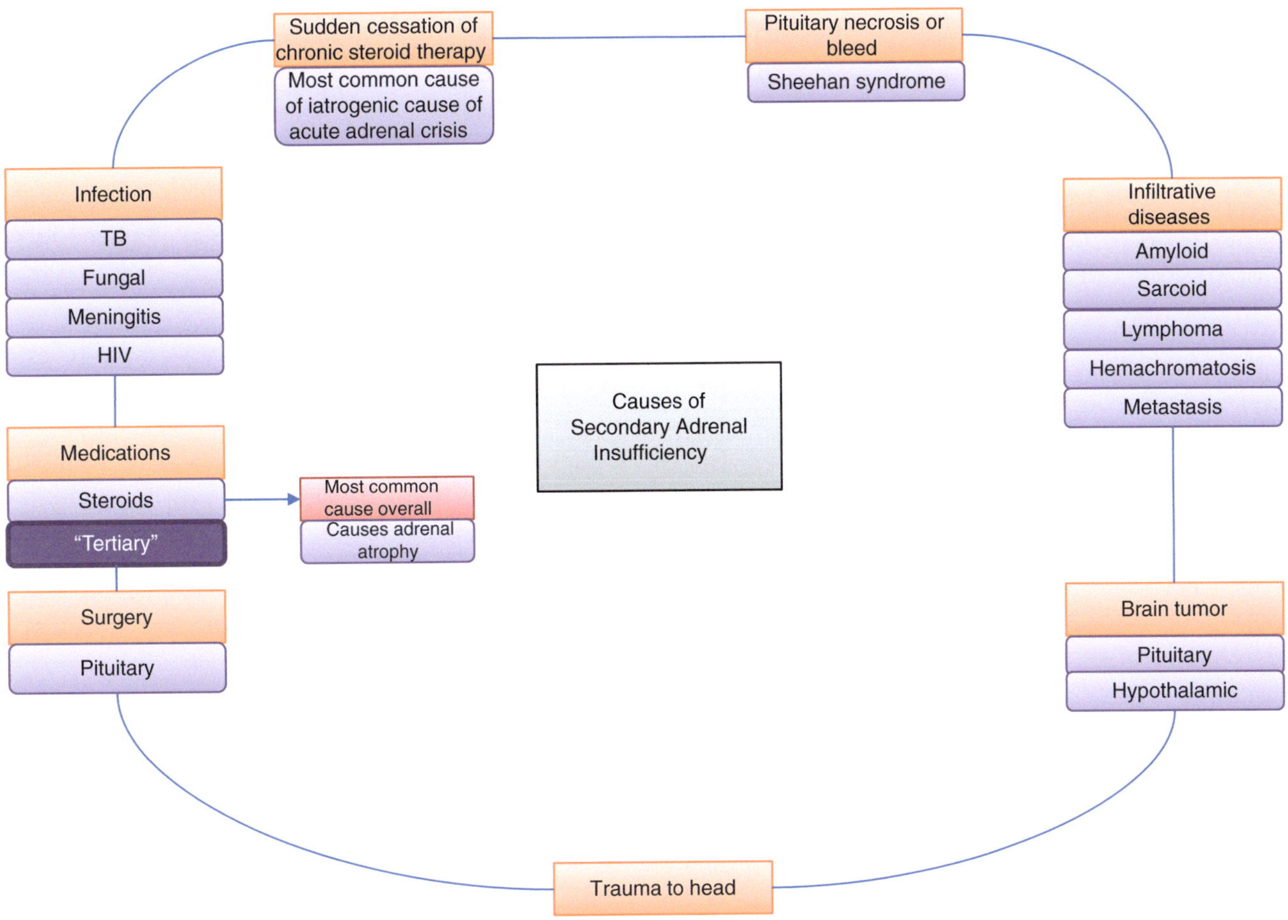

Adrenal Insufficiency: Clinical Features

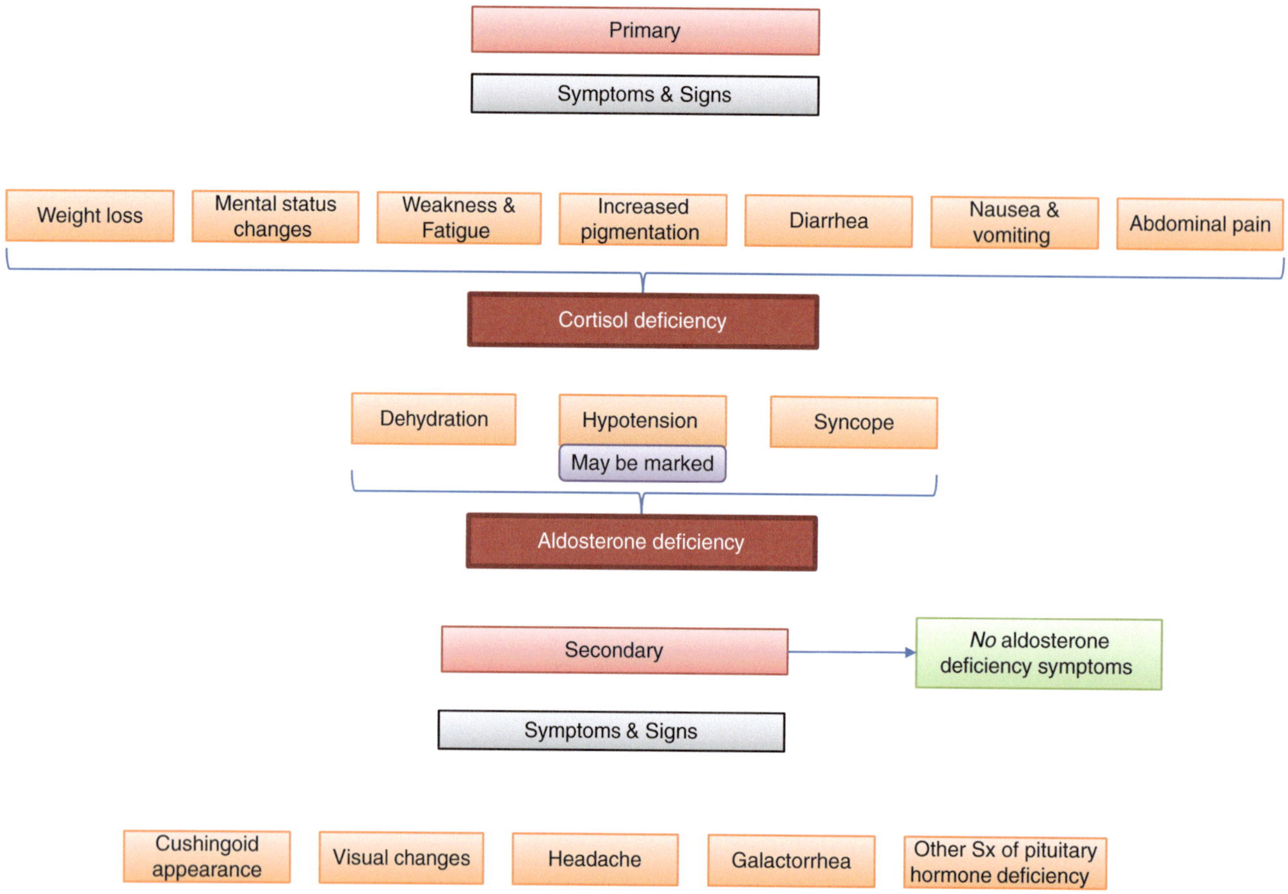

Adrenal Crisis: Clinical Features

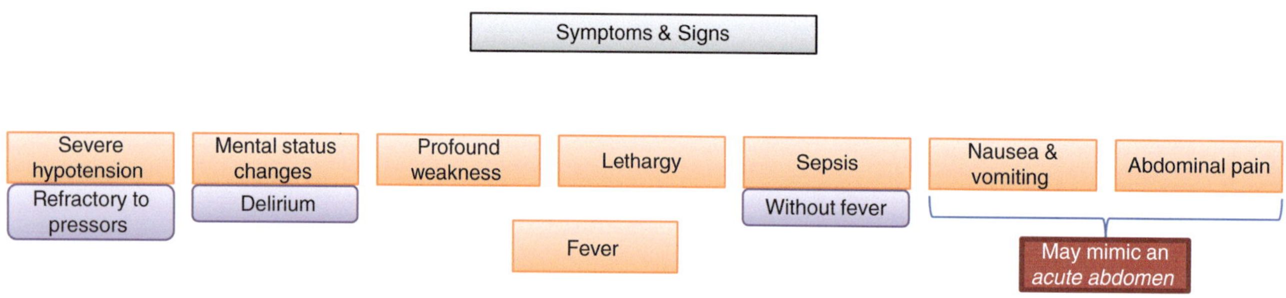

Laboratory Abnormalities and Testing Considerations

Diagnosis of Adrenal Insufficiency = *High index of suspicion* → *Especially in those with unexplained hypotension* + Those with predisposing features

***Hyper**kalemia* + ***Hypo**natremia* + Hypoglycemia = *Primary* adrenal insufficiency

***Hypo**kalemia* + ***Hypo**natremia **OR** **hyper**natremia* + Hypoglycemia = *Secondary* adrenal insufficiency

Other common laboratory findings = Hypoglycemia (Due to cortisol deficiency) + Metabolic acidosis (Due to *hypotension* & *hypovolemia*) + Eosinophilia (*Chronic insufficiency*)

EKG findings = May show evidence of K+ problems = Depends on *hyper* - or *hypokalemia*

Consider → Cortisol level + ACTH stimulation test + Other laboratories and imaging as needed (Looking for *precipitating factors*)

Treatment

Consideration of Adrenal Insufficiency? = Supportive care (IVF = D_5NS; Corrects *hypoglycemia& hyponatremia*) + Steroids (Hydrocortisone; Drug of choice; Provides mineralo - & glucocorticoid effects) + Treatment of precipitating factors

Drug of choice → ***Dexamethasone*** Can be given if ACTH simulation test will be done

Hypotension or shock? = Steroids (Give 1st) + *Consider* Vasopressors (Not effective without steroids!)

High mortality = Due to *underlying precipitant* ± Dysrhythmias (Hyperkalemia) ± Shock

Disposition

Introduction: Hyperadrenalism (Cushing's Syndrome)

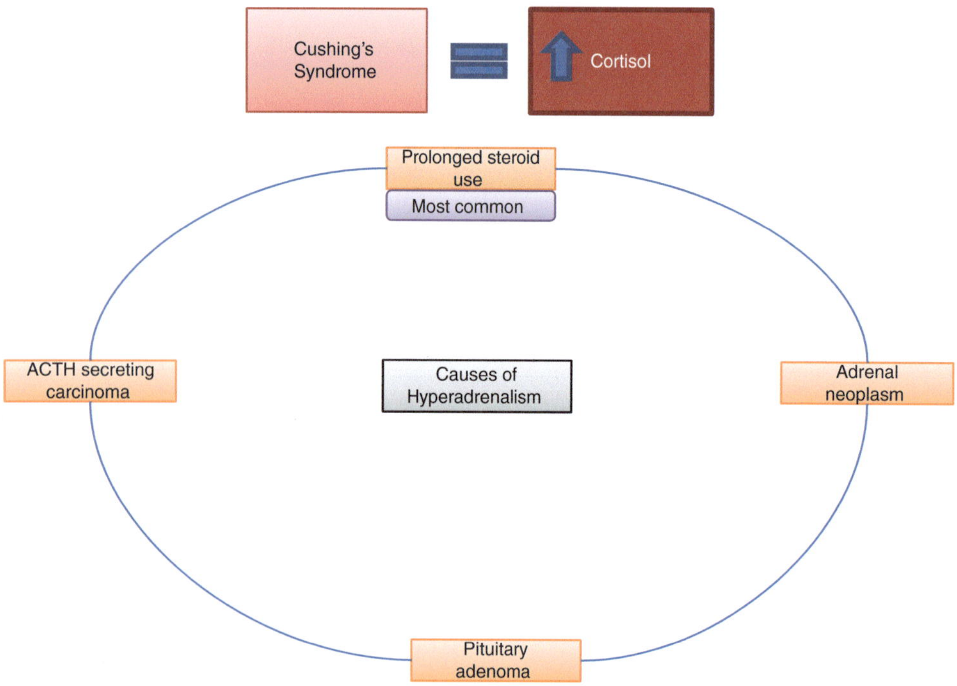

Hyperadrenalism: Clinical Features

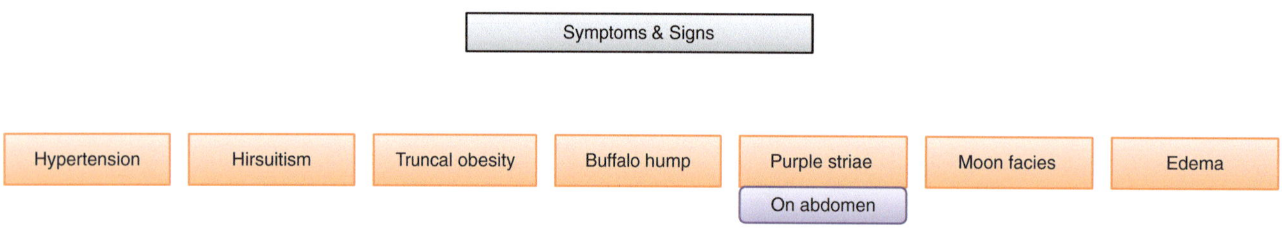

Laboratory Abnormalities and Testing Considerations

Diagnosis of Hyperadrenalism = *High index of suspicion* + Those with predisposing features

Common laboratory findings = Hypernatremia (Due to cortisol deficiency) + Hyperglycemia (Due to *hypotension & hypovolemia*) + Glucosuria (*Chronic insufficiency*)

Treatment

Consideration of Hyperadrenalism? = Supportive care + Stop steroids + Treatment of precipitating factors

Disposition

Hyperadrenalism = Depends on clinical scenario

Pheochromocytoma

Introduction

Pheochromocytoma = Rare cause of hypertension (Treatable!) + Tumor of adrenal medulla (Usually benign but can be malignant) = Secretes norepinephrine

Pheochromocytoma: Clinical Features

Symptoms & Signs → 5 P's

- Pallor
- Palpitations
- Pressure
  - Increased BP
- Pain
  - Abd pain
  - Headache
  - Chest pain
- Perspiration

Diagnosis

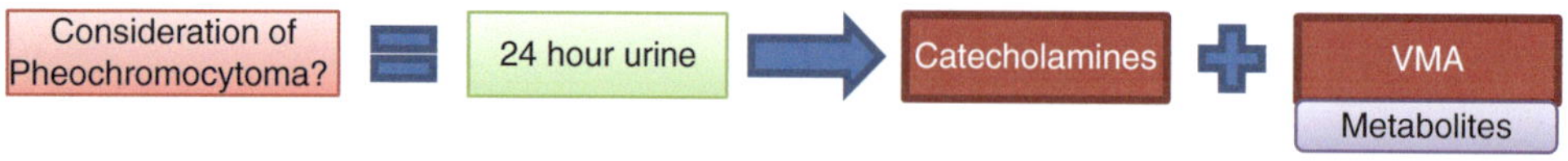

Treatment and Disposition

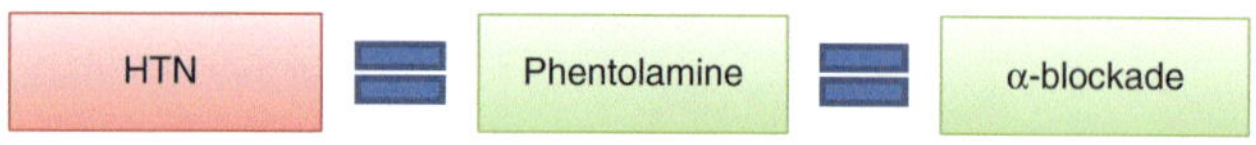

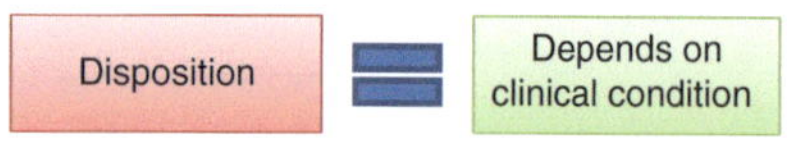

ADH-Related Diseases

Antidiuretic Hormone

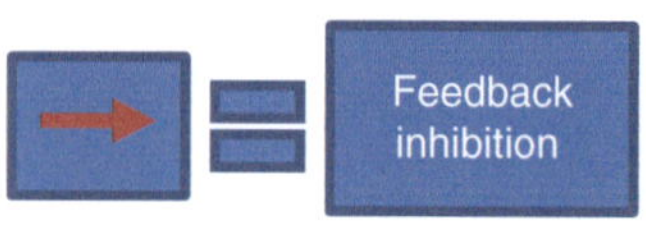

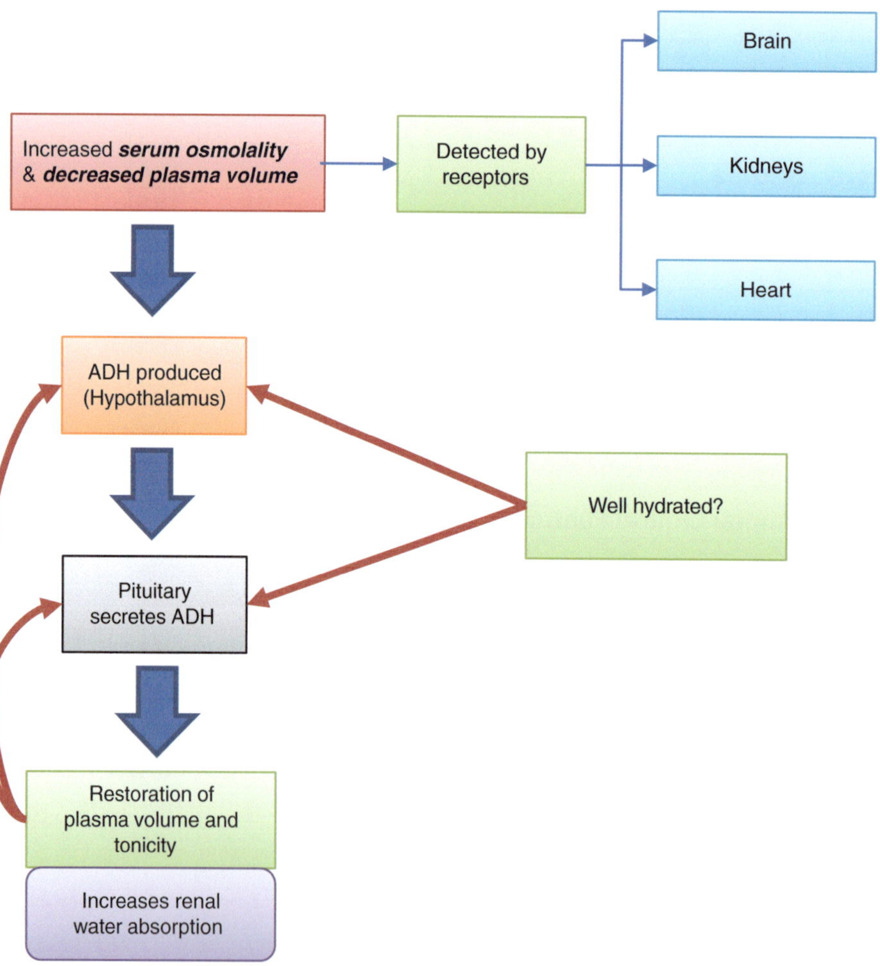

Introduction: Syndrome of Inappropriate Antidiuretic Hormone Secretion (SIADH)

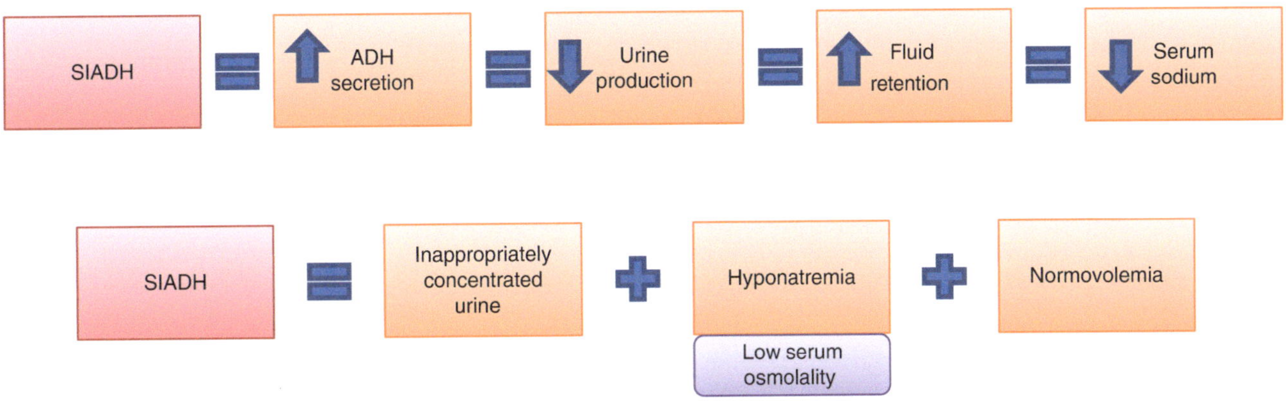

Some Causes of SIADH

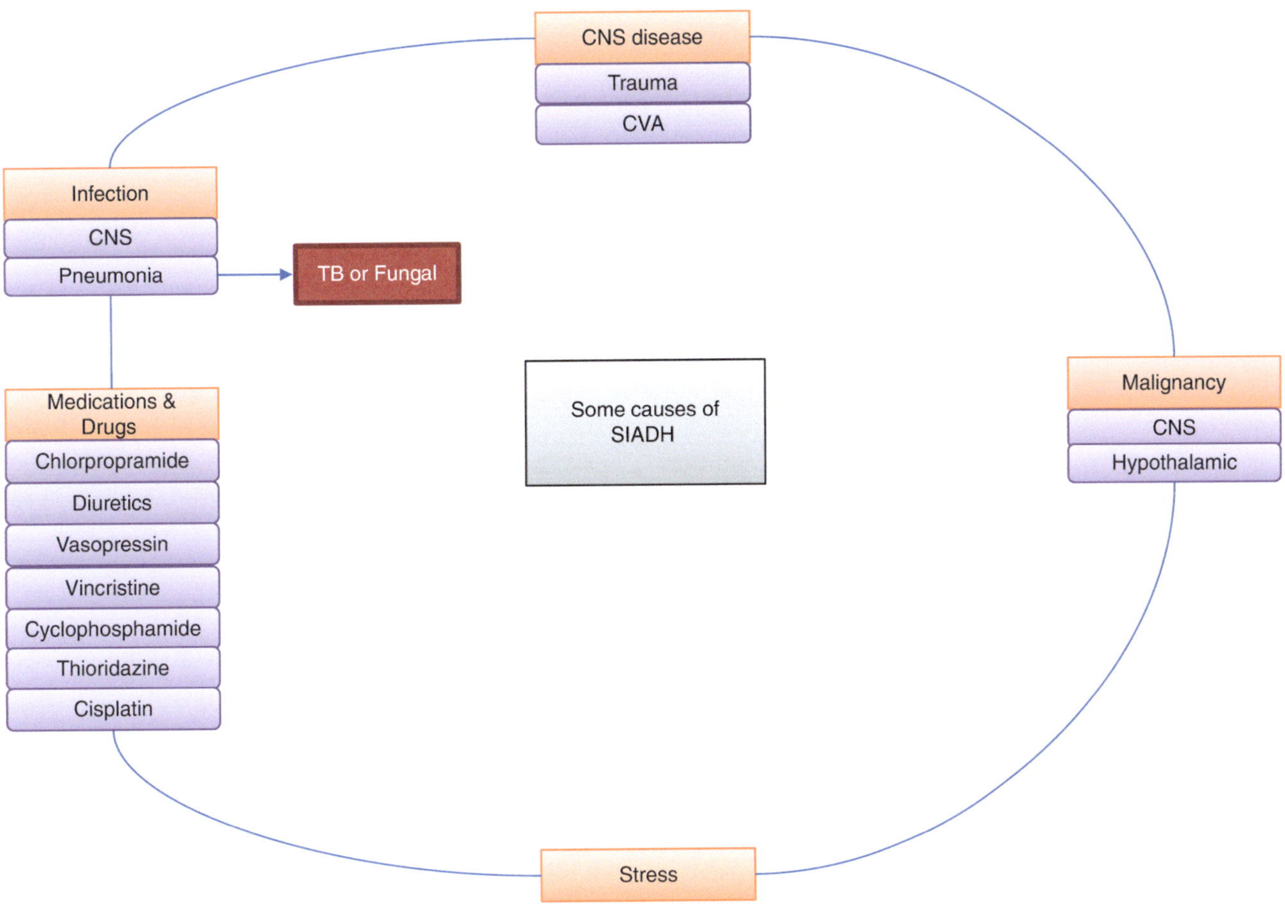

SIADH: Clinical Features

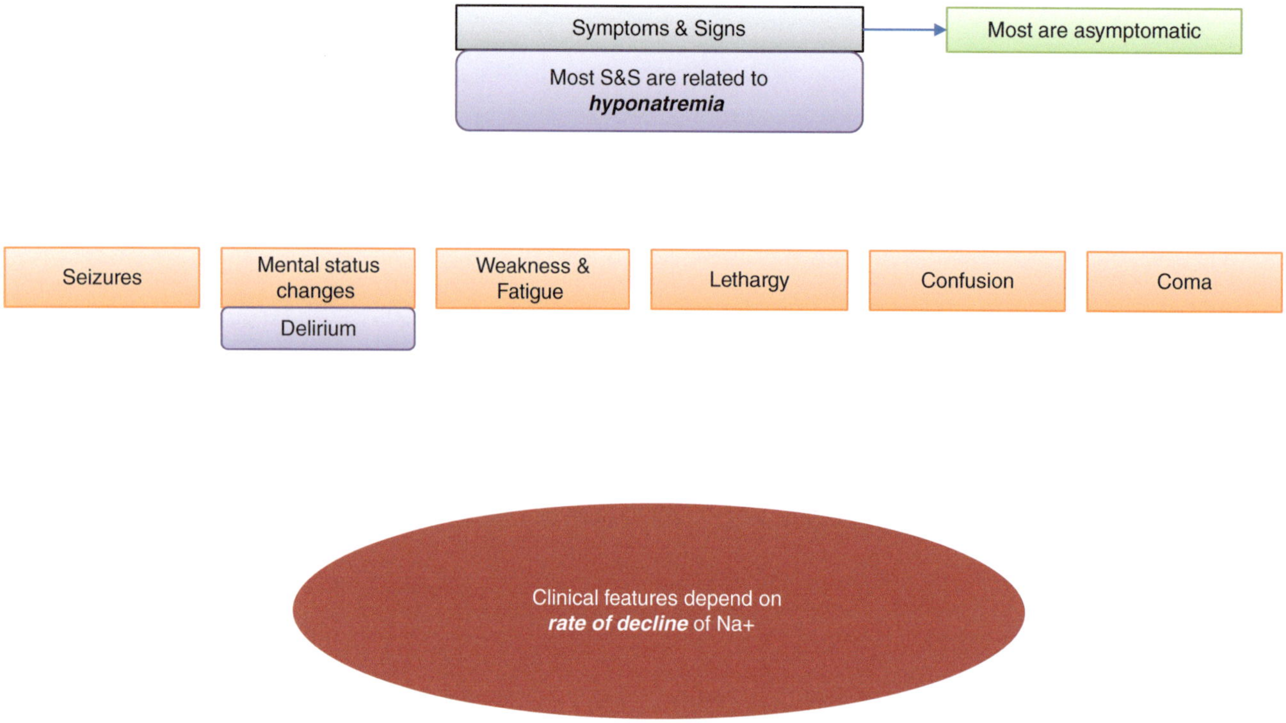

Laboratory Abnormalities and Testing Considerations

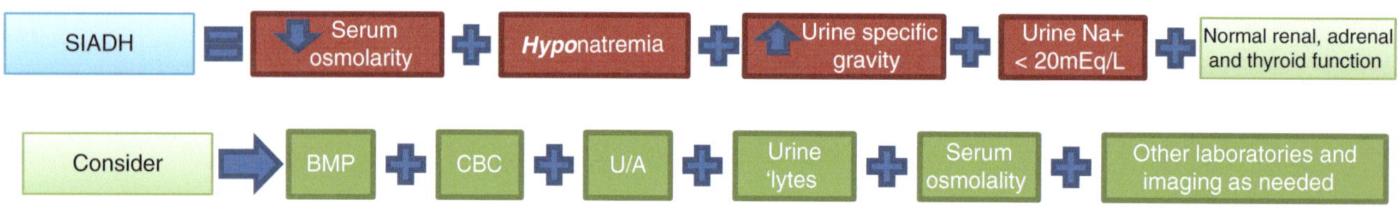

Treatment and Disposition

Consideration of SIADH? = Supportive care + Treatment of precipitating factors

Mild hyponatremia? (125 –134 mEq/L) = Fluid restriction → Slow correction over 24–48 hours (Admit) → Prevents → Central pontine myelinolysis

Severe hyponatremia? (<115 mEq/L) + Seizures or Coma = Fluid restriction + 4–6 cc/kg *3 % normal saline* (Stop when seizures subside) + Furosemide

Goal = $Na^+ > 120$ mEq/L

High morbidity = Serum $Na^+ < 120$

Serum Na+ levels can be safely raised at a rate of 1–2 mEq/L/hr

Central Pontine Myelinolysis

Central Pontine Myelinolysis = Hyponatremia corrected too rapidly

Central Pontine Myelinolysis = Confusion → Cranial nerve deficits → Quadriparesis → Locked in syndrome

Other Symptoms & Signs

- Seizures
- Mental status changes (Delirium)
- Dysarthria
- Dysphagia
- Pseudobulbar palsy
- Coma

Other risk factors for CPM = Alcoholism + Other electrolyte imbalances + Malnutrition

Concomitant use of ***furosemide*** can decrease incidence of CPM

Introduction: Diabetes Insipidus

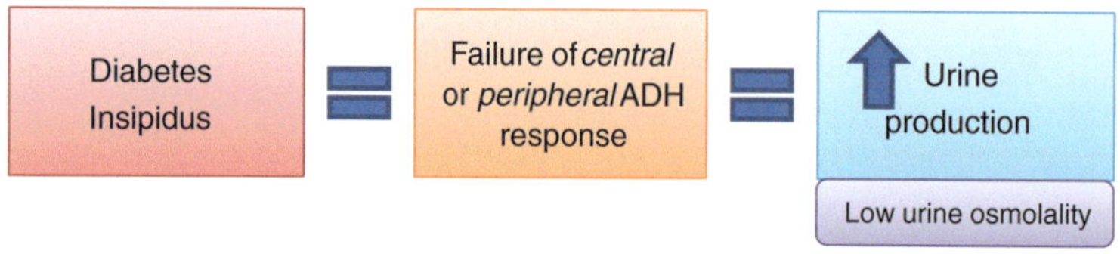

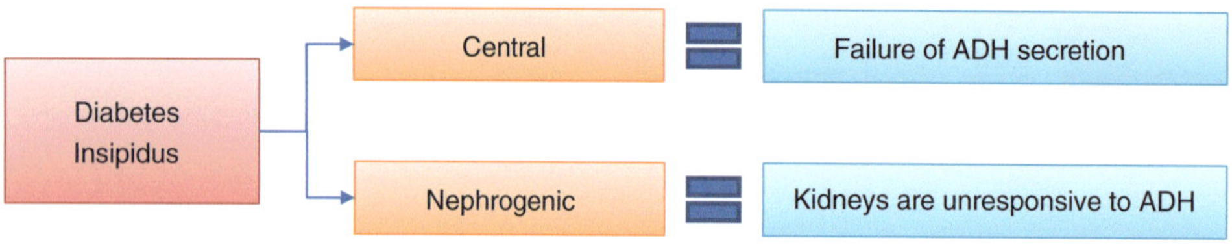

Some Causes of Central DI

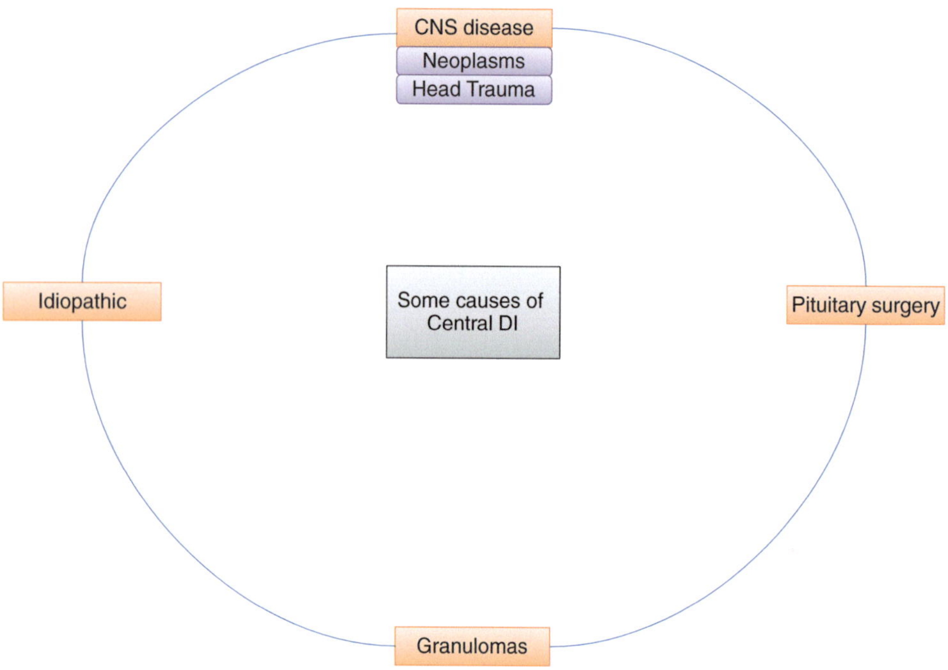

Some Causes of Nephrogenic DI

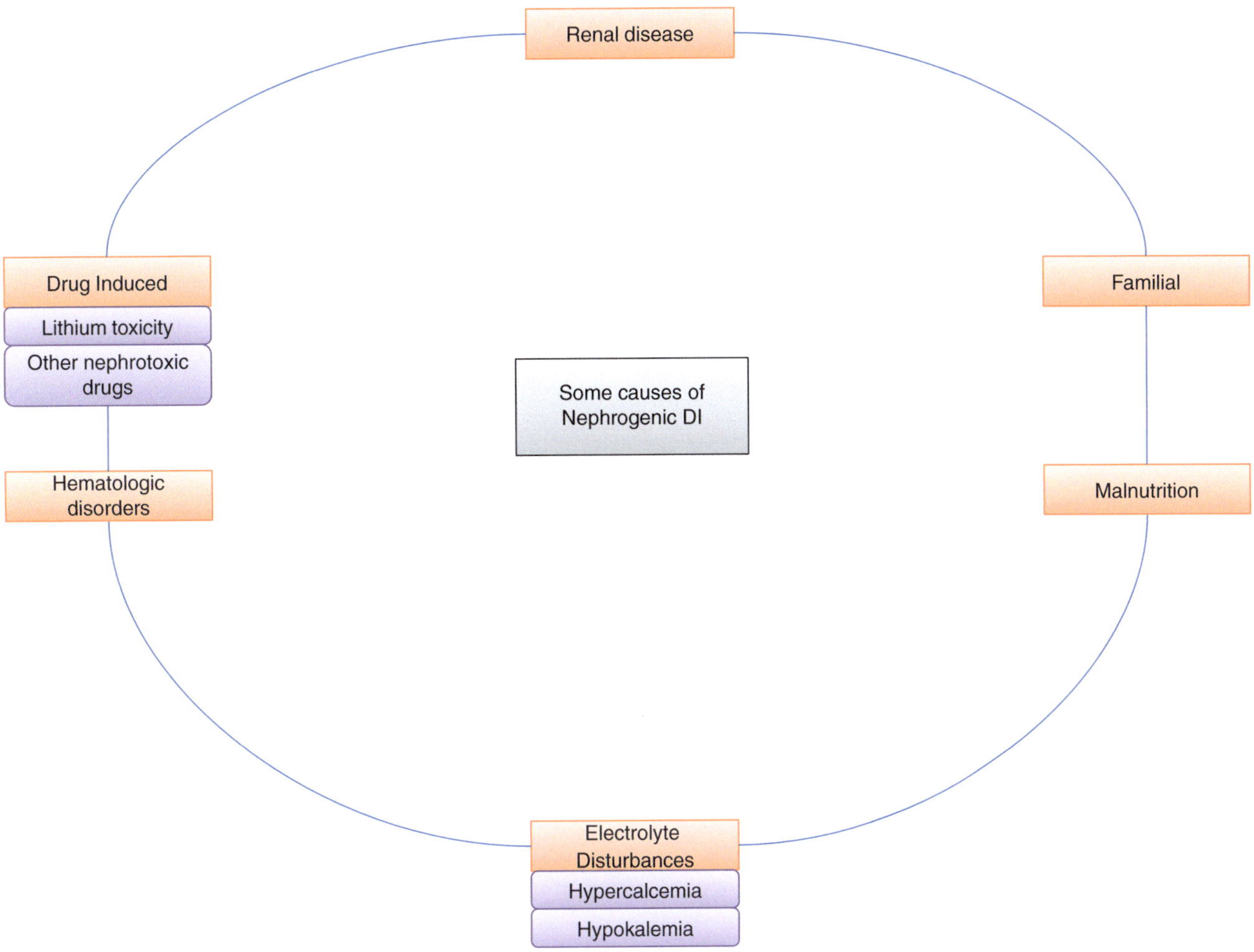

DI: Clinical Features

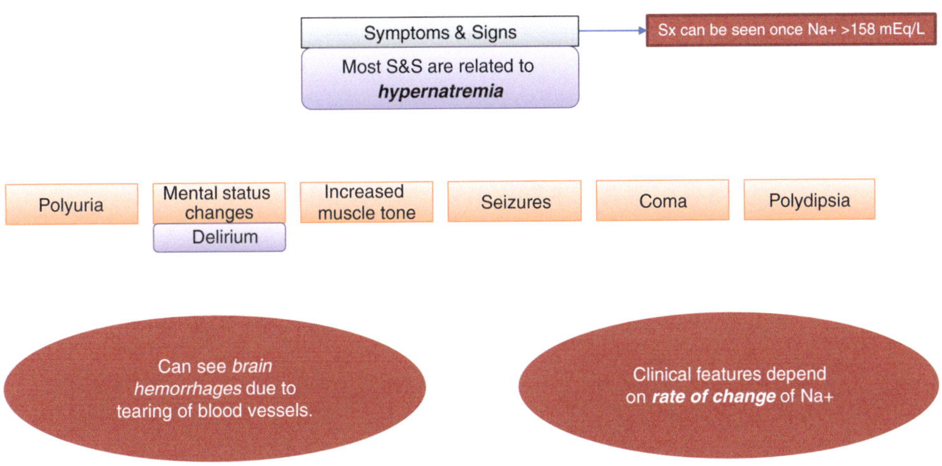

Laboratory Abnormalities and Testing Considerations

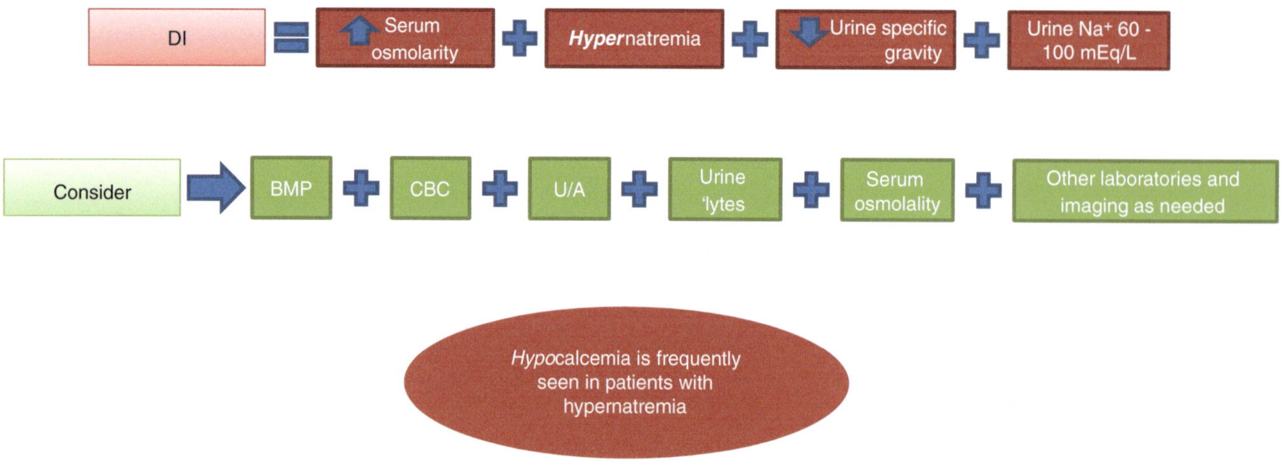

Treatment and Disposition

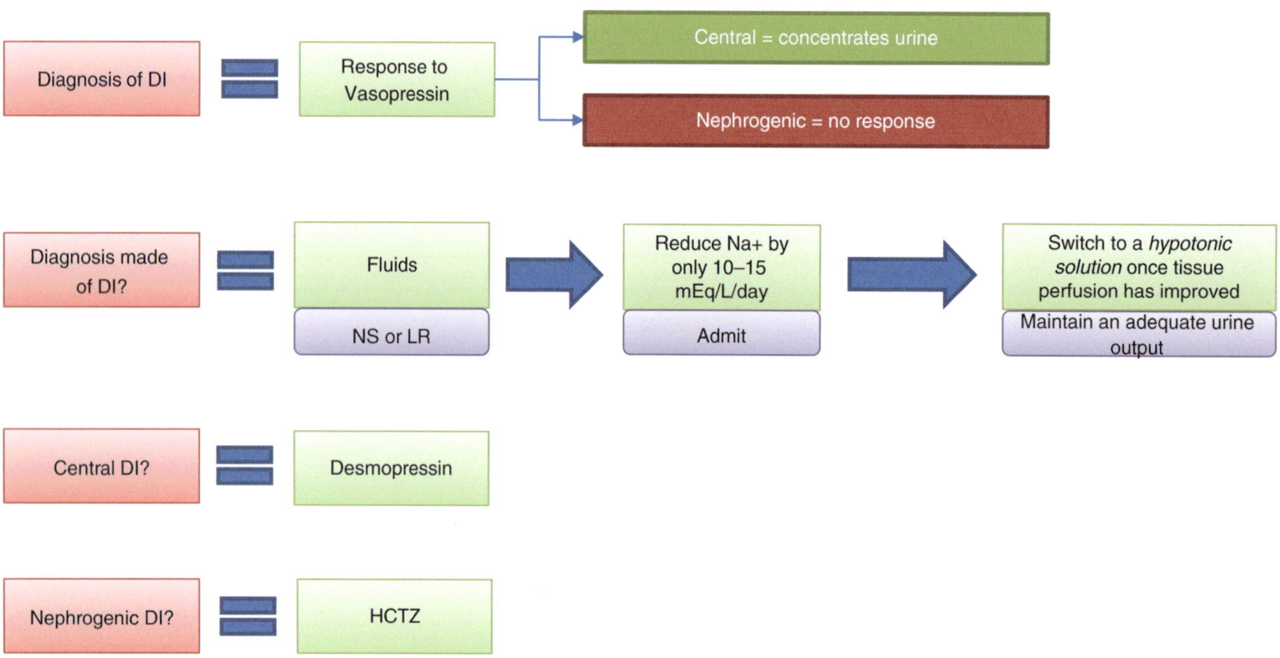

Electrolytes and Acid-Base

Sodium

Introduction: Hyponatremia

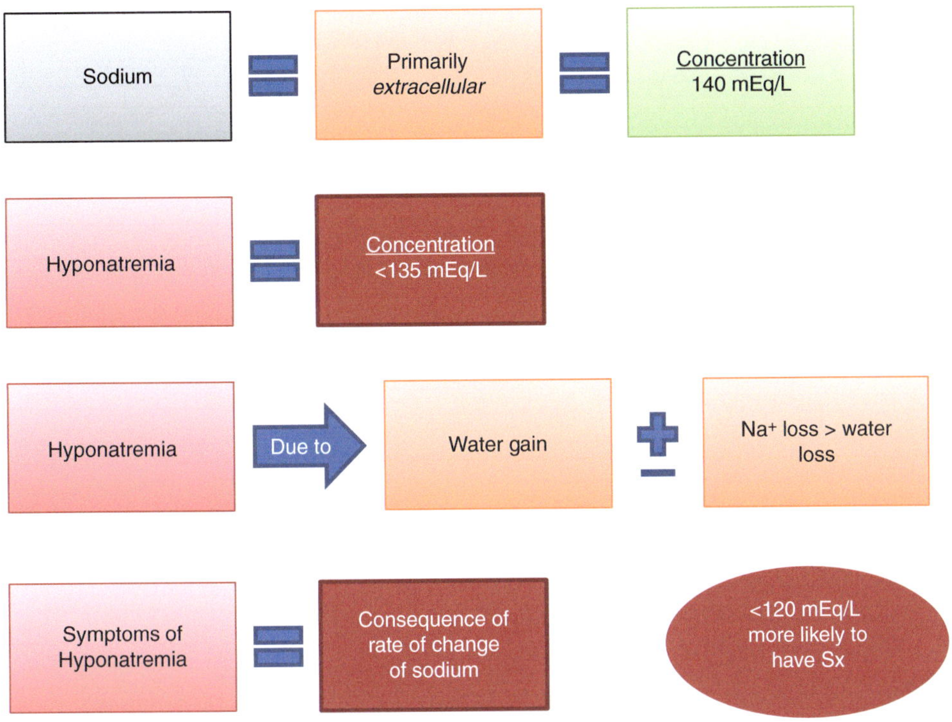

Hyponatremia

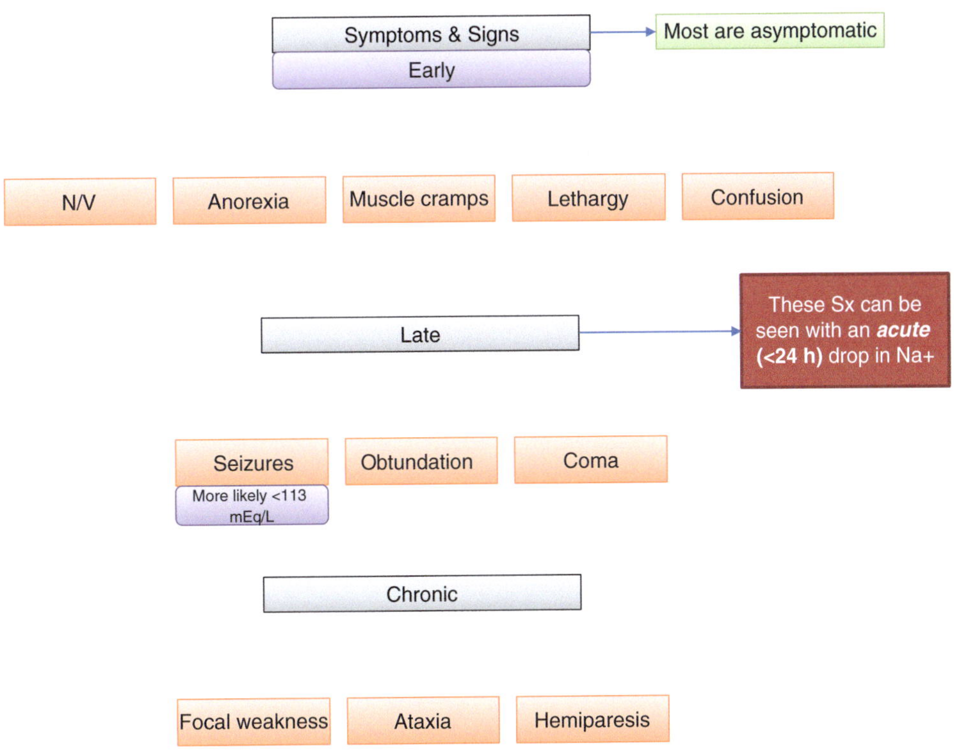

Diagnosis + Treatment

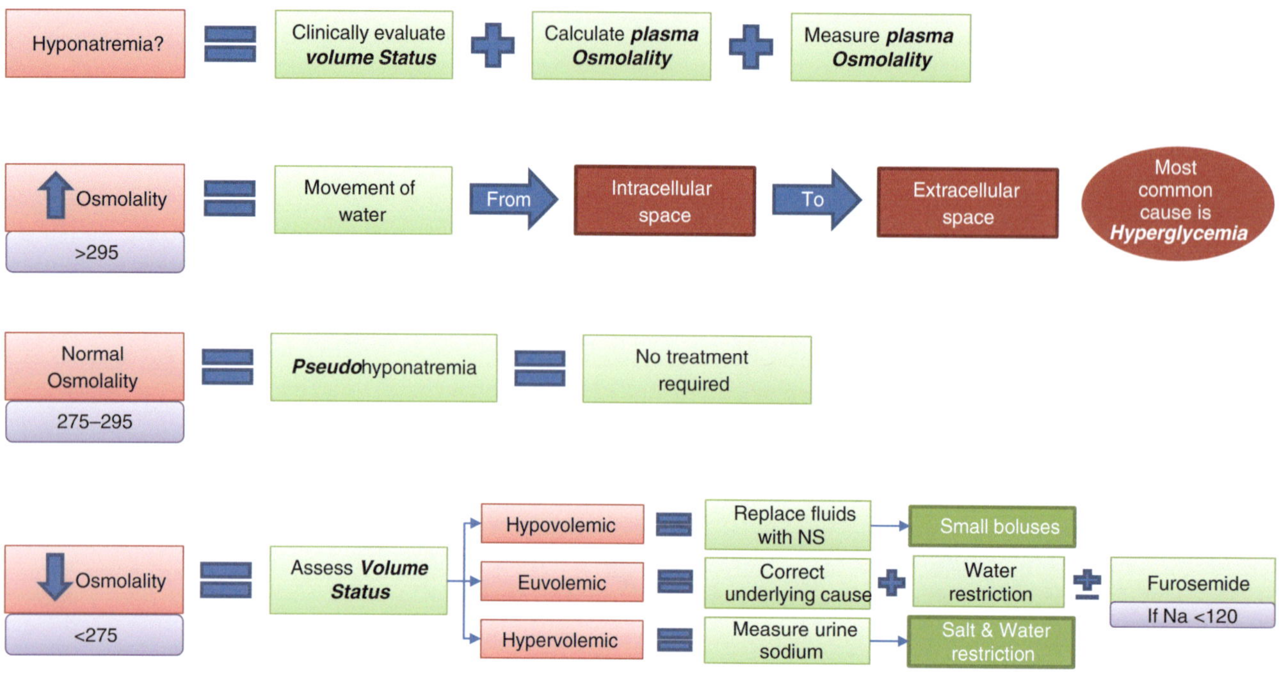

Causes of Hyponatremia

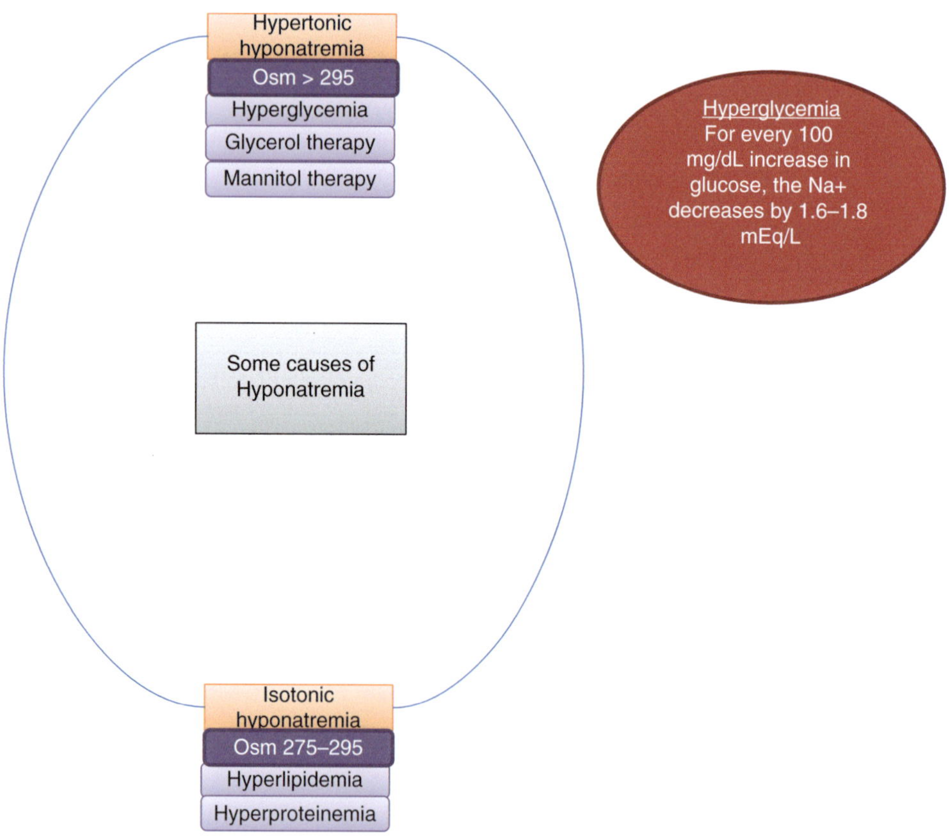

Causes of Hypotonic Hyponatremia (Osm < 275)

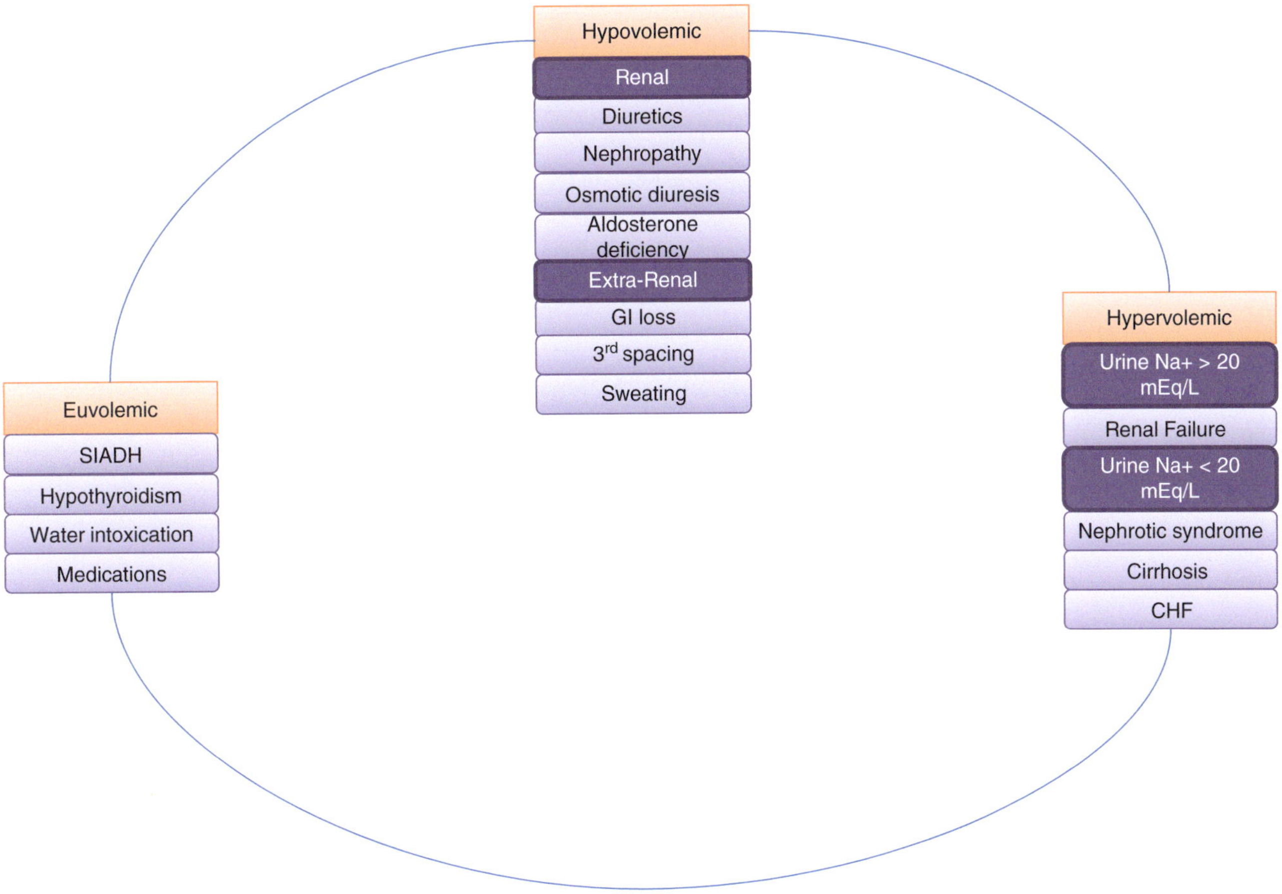

Introduction: Hypernatremia

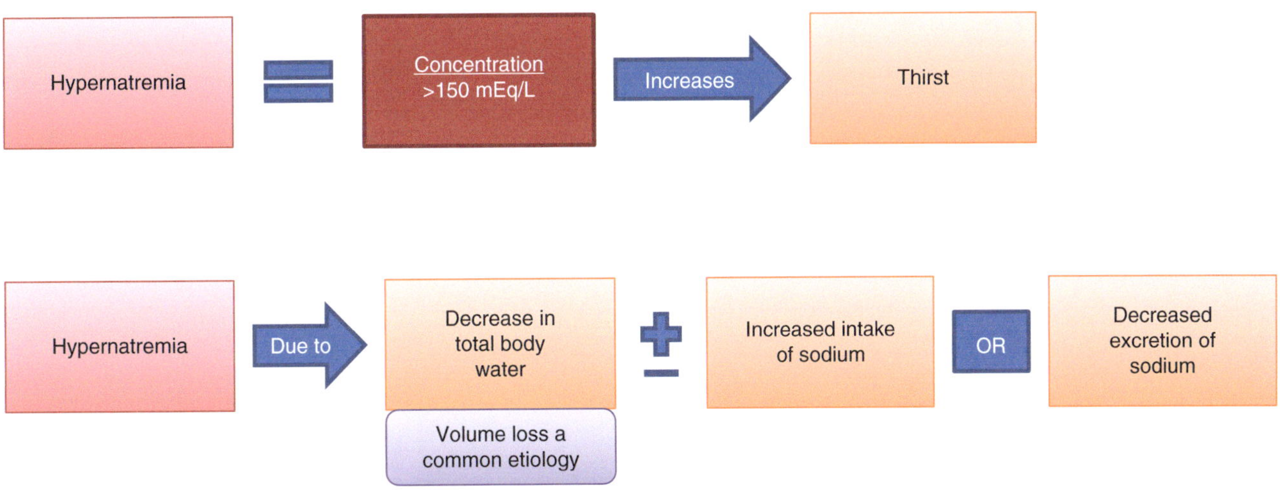

Some Causes of Hypernatremia

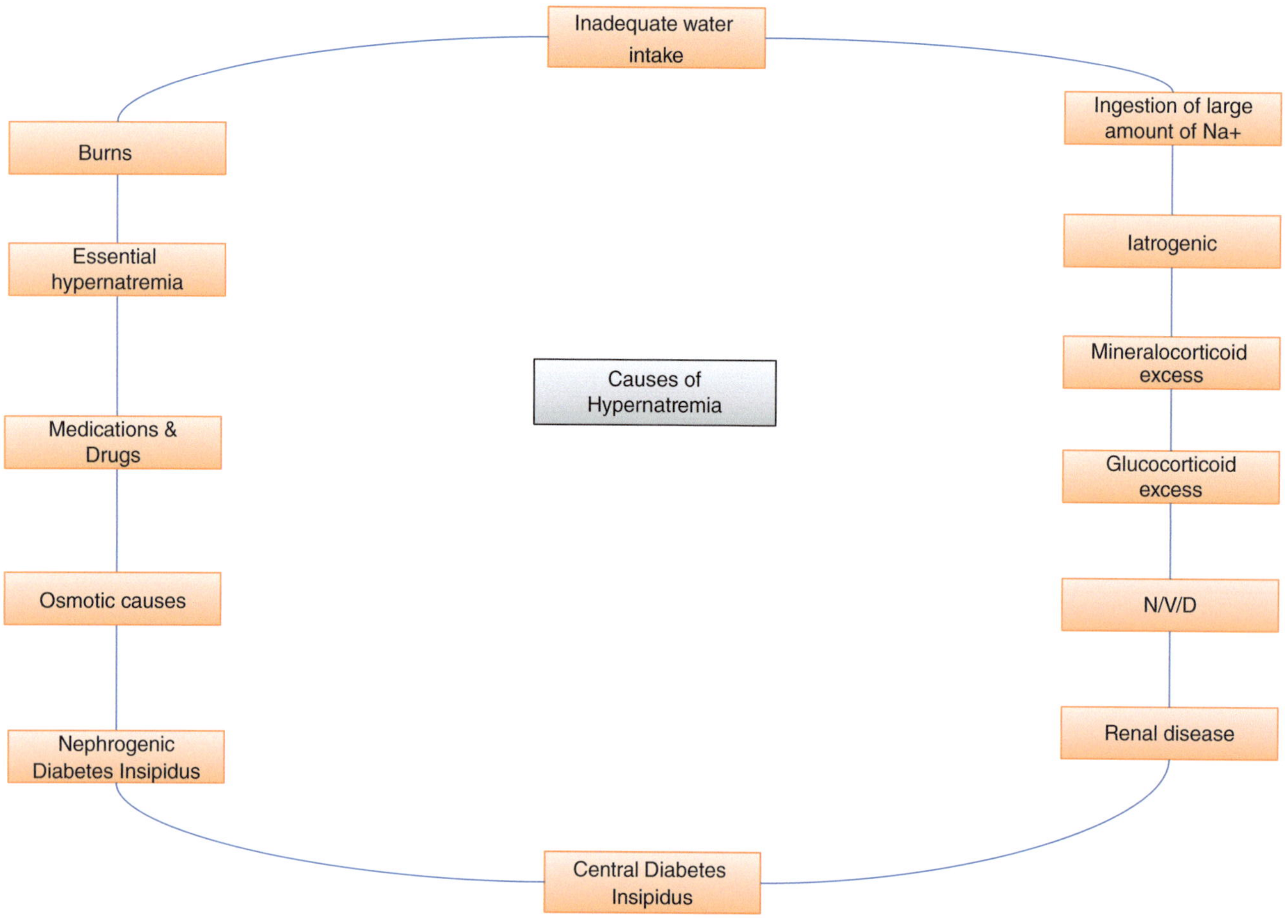

Hypernatremia Symptoms

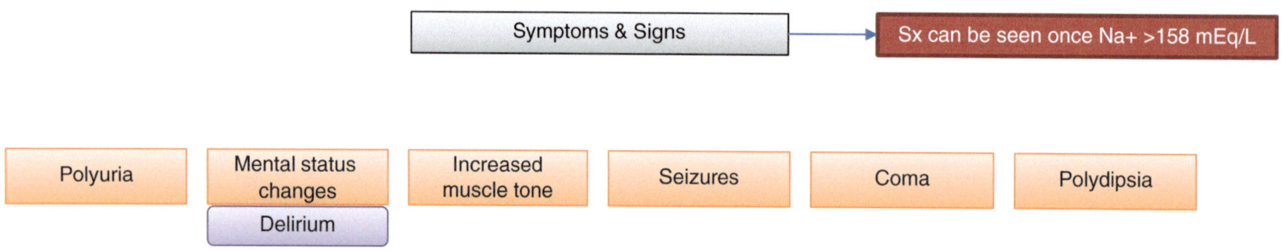

Treatment

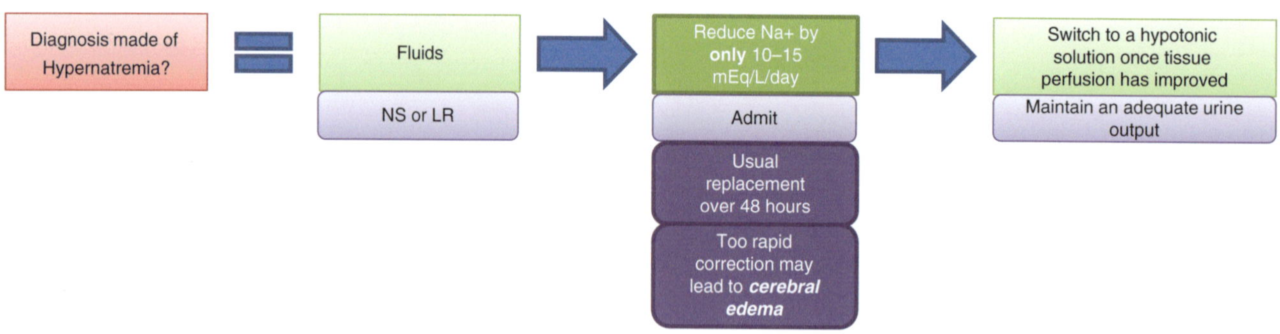

Potassium

Introduction: Hypokalemia

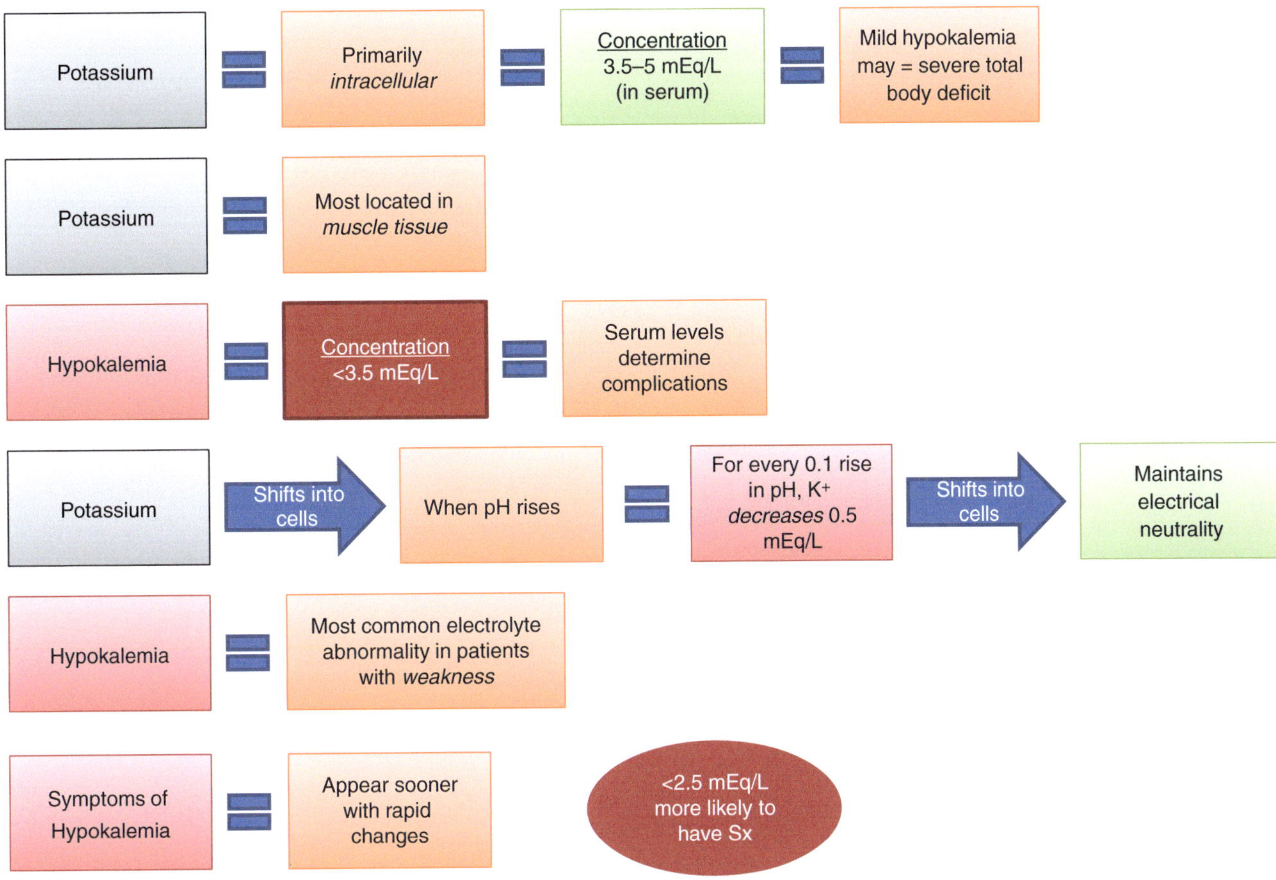

Causes of Hypokalemia

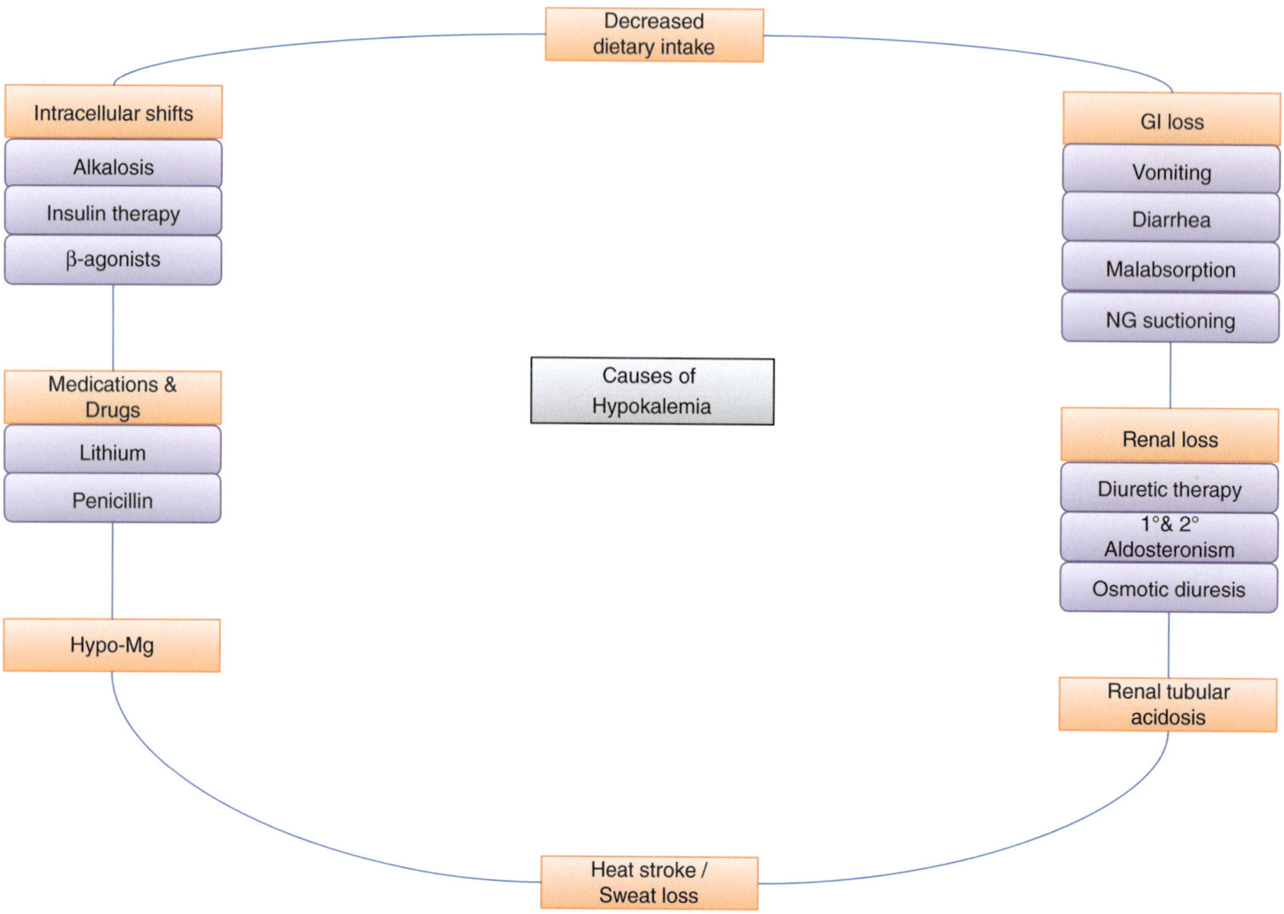

Hypokalemia Symptoms and Signs

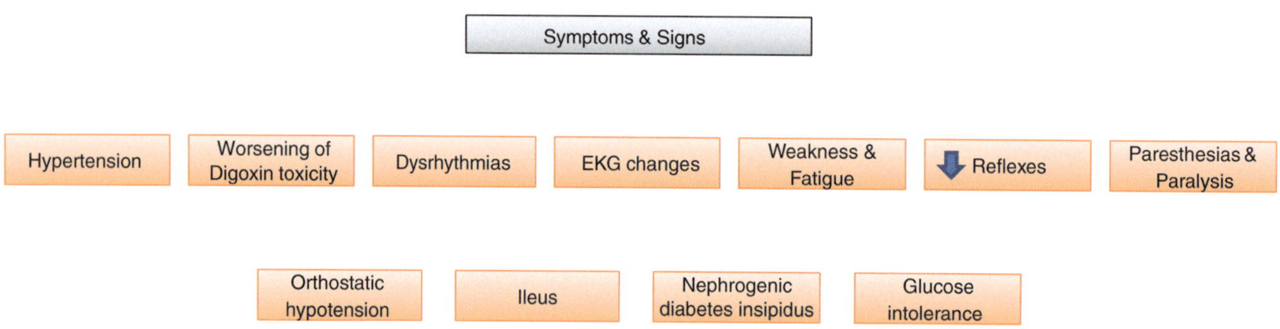

Diagnosis + Treatment

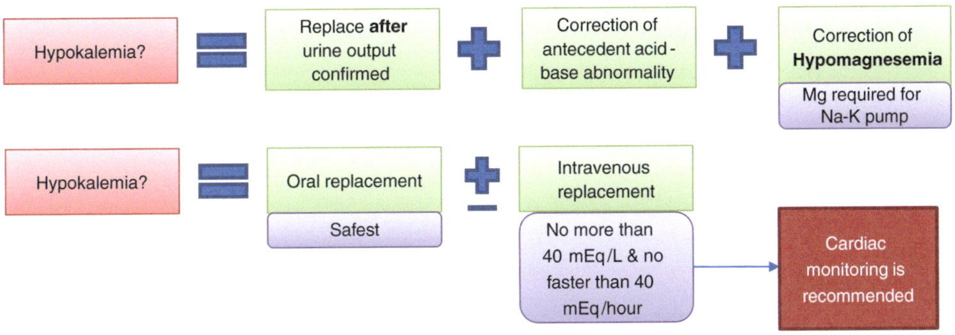

Introduction: Hyperkalemia

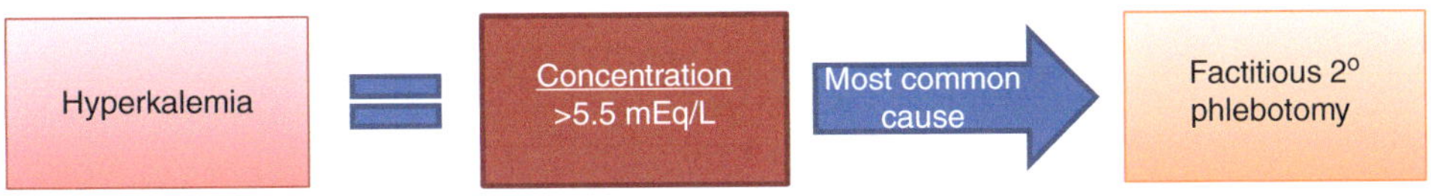

Causes of Hyperkalemia

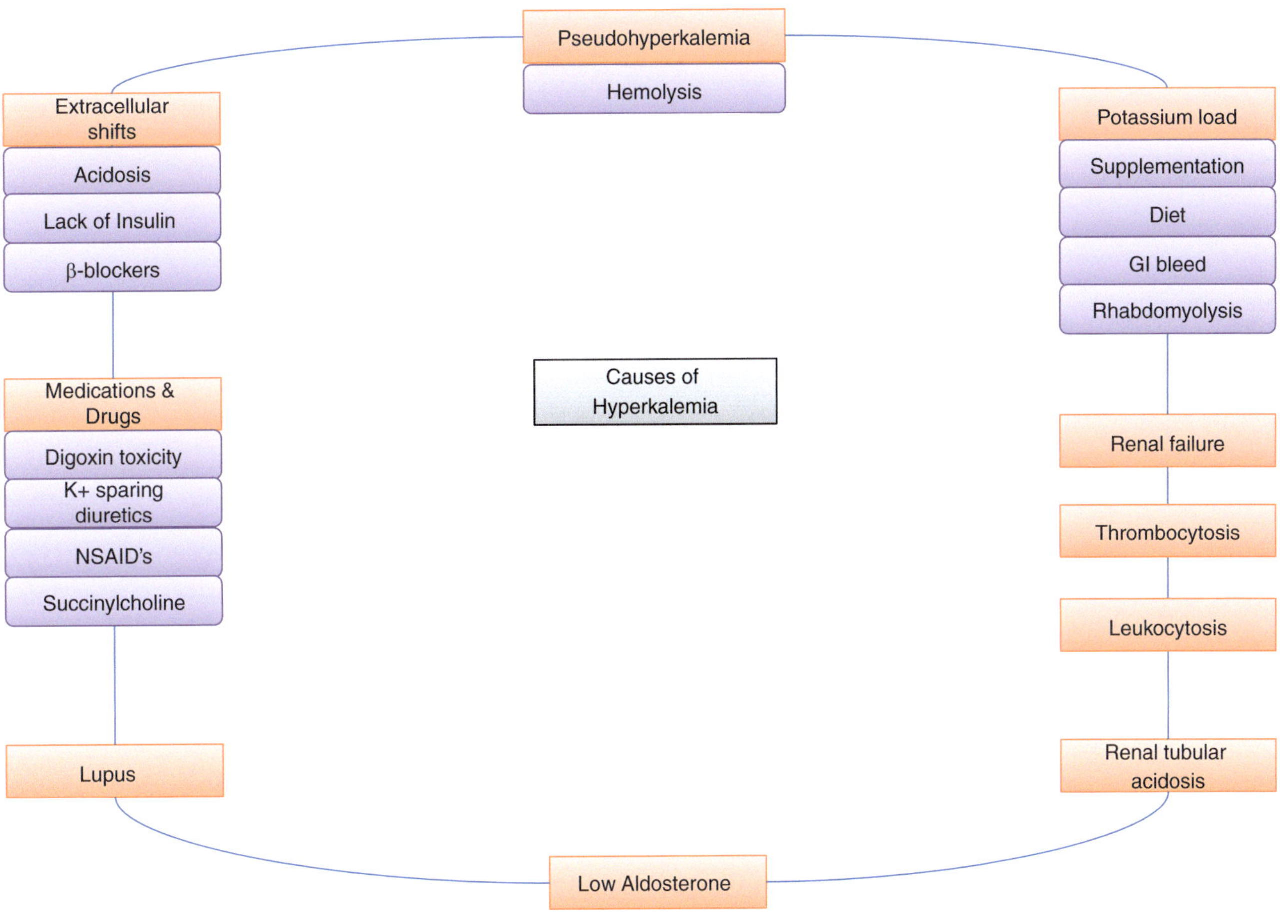

Hyperkalemia Symptoms and Signs

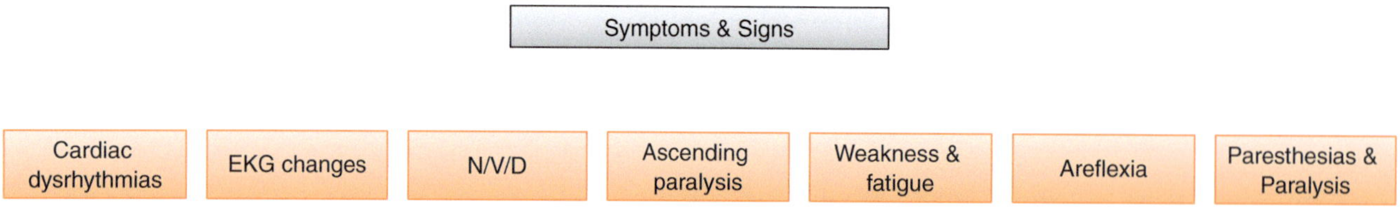

Diagnosis + Treatment

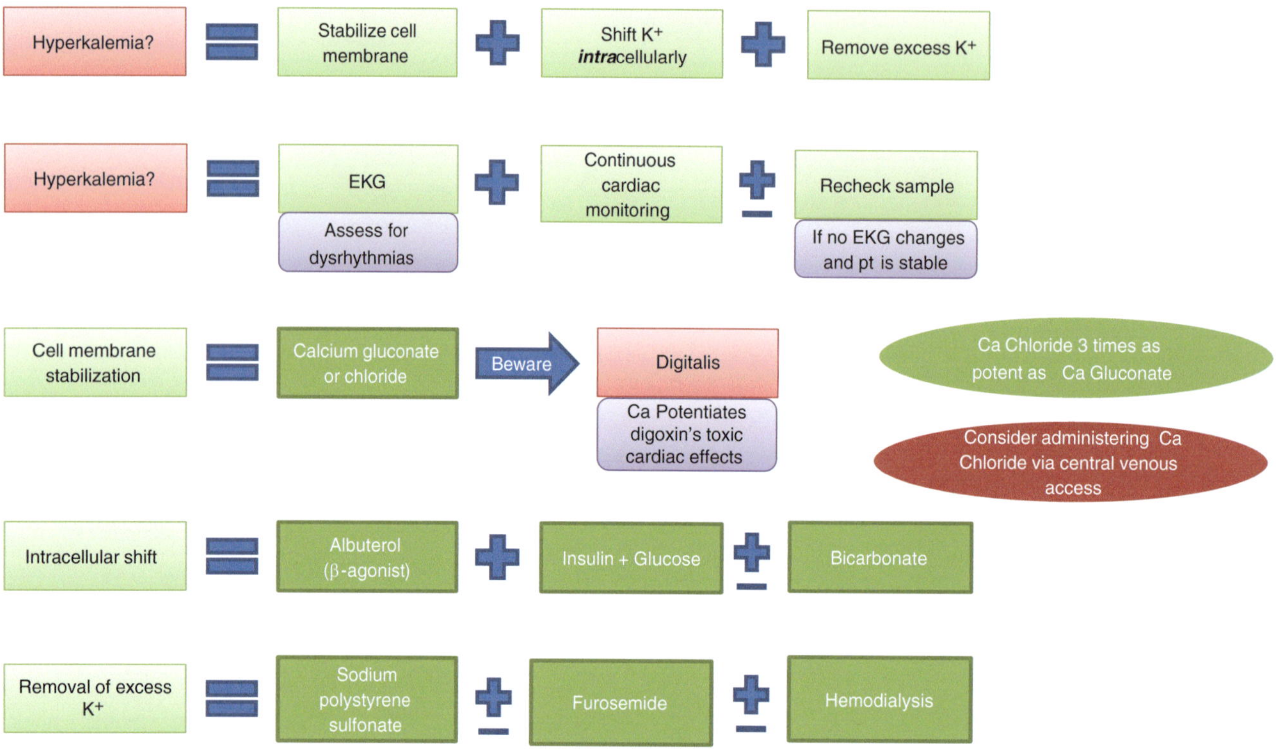

Calcium

Introduction: Calcium

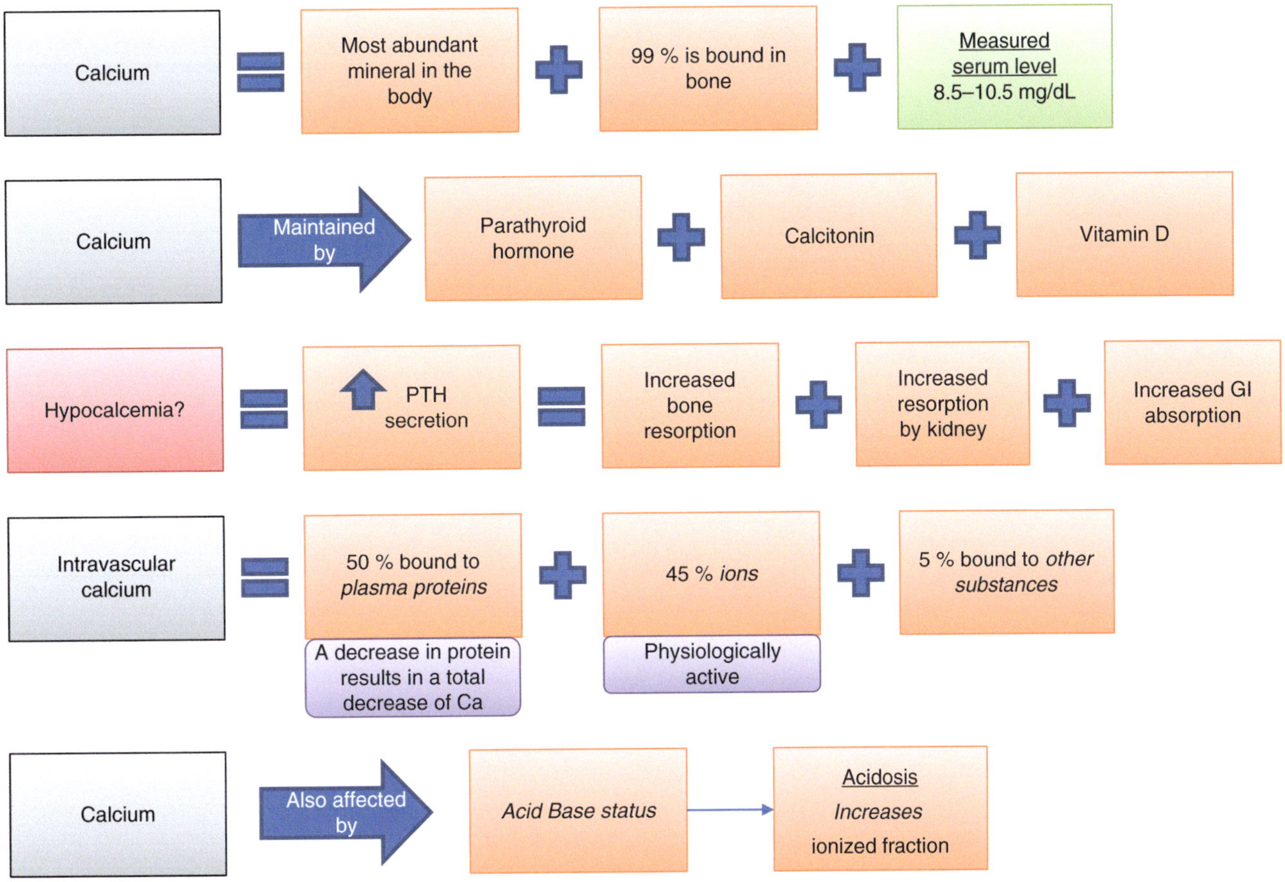

Introduction: Hypocalcemia

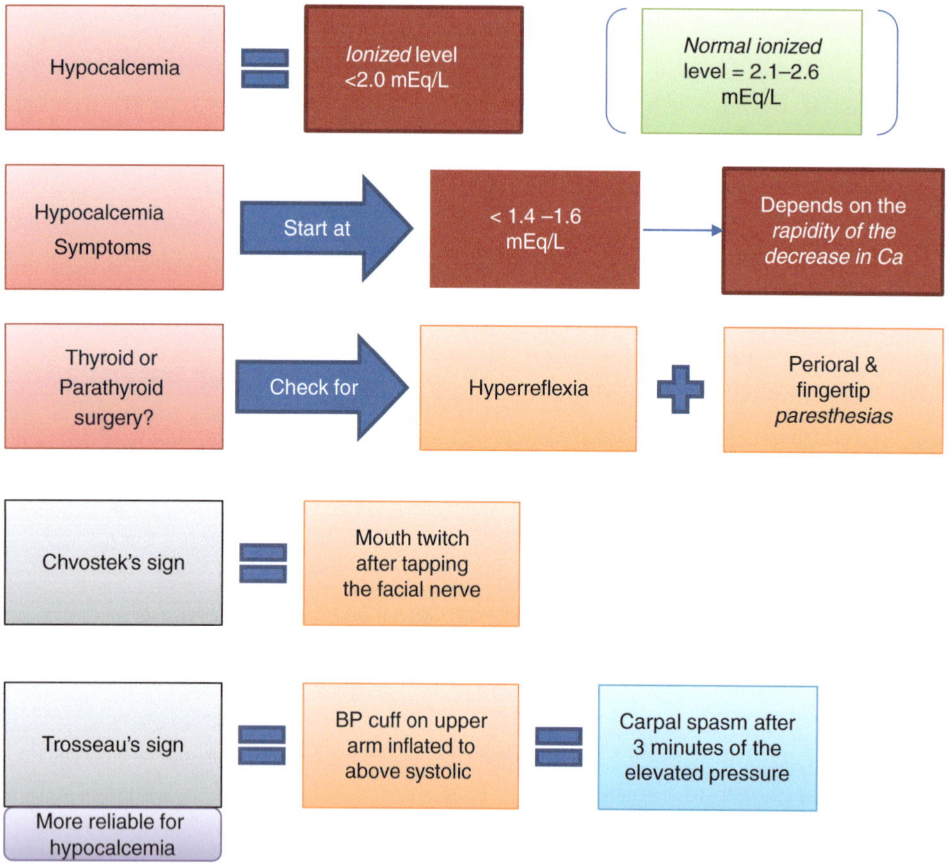

Causes of Hypocalcemia

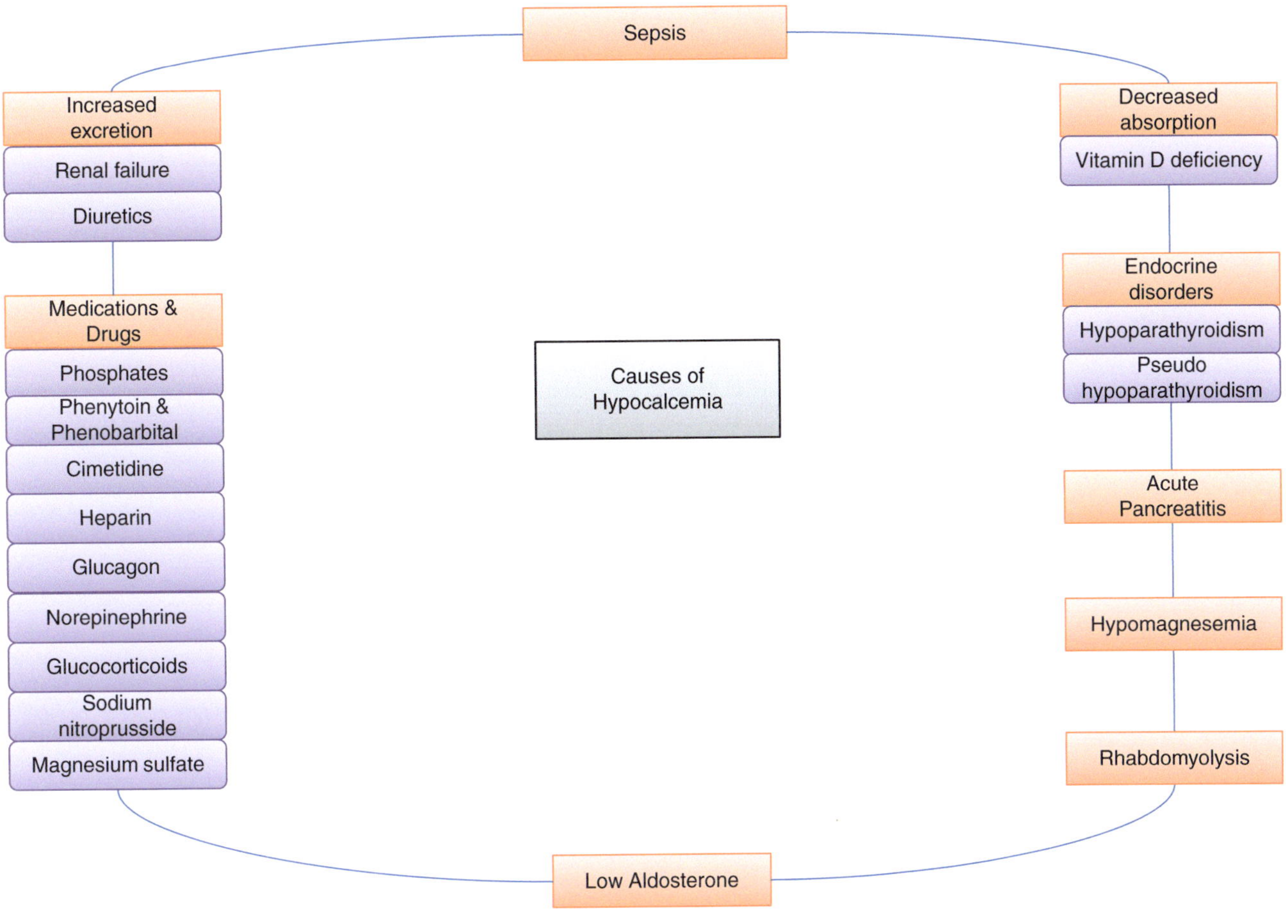

Hypocalcemia Symptoms and Signs

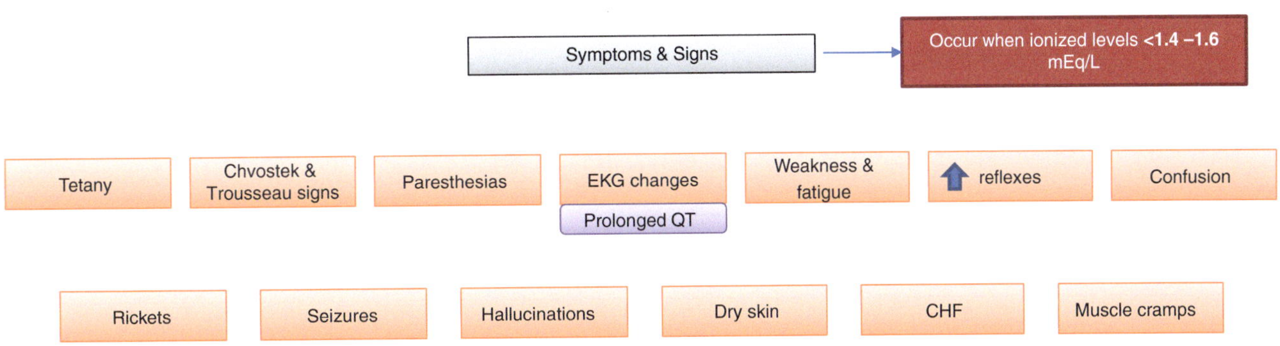

Diagnosis + Treatment

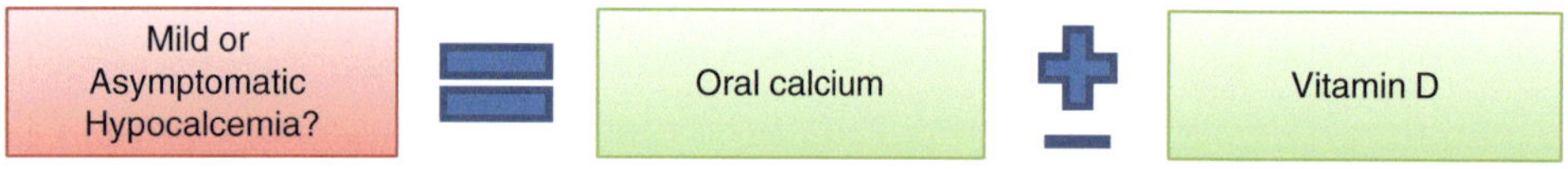

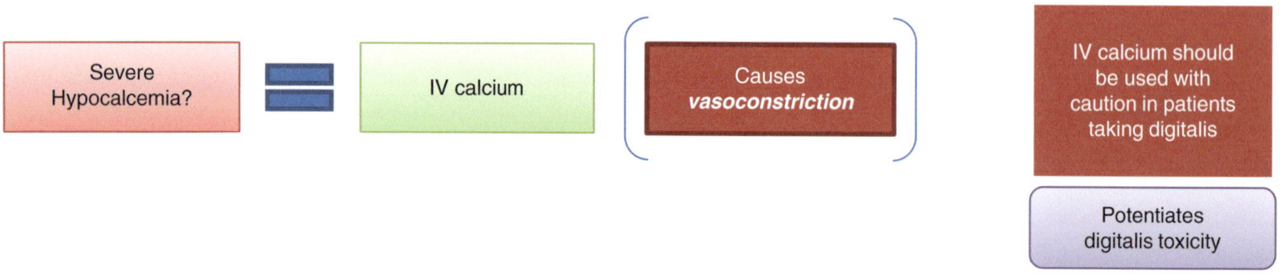

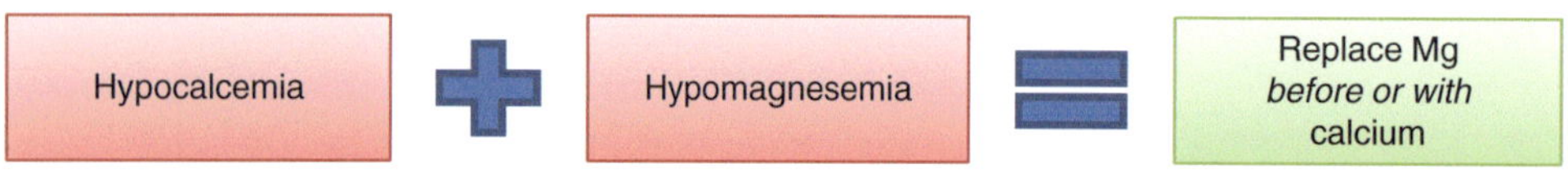

Introduction: Hypercalcemia

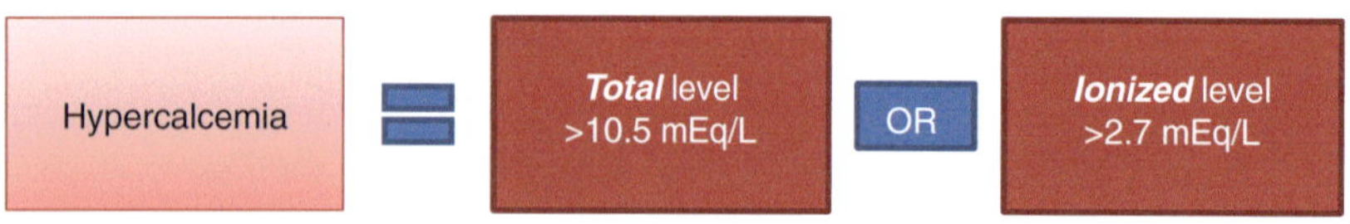

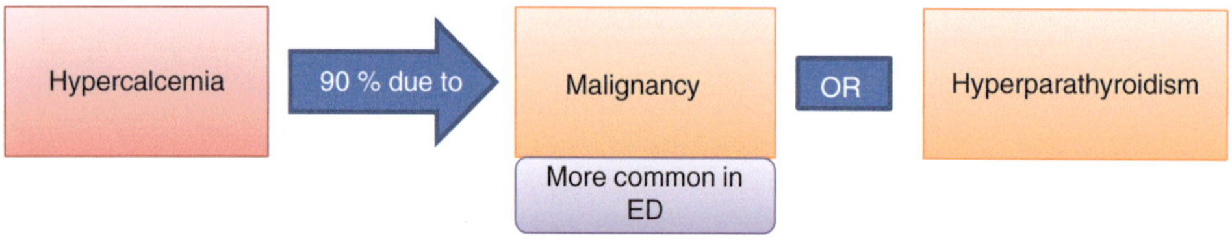

Causes of Hypercalcemia

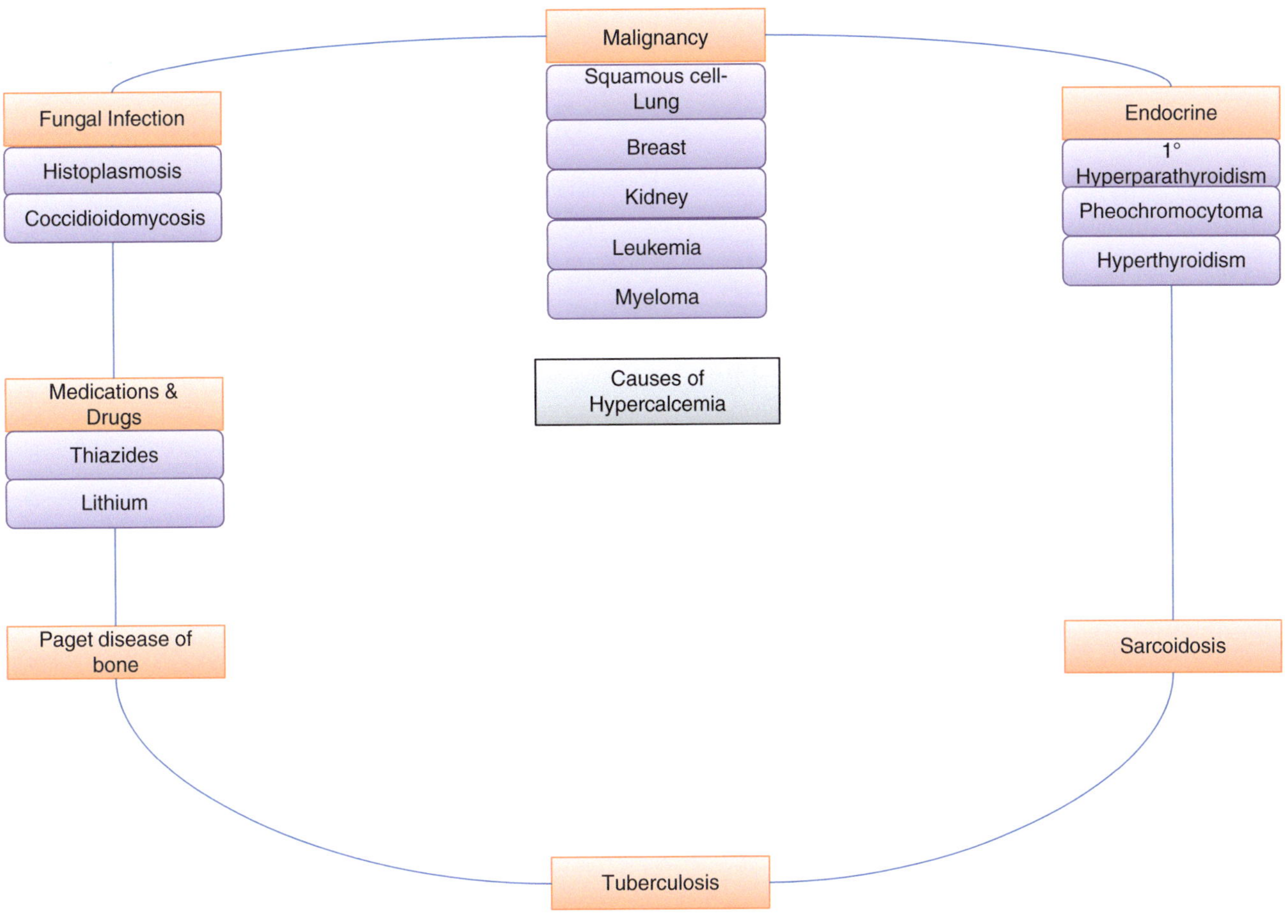

Hypercalcemia Symptoms and Signs

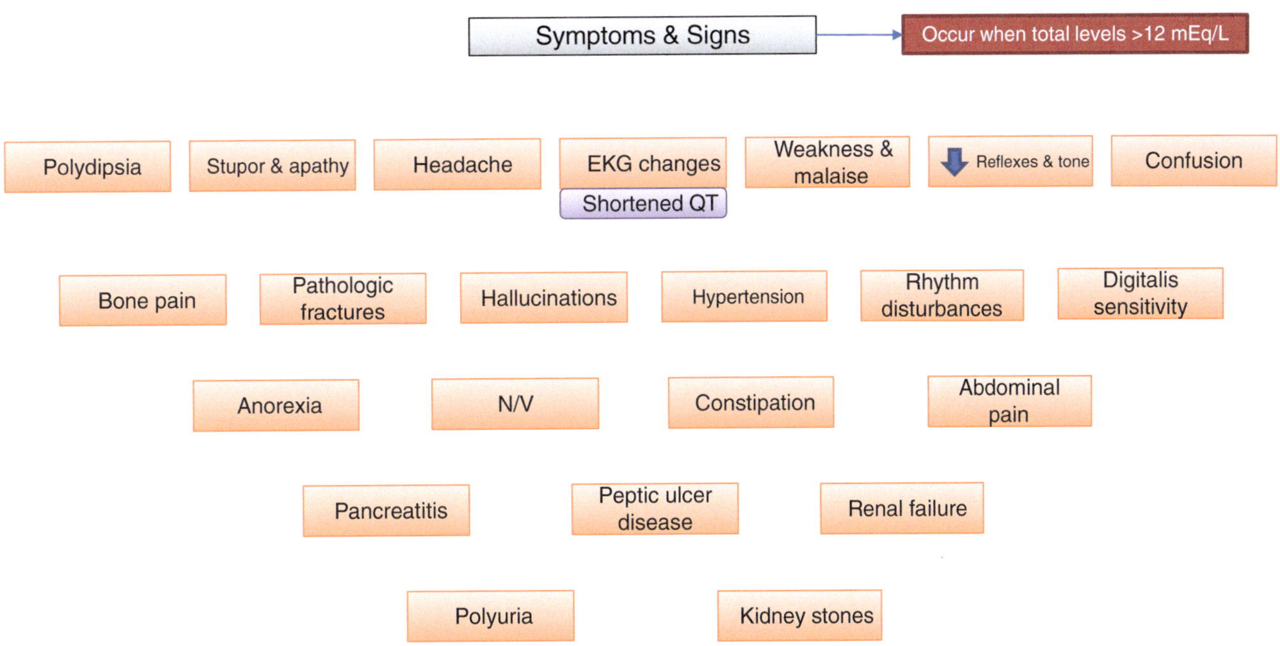

Diagnosis + Treatment

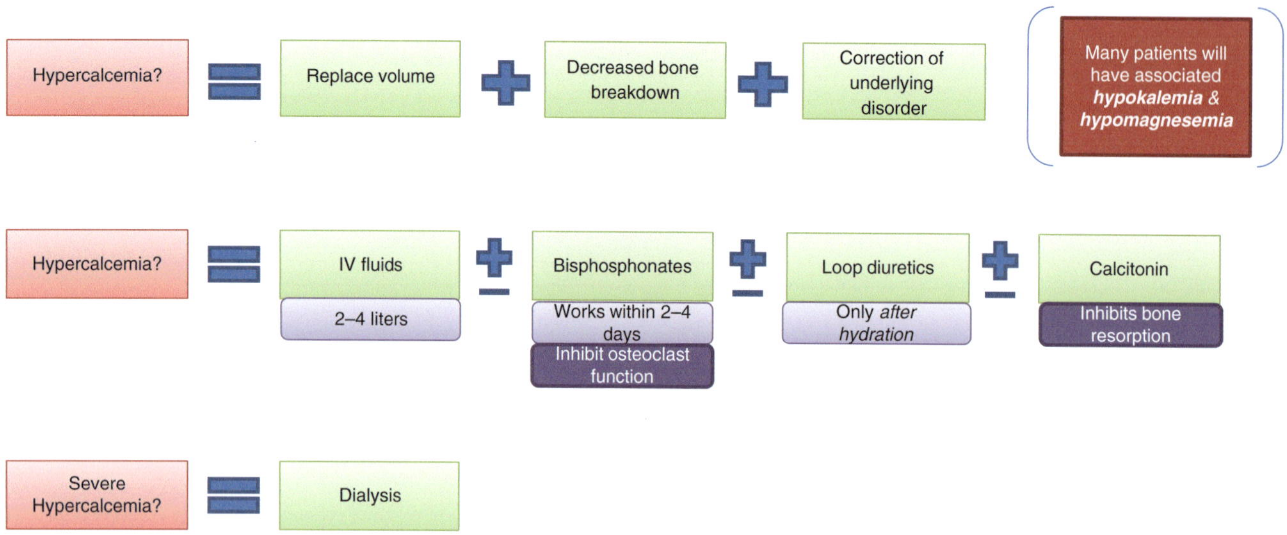

Magnesium

Introduction

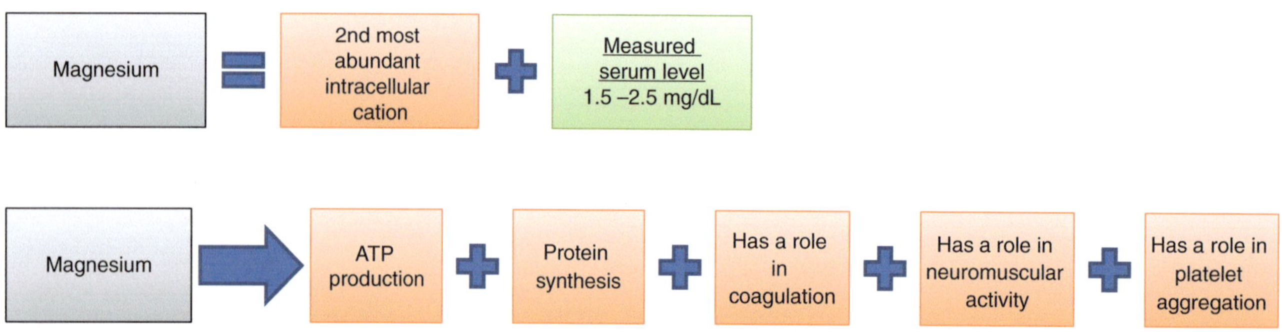

Introduction: Hypomagnesemia

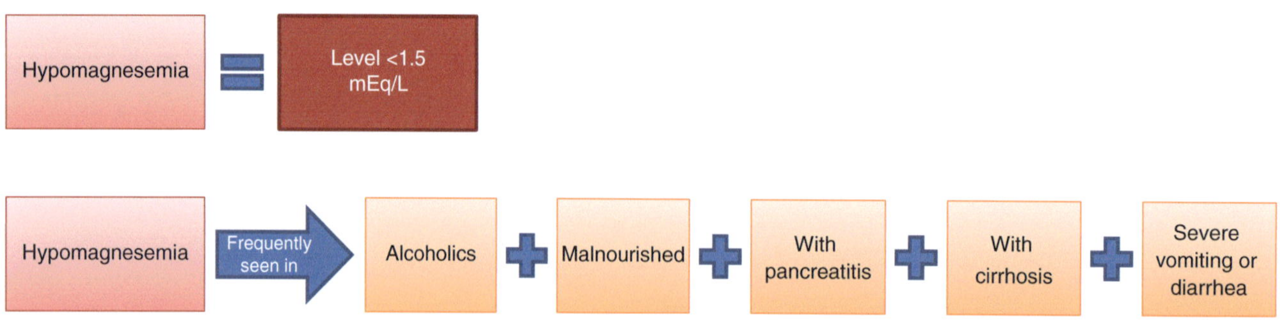

Causes of Hypomagnesemia

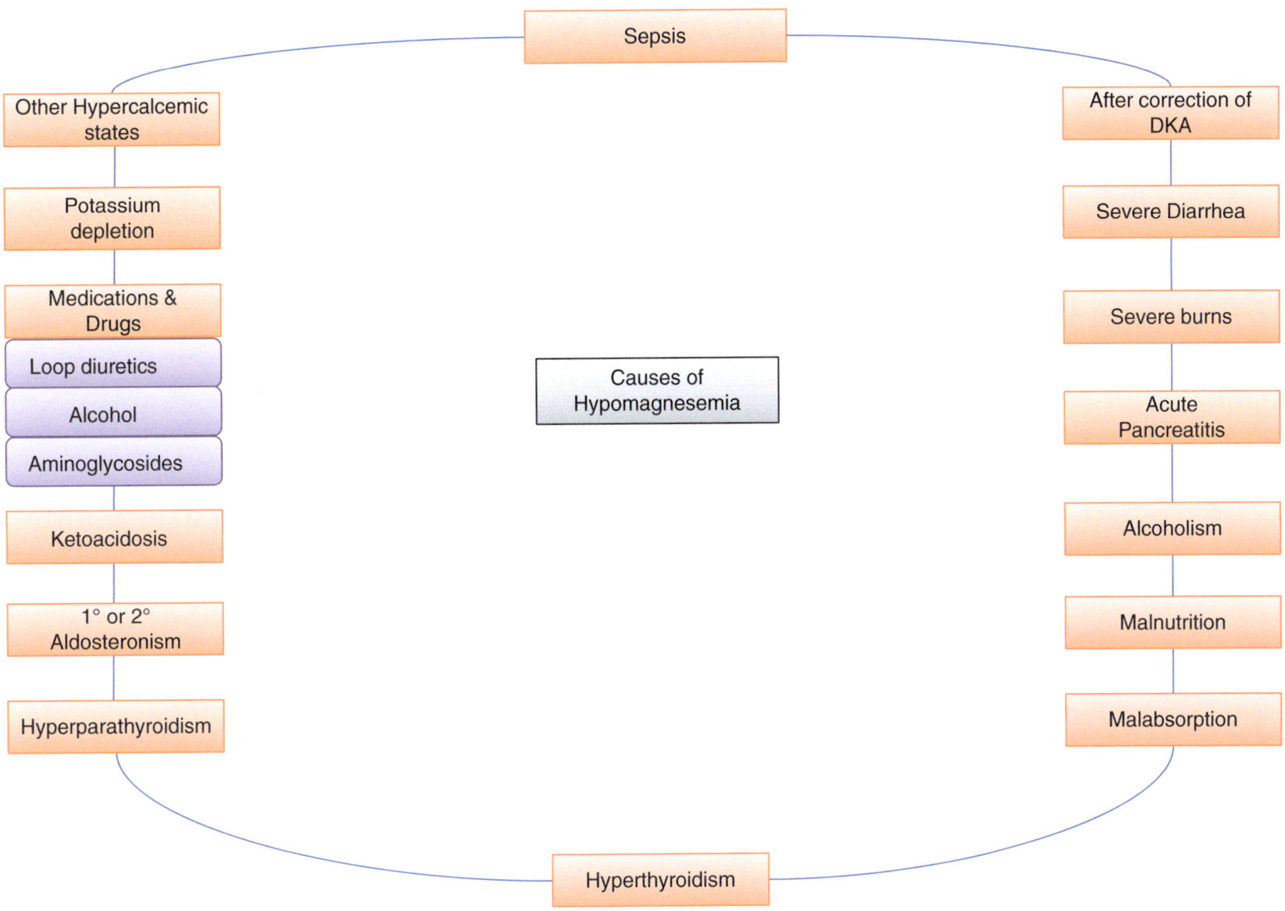

Hypomagnesemia Symptoms and Signs

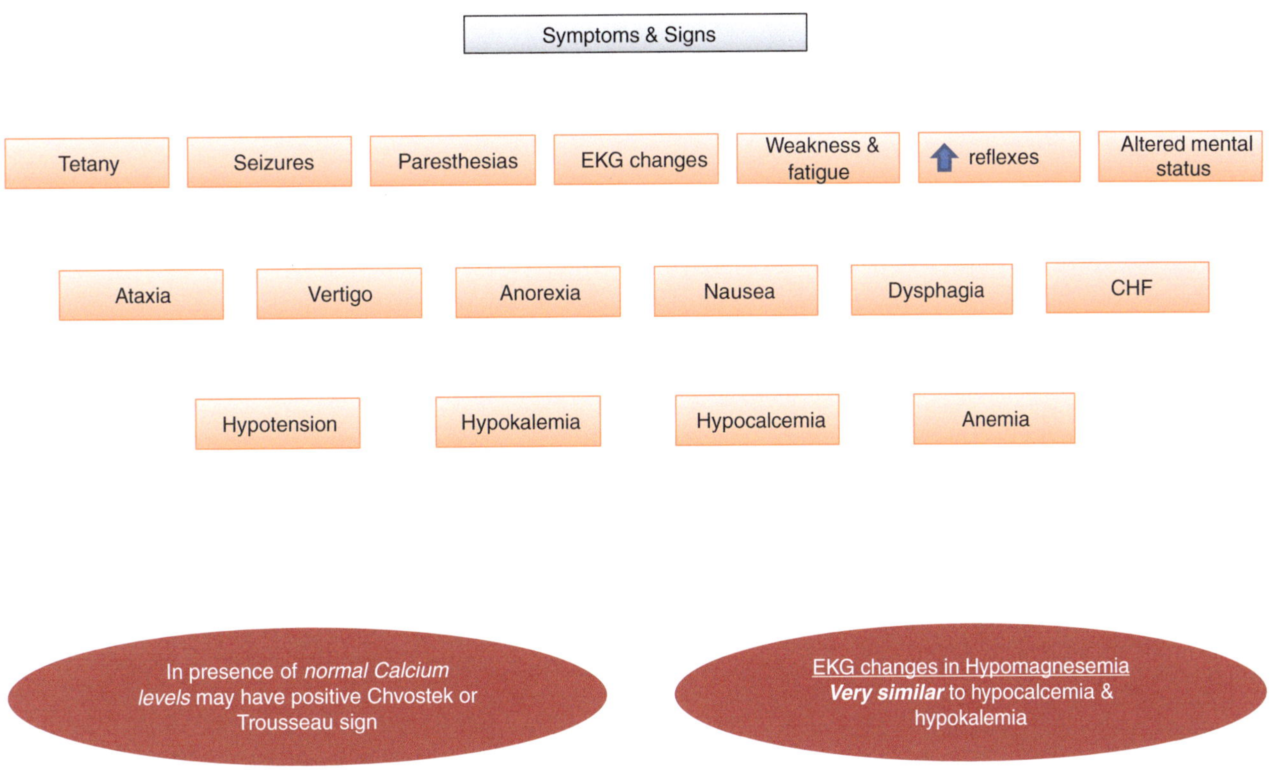

Diagnosis + Treatment

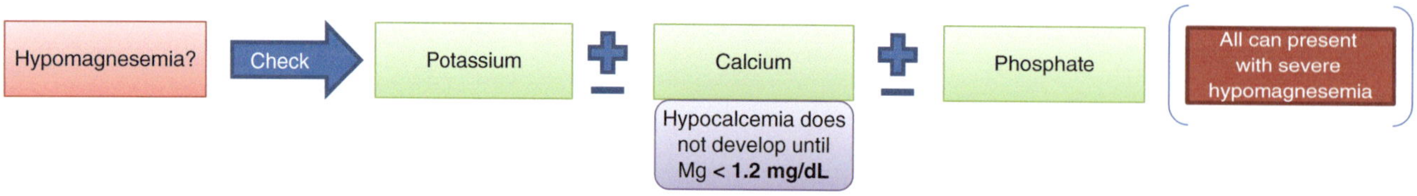

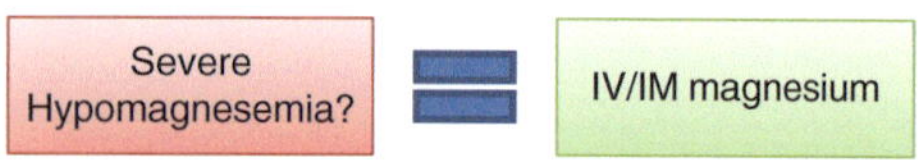

Introduction: Hypermagnesemia

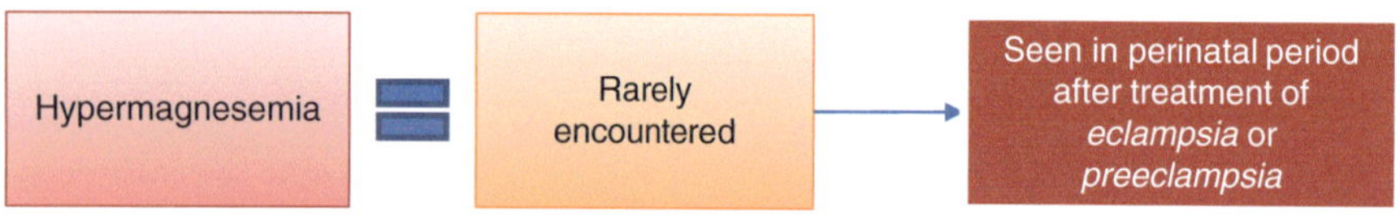

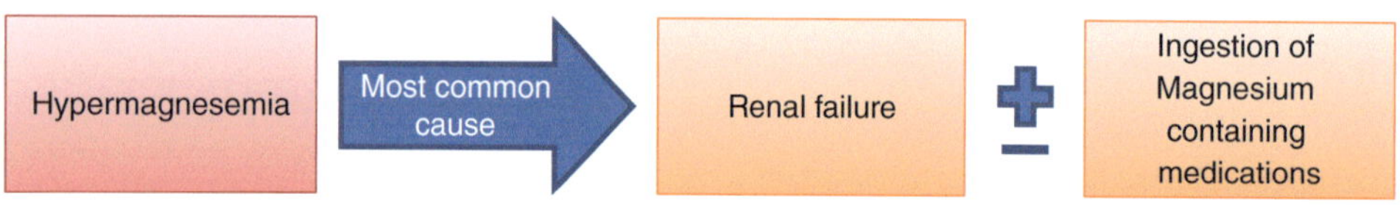

Causes of Hypermagnesemia

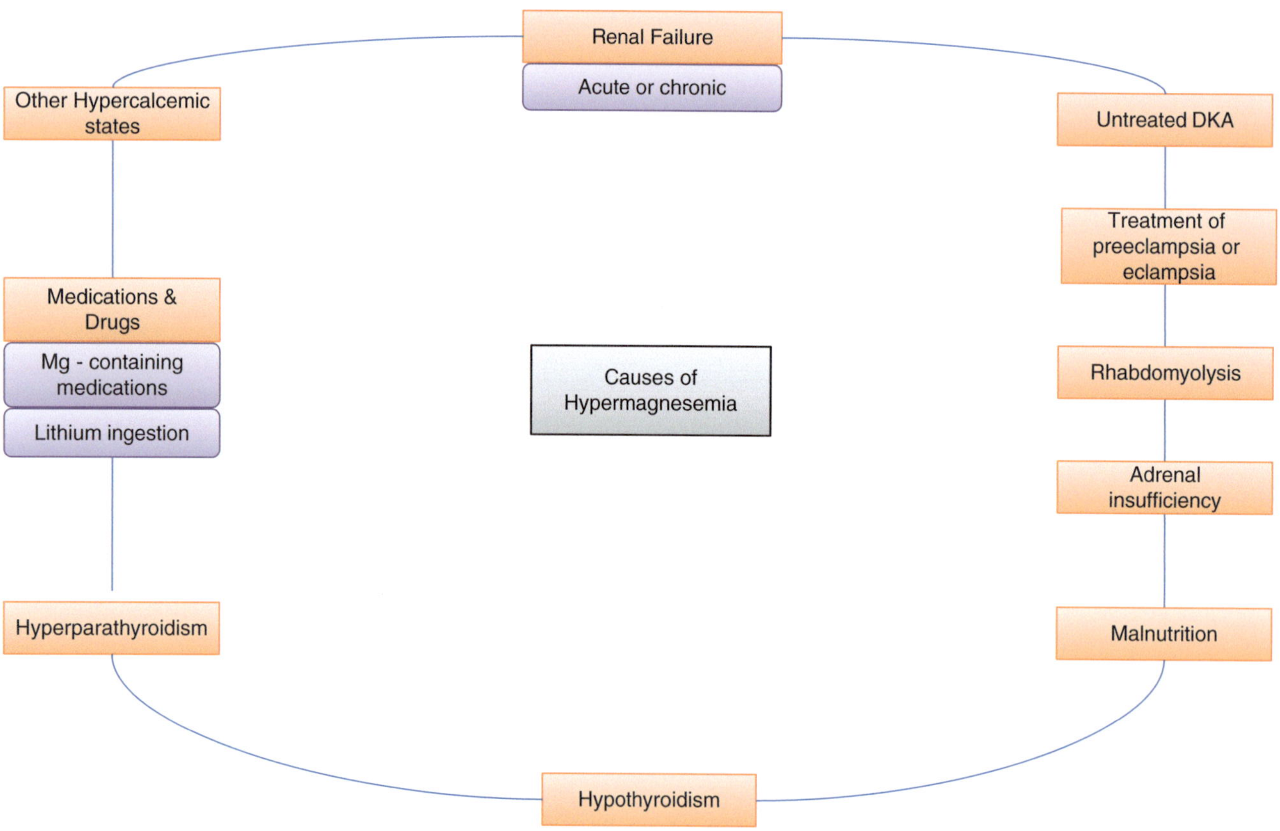

Hypermagnesemia Symptoms and Signs

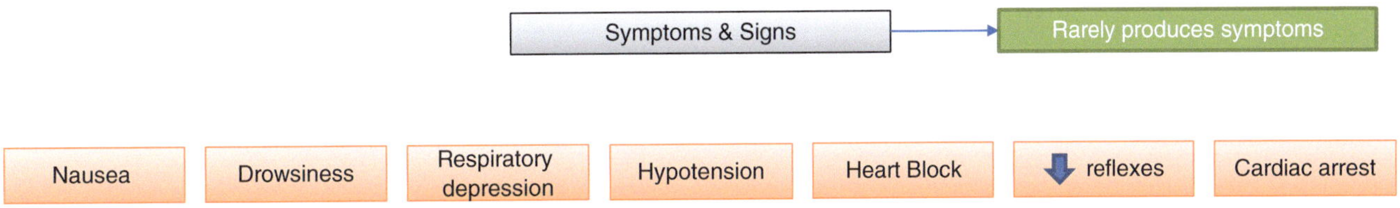

Diagnosis + Treatment

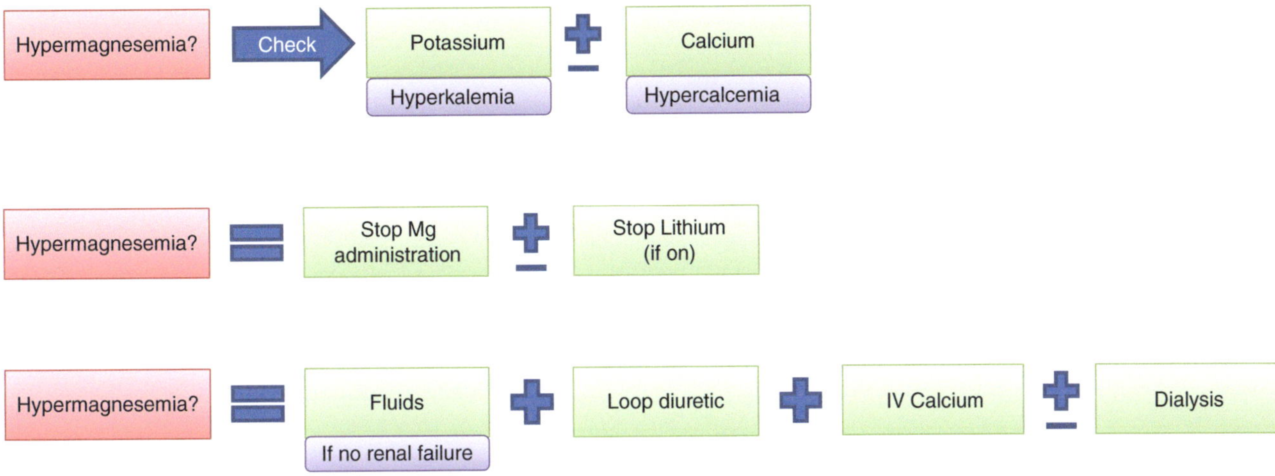

Phosphorus

Introduction

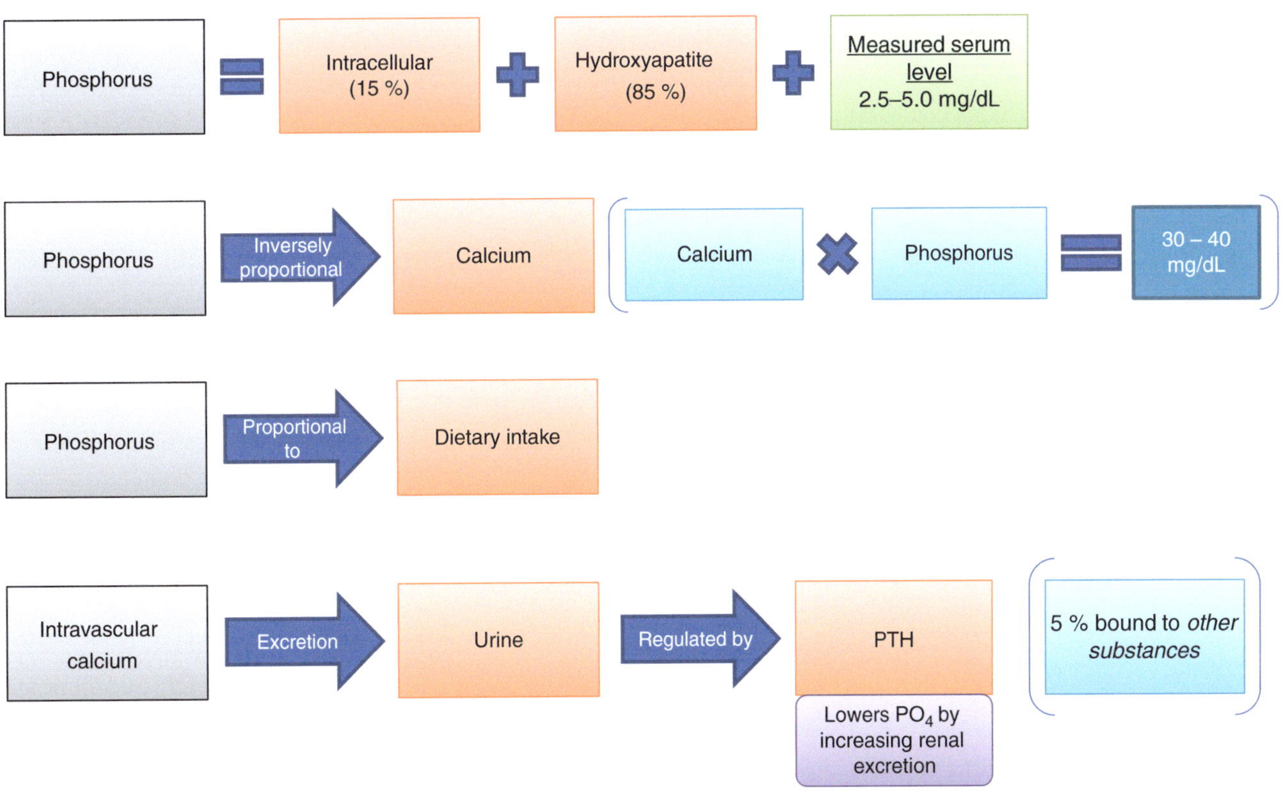

Introduction: Hypophosphatemia

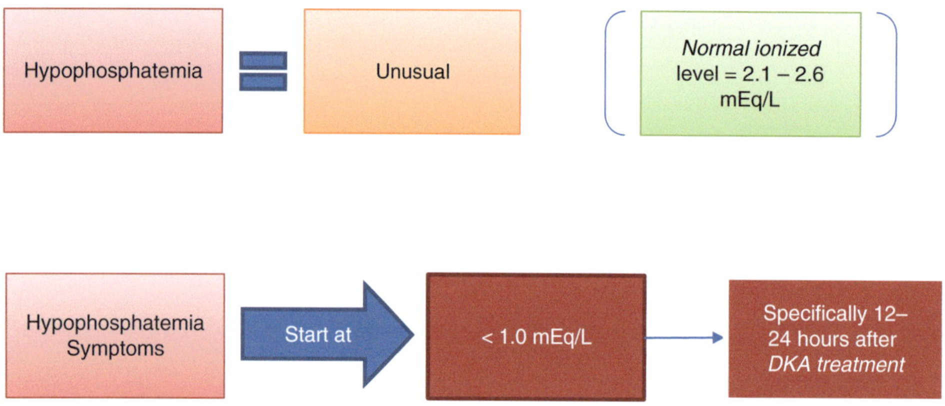

Causes of Hypophosphatemia

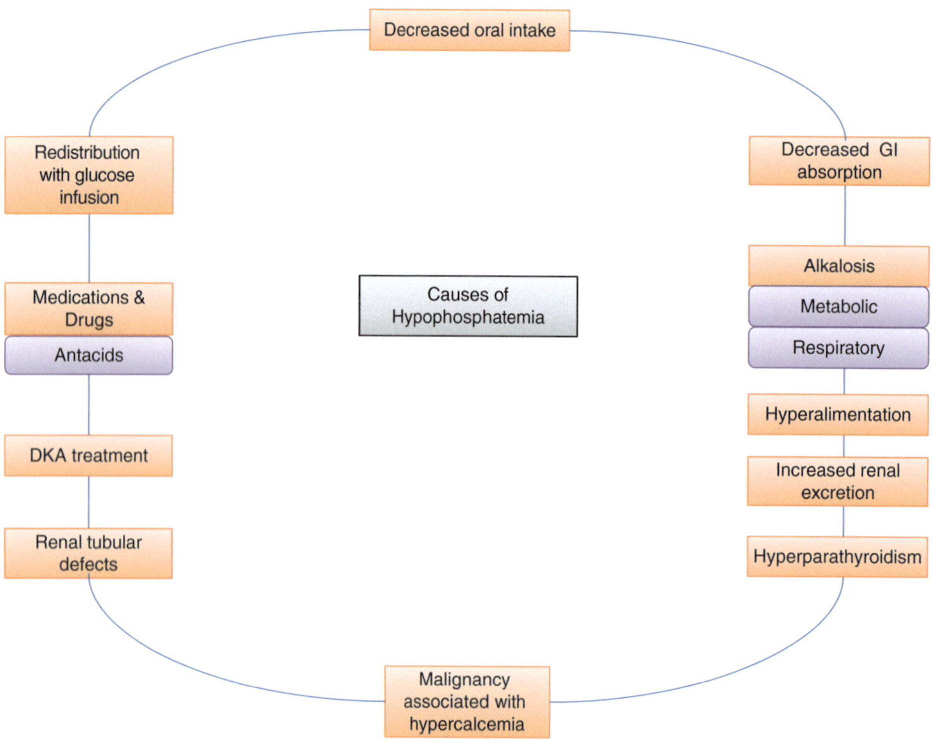

Hypophosphatemia Symptoms and Signs

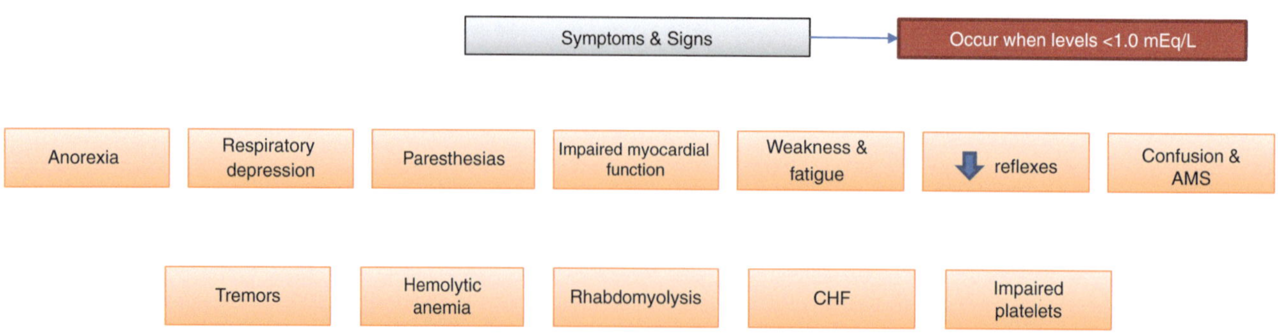

Diagnosis + Treatment

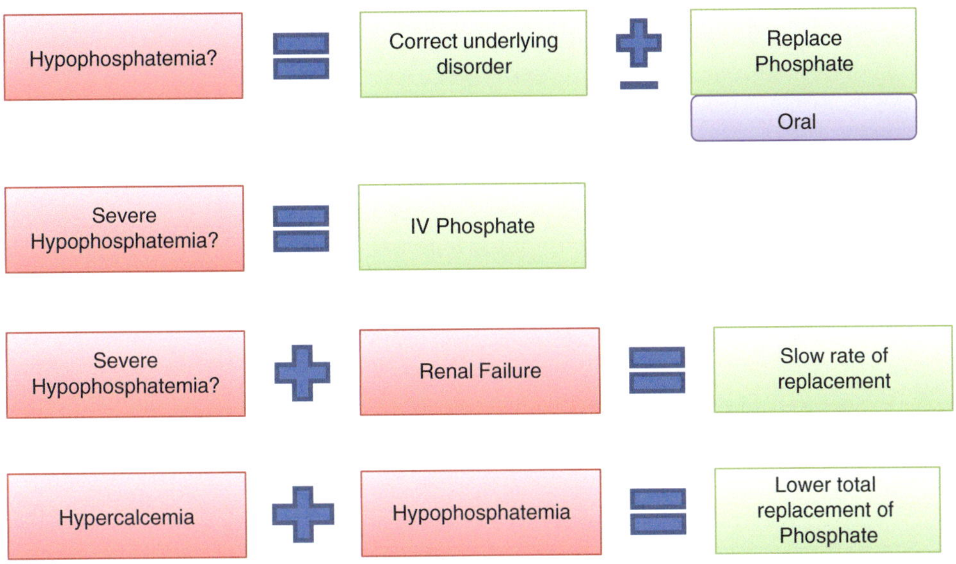

Introduction: Hyperphosphatemia

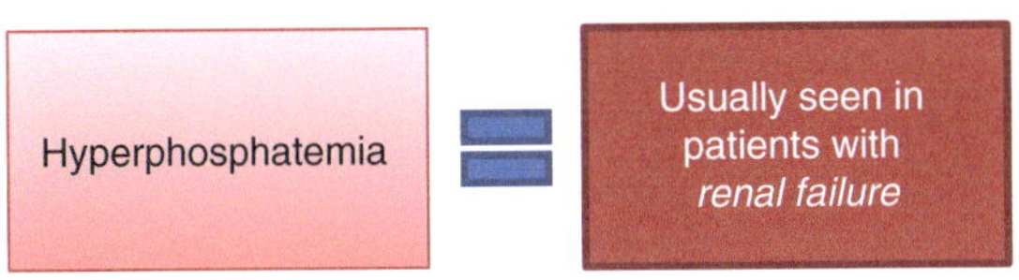

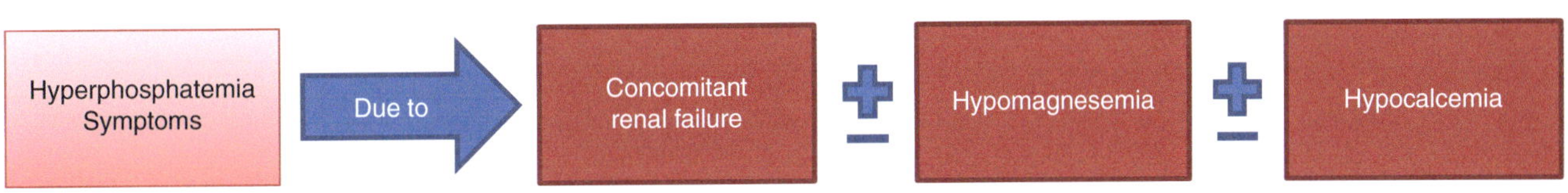

Causes of Hyperphosphatemia

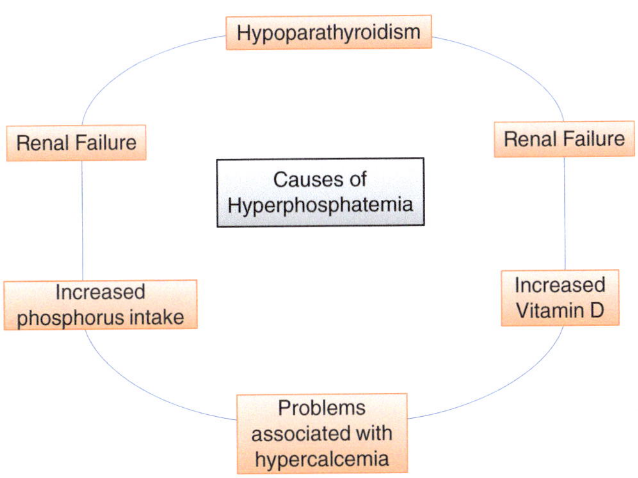

Diagnosis + Treatment

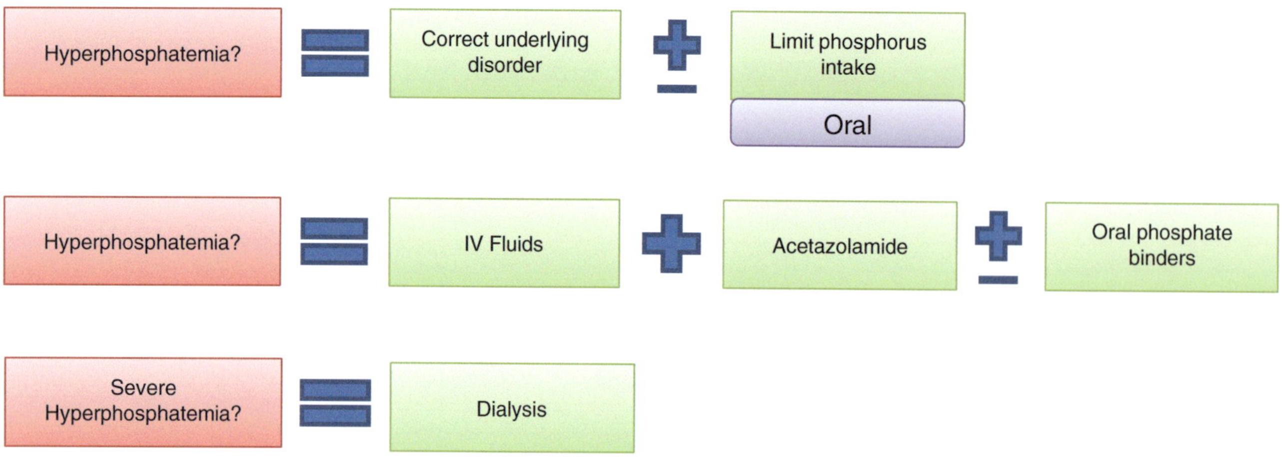

Metabolic Derangements

Introduction

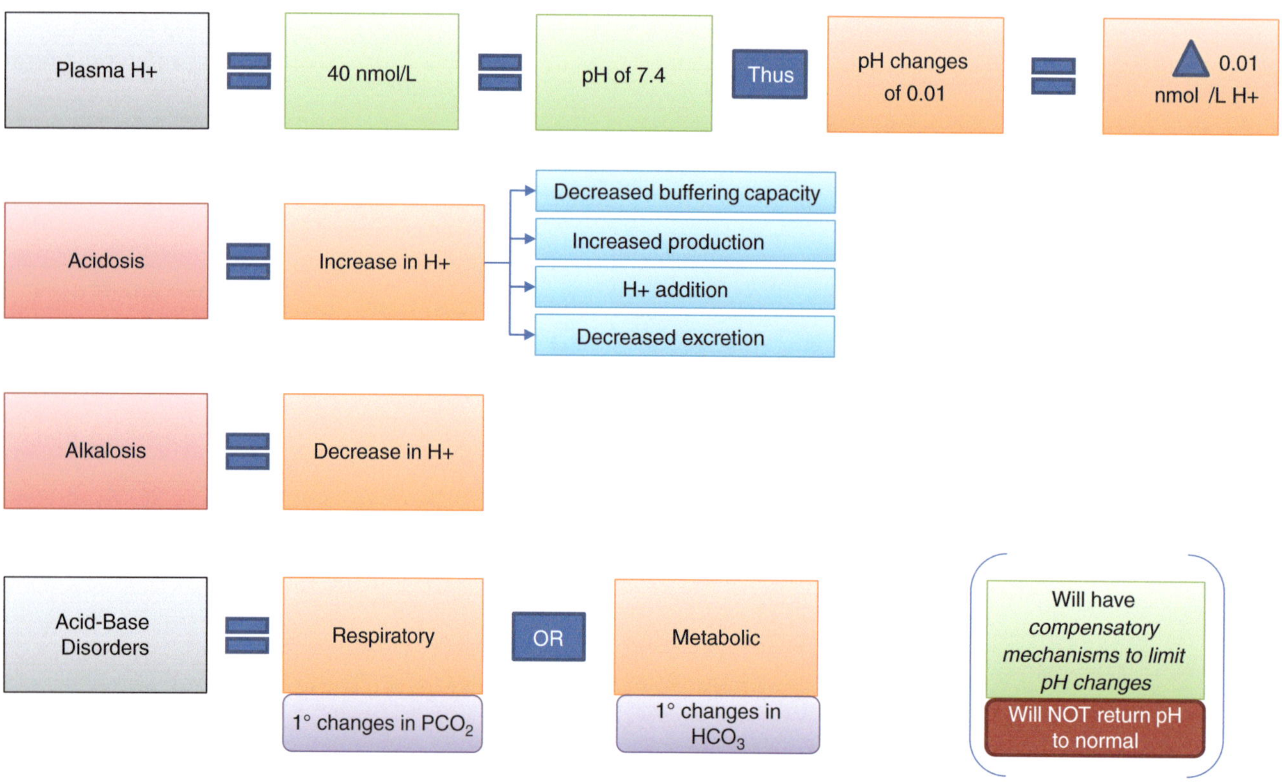

History and Physical

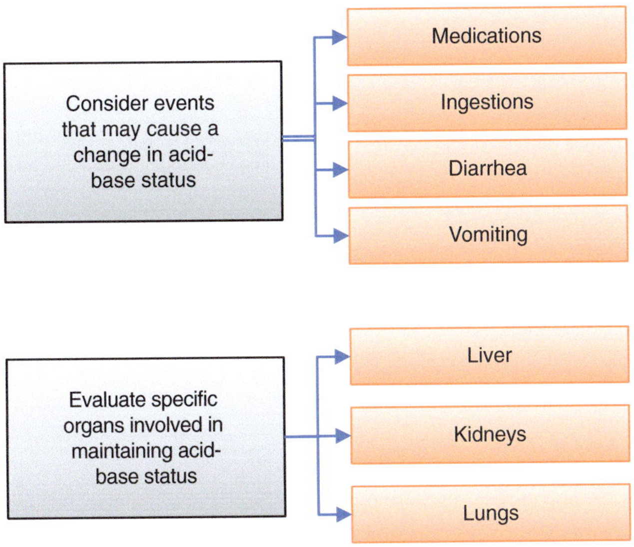

Laboratory Investigations

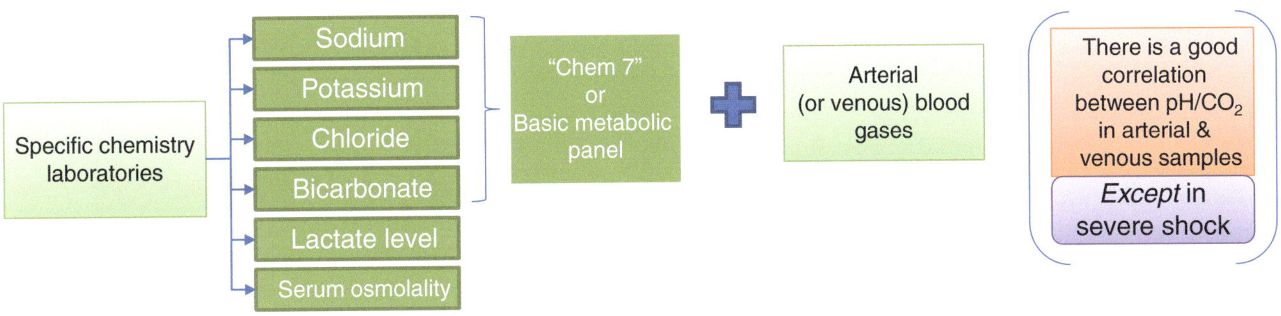

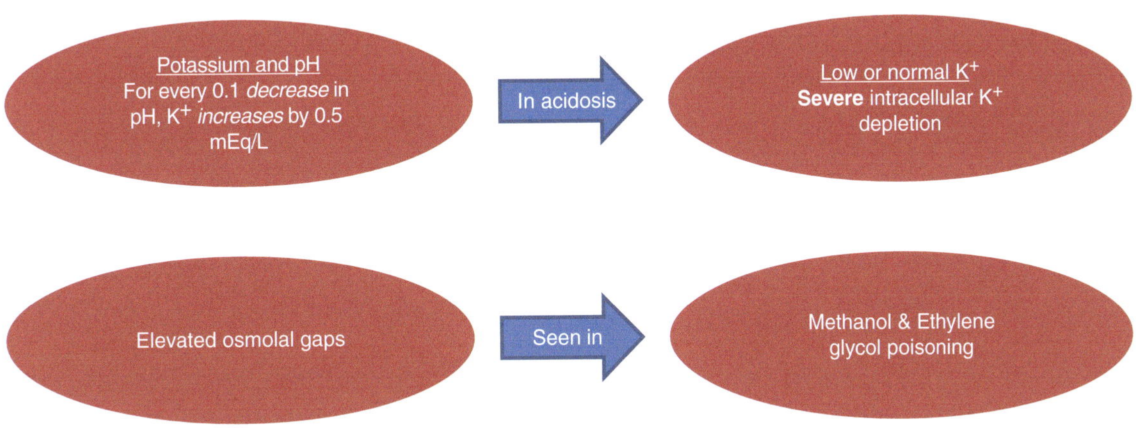

Metabolic Acidosis

Anion Gap

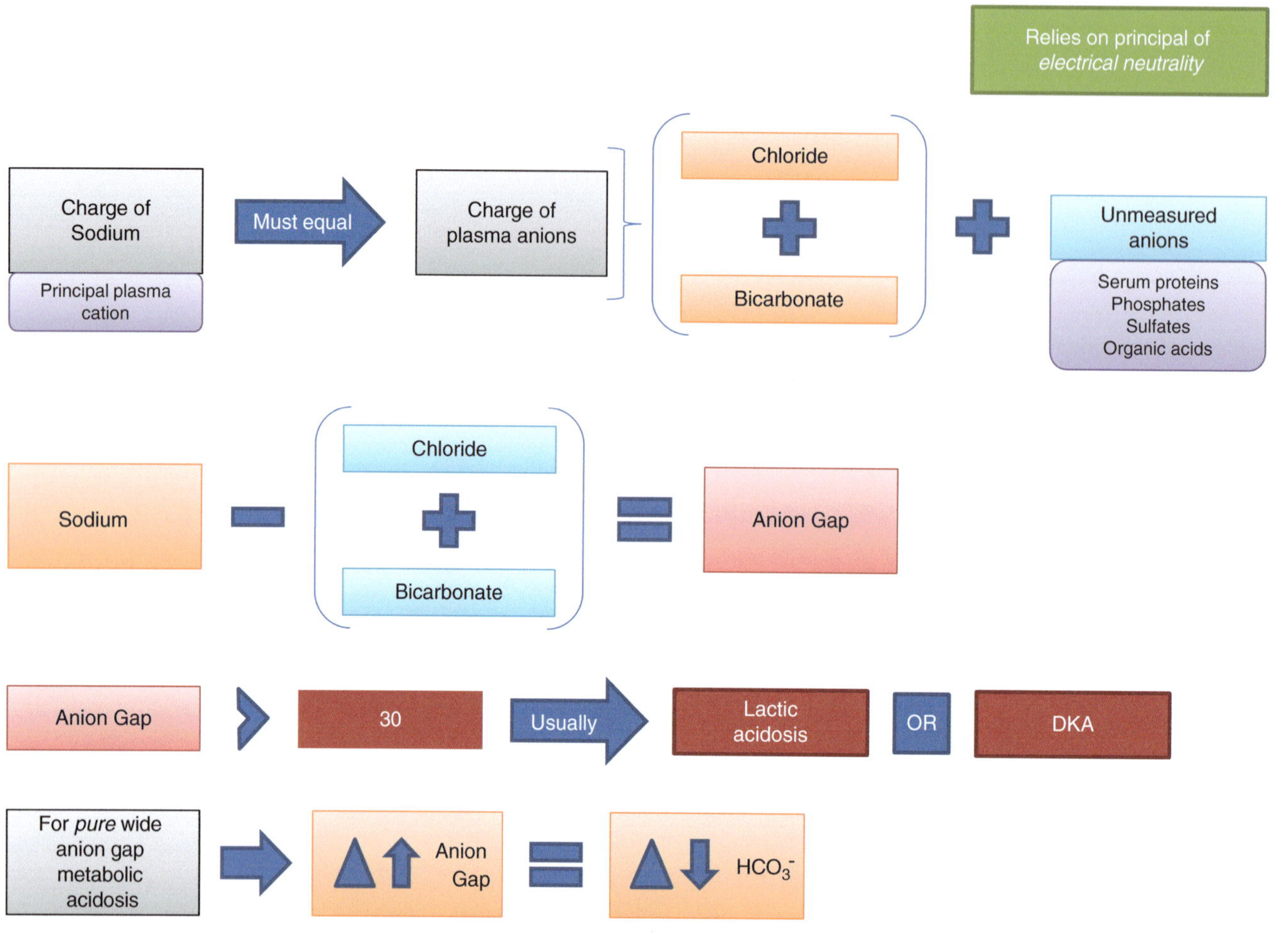

Abnormal Anion Gap Without Acid-Base Disturbance

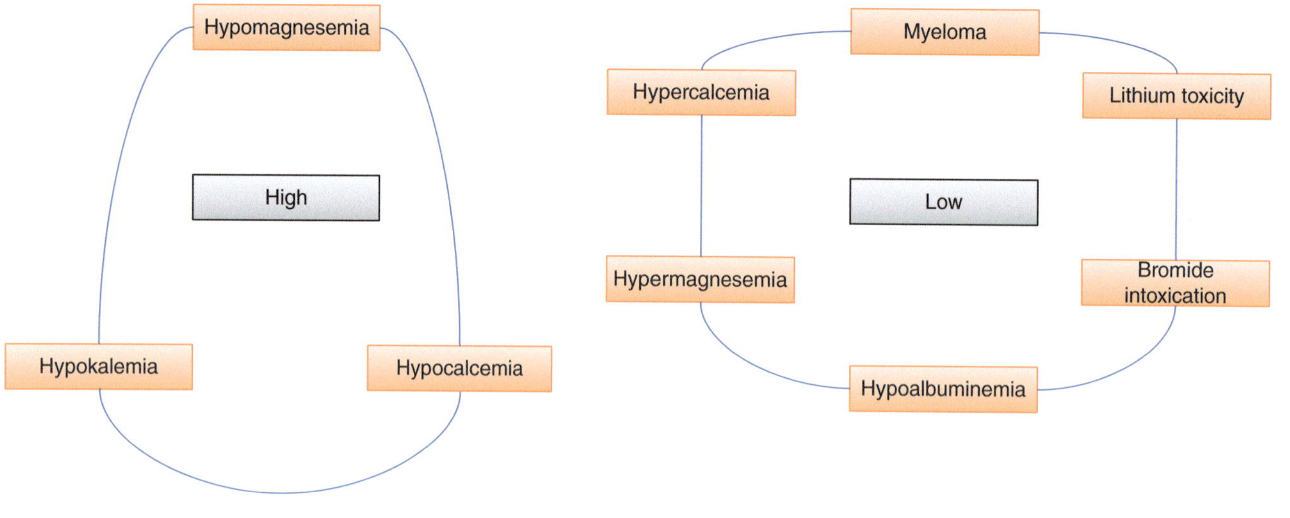

Anion Gap Causes

	Cause		Mechanism		Result
A	AKA	=	Abrupt cessation of alcohol + malnourishment	=	Ketoacidosis
C	Cyanide, Carbon monoxide	=	Toxic	=	Lactic acidosis
A	Aspirin	=	Ingestion		
T	Toluene	=	Toxic		
M	Methanol	=	Ingestion		
U	Uremia	=	Renal failure		
D	DKA	=	Ketoacidosis		
P	Propylene Glycol, Paraldehyde	=	Ingestion		
I	Iron, Isoniazid	=	Ingestion	=	Lactic acidosis
L	Lactic acidosis	=	Most common cause		
E	Ethylene Glycol, Ethanol	=	Ingestion		
S	Salicylates	=	Ingestion		

Metabolic Acidosis

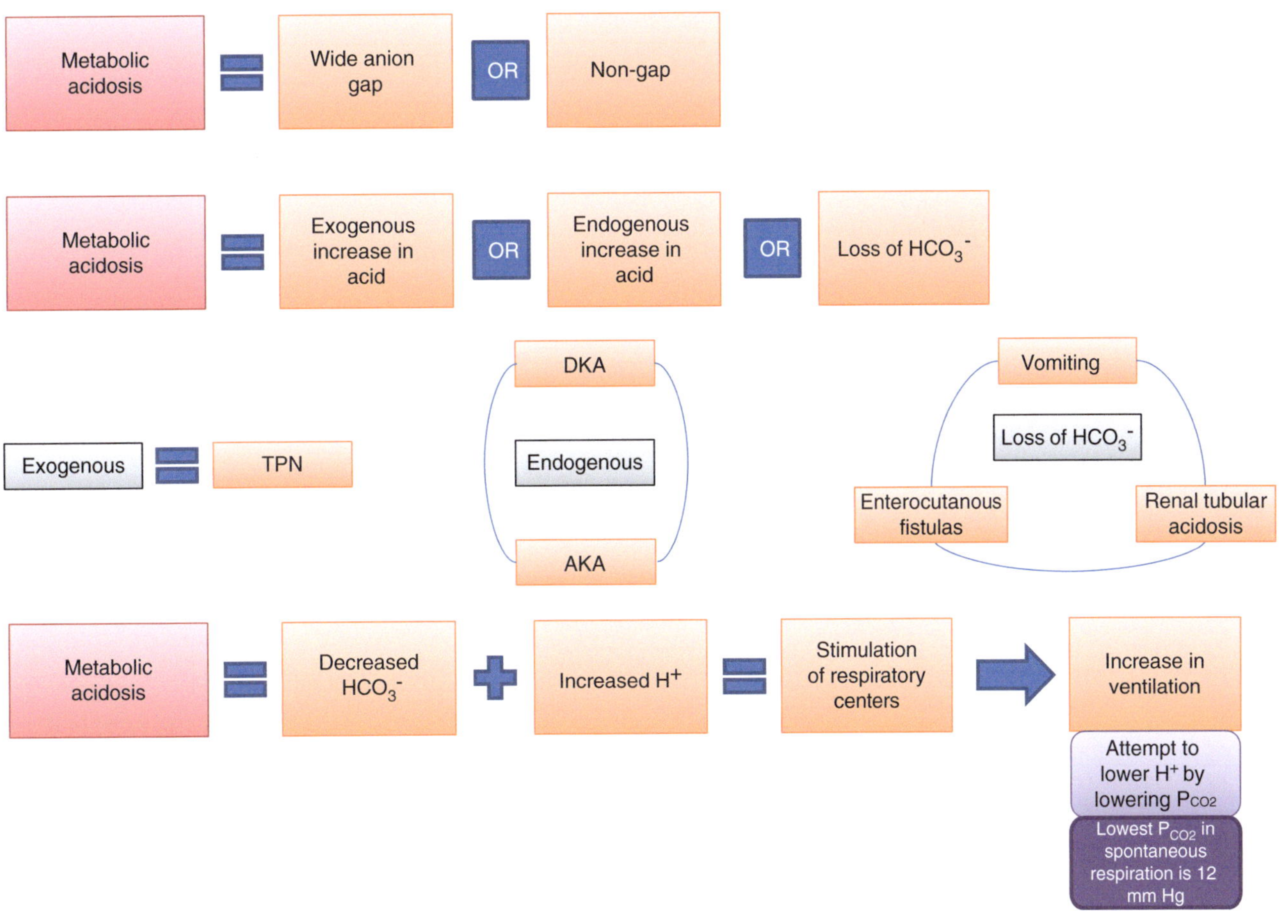

Lactic Acidosis

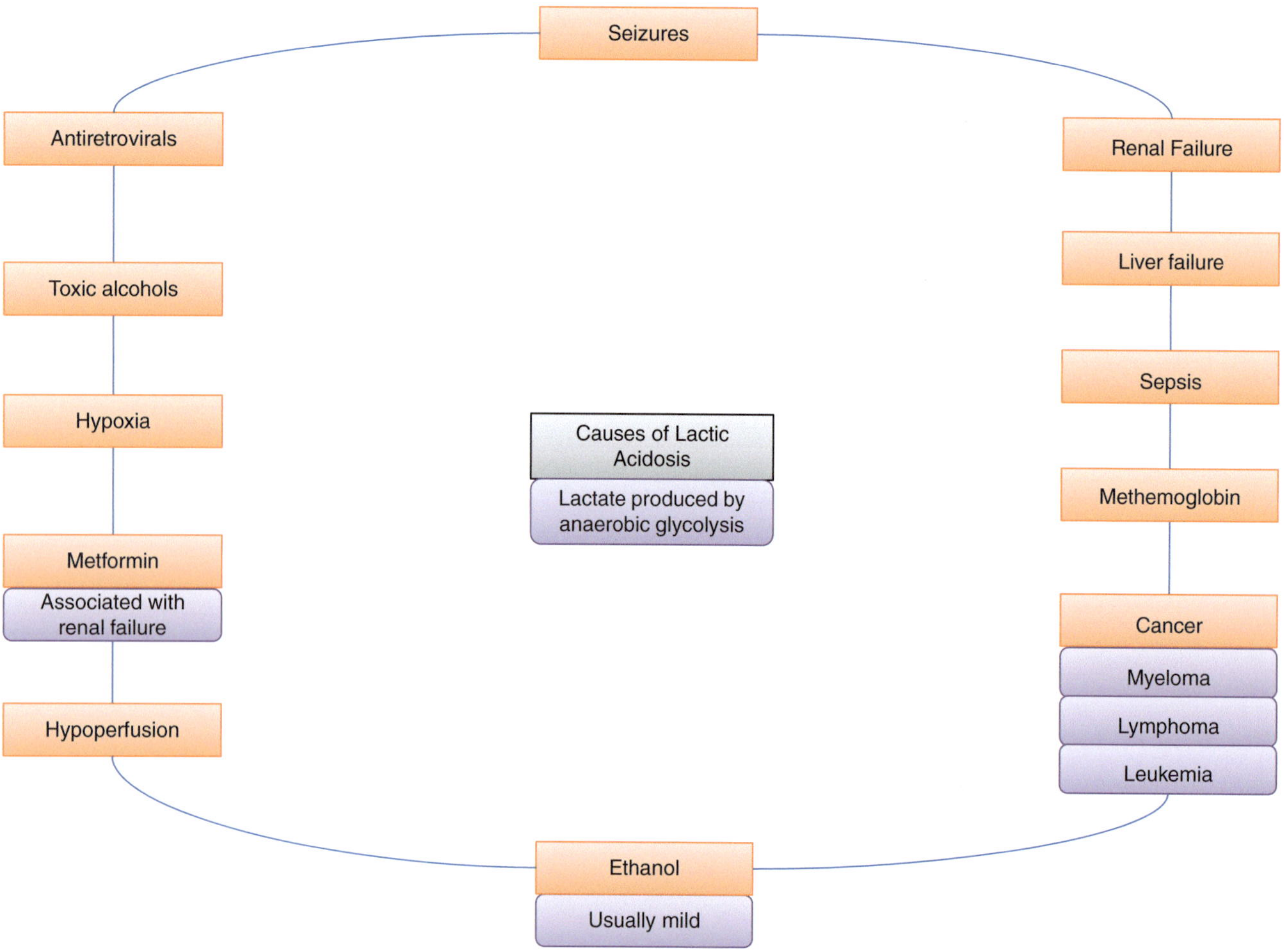

Non-anion Gap Metabolic Acidosis Causes

- **H** – Hypoaldosteronism (Addison disease)
- **A** – Acetazolamide
- **R** – Renal tubular acidosis
- **D** – Diarrhea
- **U** – Uterosigmoidostomy
- **P** – Pancreatic fistula

Usually a loss of HCO_3^- with loss of Na^+

Some may have a tendency to *Hyperkalemia*, while others have a tendency to *Hypokalemia*

Other causes

- Improving DKA
- Early Uremia
- Early obstructive uropathy
- Other potassium sparing diuretics

Effects of Acidosis

- Cardiac = Decreased contractility + Decreased ventricular fibrillation threshold + Increased energy requirement for defibrillation
- Liver = Decreased perfusion
- Kidney = Decreased perfusion + Decreased systemic blood pressure
- Lungs = Increased pulmonary vascular resistance
- Adrenals = Attenuation of catecholamine effect = Potential for systemic vascular collapse
- General = Increased metabolism
- Pancreas = Insulin resistance

Treatment

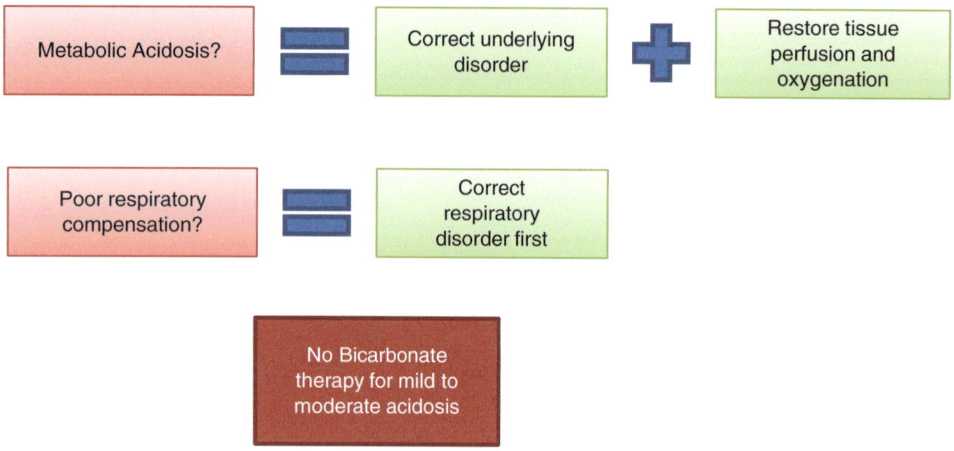

Metabolic Alkalosis

Introduction

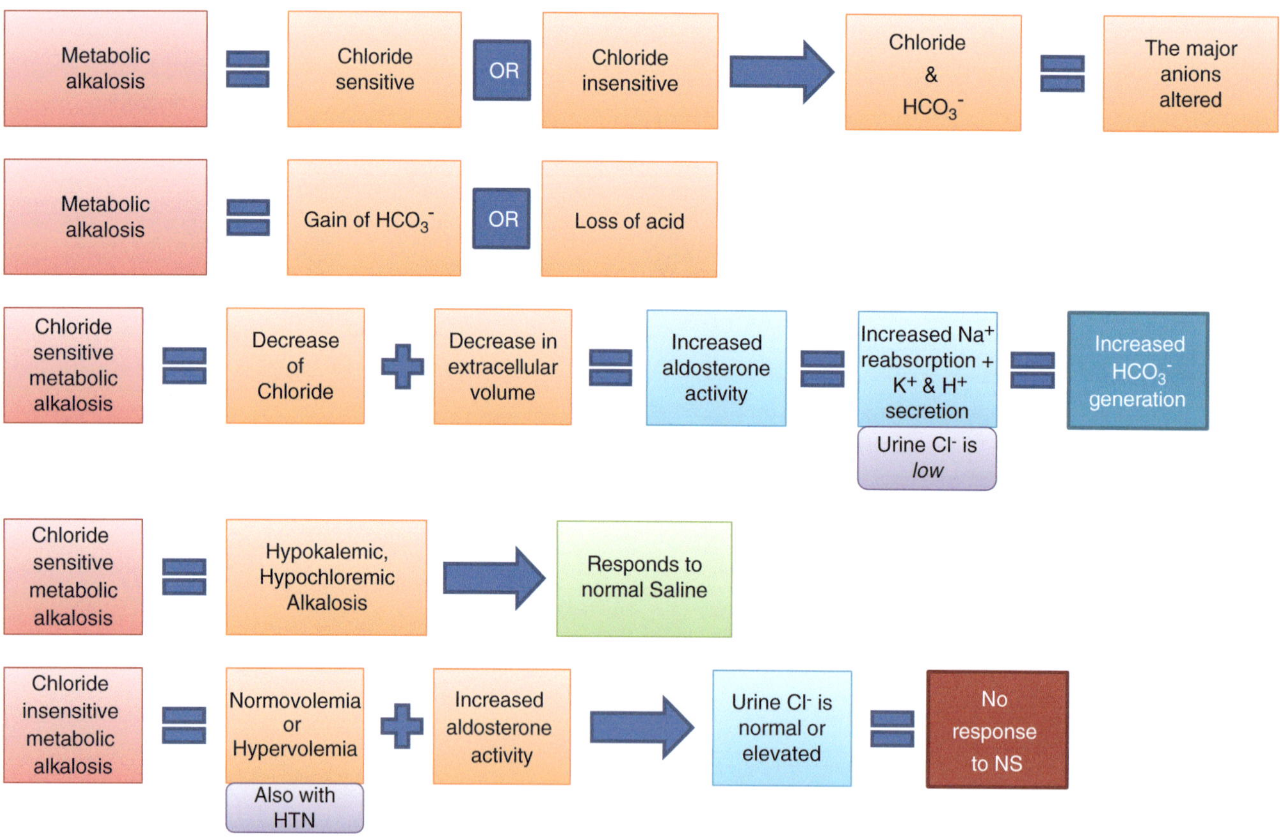

Causes of Metabolic Alkalosis

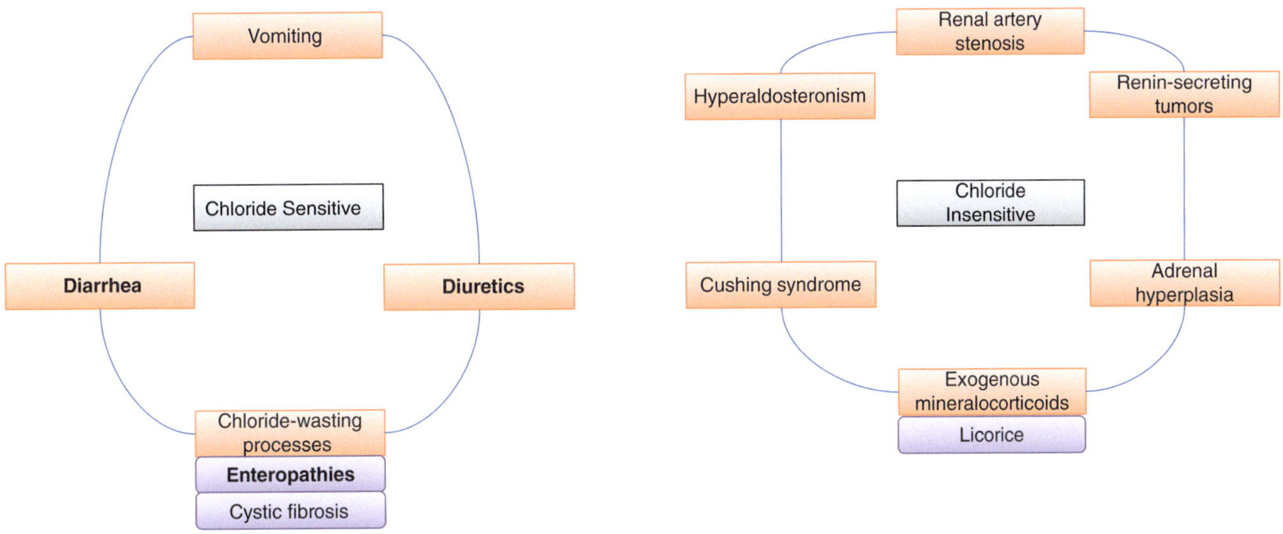

Effects of Alkalosis

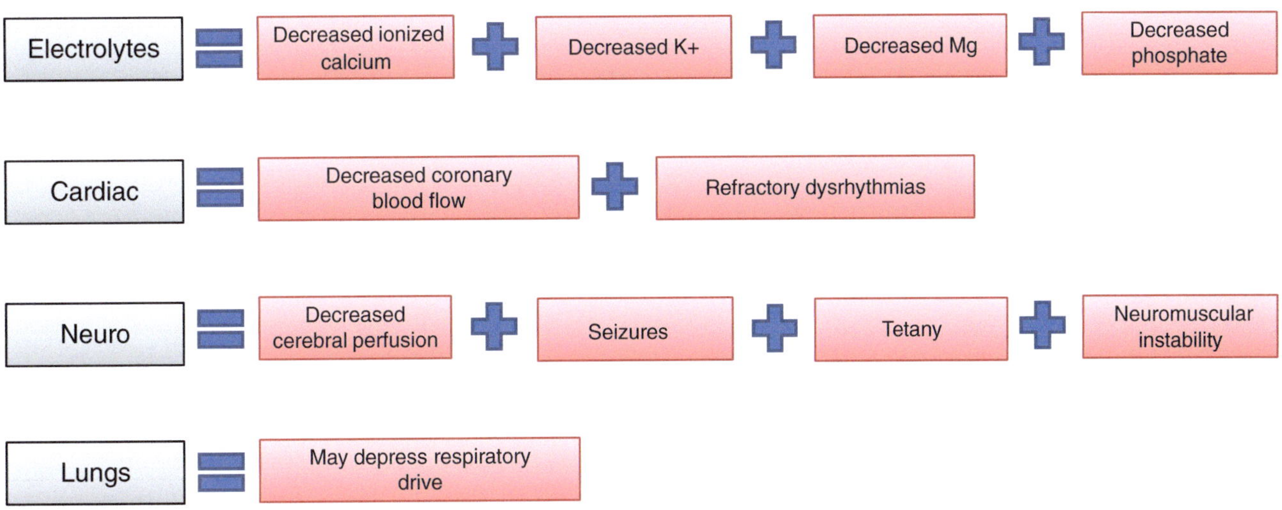

Treatment

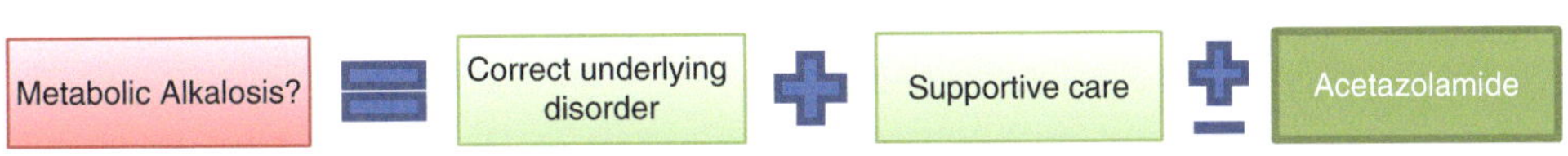

Respiratory Acidosis

Introduction

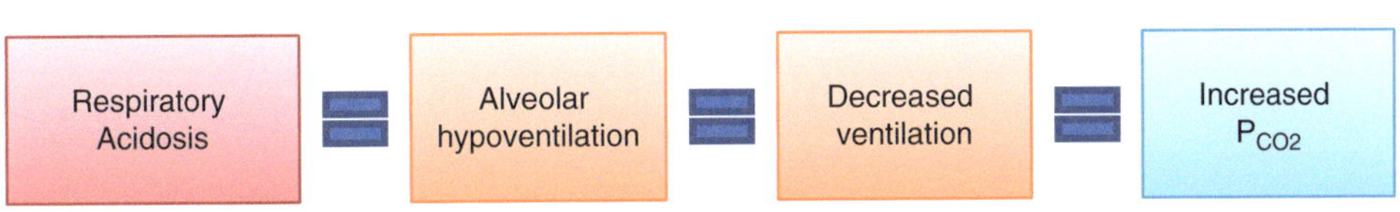

Causes of Respiratory Acidosis

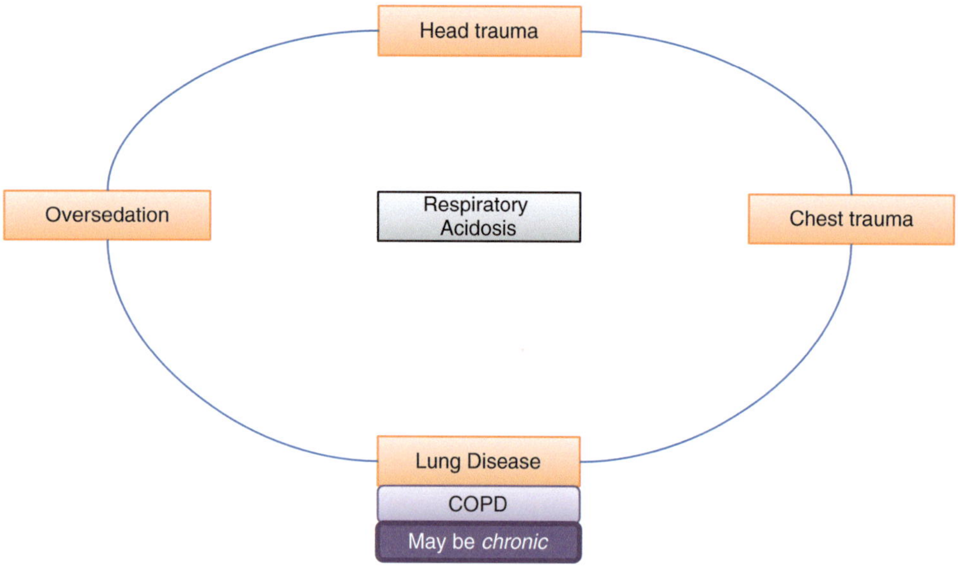

Treatment

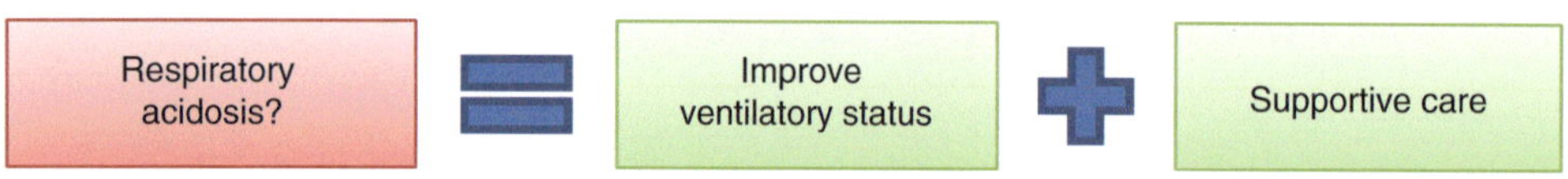

Respiratory Alkalosis

Introduction

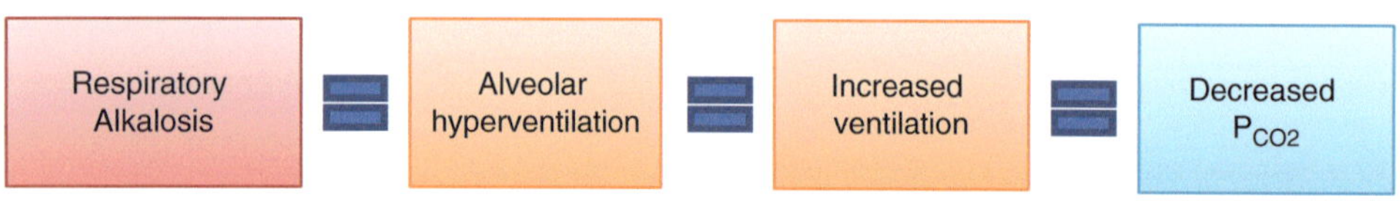

Causes of Respiratory Alkalosis

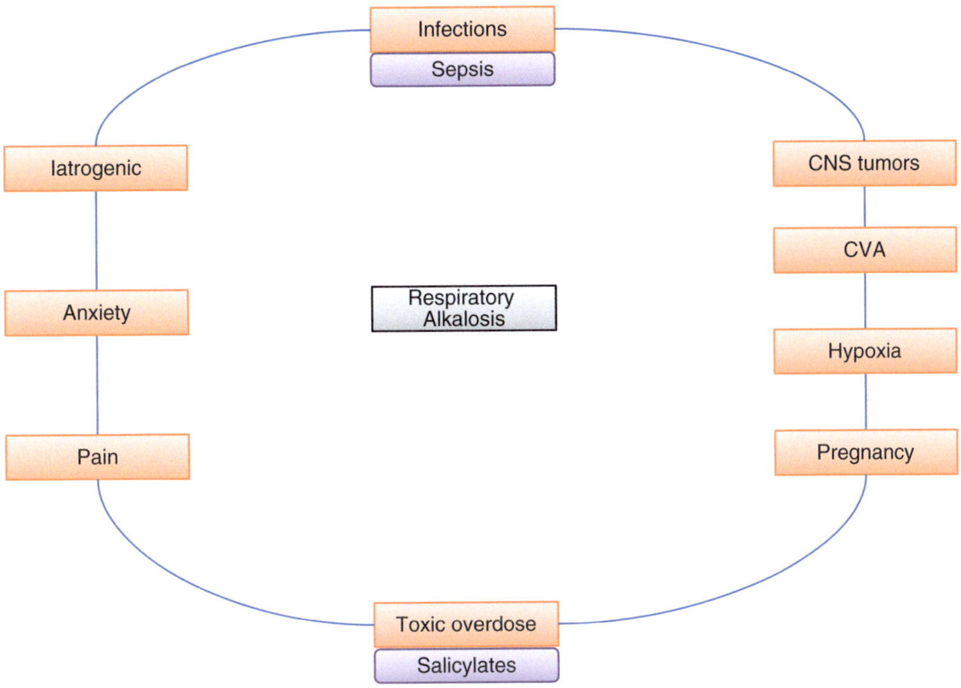

Treatment

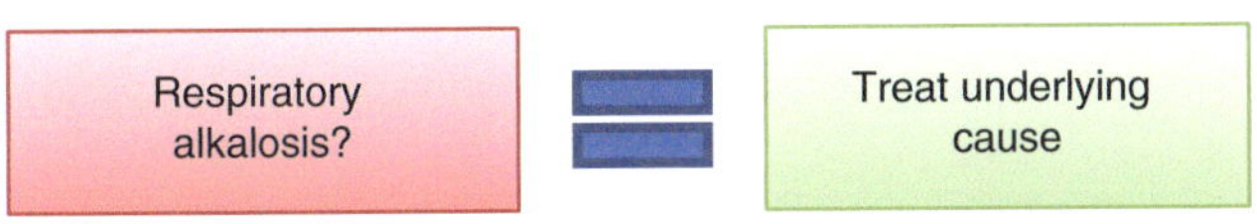

The Osmolal Gap

Introduction

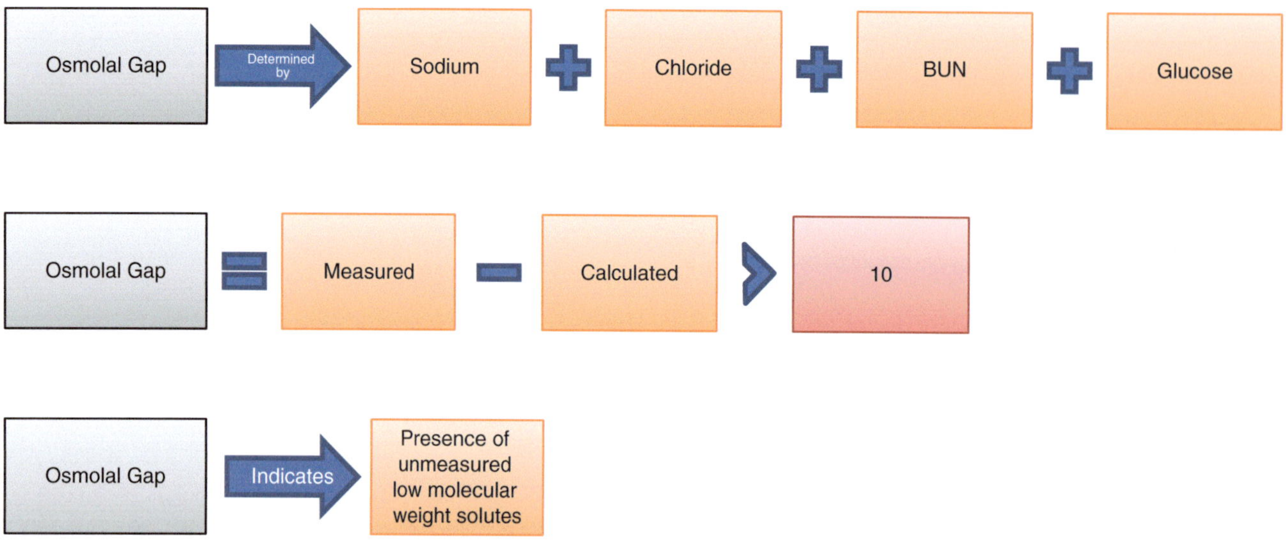

$2 \times Na^{+} + Glucose / 18 + BUN / 2.8 = \mathbf{280–295}$

Causes of Elevated Osmolal Gap

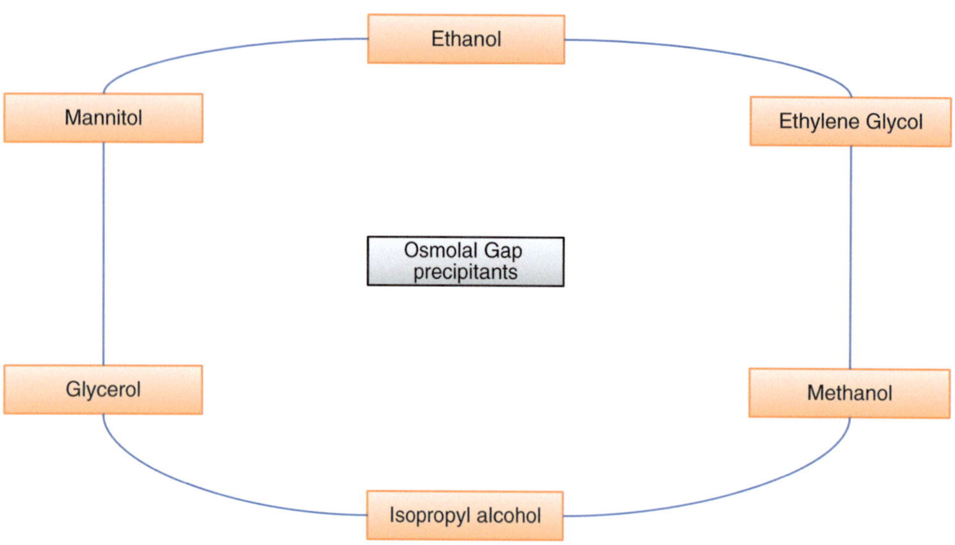

Ears, Nose, and Throat

Bobby Desai

Contents

Ear 468
Nose 478
Facial Fractures 482
Throat/Neck/Upper Airway Infections 484
Dental Emergencies 490
Neck Masses 494
Edema of Upper Airway 496
Soft Tissue Lesions 497
Intraoral and Tongue Lesions 499
Salivary Gland Disorders 501
Facial Infections 503
Other ENT Emergencies 504
Vertigo 508

B. Desai, MD, MEd
Department of Emergency Medicine, University of Florida,
Gainesville, FL, USA
e-mail: bdesai@ufl.edu

B. Desai, B.R. Allen (eds.), *Nailing the Written Emergency Medicine Board Examination*,
DOI 10.1007/978-3-319-30838-8_8

Ear

Introduction: Otalgia

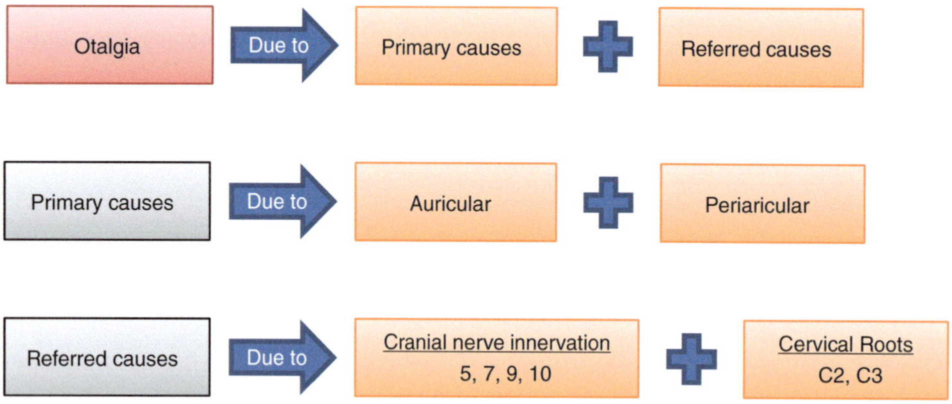

Primary and Referred Causes of Otalgia

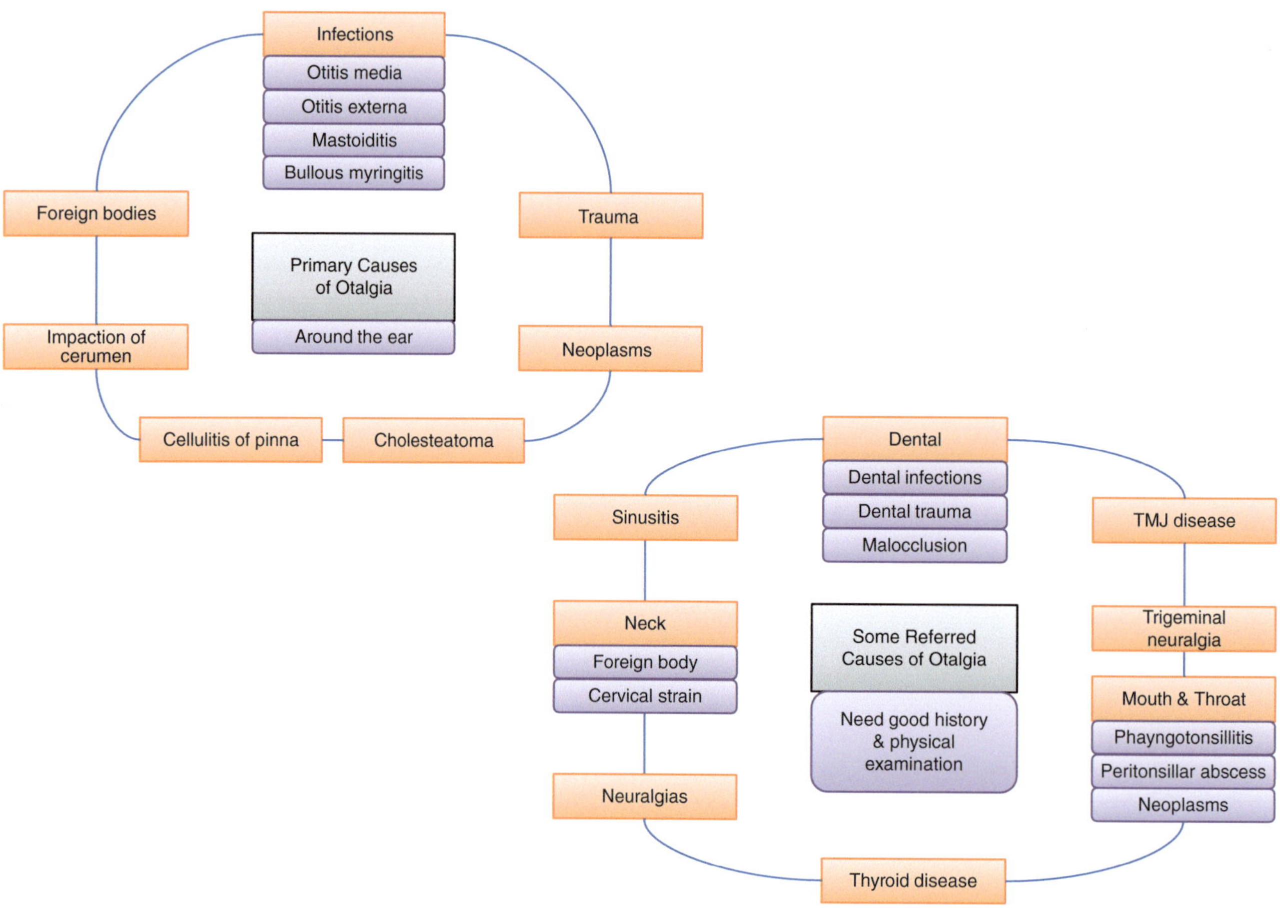

Introduction: Tinnitus

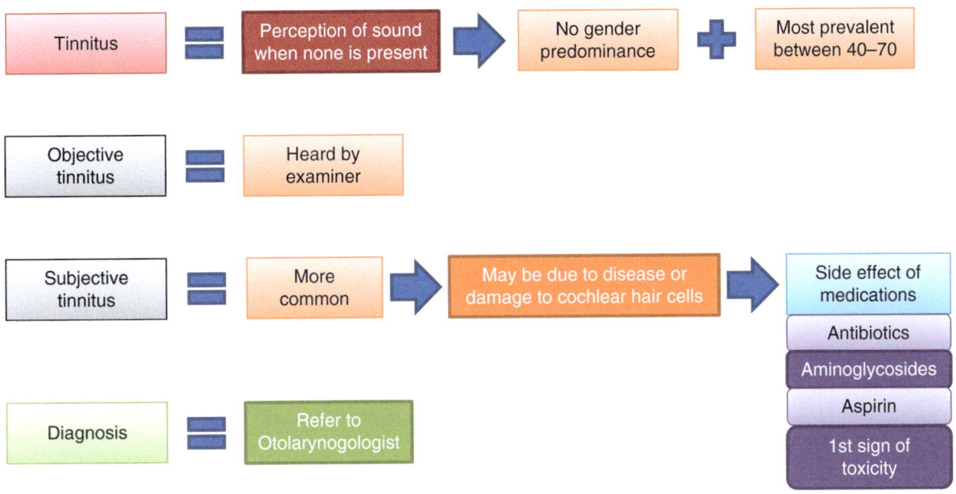

Introduction: Hearing Loss

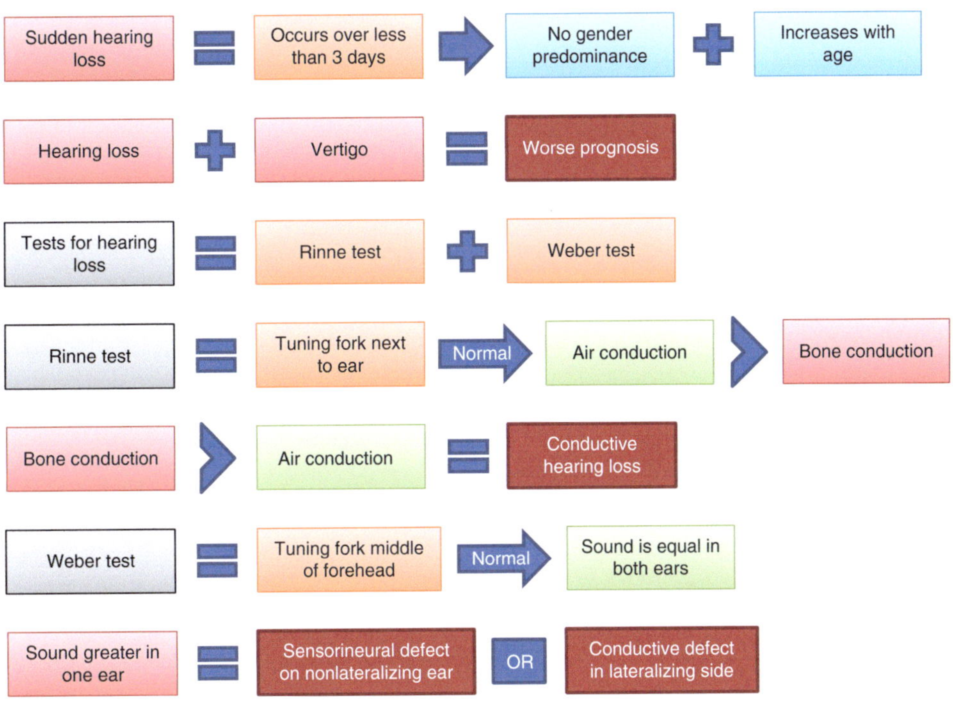

Causes of Sudden Hearing Loss

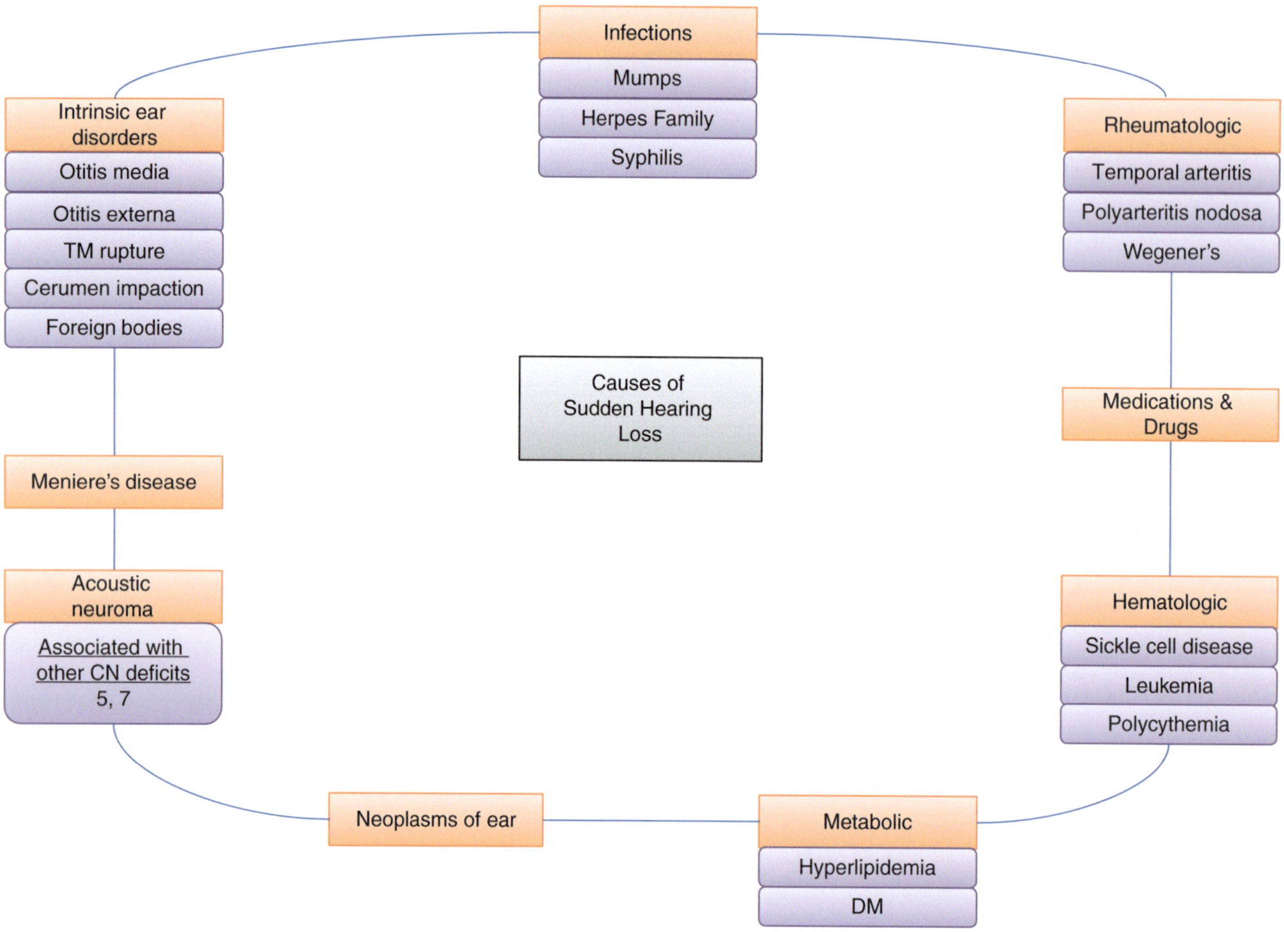

Medications and Drugs Causing Sudden Hearing Loss

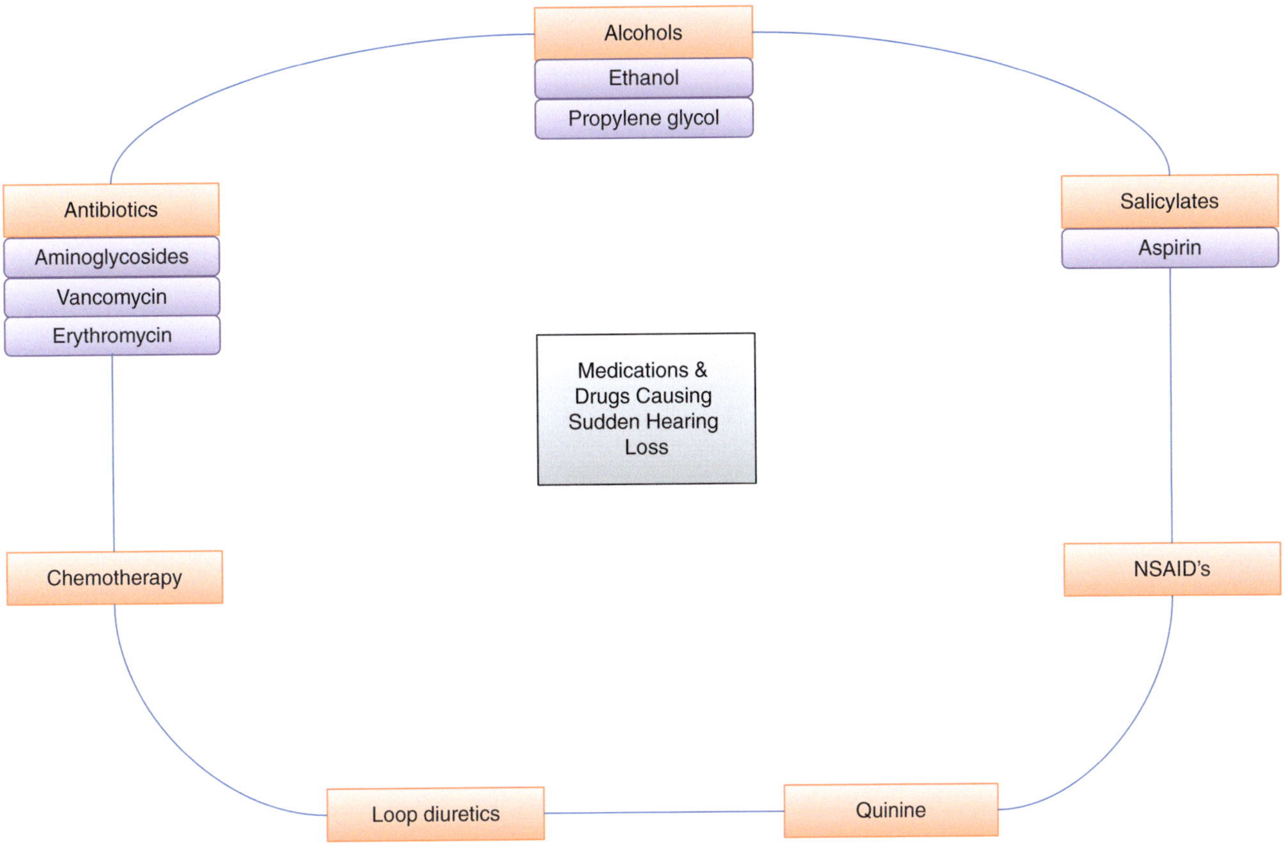

Ear Infections

Perichondritis

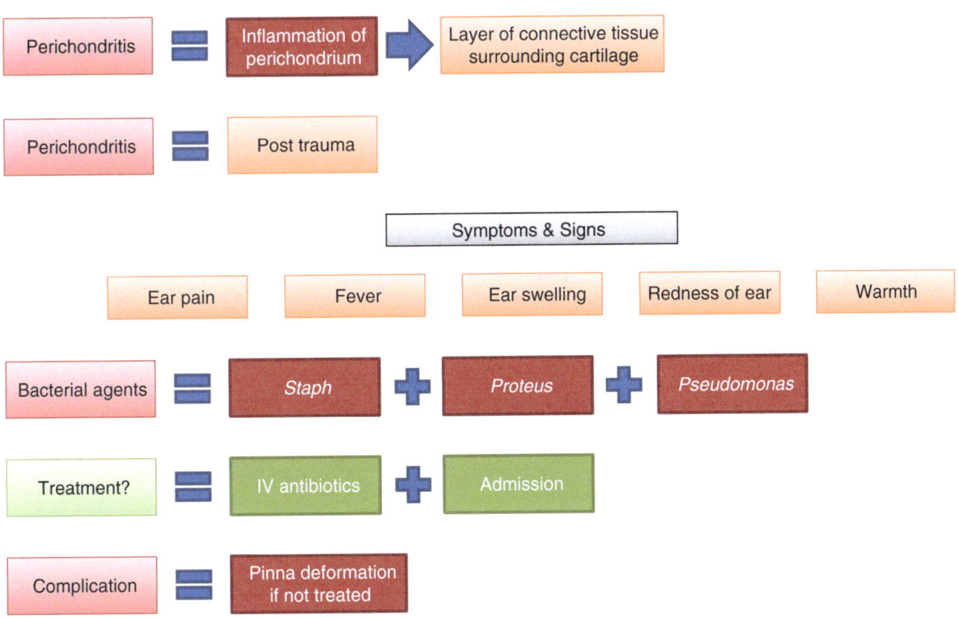

Otitis Externa (OE)

Otitis externa = Infection & inflammation of external auditory canal → Swimmer's ear OR Malignant OE

Symptoms & Signs

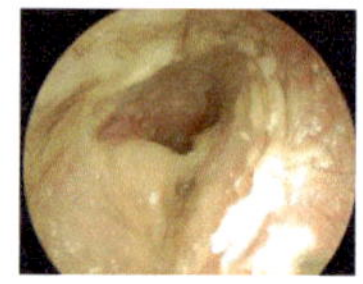

Erythema of ear canal | Edema of ear canal | Pus from ear canal | Hearing impairment if untreated | Ear pain

Predisposing factors for OE = Elevation of local pH → Frequent contact with water + Trauma to external auditory canal (EAC)

Bacterial agents = *Staph* + *Proteus* + *Pseudomonas* + *Enterobacteriaceae*

Fungal agents → Humid climates + Immune compromised = *Aspergillus* + *Candida*

Noninfectious = Contact dermatitis

Treatment? = Topical antibiotics ± steroids (Fluoroquinolones) + Gentle cleansing of EAC + Pain control + Avoidance of water in ear (Ear plugs)

Center right image (Reprinted from Önerci TM. External ear canal. In: Önerci TM, editors. Diagnosis in otorhinolaryngology: an illustrated guide. Heidelberg: Springer Verlag; 2010. p. 18–23. With permission from Springer Verlag)

Malignant Otitis Externa (MOE)

Malignant Otitis externa = Life threatening Infection of external auditory canal → Involves → Soft tissue around the pinna + May extend into the skull → *Pseudomonas* > 90 % of time

Pathophysiology = Simple OE → Cellulitis of EAC → Chondritis of outer ear → Osteomyelitis of bone

Spread of infection = Mastoid air cells + Parotid + Skull base + 7th cranial nerve (1st CN to be affected with cranial extension of infection) + 9th, 10th, & 11th cranial nerves (More severe disease)

Predisposing factors = Diabetics + Elderly + Immune suppressed

Agents = *Pseudomonas* + *Staph* + *Strep* + Fungal

Diagnosis? = CT of head (Specifically *Temporal bone*)

Treatment? = Topical antibiotics ± steroids (Fluoroquinolones) + IV antibiotics (Broad spectrum to cover *Pseudomonas*) + Pain control ± Surgical debridement

Signs and Symptoms of Malignant Otitis Externa

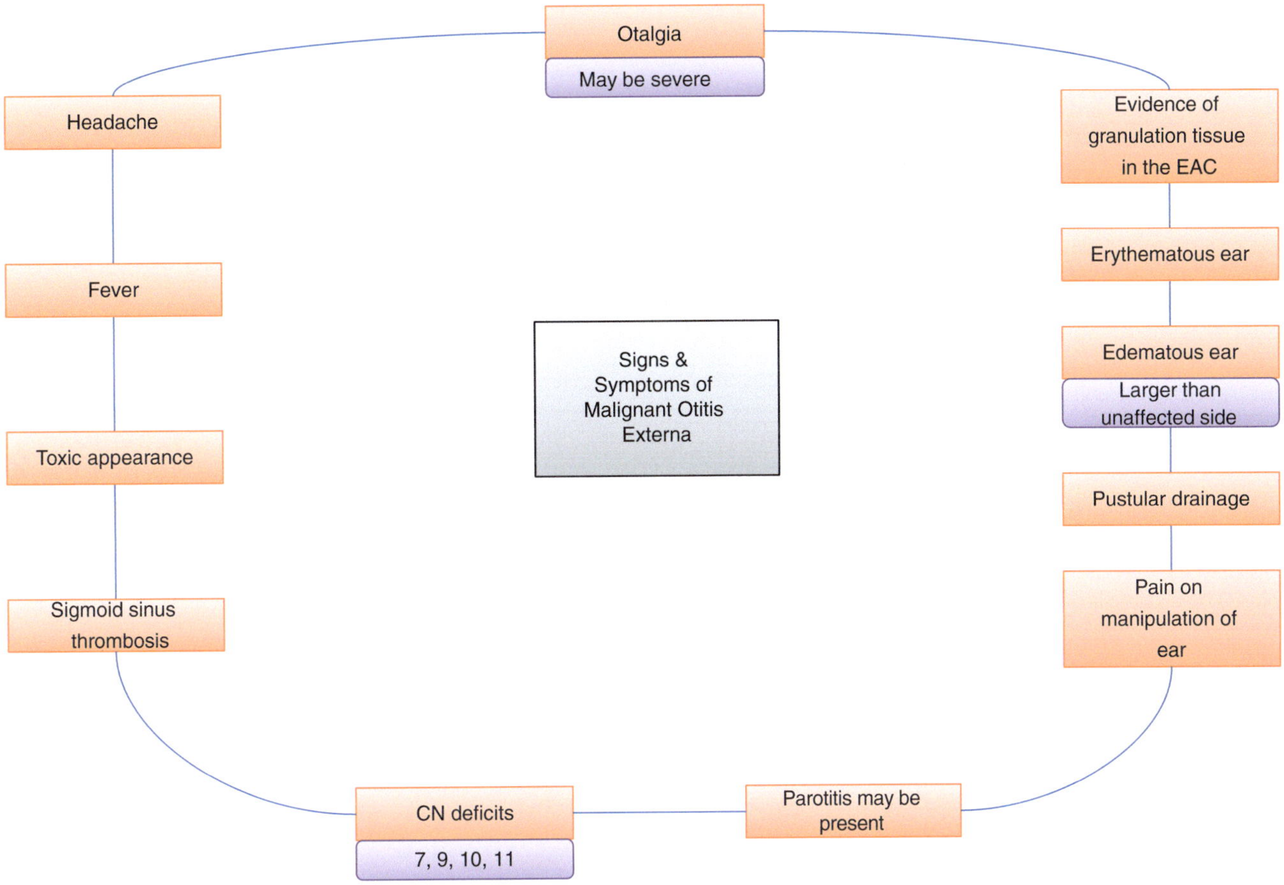

Otitis Media (OM)

PEDIATRICS

Otitis Media = Infection & inflammation of inner ear

Symptoms & Signs

- Bulging TM
- May have fluid behind TM
- ± Fever
- ± Otorrhea
  - Red, yellow or white TM
- Ear pain
- ± Hearing loss
  - Conductive if TM perforation
- Loss of light reflex

Most sensitive sign = Decreased movement of TM on insufflation

Bacterial agents = *Streptococcus pneumoniae* + *Hemophilus influenza* + *Moraxella catarrhalis* + Viral

Treatment? = Analgesia + "Watchful waiting" (Tympanostomy for recurrent serous OM)

No improvement in 48 hours? = Antibiotics → High dose Amoxicillin

Complications = TM perforation + Mastoiditis + Facial nerve palsy (Due to proximity to middle ear) + Labyrinthitis + Intracranial infections (Brain abscess, Meningitis)

Bullous Myringitis

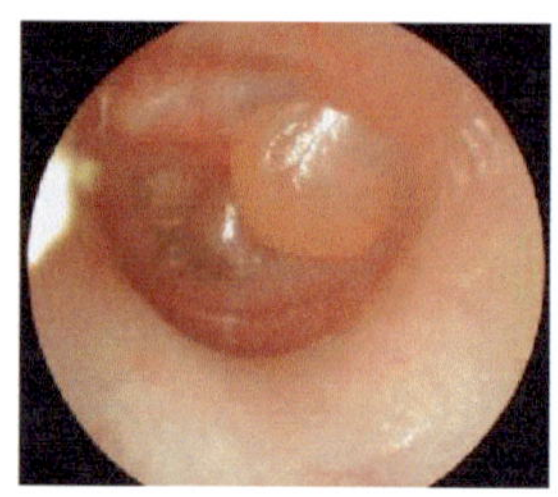

Bullous Myringitis = Characterized by bulla formation on the TM → Bloody, serous or serosangineous

Symptoms & Signs

- Ear pain
- Bullae
- Middle ear effusions
- ± Otorrhea
- ± Hearing loss

Agents = *Mycoplasma pneumoniae* + *Chlamydia psittaci* + Viral → No clear association with any one agent (Usually the same agents that cause OM)

Treatment? = Analgesia + Antibiotic drops + Oral antibiotics (For concomitant OM) ± Admission

Top right image (Reprinted from Önerci TM. Acute otitis media. In: Önerci TM, editors. Diagnosis in otorhinolaryngology: an illustrated guide. Heidelberg: Springer Verlag; 2010. p. 28–33. With permission from Springer Verlag)

Acute Mastoiditis

Acute Mastoiditis = Complication of Otitis media = Spread of middle ear infection → Mastoid air cells

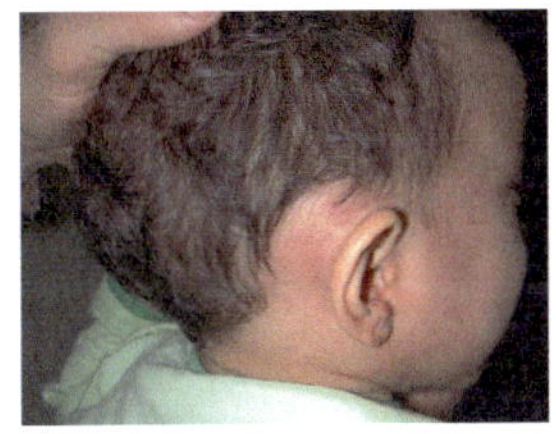

Symptoms & Signs

- Ear pain
- Erythema behind ear
- Fever
- Swelling behind ear
- Tenderness behind ear
- Downward displacement of ear

Diagnosis = CT scan (Specifically *Temporal bone*)

Treatment? = IV antibiotics + Myringotomy + Tympanocentesis ± Admission

Top right image (Reprinted from Önerci TM. Complications of otitis media. In: Önerci TM, editors. Diagnosis in otorhinolaryngology: an illustrated guide. Heidelberg: Springer Verlag; 2010. p. 43–4. With permission from Springer Verlag)

Cholesteatoma

Cholesteatoma = Epidermal collections within the middle ear → May be associated with chronic TM perforation

Symptoms & Signs

- Collection of tissue in EAC
- Foul smelling drainage
- Abnormal inner ear structure
  - Due to bone absorbing substances
- Ear pain
- ± Hearing loss

Treatment? = Surgery

Ear Trauma

Auricular Hematoma

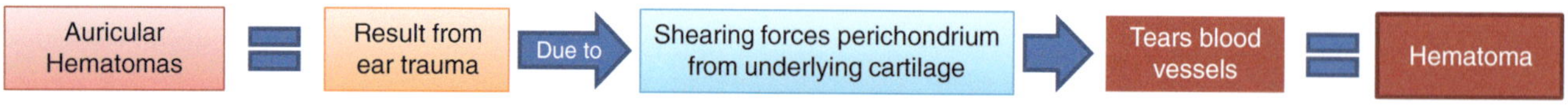

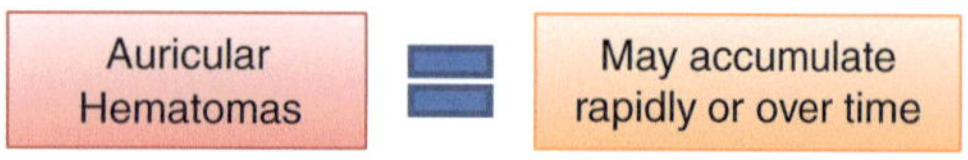

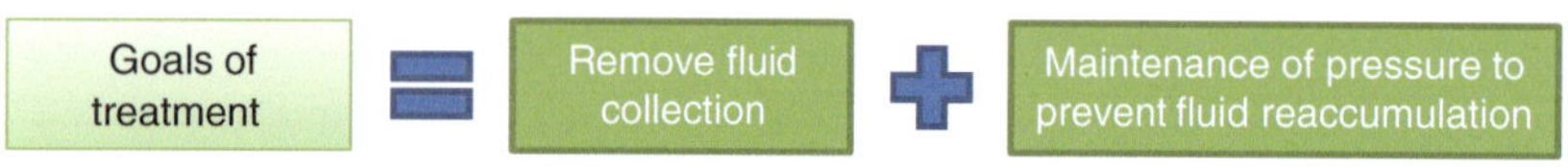

Cauliflower Ear

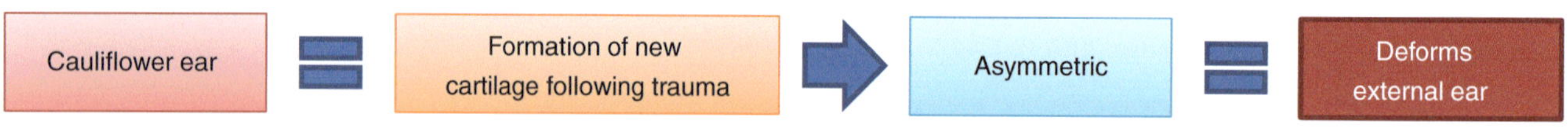

Tympanic Membrane Perforation

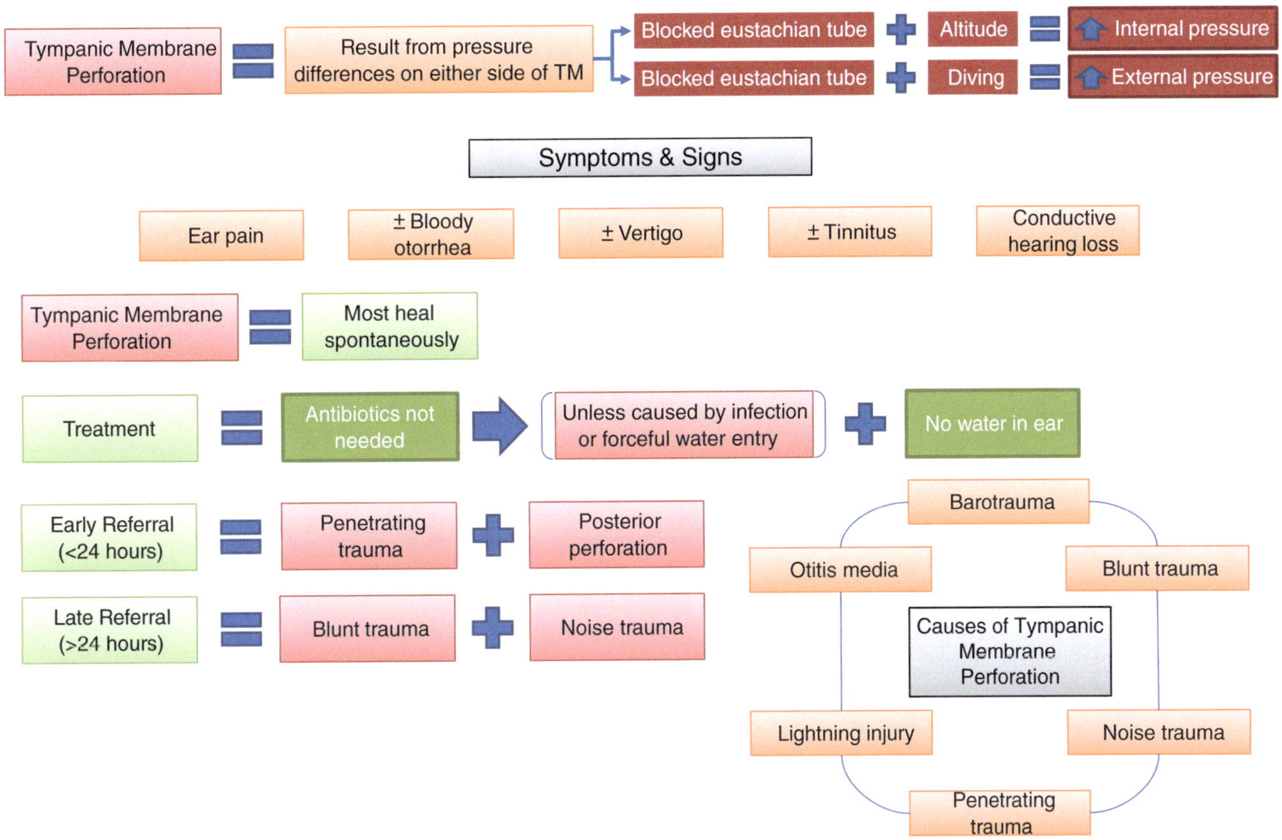

Nose

Epistaxis

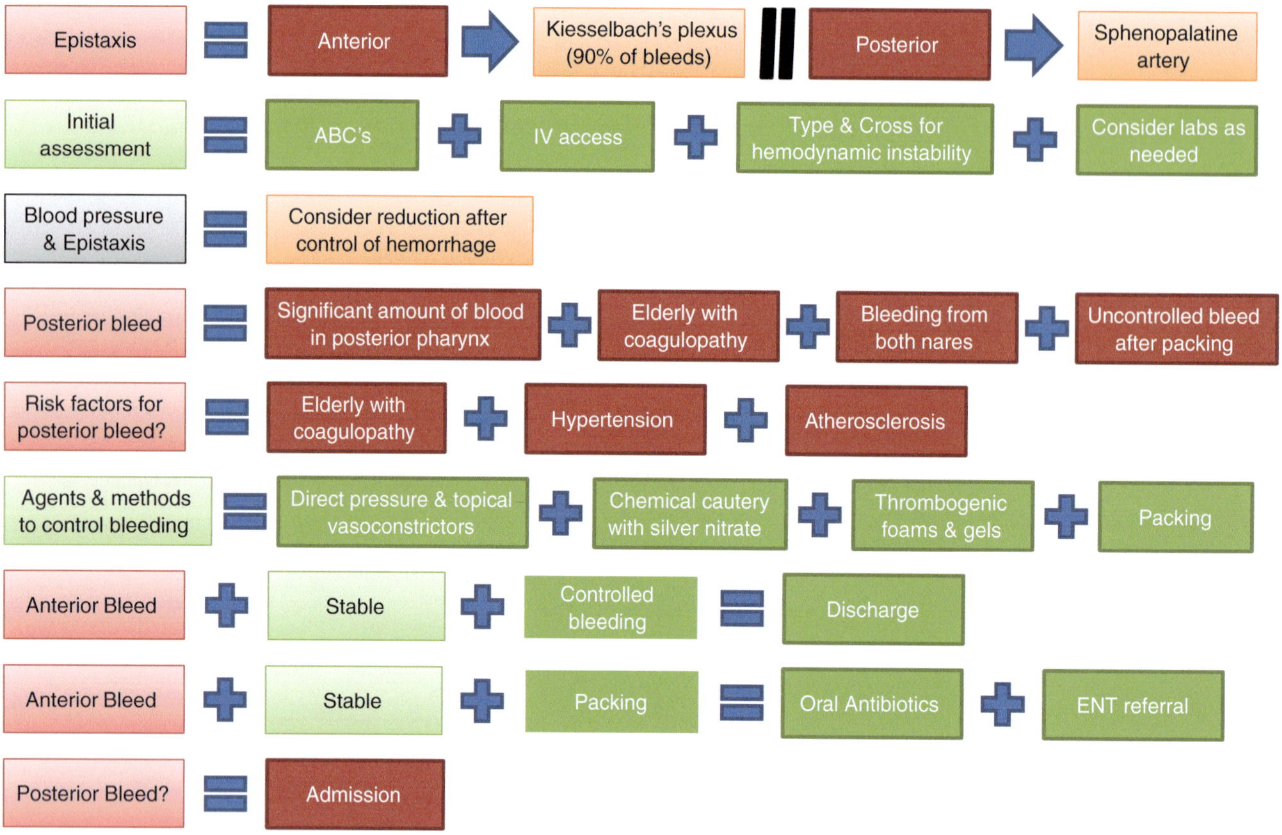

Causes of Epistaxis

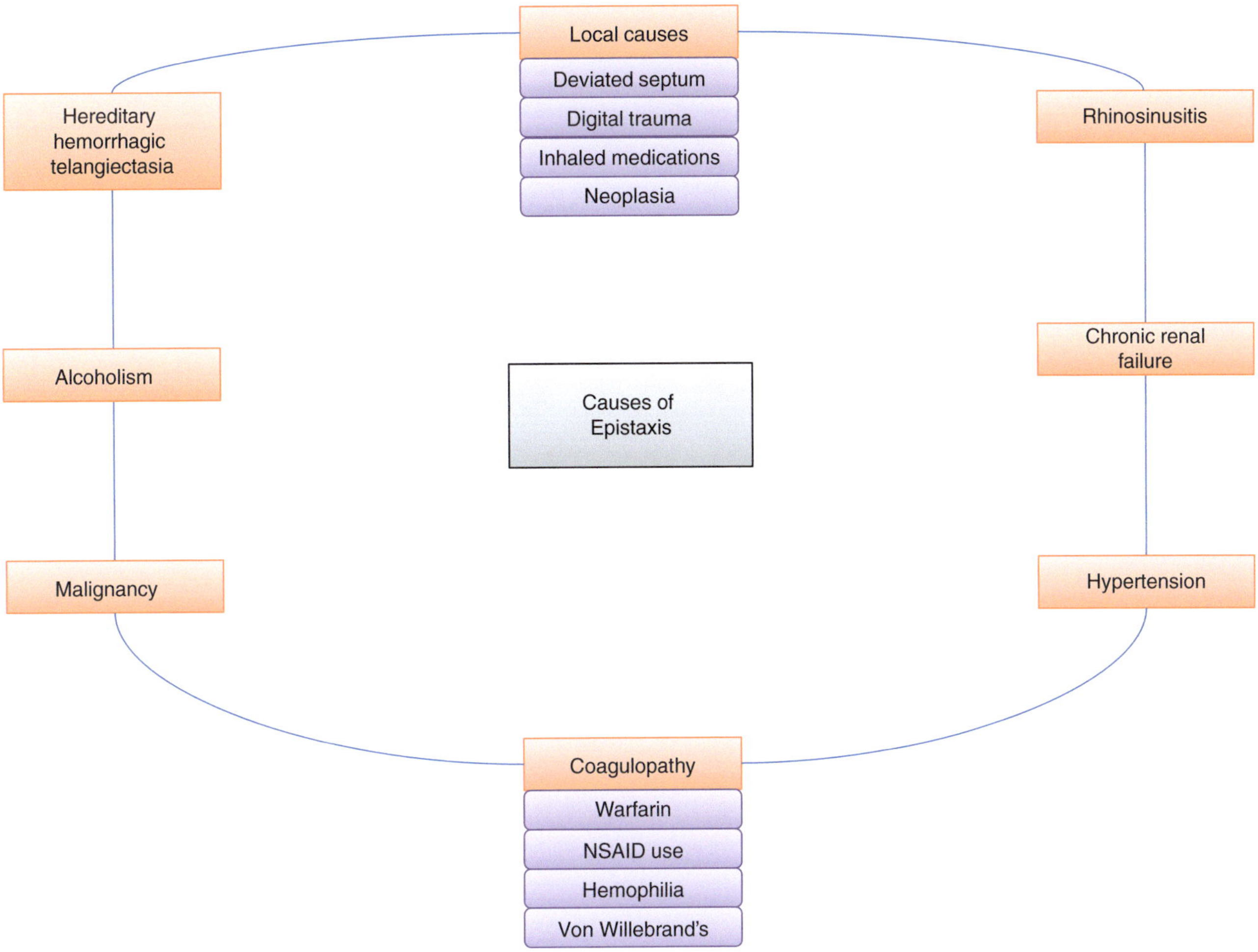

Complications of Posterior Nasal Packing

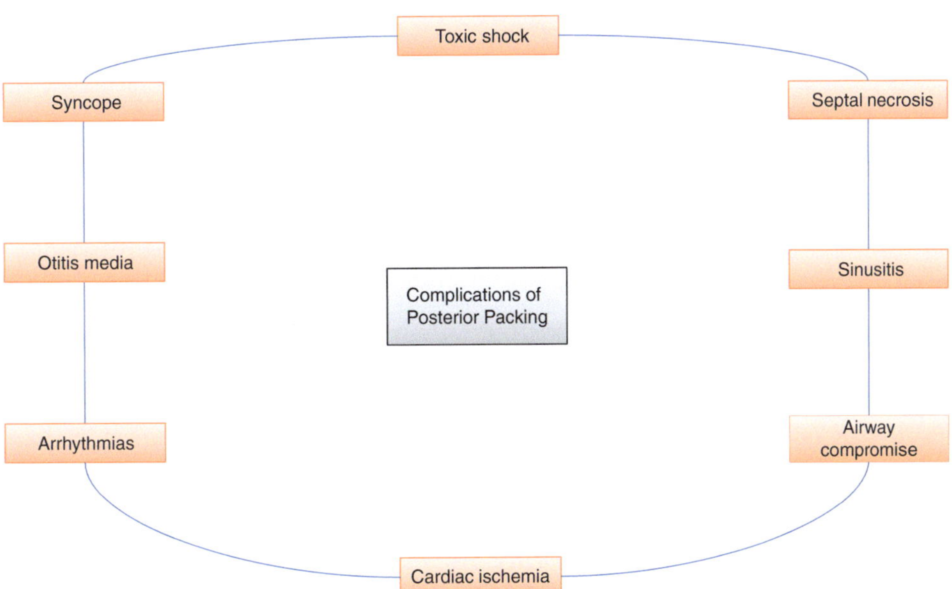

Nasal Fractures

Nasal Fractures = Most common facial fractures → Most are isolated → Have potential for associated injuries

Initial assessment = Look for deformity + Edema + Crepitus + Epistaxis + Septal hematoma

Imaging = Insensitive + Unnecessary → Clinical exam is the best indicator

Fracture of cribiform plate = CSF rhinorrhea → Dx by CT scan

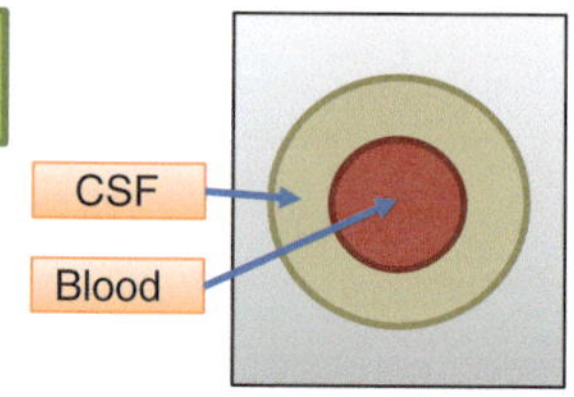

CSF Rhinorrhea = Dipstick glucose > 30 mg/dL + Ring sign on coffee filter + Worse when leaning forward

Septal hematoma = Appears as a boggy blue swelling to nasal septum → Tender to palpation → I&D → Prevents cartilage destruction & saddle nose deformity

Septal Abscess? = Intranasal drainage

Septal Perforation = Requires repair by ENT || Untreated? = Saddle nose deformity

Untreated infected hematomas = Contiguous spread → Intracranial abscess + Meningitis + Osteomyelitis + Cavernous sinus thrombosis

Allergic Rhinitis

PEDIATRICS

Allergic Rhinitis = IgE mediated response of nasal mucosa to allergen → Affects children >2 → 80 % of children with asthma have this → Makes asthma more difficult to control

Symptoms & Signs

- Clear rhinorrhea
- Sneezing
- Nasal pruritis
- Eye itching
- Conjunctival hyperemia
- Hyposmia
- Purulent nasal discharge
- Hypertrophy of nasal turbinates
- Clear secretion from nares

Treatment = Avoidance of precipitating factors + Nasal saline sprays + Antihistamines + Nasal steroids

Sinusitis – Introduction

Sinusitis = Inflammation of the mucosal lining of the paranasal sinuses || Rhinosinusitis = Inflammation of the paranasal sinuses and nasal cavity

Symptoms & Signs

Facial pain · ± Fever · Facial pressure · Ear pain · Hyposmia · Purulent nasal discharge · Blockage and congestion of nose · Tooth pain · Sinus pain when changing head position

Agents of acute sinusitis = *Streptococcus pneumoniae* + *Hemophilus influenza* + *Moraxella catarrhalis* + Viral (most common predisposing factors for bacterial sinusitis)

Agents of chronic sinusitis = *Staph aureus* + Anaerobes + Gram-(-) bacteria + Fungal in immune compromised

Diagnosis = Clinical → Imaging not needed → Use CT for potential complications of acute disease or for chronic disease

Treatment for Acute Sinusitis? = Saline irrigation + Nasal decongestants ± Intranasal steroids

Antibiotics for Acute sinusitis? = Purulent nasal secretions + Severe Sx > 7 days

Complications = Cavernous sinus thrombosis + Skull osteomyelitis (Pott's puffy tumor) + Orbital cellulitis + Intracranial infections (Brain abscess, Meningitis)

Sinusitis

PEDIATRICS

Sinusitis in children = Commonly involves the ethmoid & maxillary sinuses

Sphenoid sinus = Form at 3–5 years of age

Frontal sinus = Does not appear until 7–8 years of age

Chronic sinusitis = > 90 days → Treat for anaerobes as well → Give for 4 weeks + Refer to ENT

Facial Fractures

Frontal and Zygoma Fractures

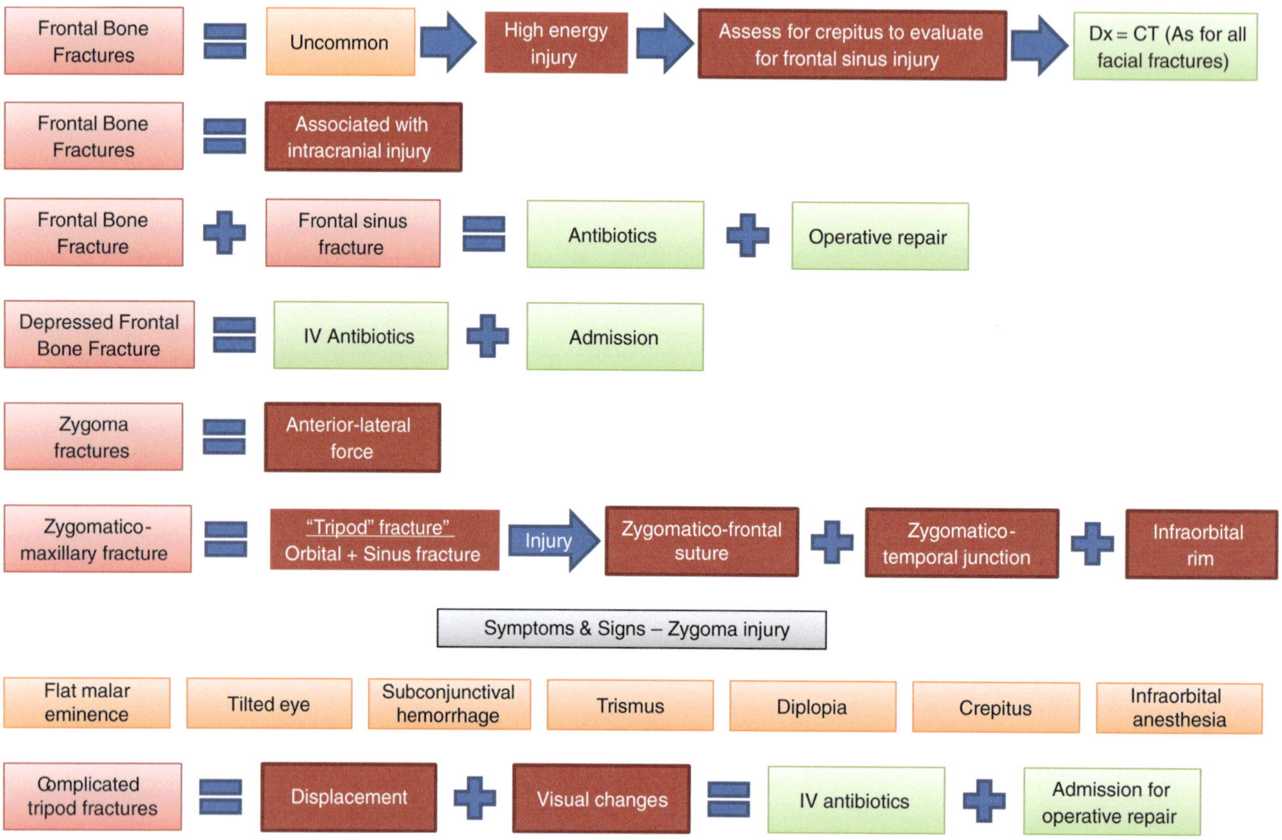

Midface Fractures

Midface fractures = LeFort classification → I, II, III → Dx= CT

Symptoms & Signs

- Hemorrhage
- Bilateral orbital ecchymosis
- Significant swelling
- CSF leaks in II & III

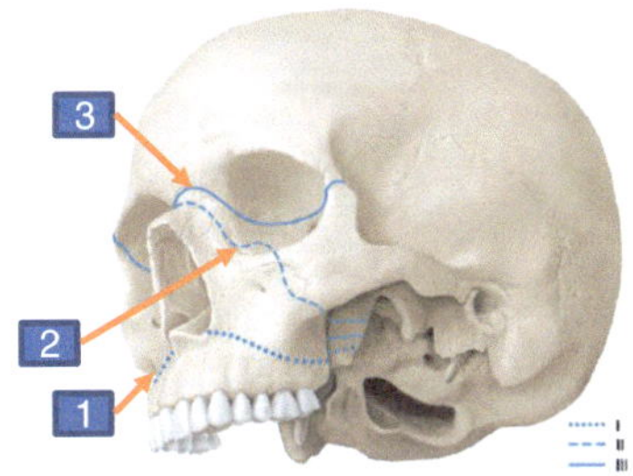

Hardt, N., & Kuttenberger, J. (2010). *Craniofacial trauma: diagnosis and management*. Springer. Fig 3.4, p. 33

LeFort I = Horizontal maxillary fracture → *Hard palate & teeth* move on exam

LeFort II = Pyramidal fracture → *Hard palate & nose* are free floating on exam

LeFort III = Craniofacial malunion → *Entire face* is mobile → Globes held in place by optic nerves

Treatment = Admission + IV antibiotics

Complications (> in II & III) = C-spine injury or fracture + Airway compromise (Retrophayngeal hematoma; Consider awake intubation) + Bleeding (May require nasal packing) + CSF rhinorrhea + Dental malocclusion

Mandible Fractures

Mandible fractures = 2nd most common facial fracture → Look for fracture on opposite side of ring → Assume open fracture

Severe Mandible fracture? = Beware tongue displacement → Causes upper airway obstruction

Symptoms & Signs

- Malocclusion
- Pain on movement
- Jaw deviates to side of fracture
- Mandible displacement
- Anesthesia in inferior alveolar or mental nerve distribution

Bedside testing = Tongue blade test → Assess in low risk patients → Bite on tongue blade while MD twists blade → Blade breaks & patient tolerates? → Unlikely fracture (95% sensitive)

Blood in mouth = Open fracture

Children 4–11 = Risk for facial growth disturbances if missed → Consider in cases with facial trauma with trismus and TMJ pain

Imaging? = Panorex + CT (complicated injury)

Treatment for stable patient? = Ace wrap over head and under mandible + Analgesia + Antibiotics + Outpatient followup

Open fracture? = Admission + Operative repair

Throat/Neck/Upper Airway Infections

Pharyngitis and Tonsillitis

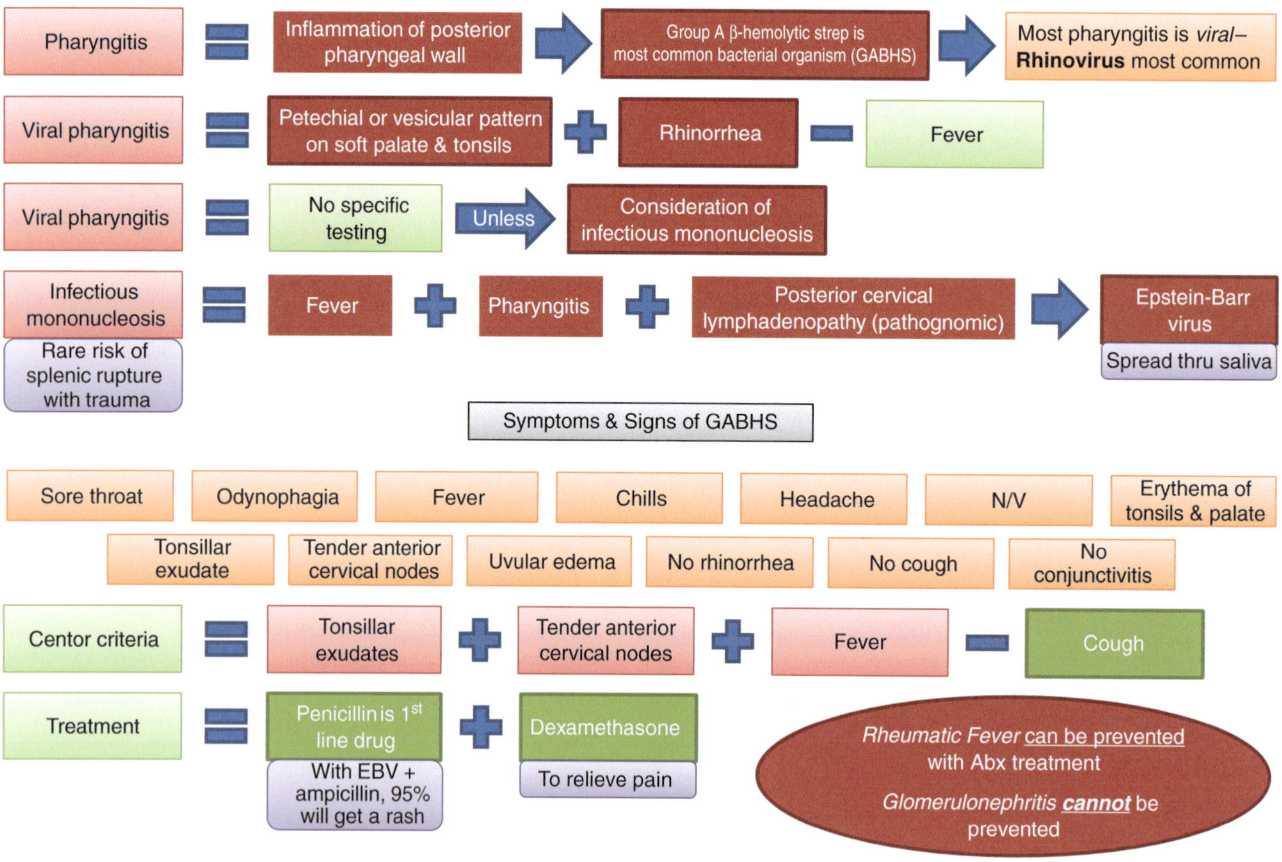

Peritonsillar Abscess (PTA)

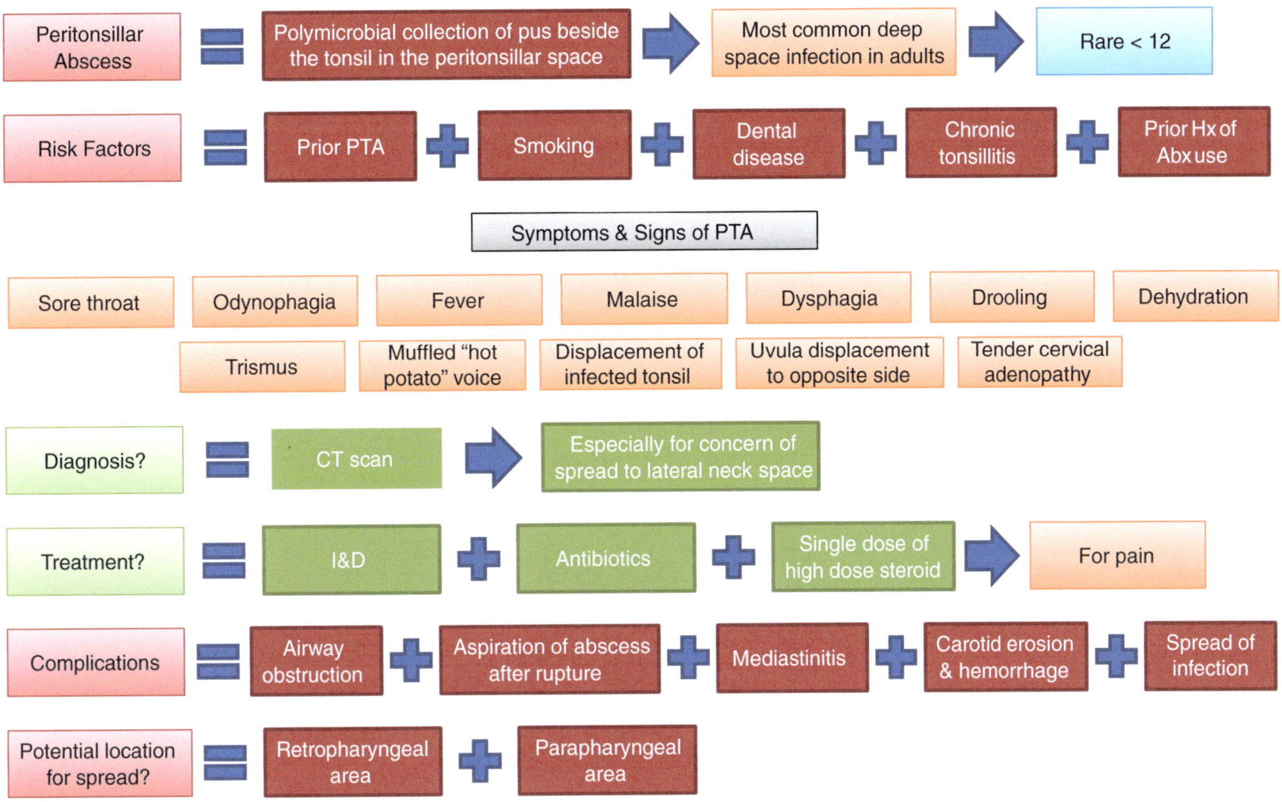

Epiglottitis

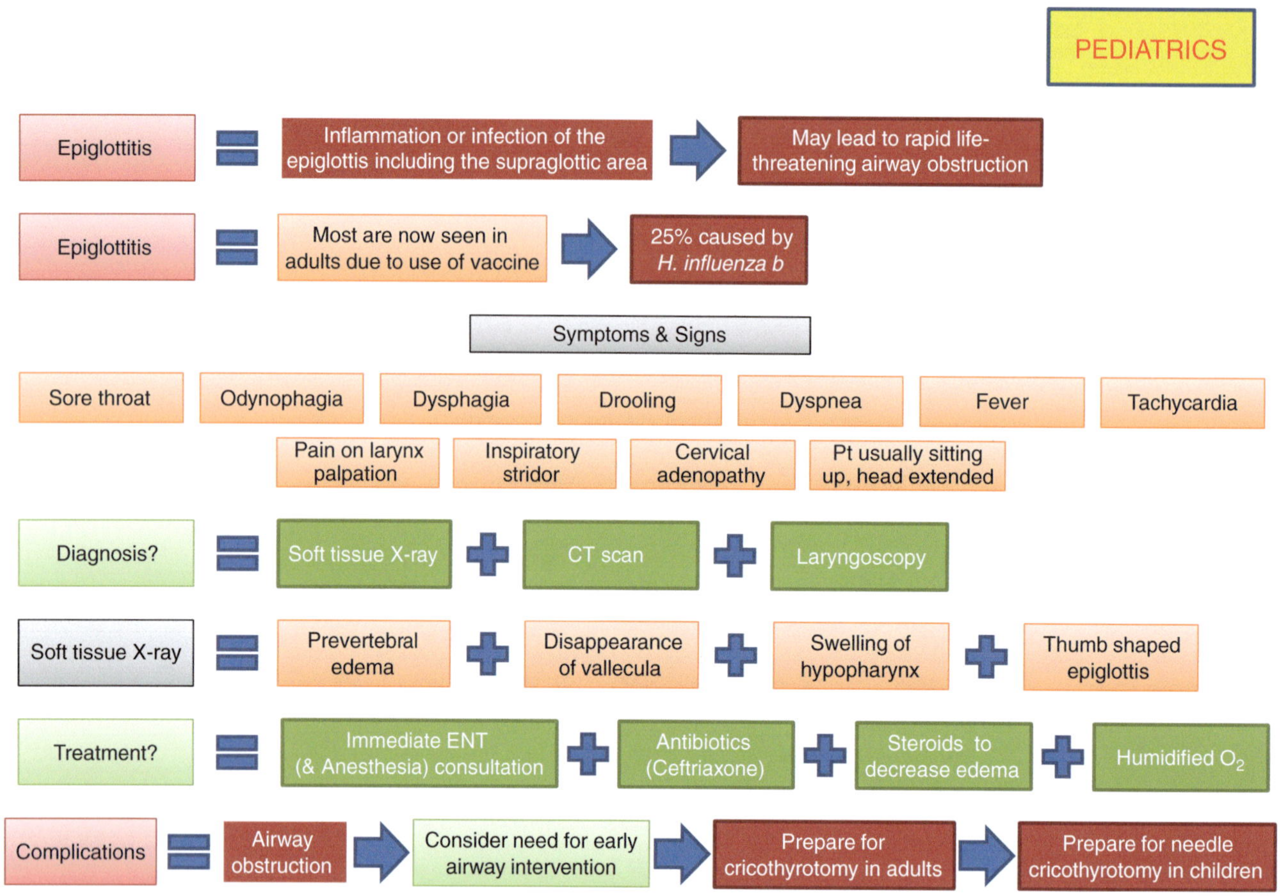

Retropharyngeal Abscess

PEDIATRICS

Retropharyngeal Abscess = Deep inflammation or infection behind the posterior pharyngeal wall → In children the primary infection is elsewhere in the head & neck

Retropharyngeal Abscess in adults = In adults, the infection is due to extension from a nearby site → More likely to extend into the mediastinum

Symptoms & Signs

- Sore throat
- Fever
- Torticollis
- Dysphagia
- Neck pain
- Cervical adenopathy
- Neck edema
- Odynophagia
- Muffled or hoarse voice ("Cri du canard" = duck like voice)
- Stridor
- Anterior displacement of posterior pharyngeal wall

Diagnosis? = Soft tissue X-ray + CT scan (Gold standard)

Soft tissue X-ray = Protrusion of retropharyngeal wall → Neck flexion may cause bulge of posterior wall

Treatment? = Immediate ENT consultation + Antibiotics + IV hydration + Surgical intervention

Complications = Airway compromise + Extension into mediastinum

Ludwig's Angina

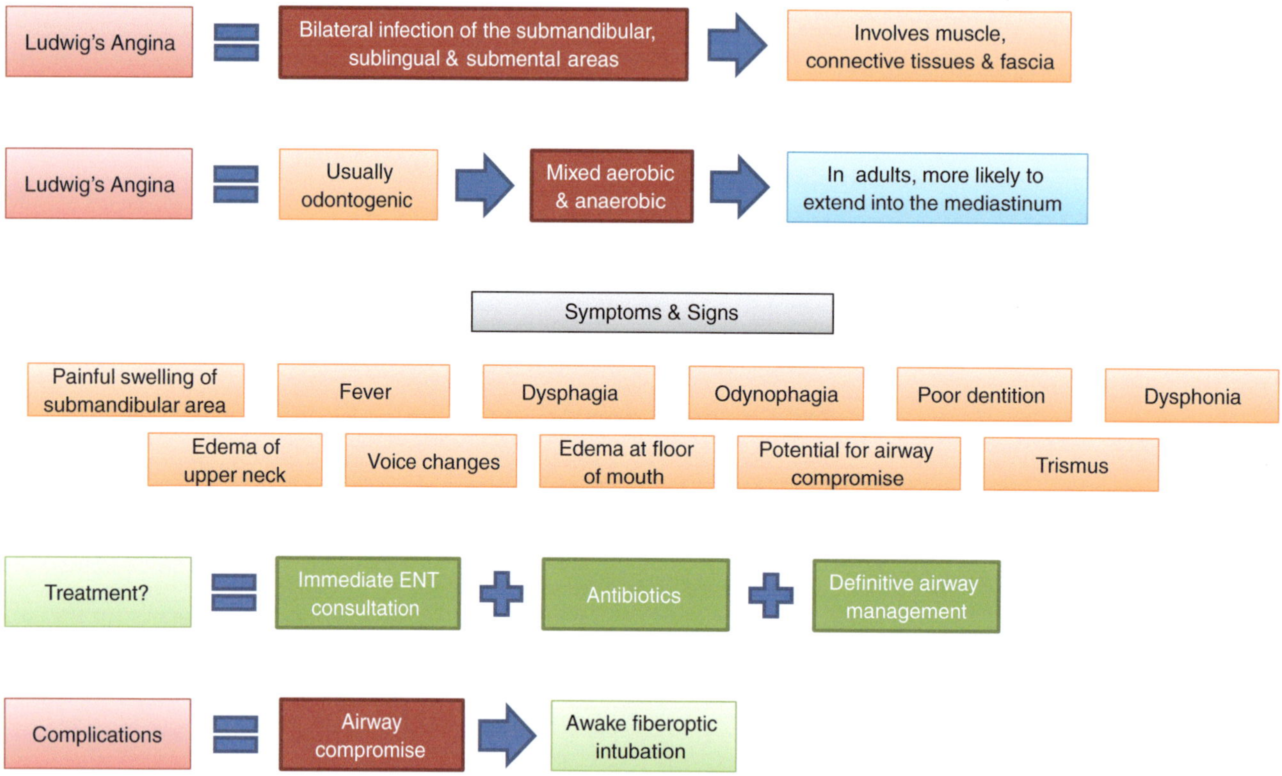

Necrotizing Infections

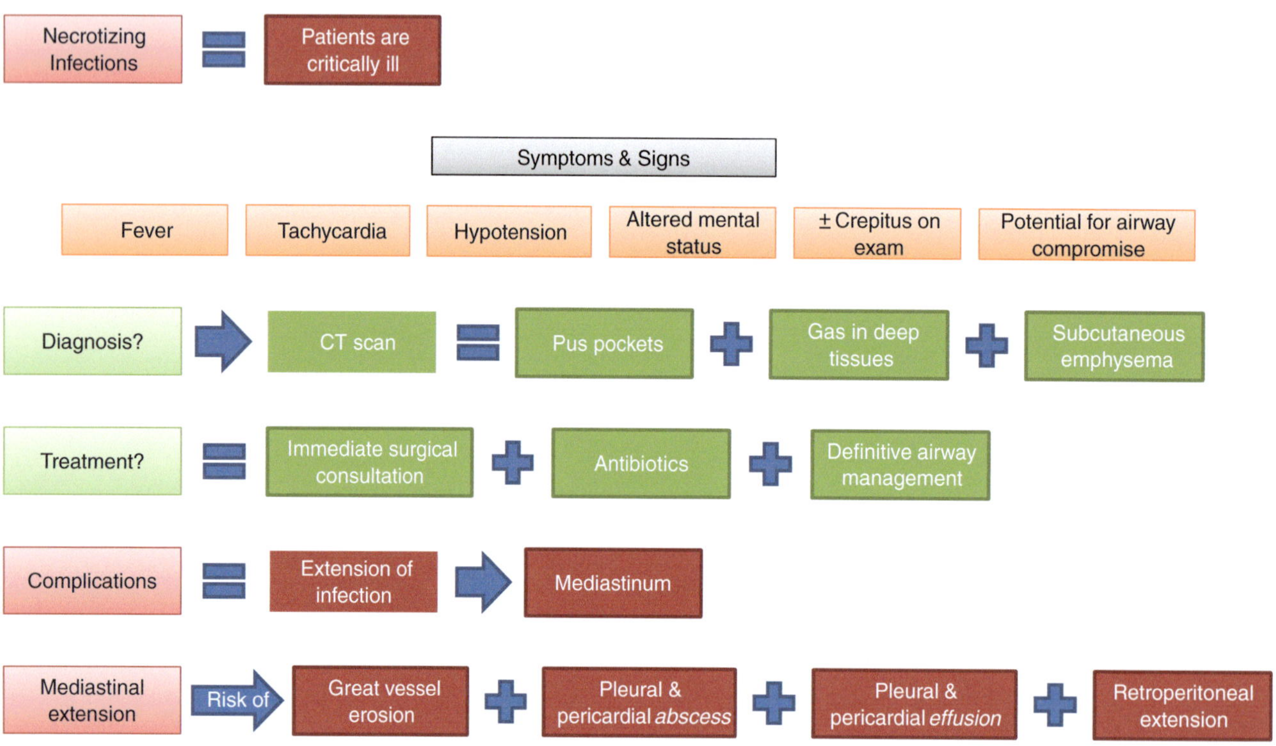

Croup

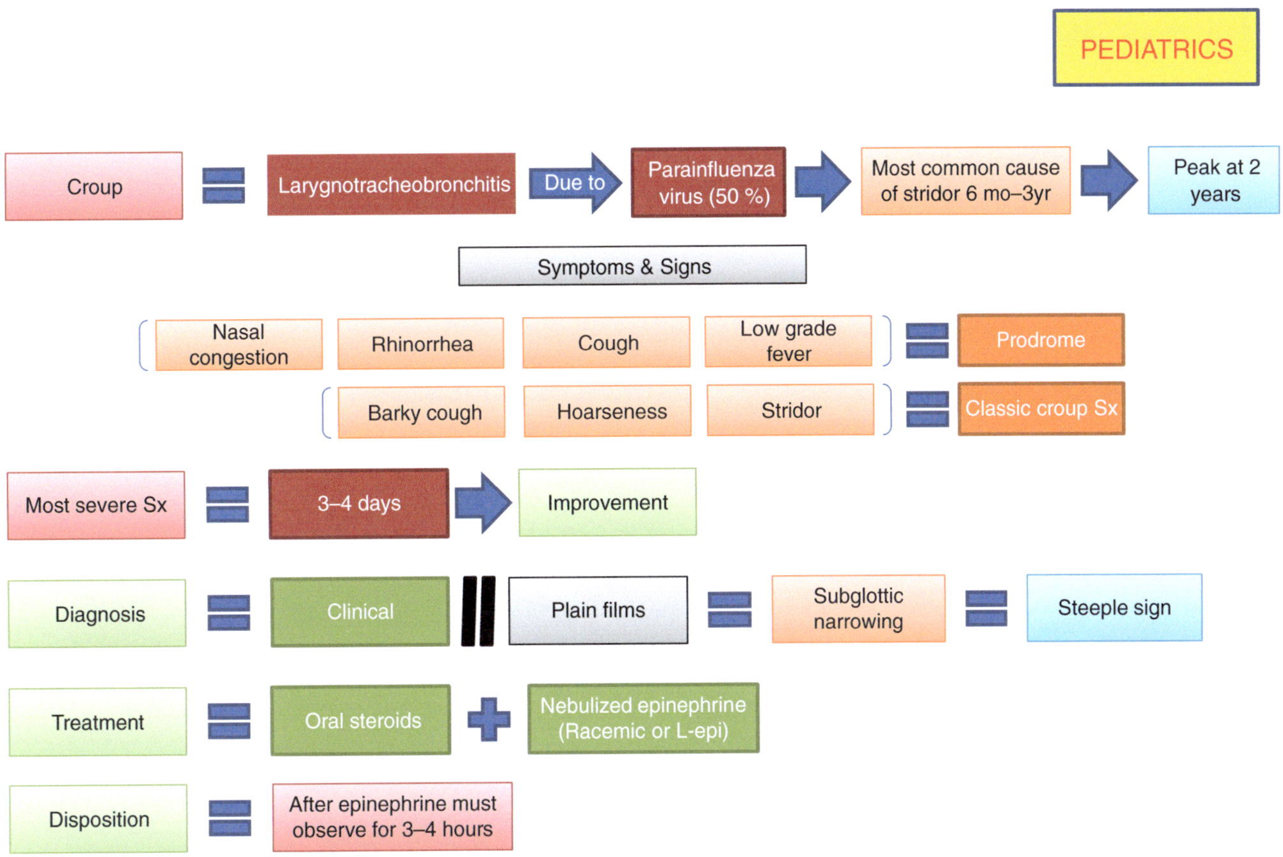

Bacterial Tracheitis

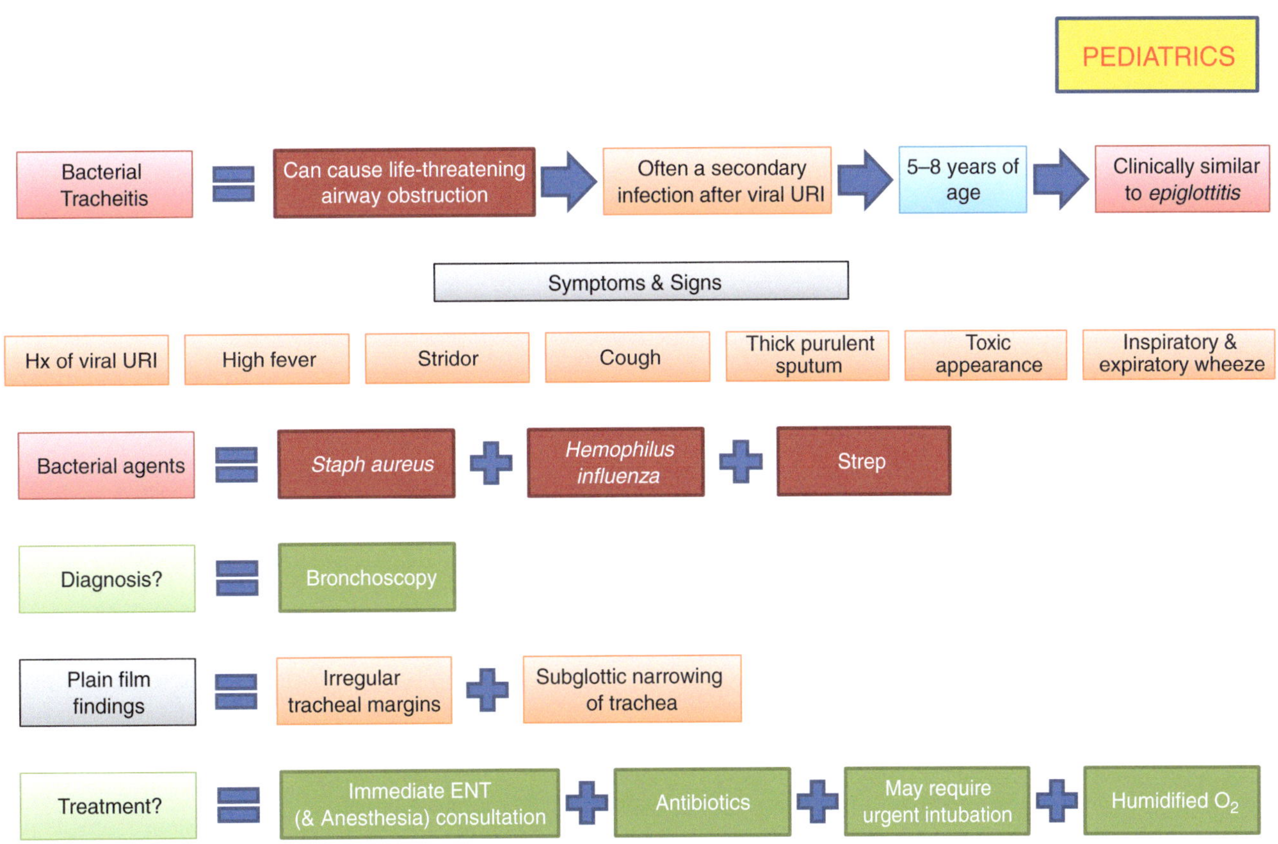

Dental Emergencies

Odontogenic Infections

Odontogenic Abscess = From infected tooth (1-21 days after onset of pain) + Following tooth extraction → Polymicrobial (aerobes & anaerobes)

Deep neck infection tidbits = Most deep neck infections arise from dental source (esp. *mandibular teeth*) = Fascial layers of head & neck have potential spaces for spread of infection

Localized dental pain = Pulpitis *or* dental caries = Intermittent pain worse with extremes of temperature → Rx = root canal or extraction

Pericoronitis = Inflammation of gum overlying tooth → Due to → Inflammation of soft tissues surrounding the crown of partially erupted teeth esp. 3rd molars → Rx = irrigation ± antibiotics

Periapical abscess = Most common cause of severe dental pain = Inflammation & infection of apical aspect of tooth → Can erode into cortical bone

Parulis = Periapical abscess draining externally on gums

Infections of molar teeth → May spread to masticator space → Parapharyngeal space → Neck → Mediastinum

Infections of anterior mandibular teeth → Spread to neck

Infections of other mandibular teeth → Spread sublingually

Treatment = Penicillin is 1st line drug + Clindamycin OR Metronidazole + I&D

Periostitis and Alveolar Osteitis and Post-extraction Bleeding

Periosteitis = 1-2 days after extraction → Due to → Trauma of surgery → Rx → Ice packs & Head elevation + NSAID's ± Narcotics

Complications = Trismus → Due to → TMJ injury + Infection + Muscular injury during anesthesia

Alveolar osteitis = 2-5 days after extraction → Due to → Dislodgement of clot from socket → Leads to → Localized osteomyelitis

Risk factors = Preexisting pericoronitis or other dental process + Smoking + Hormone replacement therapy + Traumatic extraction

Treatment? = Local & topical anesthesia + Irrigation + Ribbon gauze pack with oil of cloves or eugenol + Antibiotics

Disposition? = Referral to dentist within 24 hours

Post-extraction Bleeding = Displacement of clot

Treatment? = Firm pressure to extraction site ± Topical thrombin/ Gel foam OR Cautery with silver nitrate ± Injection of Lidocaine with epinephrine may tamponade the bleeding

Periodontal Pathology

Gingivitis = Gingival inflammation + Bleeding Due to → Plaque along gingiva

Periodontitis = Progression of gingival inflammation → Forms sulci and periodontal pockets → Tooth loss Due to → *Bacteriodes gingivalis*

Risk factors for severe Periodontitis = HIV + Down's syndrome + Diabetes mellitus

Gum disease = Most common cause of tooth loss

Periodontal abscess = Entrapment of plaque & other debris in the periodontal pocket = Severe gum pain → Warm saline rinses + Antibiotics & analgesia

Treatment = Penicillin is 1st line drug + Clindamycin OR Metronidazole + I&D

Acute Necrotizing Ulcerative Gingivitis (ANUG)

ANUG = Trench mouth → Caused by: Spirochetes & Fusobacteria → Can be very destructive → May spread from gums to tissues of face to facial bones

Risk factors = Poor oral hygiene + Immune diseases (HIV) + Prior necrotizing gingivitis

Diagnosis = Severe pain + Gingival bleeding + Ulcerated intradental papillae

Symptoms & Signs

- Red, swollen gums
- Painful gums
- Ulcerations on gums
- Foul breath
- Fever
- Malaise
- Abnormal tooth mobility
- Pseudomembrane formation
- Lymphadenopathy

Treatment = Clindamycin OR Metronidazole

Gingival Hyperplasia

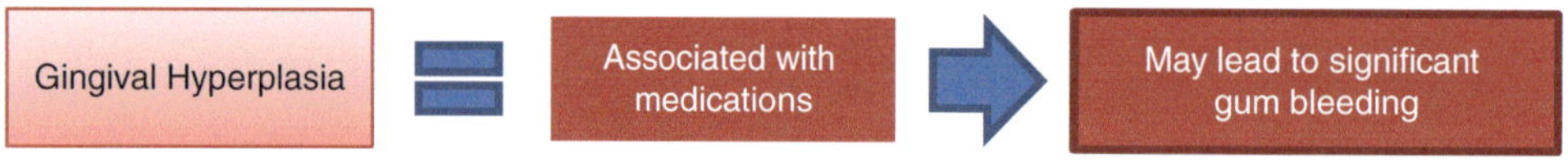

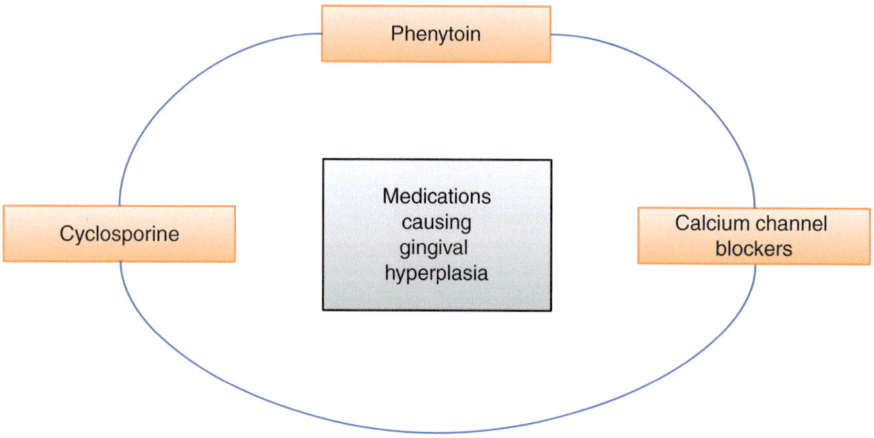

Dental Trauma: Introduction

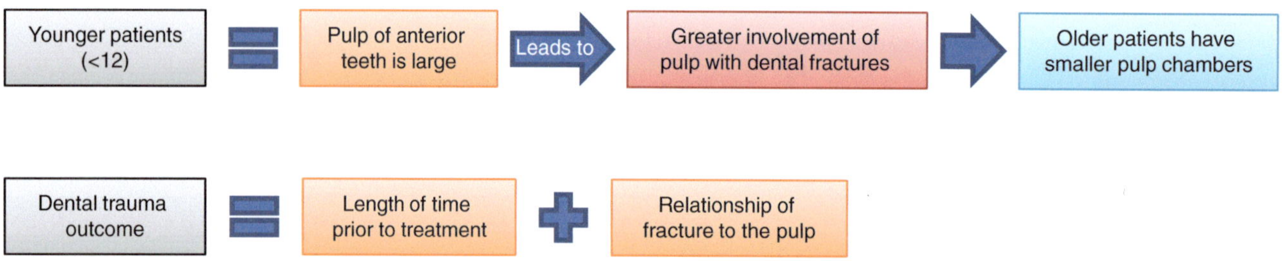

Ellis Fractures

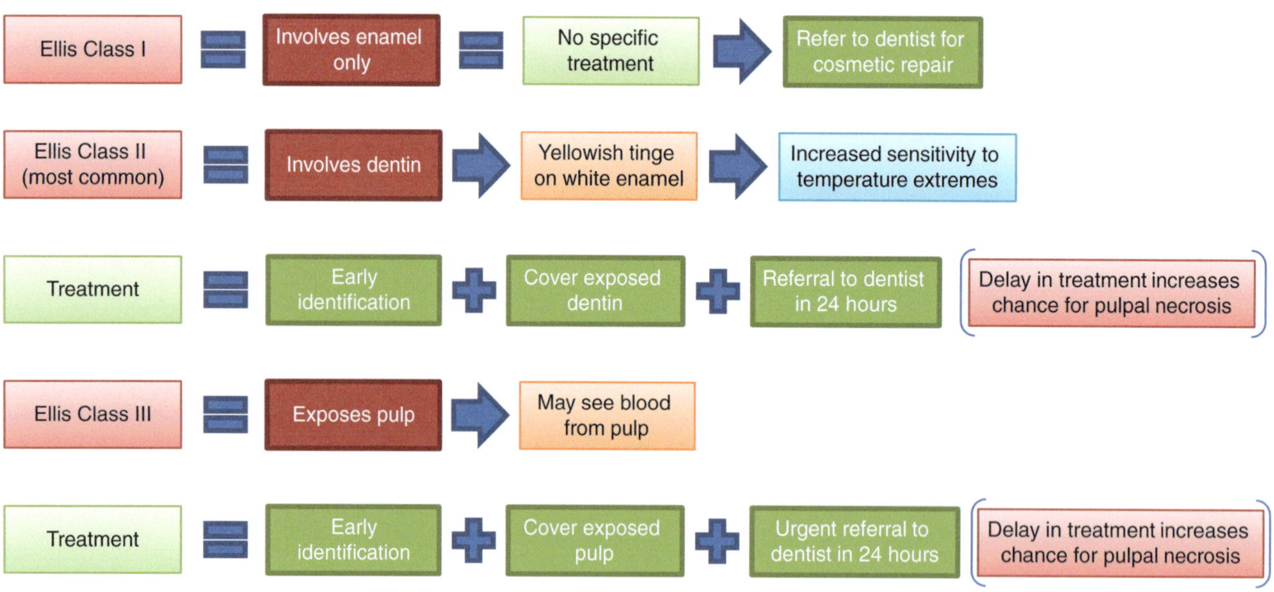

Dental Trauma

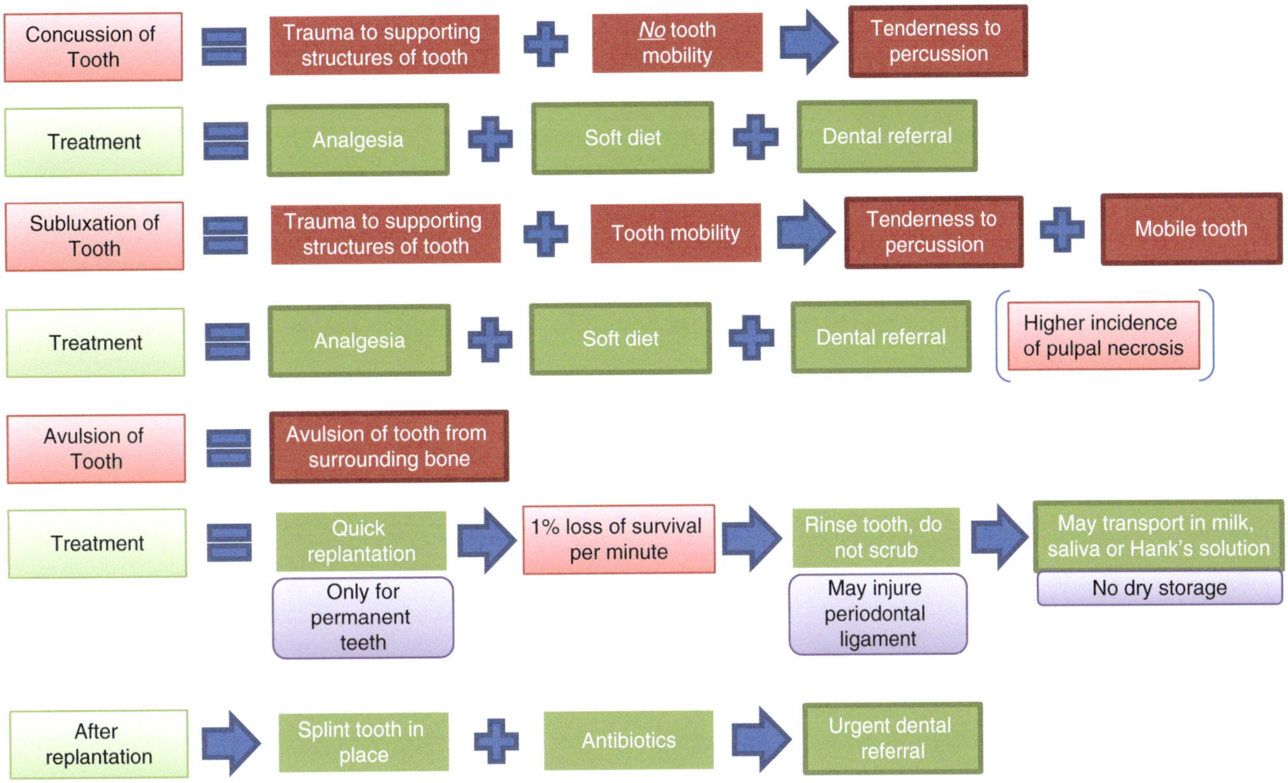

Neck Masses

Neck

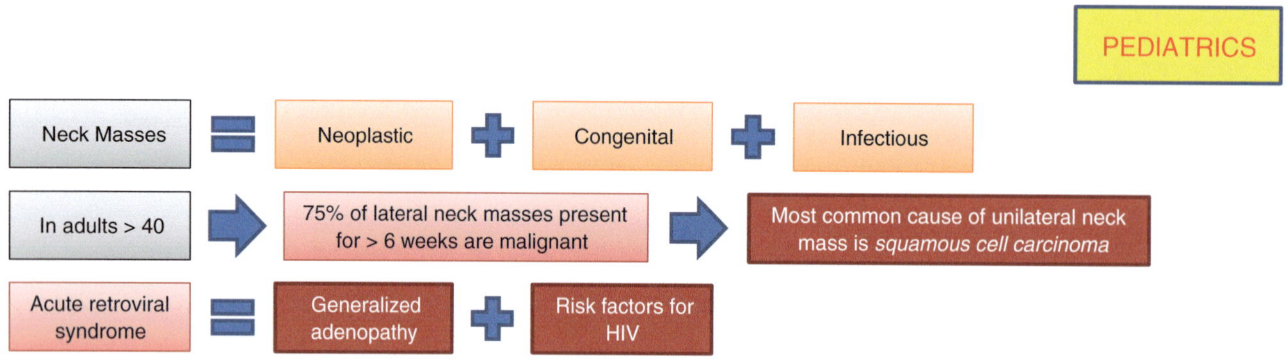

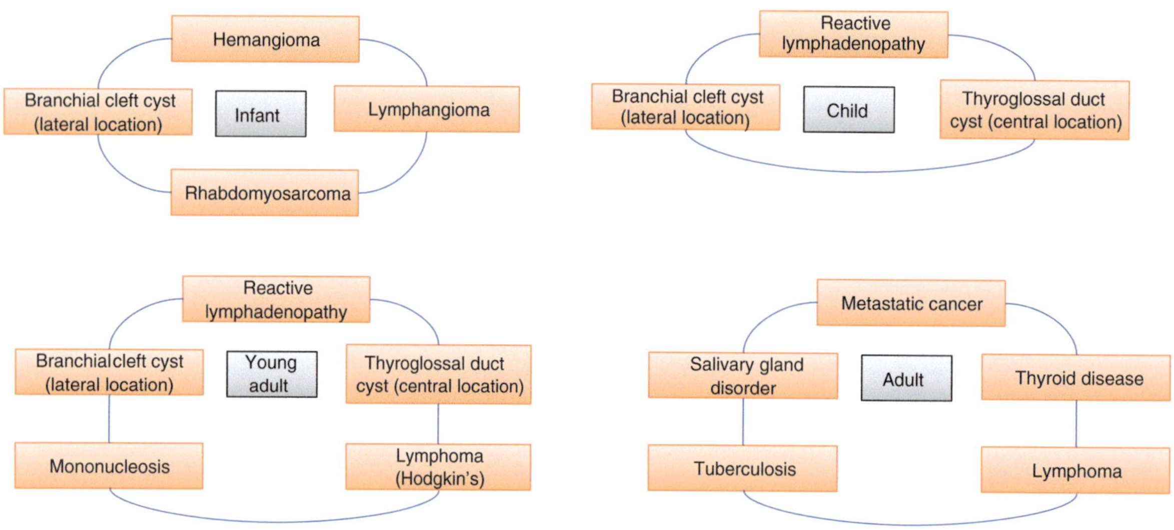

Branchial Cleft Cysts

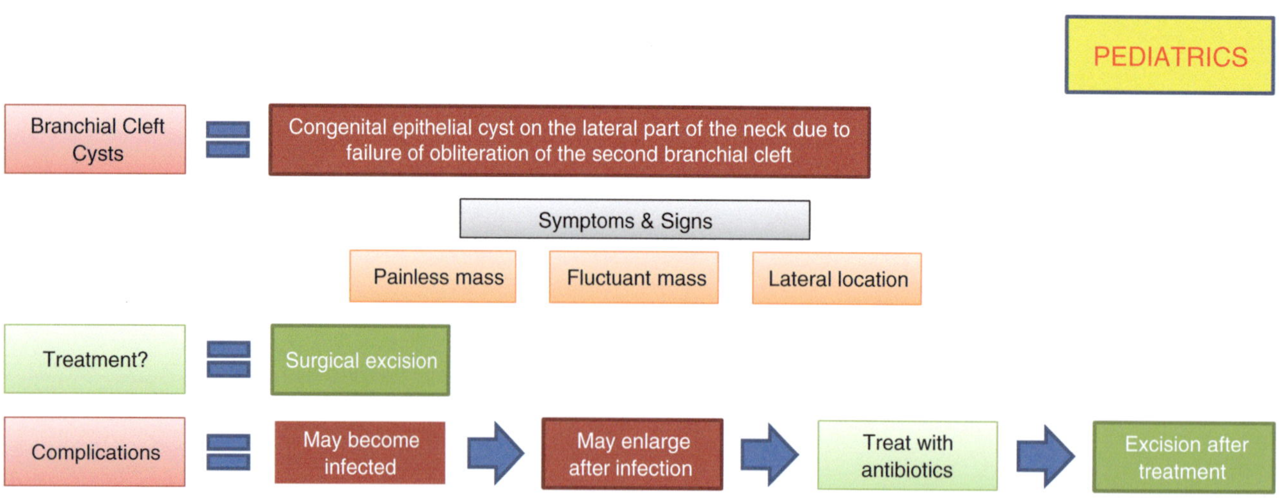

Thyroglossal Duct Cysts

PEDIATRIC

Thyroglossal Duct Cysts = Fibrous cyst that develops from persistent thyroglossal ducts → Usually in children

Symptoms & Signs

- Usually asymptomatic mass
- Soft & mobile
- Bluish hue

Treatment? = Surgical excision

Complications = May become infected → May enlarge after infection → Treat with antibiotics → Excision after treatment

Larynx Trauma

Larynx Trauma = Compression of larynx on anterior cervical spine → Laryngotracheal separation + Cartilage fractures + Mucosal tears

Larynx Trauma = Can be due to direct trauma, hyperflexion/extension, or rotation

Clothesline injury → Motorcycle, ATV, Football → Crushes thyroid cartilage → May cause immediate asphyxiation → *Tracheostomy* required in these patients

Symptoms & Signs

- Anterior neck pain
- Hoarseness
- Dysphagia
- Stridor
- Dyspnea
- Cough
- Hemoptysis
- Subcutaneous emphysema
- Aphonia
- Apnea
- **Vascular injury** = expanding hematomas, bruits, pulse deficits

Diagnosis? = CT scan

Treatment = Maintenance of airway → Endotracheal intubation OR Tracheostomy

(Avoid cricothyrotomy)

Edema of Upper Airway

Angioedema

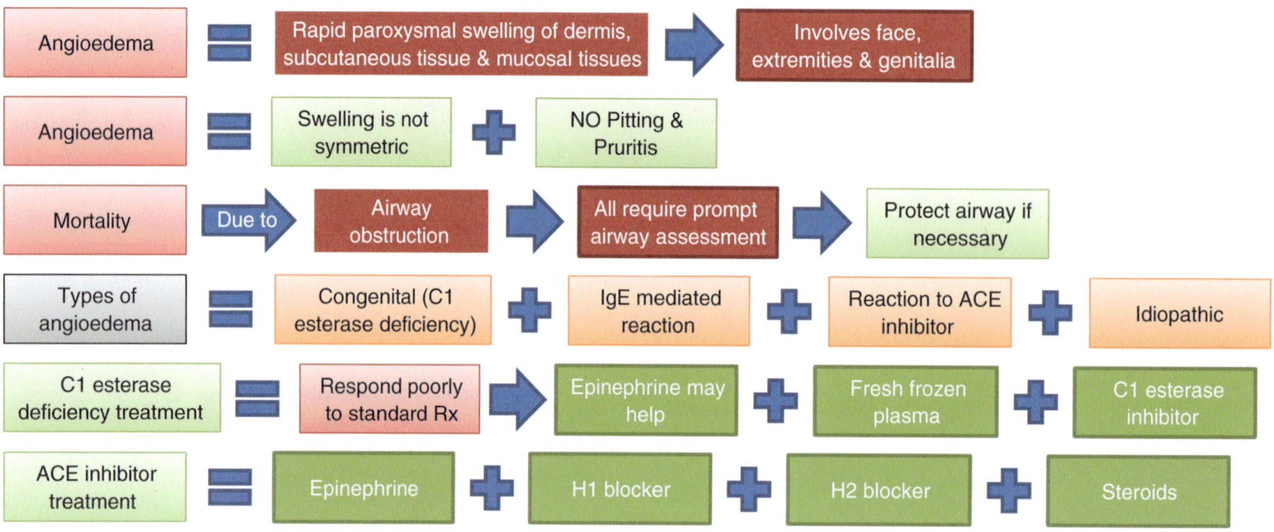

Uvular Edema

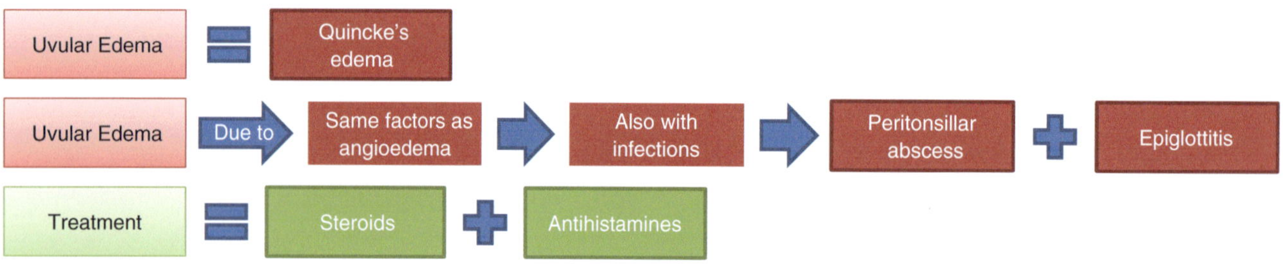

Soft Tissue Lesions

Candidiasis

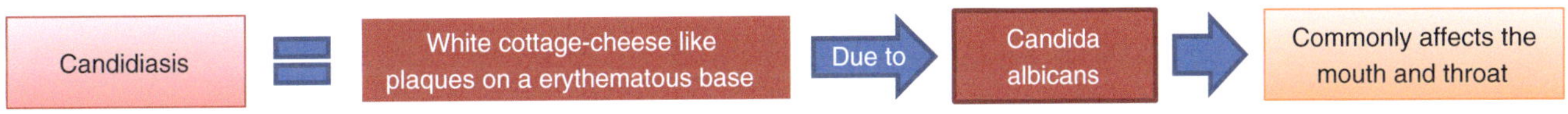

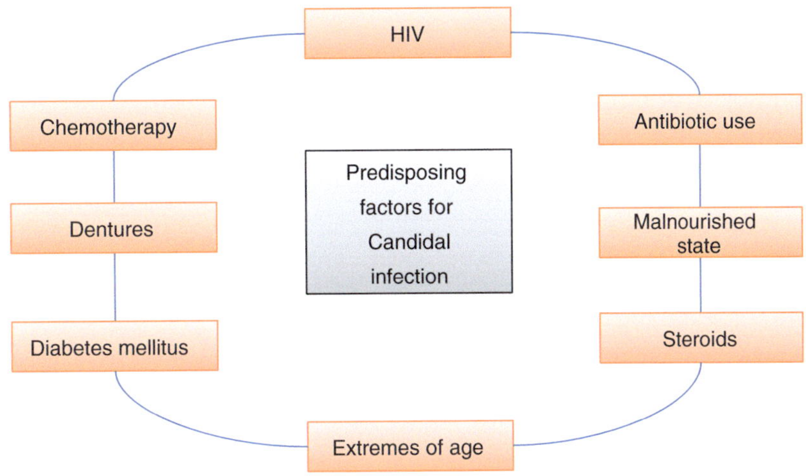

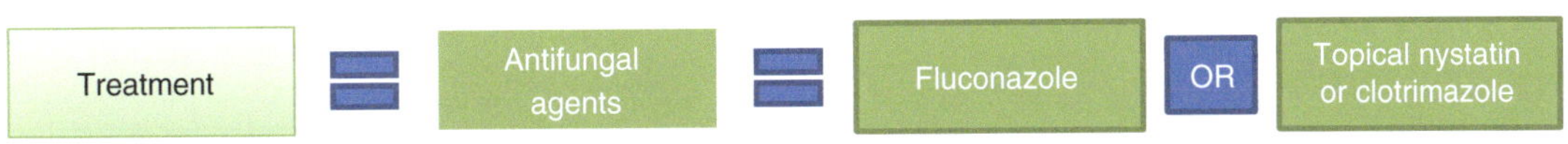

HSV infections

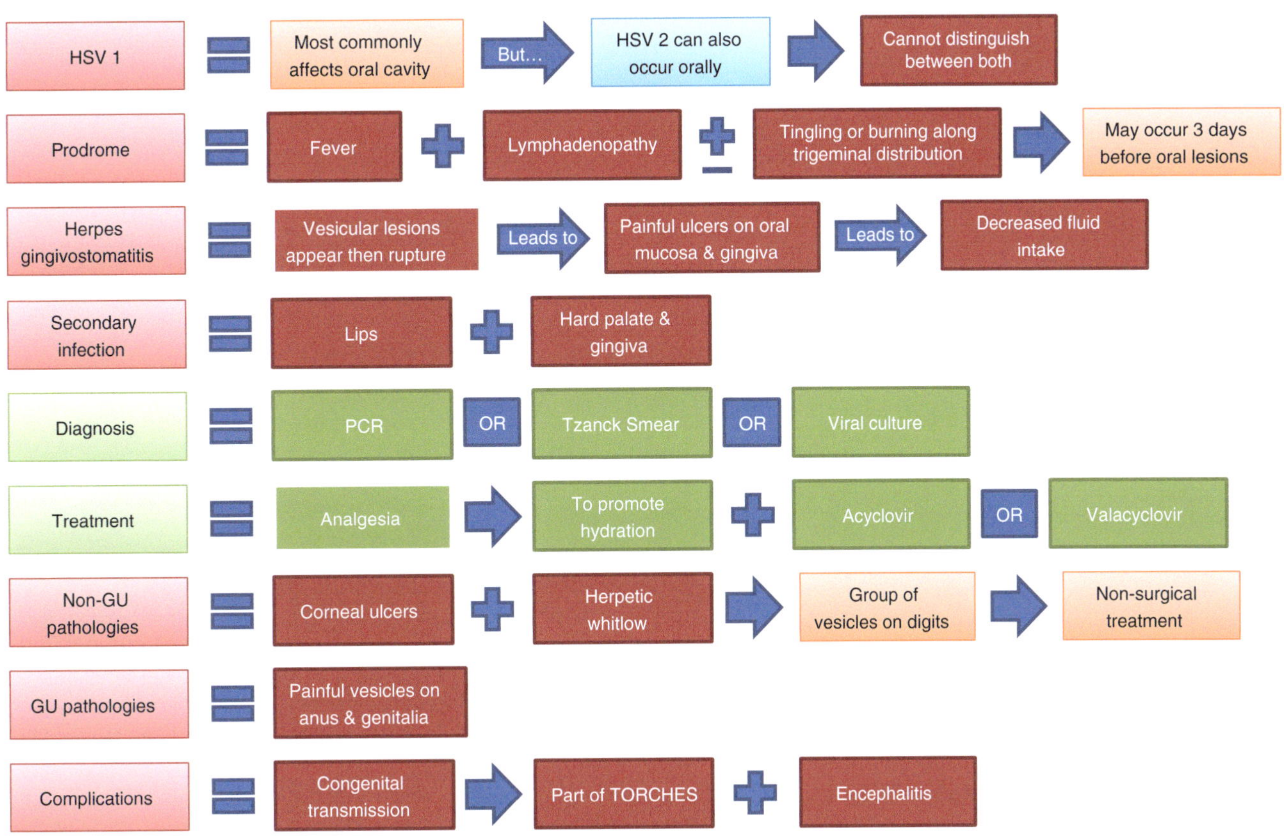

Aphthous Stomatitis

Aphthous stomatitis = Red macules that ulcerate → Leads to → Painful eschar → May be multiple

Aphthous stomatitis = Due to cell mediated immune response to an unidentified triggering agent

Aphthous stomatitis = Usually resolve in 10–14 days

Treatment = Topical steroids

Herpangina

PEDIATRIC

Herpangina = Caused by Coxsackievirus A → Fecal-oral transmission → Spreads to other children → Usually lasts 7–10 days

Symptoms & Signs

High fever | Sore throat | Headache | Malaise | Dysphagia | Vomiting | 1–2 mm oral vesicles

Natural history = Constitutional Sx → 1–2 days → Oral vesicles appear → Rupture of vesicles → Painful ulcers remain

Vesicle appearance → Tonsils + Posterior pharynx + Soft palate + Uvula

Vesicles spare → Gingiva + Tongue + Buccal mucosa

Treatment = Analgesia + Hydration

Complications? = Rare

Distinguished from Herpes gingivostomatitis which *does* affect gingiva

Intraoral and Tongue Lesions

Leukoplakia

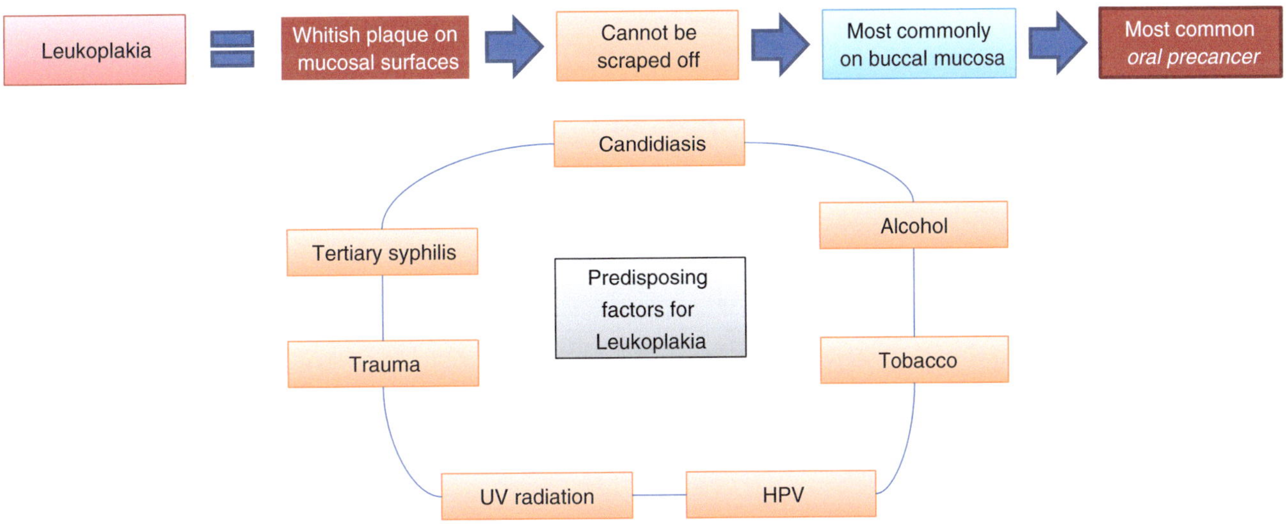

Strawberry Tongue

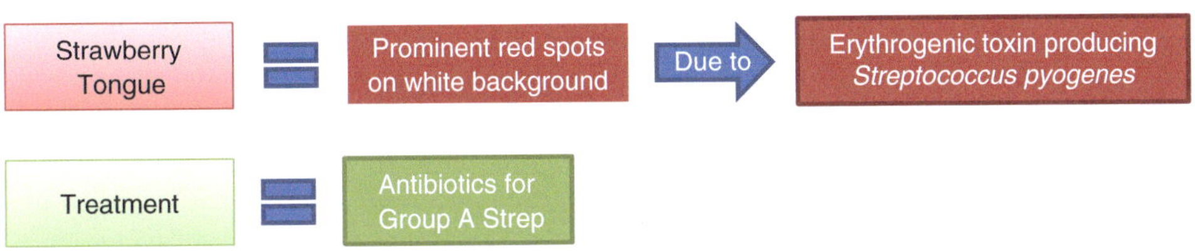

Oral Cancer

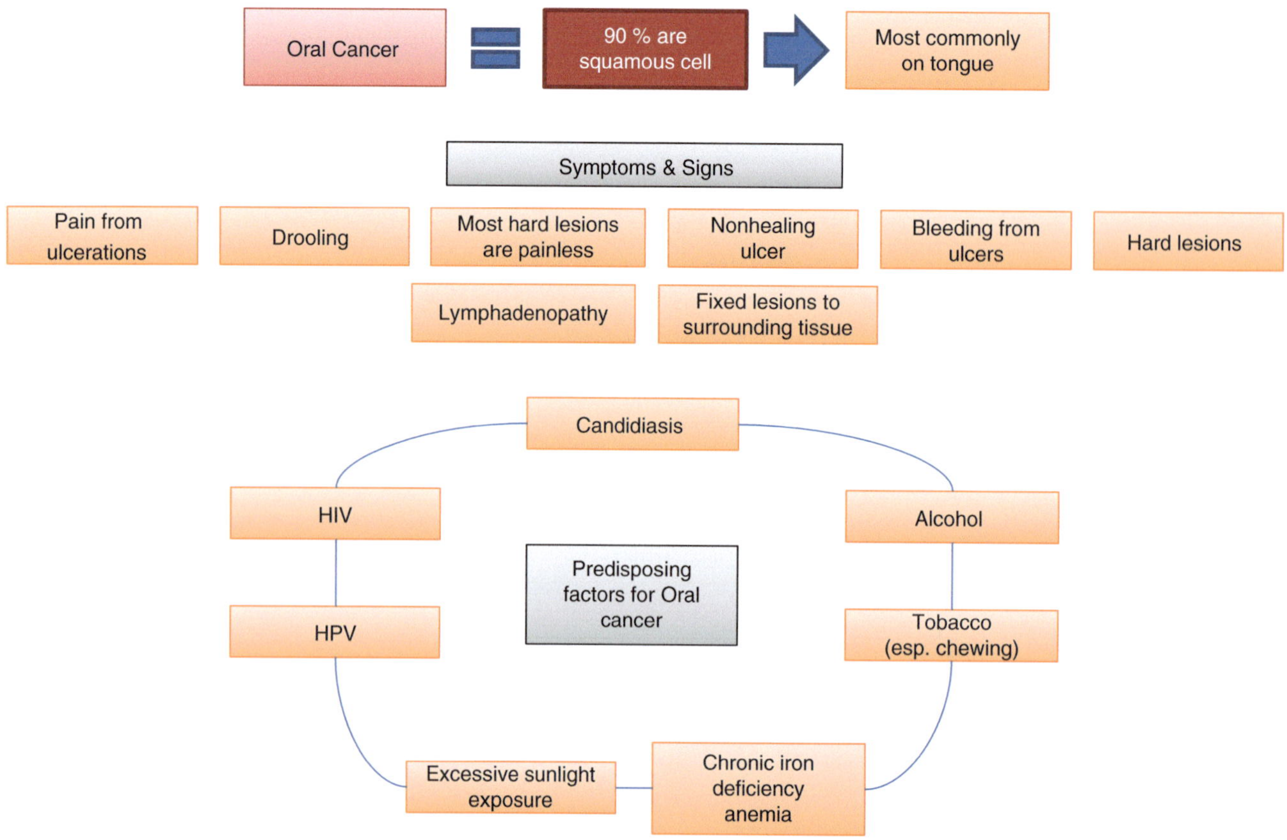
Oral Cancer
90 % are squamous cell
Most commonly on tongue
Symptoms & Signs
Pain from ulcerations
Drooling
Most hard lesions are painless
Nonhealing ulcer
Bleeding from ulcers
Hard lesions
Lymphadenopathy
Fixed lesions to surrounding tissue
Candidiasis
HIV
Alcohol
Predisposing factors for Oral cancer
HPV
Tobacco (esp. chewing)
Excessive sunlight exposure
Chronic iron deficiency anemia

Salivary Gland Disorders

Viral Parotitis (Mumps)

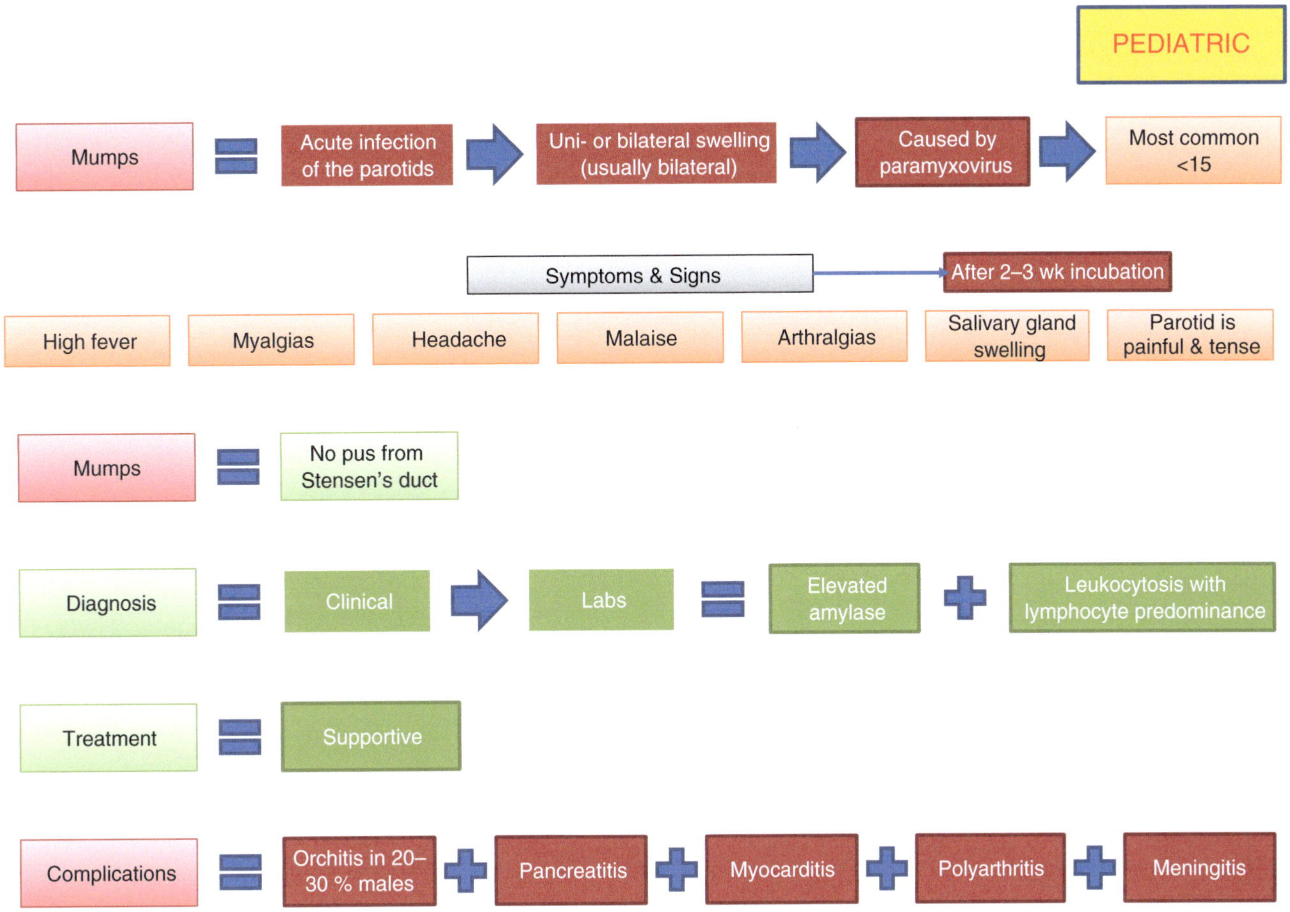

Suppurative Parotitis

Suppurative Parotitis = Bacterial infection of parotid → Due to → Impaired salivary flow → Retrograde migration of bacteria from mouth → *Staph aureus* is most common

Risk factors = Medications + Dehydration + Post-operative + Sialolithiasis + Chronic illness

Symptoms & Signs

Fever | Trismus | Skin over parotid is erythematous | Skin over parotid is tender | Pus expressed from Stensen's duct

Diagnosis = Clinical → Labs = Normal amylase + Leukocytosis with neutrophilic predominance

Imaging = U/S OR CT

Treatment = Hydration + Optimize salivary flow (lemon drops) + Massage & heat to parotid + Antibiotics

Sialolithiasis

Sialolithiasis = Formation of calcium stone in a salivary duct → Most common in men 30–60

Sialolithiasis = 80 % occur in submandibular gland → Due to ascending course & viscous secretions

Predisposition to sialolithiasis = Diabetes + Dehydration

Symptoms & Signs

Pain worse with meals | Unilateral swelling | Tenderness | Gland is firm | May palpate stone in duct

Diagnosis = Clinical → May see on X-ray or CT

Treatment = Analgesia + Sialogogues + May attempt to milk stone from duct + Antibiotics for concurrent infection

Complications = Secondary Staph infection + Recurrent obstruction + Strictures

Facial Infections

Facial Cellulitis

Facial Cellulitis = Most commonly caused by *Streptococcus pyogenes* (GABHS) & *Staph aureus* → Inciting factors of piercings

Symptoms & Signs

- Erythema
- Edema
- Warmth
- Pain at site

Diagnosis = Clinical + Imaging as needed for suspicion of deep infection

Treatment = Analgesics + Antipyretics + Removal of inciting factors + Antibiotics

Erysipelas

Erysipelas = Cellulitis affecting epidermis, upper dermis & lymphatics → Most commonly affects the LE → Can affect the face

Erysipelas = *Streptococcus pyogenes* is most common

Bullous erysipelas = More severe form → 50 % caused by MRSA

Diagnosis = Red, raised puffy skin appearance + Sharply defined border

Treatment = Antibiotics

Impetigo

Impetigo = Superficial epidermal infection → Discrete amber crusts OR Bullae → Highly infectious

Impetigo = *Staph aureus* alone OR *Staph* + *Streptococcus pyogenes* (GABHS)

Nonbullous impetigo = Start as red, moist vesicles → Have surrounding area of redness → Break down into honey-crusted lesions

Bullous impetigo = Rapidly enlarging vesicles → Become flaccid bullae with clear yellow fluid → Suggests *Staph* infection

Treatment = Antibiotics to cover Staph & Strep → Dicloxacillin Cephaloporins + Mupirocin ointment

Complication = Glomerulonephritis → **Not** prevented by antibiotics

Other ENT Emergencies

Post-tonsillectomy Bleeding

Post-tonsillectomy Bleeding = Most occurs 5–10 days after surgery Due to → Sloughing of clot or eschar from tonsil bed → Usually see a gray-white eschar

Initial stabilization = Sit upright + NPO + IV hydration + Emergent ENT consultation

Labs = CBC + Coagulation parameters + Type & Cross + Emergent ENT consultation

Treatment = Direct pressure to bleeding → Packing soaked with epinephrine or thrombin

Complications = Airway obstruction + Hemorrhagic shock

Trigeminal Neuralgia

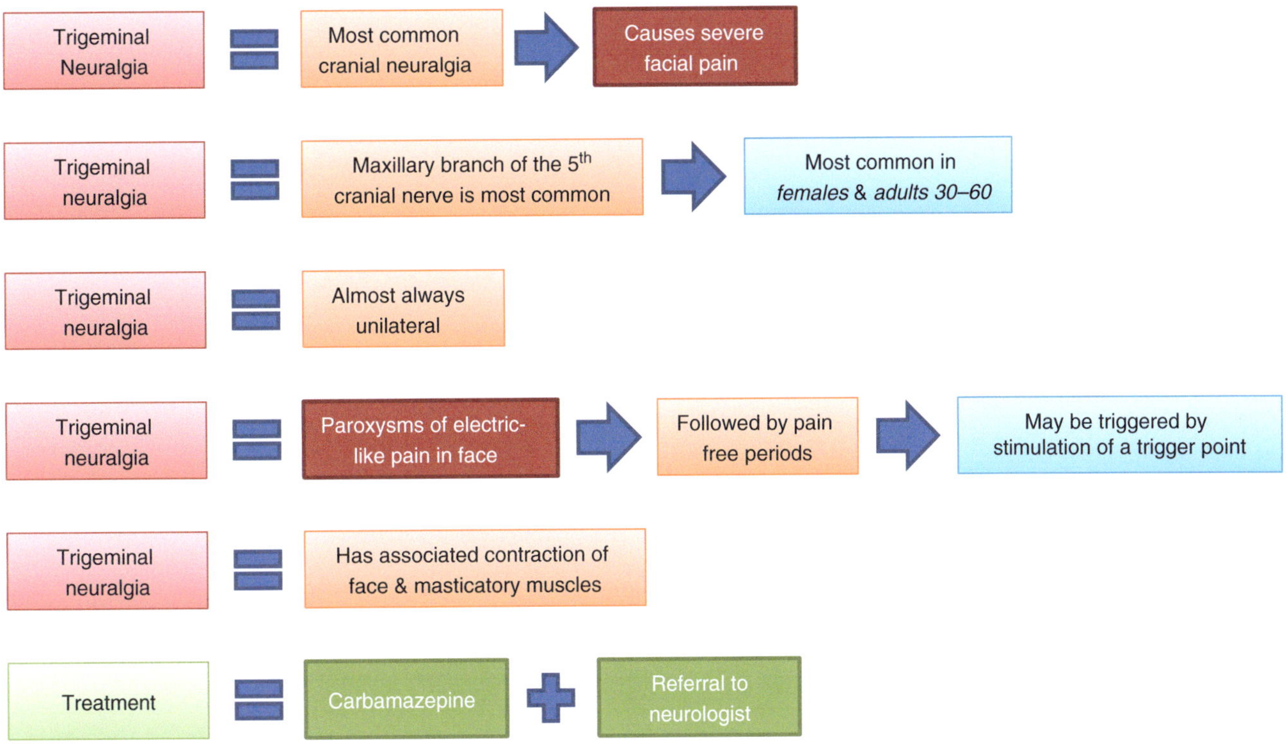

Causes of Trismus

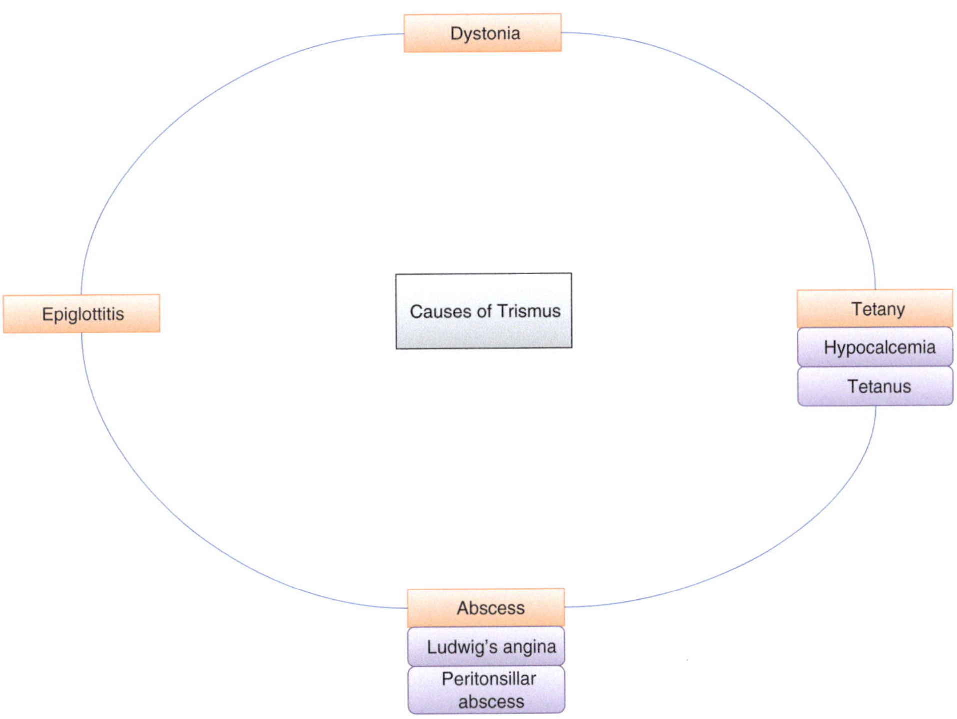

Ramsay Hunt Syndrome

Ramsay Hunt Syndrome = Reactivation of preexisting **Herpes Zoster** virus in the **Geniculate ganglion** of the Facial nerve

Geniculate ganglion = Facial movement + Touch to part of external ear and ear canal + Taste to anterior 2/3 of tongue

Symptoms & Signs

- Facial nerve paralysis
- Ear pain
- Loss of taste in anterior tongue
- Dry mouth
- Dry eyes
- Erythematous vesicular rash in ear canal, tongue &/or hard palate
- Hearing loss
- Tinnitus
- Vertigo

Treatment = Acyclovir OR Valacyclovir + Steroids

Cavernous Sinus Thrombosis

Vasculature Tidbit = Veins of face, oral cavity, middle ear & mastoid area drain to cavernous sinus

Cavernous Sinus Thrombosis = Blood clot within the cavernous sinus → Complication of a central facial infection → *Staph aureus* most common

Etiology = Nasal furuncle + Sphenoid or ethmoid sinus + Dental infection or extraction + Periorbital or orbital cellulitis

Symptoms & Signs

- Chemosis
- Ptosis
- Eyelid edema
- Facial edema
- Proptosis
- Fever
- Toxic appearance
- Pupillary dysfunction (mydriasis from III dysfunction)
- Cranial nerve dysfunction (III, IV, V, VI (most common))
- Impaired corneal reflex
- Papilledema
- Retinal hemorrhages
- Decreased visual acuity
- Headache

Diagnosis = CT or MRI

Treatment = IV antibiotics + Emergent ENT consultation

Triad

Head or neck infection + ophthalmoplegia + venous obstruction

Complications = Blindness + Oculomotor weakness + Hemiparesis + Pituitary insufficiency

Airway Foreign Body (AFB)

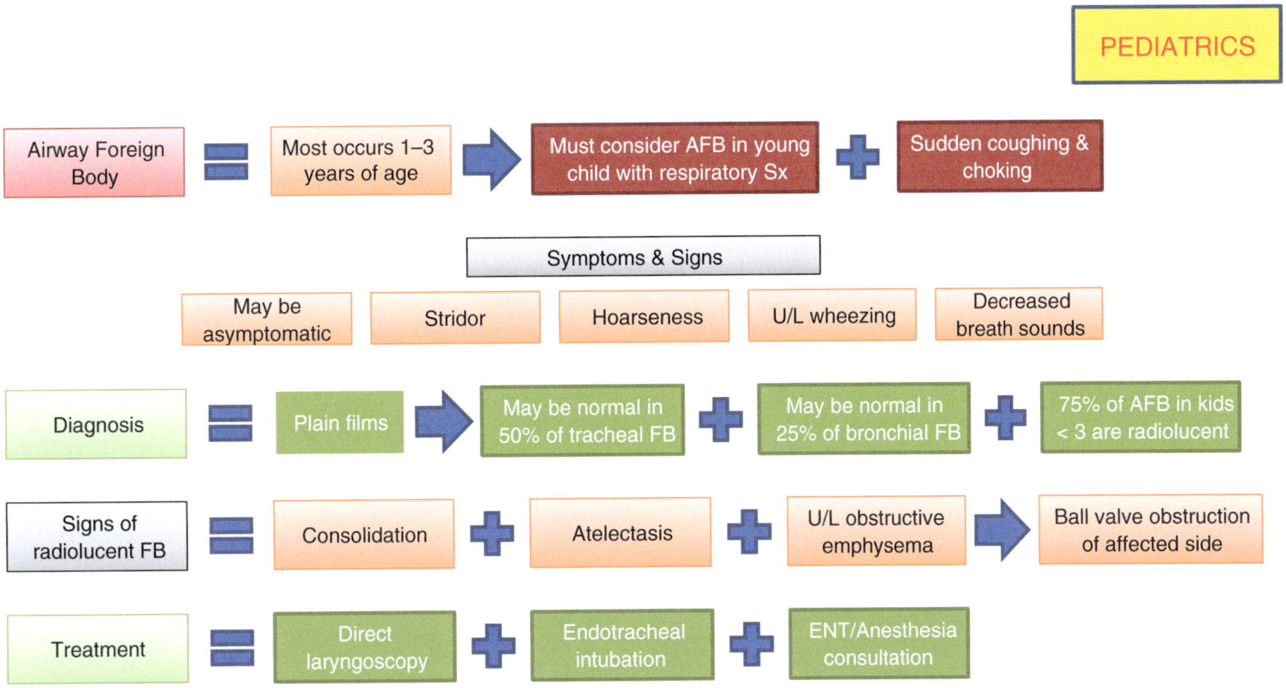

Vertigo

Introduction

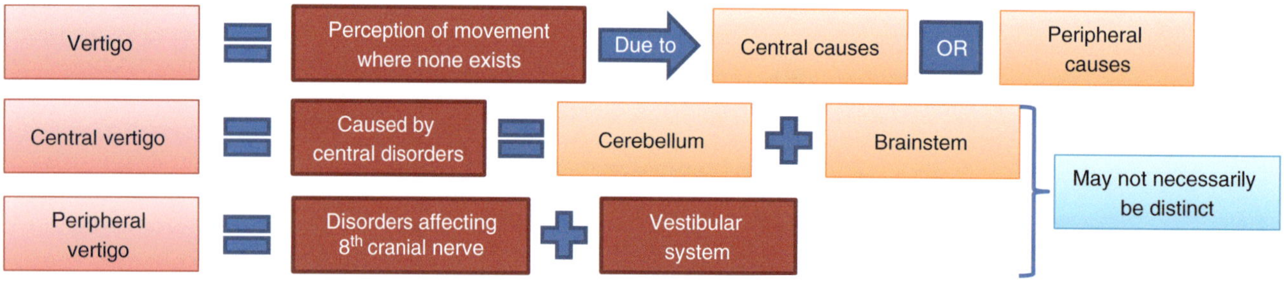

	Central	Peripheral
Onset	Slow	Sudden
Severity	Less intense	Severe spinning
Instances	Constant	Paroxysmal
Movement aggravated	No	Yes
Nausea	Infrequent	Frequent
Nystagmus	Vertical	Horizontal, rotatory-vertical
Fatiguability	No	Yes
Hearing loss	No	Possible
Tinnitus	No	Possible
TM	No	Possible
CNS Symptoms	Yes	No

Symptoms of Peripheral Vertigo

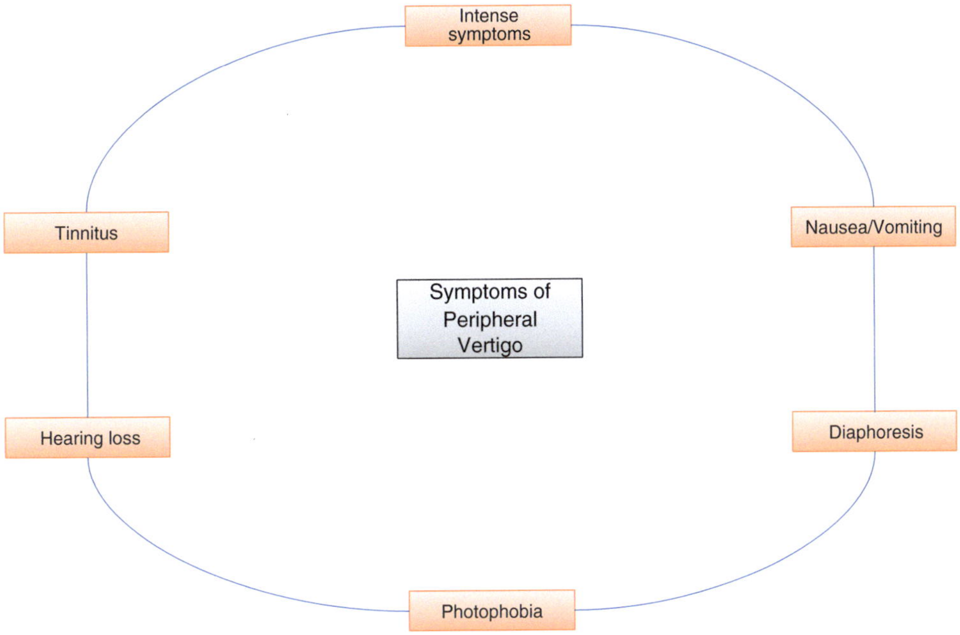

Symptoms of Central Vertigo

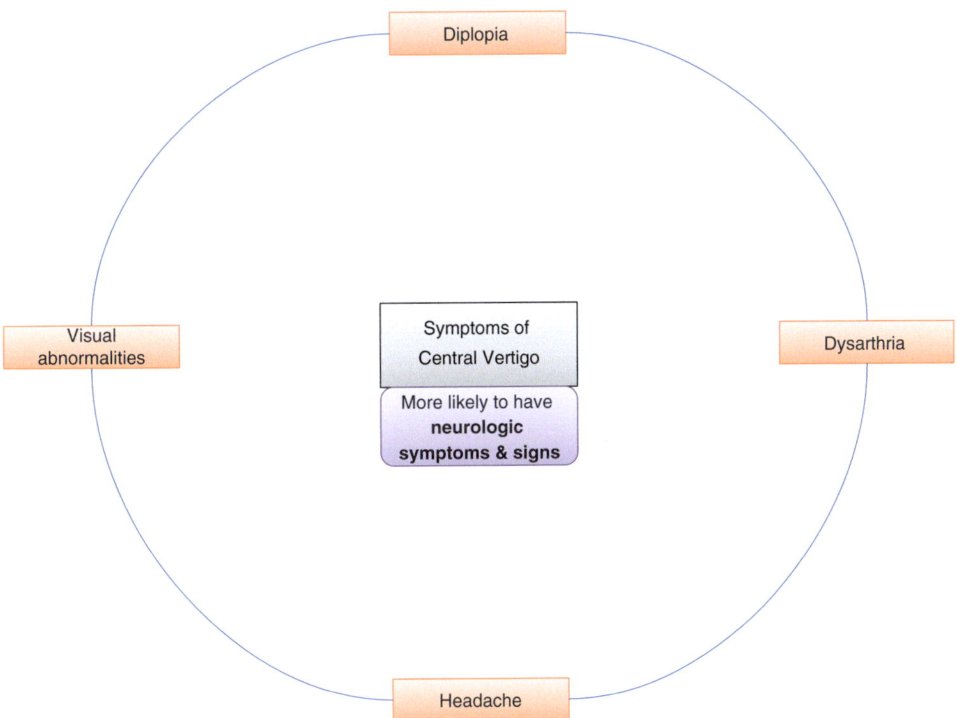

Peripheral Vertigo

Benign Paroxysmal Positional Vertigo (BPPV)

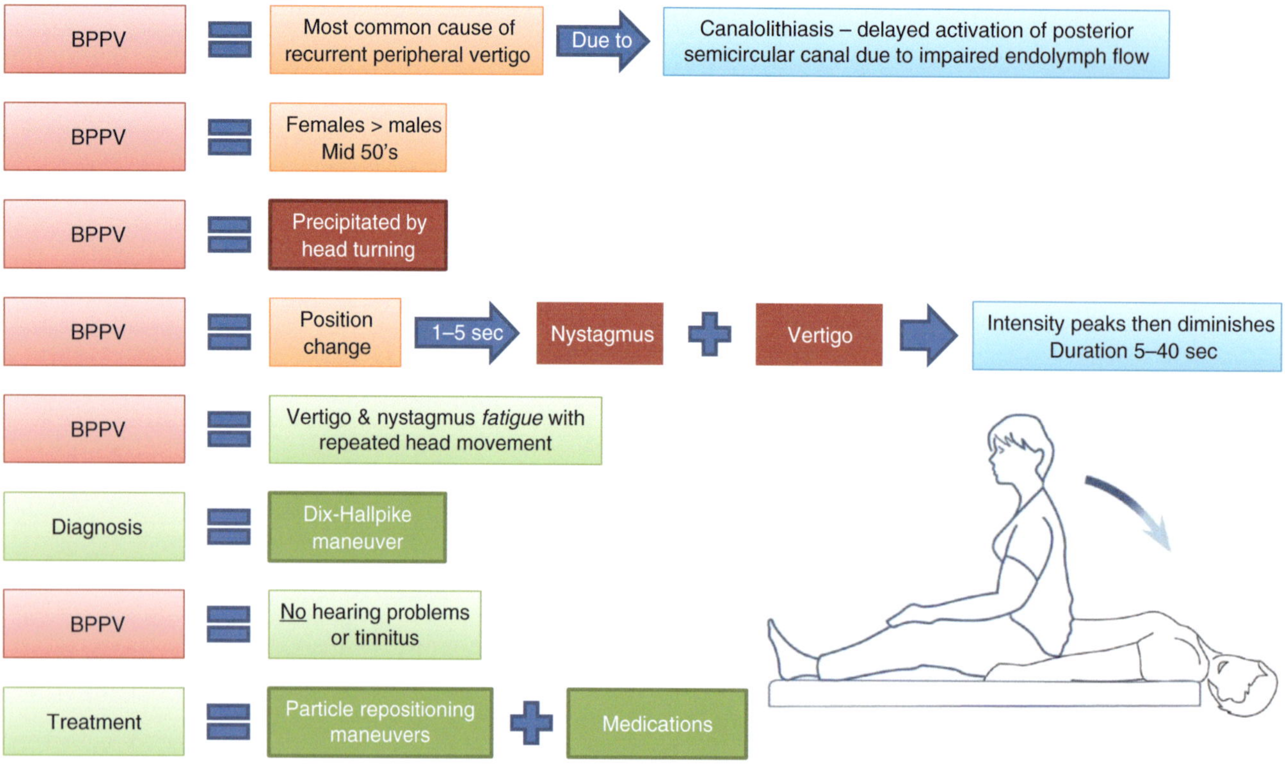

Bottom right image (Reprinted from Önerci TM. Vertigo. In: Önerci TM, editors. Diagnosis in otorhinolaryngology: an illustrated guide. Heidelberg: Springer Verlag; 2010. p. 54–6. With permission from Springer Verlag)

Meniere's Disease

Meniere's Disease = Increased endolymph within cochlea → Usually unilateral, may be bilateral → **Females = males** 1st attack usually > 65

Meniere's Disease = Sudden onset vertigo + N/V + Hearing loss + Roaring tinnitus + Unilateral ear fullness

Meniere's Disease = 20 min to 12 hours → Frequency of attacks vary from weekly to monthly

Treatment = Salt restricted diet + Medications

Vestibular Neuronitis

Vestibular Neuronitis = Acute onset → Probably viral in etiology → URI

Vestibular Neuronitis = Last several days + Does not recur

Vestibular Neuronitis = May lasts for days to weeks → Intense vertigo + Tinnitus + ± Unilateral hearing loss

Vestibular Neuronitis = Worse with change in position → Will have positional nystagmus

Vestibular Neuronitis = Patients may have unsteady gait

Treatment = Symptomatic

Perilymph Fistula

Perilymph Fistula = Opening in round window → Allows pneumatic changes to be transmitted to the vestibular system

Causes of round window pathology = Infection + Trauma + Pressure changes

Perilymph Fistula = Sudden onset of vertigo + Unilateral hearing loss

Diagnosis = Nystagmus with pneumatic otoscopy = Hennebert's sign

Treatment = Symptomatic + Bed rest

Labyrinthitis

Labyrinthitis = Infection of labyrinth → Viral in etiolgy → Associated with measles & mumps → Bacterial etiology as a sequelae of otitis media

Labyrinthitis = May be caused by ototoxic medications

Labyrinthitis = Sudden onset of vertigo + Hearing loss + Middle ear findings

Treatment = Symptomatic

Complications of bacterial labyrinthitis = Meningitis

Eighth Cranial Nerve Lesions

Eighth Cranial Nerve Lesions = Produce mild vertigo

Eighth Cranial Nerve Lesions = Acoustic schwannomas + Meningiomas

Eighth Cranial Nerve Lesions = Gradual onset of vertigo + Hearing loss precedes vertigo + Unsteady gait

Treatment = Referral to neurosurgeon

Cerebellopontine Angle Tumors

Cerebellopontine Angle Tumors = Deafness + Ipsilateral facial weakness + Ataxia + Corneal reflex deficit + Cerebellar signs

Cerebellopontine Angle Tumors = Acoustic neuromas + Meningiomas + Dermoids

Treatment = Referral to neurosurgeon

Posttraumatic Vertigo and Post-concussive Syndrome

Post Traumatic Vertigo = Direct injury to labyrinthine membrane → Immediate in onset → Associated with nauseas & vomiting

Pitfall = Failure to evaluate for temporal bone fracture

Closed head injury + Vertigo = CT/MRI → Exclude intracranial hematoma

Vertigo due to Labyrinthine trauma → Usually resolves in weeks

Post concussive syndrome = Dizziness + Gait unsteadiness + N/V

Treatment of Post Concussive = Symptomatic

Central Vertigo

Cerebellar Infarction and Hemorrhage

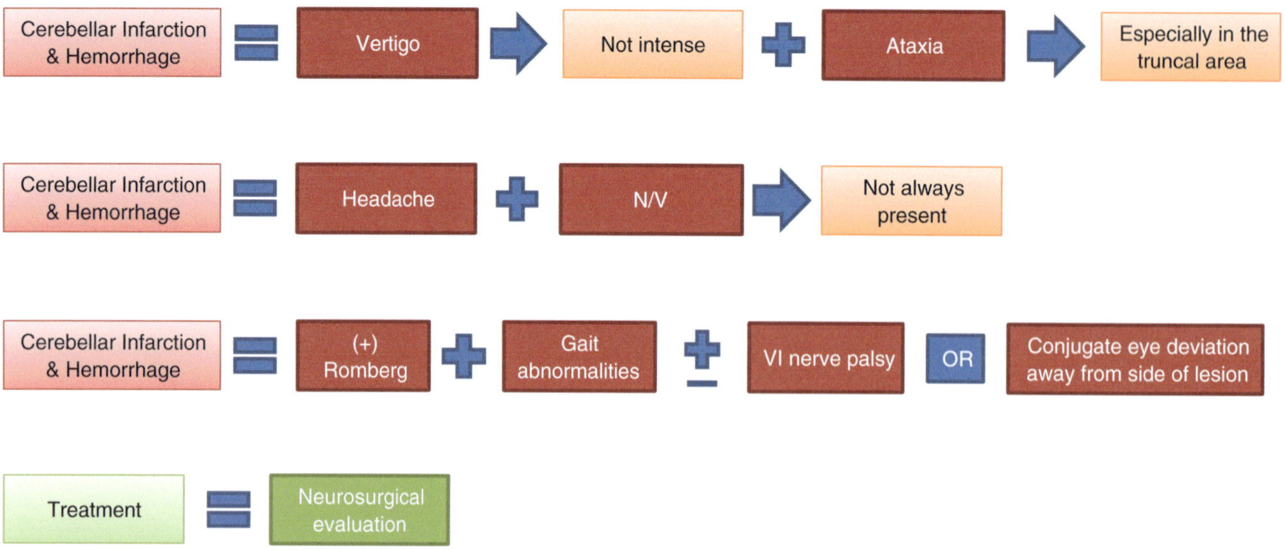

Wallenberg Syndrome

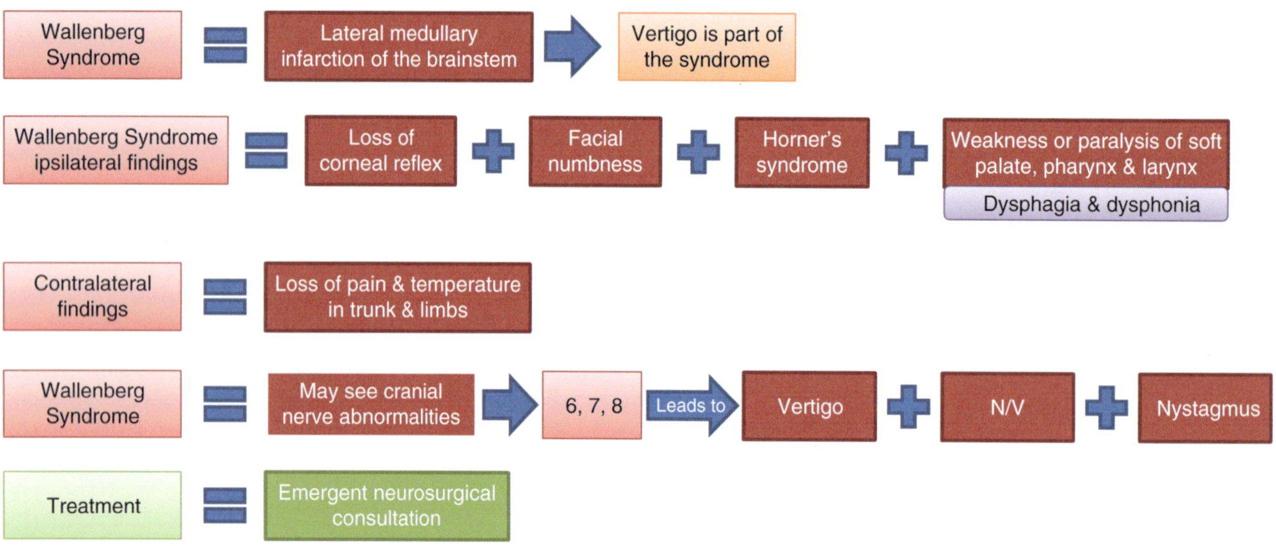

Vertebrobasilar Insufficiency

Vertebrobasilar Insufficiency = TIA of the brainstem → May cause vertigo → Usually resolve within 24 hours

Other symptoms = Bilateral blindness + Diplopia + Dysarthria + Dysphagia + Bilateral long tract signs

Vertebrobasilar Insufficiency = May be provoked by position → Turning head occludes vertebral artery

Treatment = Neurology consultation

Vertebral Artery Dissection

Vertebral Artery Dissection = Stroke involving posterior circulation → Caused by sudden rotation or extension of neck → Trauma, diving injury

Symptoms = Vertigo + Headache + Unilateral Horner's syndrome

Diagnosis = CT/MRI

Multiple Sclerosis

Multiple sclerosis = Due to demyelination → May lasts for hours to weeks → Does not usually recur

Multiple sclerosis = Vertigo is not intense + Prominent nystagmus

Multiple sclerosis = Ataxia may be present + Optic neuritis may be present

Diagnosis = MRI

Treatment = Neurology consultation + Consider steroids

Migraine-Related Vertigo

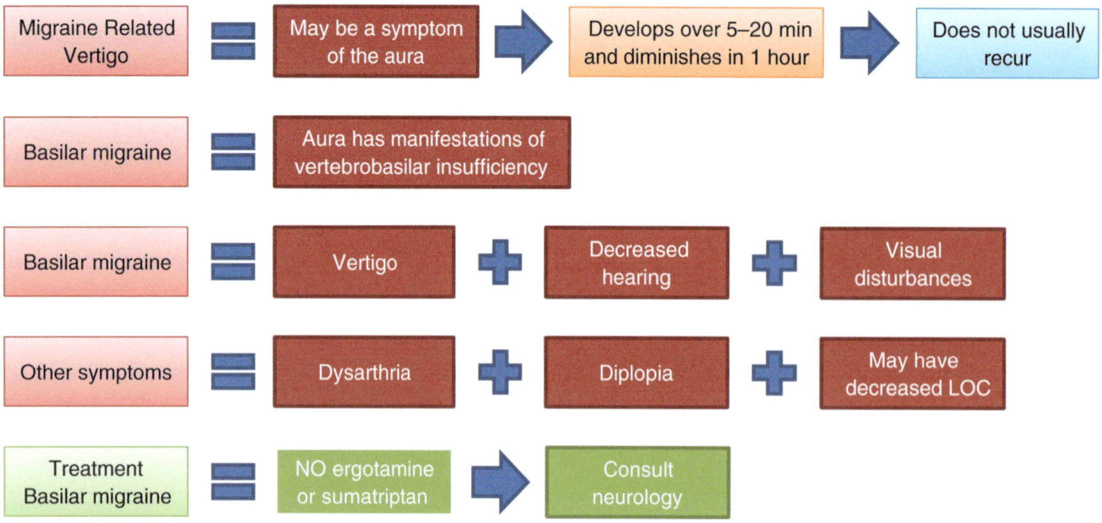

Environmental Emergencies

Michael R. Marchick and Bobby Desai

Contents

Bites and Envenomations 518
Dysbarism 526
Electrical Injuries 531
High-Altitude Illness 535
Submersion 538
Temperature-Related Illness 540
Radiation 548
Biological Weapons 548
Chemical Weapons 552
Tetanus 554

M.R. Marchick, MD
Department of Emergency Medicine,
University of Florida College of Medicine, Gainesville, FL, USA

B. Desai, MD, MEd (✉)
Department of Emergency Medicine, University of Florida,
Gainesville, FL, USA
e-mail: bdesai@ufl.edu

B. Desai, B.R. Allen (eds.), *Nailing the Written Emergency Medicine Board Examination*,
DOI 10.1007/978-3-319-30838-8_9

Bites and Envenomations

Bees/Wasps

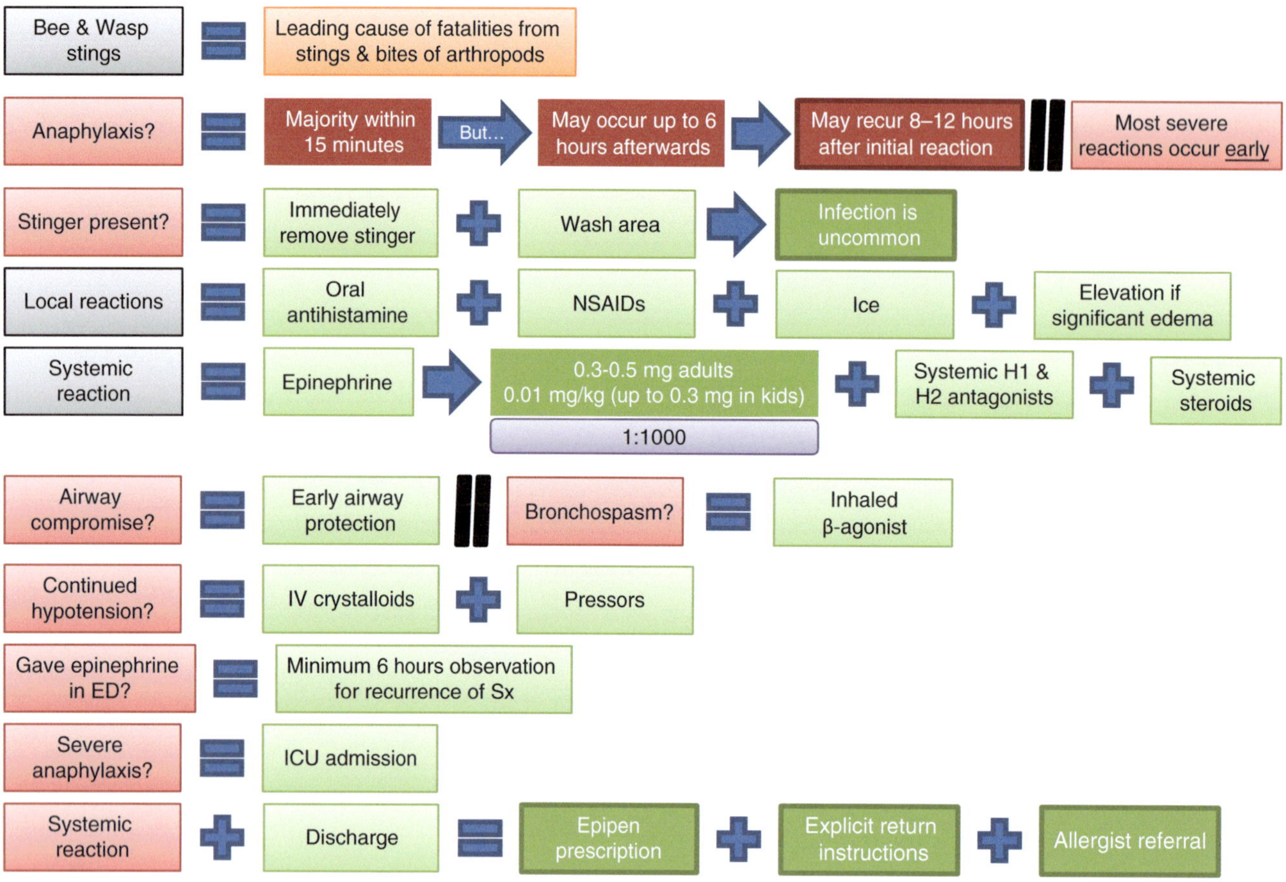

Black Widow Envenomation

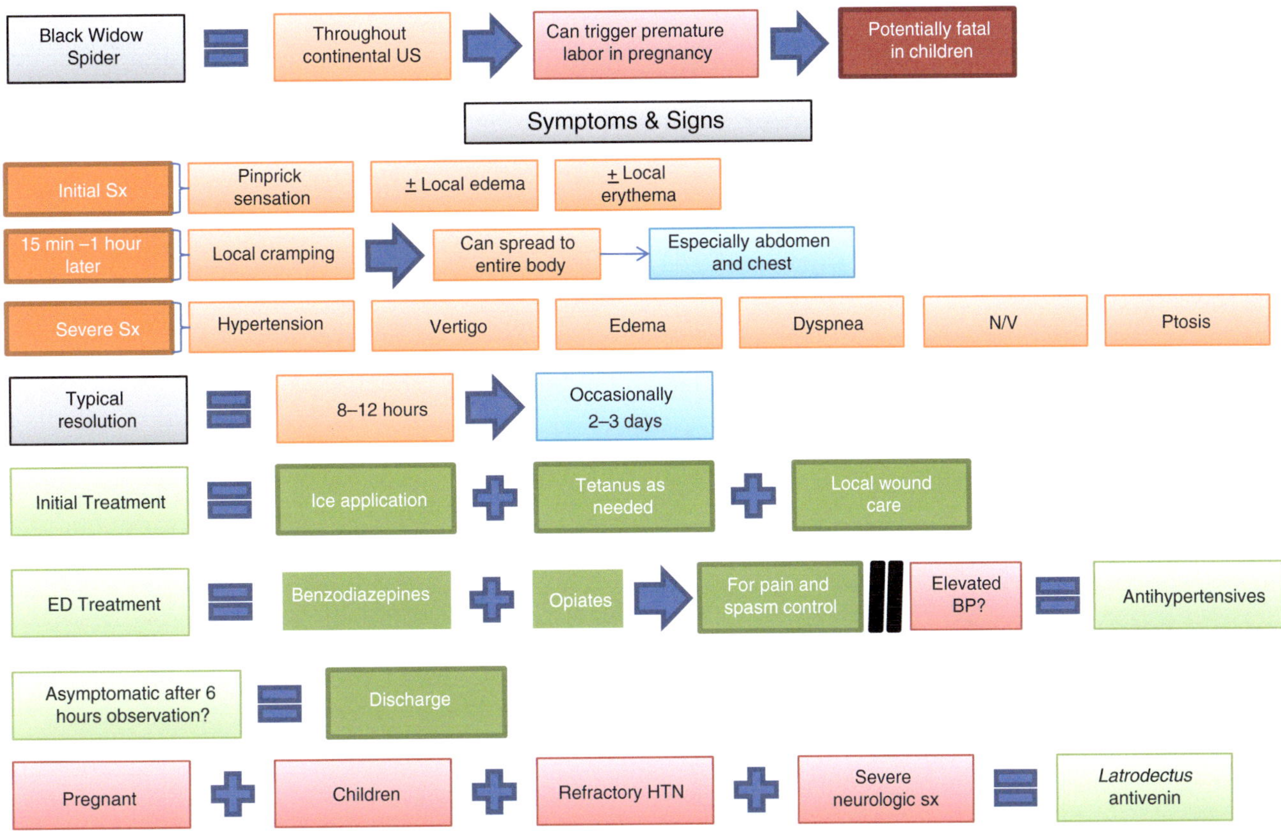

Brown Recluse Envenomation

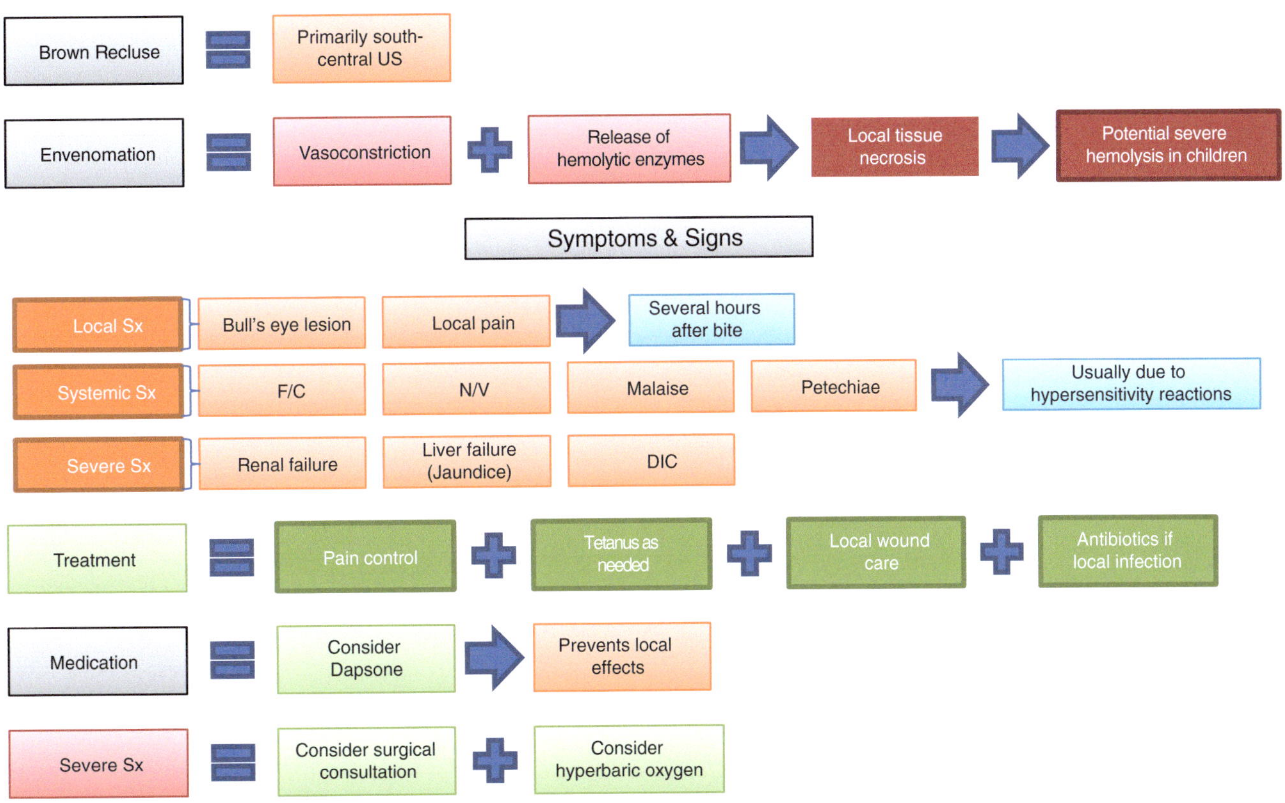

Mammalian Bites

Bites: Introduction

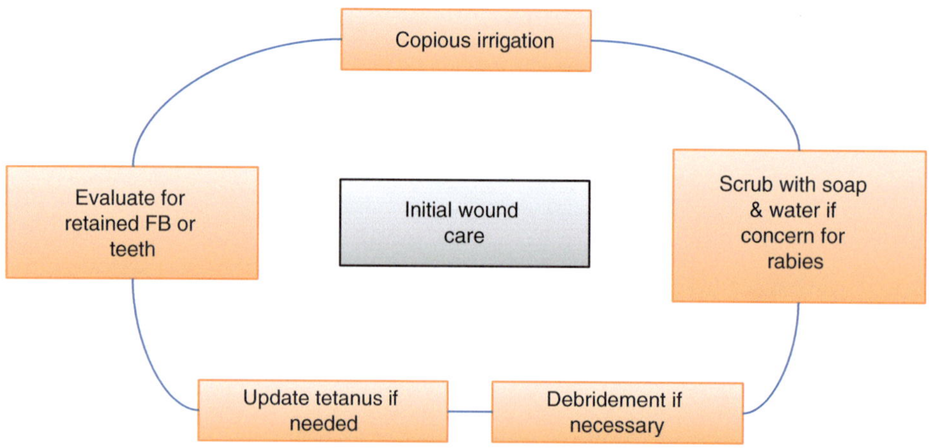

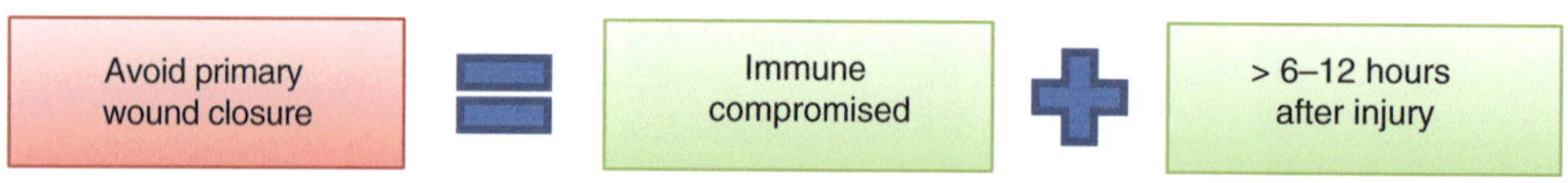

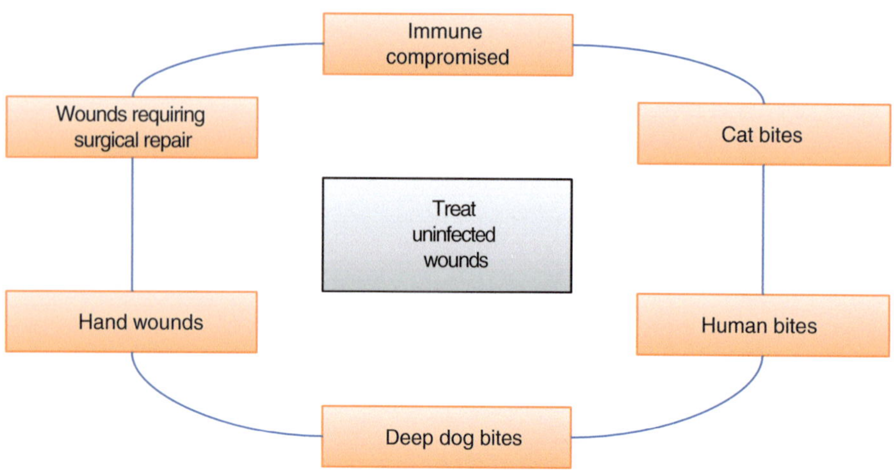

Rabies

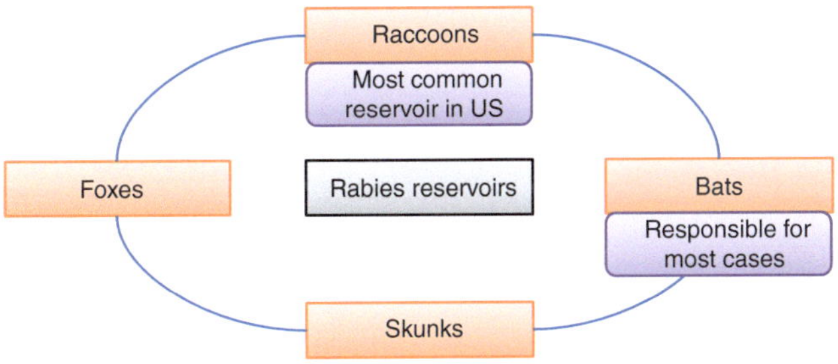

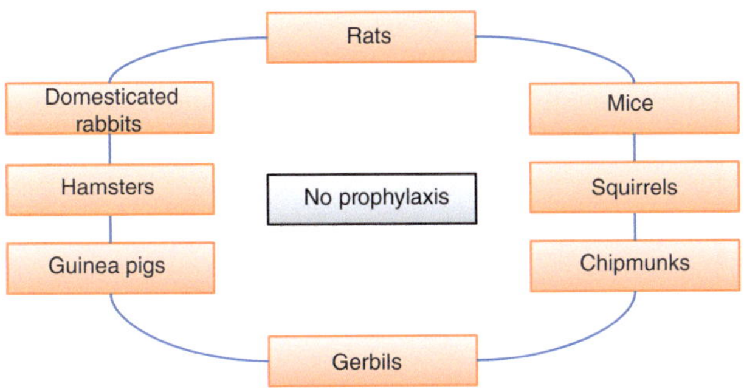

Rabies Vaccination

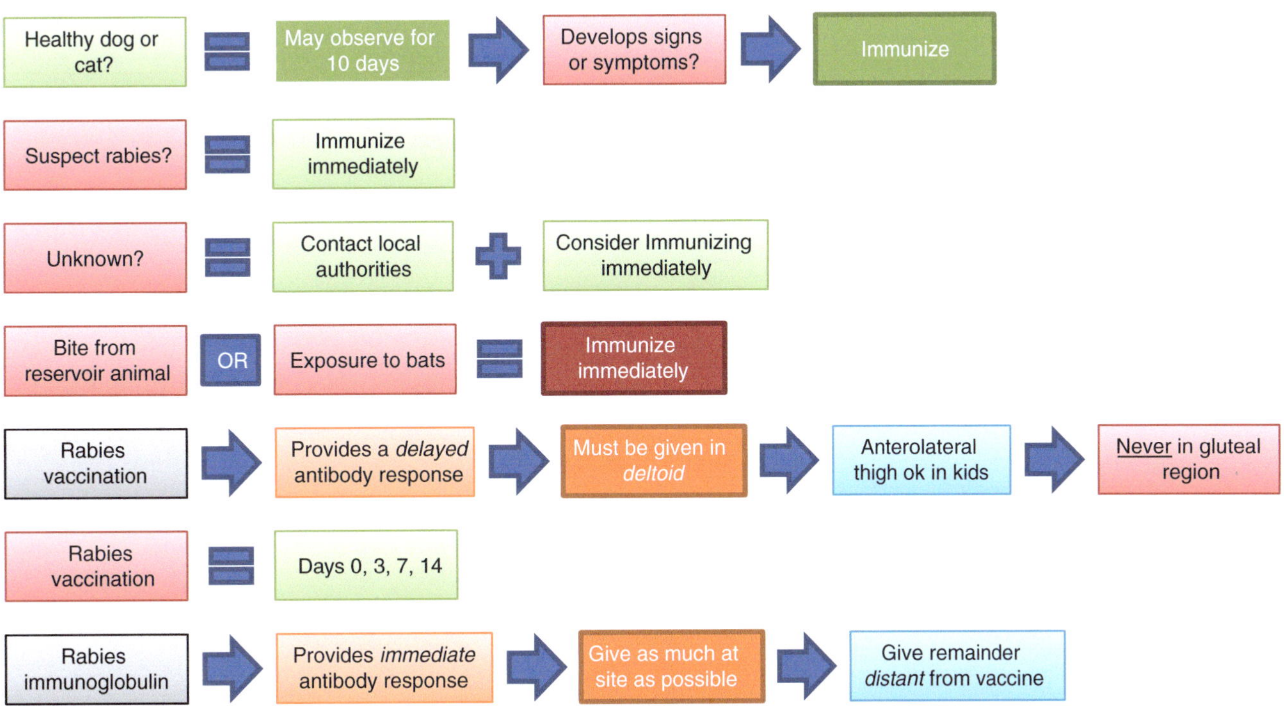

Rabies

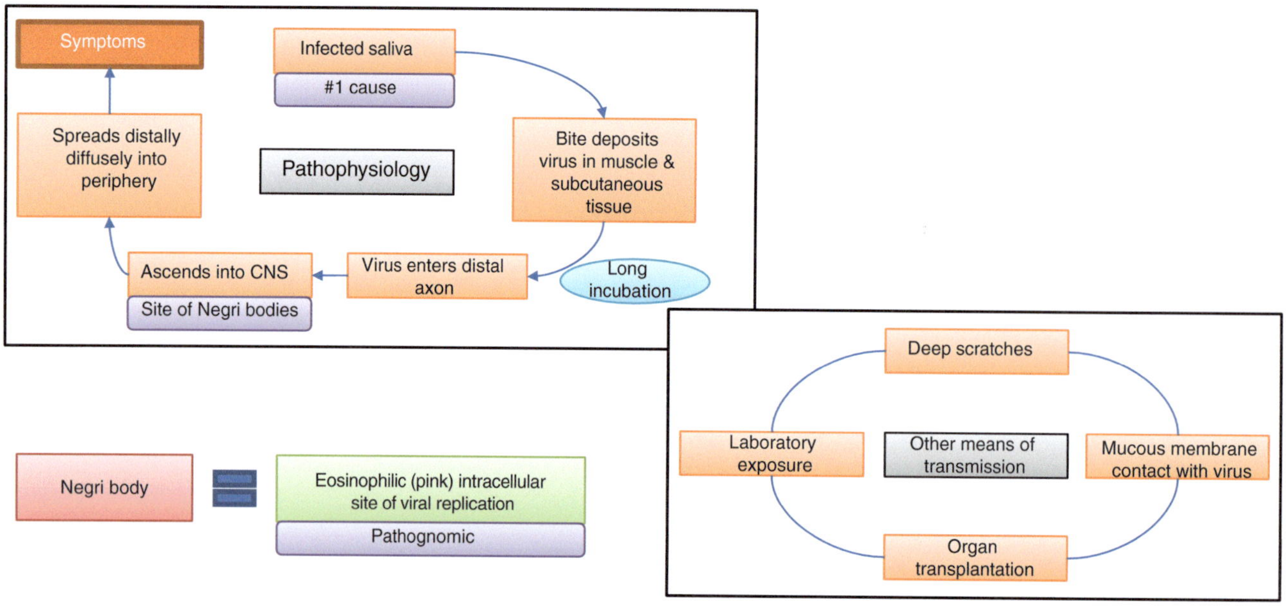

Rabies Symptoms and Signs

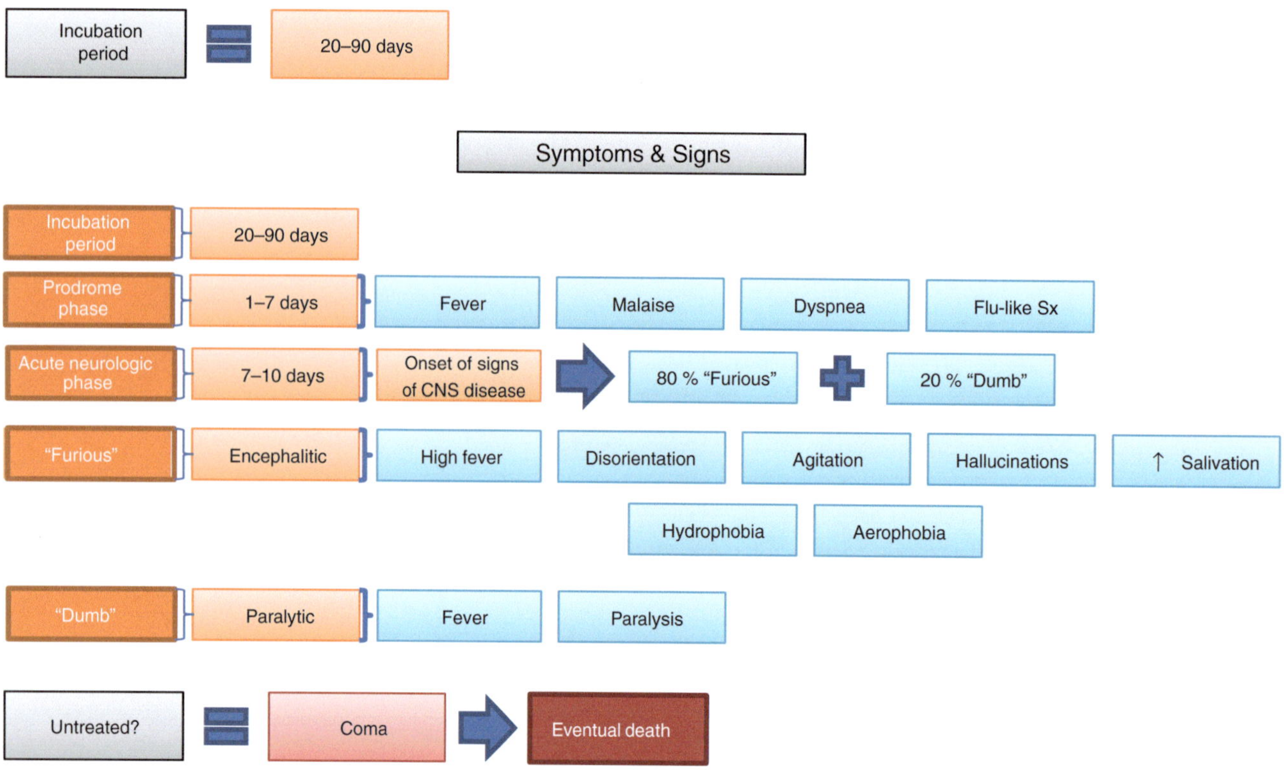

Cat Bites and Scratches

Cat Bites → Cats have sharp, narrow teeth = Deeper inoculation → Including bones, tendon sheaths → High risk of infection

Primary closure? = Avoid

Organism = *Pasteurella multocida* → Fairly rapid onset of action → Treatment = Amoxicillin-clavunate 1st line

---

Cat scratch disease = *Bartonella henselae* → 1–2 week incubation

Cat scratch disease = Region of painful, matted lymph nodes ± Flu–like symptoms → Rare severe multi-system involvement → Generally self-limited

Severe case? = Azithromycin

Pitfall = Do not I &D lesions → May cause scarring/fistulae

Dog Bites

Most common organisms = *Pasteurella* + *Streptococcus* + *Staphylococcus* + Anaerobes

Capnocytophaga canimorsus = Encapsulated bacterium

Capnocytophaga canimorsus + Immune compromised pt (Alcoholics; Post-splenectomy; Immunosuppressant) → May lead to → Sepsis; DIC; Renal failure; Death

Capnocytophaga canimorsus = Rarely after cat bites

Risk of infection increases = Hand bites + Immune compromised → Give prophylactic Abx → Amoxicillin-clavunate 1st line

Not at risk for *Capnocytophaga?* = Keflex OR TMP-SMX

Marine Envenomation

Jellyfish Stings

Jellyfish Stings = Wash area with sea water → Fresh water may cause discharge of nematocysts → Increases pain

Symptoms & Signs

Erythema | Local pain | Urticaria

Stinger or tentacles identified? = Remove tentacles with forceps

ED treatment = Wash with vinegar OR Isopropyl alcohol → Application of hot water (45°C) also effective + Update tetanus as needed

Indo-Pacific box jellyfish envenomation = Often rapidly fatal

Stingray Stings

Stingray stings = Barbed wire apparatus → Causes laceration → Followed by envenomation

Symptoms & Signs

Local injury | Local pain | Nausea | Flushing | Sweats | Diarrhea | Muscle cramps

ED treatment = Hot water → Deactivates the toxin

Snake Bites

Snake Envenomation

Pit Vipers = Rattlesnakes + Water moccasins + Copperheads

Pit Vipers = Spade-shaped head + Elliptical eyes + Presence of pit between eye and nostrils + Double row of caudal plates

Non-venomous Snakes = Rounded head + Rounded eyes + Single row of caudal plates

Elapids = Eastern coral snake (SE US) + Sonoran Coral Snake (AZ, NM) → Much less dangerous than eastern variety

Coral Snake = Red on yellow, kill a fellow ‖ King Snake = Red on black, venom lack

Pit Viper Envenomation

Envenomation = Snake bite + Tissue Injury || Dry Bite = If no evidence of tissue injury after ≥ 8 hours → Up to 25 % of bites

Symptoms & Signs

- Local: Pain, Edema, Ecchymosis → Worsening symptoms
- Systemic: AMS, Hypotension, Tachycardia, Paresthesias → Any Sx
- Coagulopathy: ↓ Platelets, ↓ Fibrinogen, ↑ INR → Abnormal?

Worsening symptoms / Any Sx / Abnormal? → Treat with antivenom

Initial Treatment = Immobilize limb in neutral position → May use constriction band → Tourniquet use contraindicated, as is suction/incision

ED Treatment = Serial measurements of limb circumference above & below bite → Mark progression of erythema/ edema every 30 min → Monitor for compartment syndrome

Laboratory investigations = Periodic measurement of **Coags, Fibrinogen, CBC**

Antivenom = Initial dose 4–6 vials IV → Give additional if local control not achieved + Additional 2 vials 6,12,18 hours after local control achieved

Antivenom for children = Same as adult dose

Active bleeding? = Consider blood products in addition to antivenom → Antivenom most effective treatment for coagulopathy

Eastern Coral Snake Envenomation

Eastern Coral Snake Envenomation = Neurotoxic venom → Little tissue injury → Can lead to respiratory failure

Definite bite? = 3–5 vials of antivenom IV → May be difficult to locate

Antivenom unavailable? = Supportive care → May need airway protection → ICU admission

Antivenom for children = Same as adult dose

Sonoran Coral Snake = Milder symptoms → Antivenom not usually needed

Dysbarism

Introduction

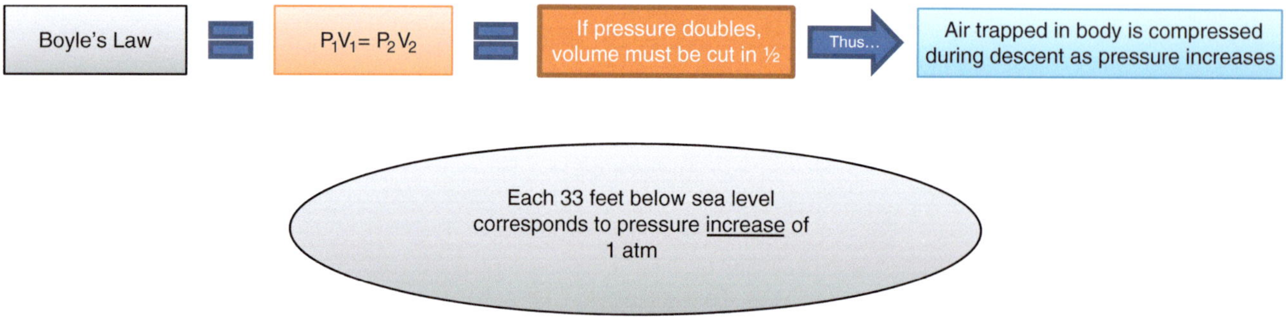

Barotrauma of Descent: Barotitis Media

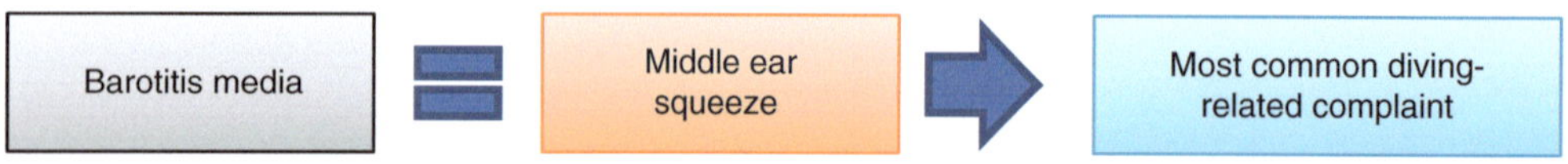

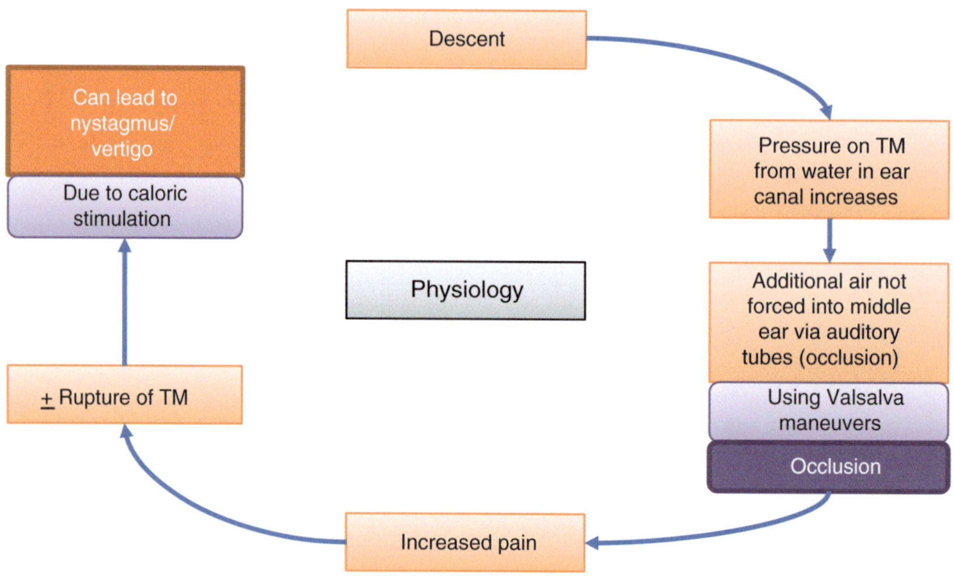

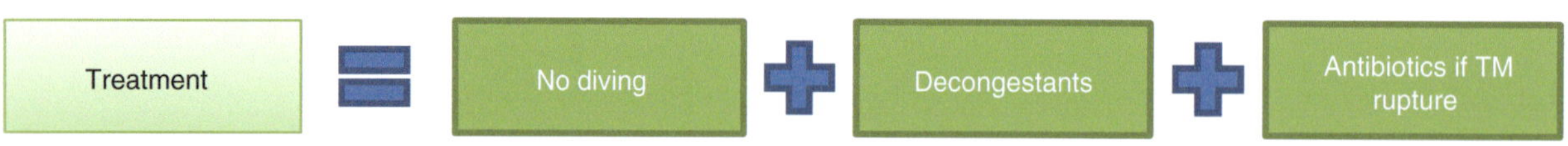

Barotrauma of Descent: Barotitis Interna

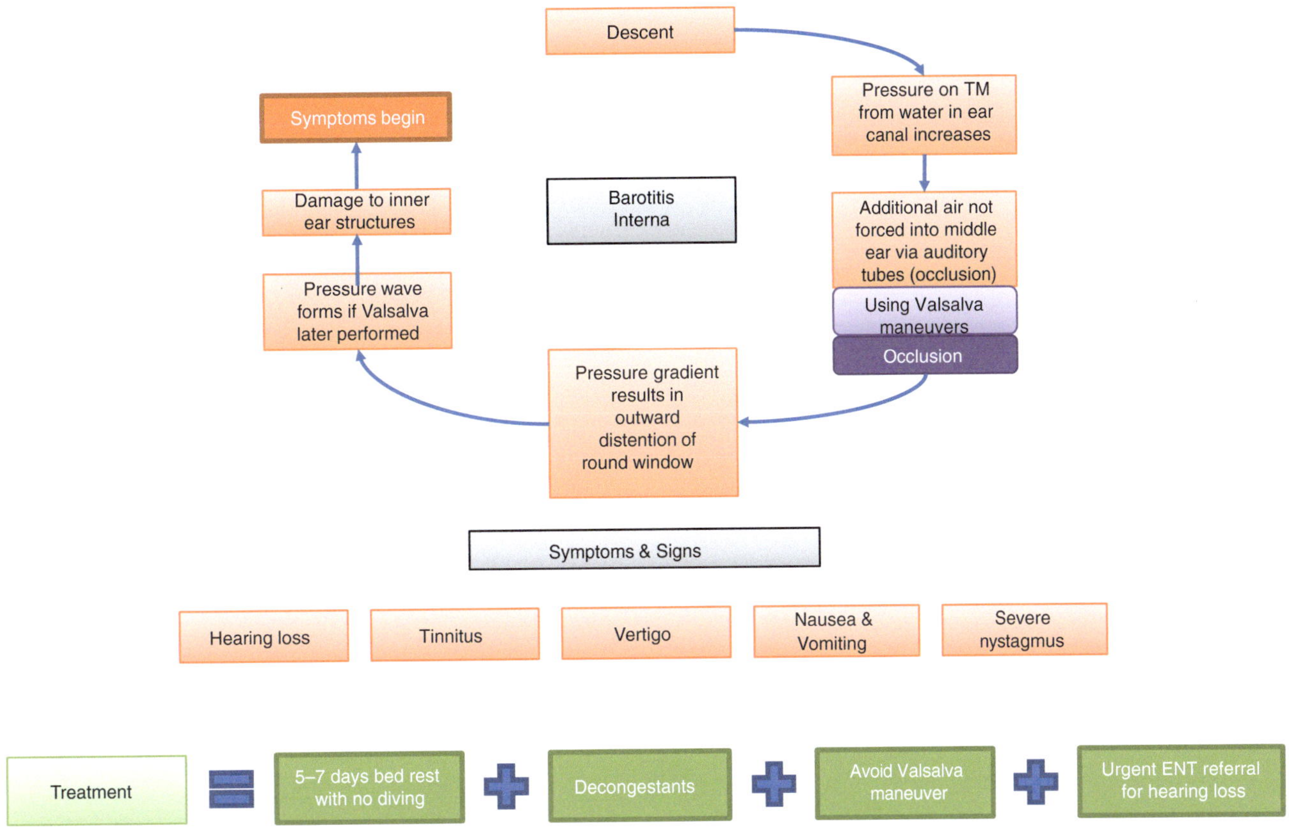

Barotrauma of Descent: Barotitis Externa

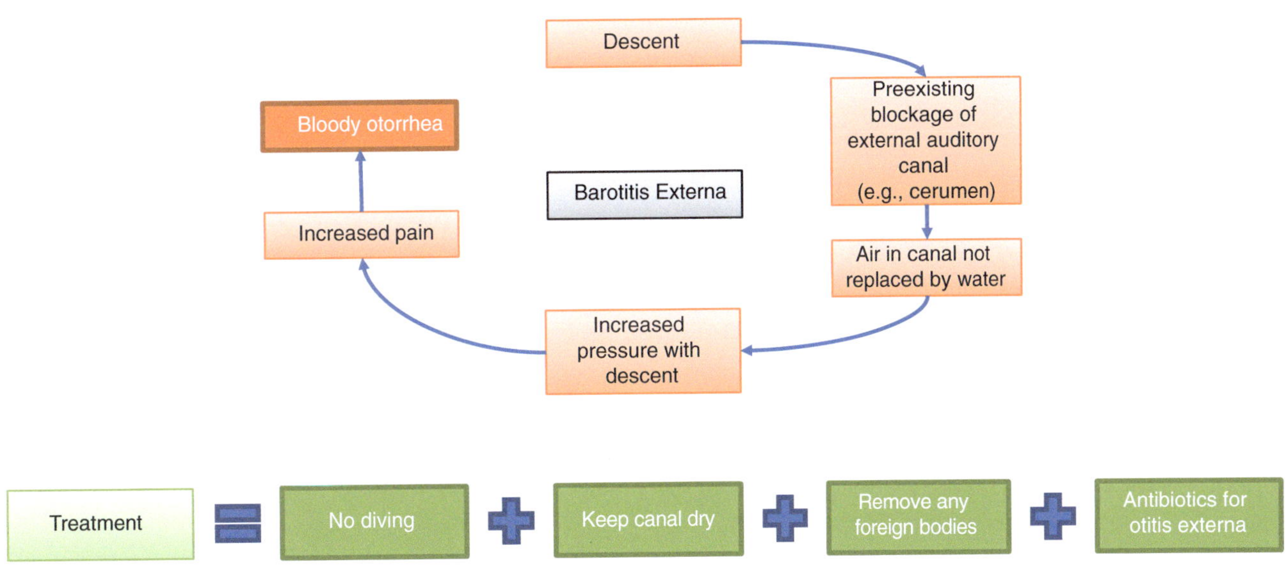

Sinus Barotrauma

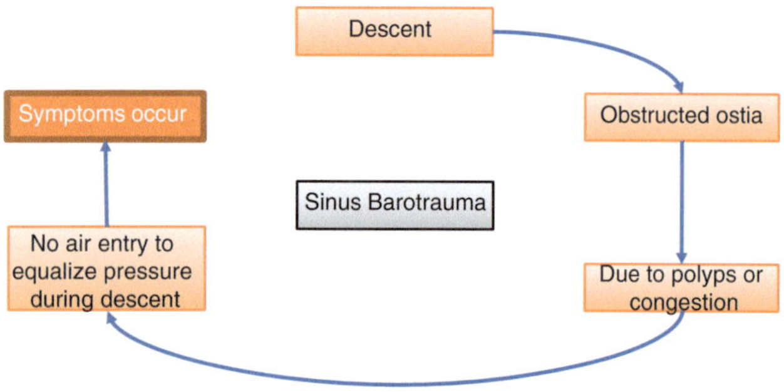

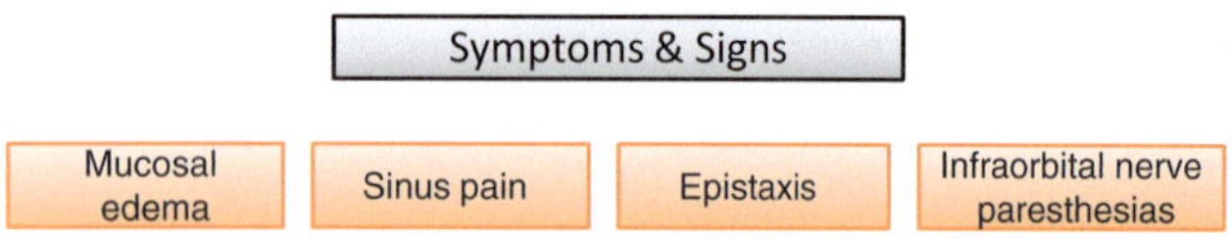

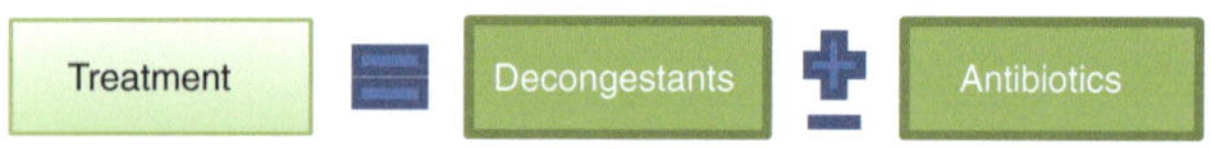

Barotrauma of Ascent

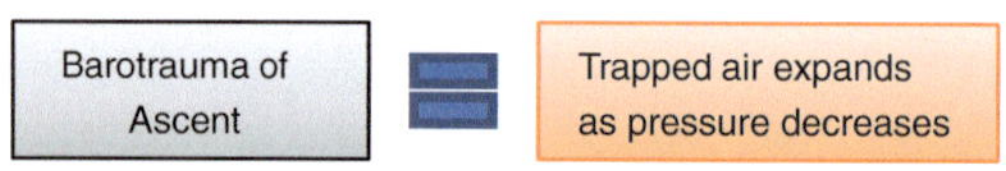

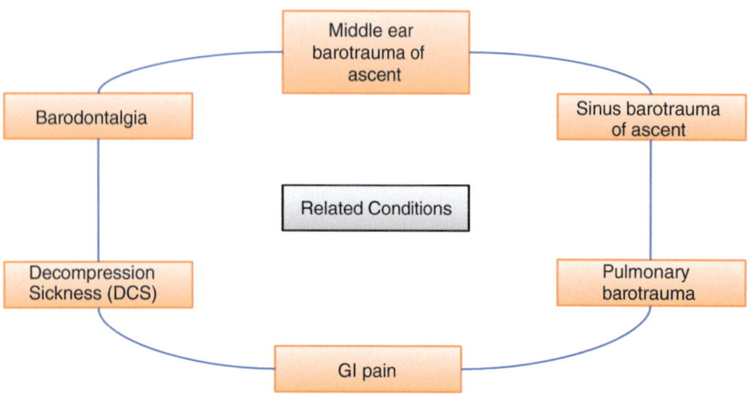

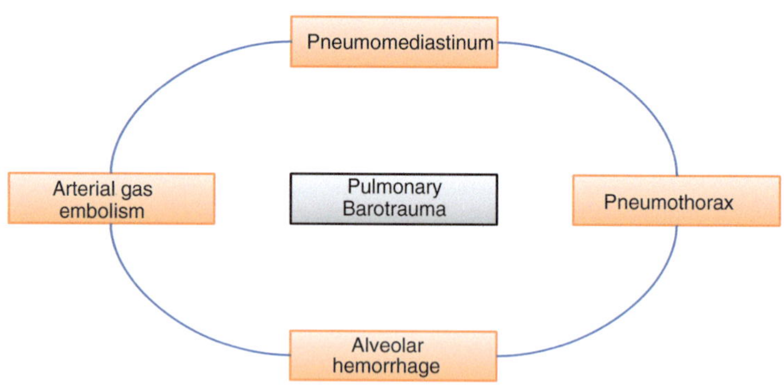

Pulmonary Barotrauma

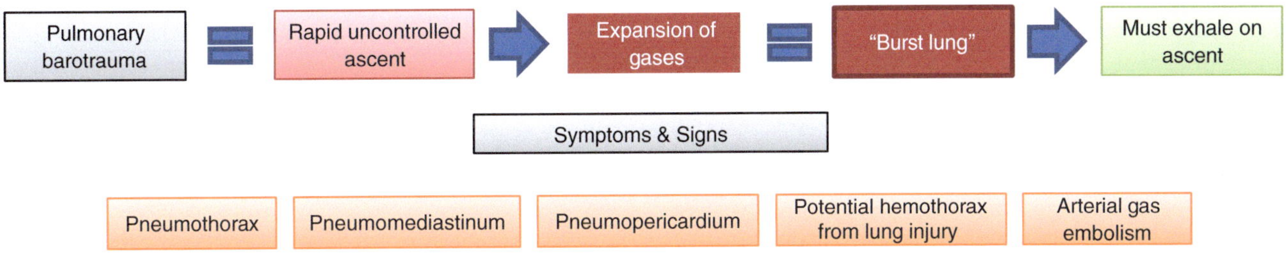

Arterial Gas Embolism

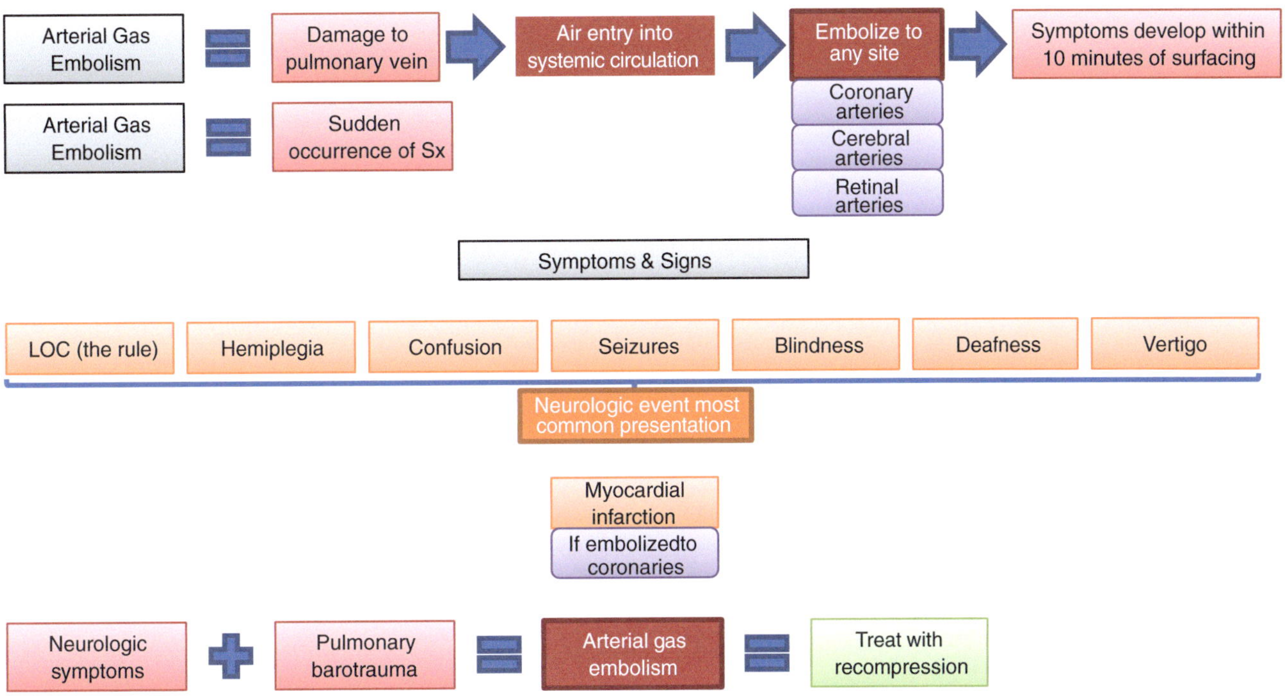

Nitrogen Narcosis

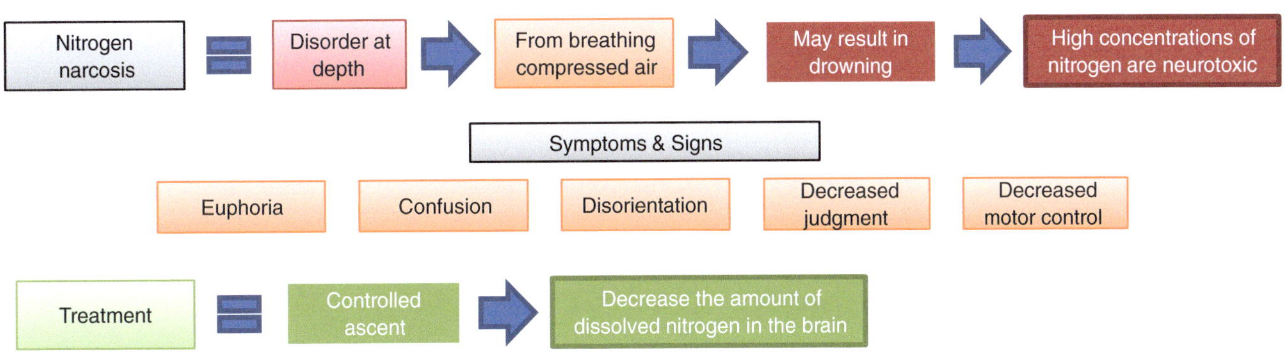

Decompression Sickness

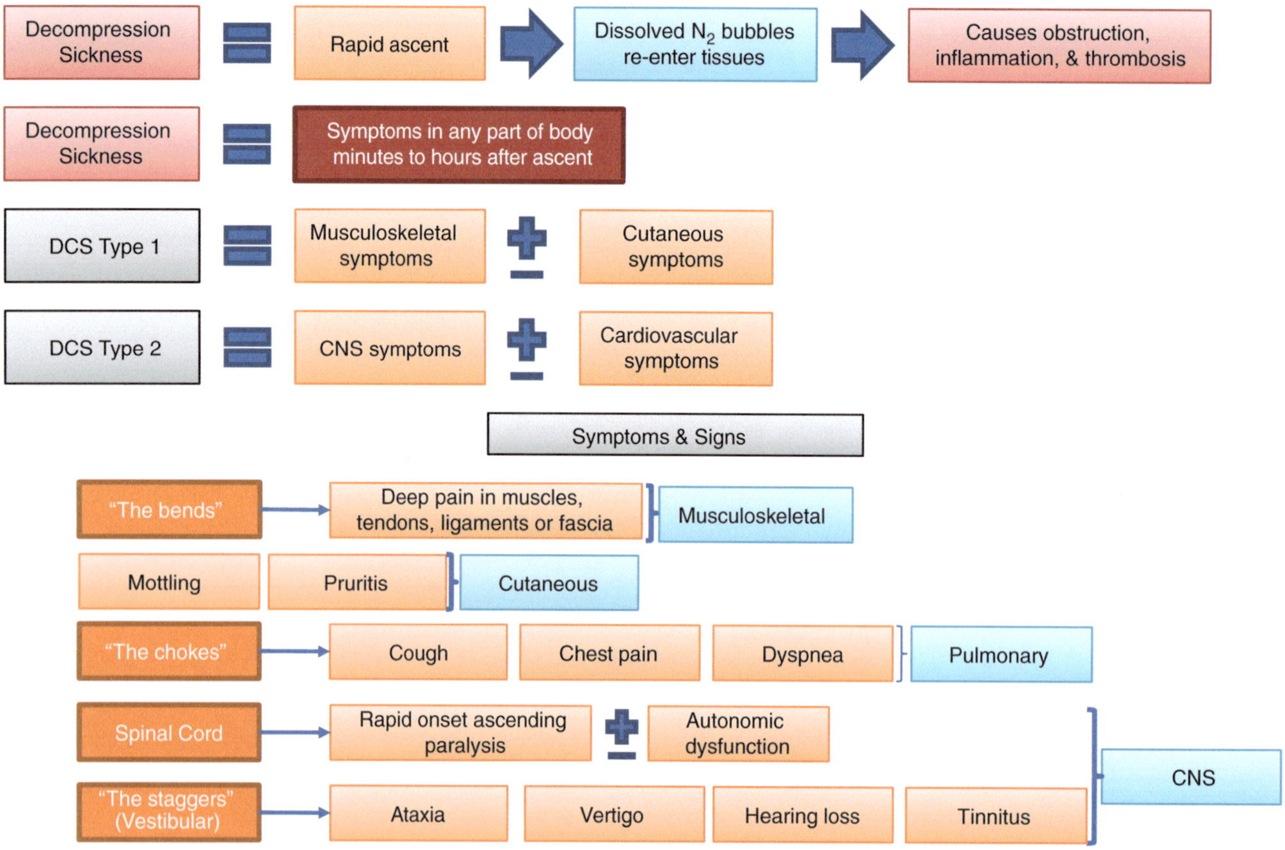

Barotrauma of Ascent Treatment

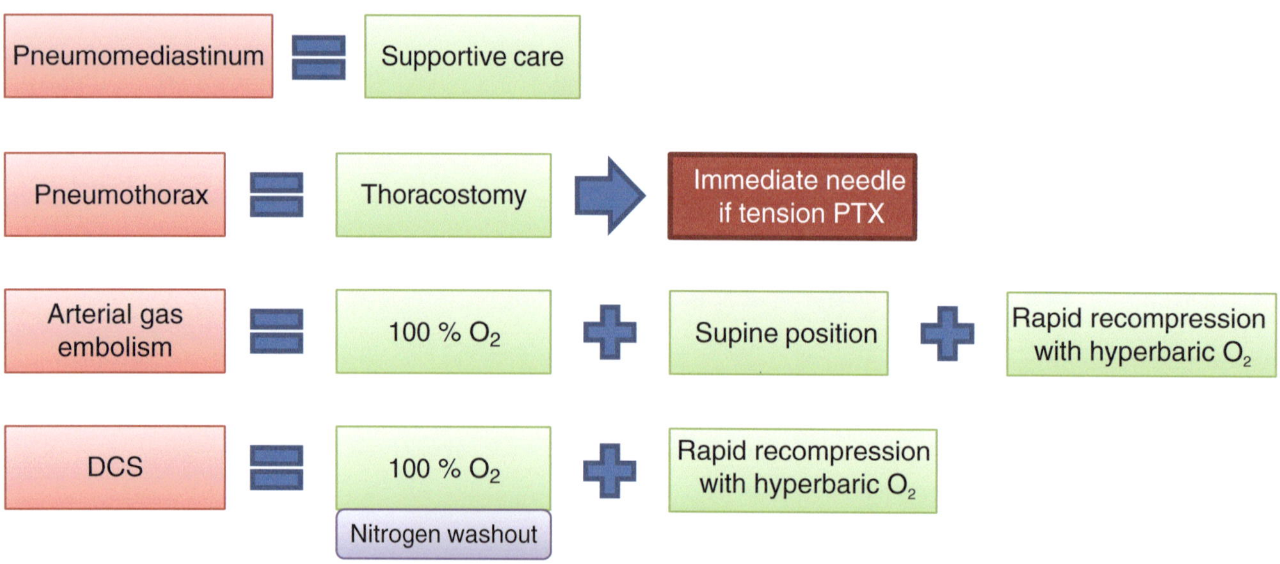

Recompression Therapy

Recompression Therapy = Definitive treatment → For → Decompression sickness + Arterial gas embolism

Pitfalls = Not having a low threshold for treatment → Due to → Subtle symptoms may develop after treatment of major symptoms + Minor symptoms may progress

Time frame for recompression? = Up to 14 days after symptom onset

Electrical Injuries

Introduction

Electrical Injuries → High voltage = ≥ 1000 Volts (Burns are severe; Significant injury & death) ‖ Low voltage = <1000 Volts (Burns are minor; More common)

Electrical Arc Burns = No passage of current through tissues → *Thermal burn ± blast injury may still occur*

Higher voltage + Longer contact time = Worsened injury = Increased trauma = Resembles **crush injury**

Alternating Current = Household electricity, power lines → Associated with *V. fib* → Can produce tetany (Victim may ***not*** be able to let go of source) → Worsened effects at a given voltage compared with DC

Direct Current = Batteries & lightning → Associated with *asystole*

Injuries? = Depend on current & tissue resistance → Increase injury with increased resistance

Pitfall = Skin & neurovascular exam may underestimate injury with deep electrical burns

Electrical Injuries

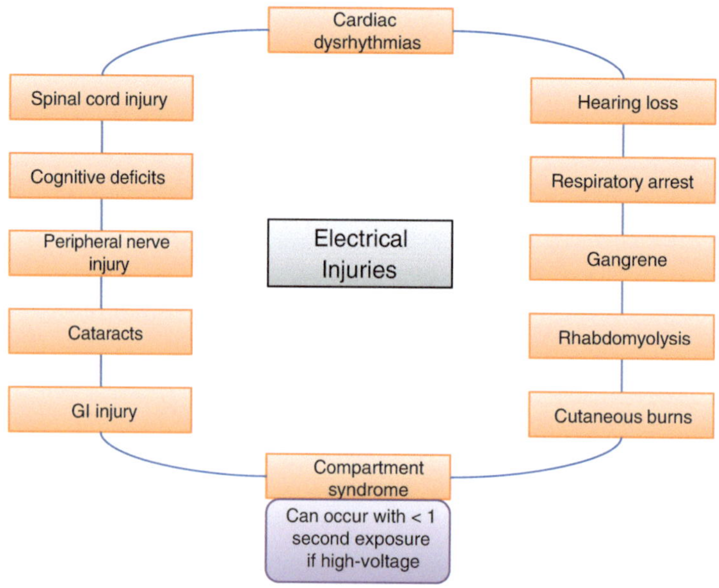

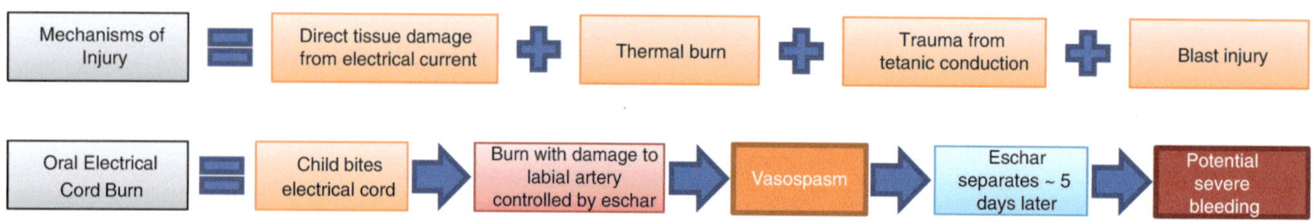

Electrical Injury Management

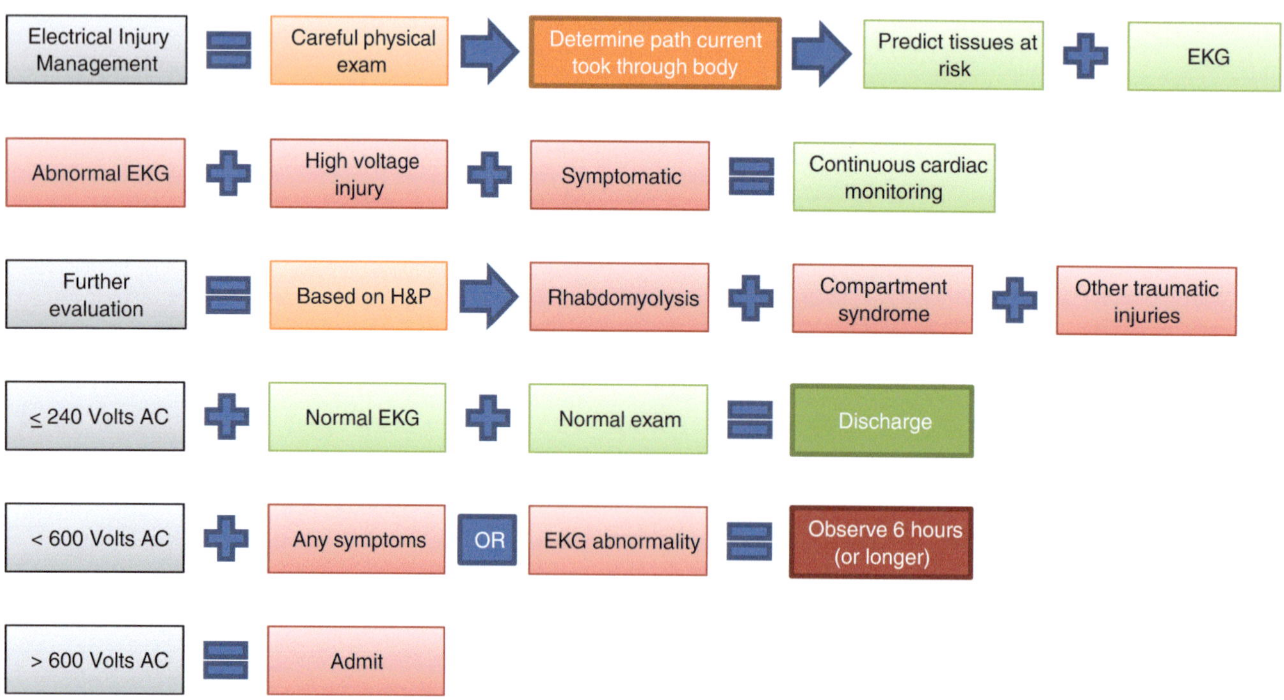

Lightning Injury

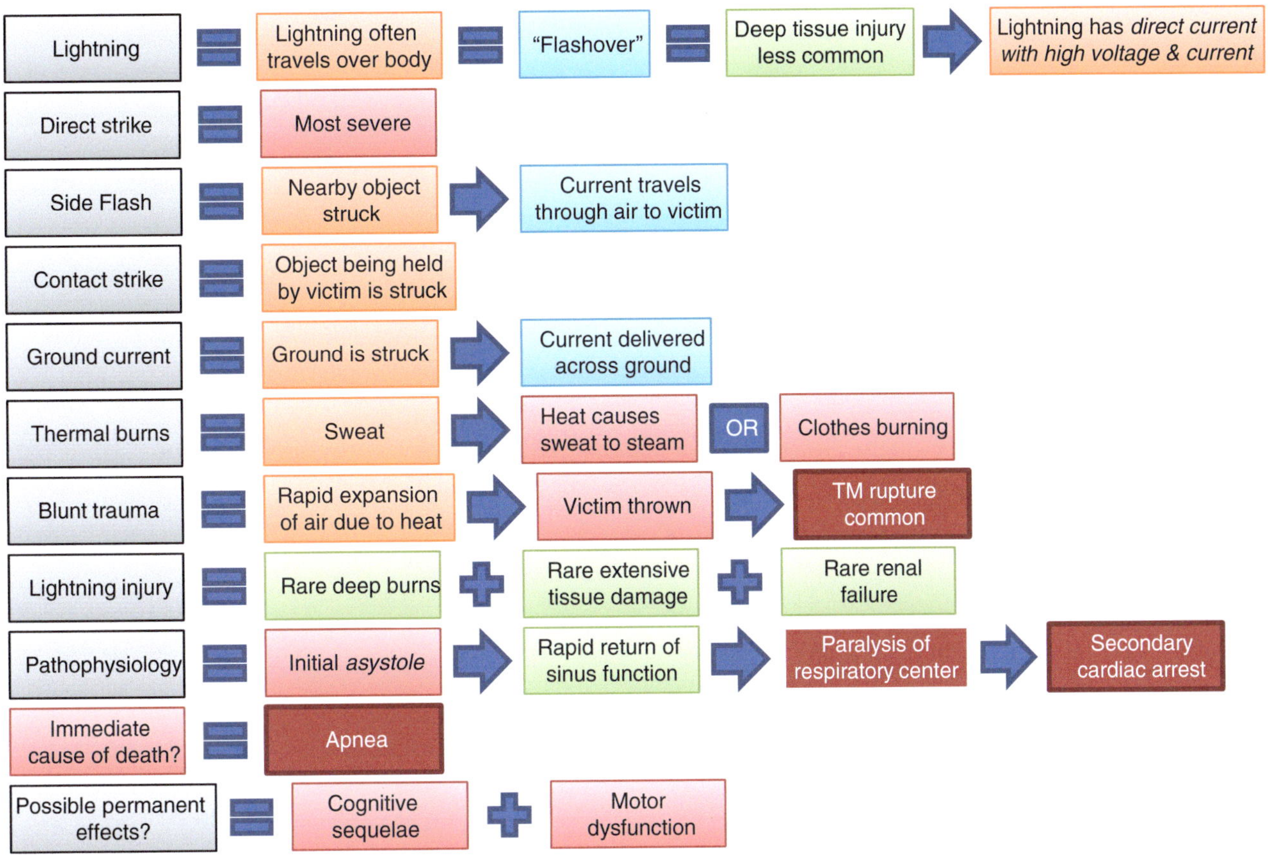

Lightning Injuries

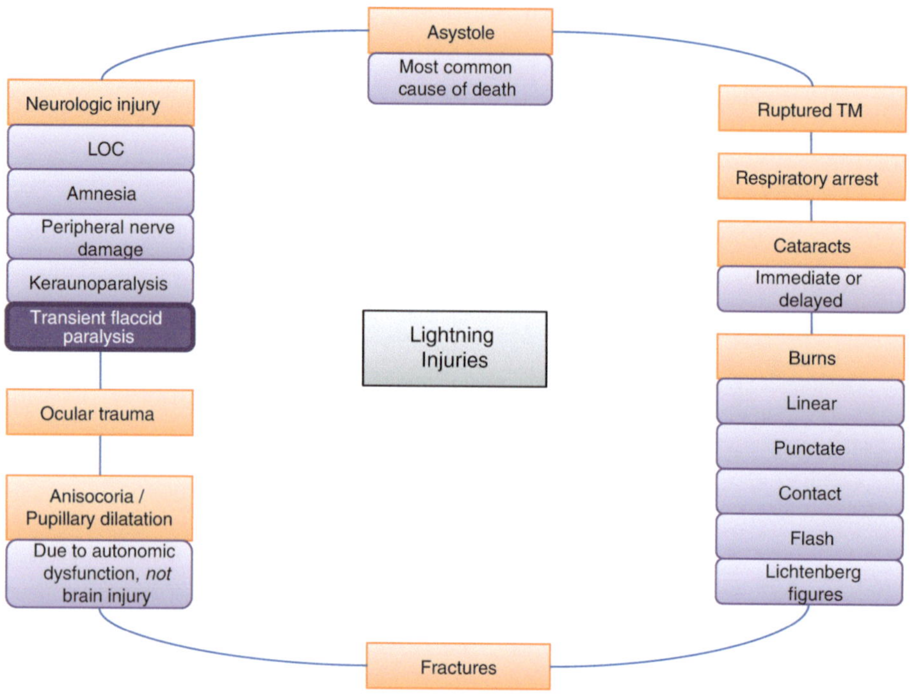

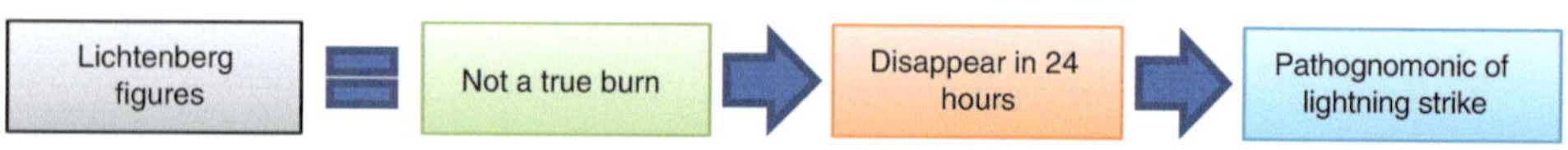

Lightning Injury Management

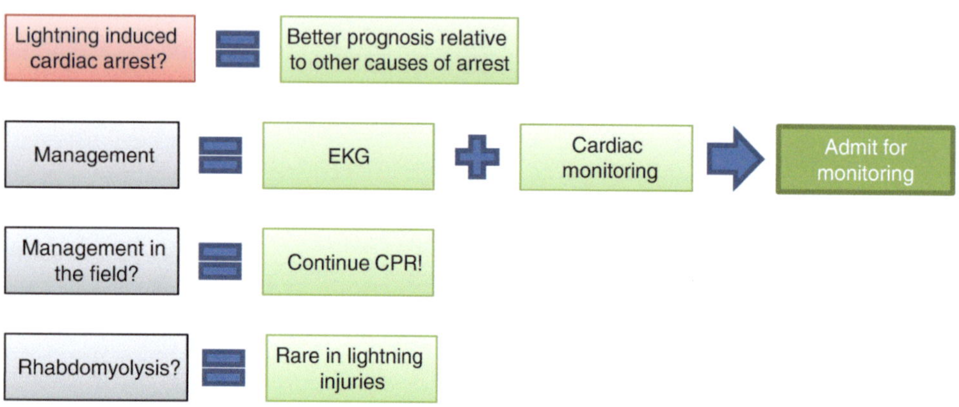

High-Altitude Illness

Introduction

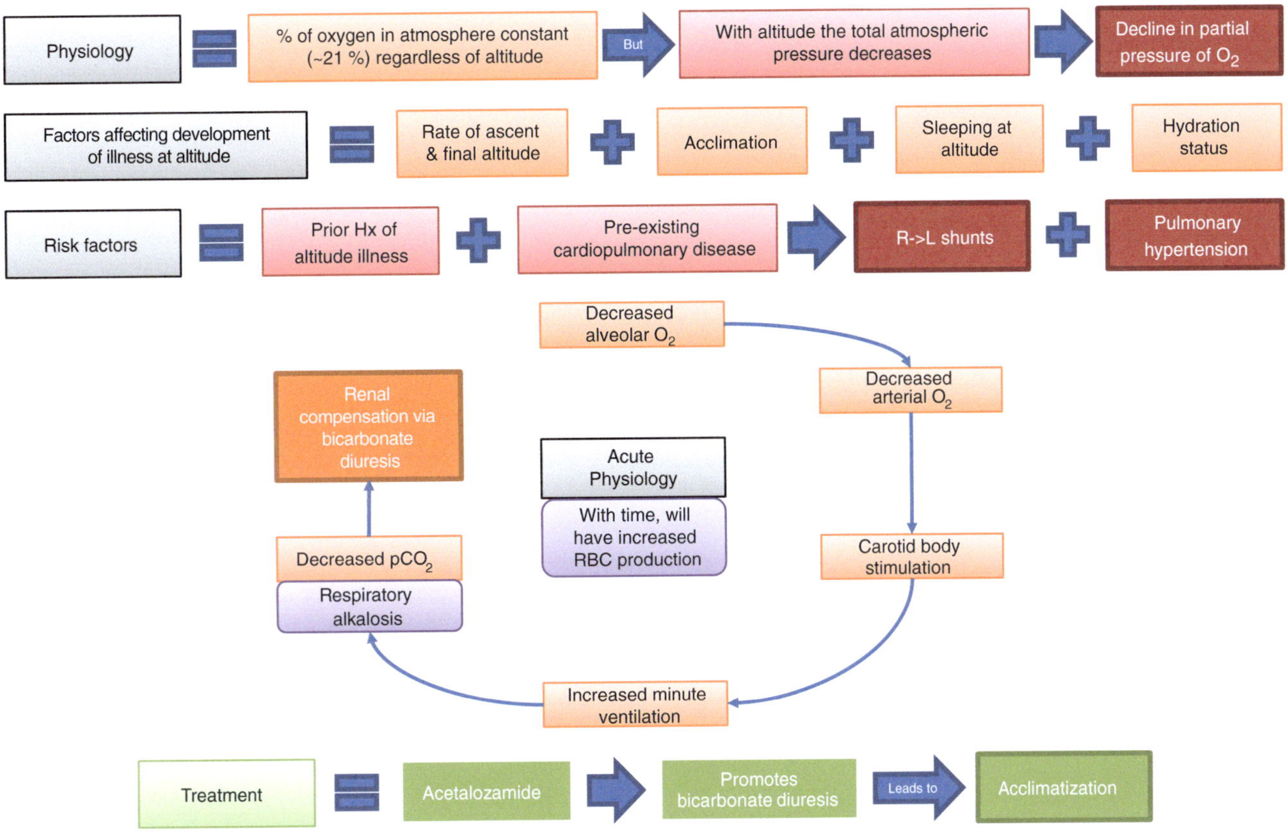

Acute Mountain Sickness

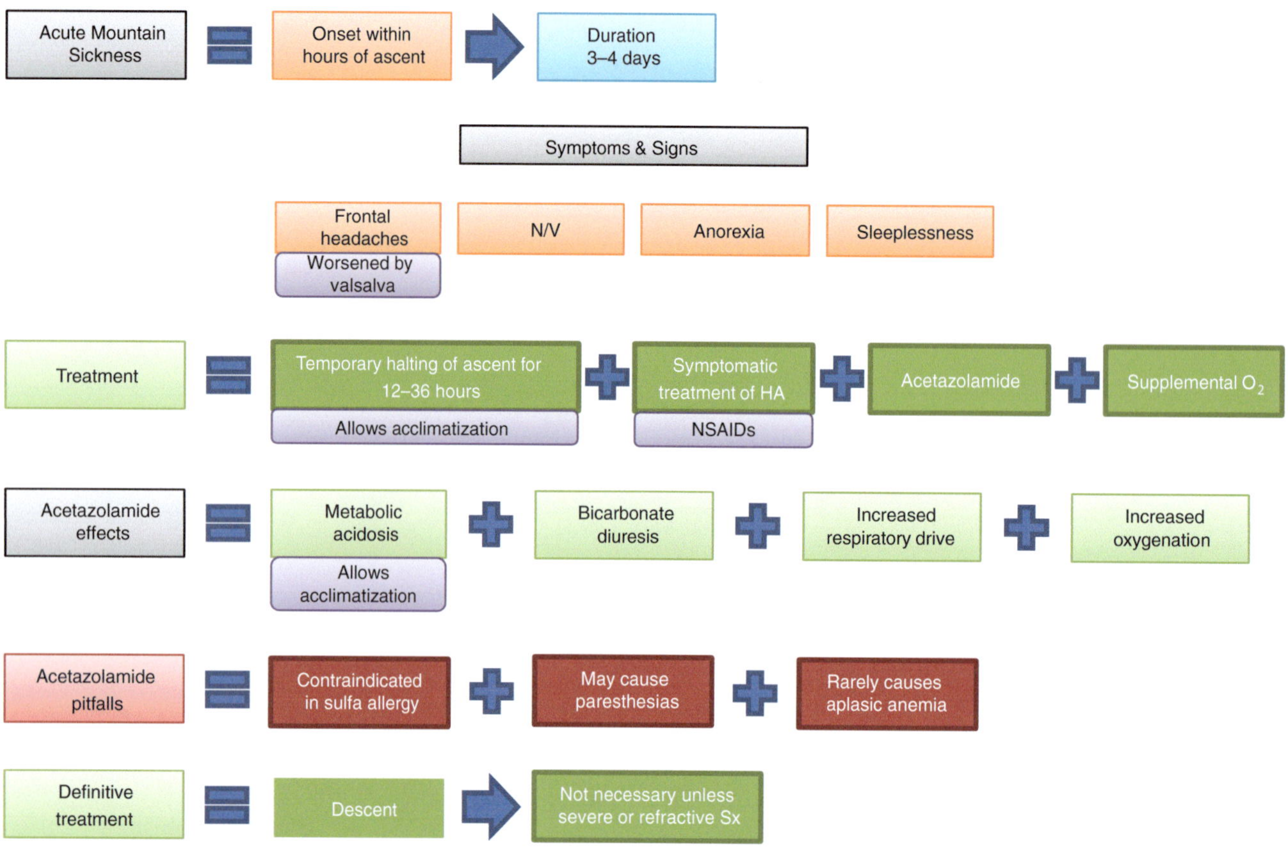

High-Altitude Cerebral Edema

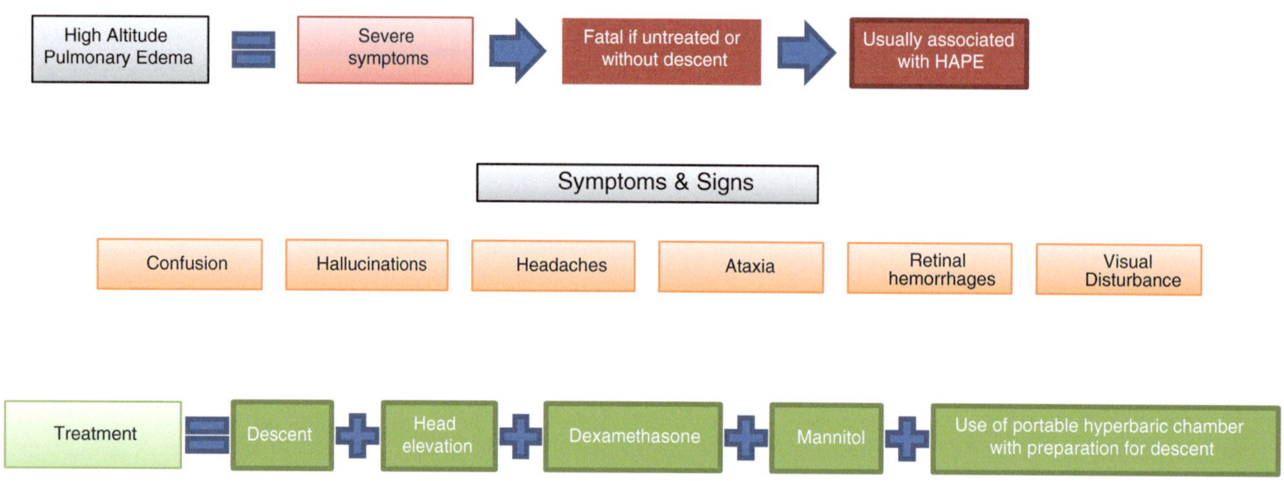

High-Altitude Pulmonary Edema

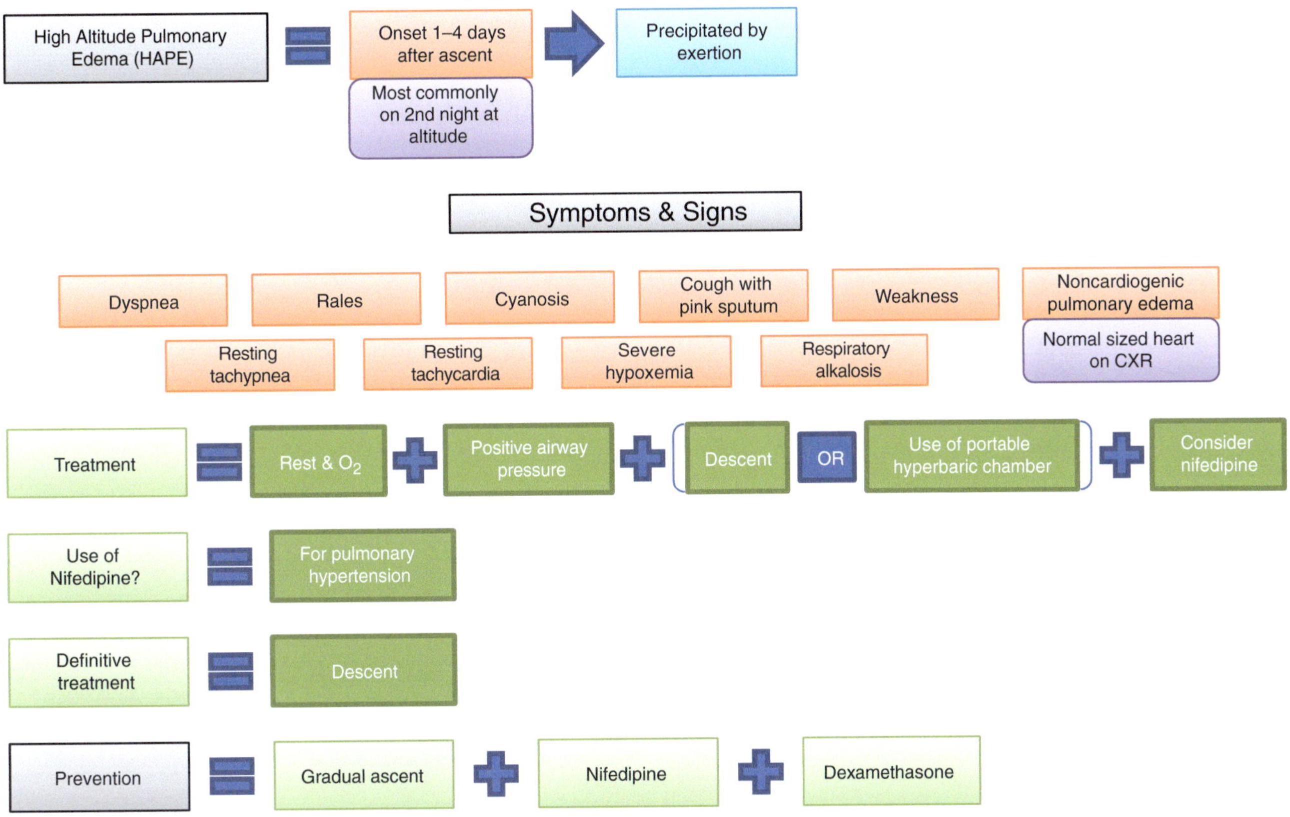

Submersion

Drowning

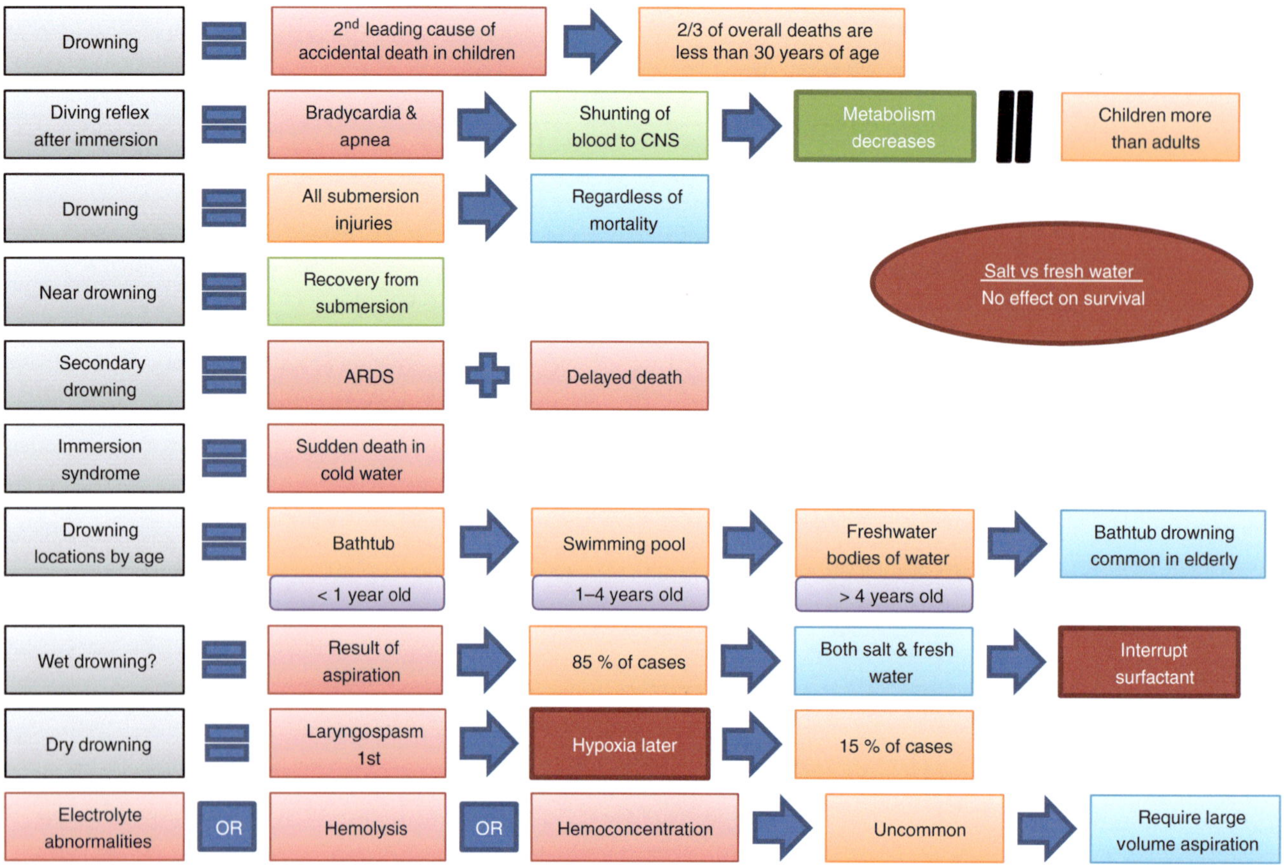

Drowning Management

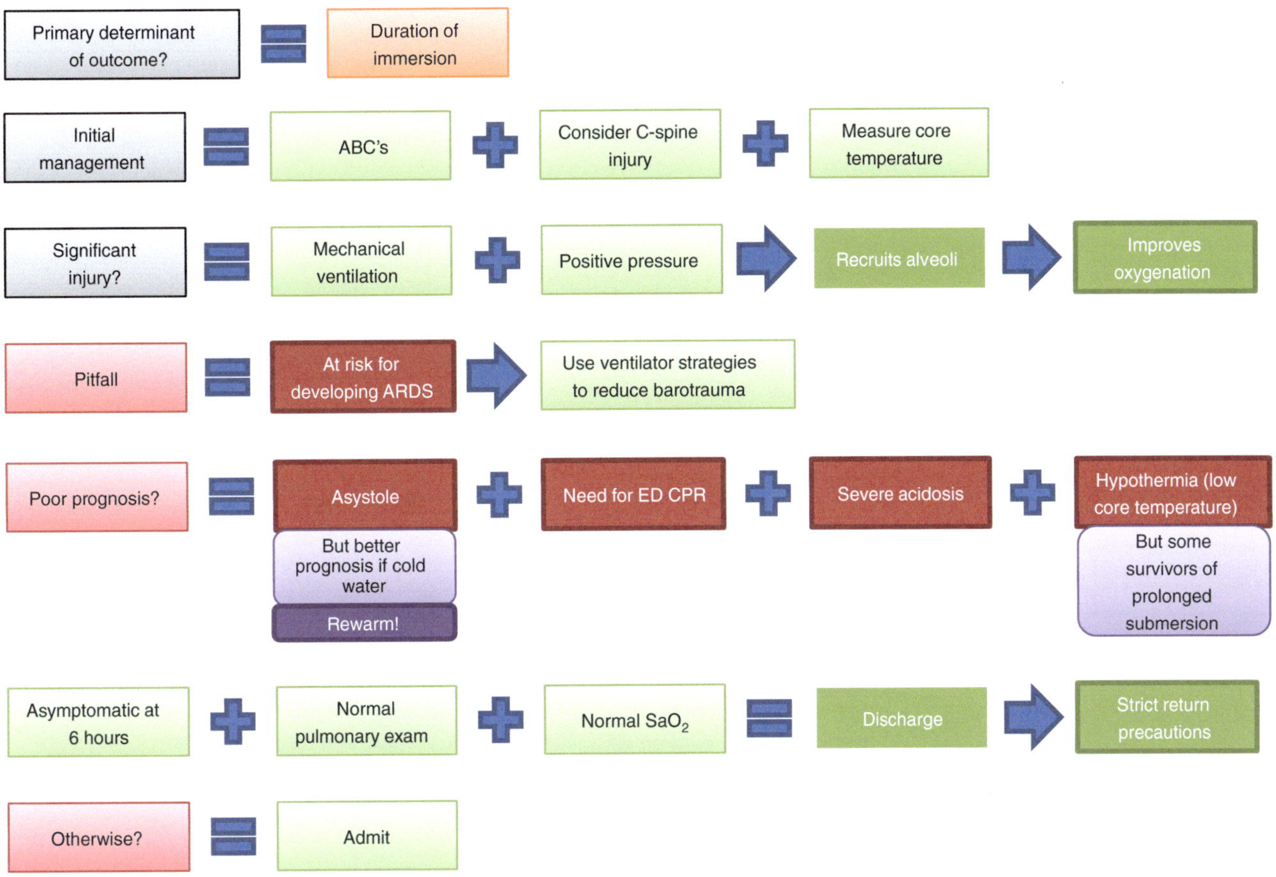

Temperature-Related Illness

Heat Dissipation Versus Generation

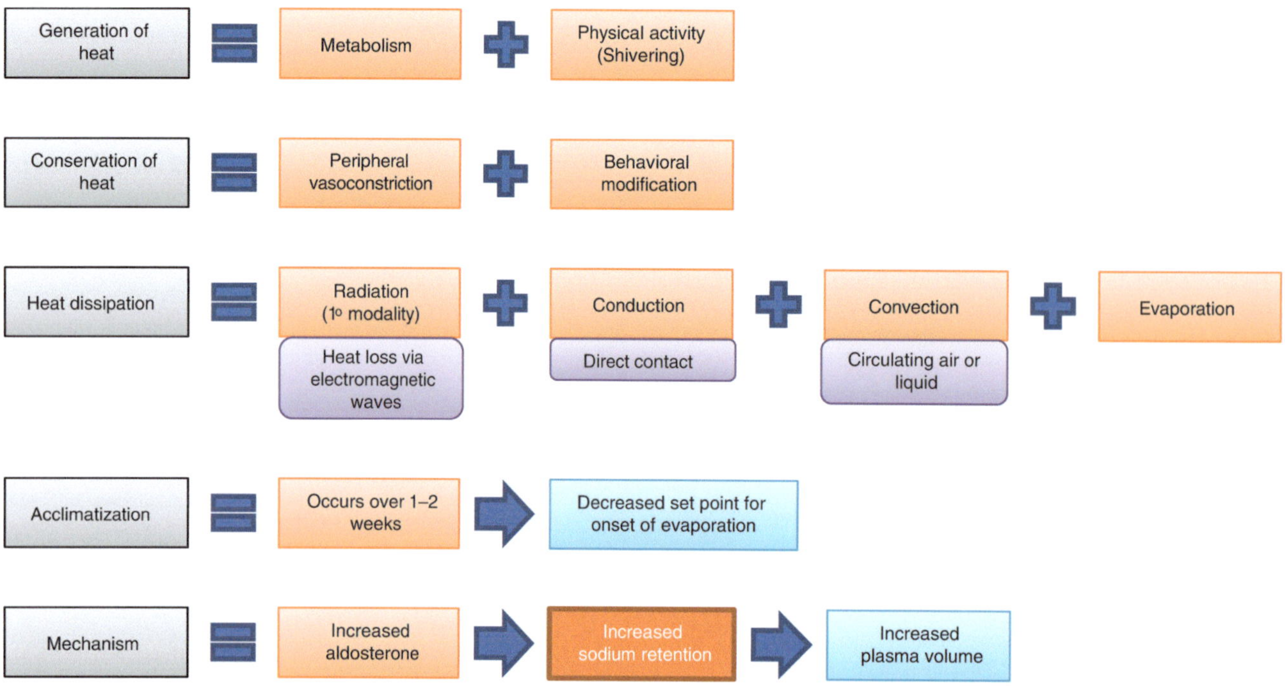

Predisposing Factors for Heat Illness

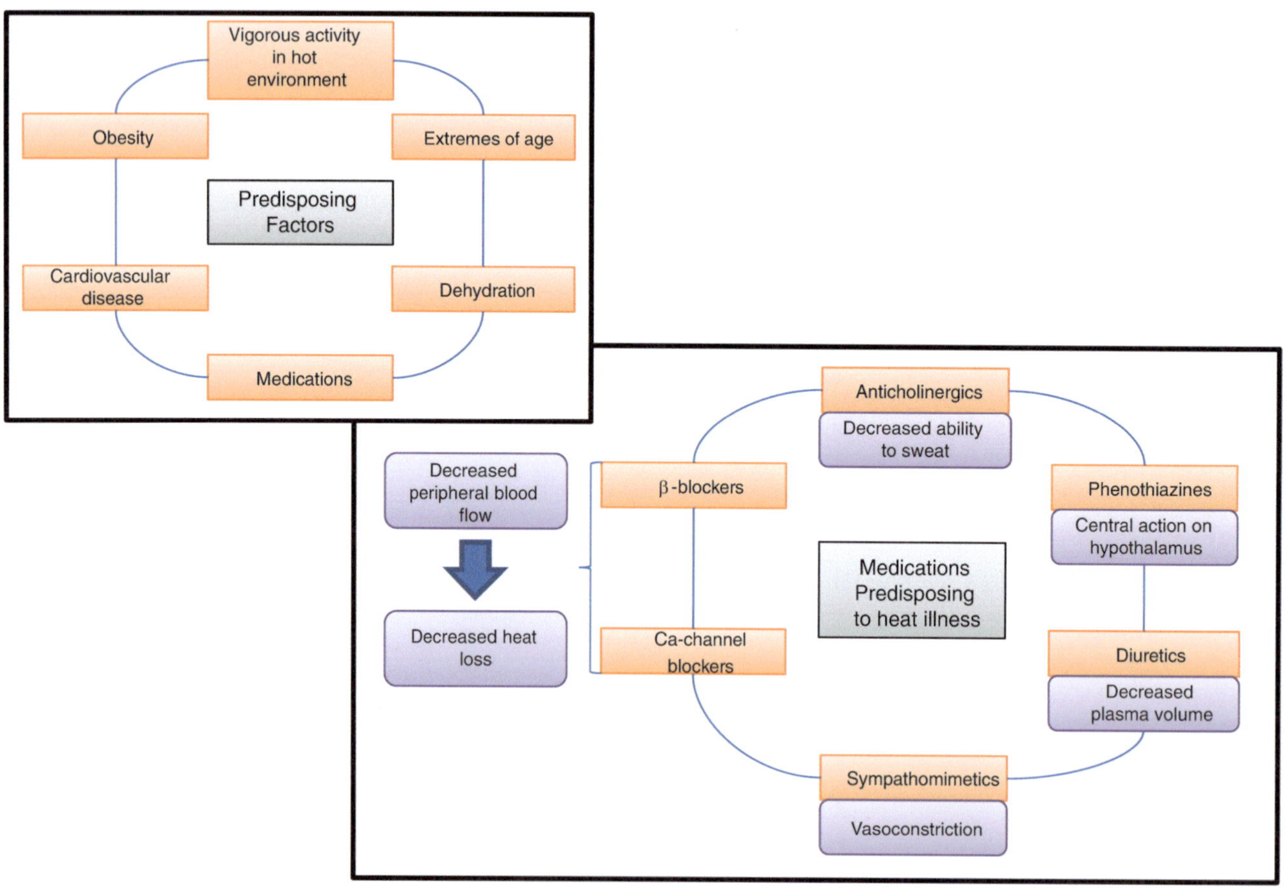

Minor/Moderate Heat Illness

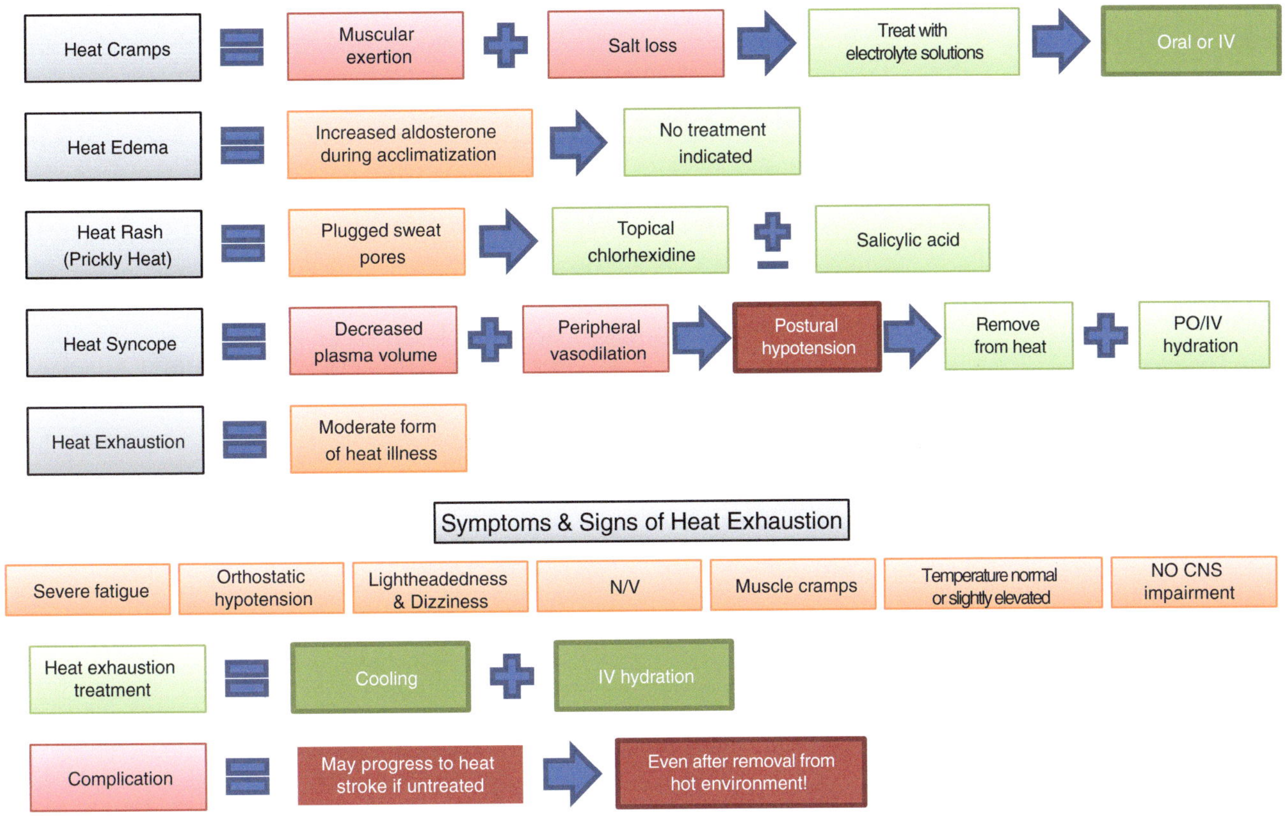

Heat Stroke

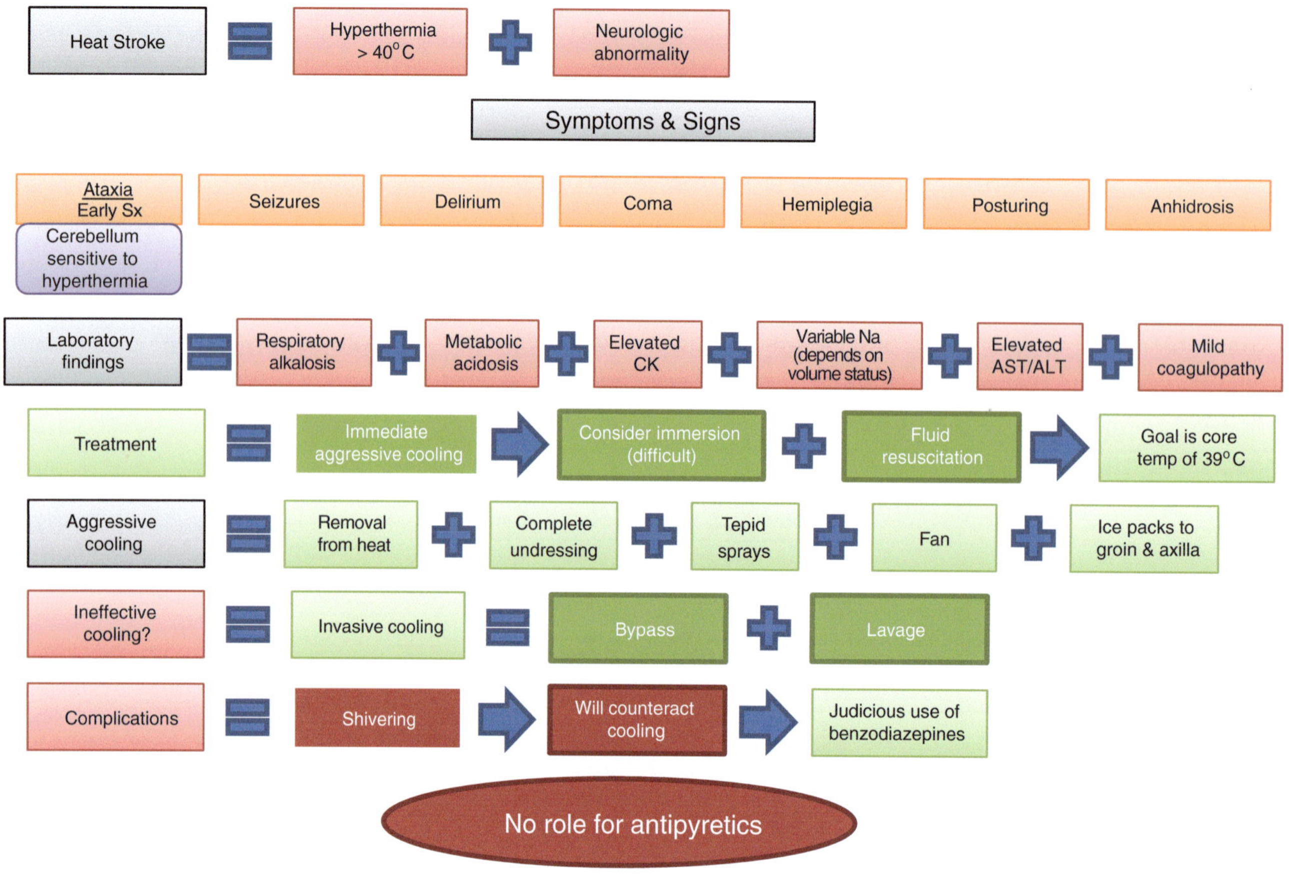
Heat Stroke
Hyperthermia > 40°C
Neurologic abnormality
Symptoms & Signs
Ataxia
Early Sx
Cerebellum sensitive to hyperthermia
Seizures
Delirium
Coma
Hemiplegia
Posturing
Anhidrosis
Laboratory findings
Respiratory alkalosis
Metabolic acidosis
Elevated CK
Variable Na (depends on volume status)
Elevated AST/ALT
Mild coagulopathy
Treatment
Immediate aggressive cooling
Consider immersion (difficult)
Fluid resuscitation
Goal is core temp of 39°C
Aggressive cooling
Removal from heat
Complete undressing
Tepid sprays
Fan
Ice packs to groin & axilla
Ineffective cooling?
Invasive cooling
Bypass
Lavage
Complications
Shivering
Will counteract cooling
Judicious use of benzodiazepines
No role for antipyretics

Cold Injury Pathophysiology

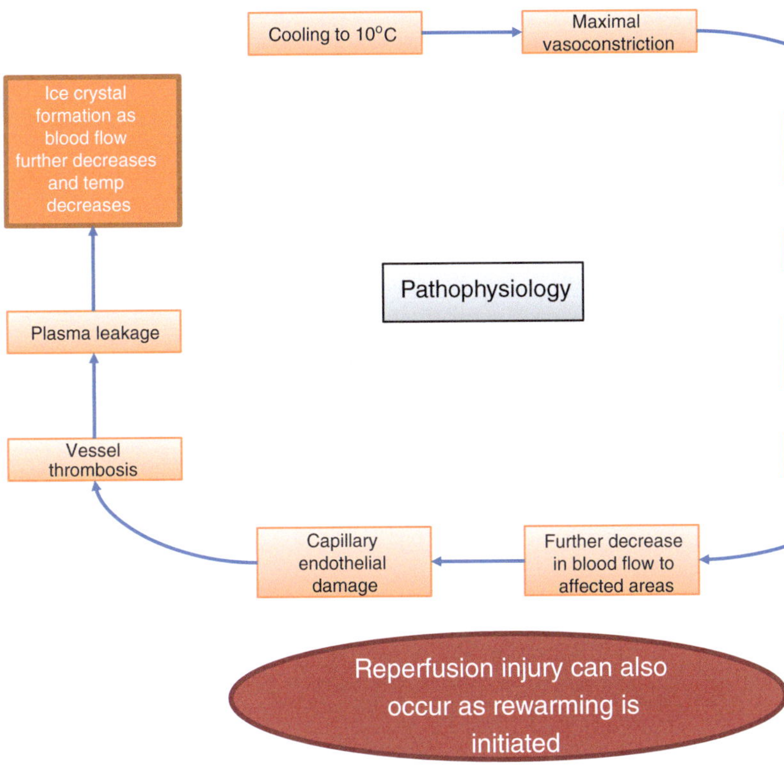

Localized Cold Injuries

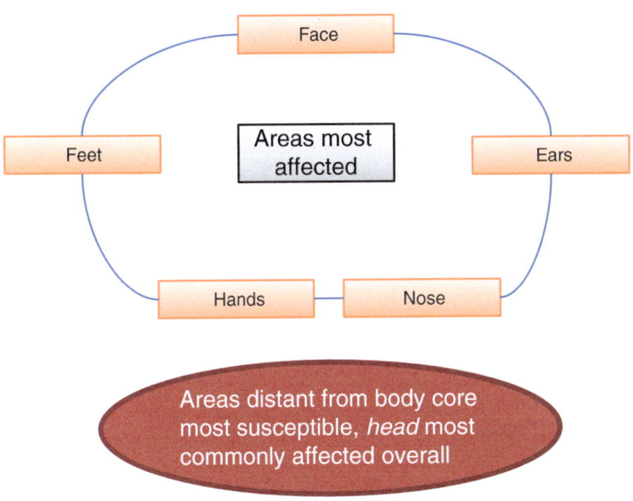

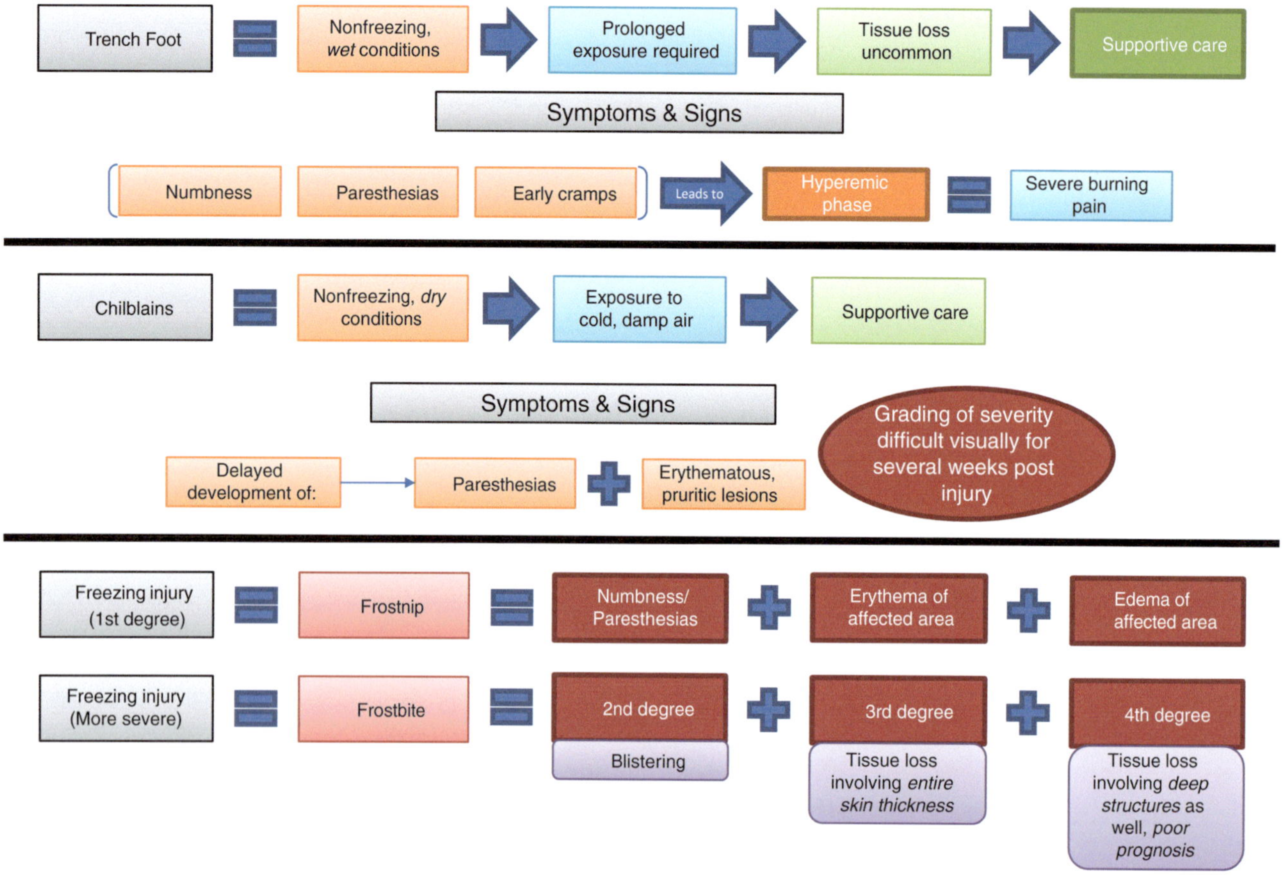
Trench Foot
Nonfreezing, wet conditions
Prolonged exposure required
Tissue loss uncommon
Supportive care
Symptoms & Signs
Numbness
Paresthesias
Early cramps
Leads to
Hyperemic phase
Severe burning pain
Chilblains
Nonfreezing, dry conditions
Exposure to cold, damp air
Supportive care
Symptoms & Signs
Delayed development of:
Paresthesias
Erythematous, pruritic lesions
Grading of severity difficult visually for several weeks post injury
Freezing injury (1st degree)
Frostnip
Numbness/ Paresthesias
Erythema of affected area
Edema of affected area
Freezing injury (More severe)
Frostbite
2nd degree
Blistering
3rd degree
Tissue loss involving entire skin thickness
4th degree
Tissue loss involving deep structures as well, poor prognosis

Management

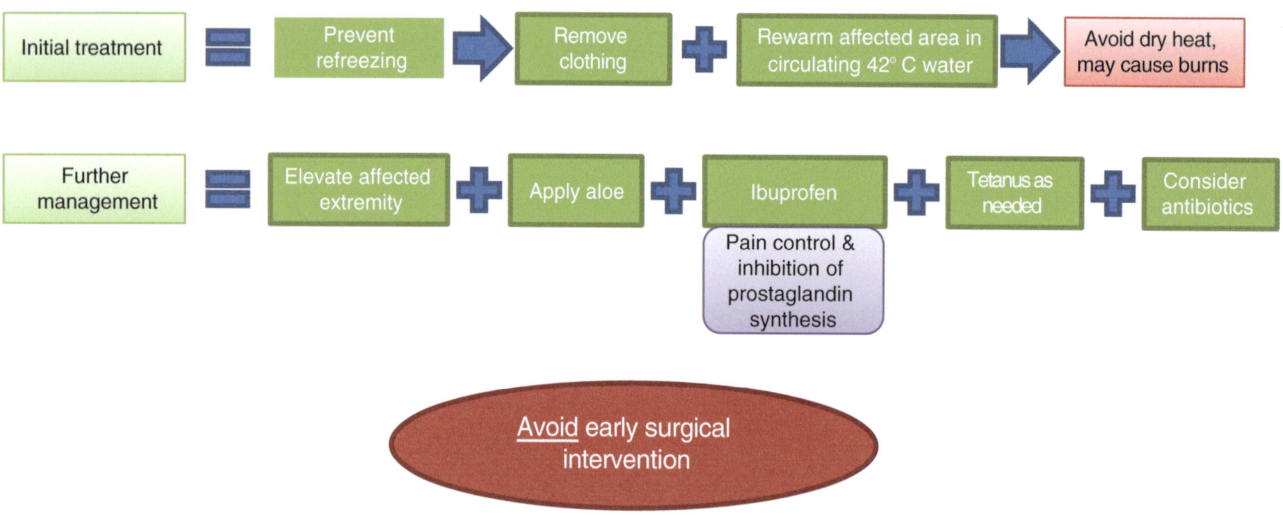
Initial treatment
Prevent refreezing
Remove clothing
Rewarm affected area in circulating 42° C water
Avoid dry heat, may cause burns
Further management
Elevate affected extremity
Apply aloe
Ibuprofen
Pain control & inhibition of prostaglandin synthesis
Tetanus as needed
Consider antibiotics
Avoid early surgical intervention

Hypothermia

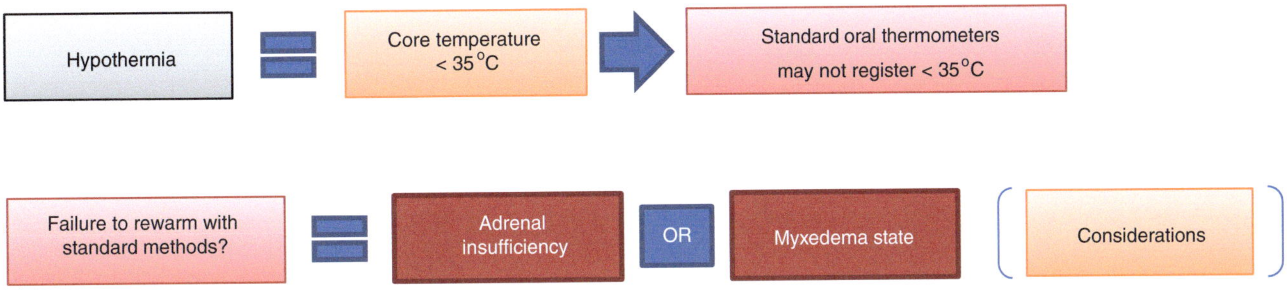

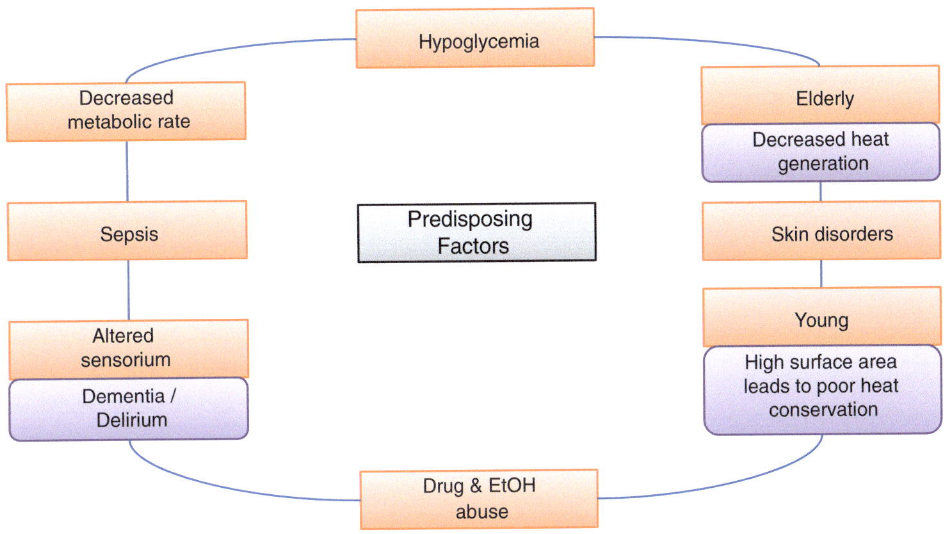

Hypothermia Manifestations

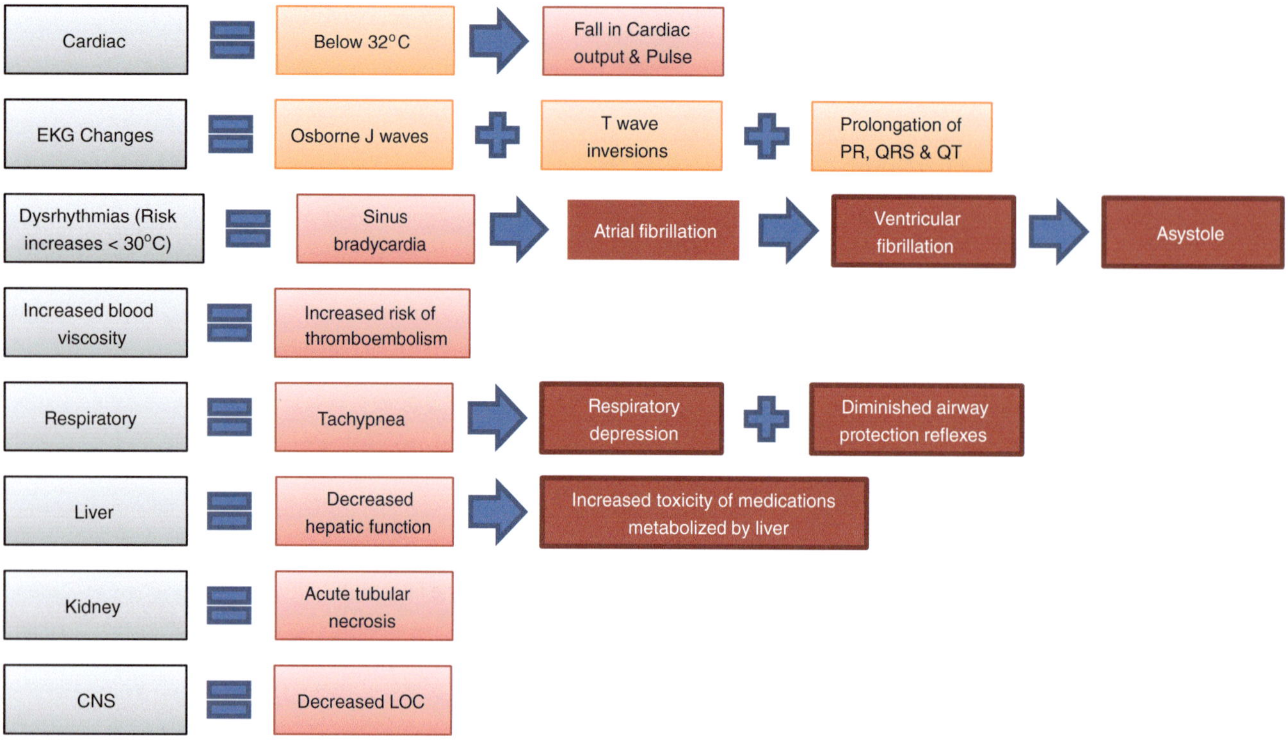

Hypothermia Treatment

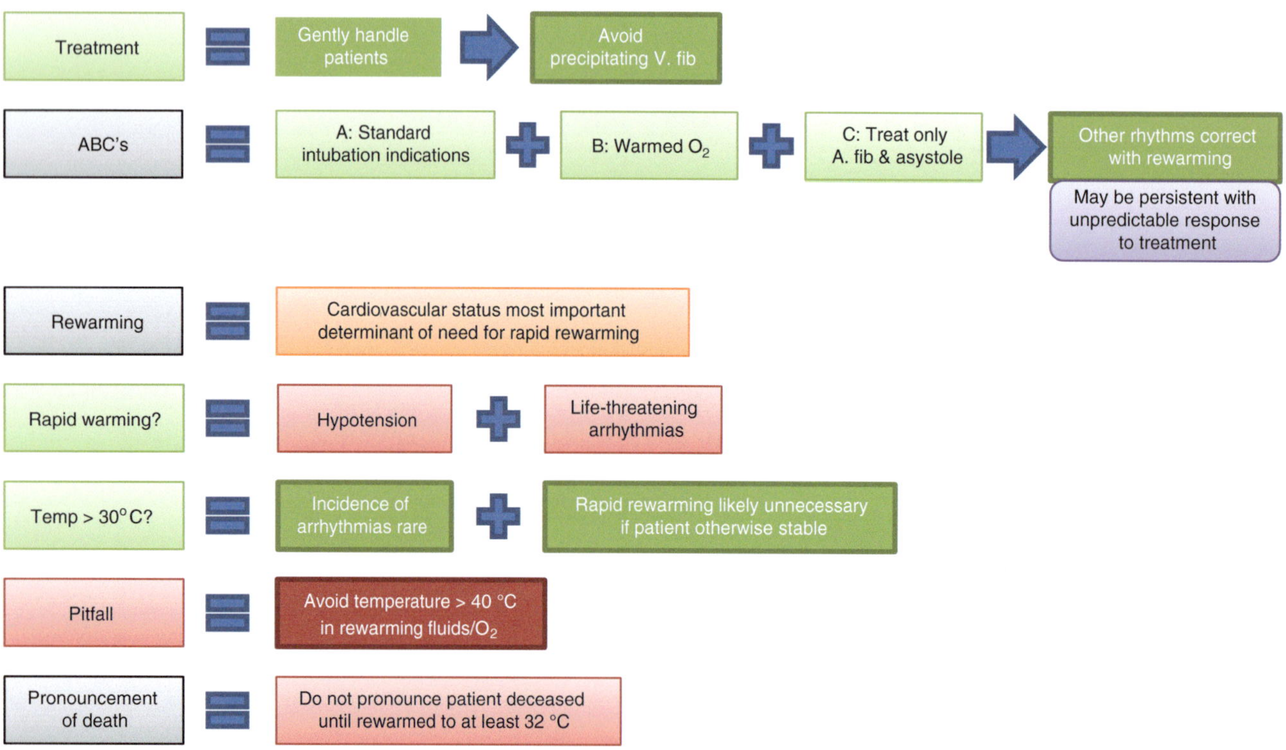

Rewarming Physiology

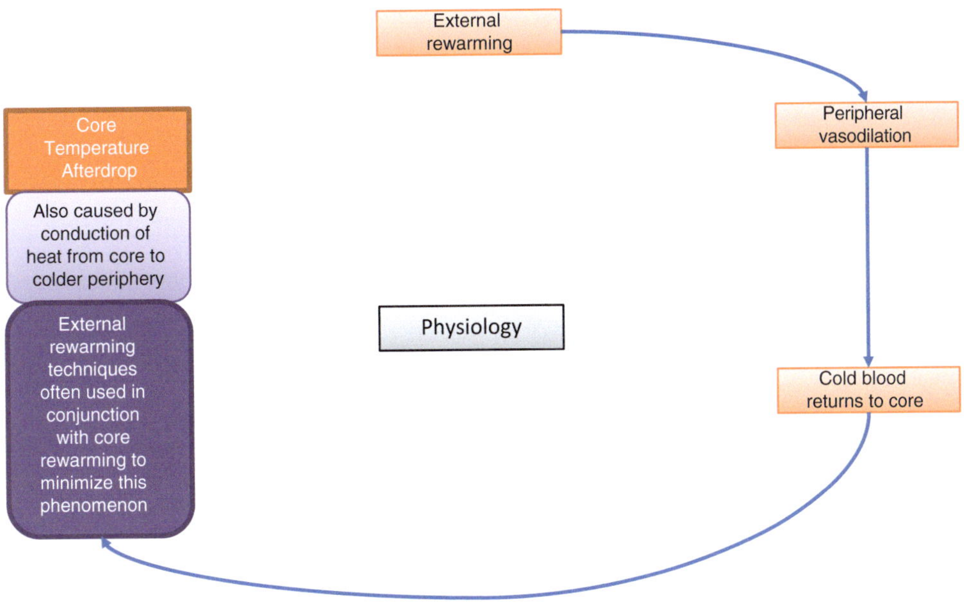

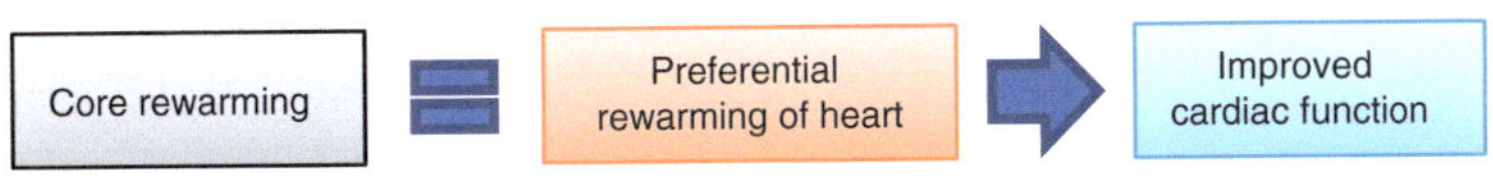

Rewarming Methods

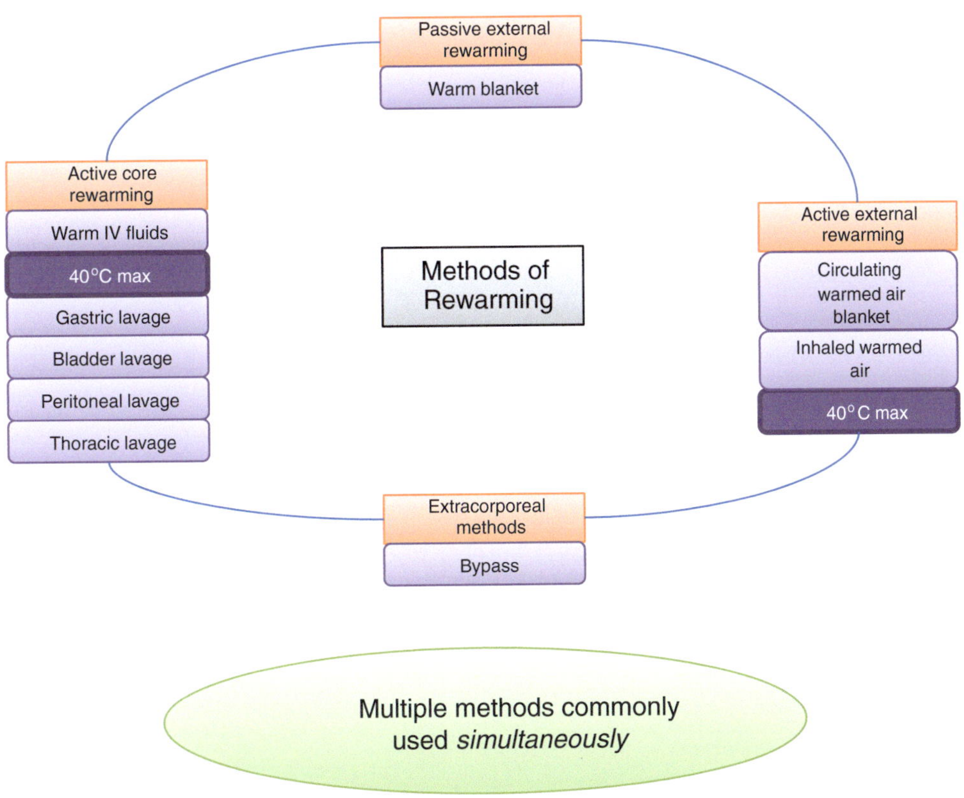

Radiation

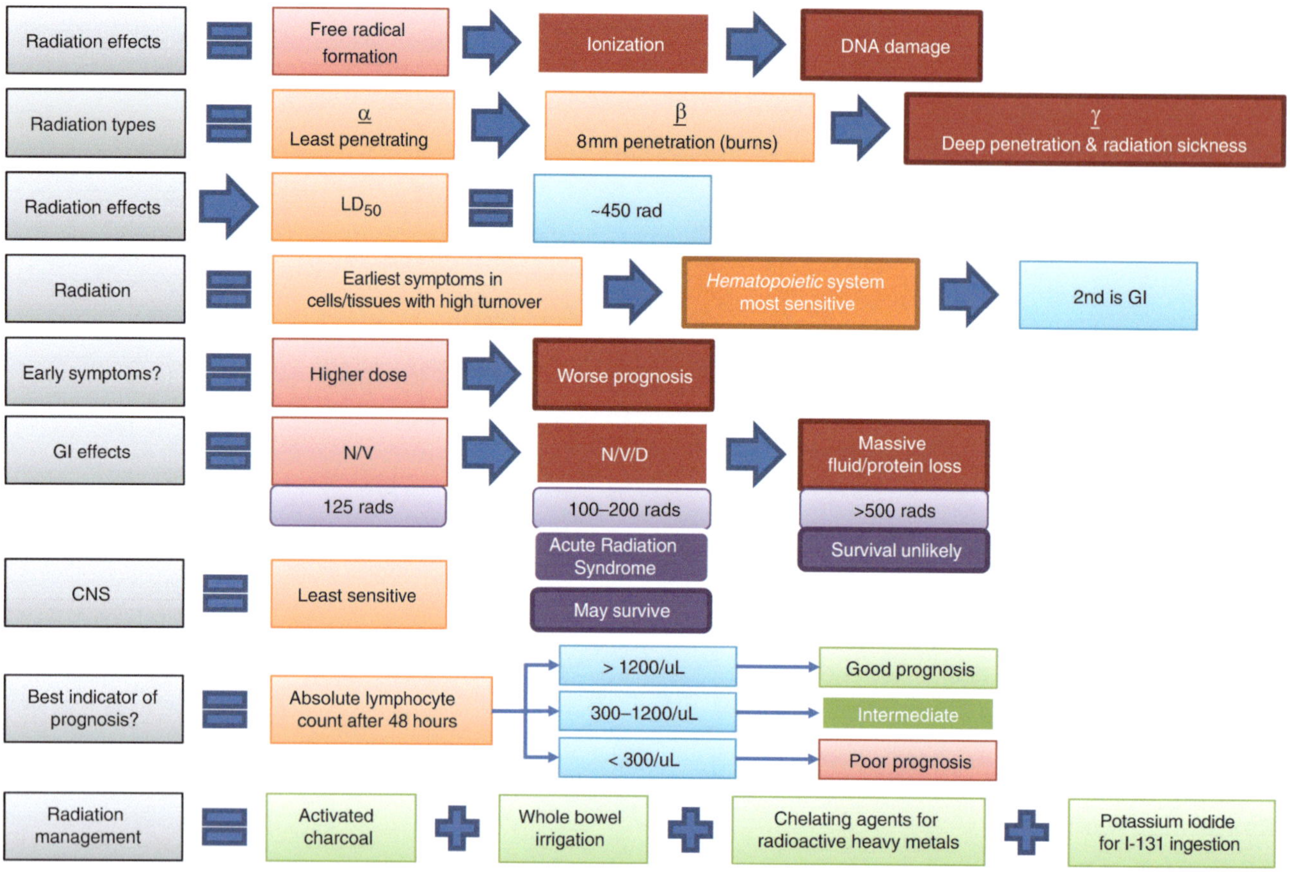

Biological Weapons

Biological Weapons Tidbits

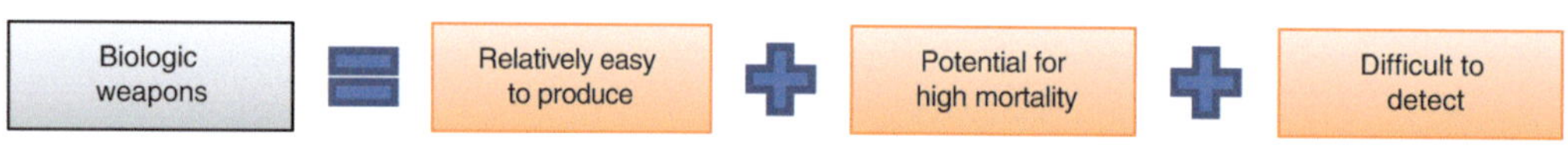

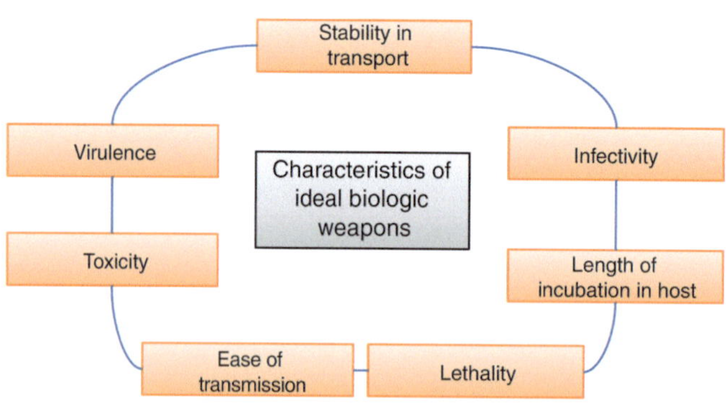

Selected Biological Agents and Toxins

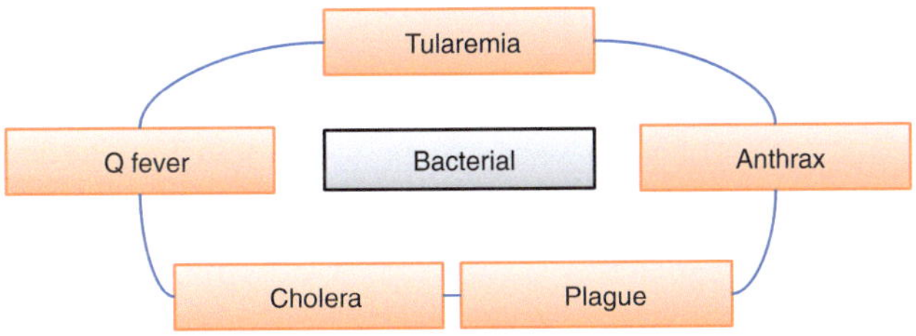

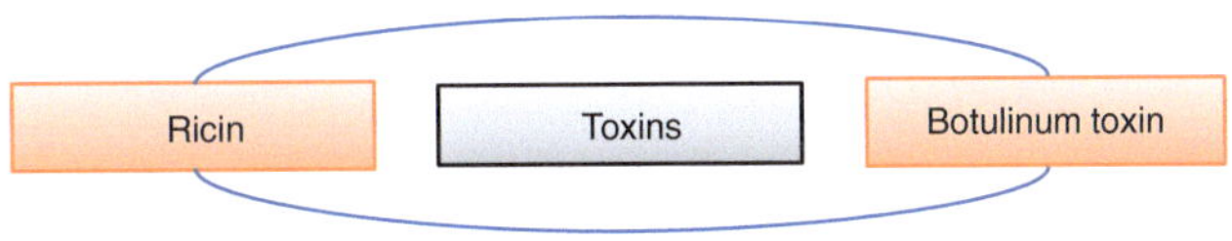

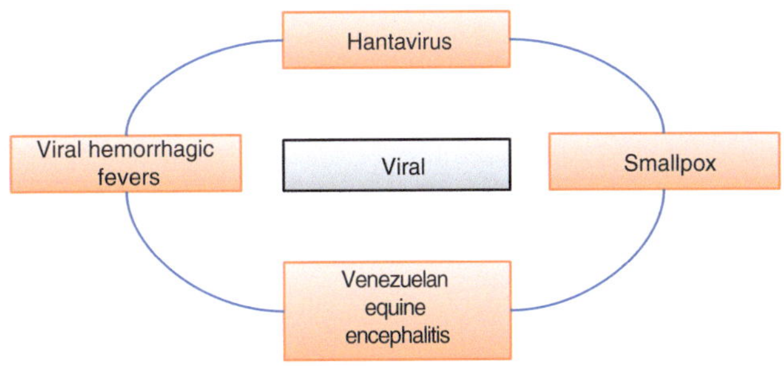

Anthrax

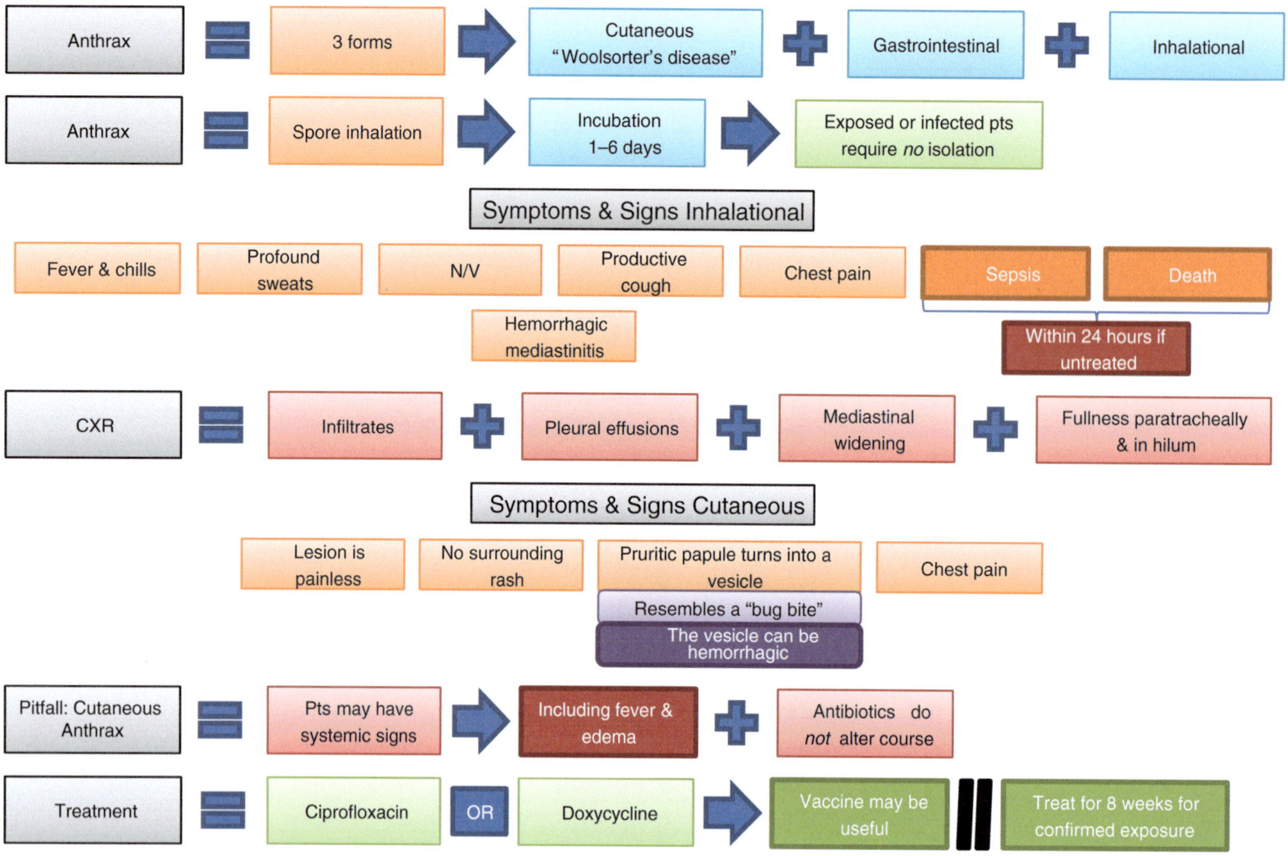
Anthrax
3 forms
Cutaneous "Woolsorter's disease"
Gastrointestinal
Inhalational
Anthrax
Spore inhalation
Incubation 1–6 days
Exposed or infected pts require *no* isolation
Symptoms & Signs Inhalational
Fever & chills
Profound sweats
N/V
Productive cough
Chest pain
Sepsis
Death
Hemorrhagic mediastinitis
Within 24 hours if untreated
CXR
Infiltrates
Pleural effusions
Mediastinal widening
Fullness paratracheally & in hilum
Symptoms & Signs Cutaneous
Lesion is painless
No surrounding rash
Pruritic papule turns into a vesicle
Chest pain
Resembles a "bug bite"
The vesicle can be hemorrhagic
Pitfall: Cutaneous Anthrax
Pts may have systemic signs
Including fever & edema
Antibiotics do *not* alter course
Treatment
Ciprofloxacin
OR
Doxycycline
Vaccine may be useful
Treat for 8 weeks for confirmed exposure

Plague

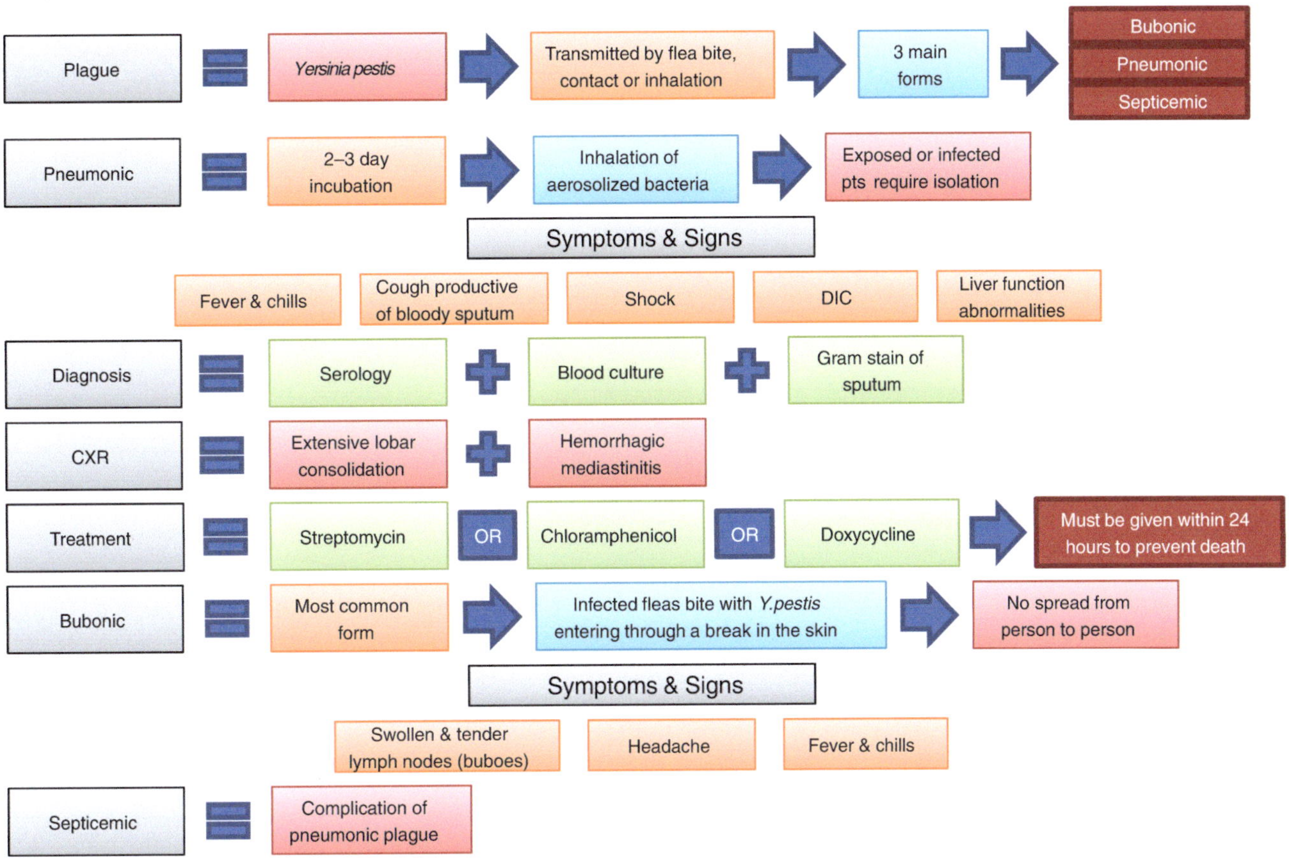

Smallpox

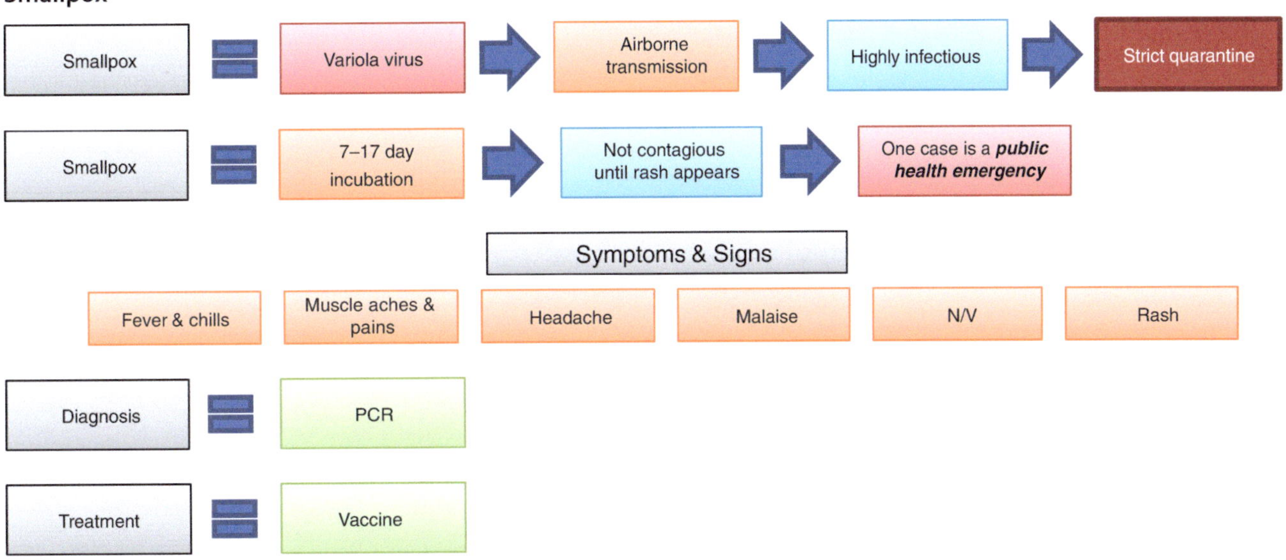

Toxins

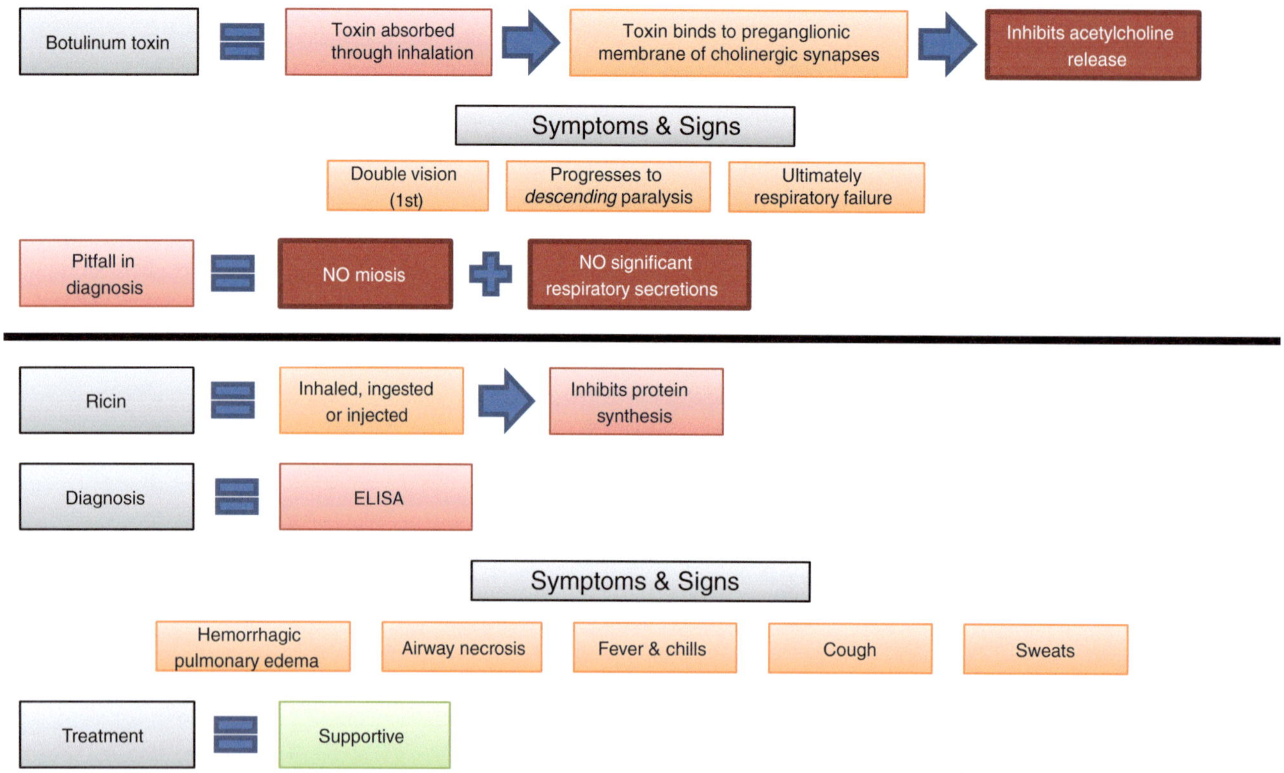

Chemical Weapons

Chemical Weapons

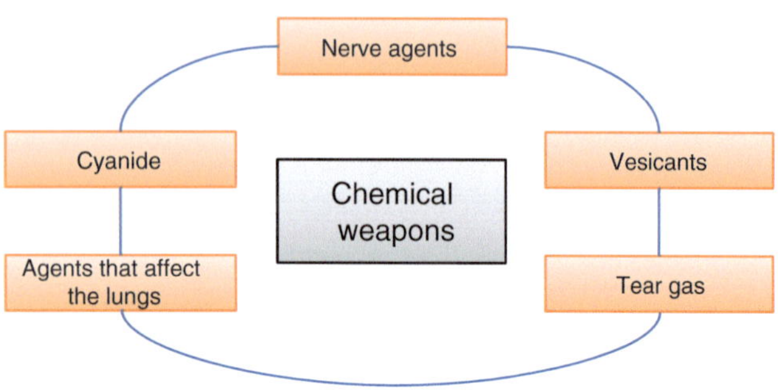

Nerve Agents

Nerve agents = Multiple → Sarin, Tabun, Soman, VX → All inhibit acetylcholinesterase

Most potent? = VX || Most volatile → Sarin

Pitfall = Secondary contamination

Symptoms & Signs – "SLUDGEM" & Killer B's"

Salivation | ***L***acrimation | ***U***rination | ***D***efecation | ***G***I Upset | ***E***mesis | ***M***iosis (& ***M***uscle spasm)

Bradycardia | ***B***ronchorrhea | ***B***ronchospasm

Treatment = Protect self - decontaminate + Oxygen + Atropine + 2-PAM

Vesicants

Vessicants = Blister the dermis

Phosgene = Not a true vessicant → Skin blanches & has wheals without blisters + May cause pulmonary edema

Mustard = Liquid or gas → Enters via inhalation or through skin – delayed pain + Causes necrotic blisters on mucus membranes and dermis

Lewisite = Liquid or gas → Causes immediate pain + Increases capillary permeability → Shock & end organ damage

Tetanus

Tetanus

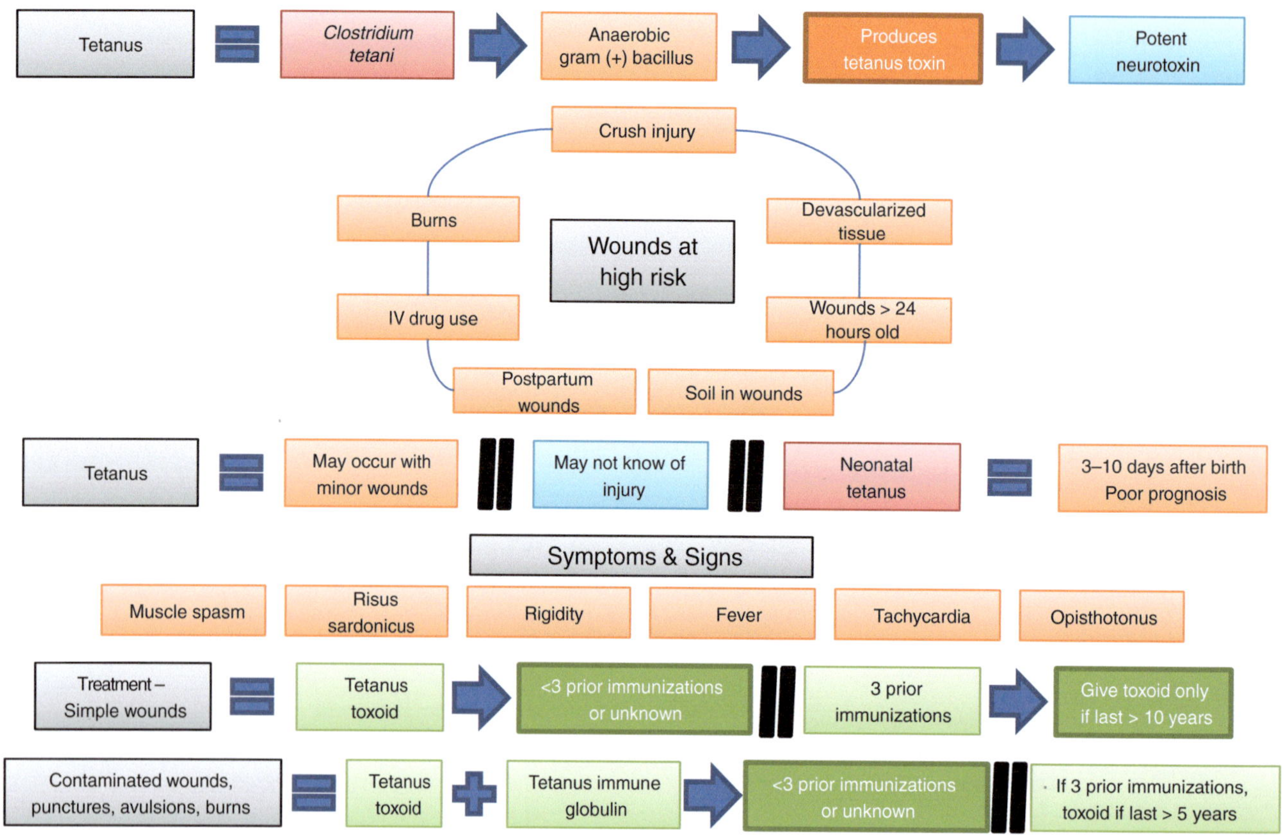

Neurologic Emergencies

Michael R. Marchick and Bobby Desai

Contents

Dermatomes and Reflexes 556
Altered Mental Status and Coma 556
Cerebrovascular Accidents 557
Seizures 565
CNS Infections 572
Encephalitis 578
Brain Abscess 580
Headache Syndromes 581
Bell's Palsy 593
Neuromuscular Disorders 594
Movement Disorders 598
Neuropathies 600
Spinal Disorders 600
Miscellaneous Disorders 601
Psychiatric Emergencies 601
Abuse/Neglect/Violence 611
Addictive Behavior and Withdrawal 613

M.R. Marchick, MD
Department of Emergency Medicine, University of Florida College of Medicine, Gainesville, FL, USA

B. Desai, MD, MEd (✉)
Department of Emergency Medicine, University of Florida, Gainesville, FL, USA
e-mail: bdesai@ufl.edu

B. Desai, B.R. Allen (eds.), *Nailing the Written Emergency Medicine Board Examination*,
DOI 10.1007/978-3-319-30838-8_10

Dermatomes and Reflexes

Dermatomes & Reflexes

Dermatome	Area
C4	Clavicle
C6	Thumb
C7	Index finger
C8	Ring Finger
T4	Nipple Line
T10	Umbilicus
L1	Inguinal ligament
L2, 3	Medial thigh
L4	Knee
L5	Lateral calf
S1	Lateral foot
S2–4	Perianal
Reflexes	**Area**
C6	Biceps
C7	Triceps
L4	Patellar
S1	Achilles

Altered Mental Status and Coma

Altered Mental Status

Altered Mental Status = Evaluate ABC's first!

Coma Cocktail = Naloxone + Glucose + Thiamine + Oxygen

AEIOU-TIPS	
A	Alcohol, Acidosis
E	Epilepsy, Endocrine, Electrolytes, Encephalopathy
I	Insulin
O	Opiates, Overdose
U	Uremia
T	Trauma, Temperature
I	Infection
P	Poisoning, Psychiatric
S	Stroke, Shock

Coma Testing

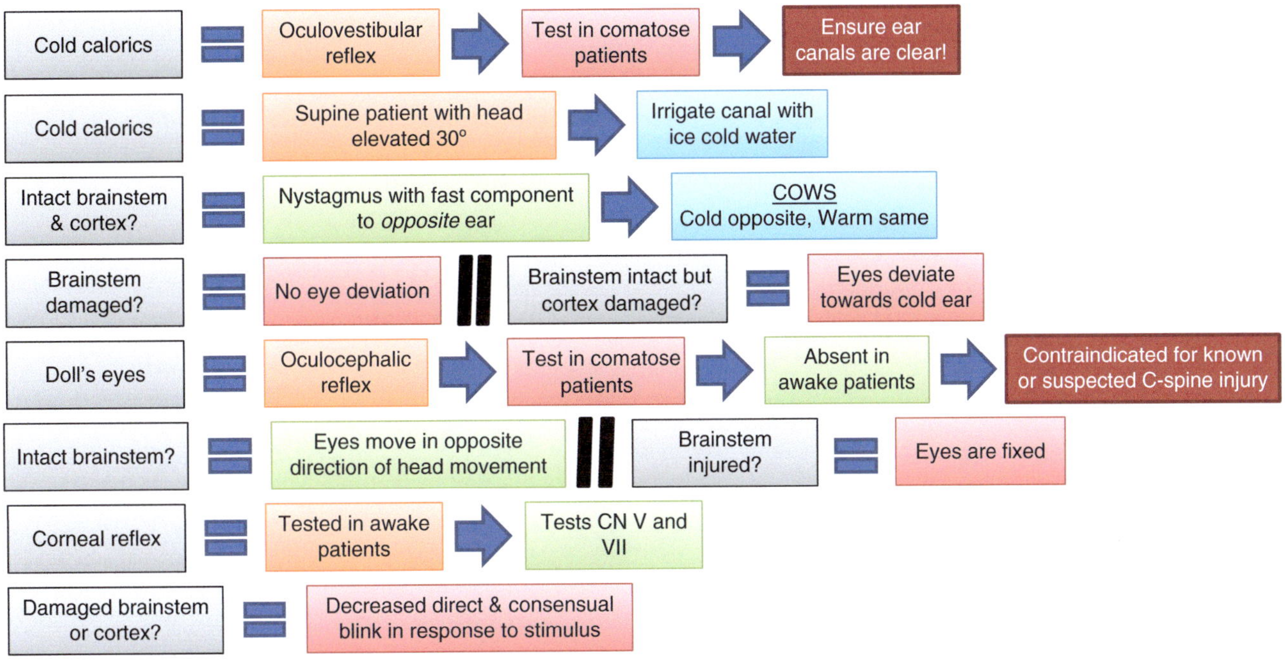

Cerebrovascular Accidents

Stroke Mimics

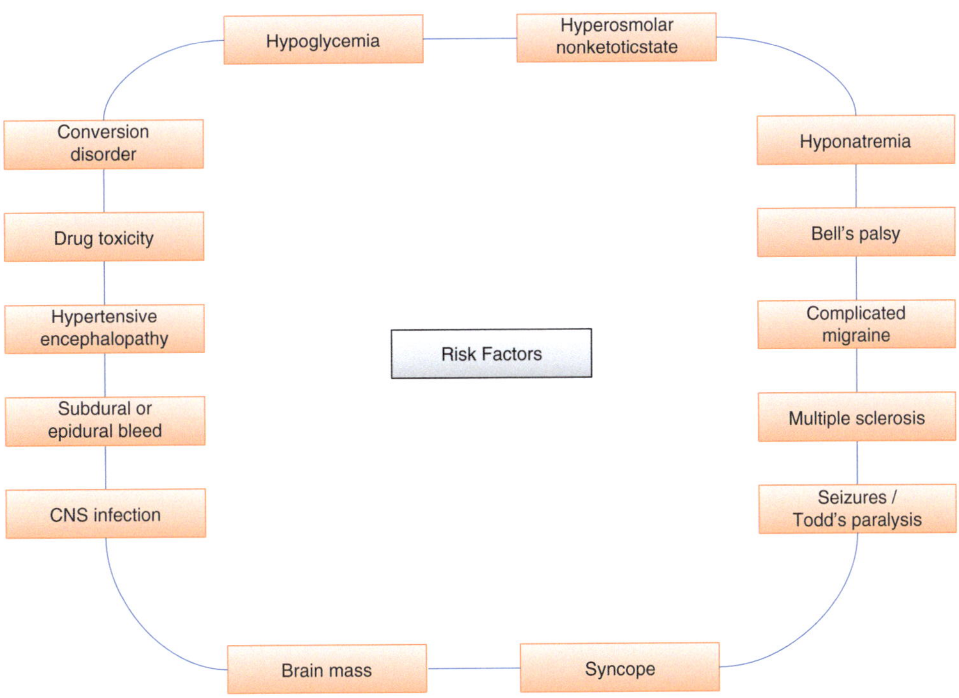

Stroke and TIA

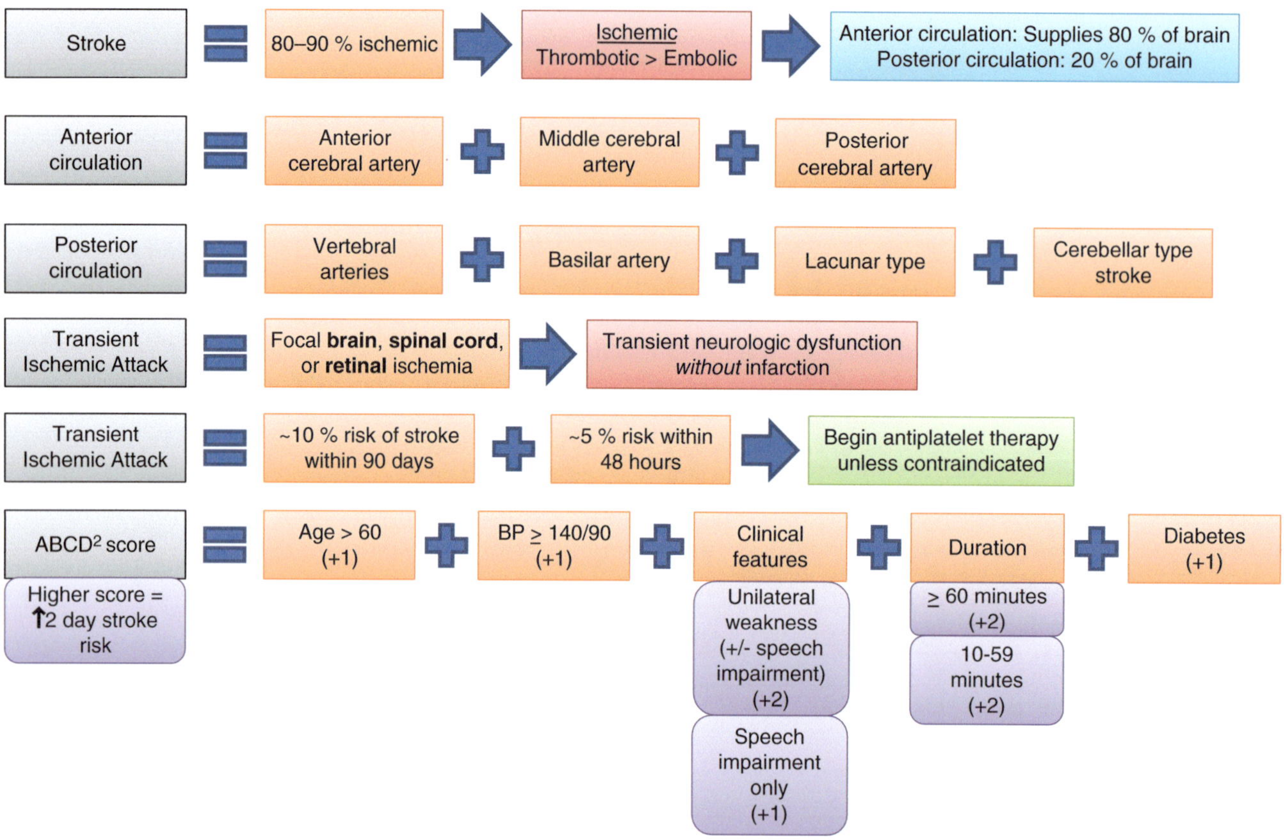

Anterior Circulation Stroke

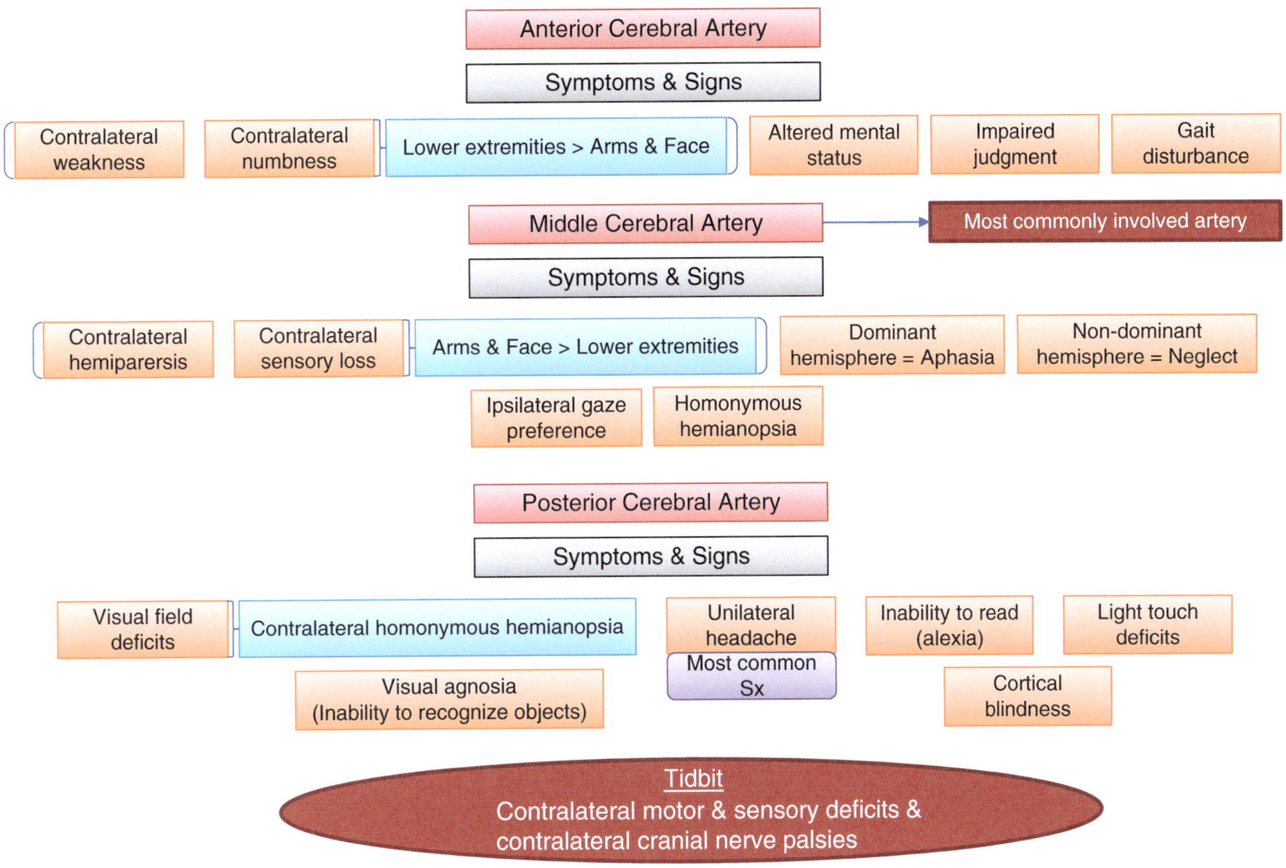

Vertebrobasilar Infarction

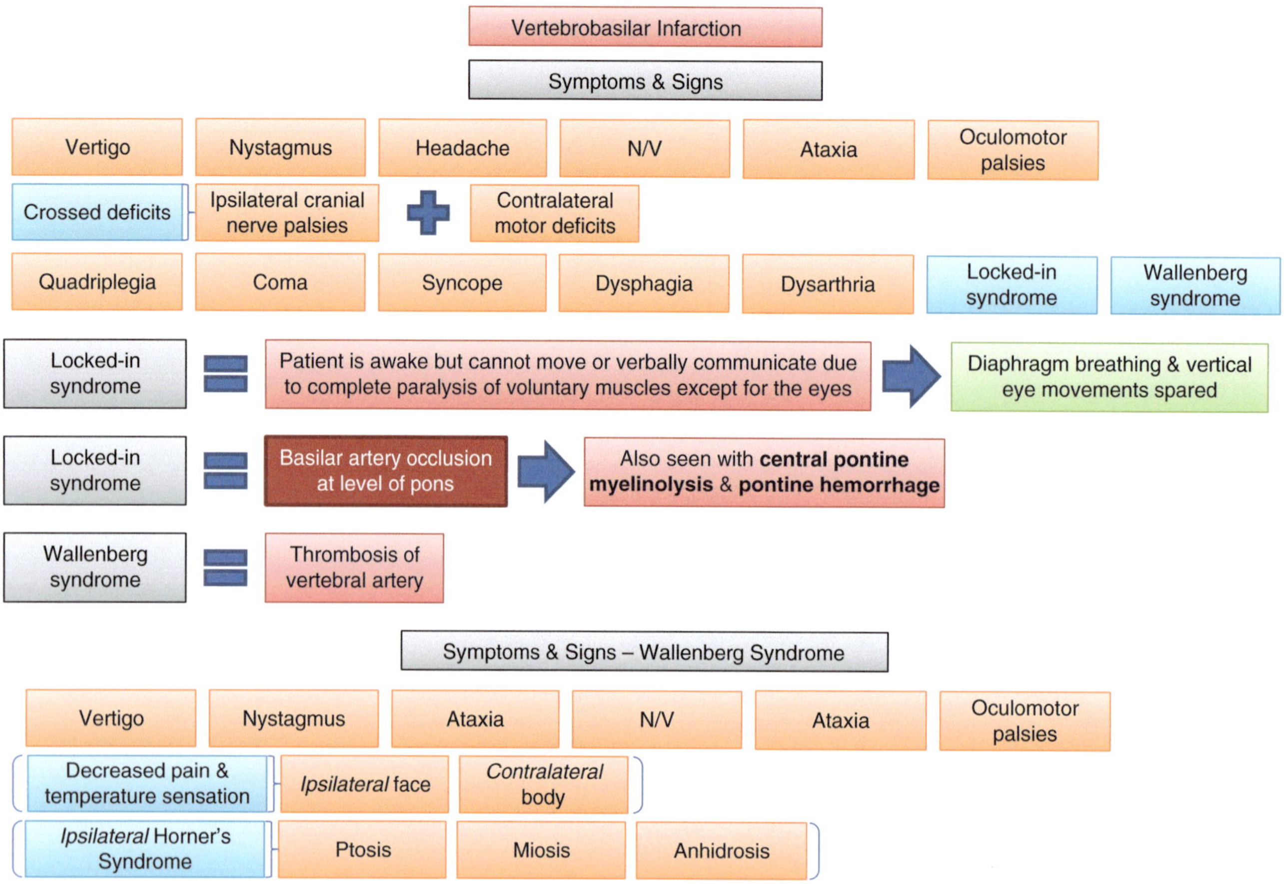

Lacunar Infarction

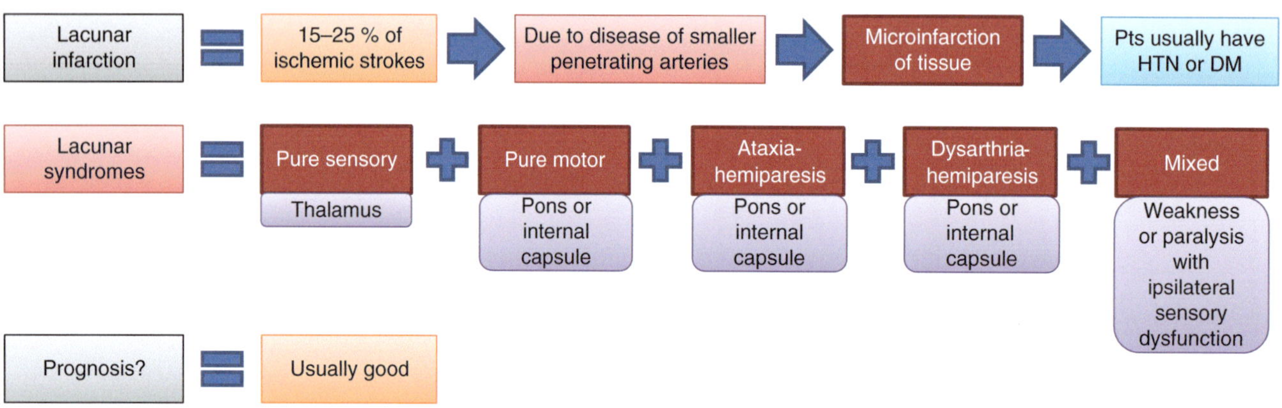

Cerebellar Infarction

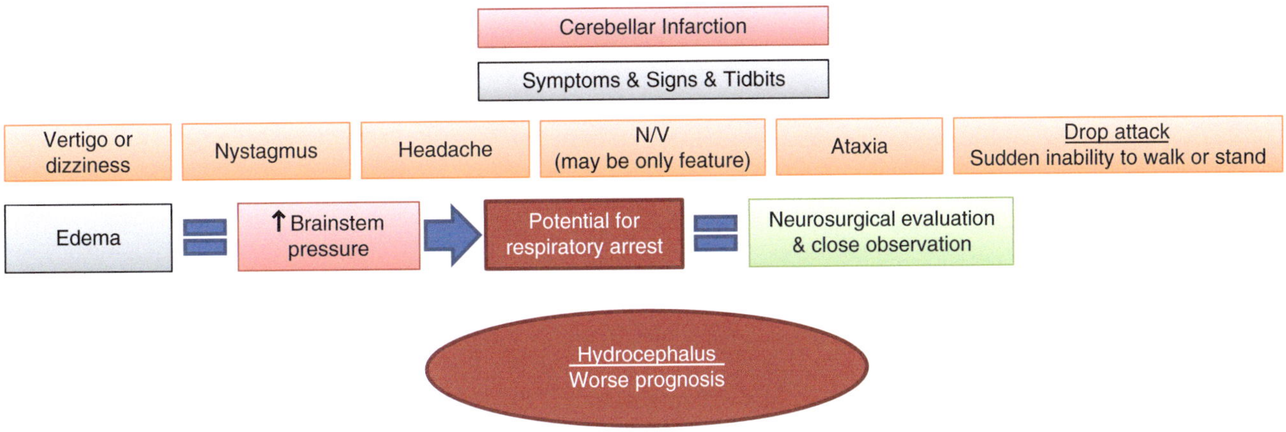

Acute Ischemic Stroke Treatment

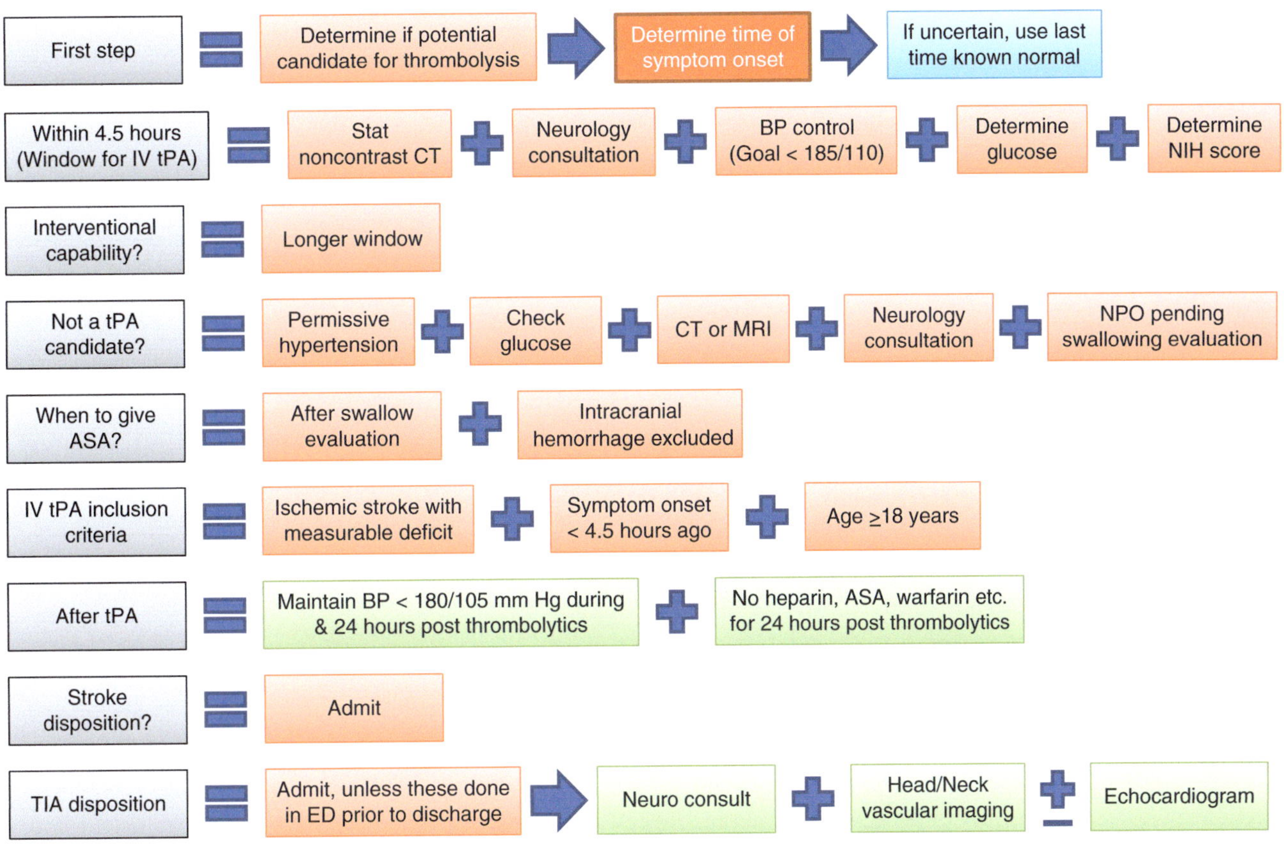

IV tPA Exclusions

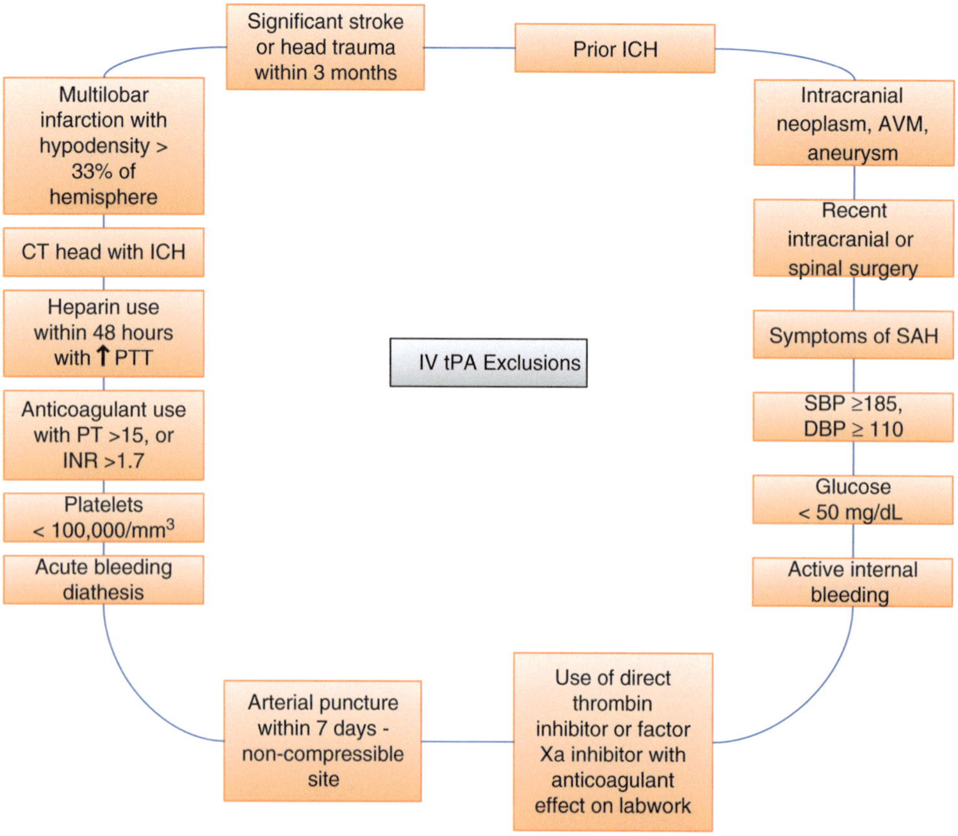

Relative Exclusions for IV tPA

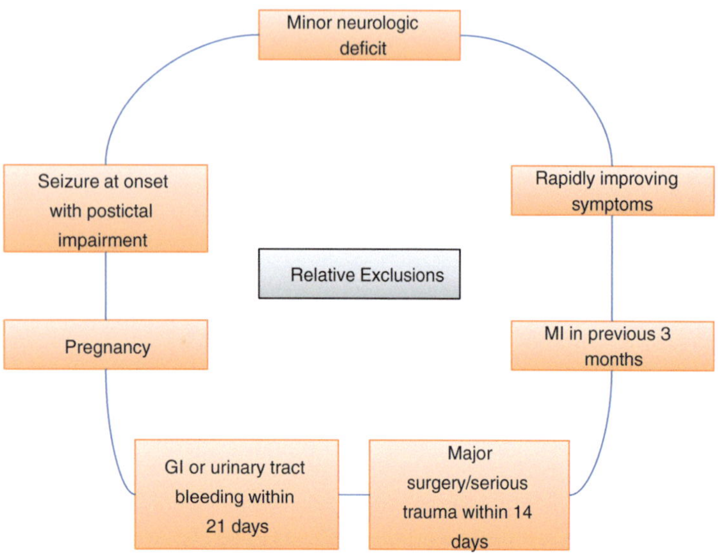

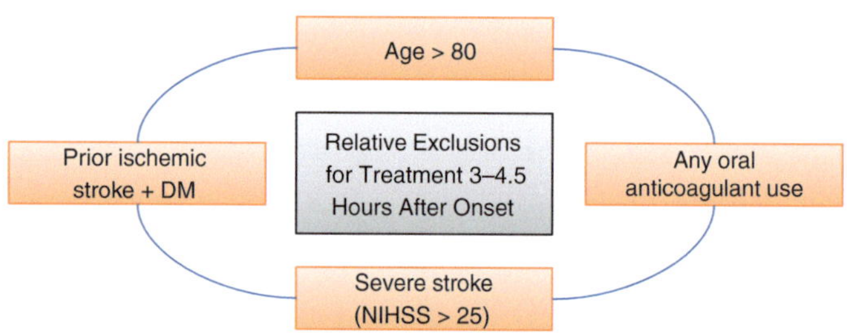

tPA Complications

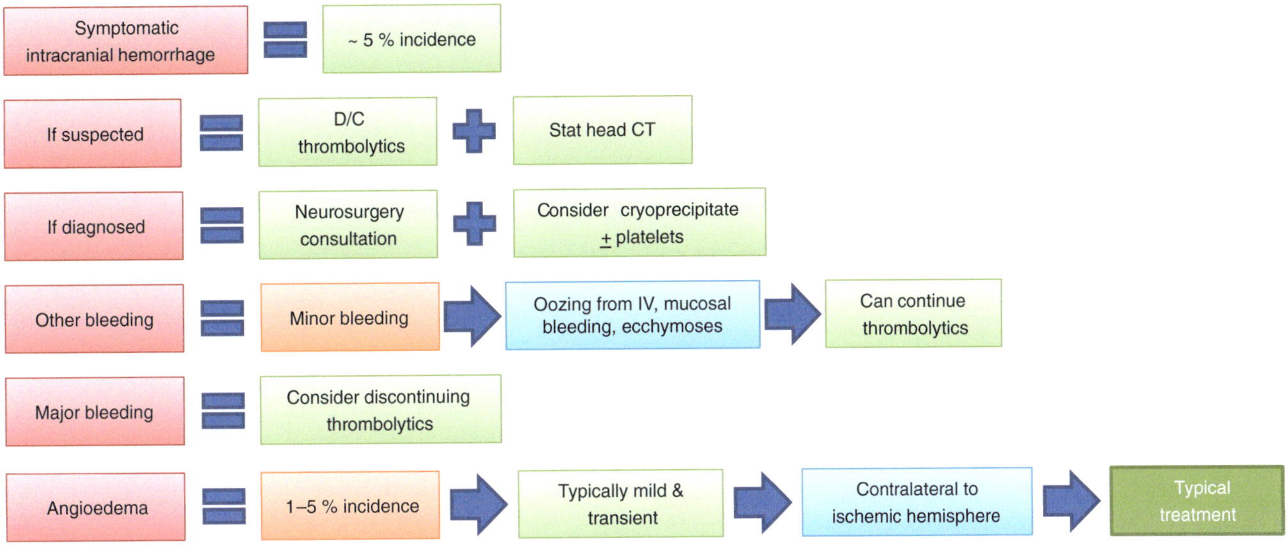

Spontaneous Intracranial Hemorrhage

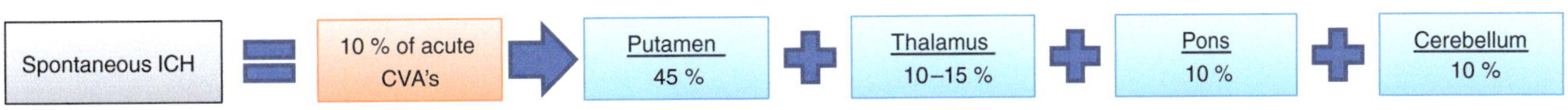

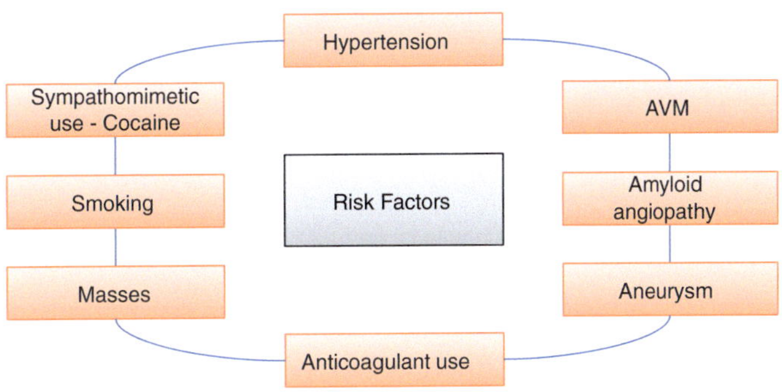

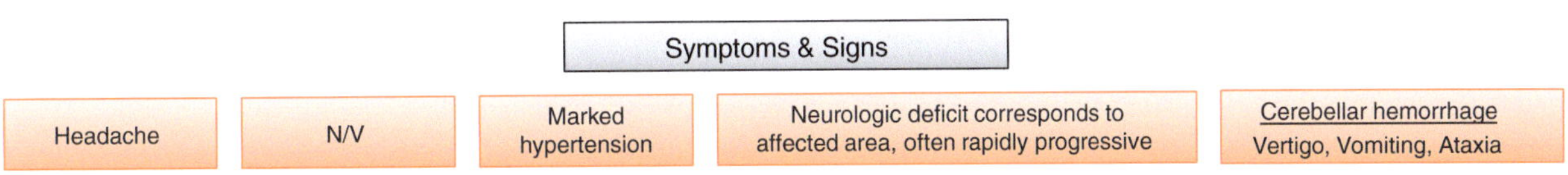

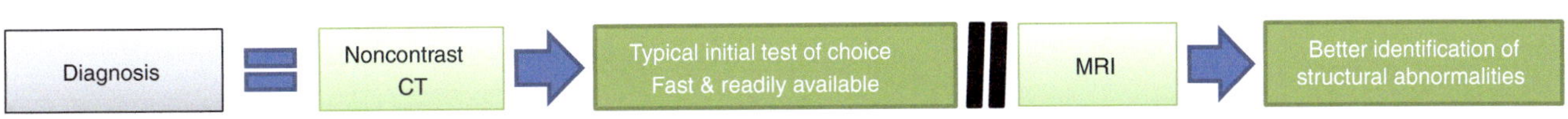

Intracranial Hemorrhage Management

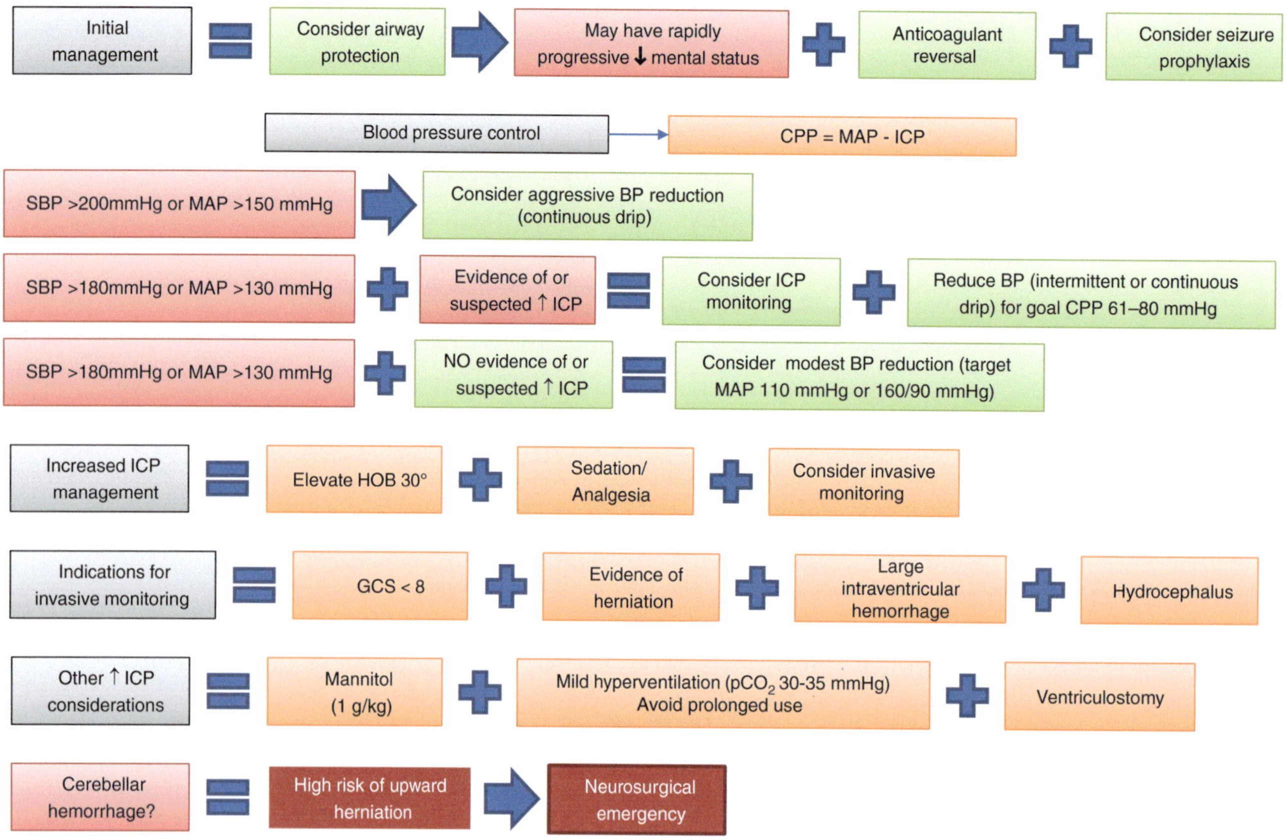

Seizures

Definitions

- Seizure = Neurologic dysfunction due to inappropriate electrical discharges of brain neurons
- Epilepsy = Recurrent seizures NOT due to secondary, reversible cause
- Primary seizure = No apparent cause identified
- Secondary seizure = Due to identifiable neurologic condition (tumor, CVA, trauma)
- Reactive seizure = Occur in otherwise normal individual exposed to insult (e.g., toxin)
- Status epilepticus = Seizure activity lasting over 5 minutes or 2 consecutive seizures without return to consciousness
- Todd's paralysis = Transient focal paralysis following seizure → Stroke mimic
- Pseudoseizure = Psychogenic nonepileptic seizures → Voluntary in nature → No loss of consciousness → No EEG changes

Seizure Classification: Generalized

- Generalized = Result of simultaneous activity involving entire cerebral cortex → Loss of consciousness without aura
- Convulsive (Grand mal) = Positive loss of consciousness → Muscle rigidity → Rhythmic, bilateral, generally symmetric contractions
- Convulsive (Grand mal) = Post-ictal state → Headache + Drowsiness
- Non-Convulsive (Petit mal) = Conscious activity suddenly ceases → Dissociated state for several seconds → Automatisms may be present
- Non-Convulsive (Petit mal) = No post-ictal confusion → Most common in children

Seizure Classification: Focal

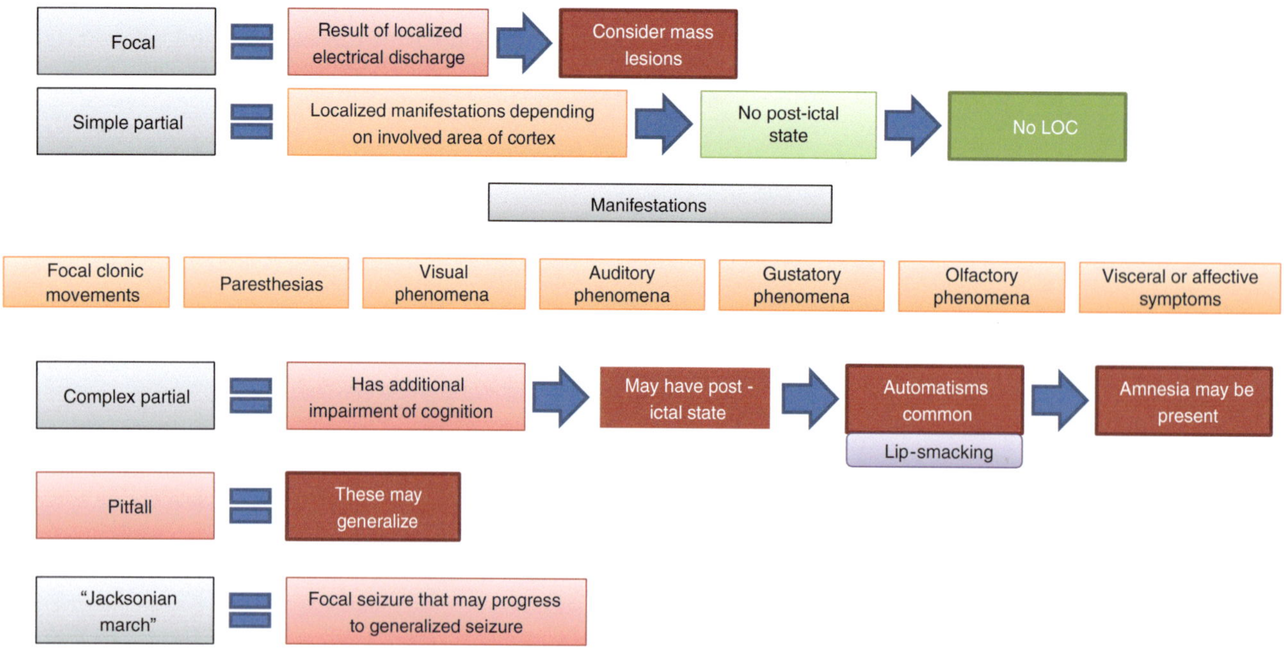

Causes of Secondary/Reactive Seizures

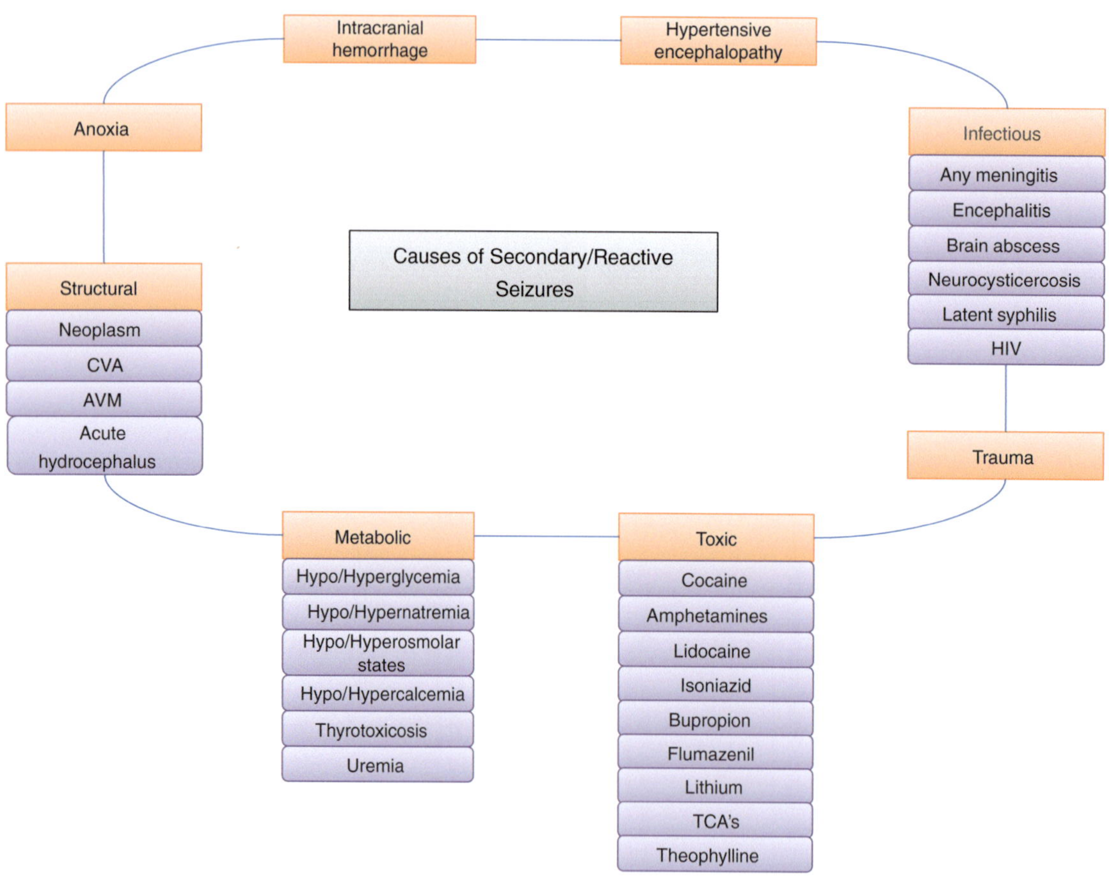

Seizure Mimics

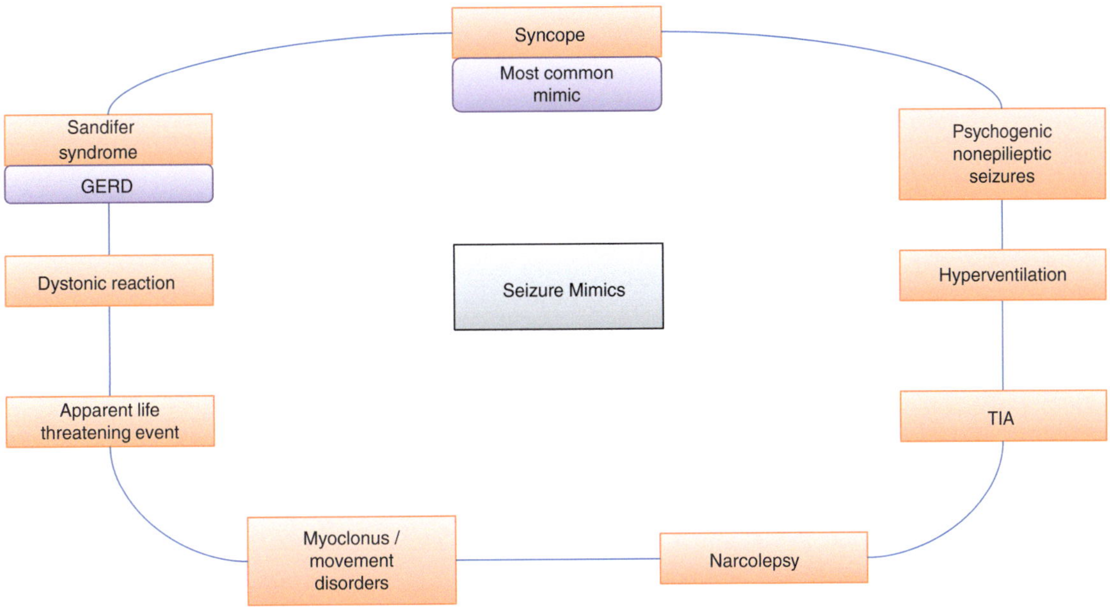

Seizure Versus Syncope

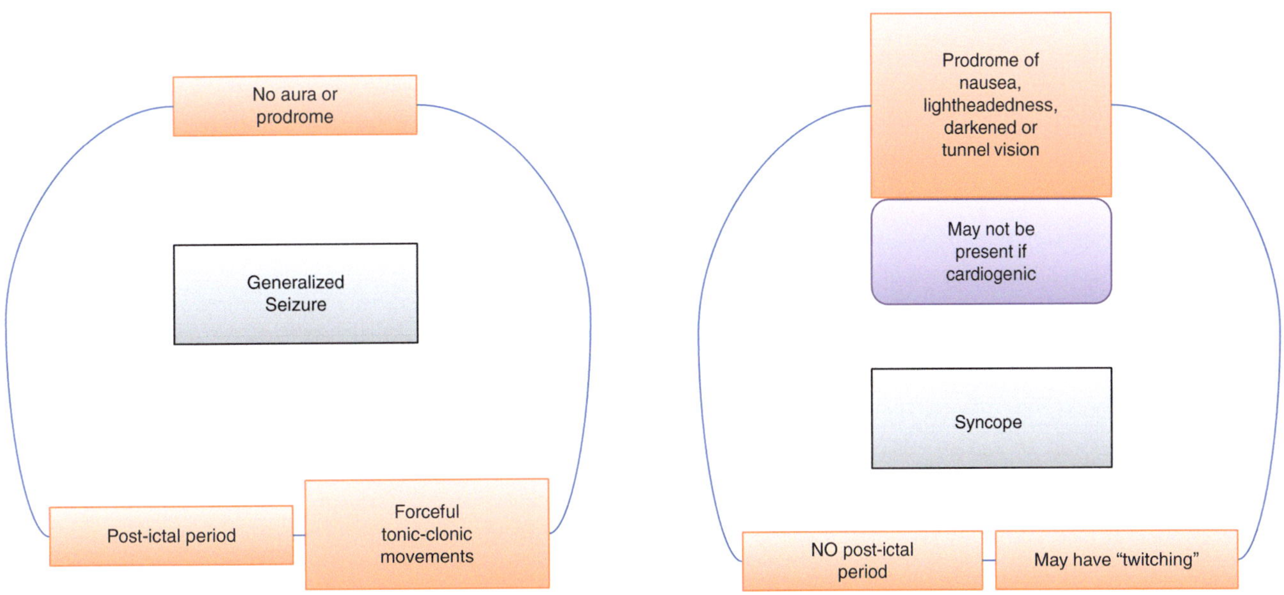

Routine First Seizure Evaluation

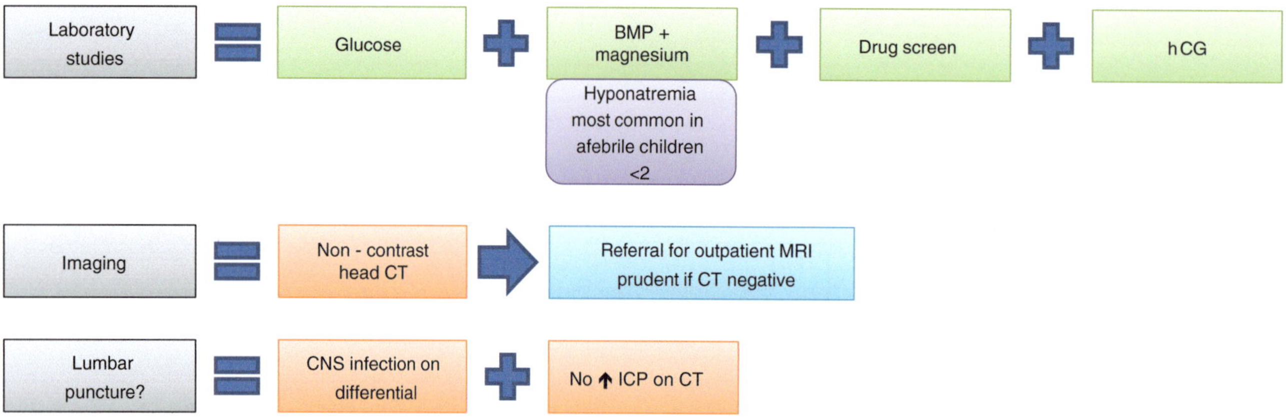

Recurrent Seizure Evaluation

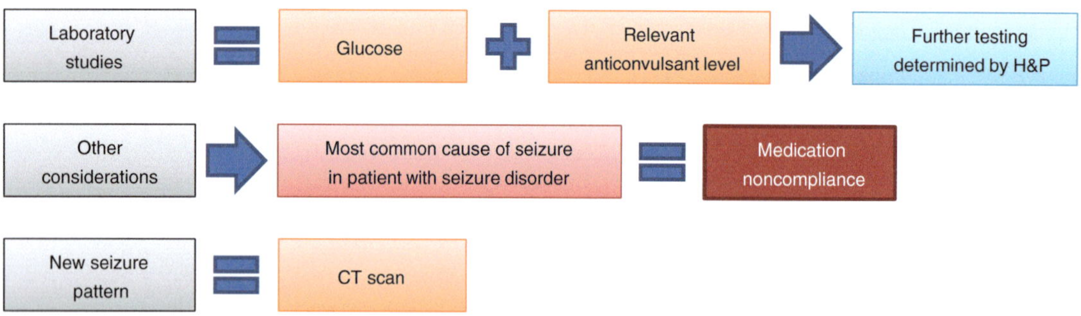

Adult Status Epilepticus Management

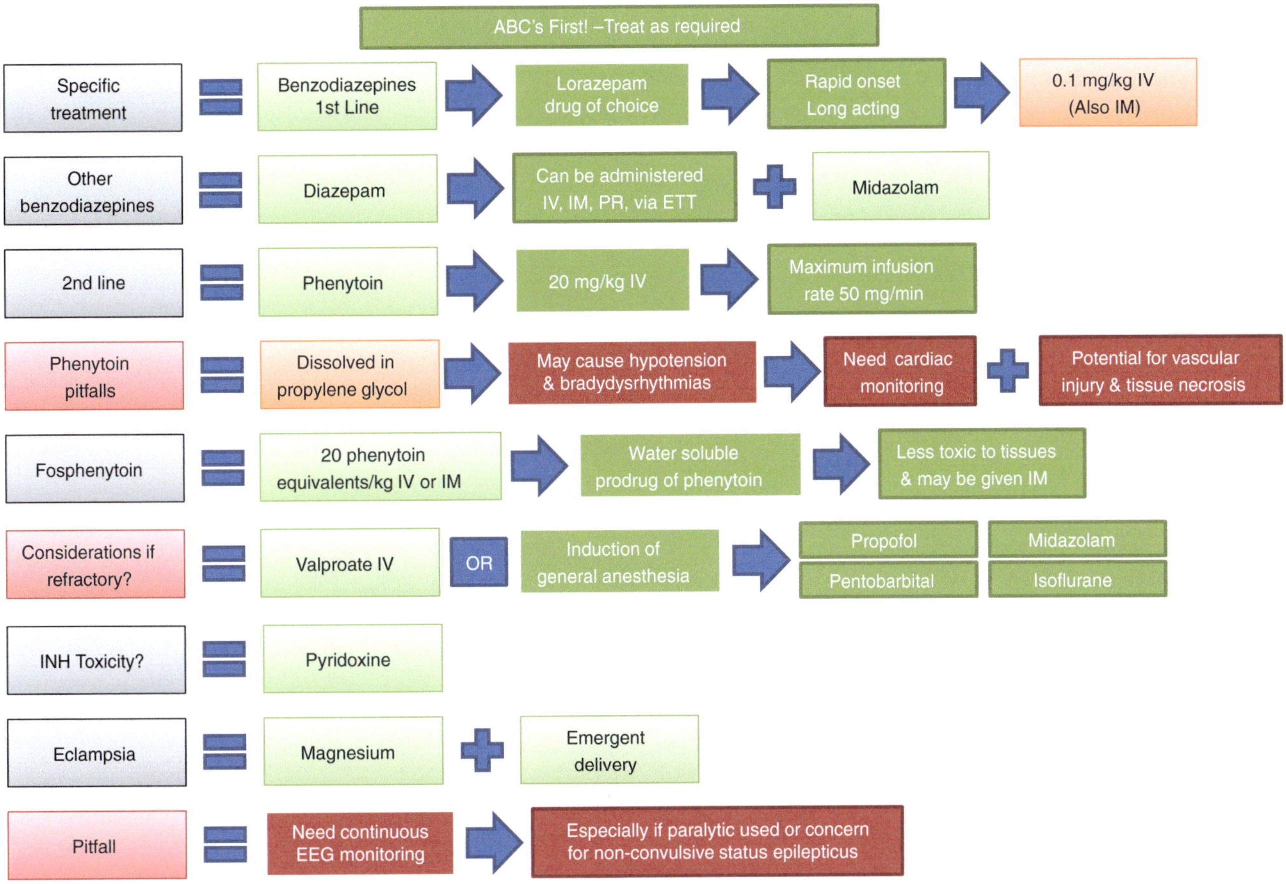

Disposition

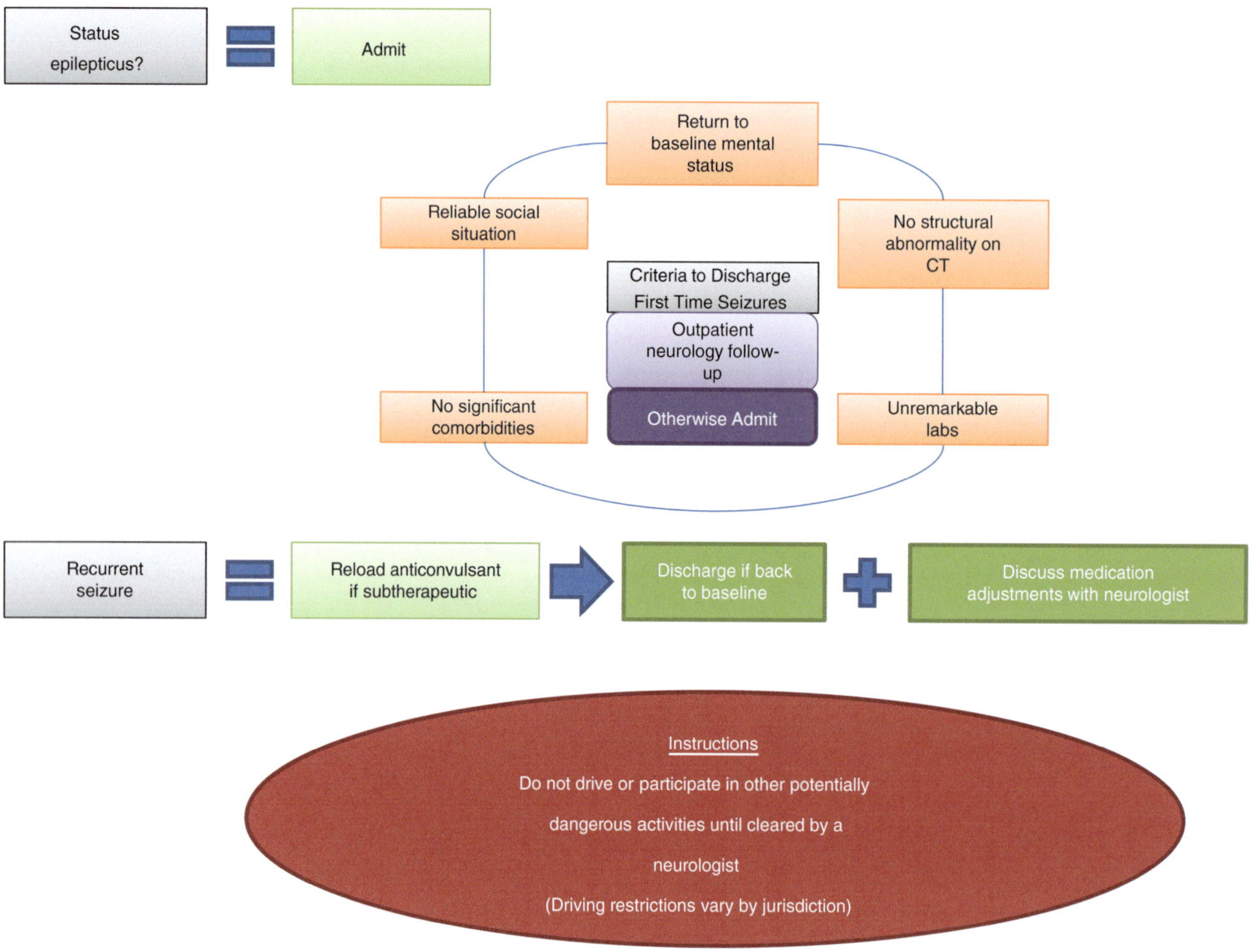

Febrile Seizures

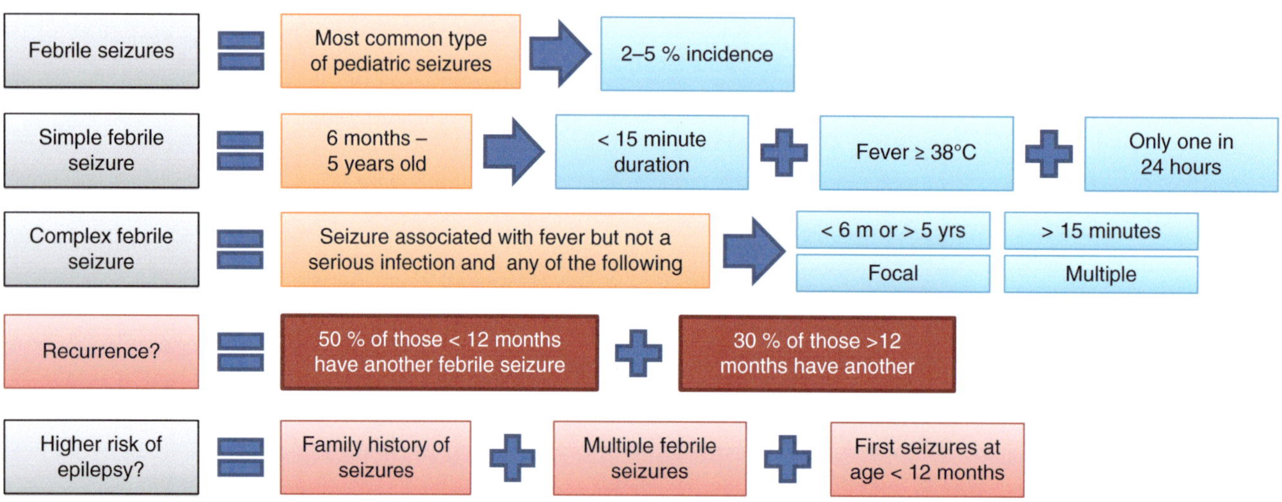

Febrile Seizure Evaluation and Management

Well appearing child? = Evaluation focuses on source of fever

Meningeal signs? = May not be present in young children → Age < 12 months Strongly consider LP + 12–18 months Consider LP

Complex febrile seizure = Consider LP + Septic workup

Prolonged seizure = LP

Ill-appearing = LP

Treatment = Diazepam per rectum if prolonged

Pitfall = Anticonvulsants not indicated

Neonatal Seizures (<28 Days)

Neonatal seizures = Often *not* a generalized tonic-clonic seizure

Neonatal Seizures: Apnea/ALTE; Eye deviation; Staring/Rhythmic blinking; Lip smacking; Bicycling

Differential: CNS infection; Intracranial hemorrhage; Hypoxic ischemic encephalopathy; Congenital brain malformations; Hypoglycemia; Hypocalcemia; Hypomagnesemia; Inborn errors of metabolism; Drug withdrawal or intoxication; Pyridoxine dependency

Evaluation = Glucose + Mg + Na + Ca + Consider ammonia & lactate if inborn error suspected + Septic workup + Neuroimaging

Specific treatment = Empirical treatment with IV antibiotics & acyclovir

Seizures? = Phenobarbital 1st Line → Pyridoxine if refractory

Background EEG abnormalities? = Poor prognosis

CNS Infections

Typical CSF Characteristics

	Normal	Bacterial	Viral	Fungal	TB	Abscess	Preterm Term Child Normals
WBCs	< 5	> 1000	< 1000	100-500	100-500	10-1000	0–25 7.3 ± 13.9 0–7
% PMNs	0-15	> 80	< 50	< 50	< 50	< 50	57 61–84 5
% Lymph	> 50	< 50	> 50	> 80	Inc. Mono	Varies	
Protein (mg/dL)	20-45	> 150	50-100	100-500	100-500	> 50	65–120 64.2 ± 24.2 5–40
Glucose (mg/dL)	40-65	< 40	40-65	30-45	30-45	45-60	24–63 51.2 ± 12.9 40–80
Opening pressure (cm H_2O)	6-20	> 25-30	Variable	> 20	> 20	Variable	8–11 < 20 < 20

Pitfalls = Viral profile may be seen with partially treated bacterial meningitis + CSF sterilization can occur within 2 hours of IV antibiotic administration

Meningitis Introduction

Natural history viral meningitis = Typically gradual onset of symptoms over several days

---

Mechanisms for bacterial meningitis = Entry via upper airway OR Contiguous spread

Pathophysiology of direct entry = Entry into upper airway → Hematogenous spread → Seeding of subarachnoid space

Contiguous spread? = From multiple sites → Brain abscess, otitis media, sinusitis, mastoiditis, cavernous sinus

Final common pathway = Inflammation of subarachnoid space → Violation of blood brain barrier → Edema → Ischemia

---

Mechanisms for fungal meningitis = Inhalation → Hematogenous spread

Fungal meningitis = Much more common in immunocompromised → Cryptococcus occurs in up to 10 % of HIV + patients → Generally CD4 count < 100

Meningitis

Symptoms & Signs

- Fever
- Headache
- Photophobia
- Vomiting
- Altered mental status
- Seizures
- Nuchal rigidity

Infants: Bulging fontanelle, Irritability, Poor feeding

Exam Findings

- Skin Rash: Petechiae; *N. meningitidis*; RMSF
- Brudzinski's sign: Passive neck flexion causes hip and knee flexion
- Kernig's sign: Passive knee extension while hips flexed causes pain
- Jolt accentuation test: Quick movement of head from side to side in a horizontal plane causes worsening headache

Pitfall = Common symptoms & exam findings may not be present in *infants* & *elderly*

Causes of Viral Meningitis

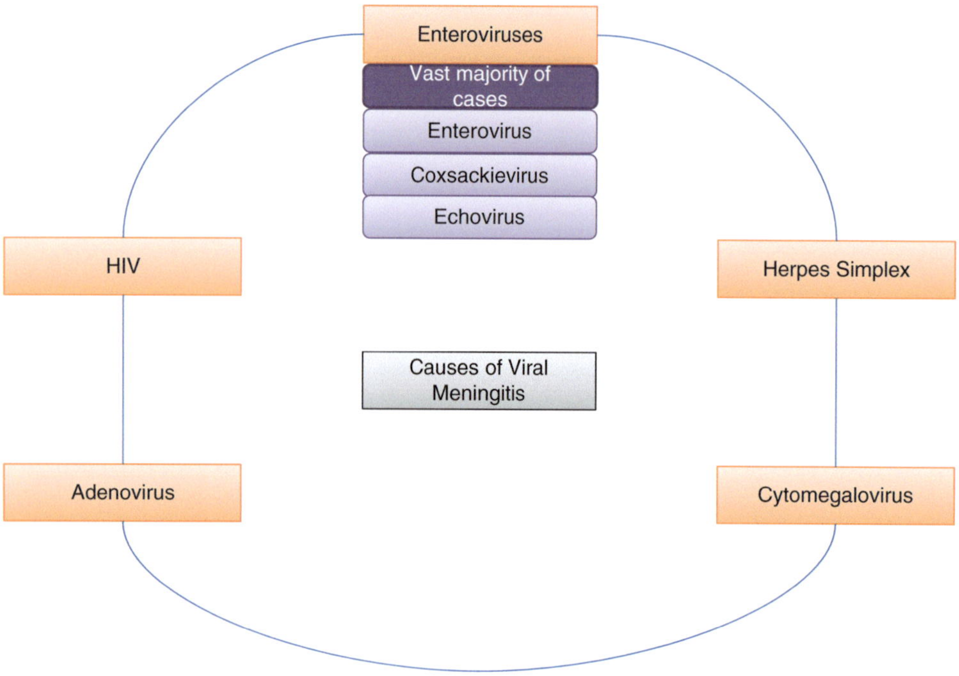

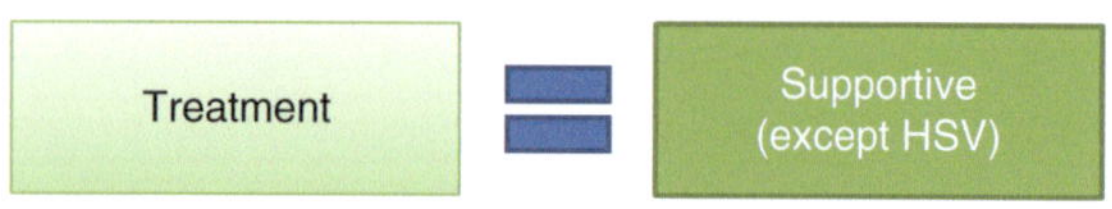

Causes of Bacterial Meningitis

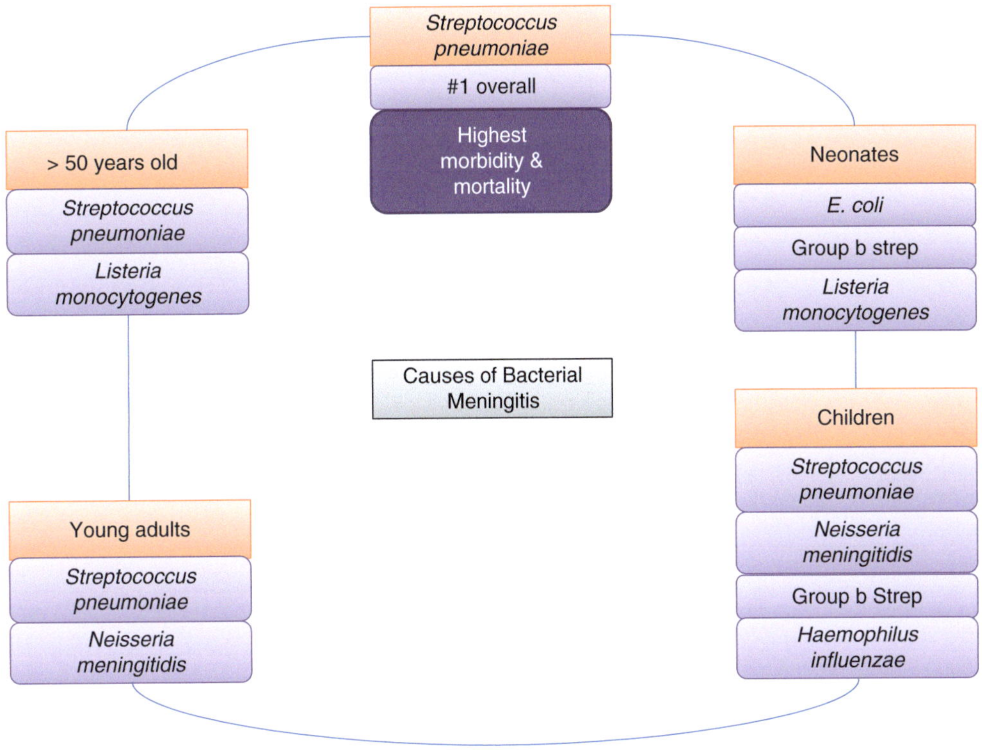

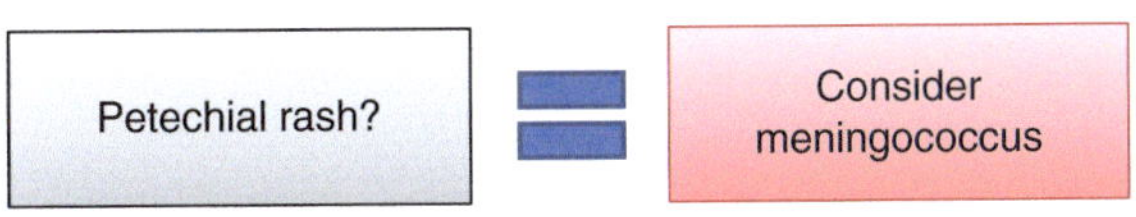

Risk Factors

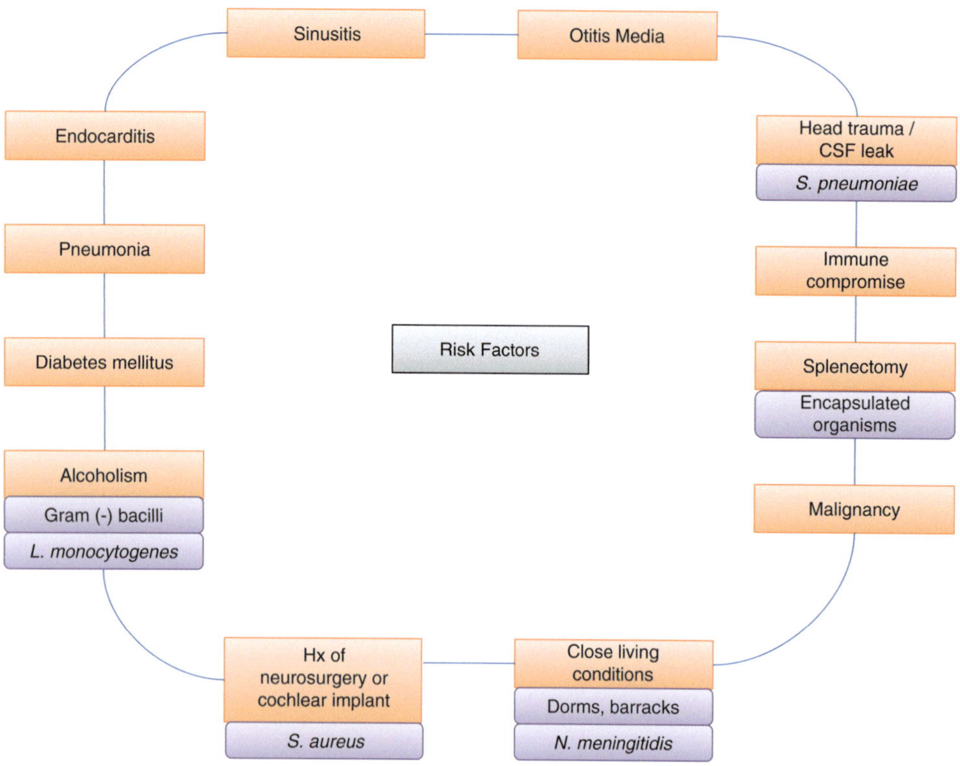

Meningitis Prophylaxis

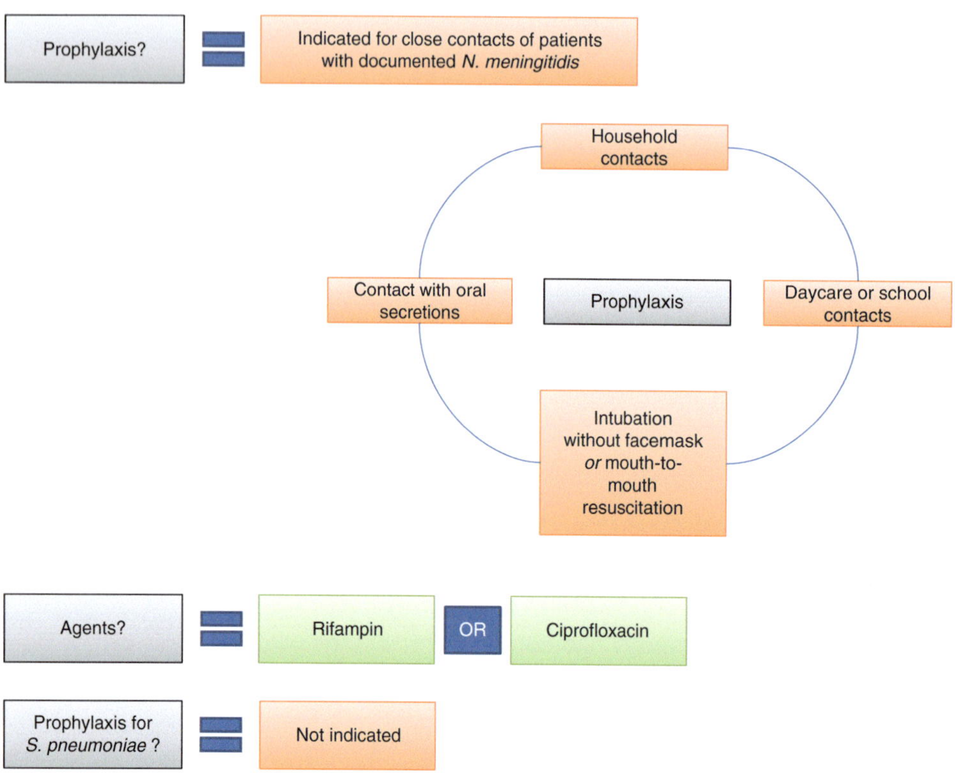

Evaluation

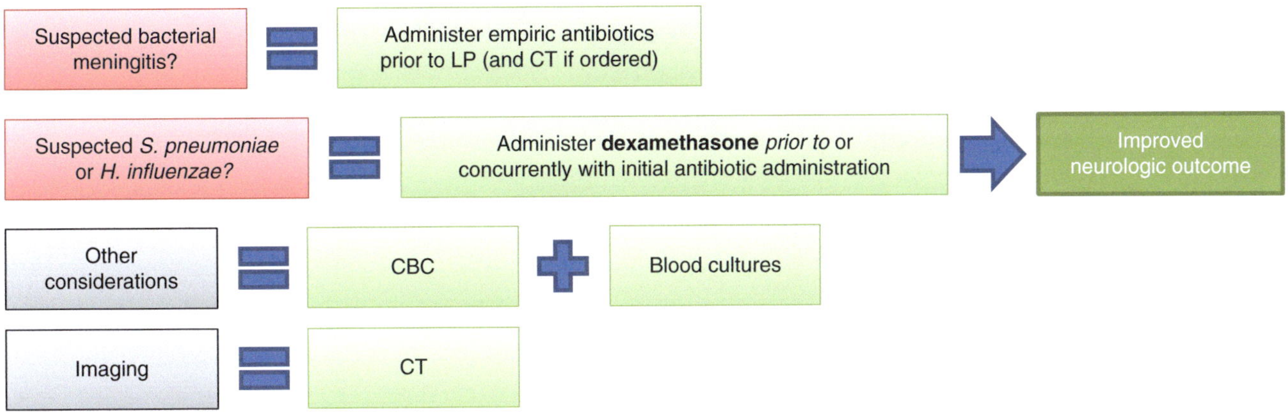

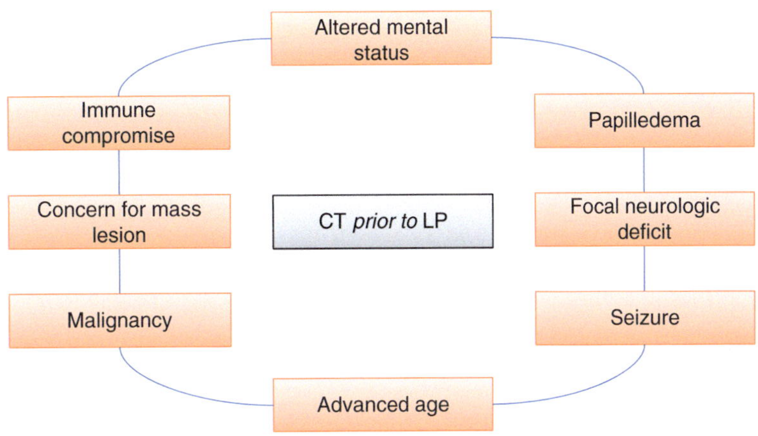

Empiric Antibiotic Treatment

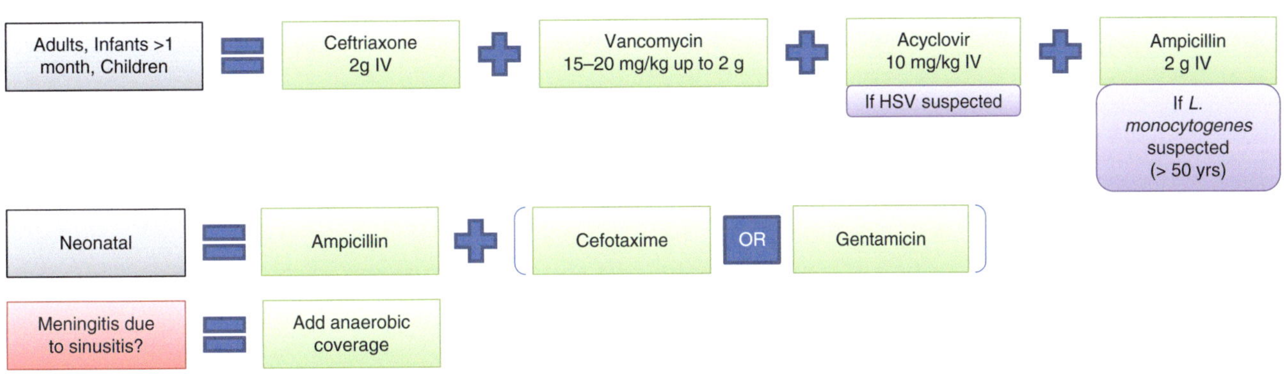

Fungal Meningitis

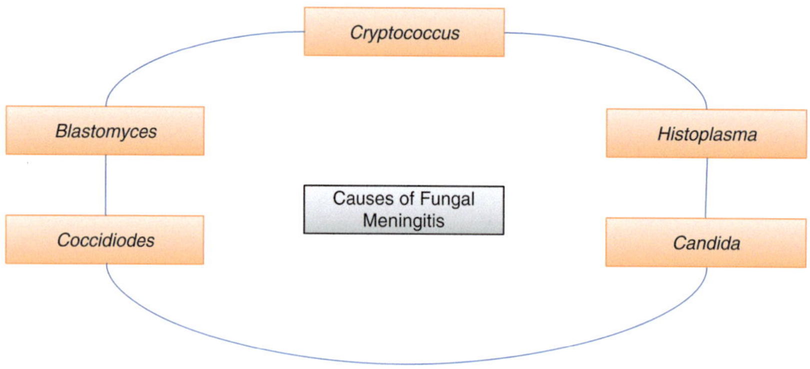

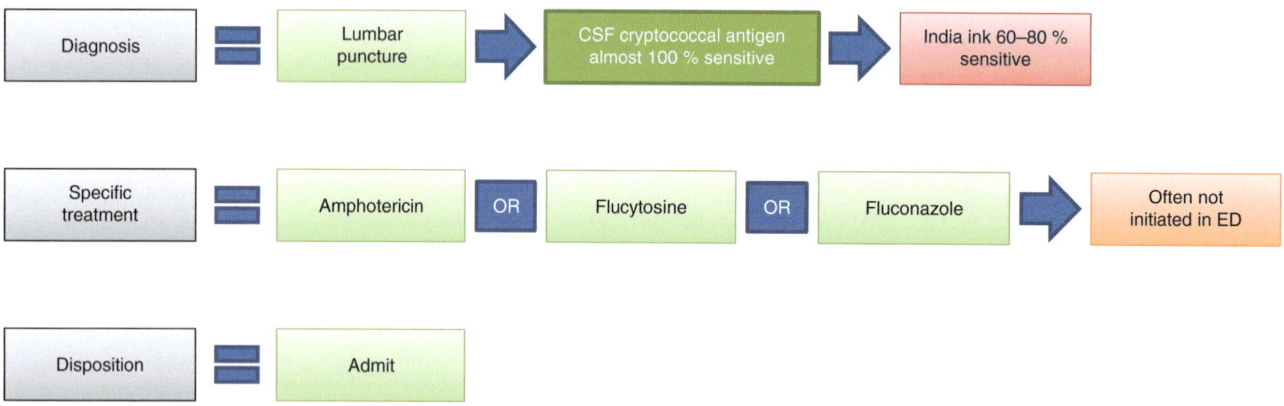

Encephalitis

Encephalitis: Introduction

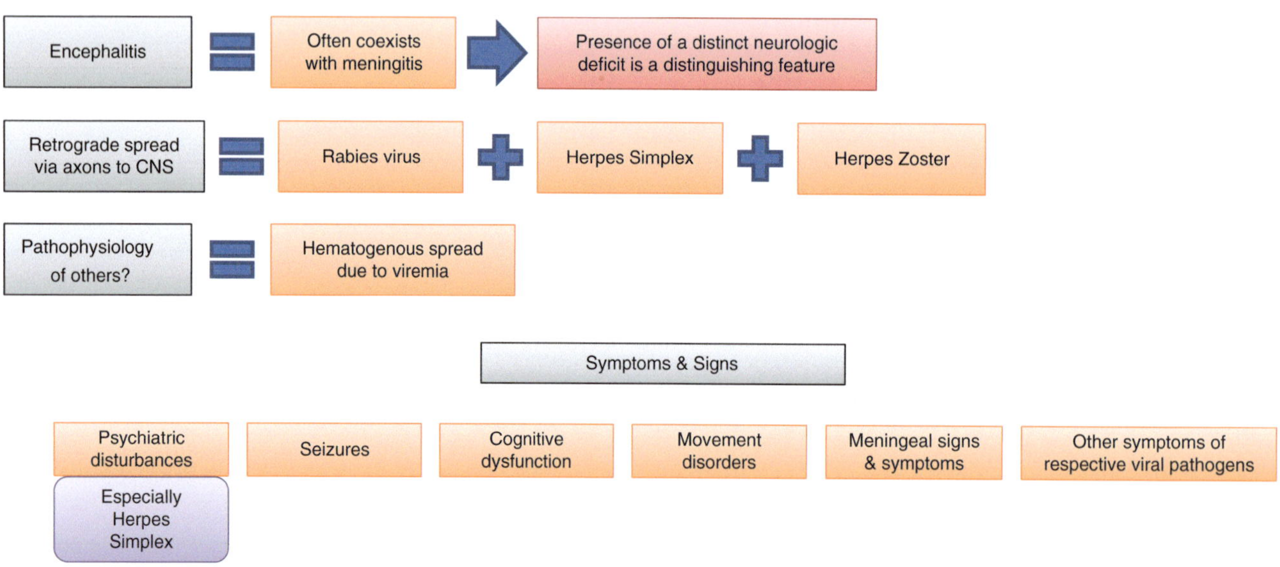

Encephalitis Causes

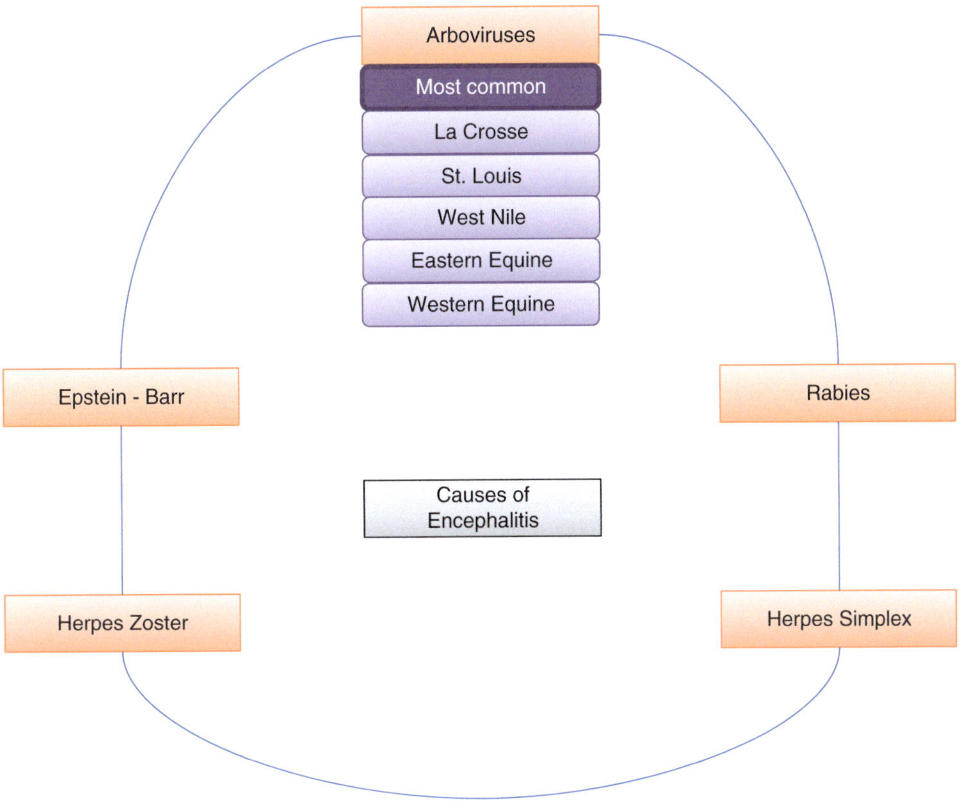

Encephalitis Diagnosis and Management

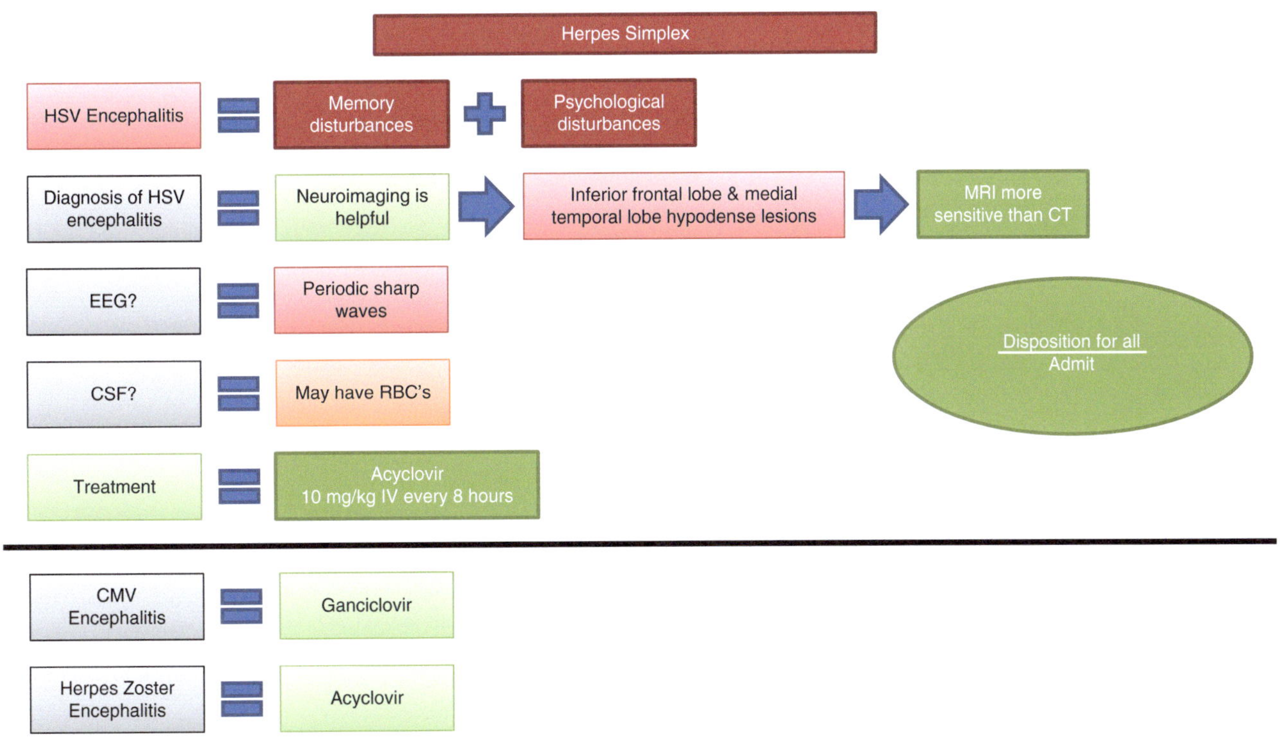

Brain Abscess

Brain Abscess Introduction

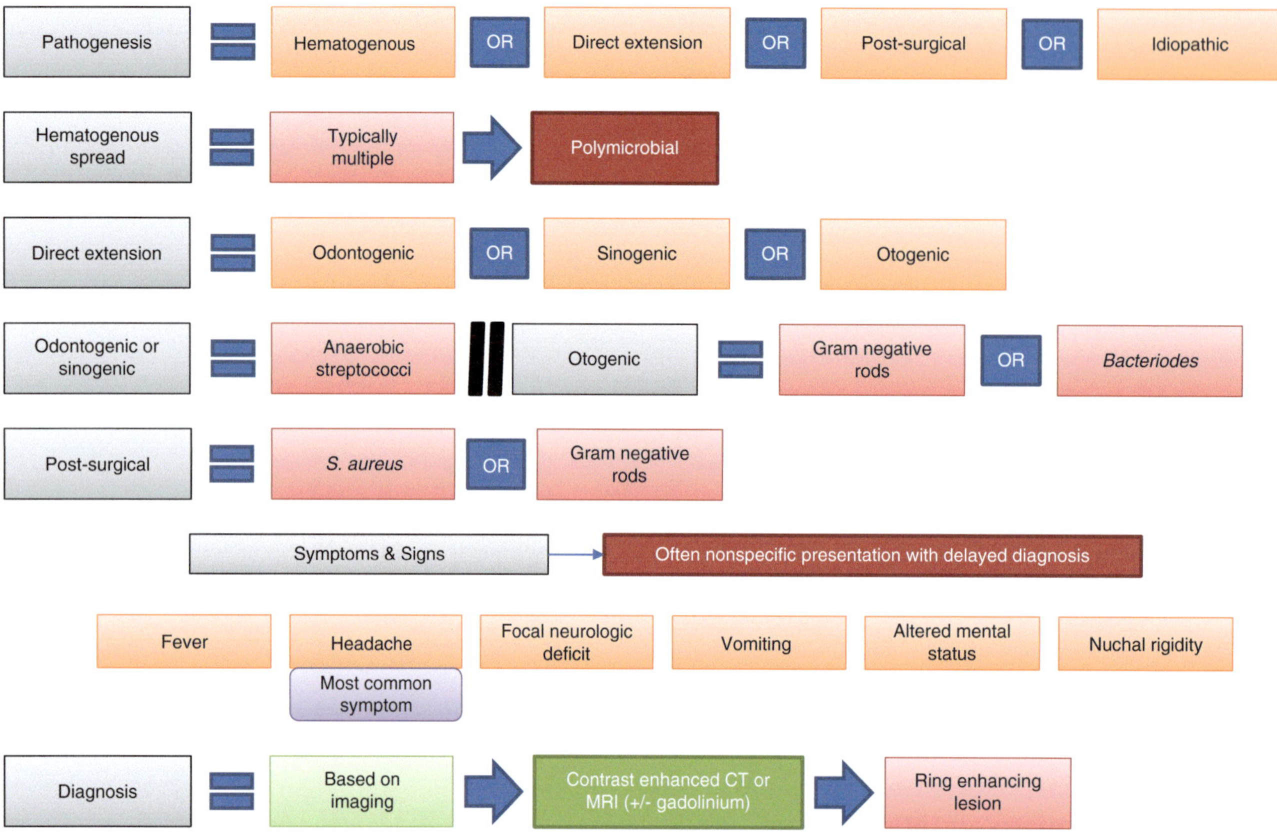

Management

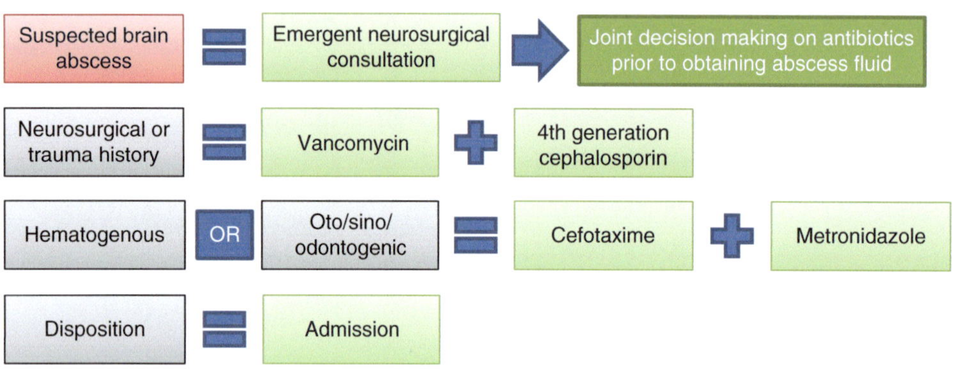

Headache Syndromes

Headache Red Flags: "SNOOP"

Odor	Agent
Systemic symptoms	Fever, weight loss
Secondary risk factors	Cancer, HIV
Neurologic symptoms	Altered mental status, focal deficits
Onset	Sudden or abrupt onset
Older	New onset headache > 50 years old
Previous history	First headache or change in headache frequency, severity or features
Eyes	Diplopia, papilledema, red eye, halos around light

Headache Classification

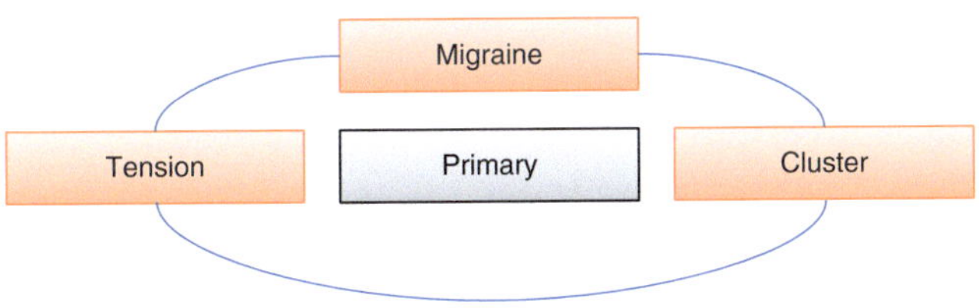

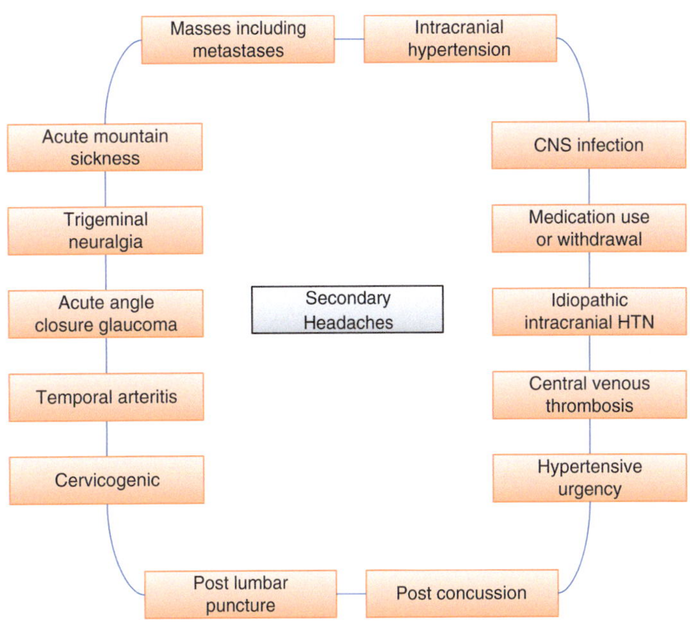

Migraine Introduction

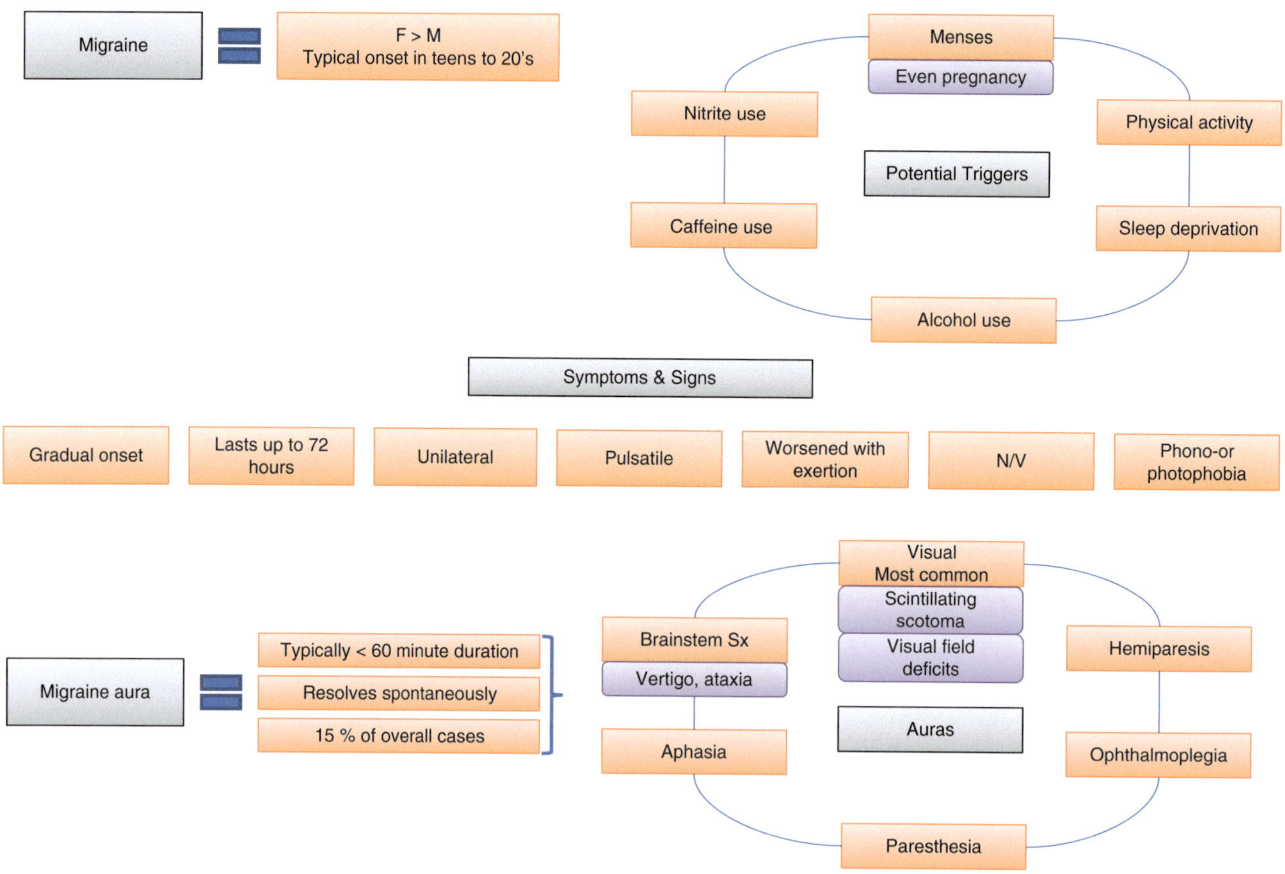

Migraine Treatment

Dopamine antagonists = Prochlorperazine OR Metoclopramide OR Droperidol

Pitfall = Potential for dystonic reactions + QTc prolongation with high doses of droperidol

DHE = Dopamine and $5HT_{1B/1D}$ agonist

DHE contraindications = Pregnancy + Patients with CAD + Basilar migraines + Hemiplegic migraines

Pitfalls = High incidence of emesis → Pretreat with antiemetic

Triptans = Selective $5HT_{1D}$ agonists → Less N/V

Triptan contraindications = Patients with HTN + Patients with CAD

Pitfall = Do not give within 24 hours of DHE + Causes increased vasoconstriction

Opioids = Can be effective for rescue analgesia But… → Frequent use may cause rebound/worsened HA

Steroids = May be effective for status migrainosus

Prophylactic Treatments
(Usually not started in ED)
Lifestyle modification
β–blockers
Ca-channel blockers
TCA's

Tension Headache

Symptoms & Signs

- Bilateral
- Band-like
- Non-pulsatile character
- Lasts minutes to days
- No aggravation with activity
- No focal deficits
- ±N/V
- NO Phono-or photophobia

Treatment = NSAIDs → If severe, consider migraine treatment

Cluster Headache

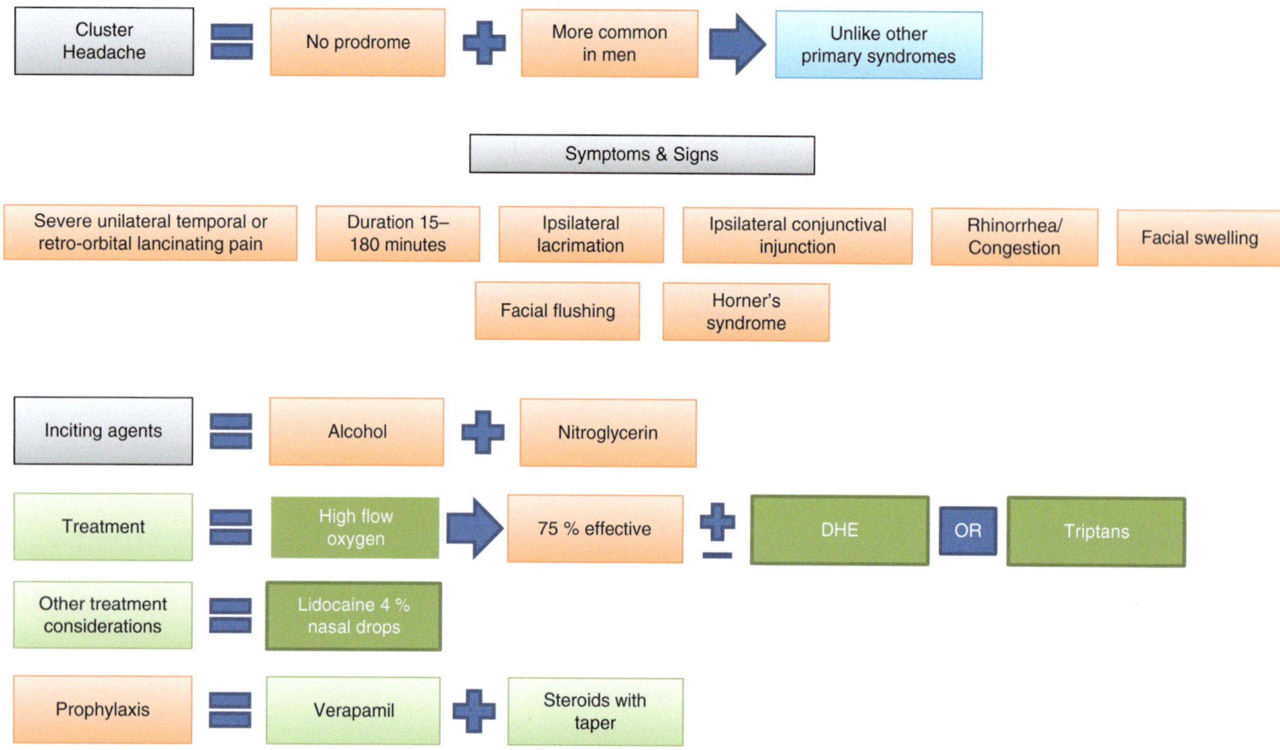

Trigeminal Neuralgia

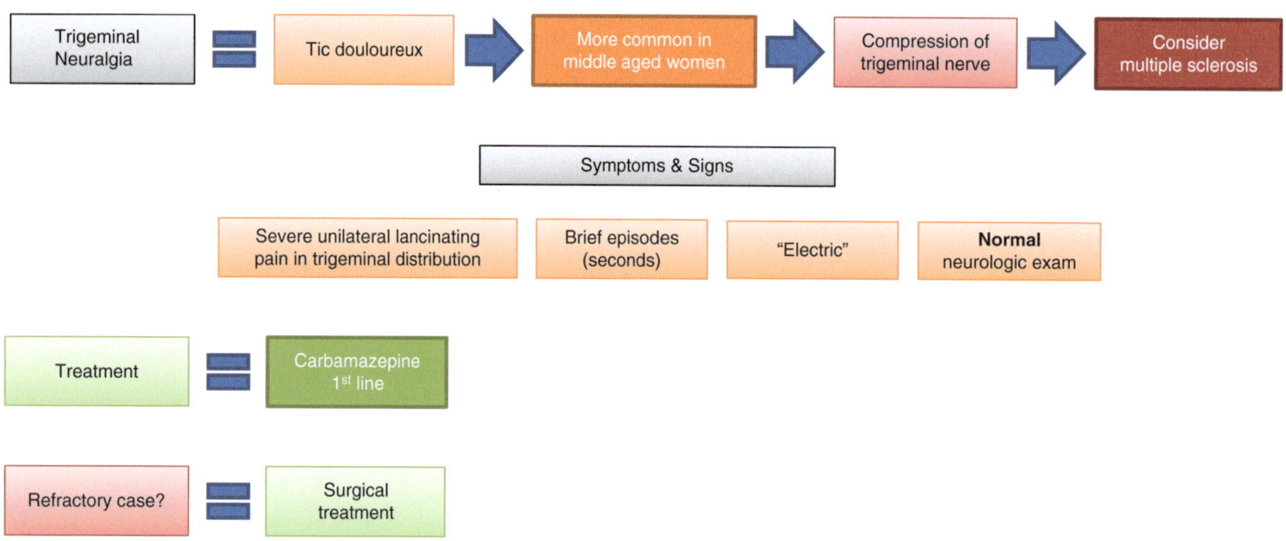

Post-lumbar Puncture Headache

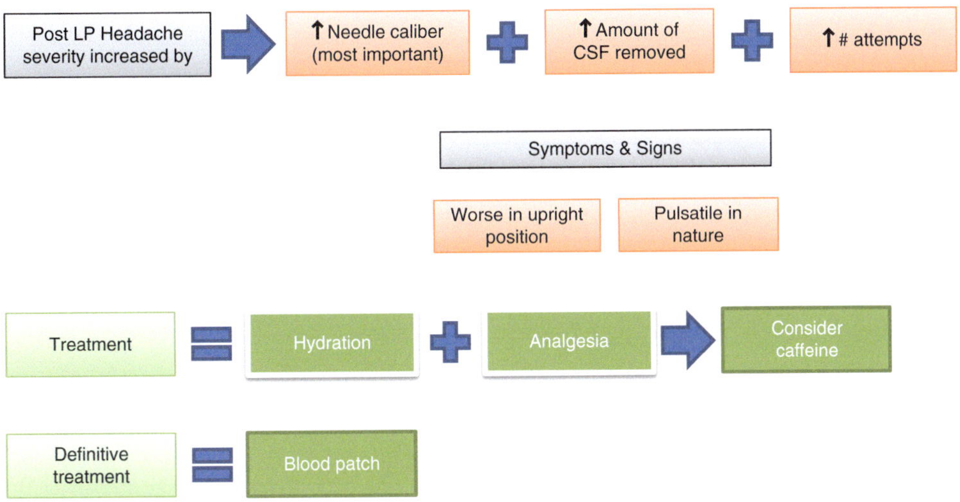

Toxic Metabolic Headache

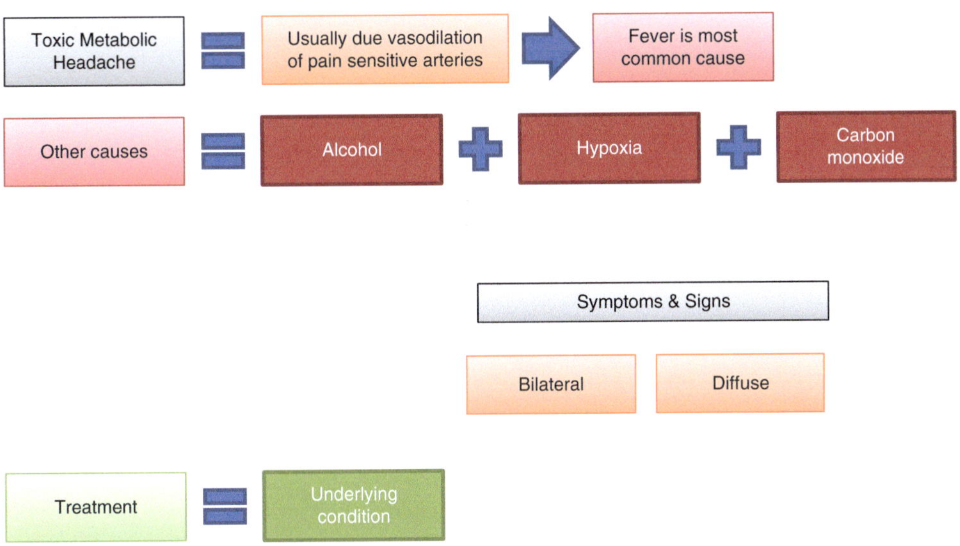

Headache Related to CNS Tumors

CNS Tumors = Headache most common Sx → Often worse at night

Symptoms & Signs

- HA may be diffuse or focal
- HA may be new onset or an increase in frequency or duration of chronic HA
- HA worse with valsalva
- HA worse with laying down
- Sleep disturbance
- Focal neurologic deficit
- N/V
- Seizures

Most common metastases to brain

- Lung
- Breast
- Melanoma
- Genitourinary
- Colon

Diagnosis = MRI test of choice → IV contrast ↑ sensitivity of CT

Treatment of acute ↑ ICP = Dexamethasone + Emergent neurosurgery consultation

Pseudotumor Cerebri (Idiopathic Intracranial Hypertension)

Pseudotumor Cerebri = Young obese females → Typically with irregular menses & amenorrhea → Due to impaired CSF absorption → ↑ CSF pressure without mass or obstruction

Symptoms & Signs

- Nausea & vomiting
- Diffuse headache
- Visual changes
- Papilledema (90 %)
- Double vision
- Pain behind eye
- Pain with eye movement
- Tinnitus
- NO focal deficits

Imaging = CT shows slit-like or normal ventricles → No mass effect

Diagnosis = Lumbar puncture shows high opening pressure

Treatment = Repeated LP's + Acetazolamide ± Shunt if refractory

Other treatment considerations = Weight loss + Steroids + Nerve sheath fenestration

Vision perimetry testing guides adequacy of treatment

Hydrocephalus

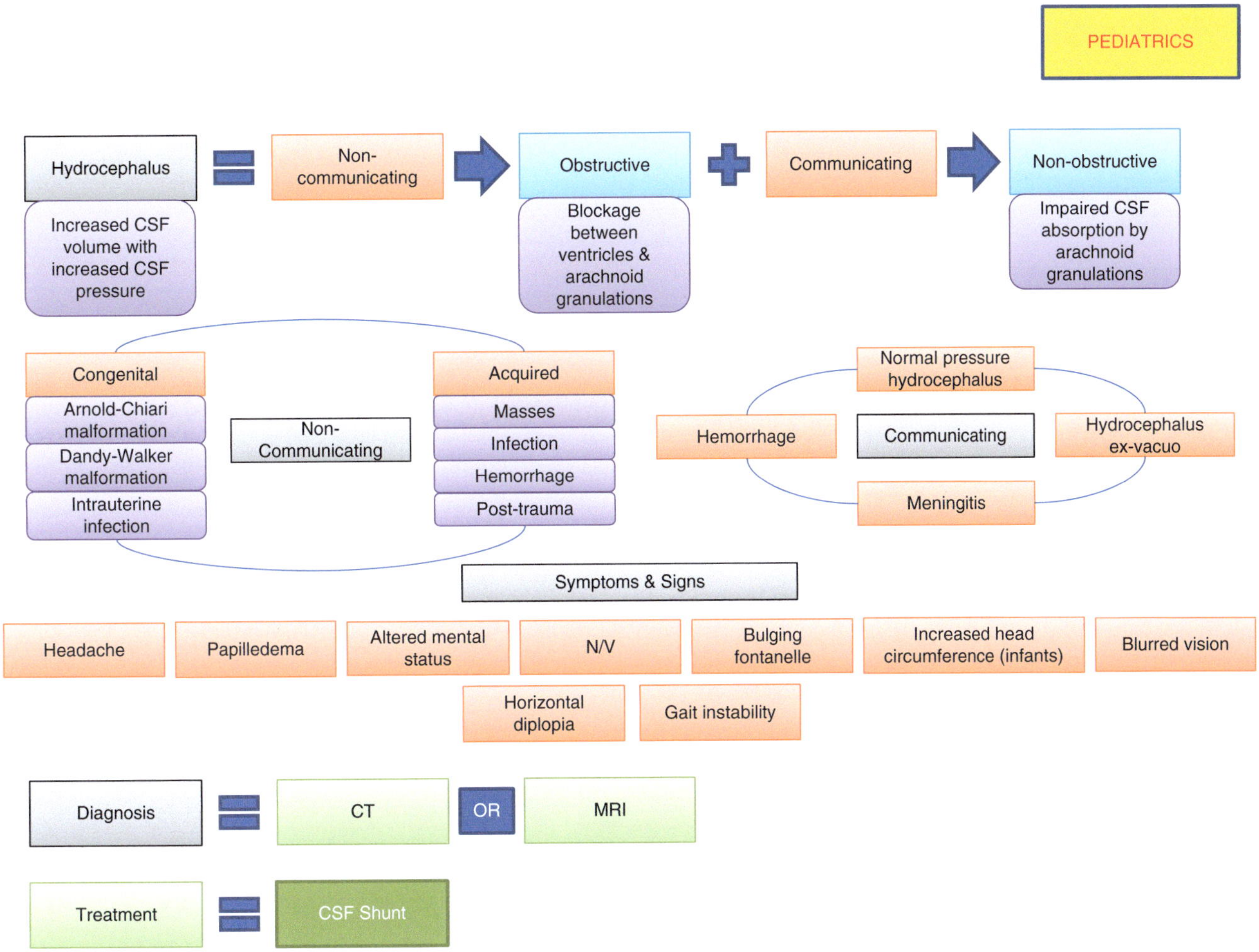

Pediatric Hydrocephalus Tidbits

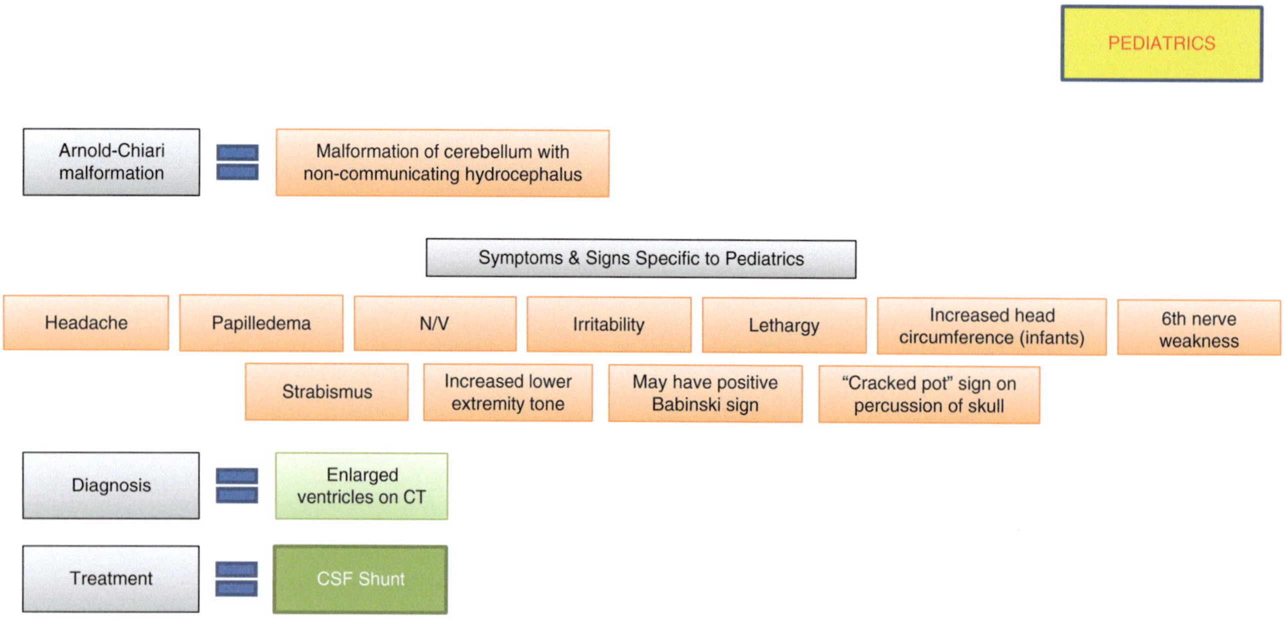

Normal Pressure Hydrocephalus

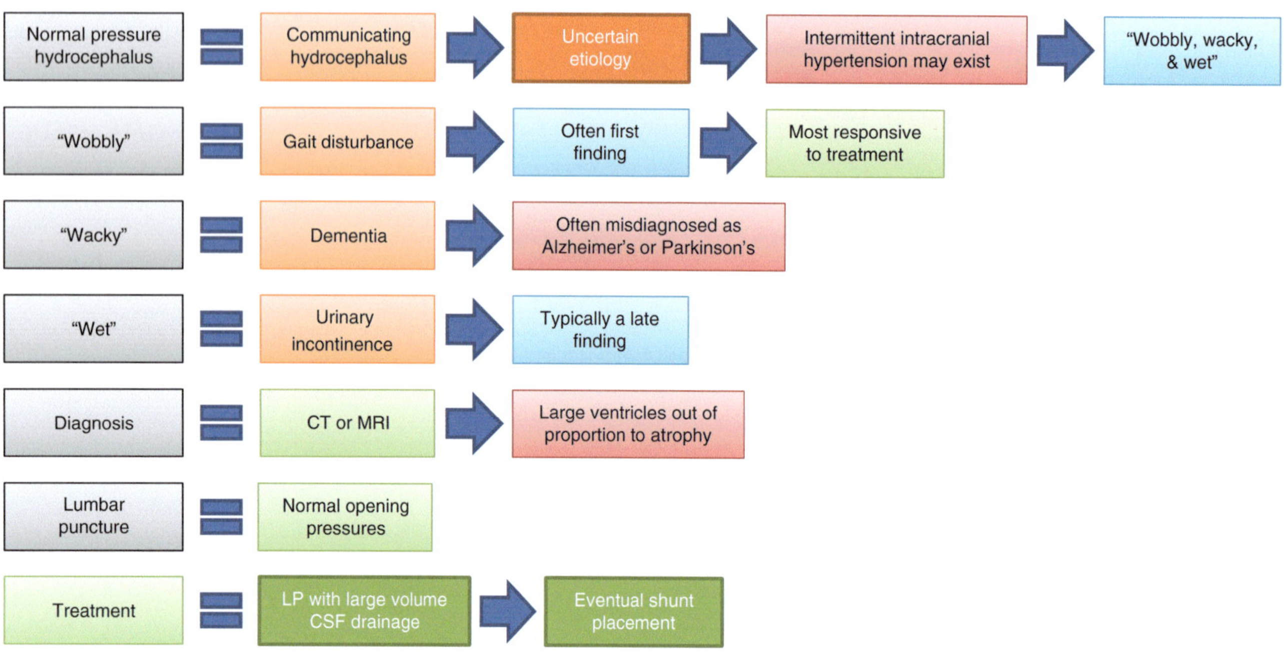

Ventricular Shunt Headache

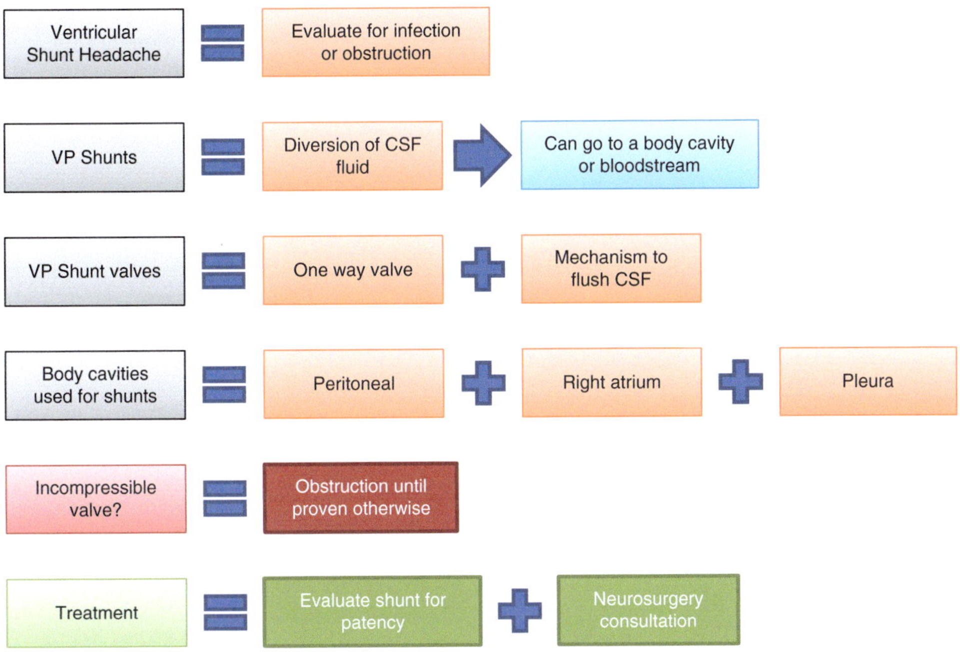

VP Shunt Complications: Malfunction

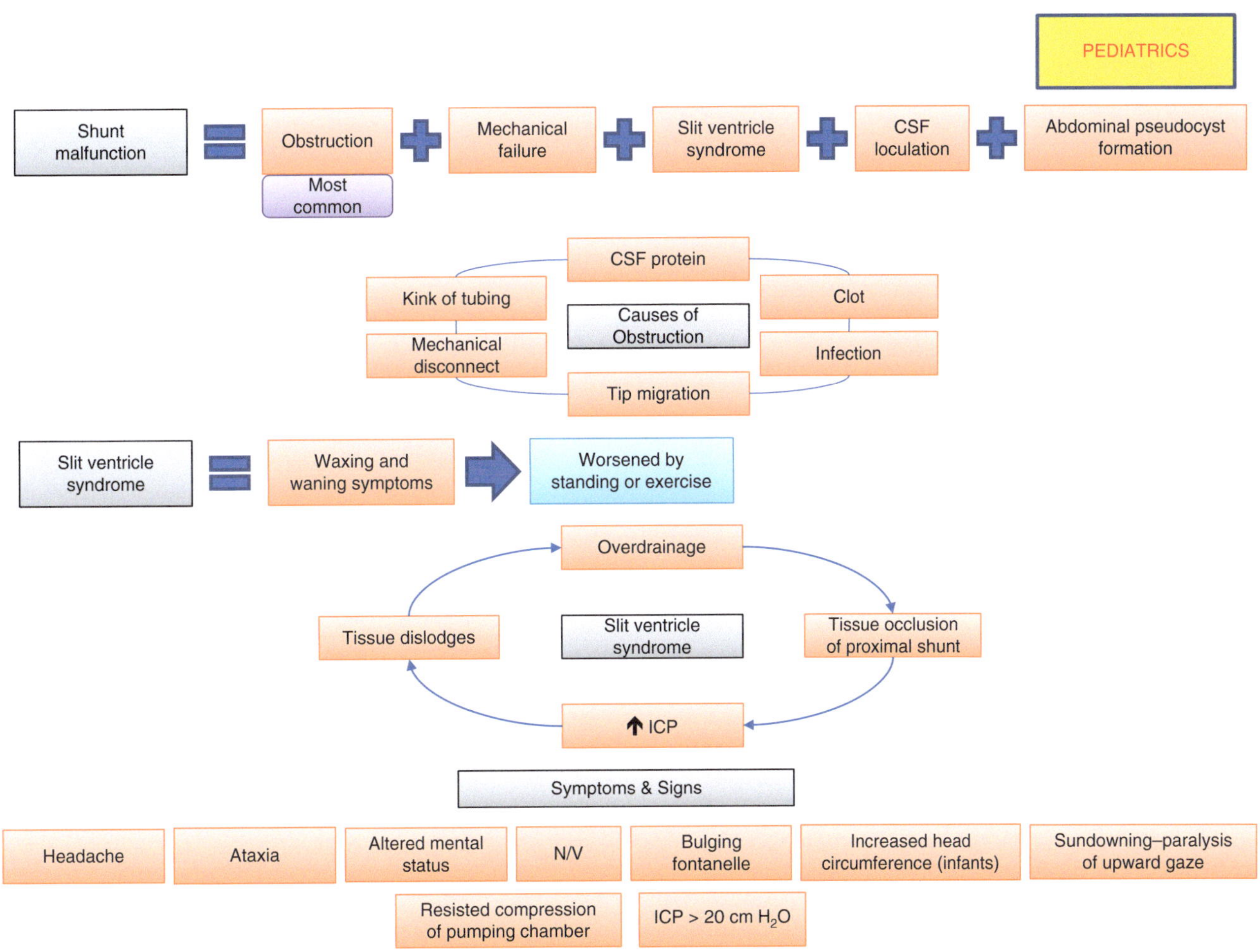

VP Shunt Complications: Infection

PEDIATRICS

Shunt infection = 50 % within 2 weeks post-op → Up to 10 % > 1 year post-op

Typical pathogens = *S. epidermidis* (#1) + *S. aureus* + *H. influenzae*

Symptoms & Signs

- Fever
- N/V
- Altered mental status
- Headache
- Abdominal pain
- Erythema/tenderness over tubing
- Meningismus
- Sepsis
- Peritonitis

Pitfall = May have peritonitis

Diagnosis and Treatment of VP Shunt Complications

Diagnosis = CT head + Shunt series → Both not 100 % sensitive & if Sx suggestive Neurosurgery consult mandatory

Suspected infection? = Shunt tap

Pitfall = Standard LP may miss shunt infection

Suspected peritonitis? = Broad spectrum antibiotics + Neurosurgery consultation

Treatment of obstruction = Elevate head + Neurosurgery consultation for potential shunt revision

Treatment of infection = Vancomycin + Ceftazidime

Coma OR Cardiopulmonary arrest OR Sudden worsening of condition = Emergent tap of shunt

Venous Sinus Thrombosis

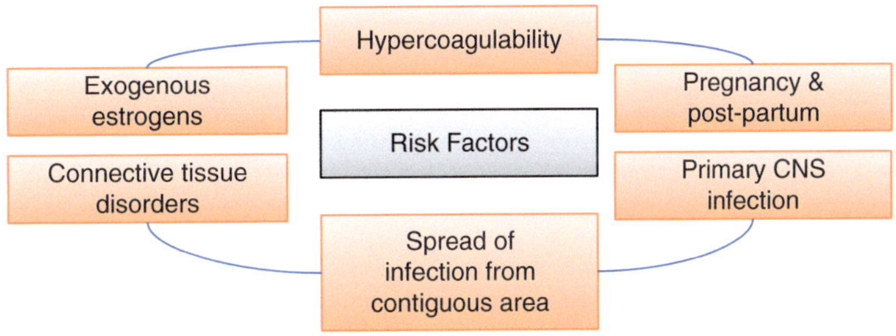

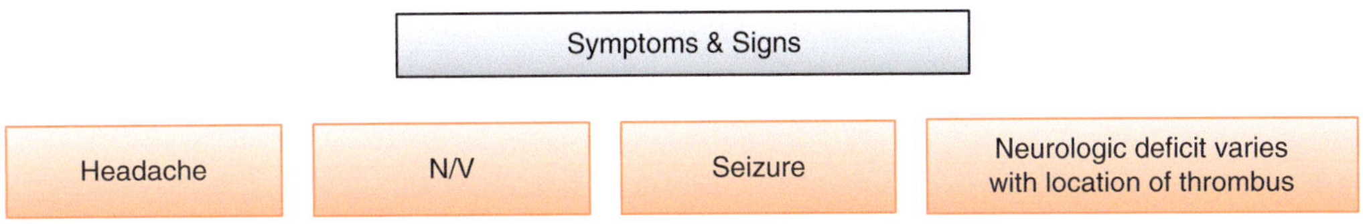

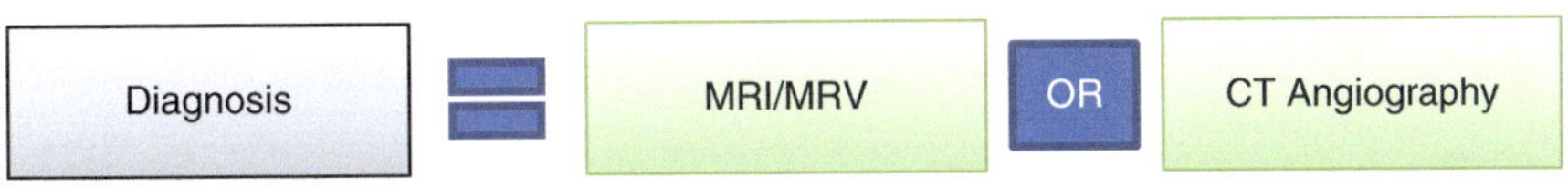

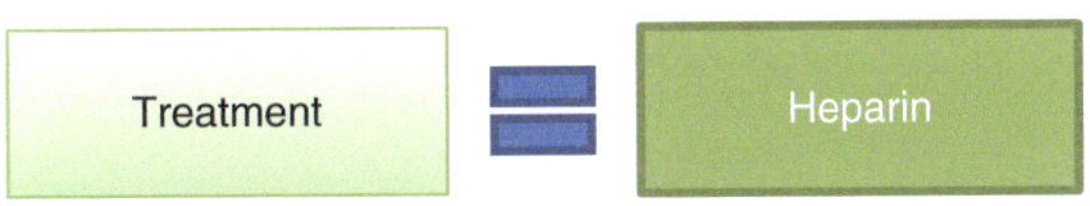

Subarachnoid Hemorrhage Introduction

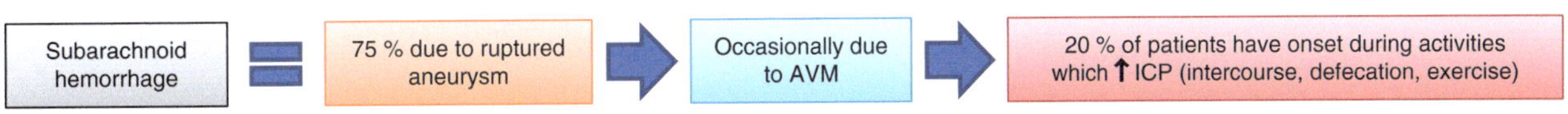

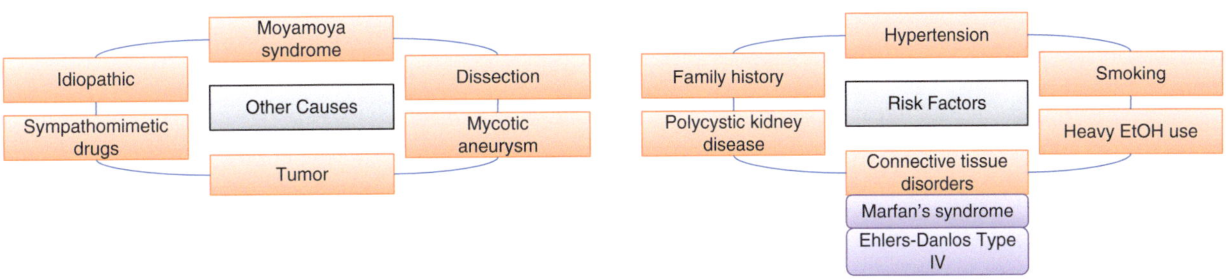

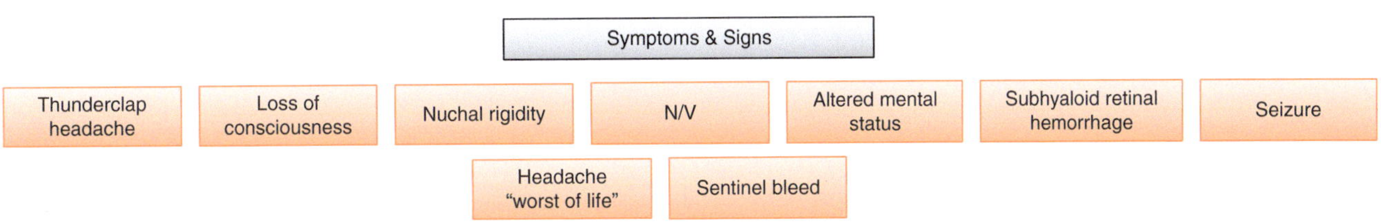

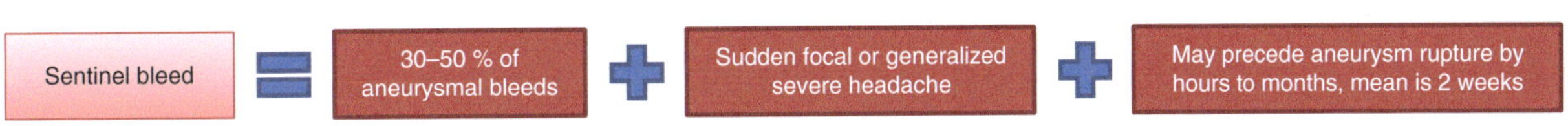

SAH Diagnosis

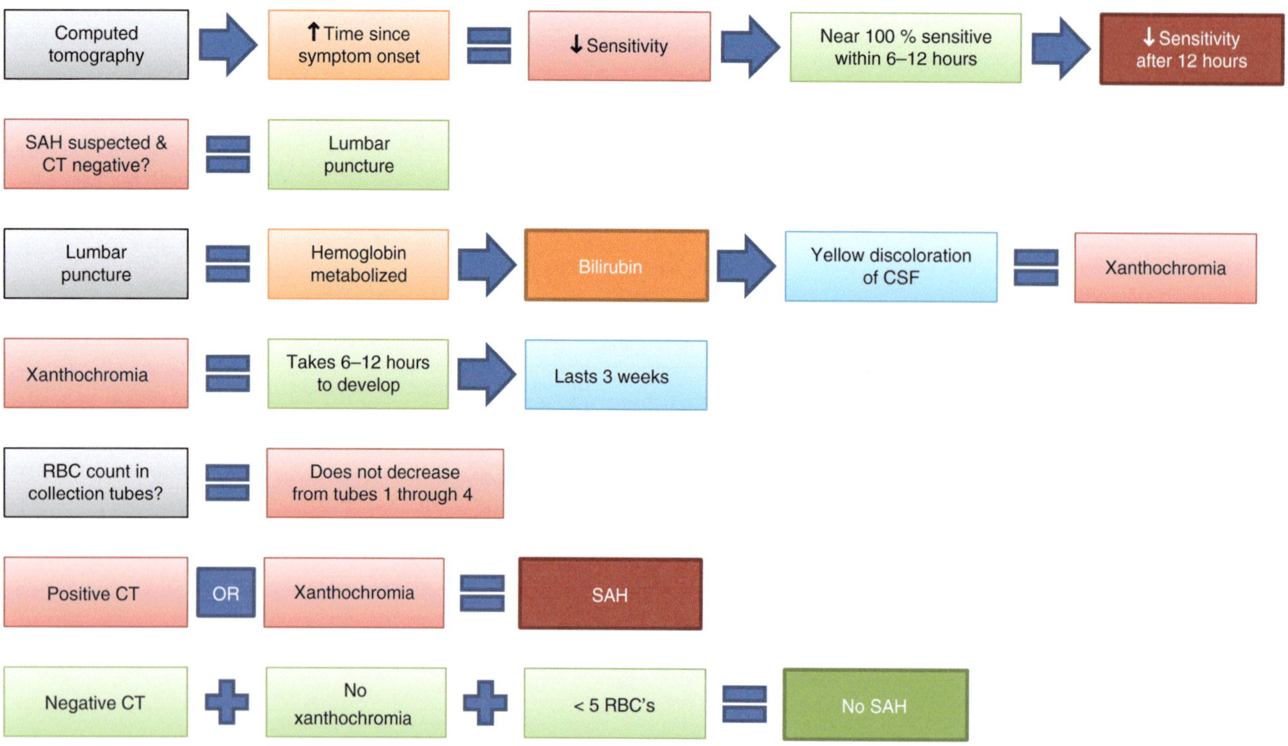

SAH Treatment and Tidbits

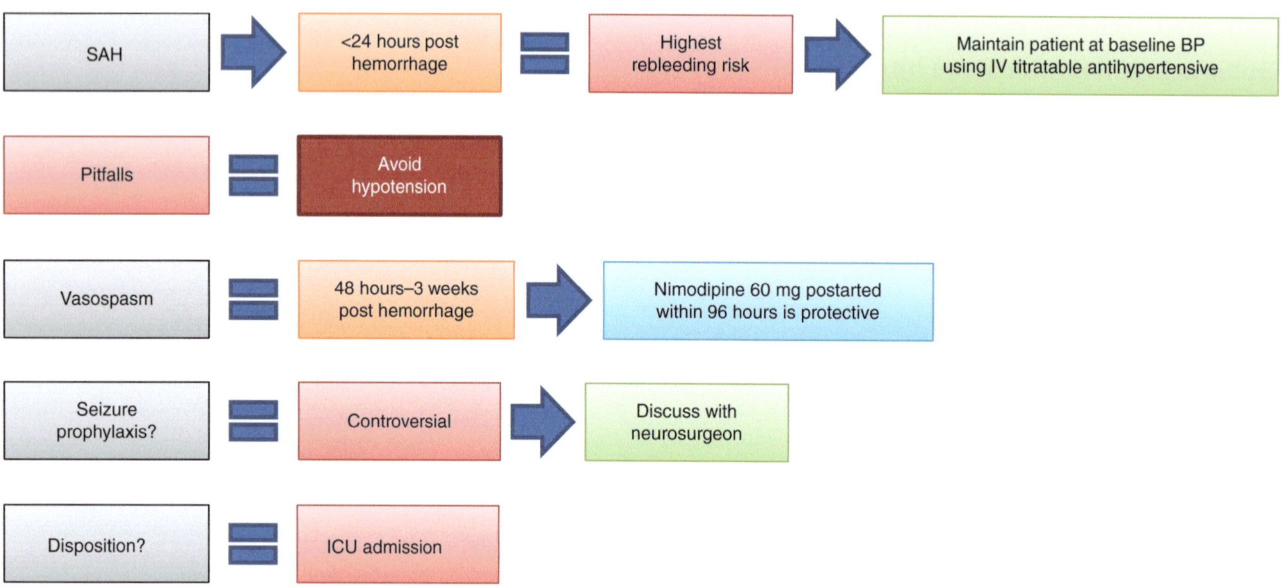

Carotid/Vertebral Artery Dissection

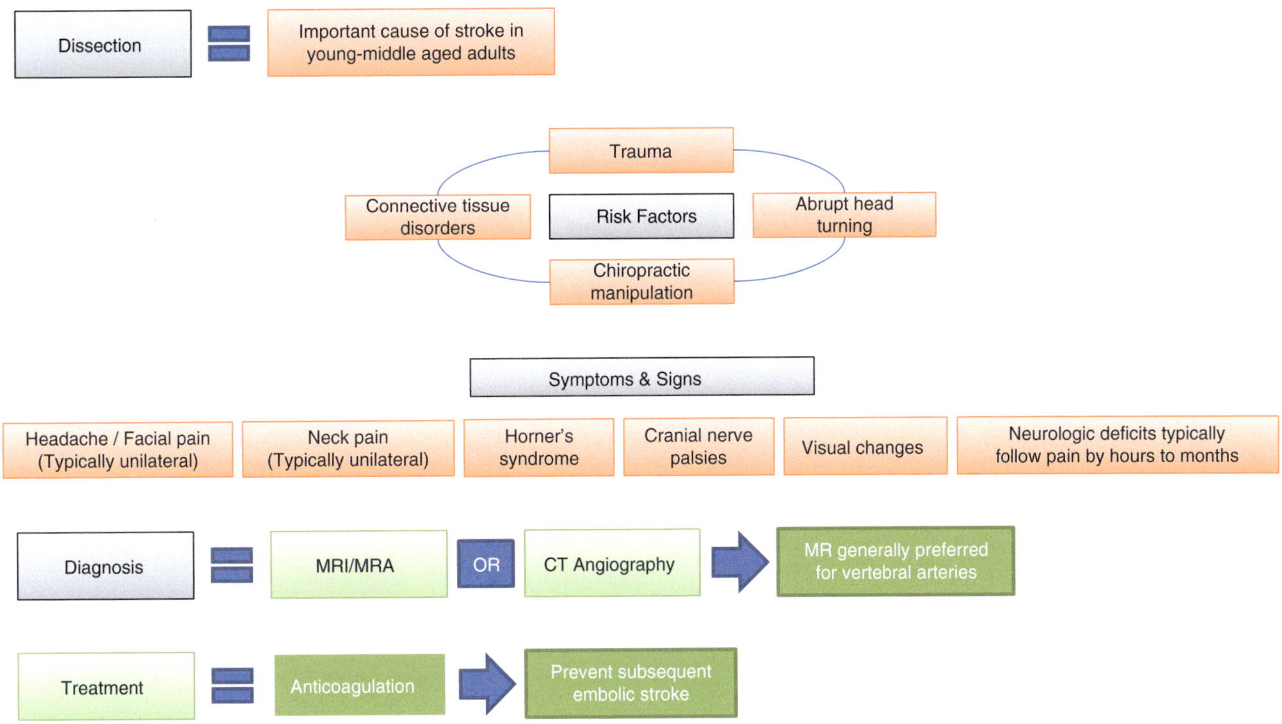

Bell's Palsy

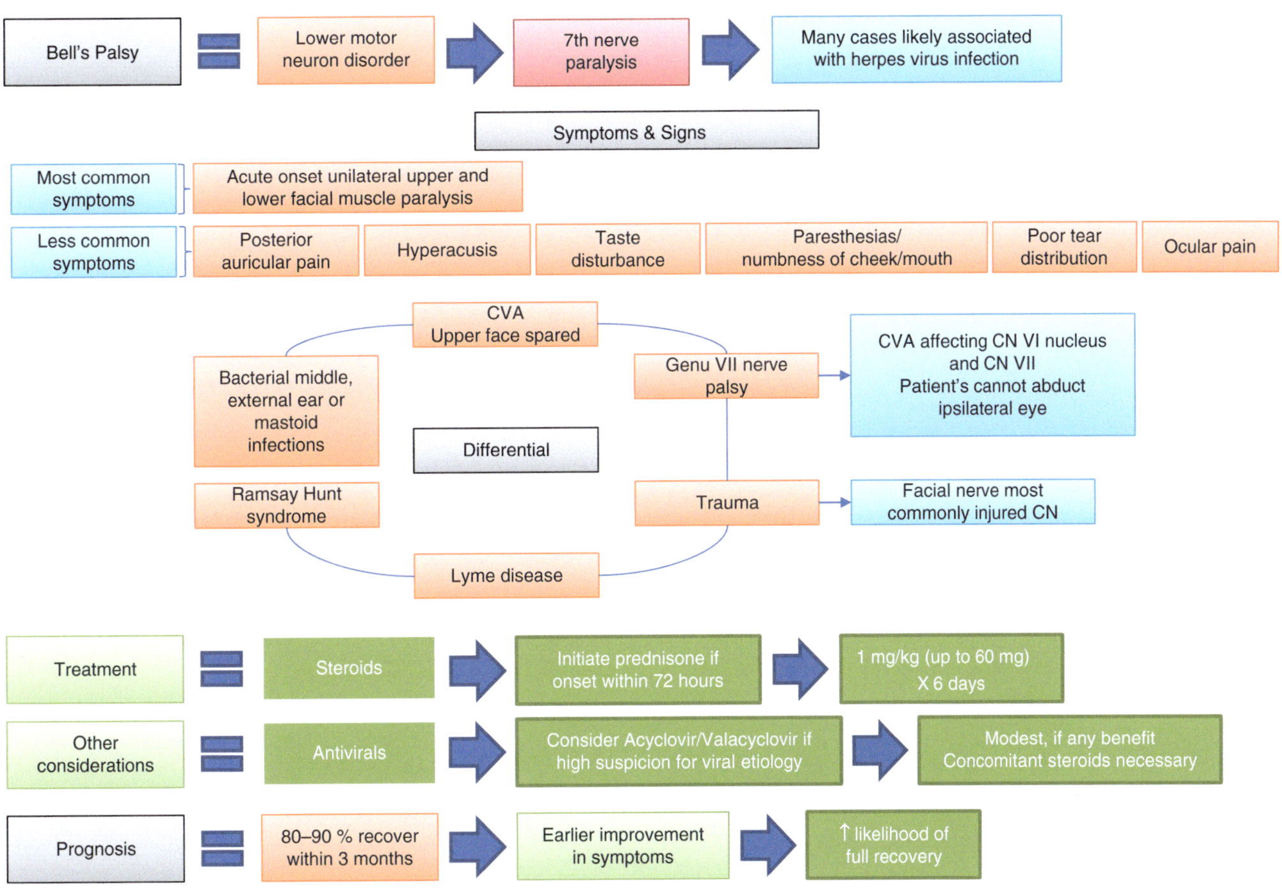

Neuromuscular Disorders

Multiple Sclerosis

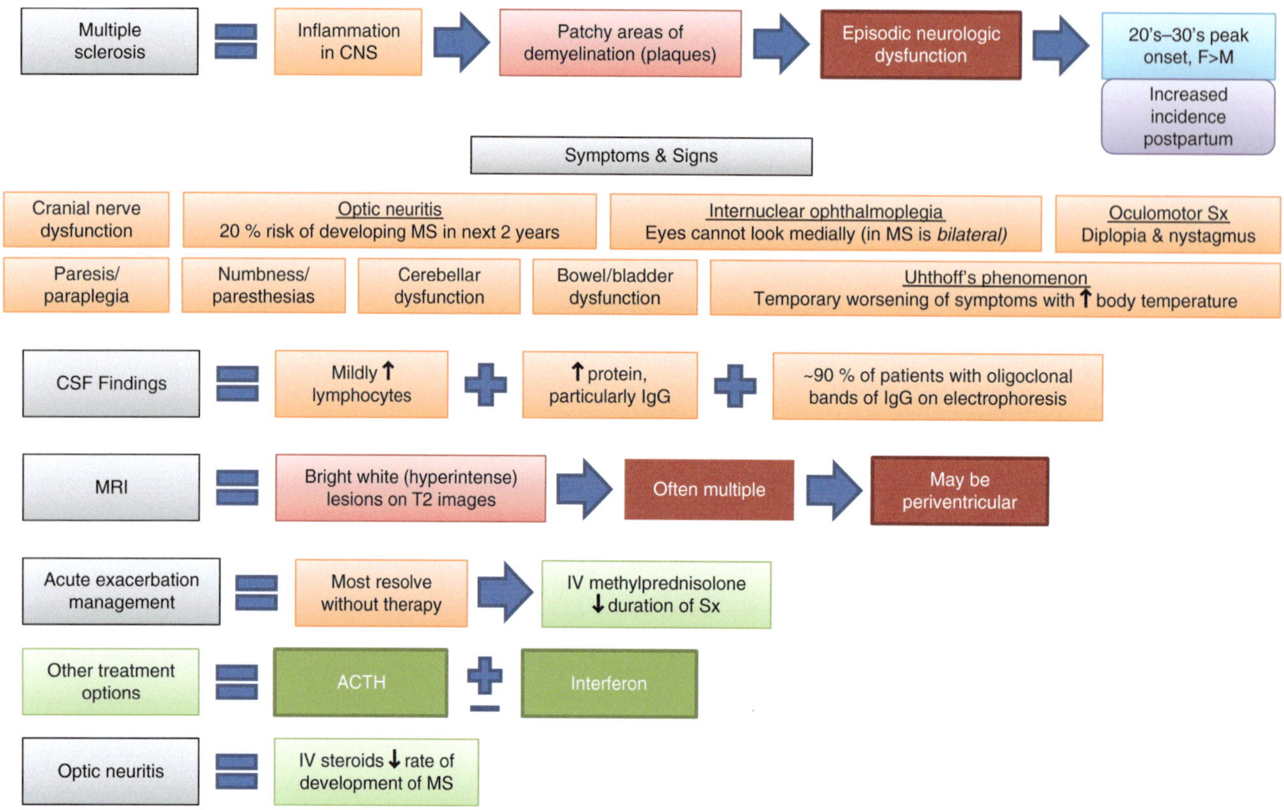

Guillain-Barre Syndrome

Guillain-Barre = Acute autoimmune demyelination of peripheral nervous system → Typically preceded by infection (rarely following vaccination)

Infectious agents implicated = *Campylobacter jejuni* + CMV + EBV + *Mycoplasma pneumoniae*

Guillain-Barre variables = Pace of progression + Severity of ventilatory compromise + Time to recovery

Symptoms & Signs

- Progressive, ascending, symmetrical weakness (Most common)
- Loss of DTR's
- Variable sensory deficits
- Signs/symptoms typically worse in lower extremities
- Ocular muscles typically spared
- 1/2 with autonomic dysfunction
- 1/3 require mechanical ventilation

Most common CSF findings = ↑↑ protein + Mildly ↑ lymphocytes → But… But may be normal

After tPA = Maintain BP < 180/105 mm Hg during & 24 hours post thrombolytics + No heparin, ASA, warfarin etc. for 24 hours post thrombolytics

More likely to need mechanical ventilation = Forced vital capacity < 20 mL/kg OR Negative inspiratory force (NIF) < 30 cm H_2O

Management = Supportive care + IVIG OR Plasma exchange

Acute Periodic Paralysis

Acute periodic paralysis = Progressive extremity weakness in young males → Typically after exercise → No pain, sensation is normal

Associations = Hypokalemia + Thyroid disease + Steroids + Renal disease + Use of alcohol

Hypokalemic periodic paralysis = Autosomal dominant variant (Most common) + Variant associated with thyrotoxicosis (Typically after exercise)

Tick Paralysis

Tick Paralysis = Rapidly ascending paralysis → Reversible → Similar to Guillain-Barre

Treatment = Find & remove tick

Myasthenia Gravis

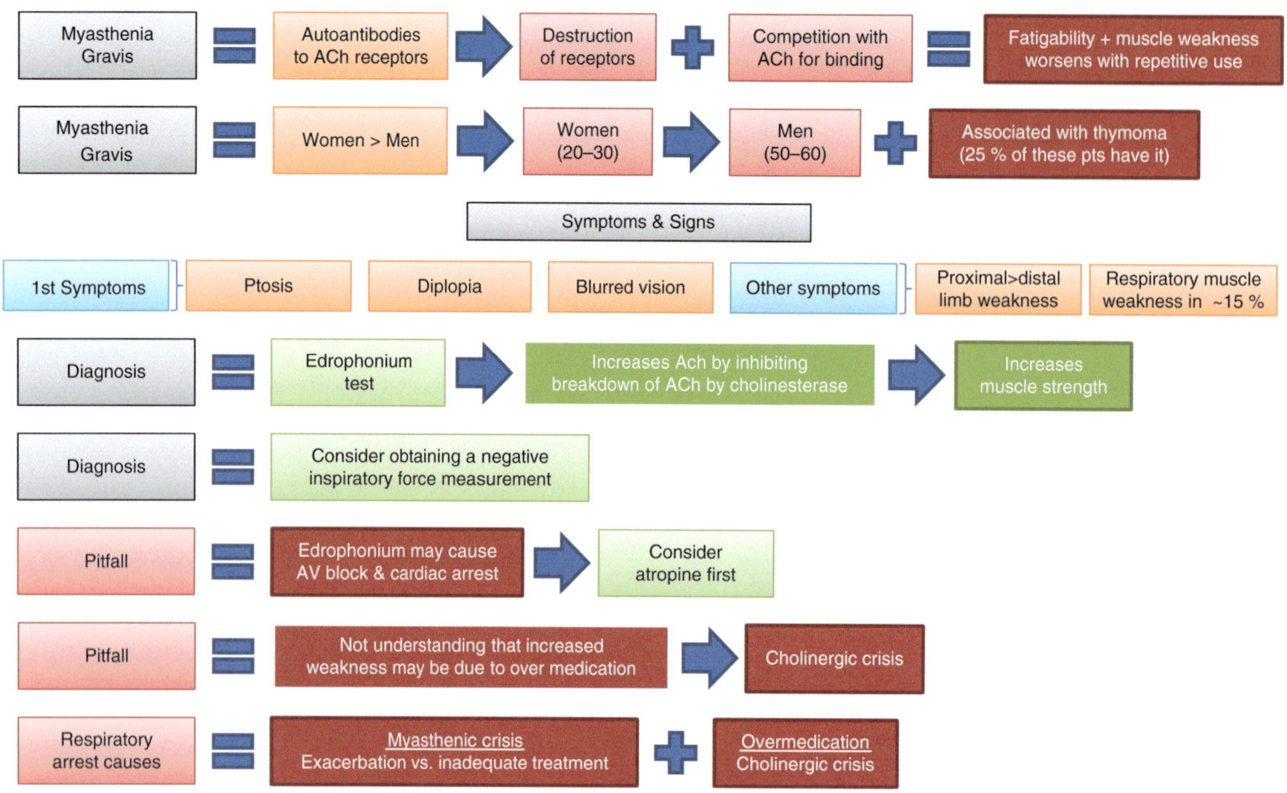

Precipitants of Myasthenic Crisis

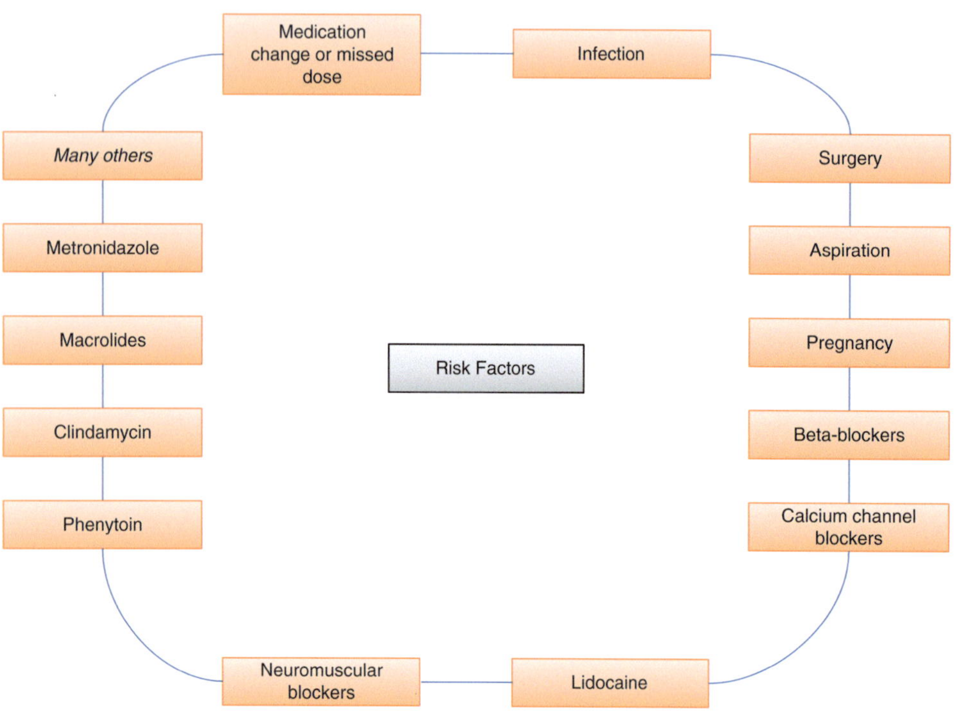

Myasthenia Gravis Treatment

Acute myasthenic crisis? = Airway protection + Plasma exchange OR IVIG

Pitfall = Avoid depolarizing & nondepolarizing paralytic agents → Very sensitive to effects → ↑ Duration of action

Pitfall = Very unpredictable response to succinylcholine

Chronic management = Pyridostigmine or neostigmine → ↑ ACh ± Immunosuppressants ± Thymectomy

Lambert-Eaton Myasthenic Syndrome

Lambert-Eaton syndrome = Clinically similar to myasthenia gravis → Autoantibodies to Ca^{2+} channels + ↓ ACh release = Proximal muscle weakness

Lambert-Eaton syndrome = Highly associated with malignancies especially small cell lung CA

Repeated stimulation = ↑ ACh release → ↑ Strength

Symptoms & Signs

- Weakness & fatigue of proximal muscles
- Especially thighs & hips
- Weakness improves with use

Treatment = Treat underlying condition + Plasmapheresis OR IVIG

Pitfall = Syndrome worsened by → **Neuromuscular blockers, Ca channel blockers, IV contrast**

Movement Disorders

Movement Disorders: Dystonic Reaction and Chorea

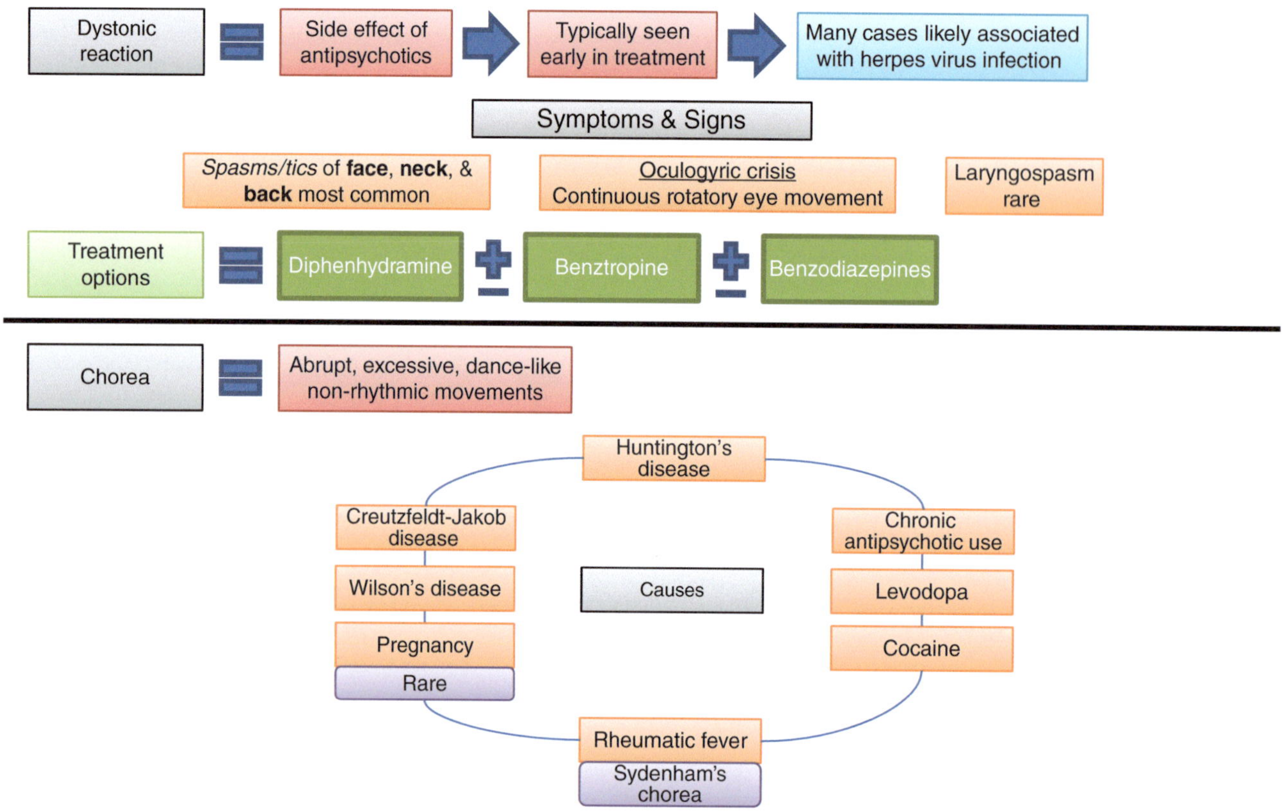

Movement Disorders: Akathisia and Tardive Dyskinesia

Akathisia = Subjective and objective motor restlessness → Typically seen early in treatment with antipsychotics → High incidence with prochloperazine

Treatment options = Diphenhydramine ± Benztropine ± Propranolol (chronic cases)

Tardive dyskinesia = Prolonged use of anitpsychotics → *Late* onset, chronic, rapid involuntary movements + Especially of face, with trunk/limb choreoathetosis

Tardive dyskinesia = Risk higher with traditional agents vs atypicals

Treatment = Psychiatrist to consider ↓ dose or alternative agent

Pitfall = Often irreversible

Parkinson's Disease

Symptoms & Signs:

- Pill-rolling tremor (decreases with purposeful movement)
- Cogwheel rigidity
- Dysequilibrium
- Posture changes
- Bradykinesia/ Akinesia

Parkinson's types = Drug induced + Idiopathic

Treatment Drug-induced = Discontinue inciting agent → e.g., metoclopramide & neuroleptics

Treatment Idiopathic = Benztropine || Amantadine || Carbidopa Levodopa

Pitfall of Carbidopa/Levodopa = Can cause **dysrhythmias**, **dystonia**, **orthostatic hypotension**

General pitfalls = Avoid haloperidol & other neuroleptics → Can precipitate tardive dyskinesia

Neuropathies

Peripheral Polyneuropathies

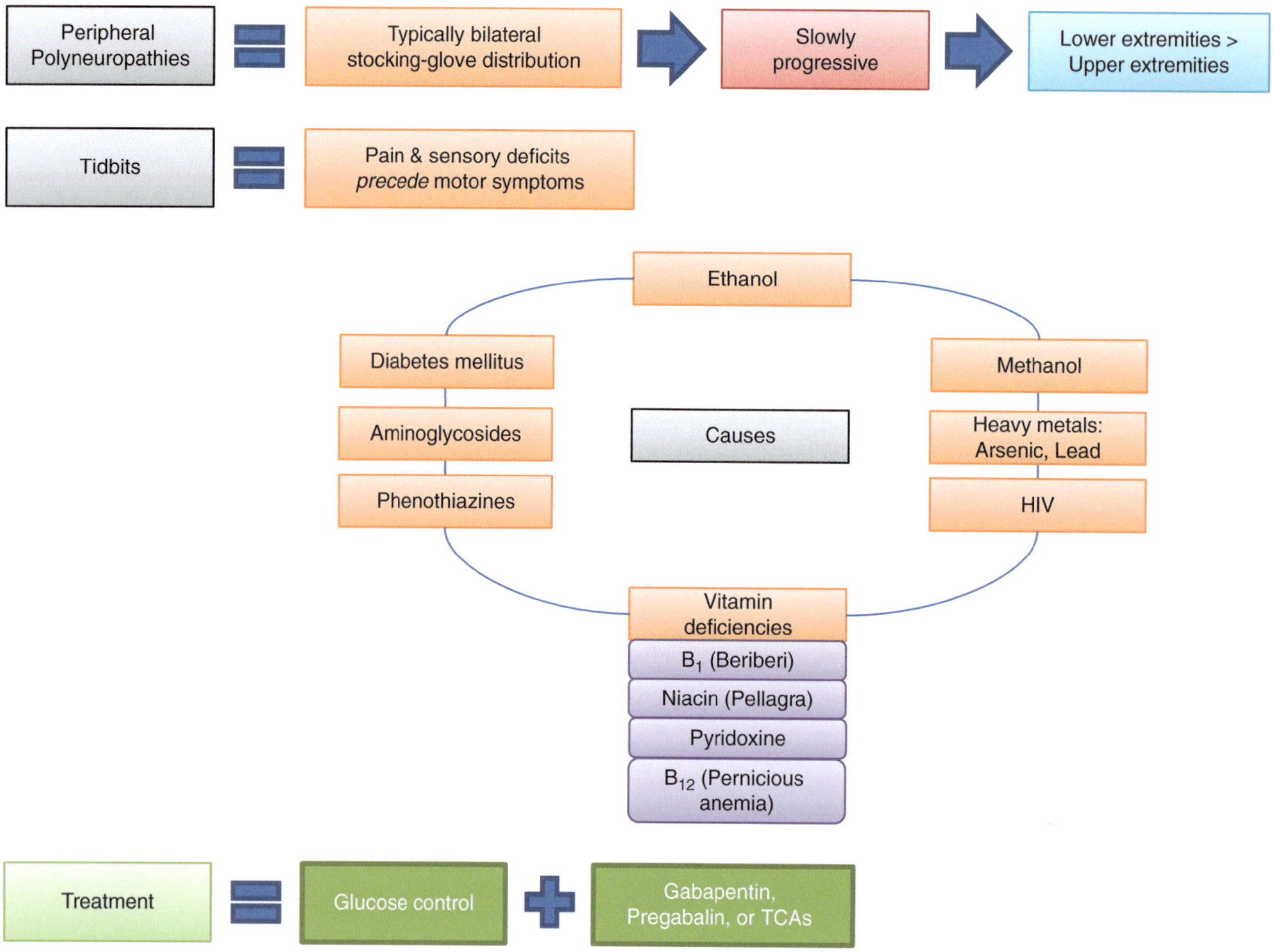

Spinal Disorders

Amyotrophic Lateral Sclerosis

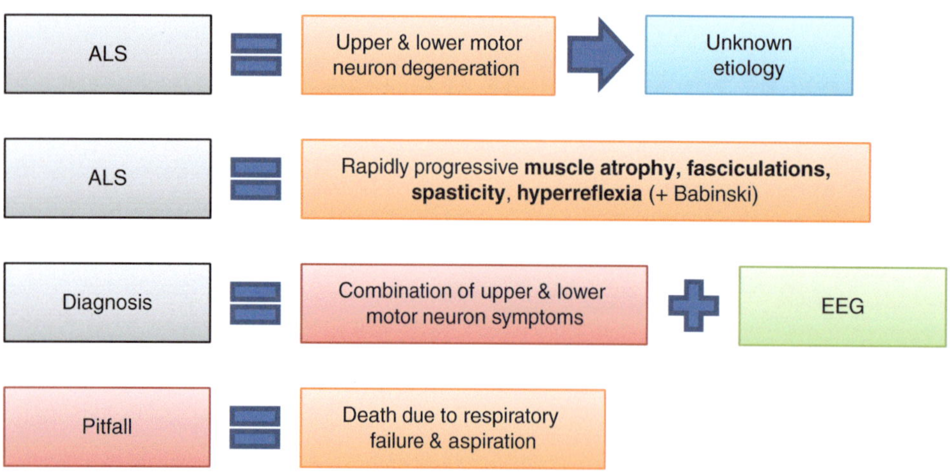

Miscellaneous Disorders

Wernicke's Encephalopathy

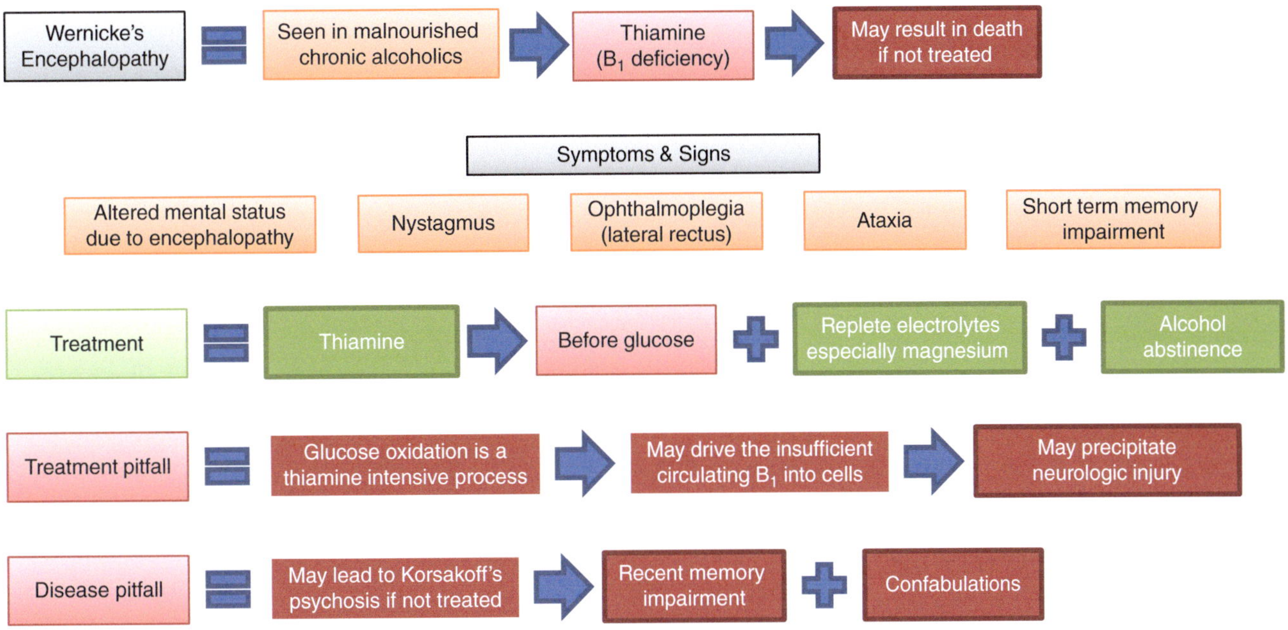

Psychiatric Emergencies

Delirium Versus Dementia

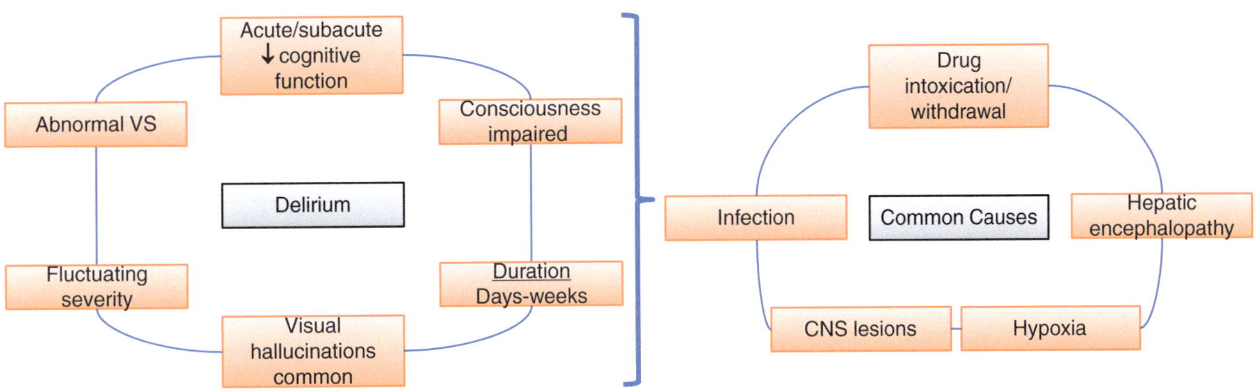

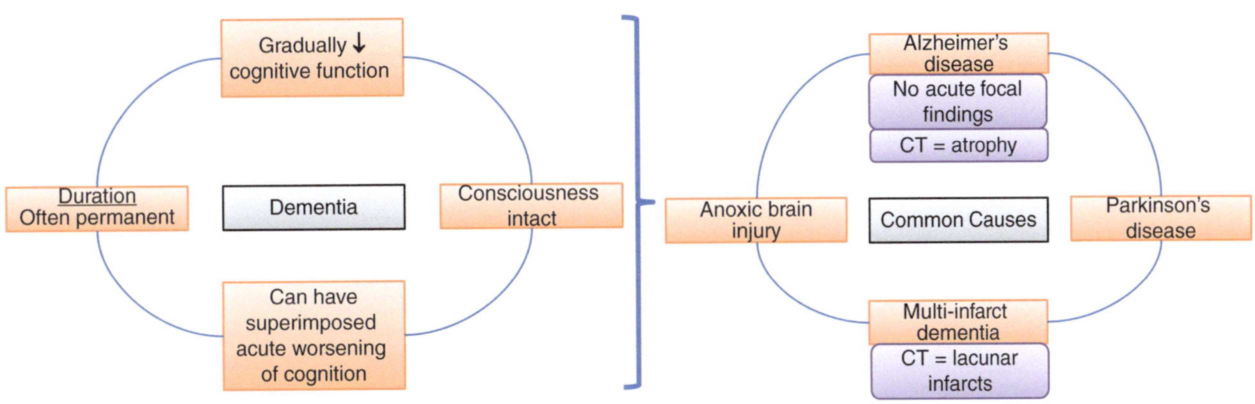

Organic Acute Psychosis Etiologies Medications/Drugs (Including Withdrawal)

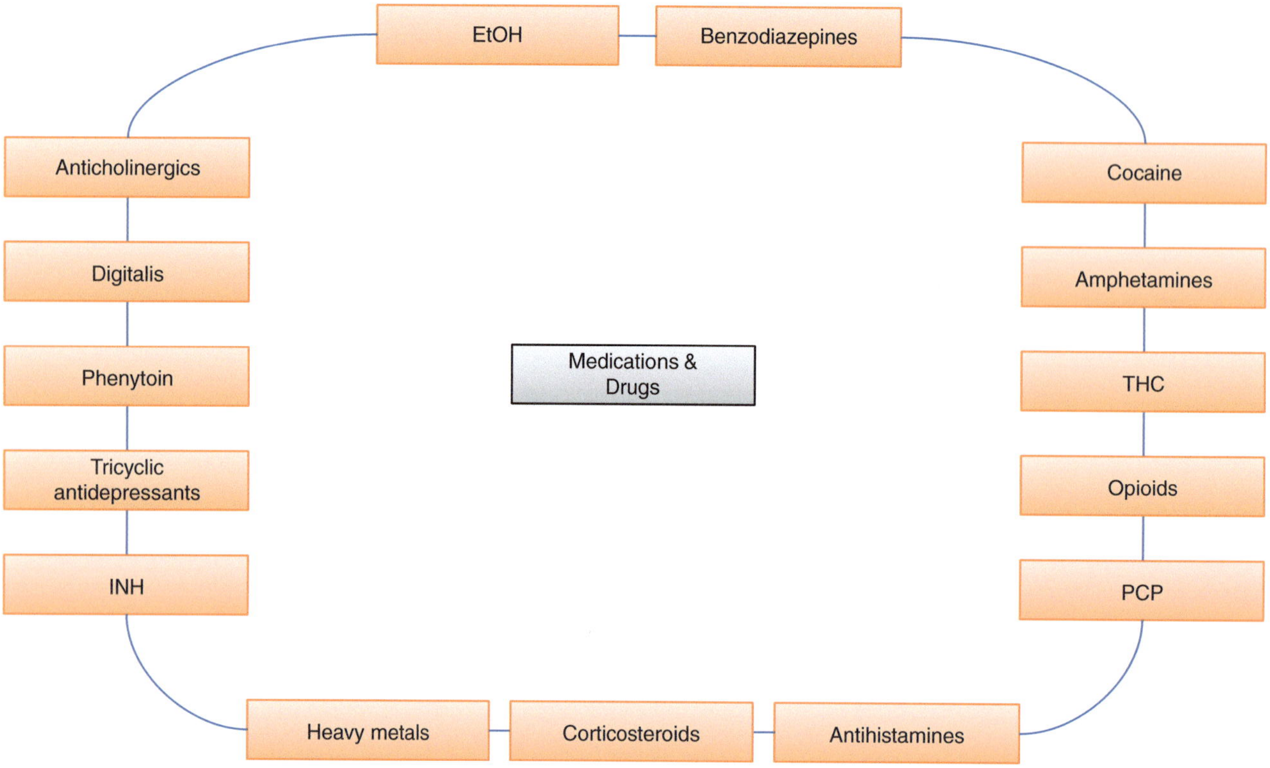

Organic Acute Psychosis Etiologies Medical Conditions

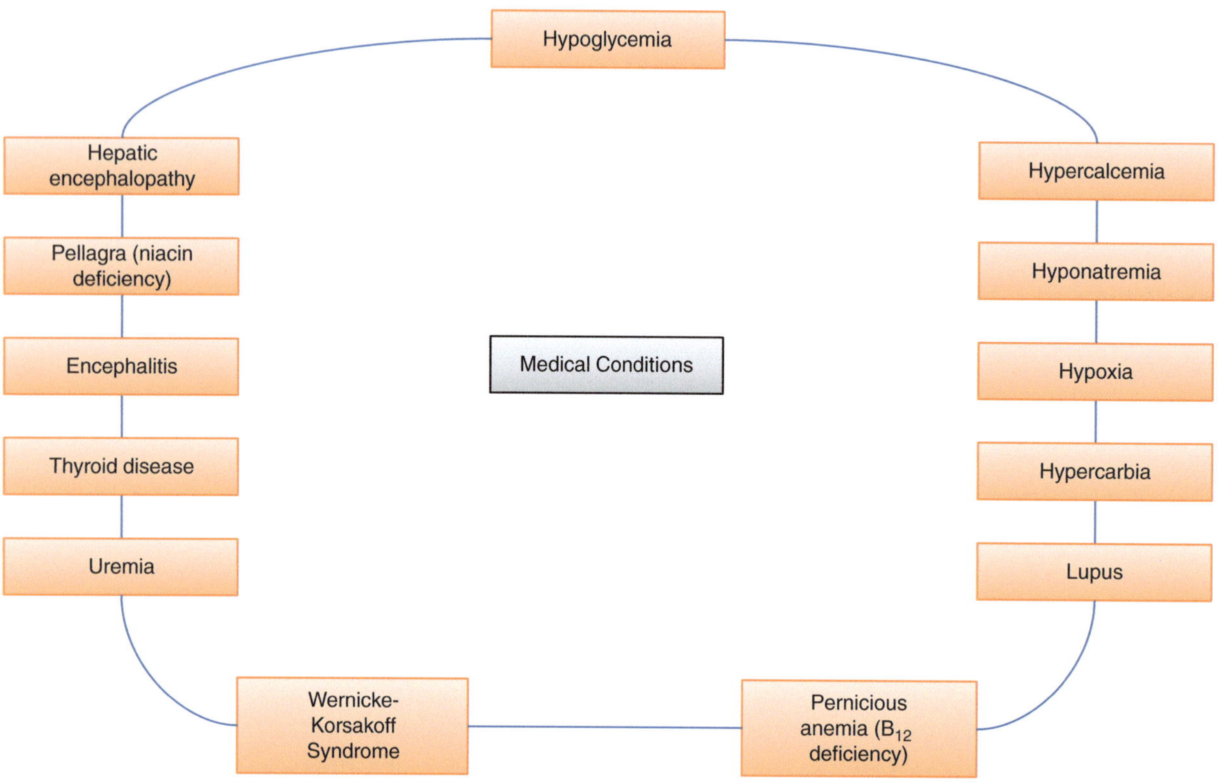

Organic Versus Functional Psychosis

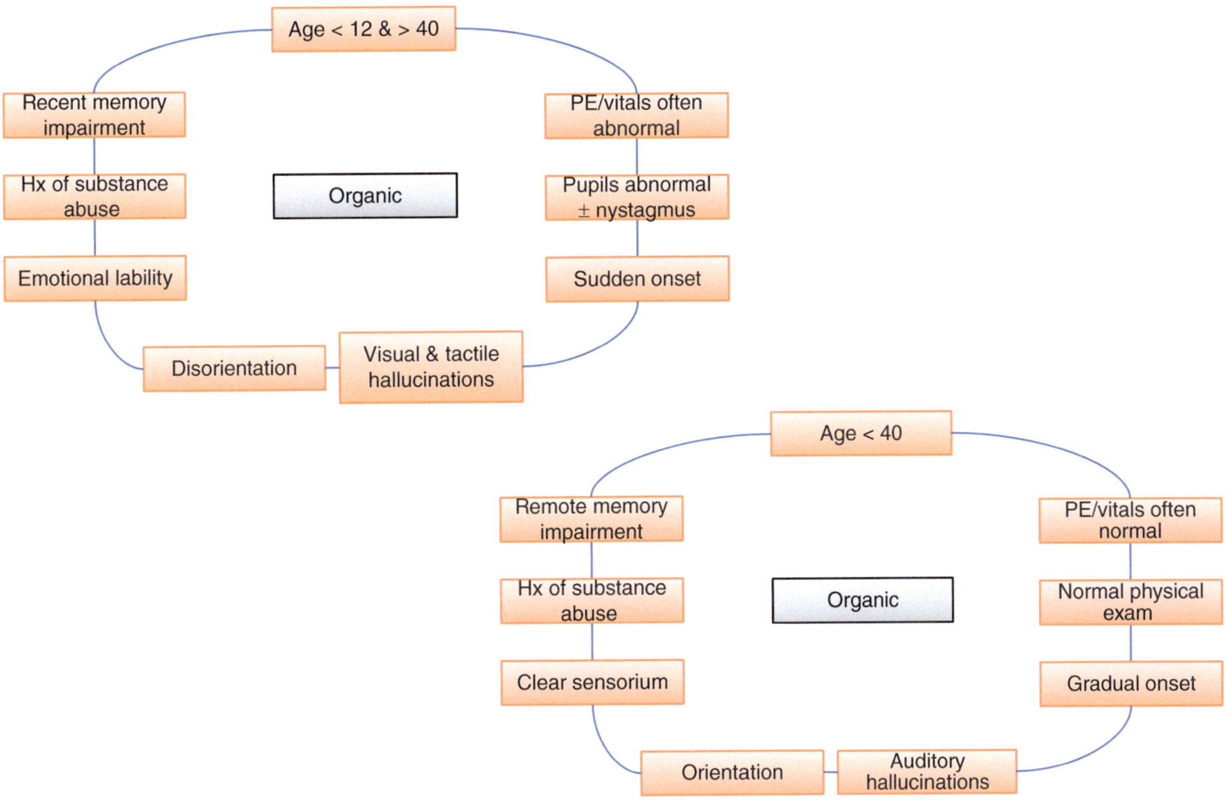

Amnesia

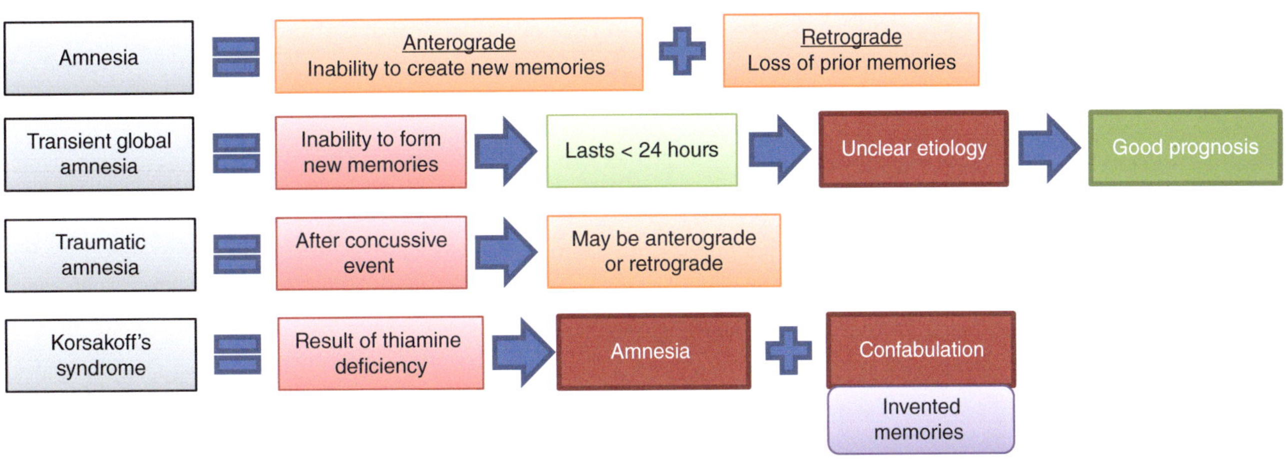

Major Depression

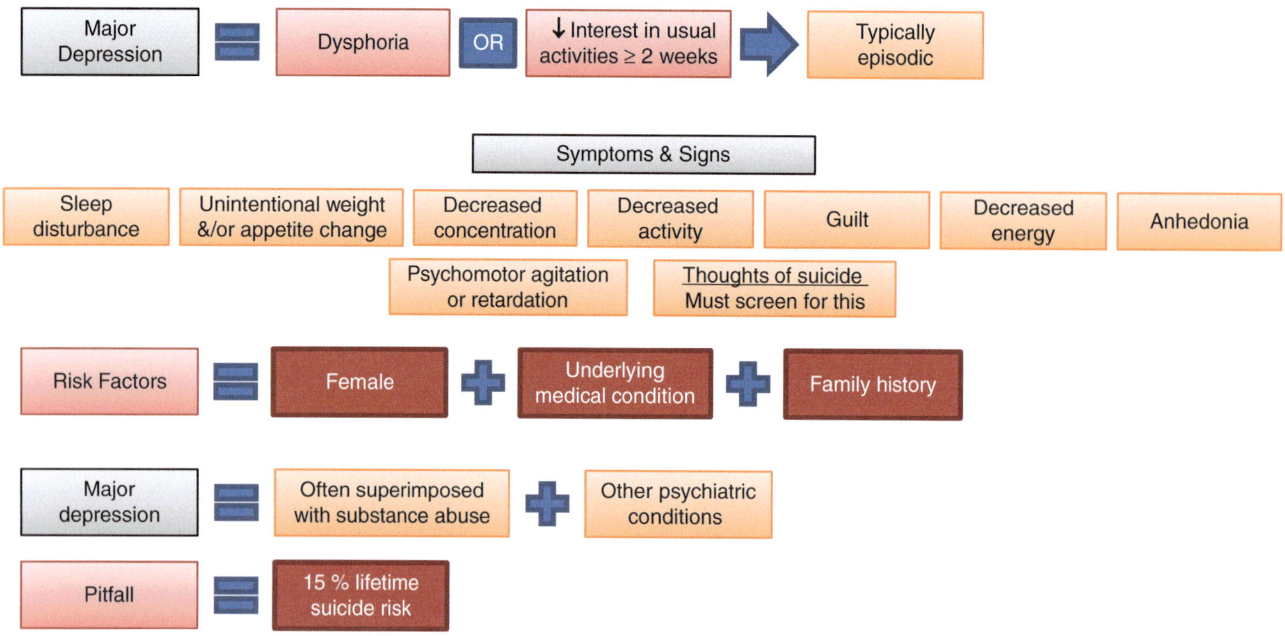

Suicide

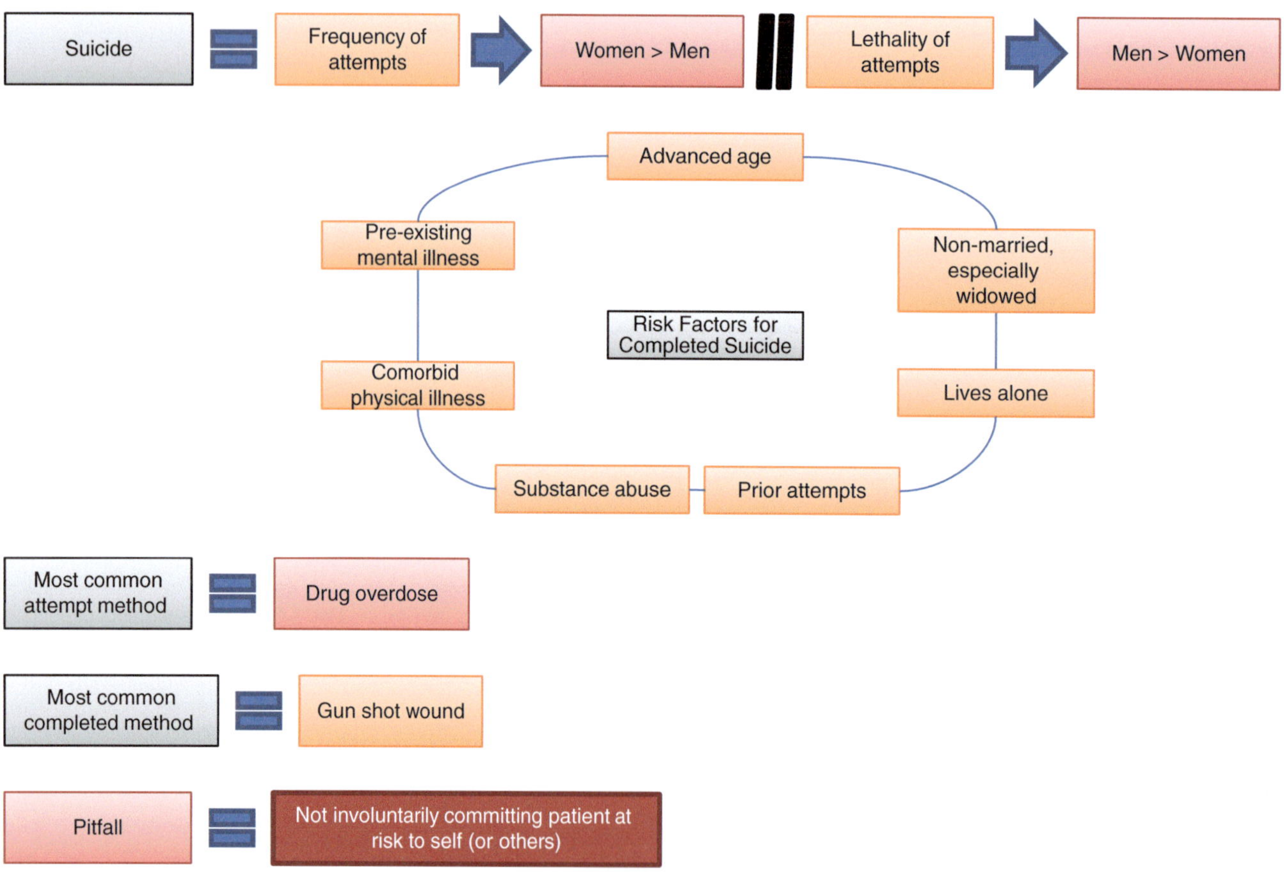

Grief Reaction

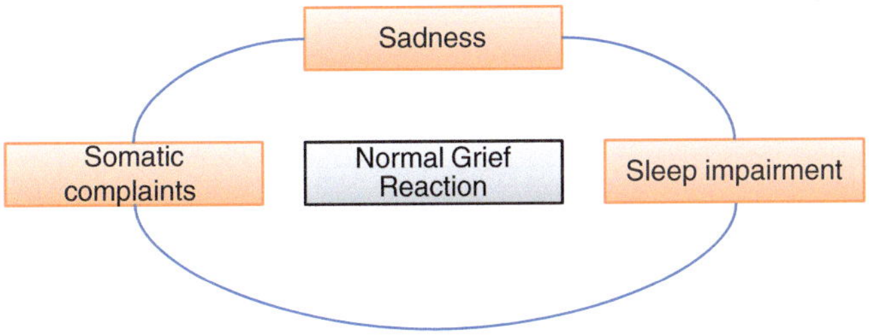

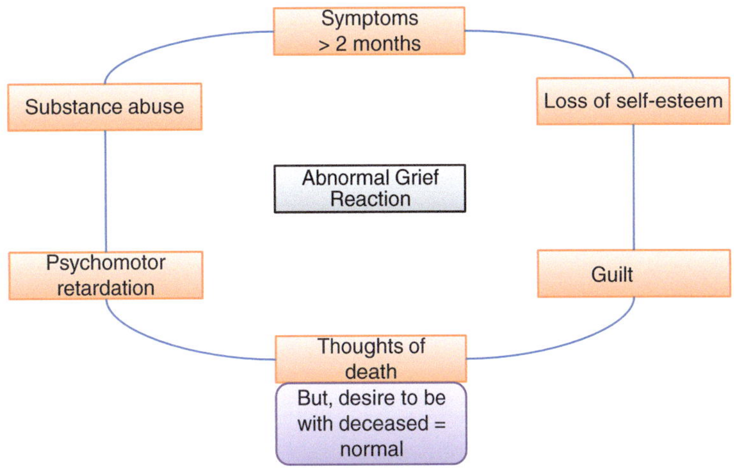

Bipolar Disorder

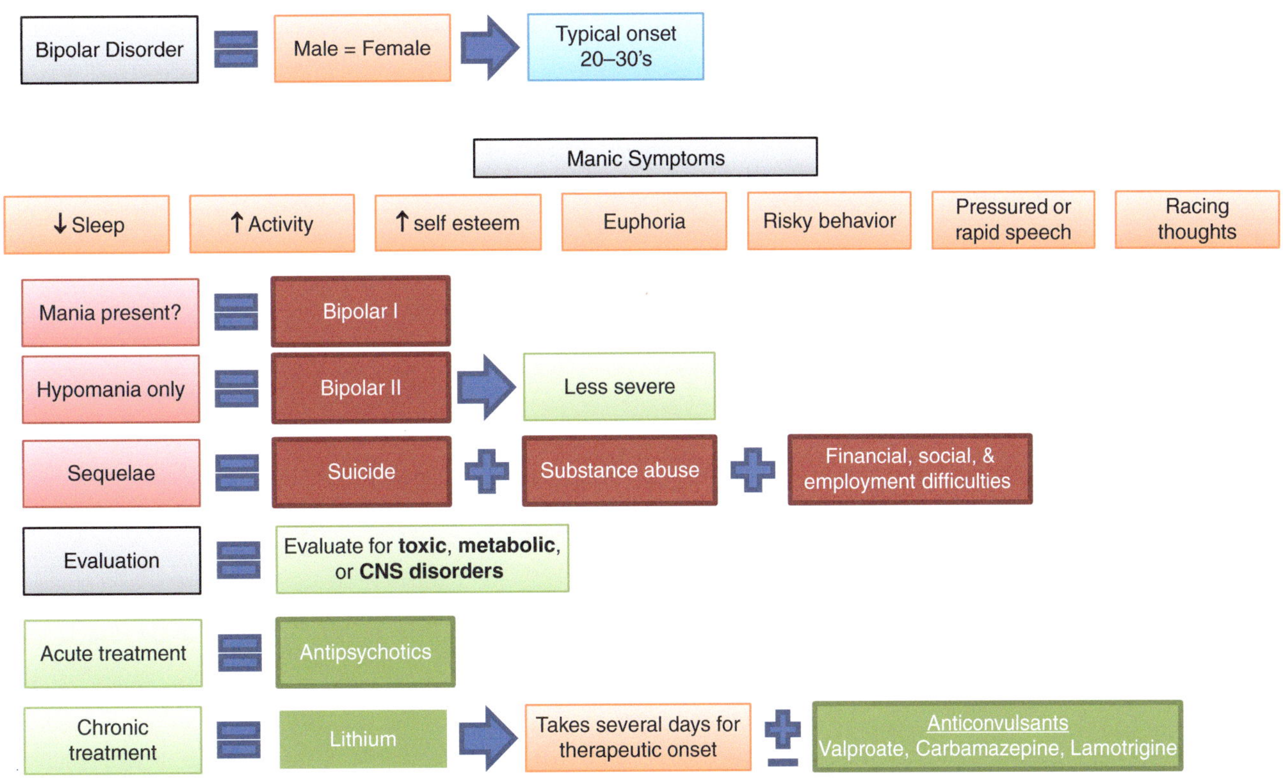

Schizophrenia

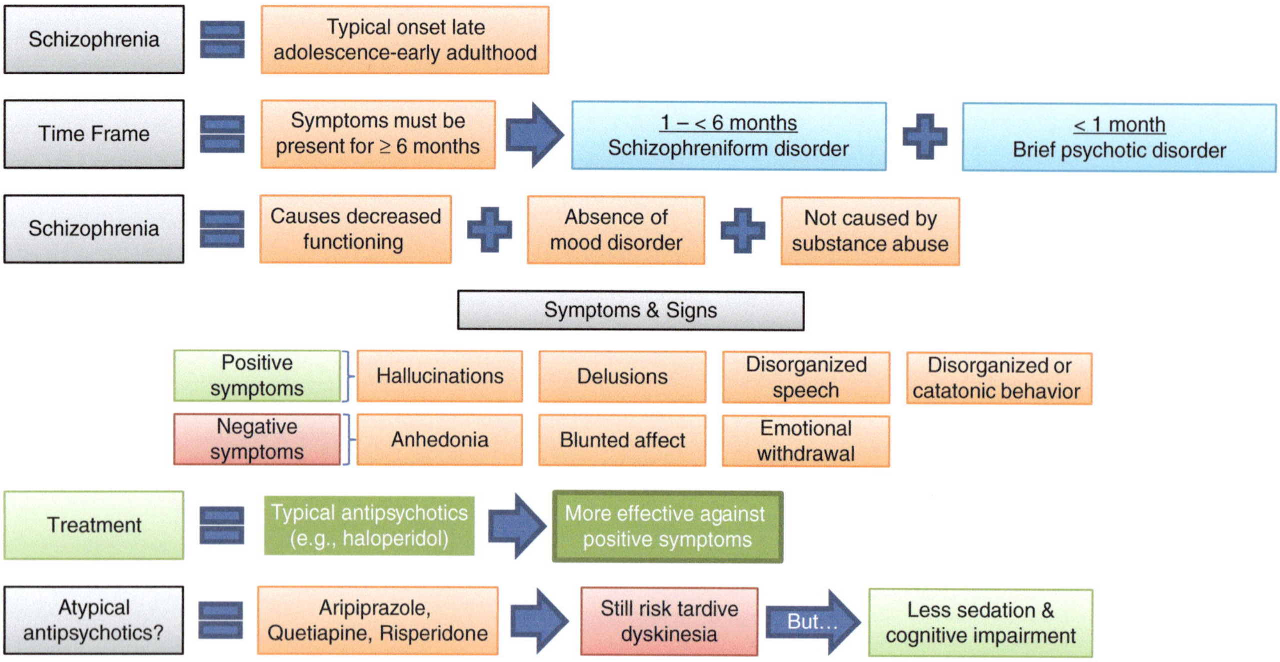

Anxiety

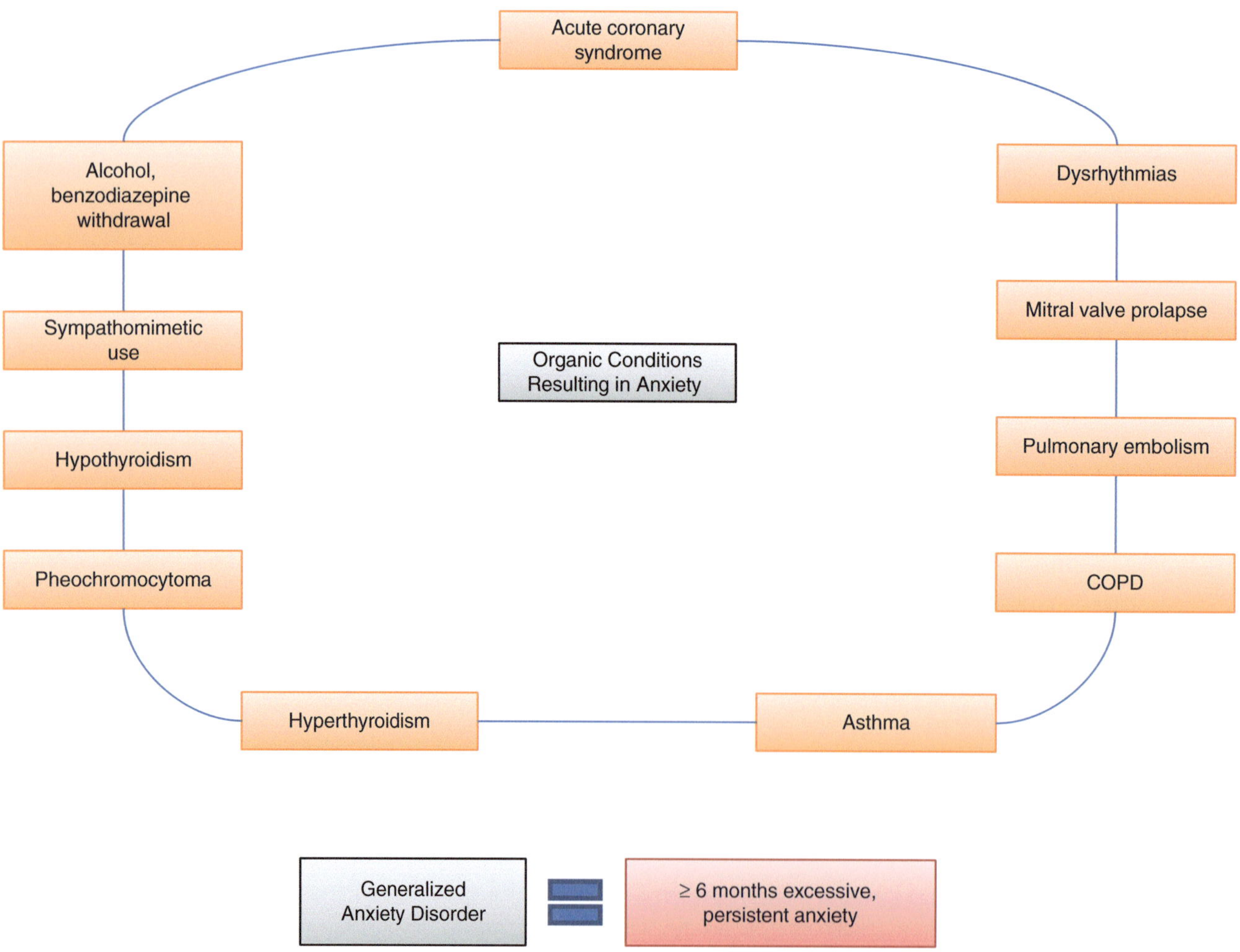

Anxiety Disorders

Panic Attack = Rapid onset of anxiety or impending doom + Autonomic symptoms: Dyspnea, chest tightness, palpitations, tachycardia, diaphoresis

Panic disorder = Recurrent panic attacks + Fear of future attacks OR Worry over panic attack consequences OR Resulting behavior change

Post-traumatic stress disorder = Intrusive memories of extremely traumatic event ± Guilt, depression, anxiety → Substance abuse often results

Phobia = Irrational fear of specific situation → Avoidance

Evaluation = Evaluate for organic etiology → Especially medications & drugs

Obsessive-Compulsive Disorder

Obsessions = Recurrent, intrusive, unwanted thoughts

Compulsions = Behaviors patient engages in to "control" thoughts → Repetitive hand washing, checking

Pitfall = May occupy significant amount of time per day → May cause a significant lifestyle disruption

Anorexia

Anorexia = Refusal to maintain normal body weight (>15 % under ideal body weight) + Fear of gaining weight + Distorted body image

Anorexia = Onset typically in teens → Female >> Male

Symptoms & Signs:

- Secondary amenorrhea
- Bradycardia
- ↓ Cardiac contractility
- Normochromic anemia
- ↓Mg > ↑QTc

Pitfall = Significant mortality → Suicide is a common cause

Treatment = Correct electrolyte abnormalities → Admission to inpatient treatment center

Bulimia Nervosa

Bulimia Nervosa = Poor impulse control → Episodes of binge eating → Unlike anorexia weight often normal → Onset typically in teens-early adulthood

Bulimia Nervosa = Binging typically followed by purging (vomiting, diuretic or laxative abuse) OR Excessive exercise OR Fasting

Symptoms & Signs

- Vomiting: ↓K, ↓Cl, Metabolic alkalosis
- Laxative Abuse: ↓Na, ↓K, Metabolic alkalosis
- Mallory-Weiss tears
- Tooth decay

Prognosis = Generally better than anorexia

Somatoform Disorders

Somatoform disorders = Physical symptoms + No medical explanation + Symptoms not voluntary

Somatization = Numerous symptoms + Multiple organ systems affected + NO medical explanation

Hypochondriasis = Preoccupying fear of serious disease → Persists despite evaluation and reassurance → ≥6 months significant distress or impairment

Hypochondriasis = No secondary gain

Conversion disorder = Single neurological symptom (e.g., paralysis, blindness, seizure) → Often triggered by stressor → Not explained by organic disease

Conversion disorder = Patient does NOT consciously produce symptom → Symptom onset typically sudden

"La belle indifference" = Patient with lack of concern regarding symptoms, common

Evaluation = Rule out organic pathology → Beware MS, SLE

Malingering, Factitious Disorders, and Munchausen's Syndrome

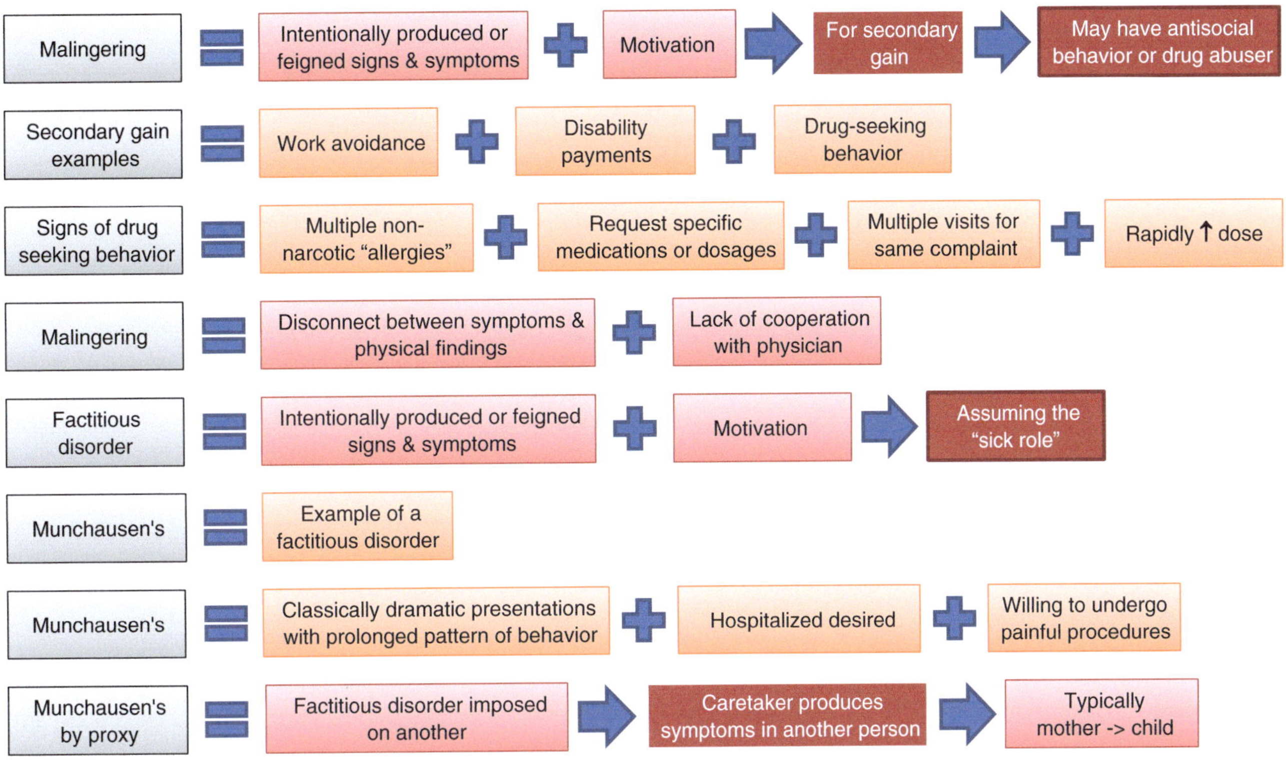

Personality Disorders

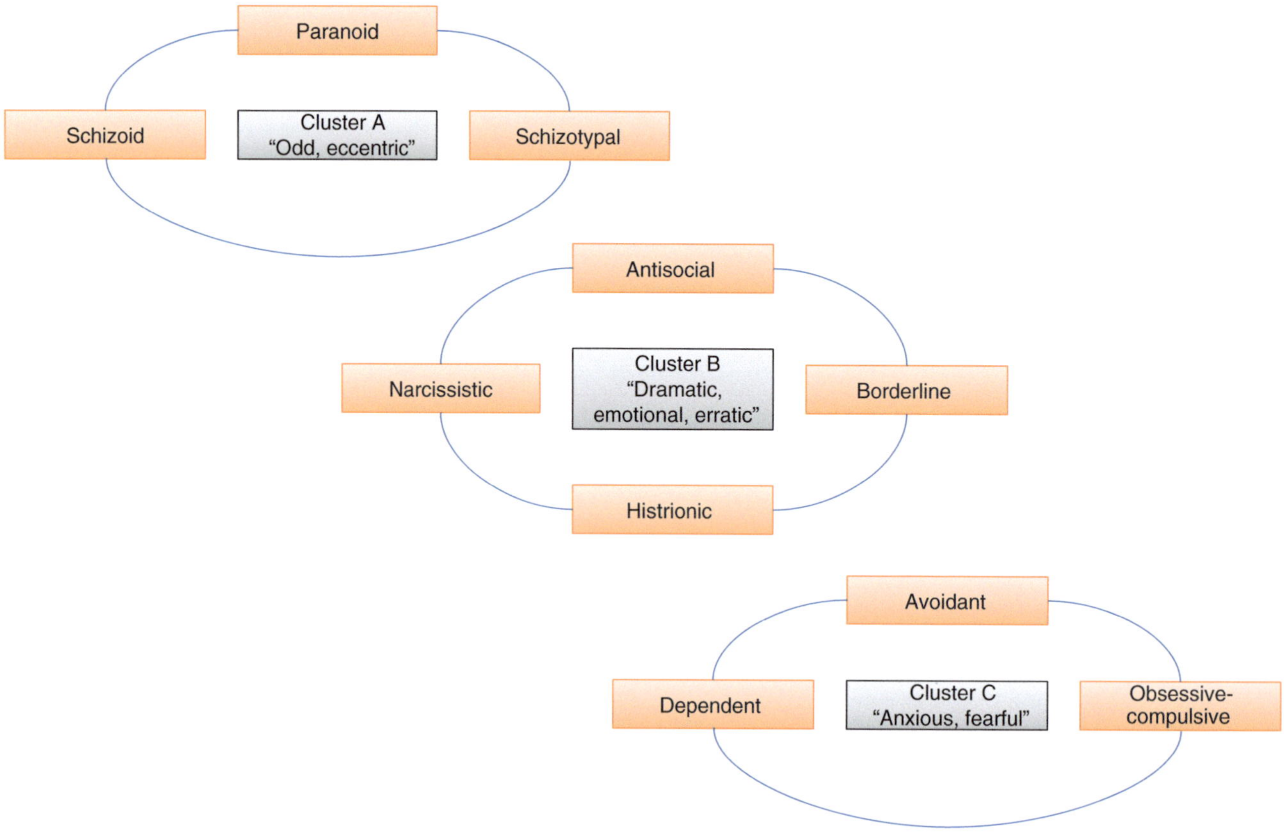

Antisocial, Borderline, Histrionic, and Narcissistic Personality Disorders

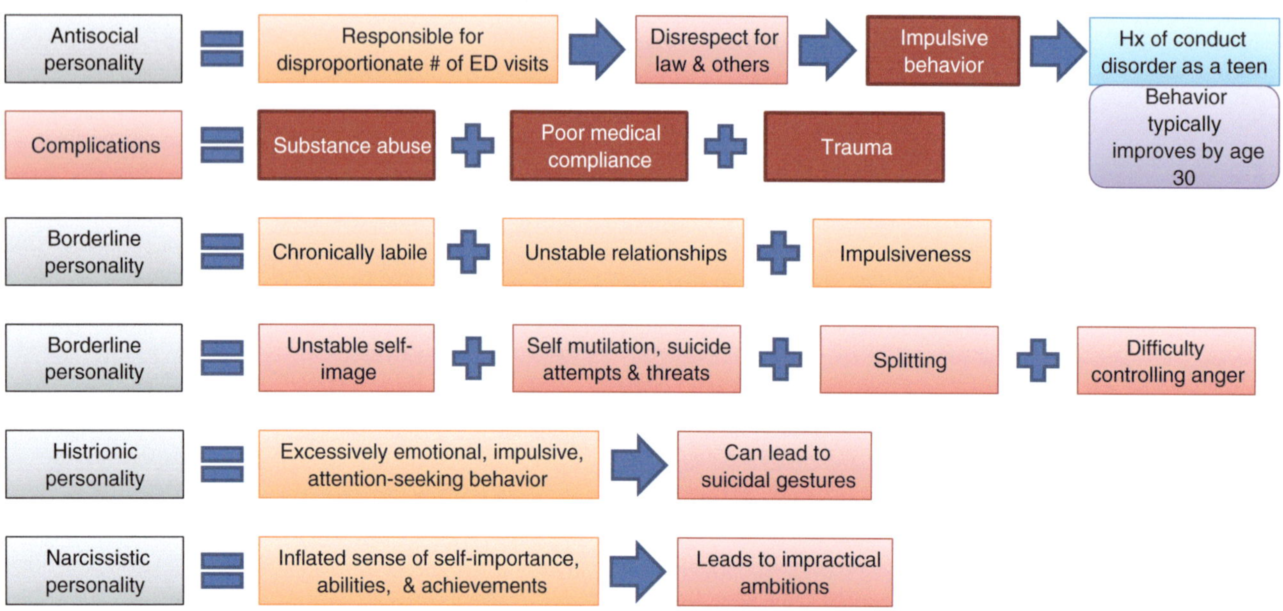

Abuse/Neglect/Violence

Intimate Partner Violence

Intimate Partner Violence = Harm (Physical, Psychological, Sexual) by current or former partner + Victims F >> M

Other risk factors = Young adulthood + Low socioeconomic status + Pregnancy

Common Patterns of Injury

- Fingernail scratches
- Broken nails
- Forearm injuries
- Injuries in multiple healing stages

Pitfall for ↑ assault risk = Victim attempts to end relationship OR When abuse reported

Management = Screen females + Ensure patient and child safety + Refer to social services & victim advocate + Report to law enforcement as appropriate

Elder Abuse

Elder Abuse = Neglect or action resulting in harm to elderly

Risk factors for Elders

- F>M
- Hx of domestic violence
- Lack of social support
- Cognitive impairment
- Physical dependency

Characteristics of Abusers

- M > F
- Substance abuse
- History of violence
- Typically primary caregiver
- Mental illness
- Financial dependence on elder

Patterns of Injury

- Decubiti
- Dehydration
- Electrolyte abnormalities
- Forearm injuries
- Rhabdomyolysis
- Rape marks

Pitfall = Chronic neurologic conditions and/or immobility may result in some of these findings

Management = Treat injuries + Replete electrolytes & fluids + Report to authorities + Social work to assist with placement vs. admission

Sexual Assault

Sexual assault = ~1/2 assaults have no visible genital injury

> 72 hours post assault? = Unlikely to find evidence + Consider deferring forensic exam → Shared decision making with victim & victim advocate

Pitfall = Must maintain chain of custody of evidence

Post evaluation = Offer pregnancy, STD, HIV prophylaxis

ED Staff/Patient Safety

Chemical restraints = Typical antipsychotics (Droperidol; Haloperidol) + Atypical antipsychotics + Benzodiazepines + Antipsychotic + benzodiazepine (Synergism; Reduced side effects)

Pitfall of physical restraints = Failure to reassess physically restrained patients frequent & document neurovascular status

Potential injuries = Neurovascular injury + Rhabdomyolysis + Asphyxia

Violence prevention methods = Screening for weapons + Visible and responsive security + Limited ED access + Alarm systems

Addictive Behavior and Withdrawal

Substance Abuse/Dependence

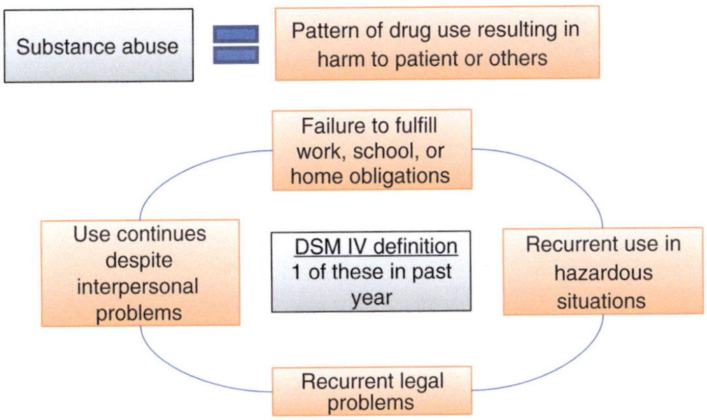

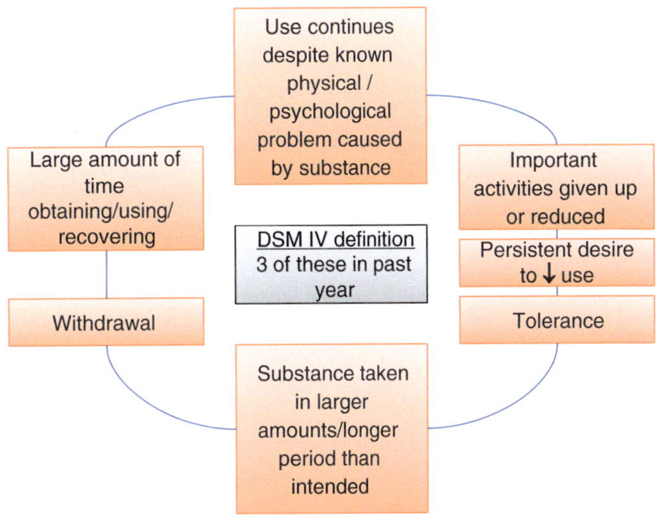

Alcohol Withdrawal

Alcohol Withdrawal = Onset 6–48 hours after last use ≠ Delirium Tremens = 48–120 hours after last use = Potentially fatal

Symptoms & Signs Withdrawal

- Generalized tonic-clonic seizures
- Tremulousness
- Tongue fasciculations
- Irritability
- Tachycardia
- Hypertension

Pitfall = Must consider trauma or SDH as etiology of seizure

Symptoms & Signs Delirium Tremens

- Visual hallucinations
- Paranoia
- Diaphoresis
- Irritability
- Tachycardia
- Hypertension
- Elevated temperature

Uncomplicated withdrawal or seizures? = Long acting benzodiazepine (lorazepam, diazepam or chlordiazepoxide) → ***Lorazepam*** preferred if hepatic impairment, elderly due to no active metabolites

Pitfall = Phenytoin not useful for EtOH withdrawal seizures

Delirium tremens? = High doses of benzodiazepines → If refractory consider ***Propofol*** & **airway protection**

Chronic alcoholics? = IV thiamine, glucose, fluids → K^{+}, Mg^{++} often depleted in chronic alcoholics

Benzodiazepine Withdrawal

Benzodiazepine Withdrawal = Similar symptoms to EtOH withdrawal → But… → Rarely fatal

Pitfall = Withdrawal may be delayed → Depends on agent half-life → Symptoms may not develop for 7–10 days

Management = Gradual taper of agent over up to 10 weeks

Opiate Withdrawal

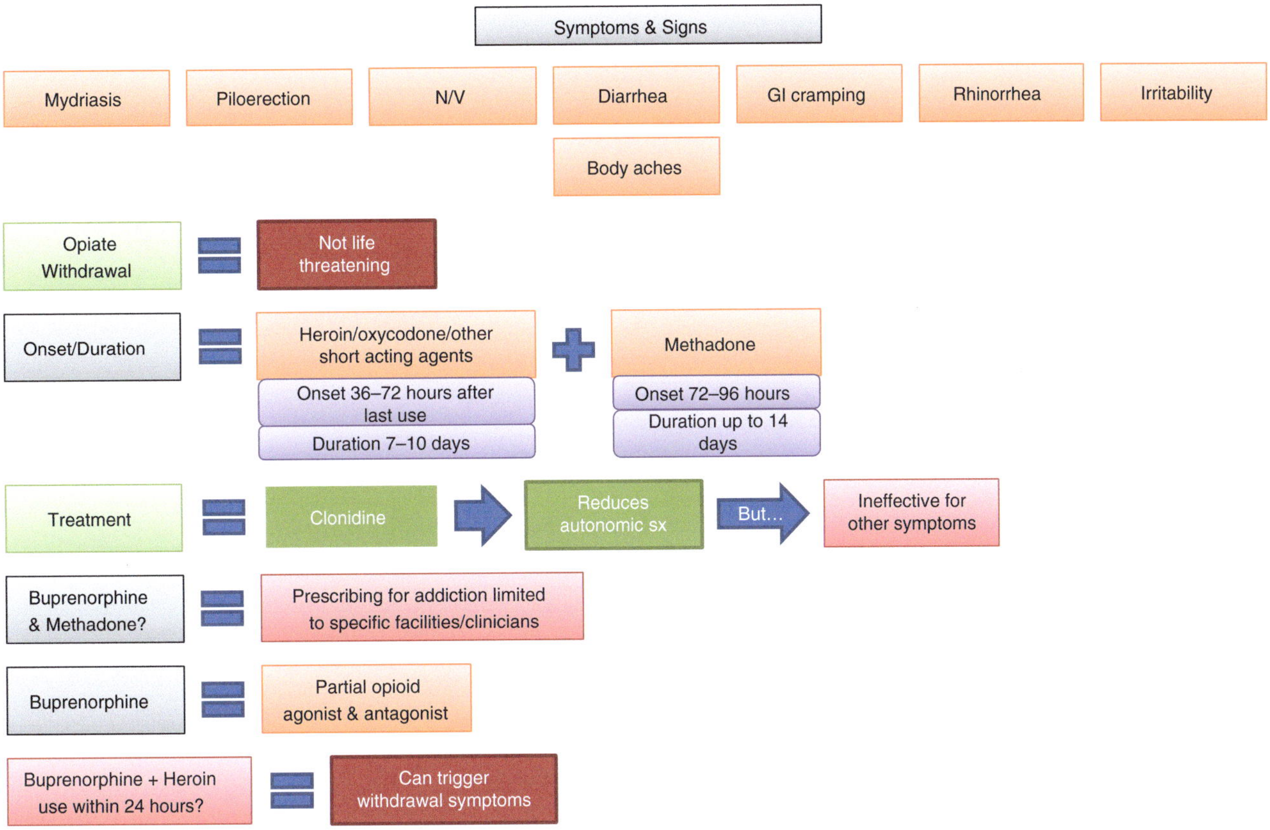

Cocaine/Sympathomimetic Withdrawal

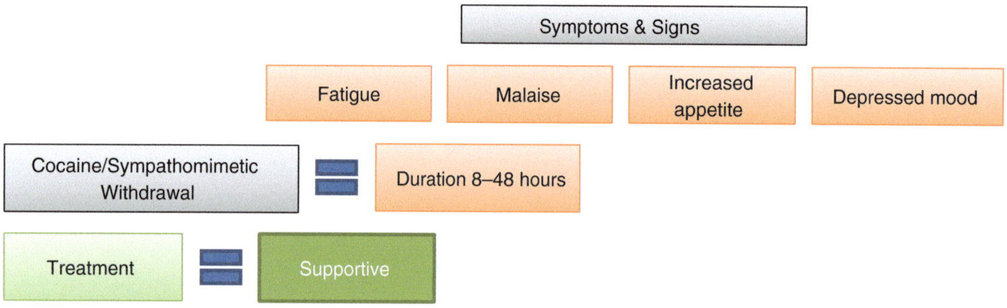

THC Withdrawal

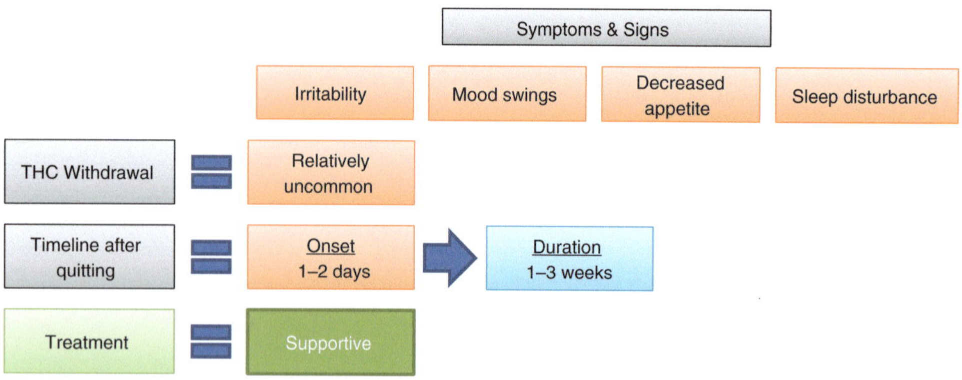

Obstetrics and Gynecology

Bobby Desai and Alpa Desai

Contents

Infections ... 618

Gynecologic Oncology ... 627

Obstetrics ... 629

B. Desai, MD, MEd (✉)
Department of Emergency Medicine, University of Florida,
Gainesville, FL, USA
e-mail: bdesai@ufl.edu

A. Desai, DO
Community Health and Family Medicine,
University of Florida College of Medicine, Gainesville, FL, USA

B. Desai, B.R. Allen (eds.), *Nailing the Written Emergency Medicine Board Examination*,
DOI 10.1007/978-3-319-30838-8_11

Infections

Pelvic Inflammatory Disease

Introduction

PID = Infections of the upper reproductive tract → Ascending from the vagina & cervix → Includes a spectrum of diseases → Most common gynecologic cause of ED visits

PID Due to → *Chlamydia* (Most common) OR Gonorrhea OR Polymicrobial (30–40 %) Including anaerobes

Risk factors = Prior PID or STD + Multiple sexual partners + Younger age + IUD in 1st month + Hx of sexual abuse

Decreased risk of PID = Pregnancy + Use of barrier contraceptives

General Symptoms & Signs → Most commonly occur early in or at the end of menstrual cycle due to thinning of cervical mucosal barrier

- Lower abdominal pain
- Vaginal discharge
- Vaginal or postcoital bleeding
- Dysuria
- Fever
- Malaise
- N/V
- Cervical motion tenderness
- Uterine tenderness
- Adnexal tenderness (most sensitive finding)
- Mucopurulent cervicitis
- Abdominal guarding & rebound → Associated peritonitis

(RUQ pain + Jaundice = Fitz-Hugh-Curtis syndrome)

Diagnosis and Treatment

Diagnostic tests = Ultrasound OR CT OR Laparoscopy (Gold standard) ± Laboratory evaluation

Ultrasound utility = Thickened fluid filled fallopian tubes + Free pelvic fluid + Dx of TOA

CT utility = Rule out other surgical causes

Other diagnostic criteria = Temp > 38 + Mucopurulent cervicitis + Elevated ESR/CRP + Confirmation of GC or Chlamydia

Empiric therapy For → Uterine tenderness OR Adnexal tenderness + Cervical motion tenderness

Inpatient treatment = Cefotetan or Cefoxitin + Doxycycline ‖ Clindamycin + Gentamicin ‖ Ampicillin/Sulbactam + Doxycycline

Outpatient treatment = Cefotetan or Cefoxitin + Doxycycline ± Metronidazole OR Levofloxacin or Ofloxacin ± Metronidazole

IUD? = Remove IUD

Admission Criteria for PID

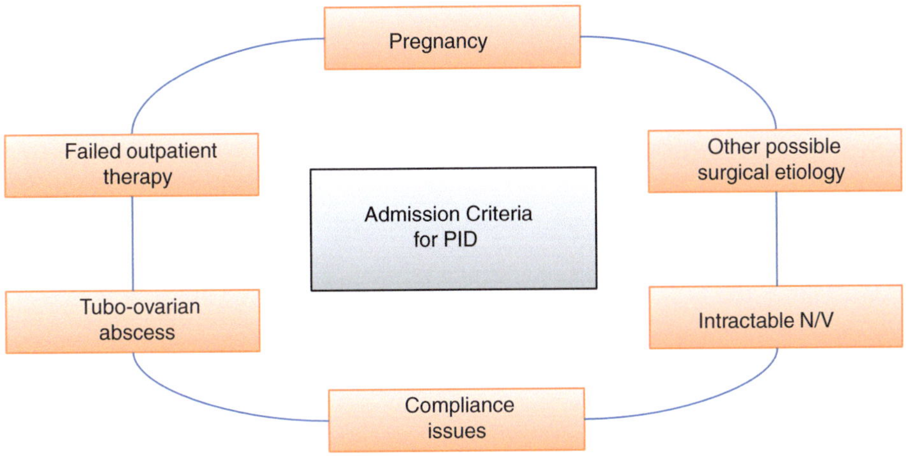

Complications of PID

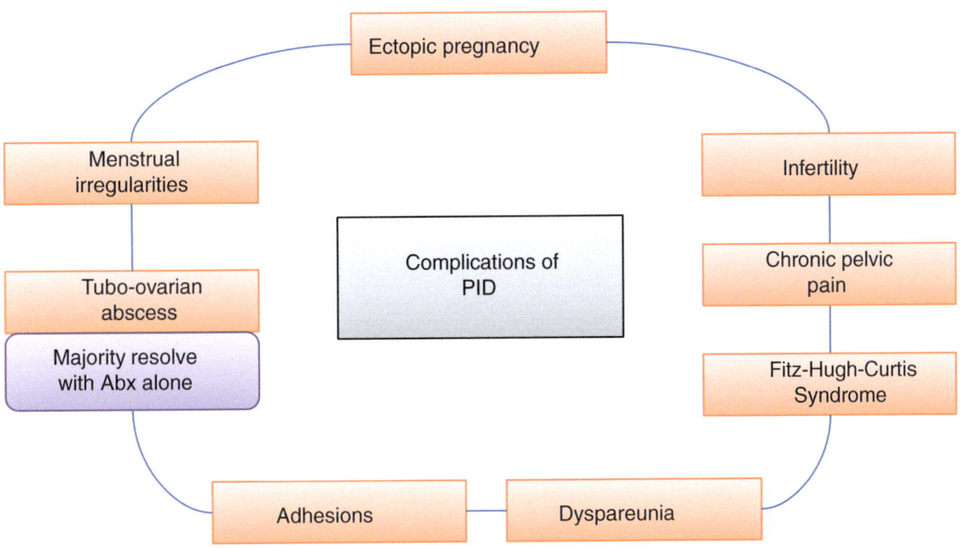

Fitz-Hugh-Curtis Syndrome

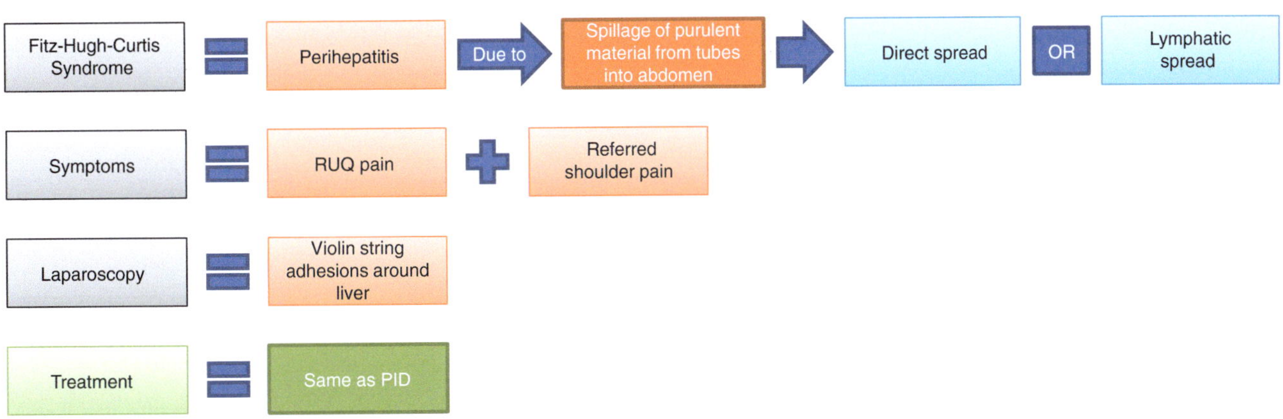

Vulvovaginitis

Introduction

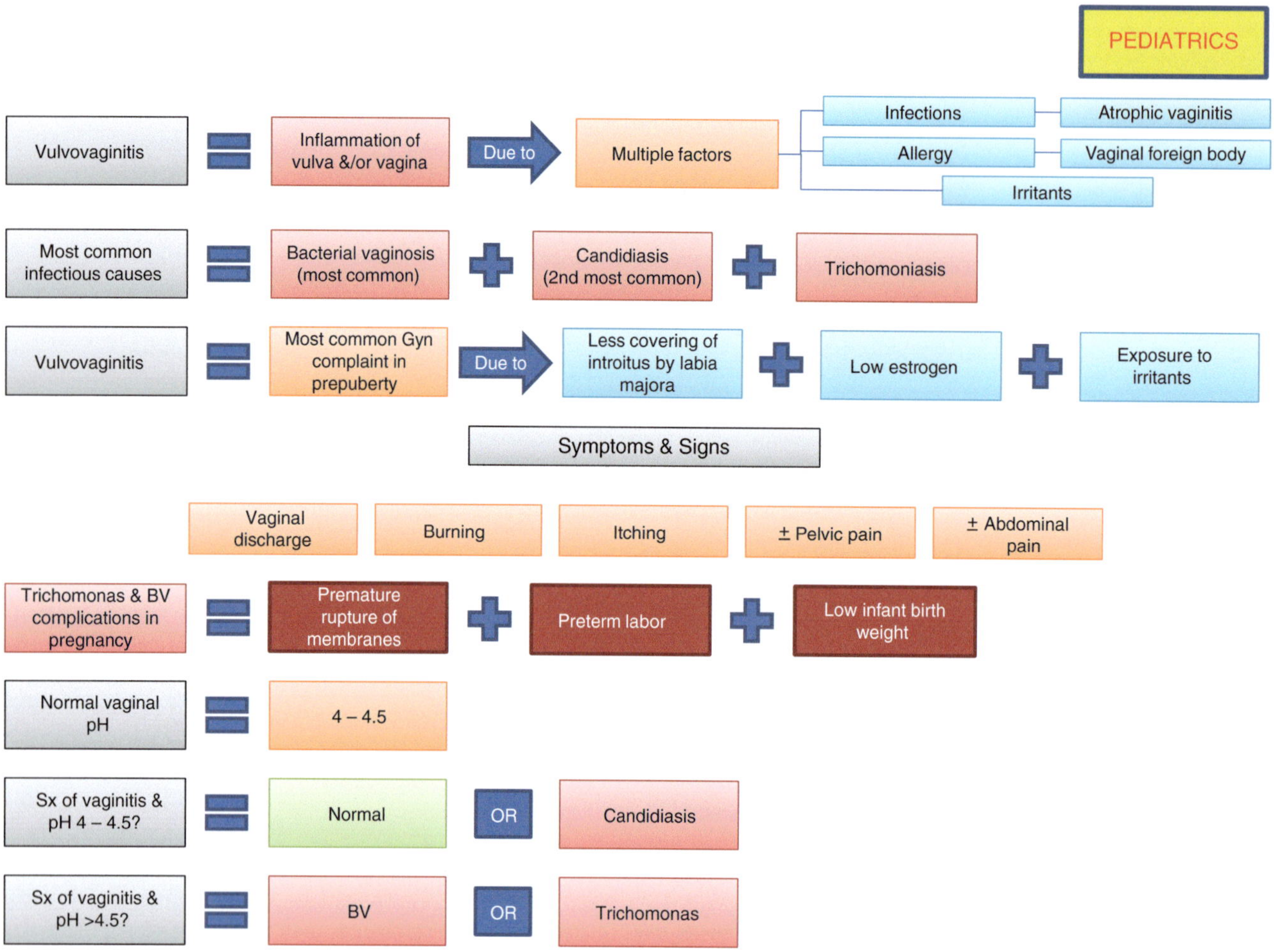

Bacterial Vaginosis (BV)

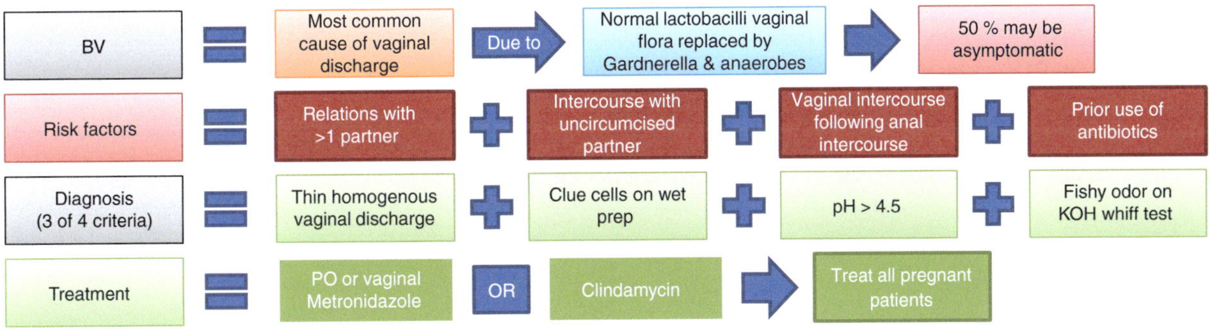

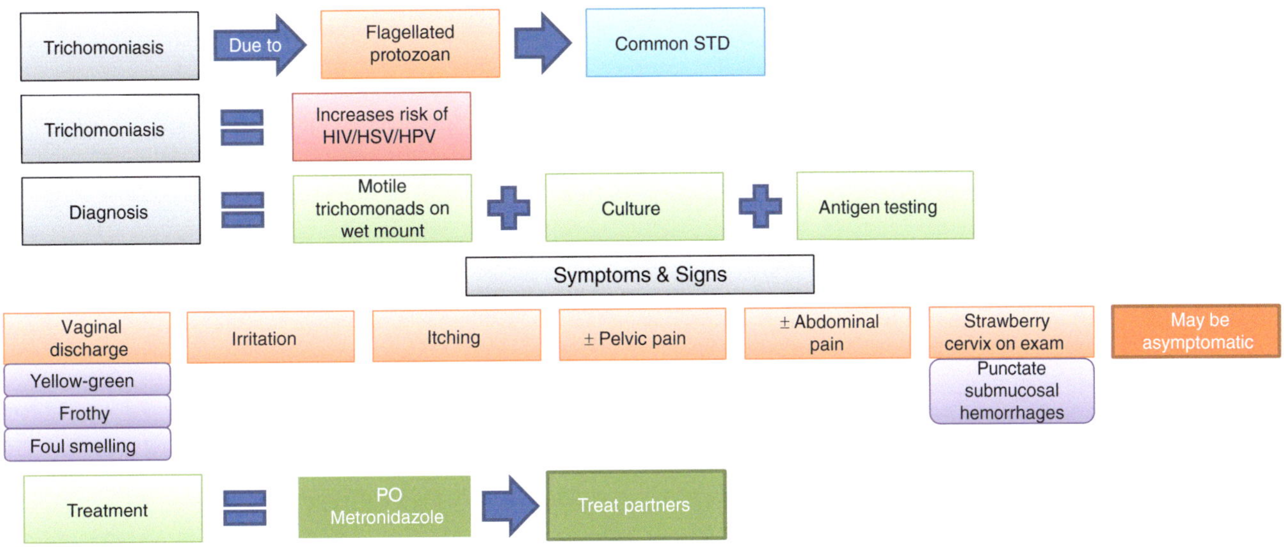

Trichomoniasis

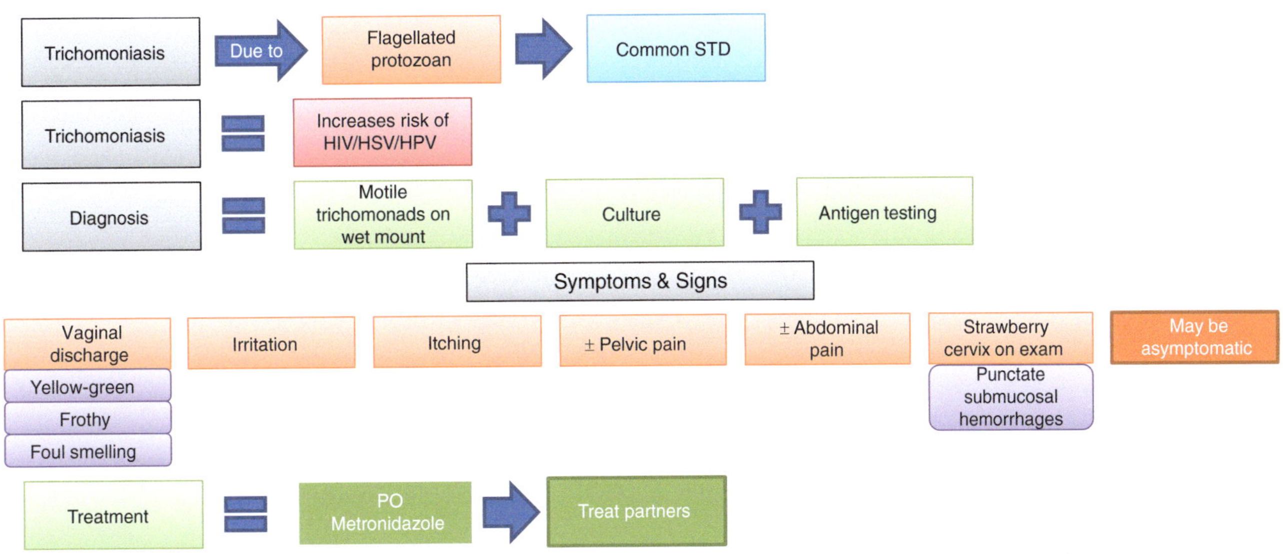

Candida Vaginitis

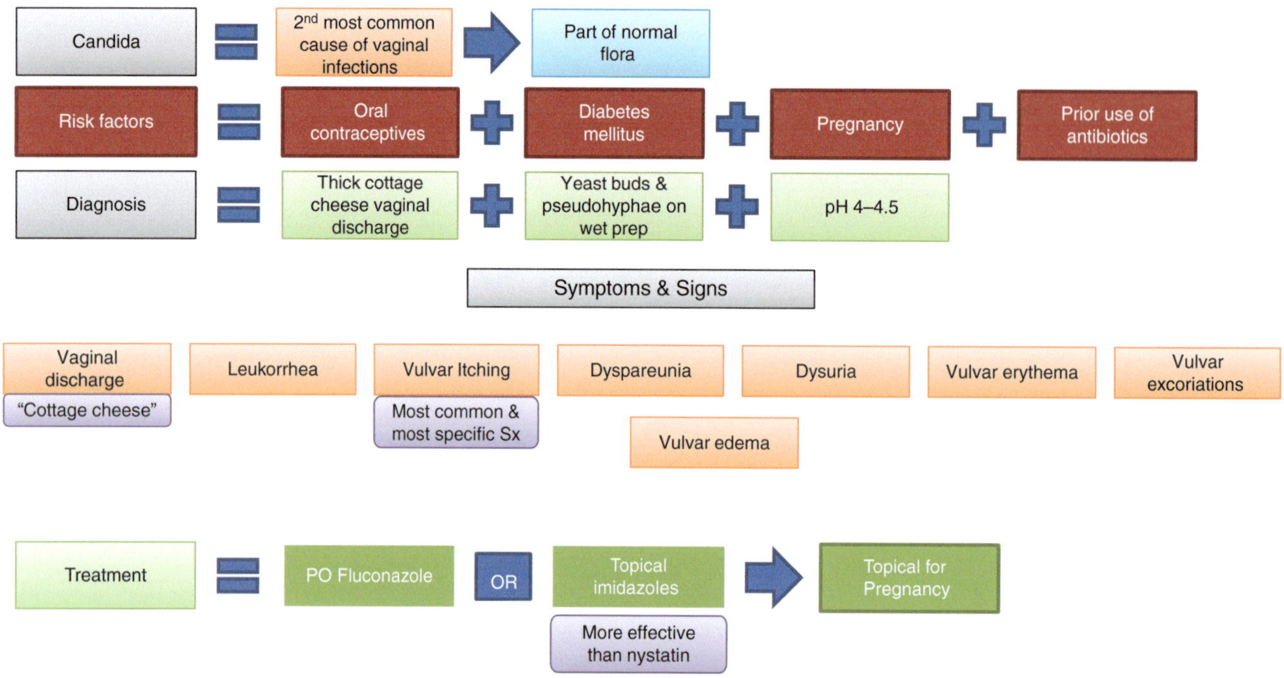

Bartholin Cyst and Abscess

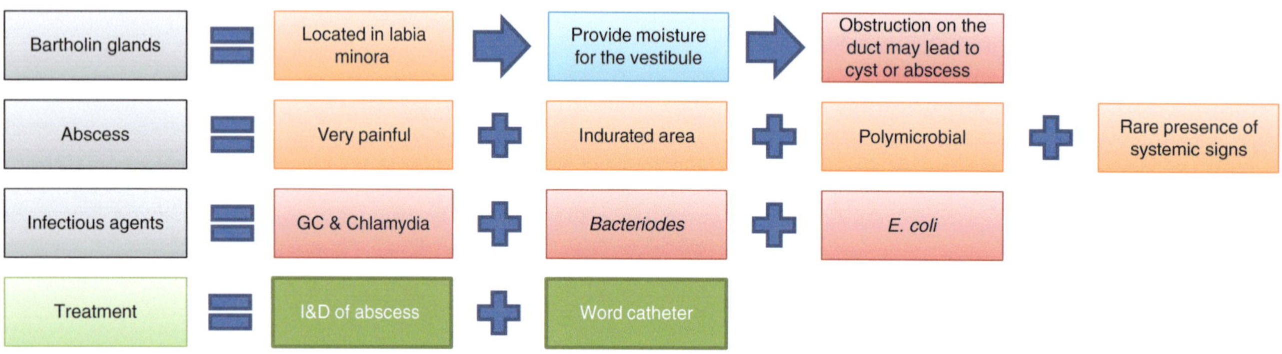

Abdominal and Pelvic Pain in the Nonpregnant Patient

Ovarian Cysts

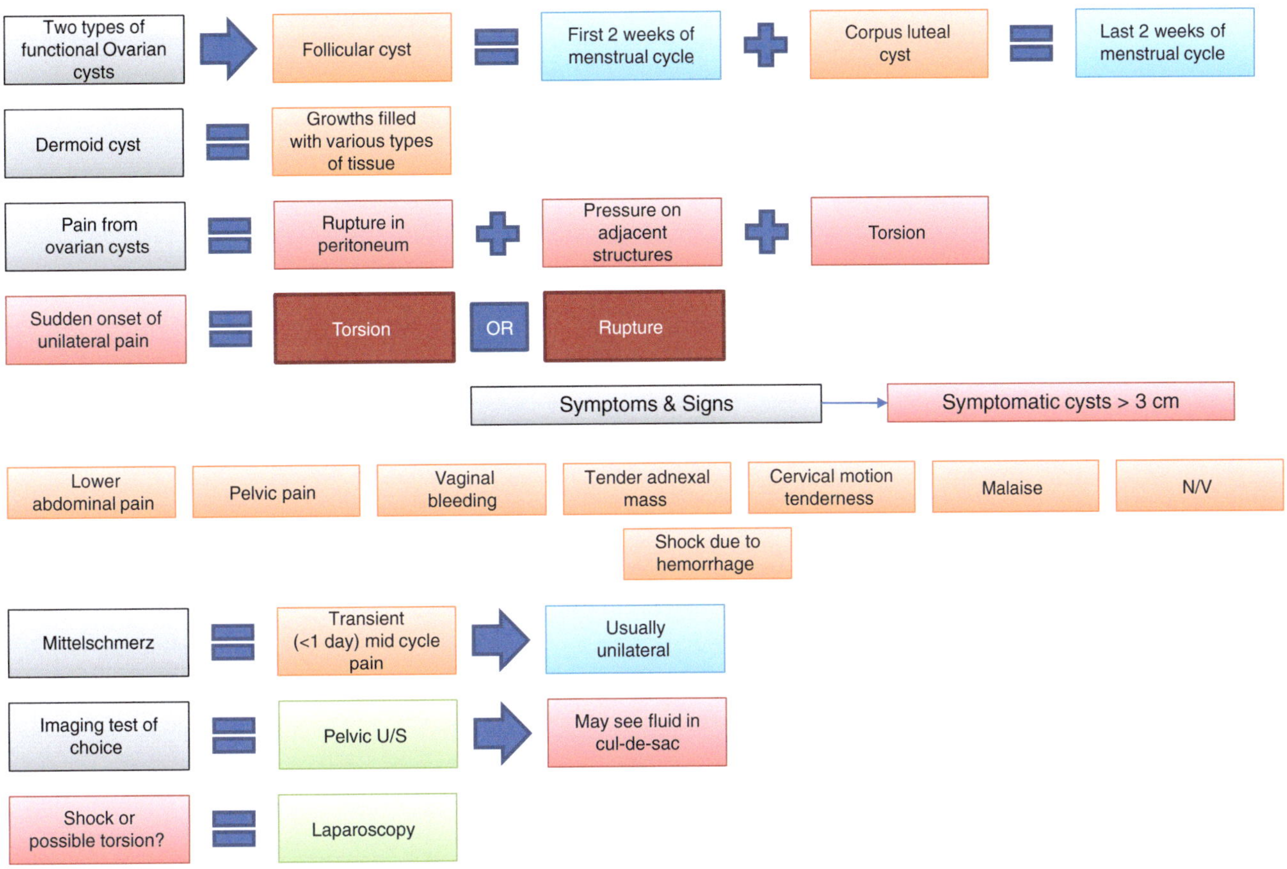

Ovarian or Adnexal Torsion

Torsion = Ovary twists on oviduct (Adnexa) → Due to Ovarian enlargement = Surgical emergency → Adenexal > Ovarian torsion

Pathophysiology = Venous blockage → Congestion of ovary → Arterial blockage → Ischemia and potential necrosis

Torsion = >50 % on the *Right* + Most associated with benign tumors or cysts → Dermoid cyst most common

Risk factors = Pregnancy (Corpus luteum) + Large cysts or tumors + Chemical induction of ovulation

Symptoms & Signs

- Unilateral constant lower abdominal pain
- N/V
- Vaginal bleeding is *not common*
- Tender adnexal mass
- Cervical motion tenderness

Imaging test of choice = Pelvic U/S with Doppler → Low flow to ovary

Treatment = Laparoscopy

Endometriosis

Endometriosis = Common cause of infertility & pelvic pain → Due to Endometrial tissue outside of uterus = Chronic inflammatory reaction → Mostly in reproductive age

Adenomyosis = Endometrial tissue in uterine wall

Common locations = Ovary (most common) + Fallopian tubes + Bladder + Abdominal cavity + Lungs (May cause *catamenial pneumothorax*)

Symptoms & Signs

- Chronic lower abdominal pain
- Pain is cyclical, associated with menses
- Dysmenorrhea (most common symptom)
- Dyspareunia
- Hypermenorrhea
- Pelvic pain
- Enlarged adherent uterus
- Ovarian mass (Chocolate cyst)
- Infertility

Imaging test of choice = Pelvic U/S

Diagnosis = Laparoscopy

Treatment = Analgesia + Referral

Leiomyomas

Leiomyomas = Uterine fibroids = Benign tumors of uterine muscle = Most common pelvic tumor in African Americans

Complications = May outgrow blood supply + May torse if on a pedicle + Pregnancy results in growth and loss of blood supply = Pain

Symptoms & Signs

Pelvic pain | Hypermenorrhea | Lower abdominal pain | Mass on examination

Imaging test of choice = Pelvic U/S

Treatment = Analgesia + Referral

Abnormal Vaginal Bleeding

Abnormal Vaginal Bleeding

Vaginal bleeding = Premenstrual + Midcycle + Menstrual + Postmenstrual

Menorrhagia = Heavy bleeding | Metrorrhagia = Bleeding outside normal cycle | Menometrorrhagia = Excessive irregular bleeding

Abnormal vaginal bleeding in non-pregnant females = Nonuterine bleeding + Ovulatory bleeding + Anovulatory bleeding

Abnormal ovulatory bleeding = Metrorrhagia + Bleeding between menses

Treatment = Oral contraceptives + NSAIDs

Anovulatory bleeding = Menometrorrhagia OR Light & frequent bleeding OR Prolonged amenorrhea with intermittent metrorrhagia

Treatment = Oral contraceptives + NSAIDs

Consider *endometrial cancer* in pts > 35!

Ovulatory Bleeding

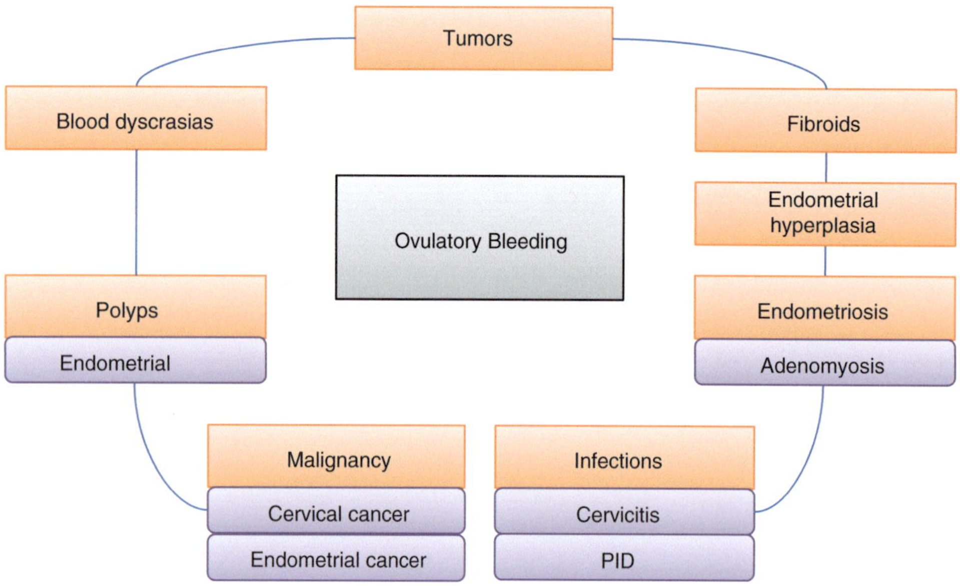

Anovulatory Bleeding

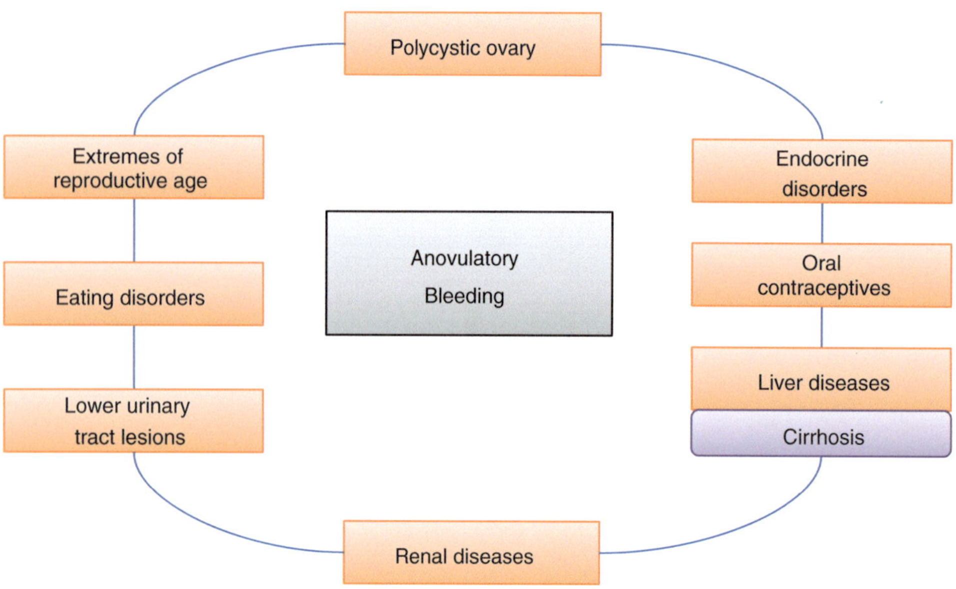

Gynecologic Oncology

Ovarian Cancer

Ovarian cancer = 2nd most common gyn malignancy → But… Has highest mortality rate of GYN malignancy → May be advanced on diagnosis → Peak incidence 55–65

Risk factors = Infertility + Low parity + Obesity (high fat diet) + Family history + Hx of breast or colon cancer

Symptoms & Signs

Abdominal pain | Bloating | Weight loss | Pleural effusion | Ascites | Urinary frequency or urgency | Early satiety

Unilateral fixed mass

Rare torsion

Unexplained ascites = Gyn neoplasm until proven otherwise

Diagnosis = Ultrasound OR CT scan

Uterine Cancer

Uterine cancer = Most common GYN malignancy → Adenocarcinoma is most common → Usually caught early → Average age 55–58

Sarcoma? = More aggressive = Worse prognosis

Risk factors = Continuous estrogen + Nulliparity + Obesity (high fat diet) + DM HTN + Early menses Late menopause

Symptoms & Signs

Abnormal vaginal bleeding | Uterine enlargement | Weight loss

Diagnosis = D&C OR Endometrial biopsy OR Transvaginal U/S in postmenopause

Cervical Cancer

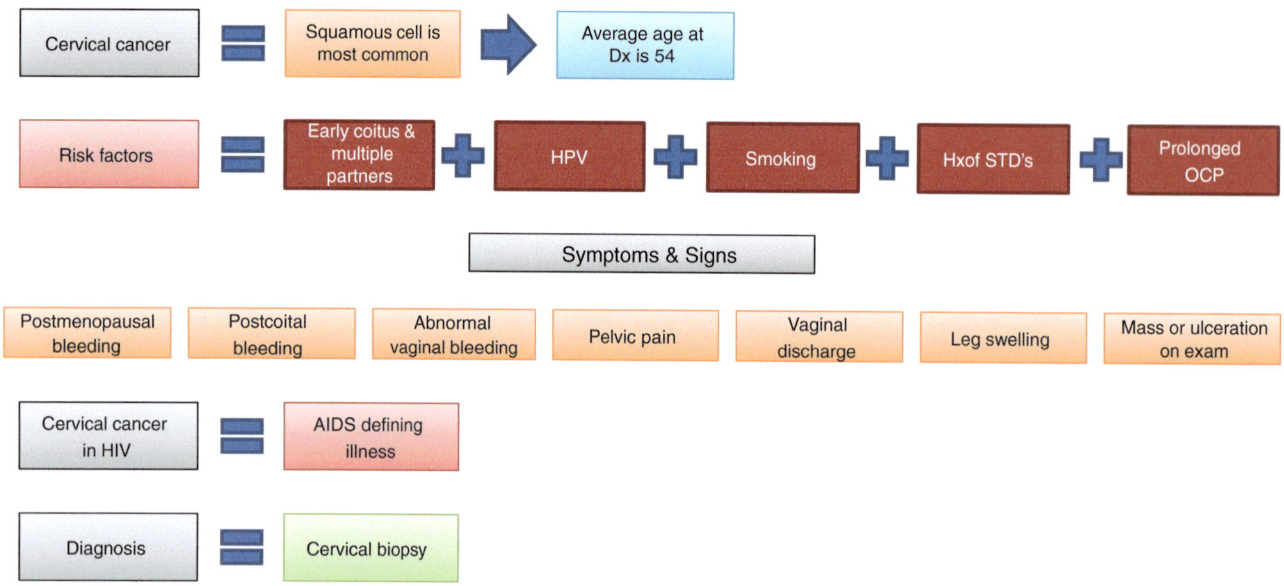

Obstetrics

Ectopic Pregnancy

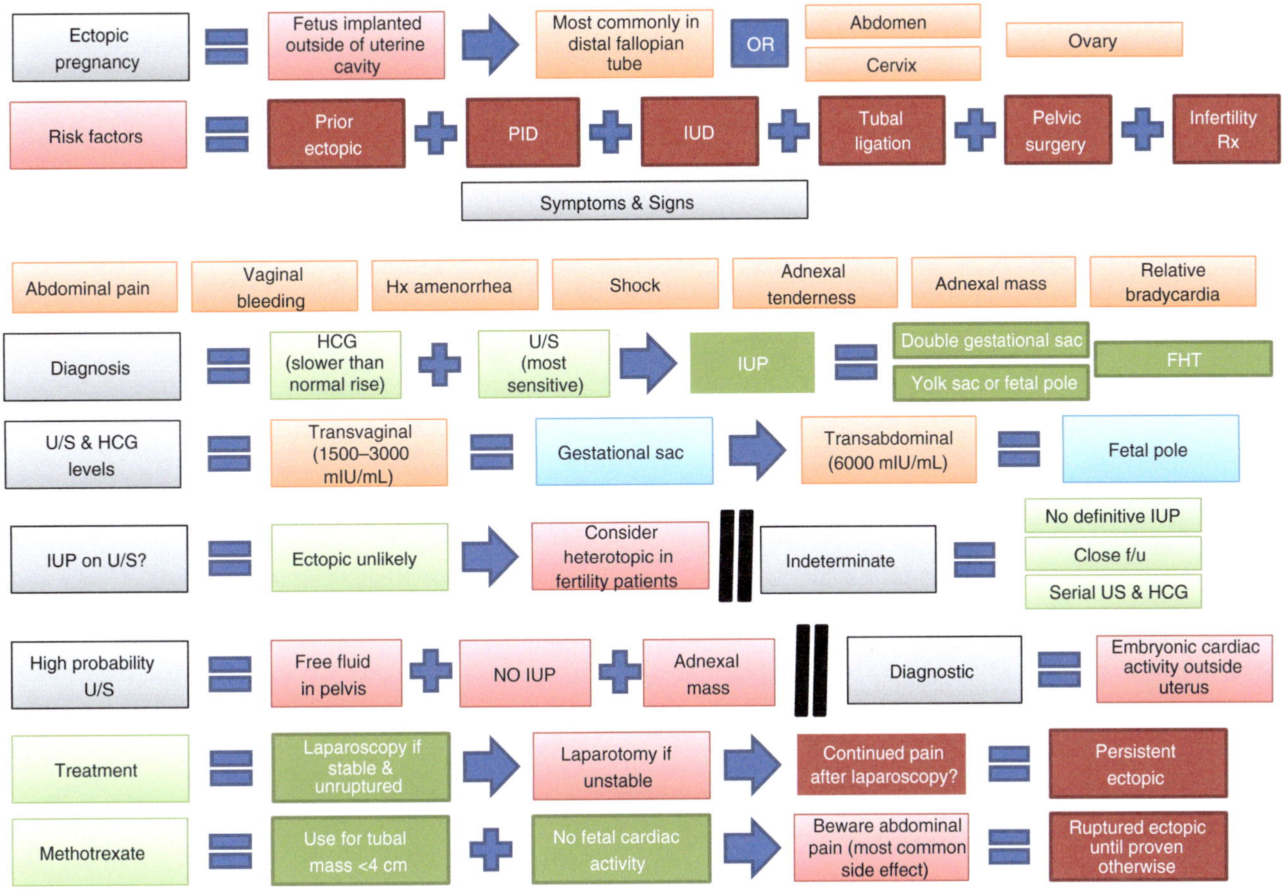

Abortions

Threatened = < 20 weeks gestation + Abdominal cramps or pain + Vaginal bleeding + Closed os

Treatment = Vaginal rest

Inevitable = < 20 weeks gestation + Abdominal cramps or pain + Vaginal bleeding + Open os

Treatment = D&C

Incomplete = Vaginal bleeding + Tissue noted as cervical os → Likely to occur at 6–14 weeks

Treatment = D&C

Complete = Vaginal bleeding + Passage of all fetal tissue + <20 weeks + Closed os

Missed = Fetal death <20 weeks + No passage of tissue = D&C

Septic = Infection during abortion

Treatment = Fluids + Antibiotics + D&C

RhoGAM

Rhogam = Anti-D IgG

Immunization = 0.1 mL of fetal blood mixing with mother's → Also can occur with ectopics

Pathophysiology = Destruction of Rh+ fetal RBC in maternal circulation → Immunization → Antibodies to Rh+ fetal RBC which cross placenta

Complications = Fetal hemolytic anemia + Splenomegaly + Erythroblastosis + Potential death of fetus

Indications in Rh (-) mother = Ectopic + Any type of abortion + Placenta abruption + Antepartum hemorrhage + Trauma

Dose = <12 weeks → 50 mcg | >12 weeks → 300 mcg

Gestational Trophoblastic Disease

Gestational trophoblastic disease = Spectrum of processes → Partial hydatidiform mole OR Choriocarcinoma

Gestational trophoblastic disease = Arises in trophoblastic cells of the placenta

Hydatidiform mole = Noninvasive → Partial OR Complete → Complete is more common

Complete = No fetus || Incomplete = Deformed nonviable fetus present

Symptoms & Signs

- 1st Trimester: Vaginal bleeding (75–95 %), Hyperemesis
- 2nd Trimester: Preeclampsia, Large uterus
- Passage of "grape like" clusters

Diagnosis = Ultrasound → Lucent areas & brighter areas + Elevated HCG levels

Treatment = Suction curettage

Complications = Amniotic fluid embolism + Metastases to lung, liver, brain + Preeclampsia

Hypertension, Preeclampsia, and Eclampsia

Hypertension in Pregnancy

Chronic Hypertension = Existed prior to pregnancy OR Dx < 20 weeks OR Persists > 6 weeks after delivery

Complications of chronic HTN = Abruptio placentae + Preterm birth + Preeclampsia + Low birth weight

Treatment = Labetalol OR Methyldopa + OB/GYN referral

Transient HTN = HTN during pregnancy − Proteinuria − Complications to pregnancy + Resolves within 2–4 weeks of delivery

Preeclampsia

Preeclampsia = HTN + 140/90 or SBP >20 or DBP >10 over baseline + Proteinuria ± Edema → After 20 weeks

Before 20 weeks? = Consider molar pregnancy

Pathophysiology = Vasospastic disease of unknown etiology → Causes end organ damage

Associations = Premature labor + Low birth weight + Intrauterine growth retardation + Abruptio placenta

Risk factors = Nulliparous + DM HTN Renal dis. + <20 >40 + Multiple gestation + Obesity + FHx + Molar pregnancy

Symptoms & Signs

Headache | Visual symptoms | Abdominal pain | Edema

Treatment = Delivery of fetus

Eclampsia

Eclampsia = Preeclampsia + Seizures + >20 weeks gestational age OR <4 weeks postpartum

Symptoms & Signs

Headache | Visual symptoms | Abdominal pain | Edema | Seizures | Hyperreflexia

Treatment of Seizures = Magnesium sulfate

Magnesium toxicity? = Hyporeflexia + Decreased respiratory drive → Treatment = Calcium gluconate

Treatment of HTN = Hydralazine OR Labetalol

Complications = Liver/spleen hemorrhage + End organ failure + Abruptio placenta + Intracranial hemorrhage

HELLP Syndrome

HELLP syndrome = *Hemolysis* + Elevated *Liver* enzymes + *Low Platelets* = Clinical variant of Preeclampsia

HELLP syndrome = ± HTN + Epigastric abdominal pain OR RUQ abdominal pain

HELLP syndrome = Multigravid > Primigravid

Diagnosis = Schistocytes on peripheral smear + Platelets <100,000/mcL + Elevated AST and ALT = Calcium gluconate

Treatment = Same as Preeclampsia = Delivery of fetus + Control of BP + Magnesium

Complications = Subcapsular liver hematoma + Rupture of right lobe of liver

Placental Emergencies

Abruptio Placentae

Abruptio Placentae = Separation of placenta from uterine wall → Can occur spontaneously → 2nd most common cause of fetal death

Risk factors = HTN (most common) + Trauma + Smoking + Advanced age + Cocaine abuse + Hx of abd surgery + Prior incidence

Symptoms & Signs

Painful vaginal bleeding | Contractions | Abdominal pain | Uterine tenderness | Hypotension | N/V | Back pain

If no bleeding, then *concealed abruptio*

Fetal distress → Tachycardia then bradycardia | Fetal decelerations

Maternal complications = DIC + Hemorrhagic shock + Rupture of uterus + Multi-organ failure

Fetal complications = Death + Neurologic abnormalities + Rupture of uterus + Multi-organ failure

Ultrasound? = Not sensitive for Dx → External fetal monitoring more sensitive → Indicated for blunt trauma pts > 20 weeks

Fetal monitoring = > 8 contractions/hr for 4 hours = Risk for abruption ‖ 3–7 contractions/hr for 4 hours = Extend monitoring for 24 hours

Treatment = Fluid resuscitation + Blood products at the ready + Fetal monitoring + Emergent OB consultation

Fetal distress + > 23 weeks gestation = Consideration of emergent C - section

Placenta Previa

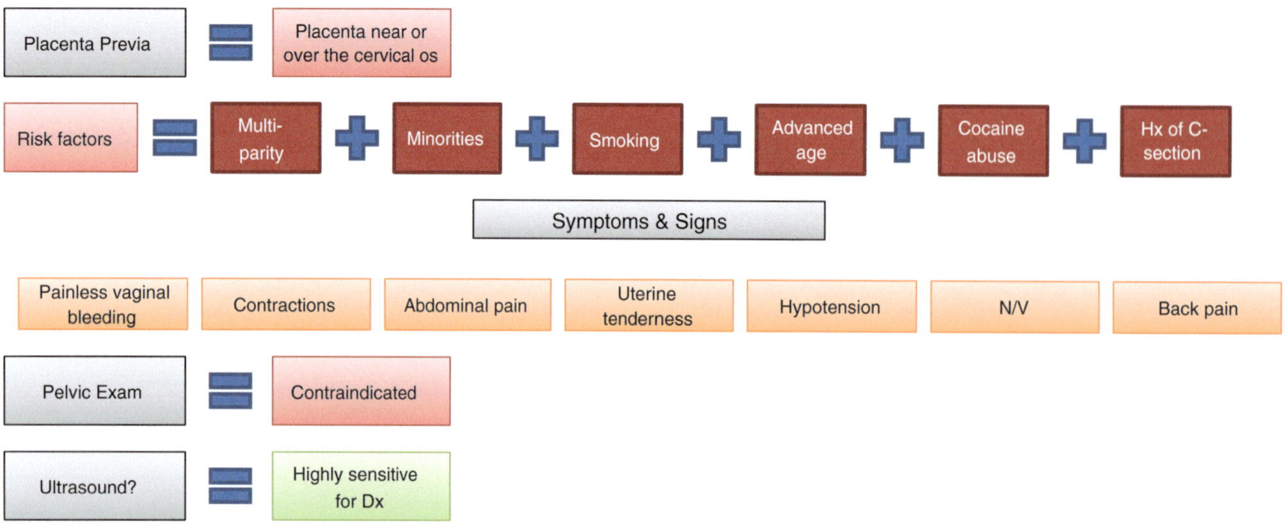

Other Emergencies of Pregnancy, Deliveries, or the Postpartum Period

Tidbits

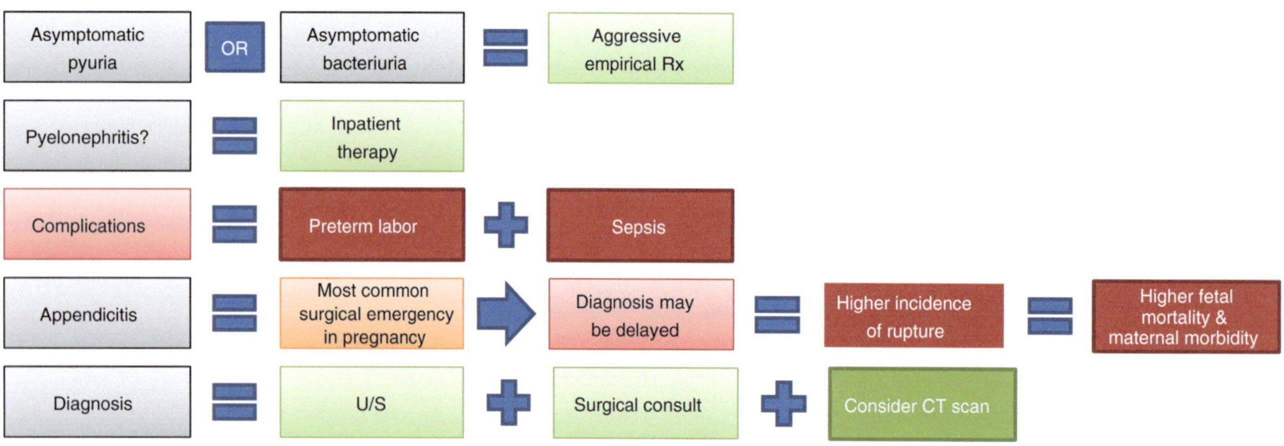

Preterm Birth and Premature Rupture of Membranes (PROM)

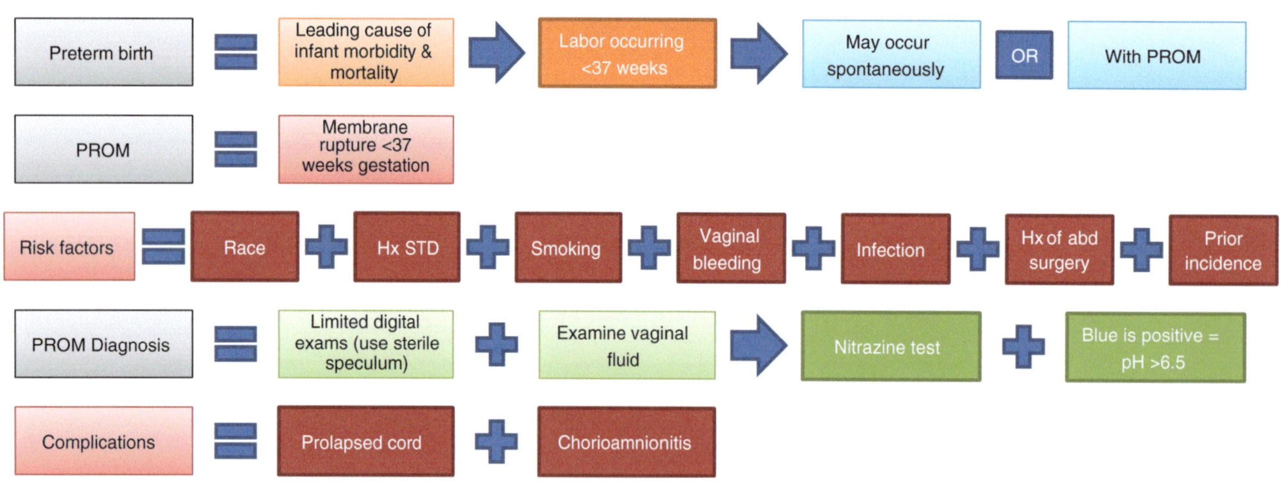

Umbilical Cord Prolapse

Prolapsed umbilical cord = High mortality

Prolapsed umbilical cord = Place mother in knee to chest position

Treatment = Elevate presenting part + Impede delivery + Emergent C-section

Postpartum Hemorrhage

Postpartum Hemorrhage = Most common cause of maternal mortality worldwide + Primary: In 1st 24 hours + Secondary: >24 hours, < 6 weeks

Primary Postpartum Hemorrhage = Uterine atony + Retained placental fragments + Lacerations of genital tract + Rupture of uterus + Inversion of uterus + Clotting problems

Uterine atony = Enlarged uterus ("Doughy") || Risk factors = Prolonged labor + Multiple gestations + Multiparity

Treatment = IV fluids + Fundal massage + Oxytocin

Uterine rupture Risks = Trauma + Cocaine + Prior C-section + High doses of Oxytocin

Symptoms & Signs = Shock + Copious bleeding + Absent FHT + Tender uterus || Treatment = C-section

Retained Products of conception = Early or delayed painless bleeding + Firm uterus || Treatment = D&C + Oxytocin

Uterine Inversion = Excessive traction on umbilical cord + Mass in vagina + Non-palpable uterus = Obstetric Emergency

Treatment = Tocolytic medications + Do not separate placenta + Manual reduction OR Emergent laparotomy

Amniotic Fluid Embolism

Amniotic Fluid Embolism = Occurs when amniotic fluid enters the maternal circulation = Immunologic response by mother = May simulate anaphylaxis = High mortality

Occurs with = C-section + Labor + Abruptio placentae + Abortion + Trauma + Amnio-centesis

Symptoms & Signs

- Acute cardiovascular collapse
- Seizures (hypoxic)
- Shock
- Dyspnea
- ARDS
- DIC
- Hypoxemia

Treatment = Supportive + Place in left lateral decubitus position + Immediate delivery of the infant

Peripartum Cardiomyopathy

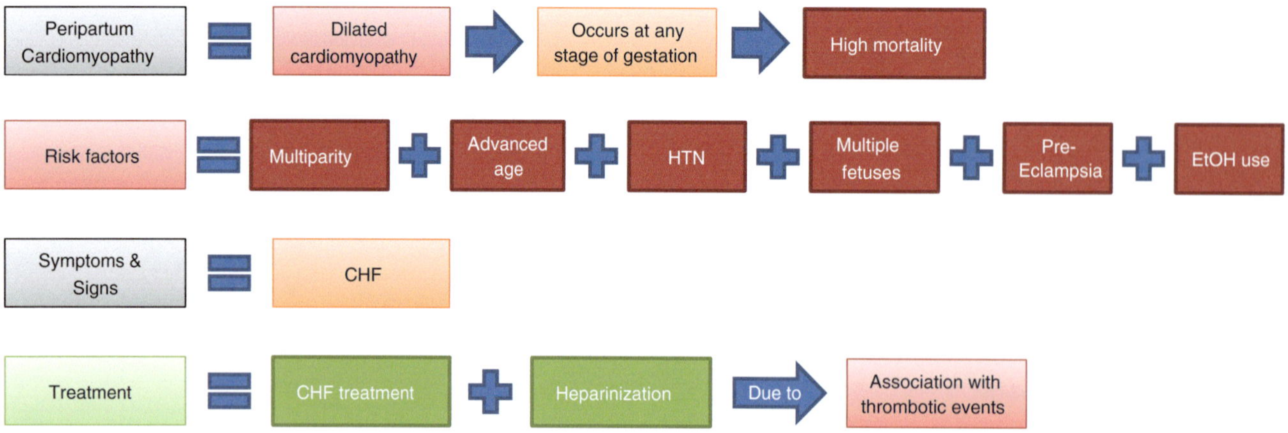

Endometritis

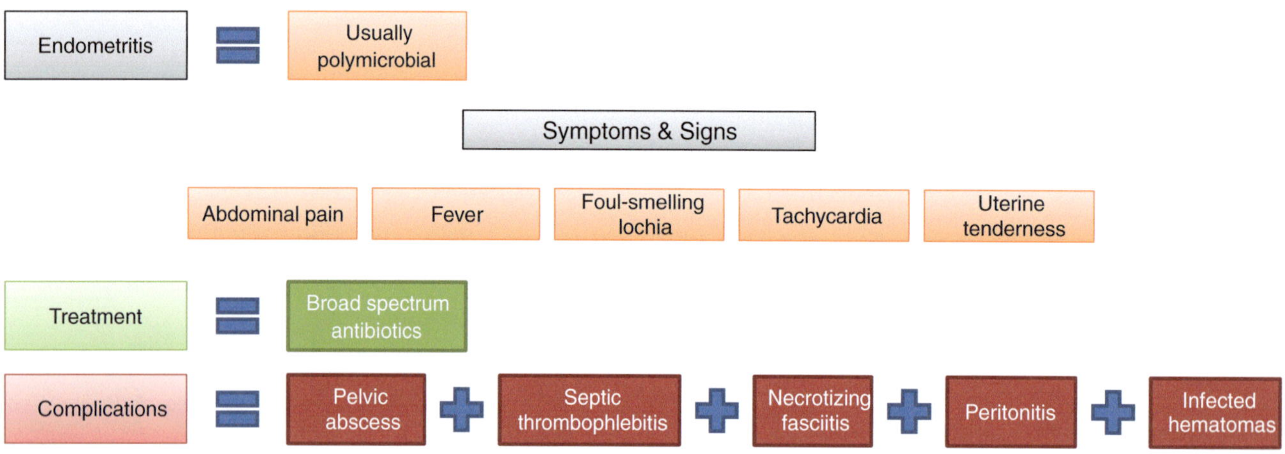

Mastitis

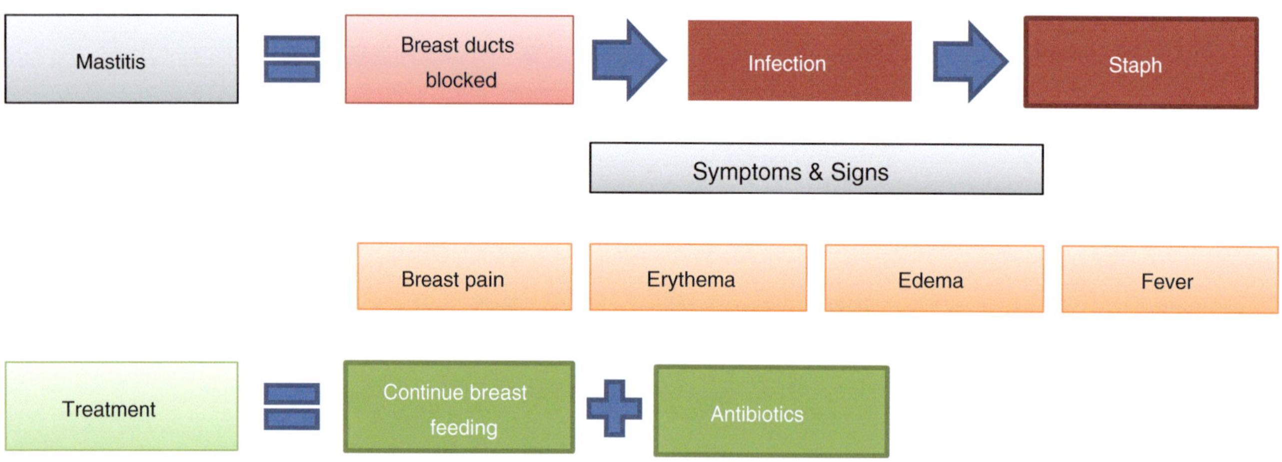

Ophthalmology

Bobby Desai

Contents

Neuro-ophthalmology ... 638
Pupil Abnormalities ... 640
Visual Field Deficits ... 641
External Eye ... 642
Conjunctiva ... 648
Cornea ... 653
Corneal Abrasion, Laceration, and Ulcers ... 657
Uveitis and Iritis ... 660
Vitreous and Intraocular Cavities ... 661
Retina ... 663
Optic Nerve ... 666
Temporal Arteritis ... 668
Glaucoma ... 669
Trauma ... 670
Blow-Out Fractures ... 673
Retrobulbar Hematoma ... 673
Chemical Burns ... 674
Lacerations to Refer ... 674

B. Desai, MD, MEd
Department of Emergency Medicine, University of Florida,
Gainesville, FL, USA
e-mail: bdesai@ufl.edu

B. Desai, B.R. Allen (eds.), *Nailing the Written Emergency Medicine Board Examination*,
DOI 10.1007/978-3-319-30838-8_12

Neuro-ophthalmology

Eye Muscles: Left Eye

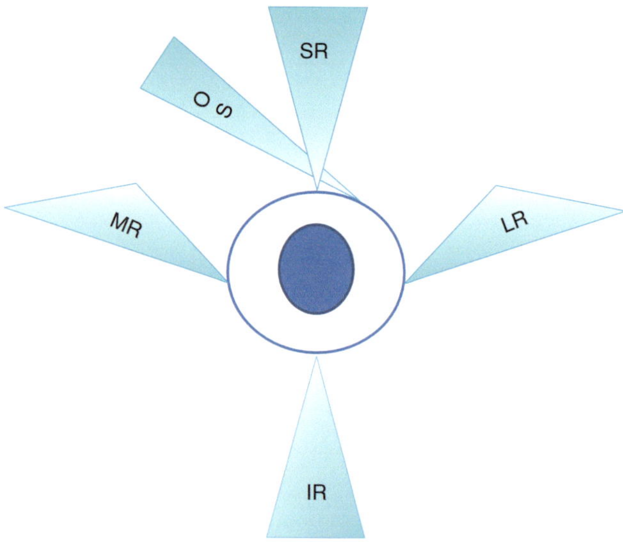

Eye Movements: Right Eye

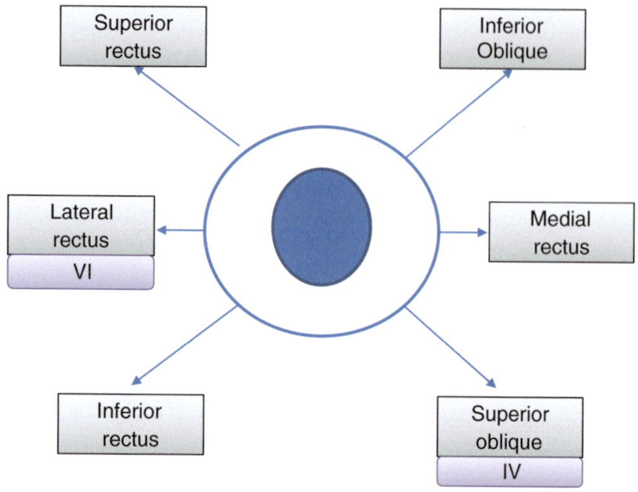

$LR_6(SO_4)_3$

Cranial Nerves

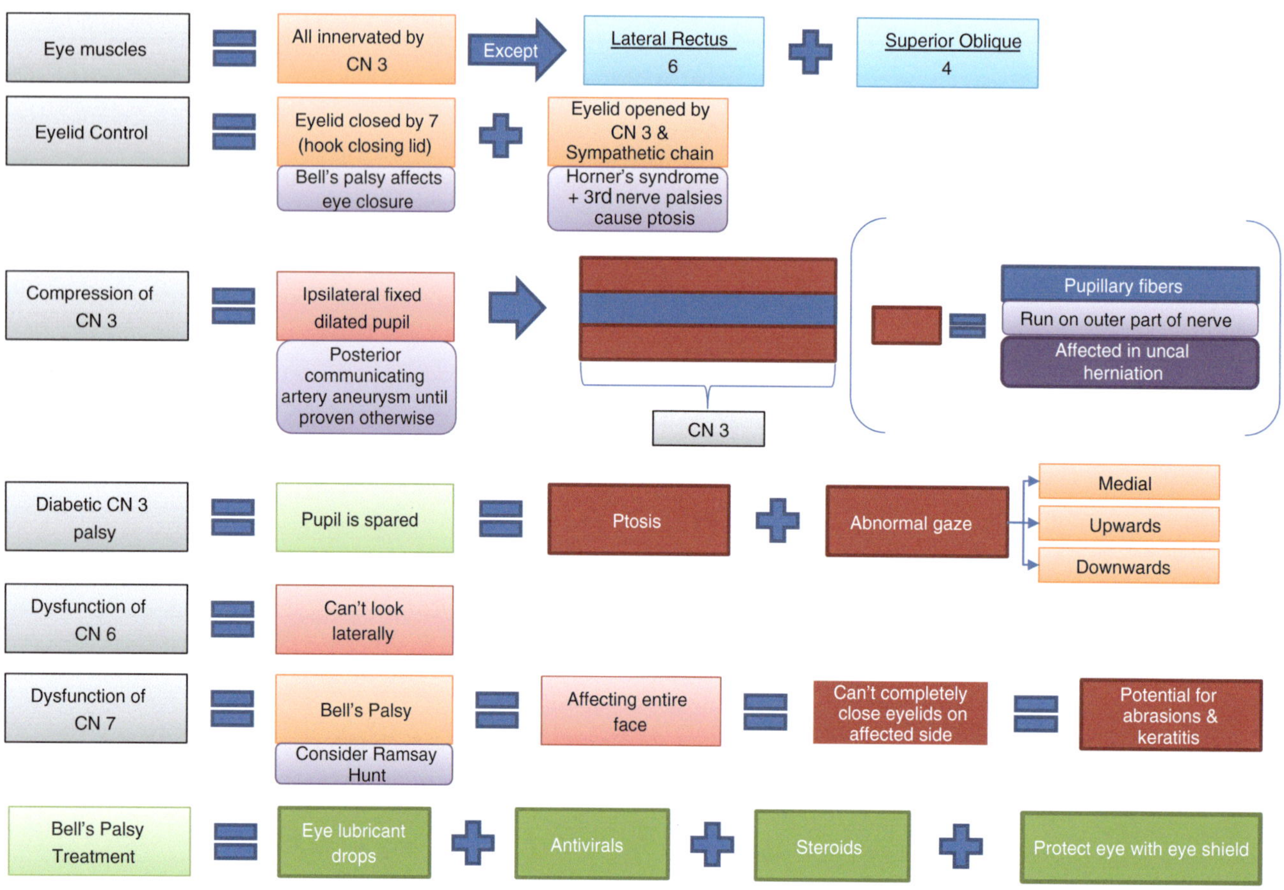

Sympathetic Chain and Horner's Syndrome

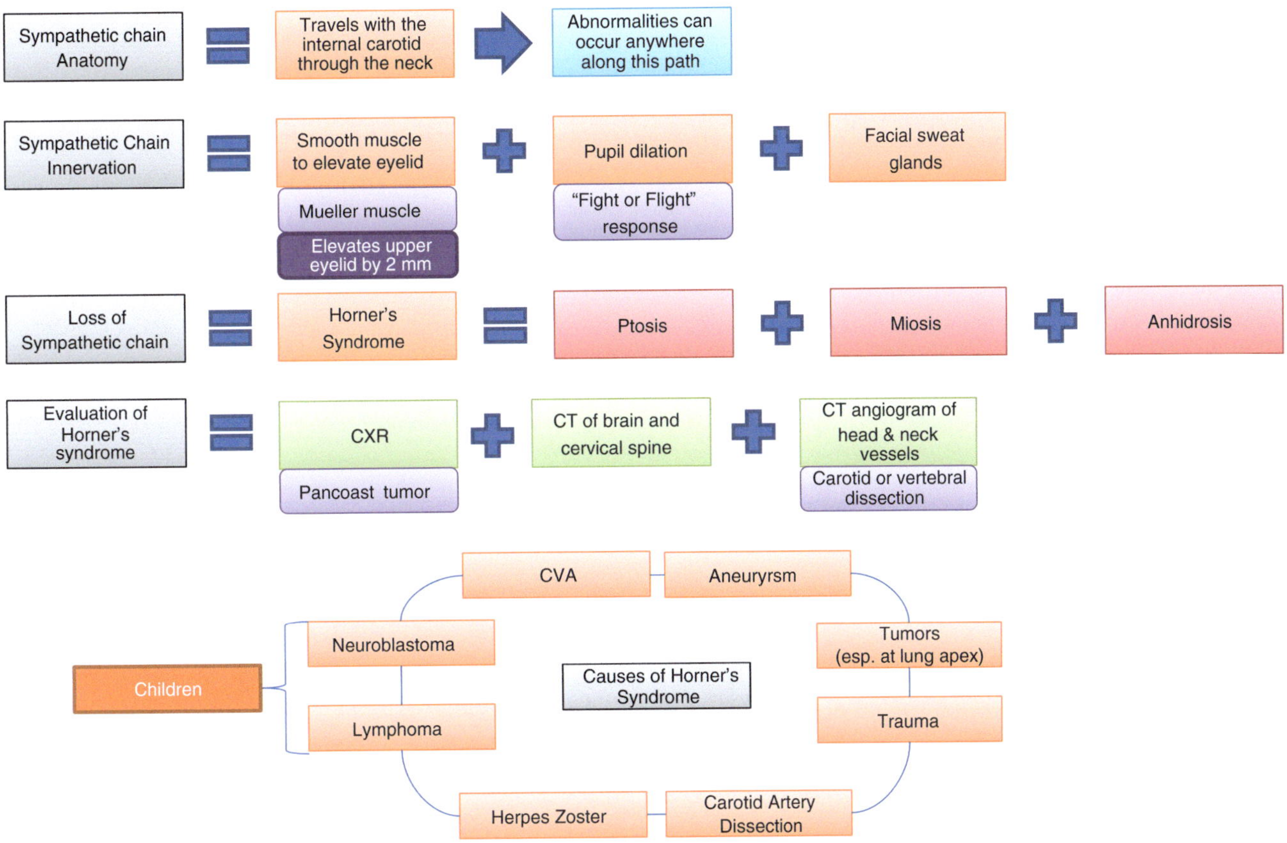

Pupil Abnormalities

Introduction

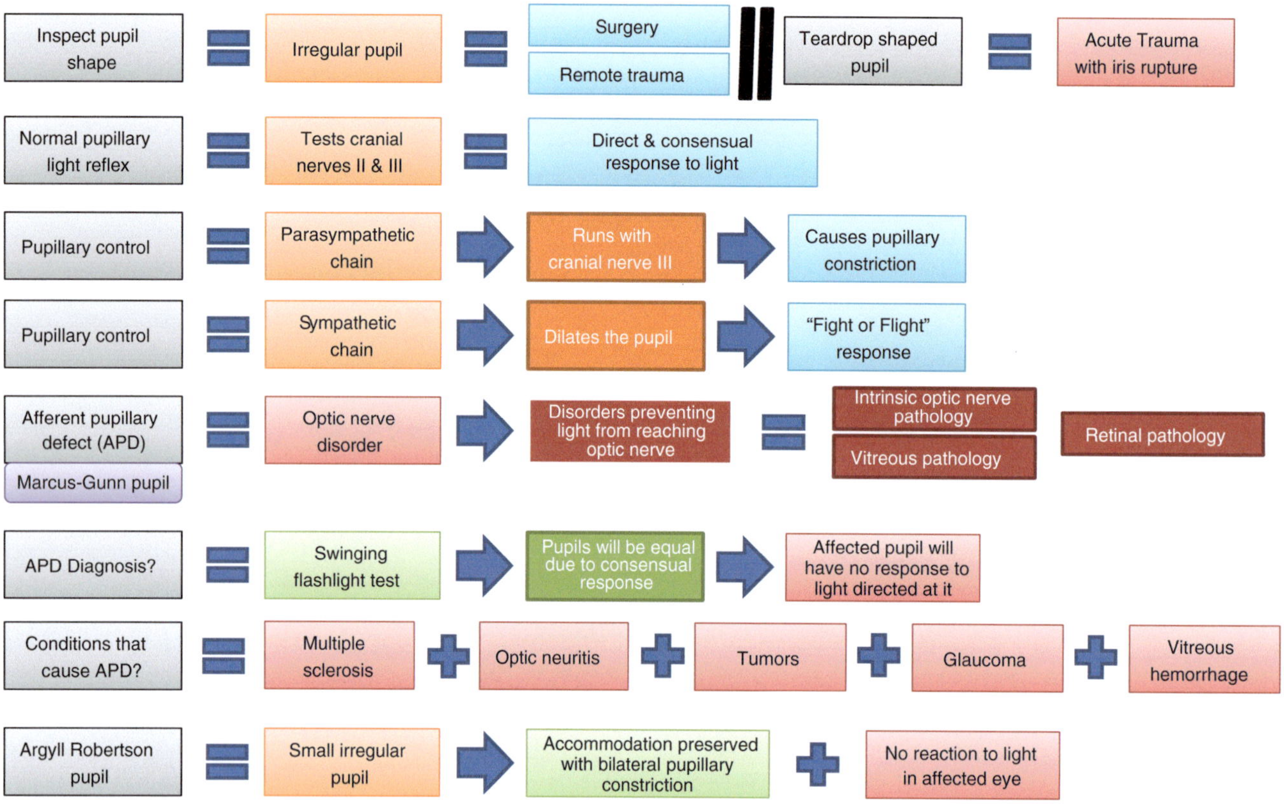

Visual Field Deficits

Visual Field Deficits

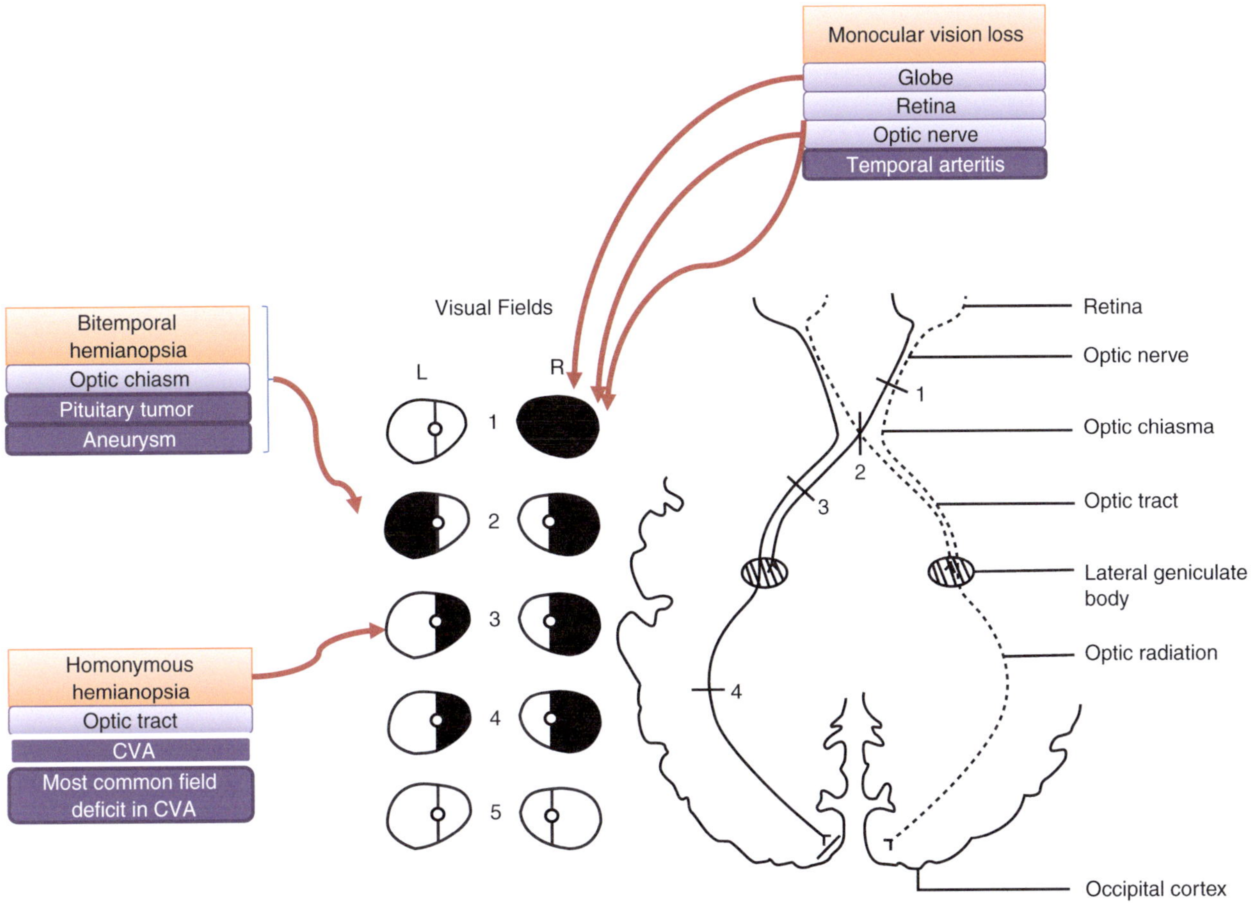

Bottom right image (Reprinted from Galloway NR, Amoaku WMK, Galloway PH, Browning AC. Neuro-ophthalmology. In: Galloway NR, Amoaku WMK, Galloway PH, Browning AC, editors. Common eye diseases and their management. London: Springer Verlag; 2006. p. 179–88. With permission from Springer Verlag)

External Eye

Lids

Hordeolum (External and Internal)

External hordeolum (Stye) = Infection of eyelash follicle & sebaceous or sweat gland (At lid margin) → Usually bacterial (Staph) = Pustule at eyelid margin

Internal hordeolum = Infection of meibomian glands → Pustule is on surface of tarsal plate

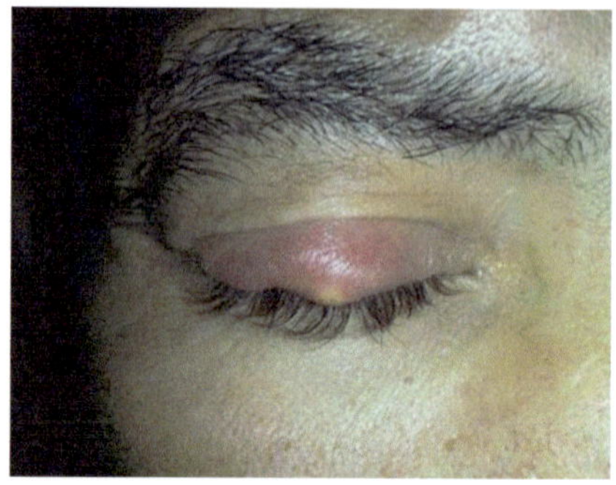

Symptoms & Signs

Pain | Redness | Eyelid swelling

Hordeolum Rx = Warm compresses + Topical ointment to prevent infection (Erythromycin)

Need I&D? = Refer to ophthalmology

Center right image (Reprinted from Khairallah M, Kahloun R. Infections of the eyelids. In: Tabbara KF, Abu El-Asrar AM, Khairallah M, editors. Ocular infections. Heidelberg: Springer Verlag; 2014. p. 51–61. With permission from Springer Verlag)

Chalazion

Chalazion = Chronic inflammation of eyelid due to blockage of Meibomian glands in the tarsal pate → Mid portion of upper lid away from margin (Lid may have mild erythema) → Usually painless

Chalazion = Difficult to distinguish from internal hordeolum → Same treatment

Chalazion = Associated with squamous cell carcinoma

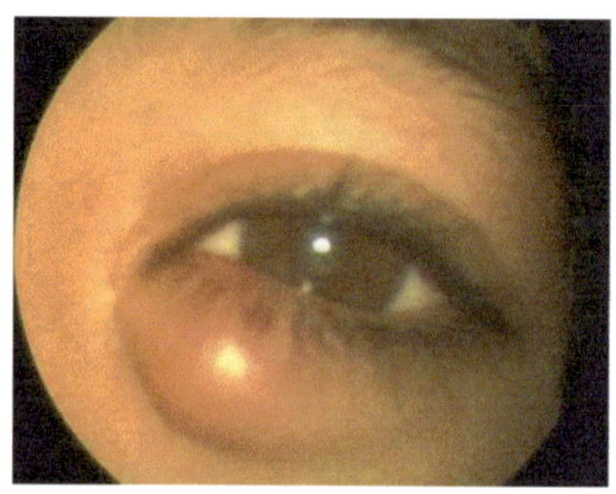

Chalazion Rx = Warm compresses + Topical ointment to prevent infection (Erythromycin) + Ophthalmology referral

Center right image (Reprinted from Khairallah M, Kahloun R. Infections of the eyelids. In: Tabbara KF, Abu El-Asrar AM, Khairallah M, editors. Ocular infections. Heidelberg: Springer Verlag; 2014. p. 51–61. With permission from Springer Verlag)

Blepharitis

Blepharitis = Inflammation of eyelid → Chronic *Staph epidermidis* infection

Symptoms & Signs

- Conjunctival injection
- Crusting around lids
- Eyelid redness + swelling
- ± Eye pain
- Pruritis
- ± Ulceration

Blepharitis Associations = Seborrheic dermatitis + Atopic dermatitis + Lice infestation + Staph aureus infection

Treatment = Daily cleansing with baby shampoo + Topical antibiotics

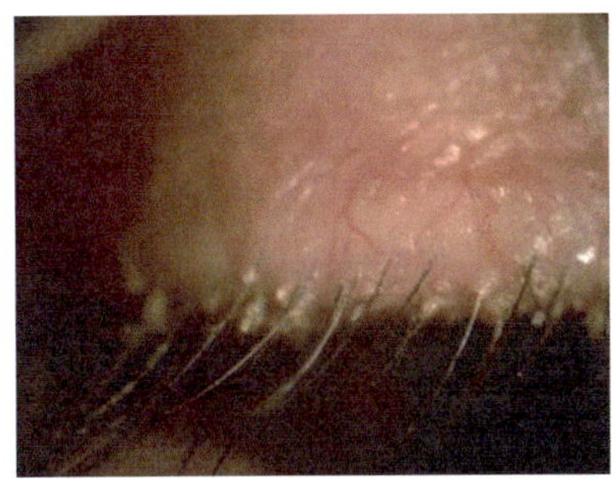

Bottom right image (Reprinted from Khairallah M, Kahloun R. Infections of the eyelids. In: Tabbara KF, Abu El-Asrar AM, Khairallah M, editors. Ocular infections. Heidelberg: Springer Verlag; 2014. p. 51–61. With permission from Springer Verlag)

Dacryocystitis

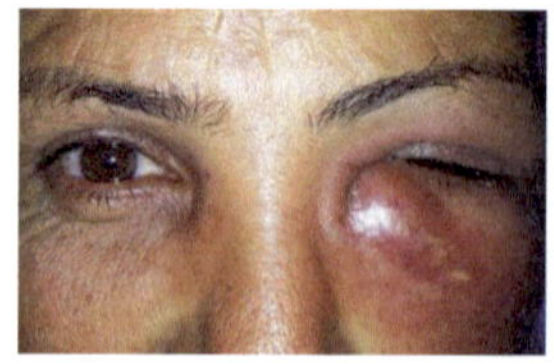

Dacryocystitis = Infection of lacrimal sac → Usually Staph OR *Strep pneumoniae*

Dacryocystitis = Red, tender swelling → Below the inner canthus → Inferior-medial

Symptoms & Signs

- Low grade fever
- Pressure over lacrimal sac = pus through punctum
- Eyelid redness + swelling — Lower eyelid
- Excess tearing
- Crusting

Dacryocystitis complication = Corneal ulceration → Associated with *Strep pneumoniae*

Treatment = Oral antibiotics + Warm compresses + Decongestants + Relief of duct obstruction (Ophthalmology consult)

Top right image (Reprinted from Khairallah M, Attia S. Infections of the orbit. In: Tabbara KF, Abu El-Asrar AM, Khairallah M, editors. Ocular infections. Heidelberg: Springer Verlag; 2014. p. 37–43. With permission from Springer Verlag)

Dacryoadenitis

Dacryoadenitis = Inflammation of lacrimal gland → Bacterial or Viral

Dacryoadenitis = Red, tender swelling → Outer portion of upper lid

Acute causes? = Mumps + EBV + Staph + Gonococcus

Chronic causes? = Sarcoid + Neoplasm + Sjogren's

Symptoms & Signs

- Tenderness
- Eyelid redness + swelling — Upper eyelid
- Excess tearing
- Preauricular lymph nodes

Treatment = Oral antibiotics + Warm compresses ± Incision & Drainage (Ophthalmology consult)

Periorbital and Orbital Cellulitis

Introduction: Orbital Infections

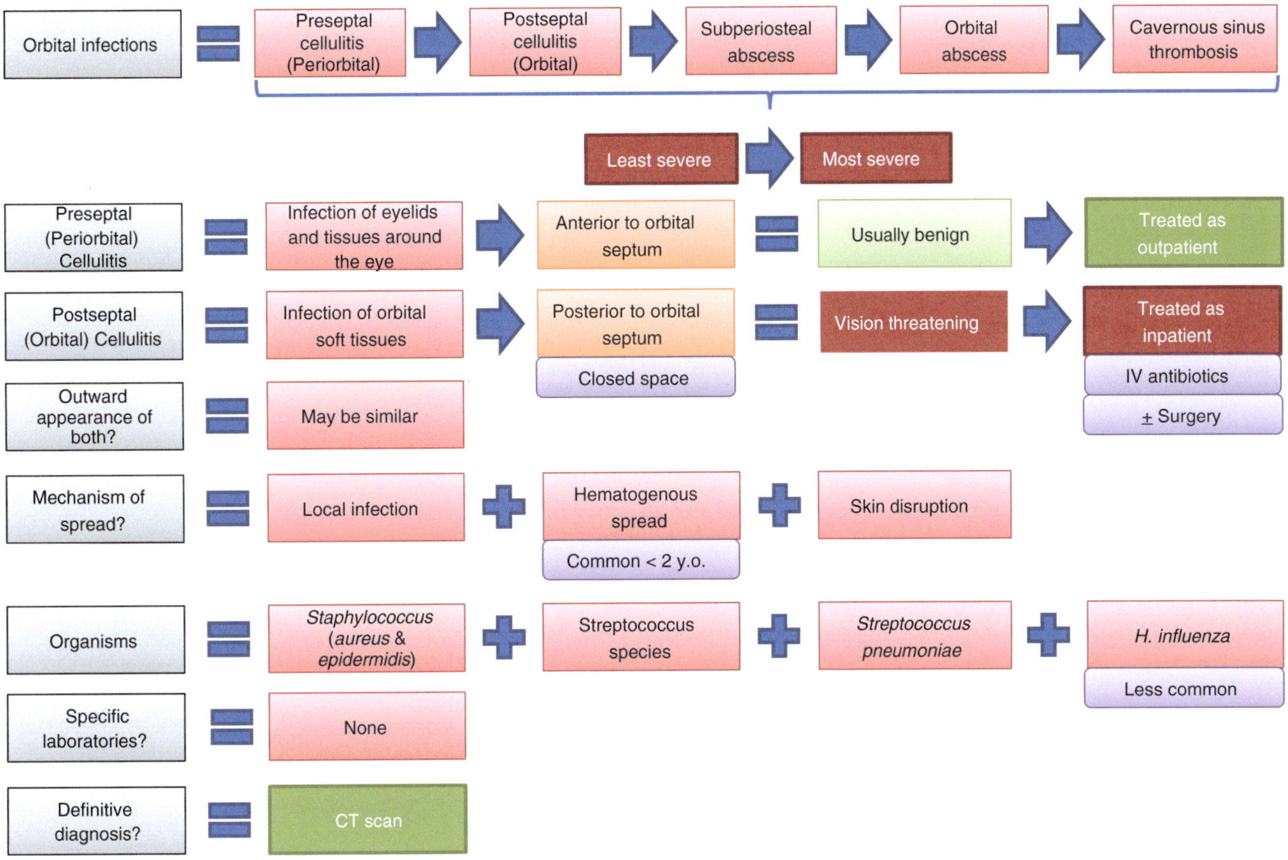

Preseptal Cellulitis

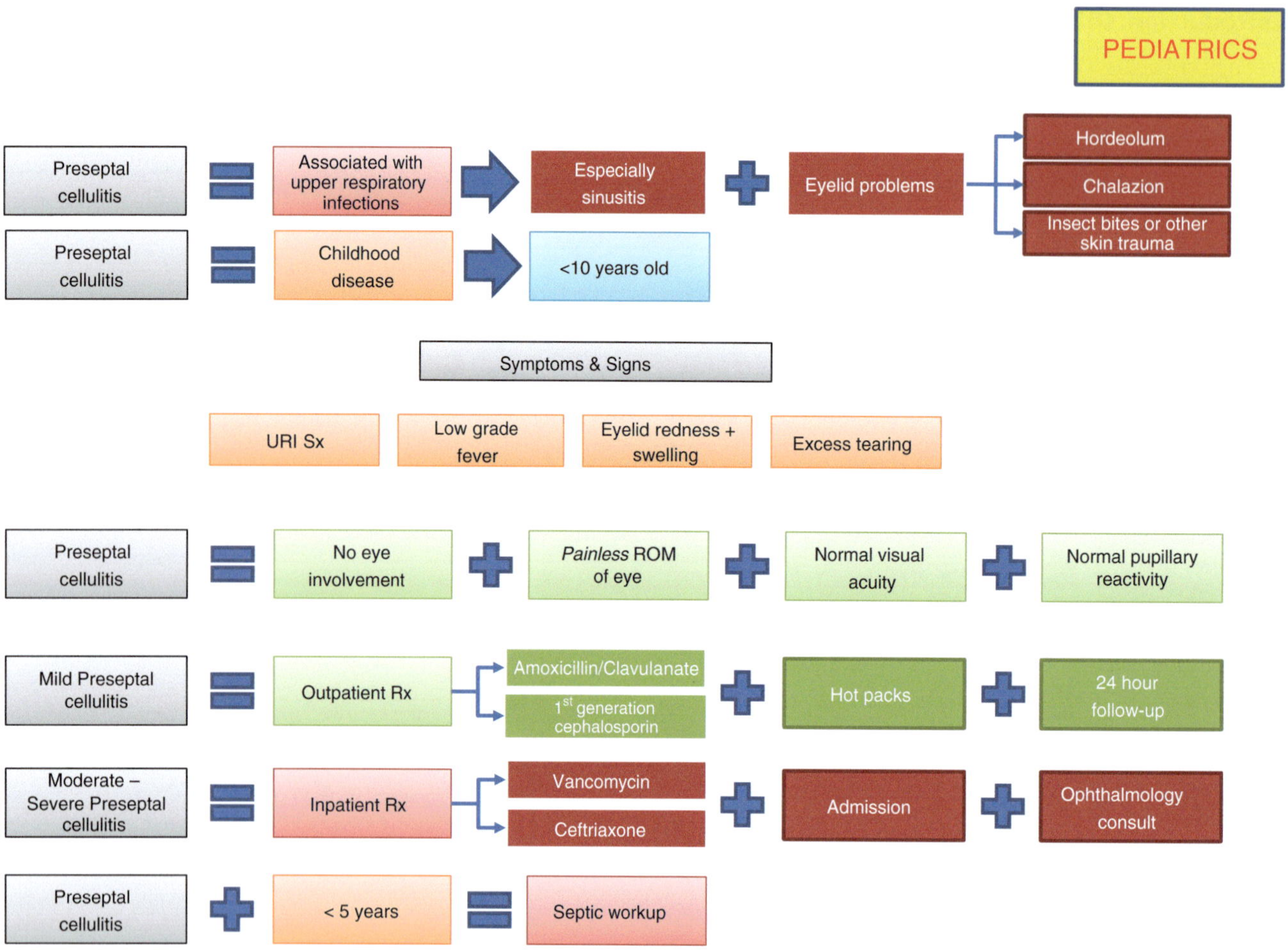

Postseptal Cellulitis

Postseptal cellulitis = Associated with sinus & dental infections → Especially *ethmoid* sinusitis (most common cause) + Other factors = Intraocular FB / Hematogenous spread / Insect bites or other skin trauma

Postseptal cellulitis = Usually polymicrobial → *Staph aureus* + *S. pneumoniae* + Anaerobes

Symptoms & Signs

- URI Sx
- Often high fever
- Eyelid is dark red + swelling
- Pain on eye movement
- Facial pressure
- Chemosis
- Proptosis

Postseptal cellulitis = Eye is involved (Elevated IOP) + ***Painful*** ROM of eye + ± Decreased visual acuity + Abnormal pupillary reactivity

Diagnosis = CT

Postseptal cellulitis = Inpatient Rx → Amoxicillin/Sulbactam or 3rd generation cephalosporin + Metronidazole + Ophthalmology consult (Debridement)

Orbital Cellulitis Complications

Orbital Cellulitis Complications — Usually seen on CT

- Meningitis — Most common
- Septicemia
- Brain abscess
- Orbital abscess
- Epidural abscess
- Frontal bone osteomyelitis — Pott's puffy tumor
- Cavernous sinus thrombosis — Involvement of CN 3, 4, or 6
- Subdural empyema
- Vision loss — Due to increased IOP decreasing retinal blood flow
- Subperiosteal abscess

Conjunctiva

Conjunctivitis

Introduction

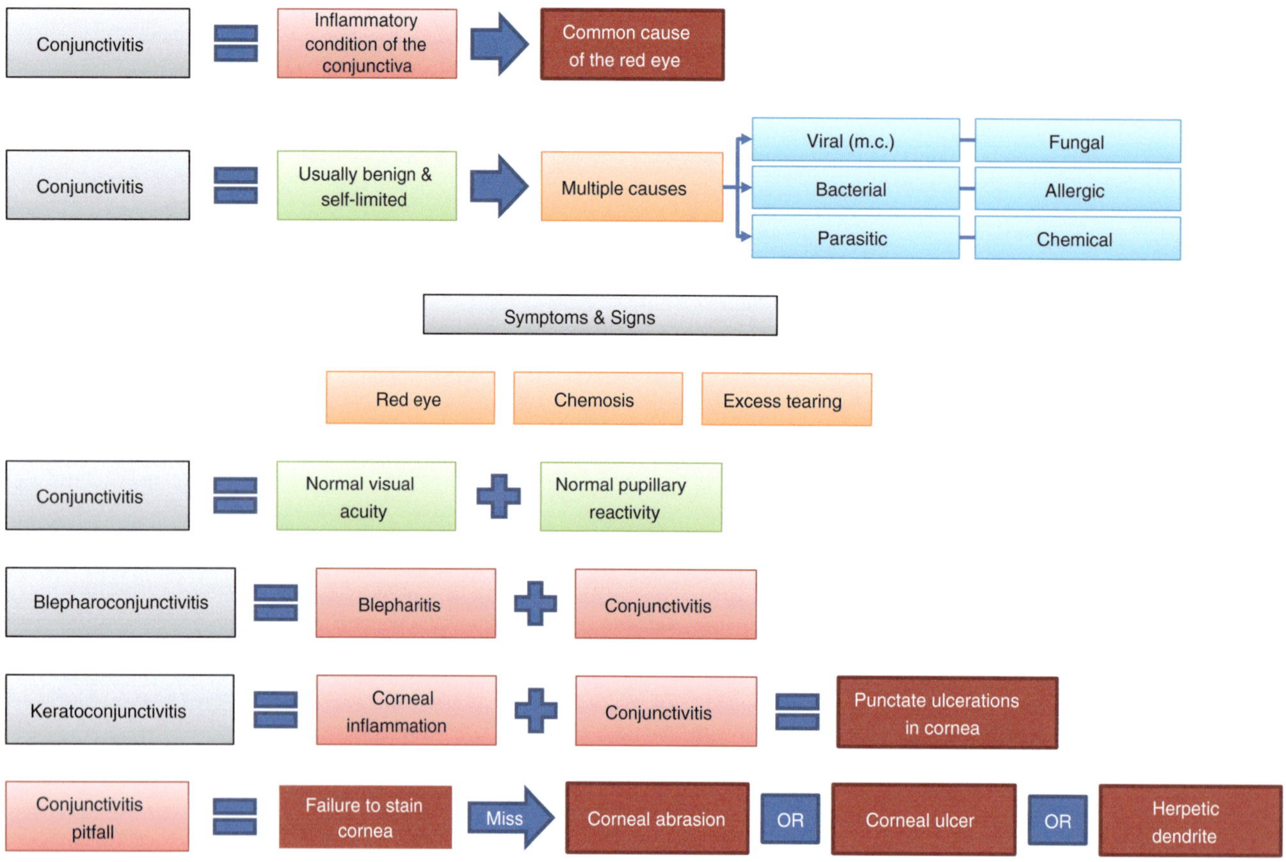

Bacterial Conjunctivitis

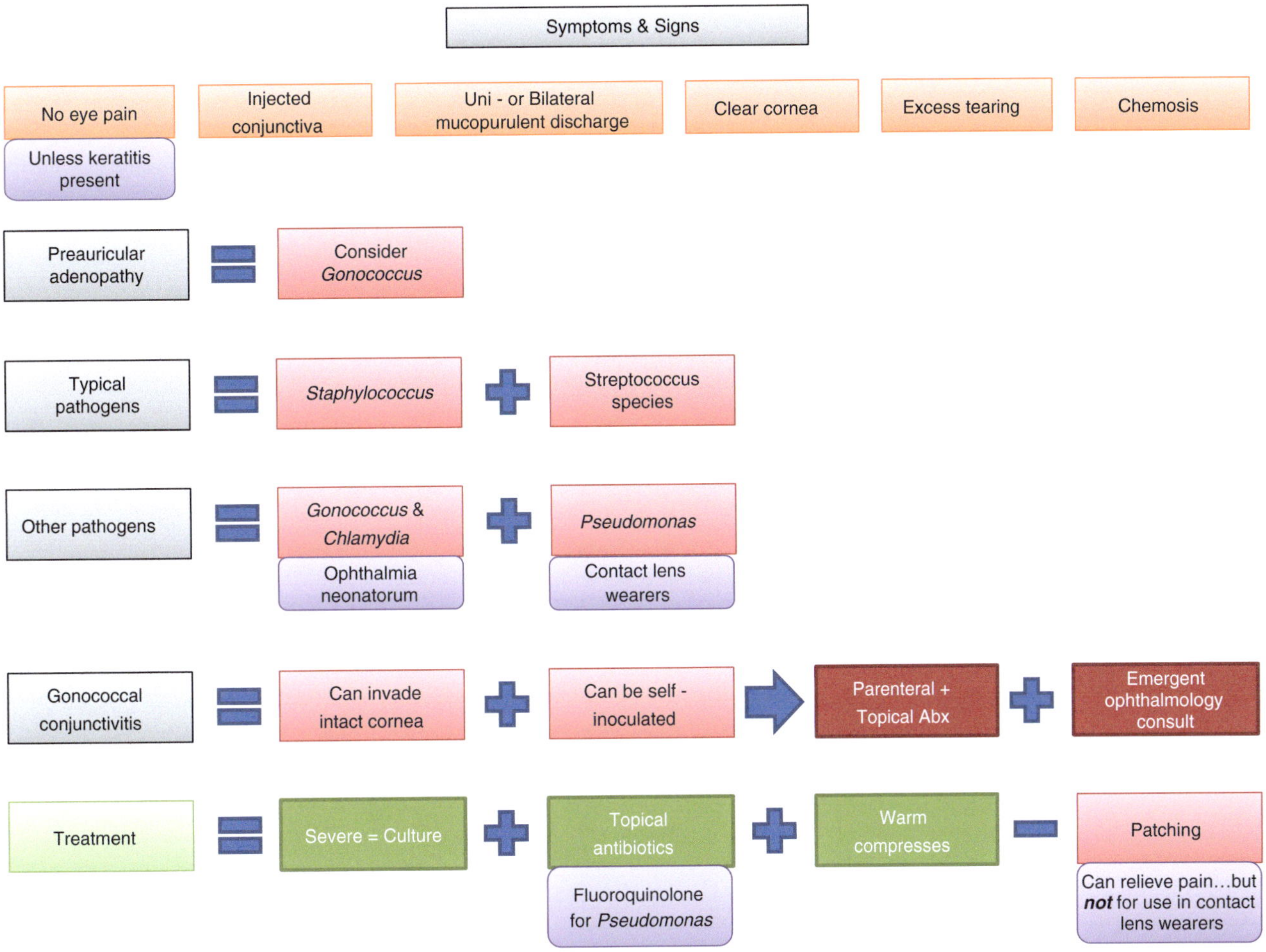

Ophthalmia Neonatorum

PEDIATRICS

Ophthalmia neonatorum = Conjunctivitis in the 1st 28 days → Chemical / Gonococcal / Other bacterial / Viral / Chlamydial

Chemical = 1st 2 days postpartum → Resolves within 48 hours → Negative gram stain

Gonococcal = 2–7 days of life → Bilateral conjunctival injection + Chemosis + Copious purulent discharge + (+) Gram stain

GC Treatment = Evaluation for disseminated disease + IV Abx

GC Complications = Corneal ulceration + Corneal perforation

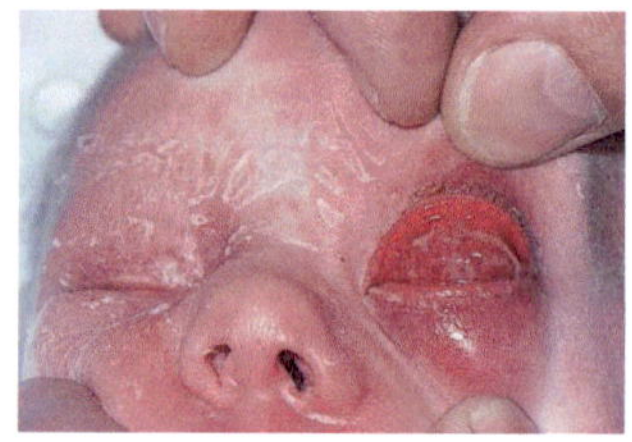

Chlamydial = Most common conjunctivitis (5–14 days of life) → Bilateral conjunctival injection + Bilateral purulent discharge

Chlamydia Treatment = PO Erythromycin

Chlamydia Complications = Associated with chlamydial pneumonia + Staccato cough + Otitis media

Trachoma = most common cause of blindness worldwide

Viral (Herpes) = 6–14 days of life → Bilateral lid edema + Conjunctival injection + Keratitis (Corneal dendrites) ± Hx of maternal herpes

Herpes Treatment = Evaluation for disseminated disease + IV & topical Acyclovir

Center right image (Reprinted from Galloway NR, Amoaku WMK, Galloway PH, Browning AC. Common diseases of the conjunctiva and cornea. In: Galloway NR, Amoaku WMK, Galloway PH, Browning AC, editors. Common eye diseases and their management. London: Springer Verlag; 2006. p. 45–60. With permission from Springer Verlag)

Viral Conjunctivitis

Symptoms & Signs

- No eye pain — Unless keratitis present
- Injected conjunctiva
- Uni - or Bilateral watery discharge — One eye followed by the other
- Clear cornea — Unless keratitis present
- Excess tearing
- Chemosis
- Preauricular adenopathy — Common — Esp. with Adenovirus

Viral conjunctivitis = Usually resolves spontaneously → Typically preceded by URI → Highly contagious

Typical pathogens = Adenovirus = Epidemic keratoconjunctivitis

Treatment = Warm compresses + Frequent hand washing − Patching

Epidemic Keratoconjunctivitis (EKC)

EKC = Virulent strain of Adenovirus → Tends to occur in epidemics → Extremely contagious

EKC Preceded by Cough + Fevers + Malaise + Muscle aches + N/V

Symptoms & Signs

- Eye pain
- Very injected conjunctiva
- Swelling & redness of eyelid
- Chemosis
- Excess tearing
- FB sensation
- Preauricular adenopathy — Ipsilateral
- Papillae of inferior conjunctiva
- Subconjunctival hemorrhages
- Corneal stippling on slit lamp exam

EKC = Sx may persist for 2–3 weeks

EKC Treatment = Artificial tears + Cool compresses ± Cycloplegic agents (Severe photophobia) + Ophthalmology consult

Allergic Conjunctivitis (AC)

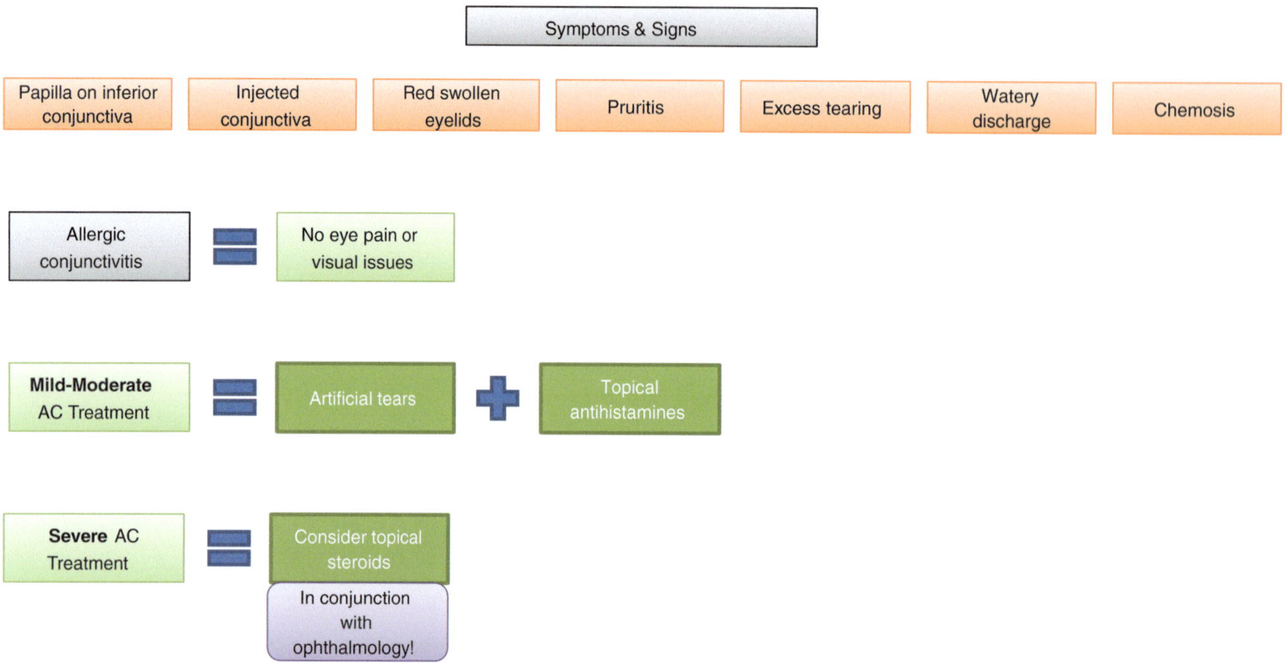

Subconjunctival Hemorrhage

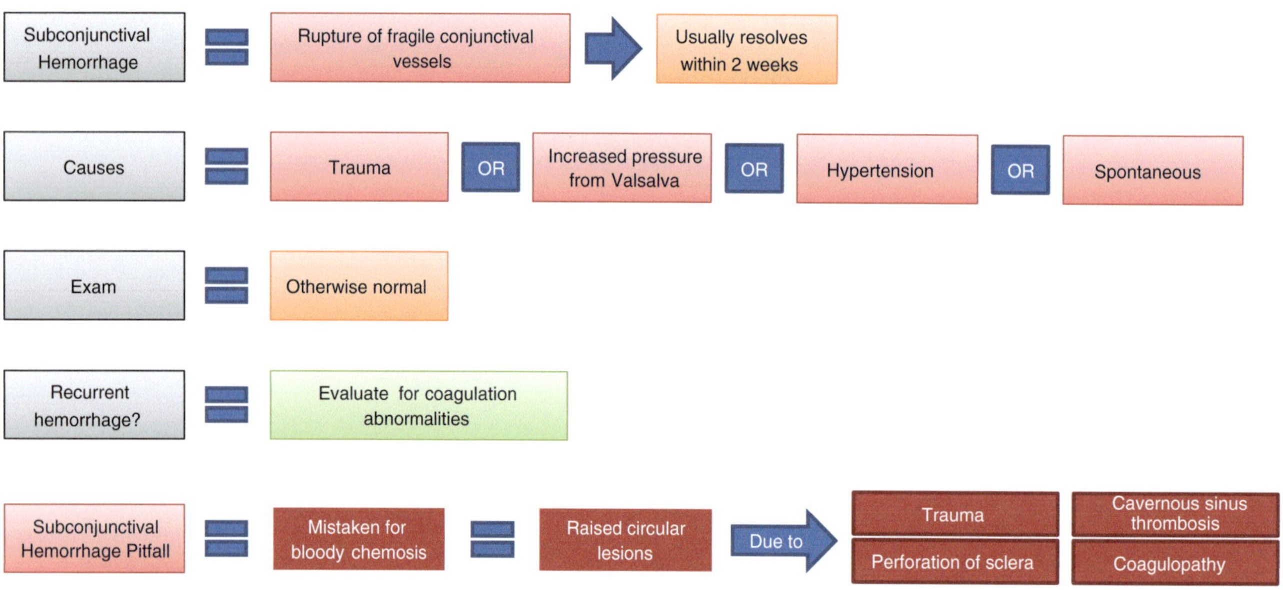

Cornea

Keratitis

Introduction

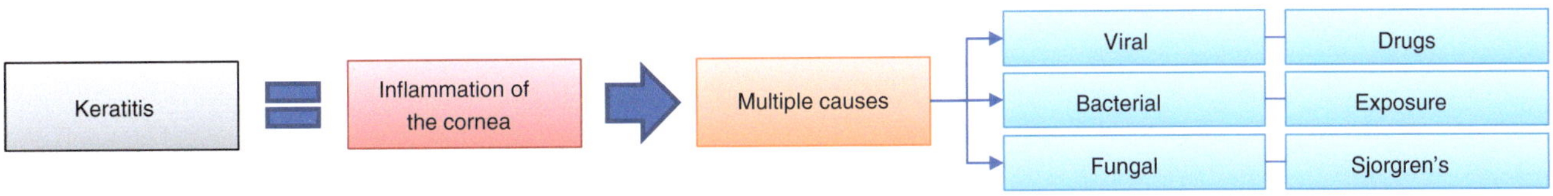

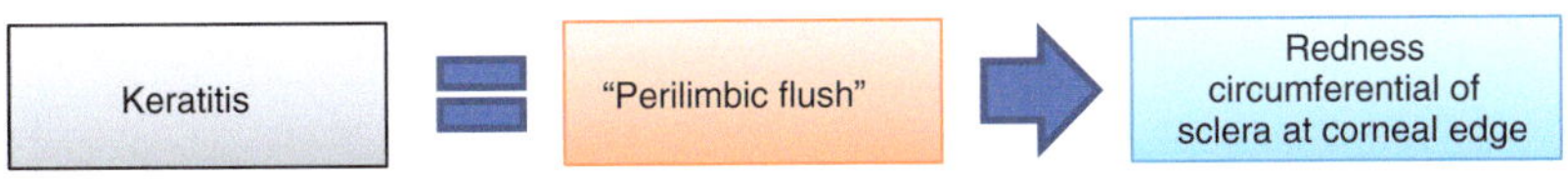

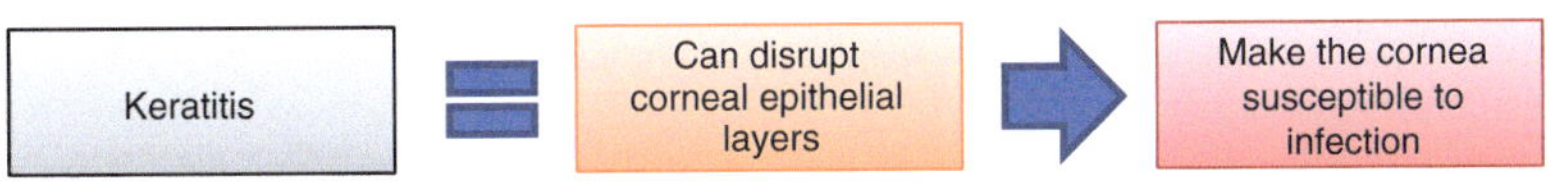

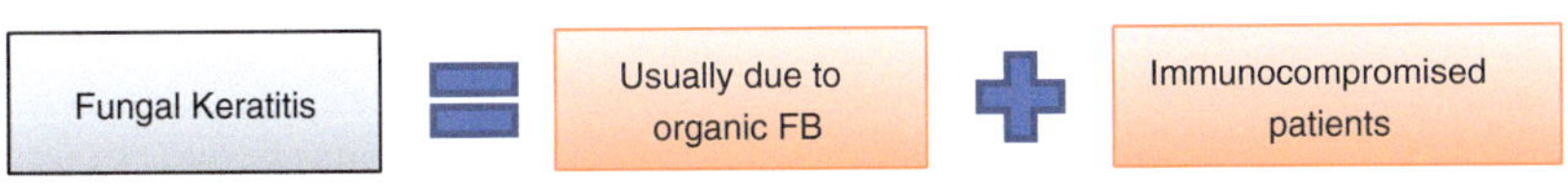

Bacterial Keratitis

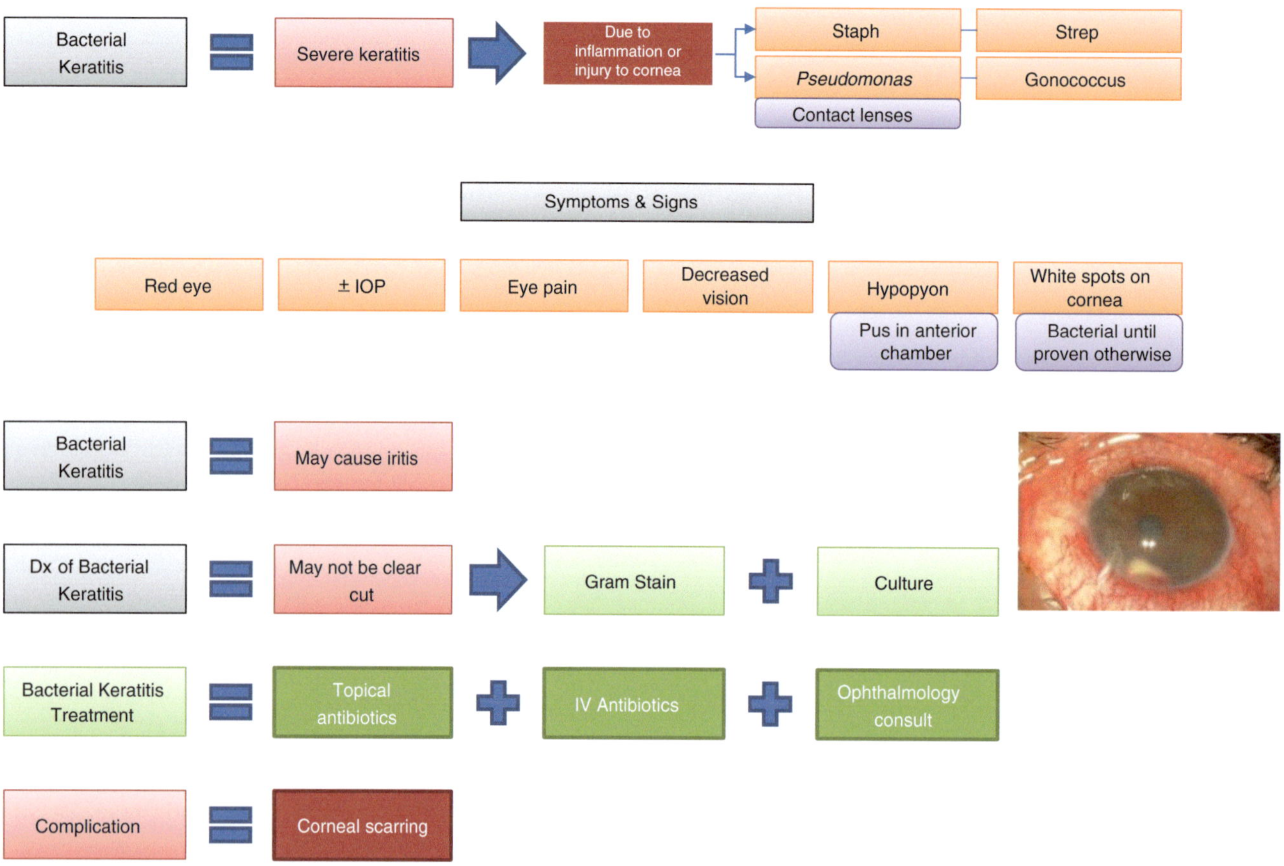

Center right image (Reprinted from Mete G, Turgut Y, Osman A, Gülşen Ü, Hakan A. Anterior segment intraocular metallic foreign body causing chronic hypopyon uveitis. J Ophthalmic Inflamm Infect. 2011;1(2):85–7. With permission from Springer Verlag)

HSV Keratitis

Herpes Simplex = Can affect eyelids, conjunctivitis & cornea → Hx of cold sores OR Genital herpes

Symptoms & Signs

- Red eye
- ± IOP
- Eye pain
- Decreased vision
- Photophobia
- ± Skin involvement (Typical vesicular eruptions)
- Decreased corneal sensation

Dx of HSV Keratitis = Fluorescein staining → Herpetic dendrites → Linear branching pattern OR Geographic ulcer ("Amoeba -like")

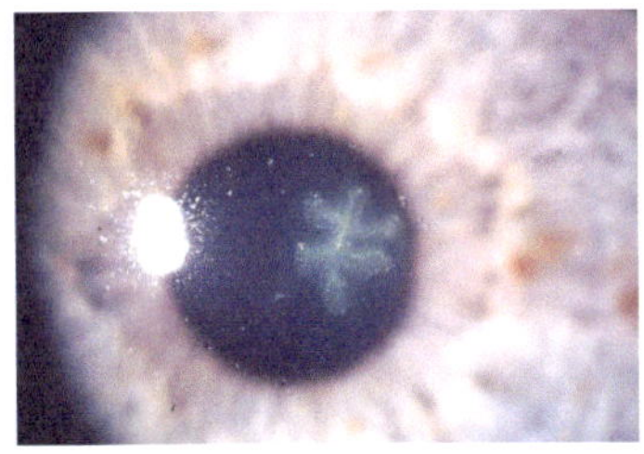

Dx of HSV Keratitis = May not be clear cut → May not see the dendrites

HSV Affecting Lids? = Oral Acyclovir

HSV Affecting Conjunctiva? = Topical Trifluridine

HSV Keratitis Treatment = Topical Trifluridine ± Erythromycin ointment (To prevent 2° bacterial infection) + Cycloplegics + Ophthalmology consult

HSV Keratitis Complication = Corneal scarring

Center right image (Reprinted from Sundmacher R. Herpes simplex virus (HSV) diseases of the anterior segment and the adnexa. In: Sundmacher R, editor. Color atlas of herpetic eye disease: a practical guide to clinical management. Heidelberg: Springer Verlag; 2008. p. 5–112. With permission from Springer Verlag)

Herpes Zoster Ophthalmicus

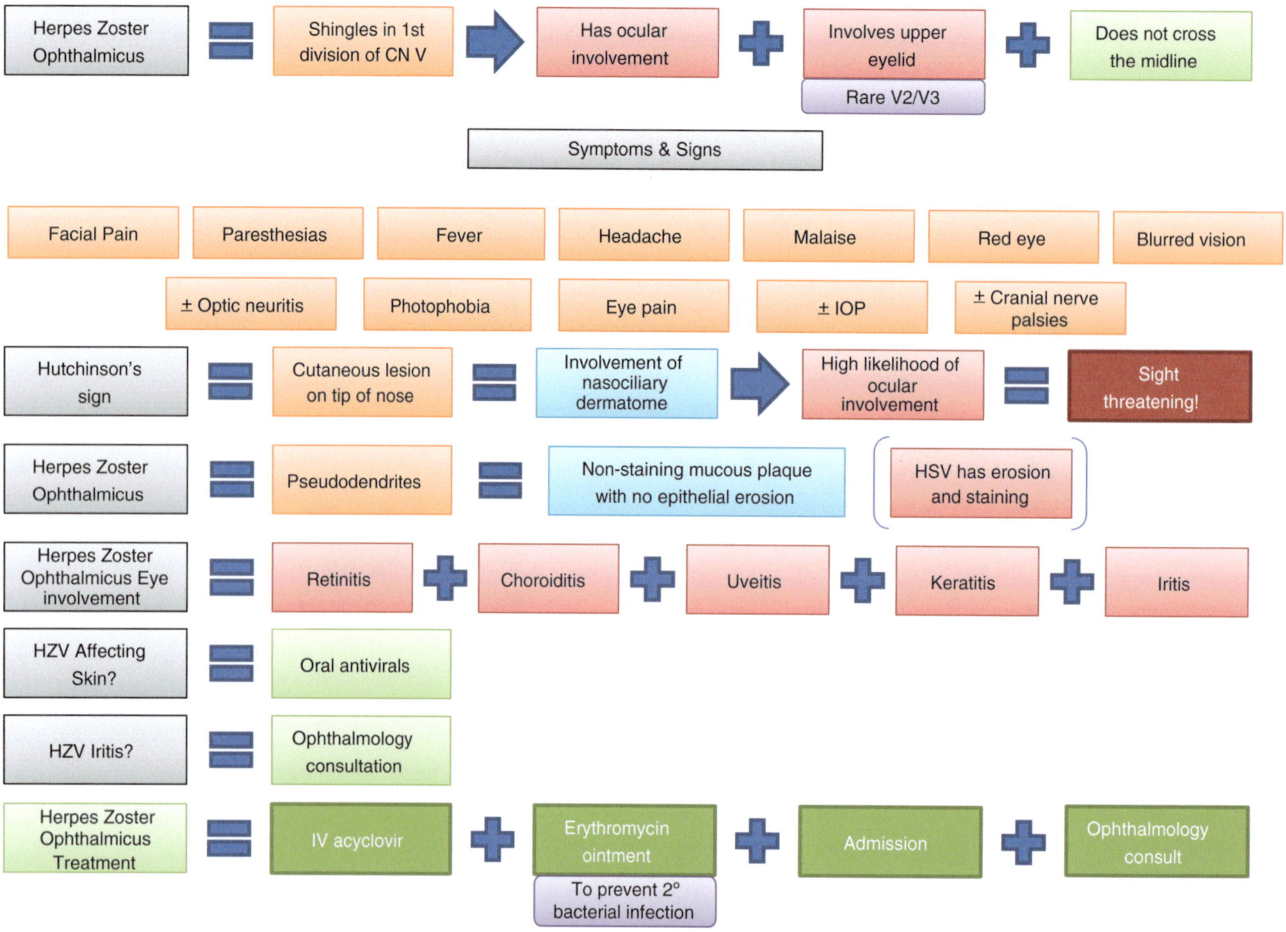

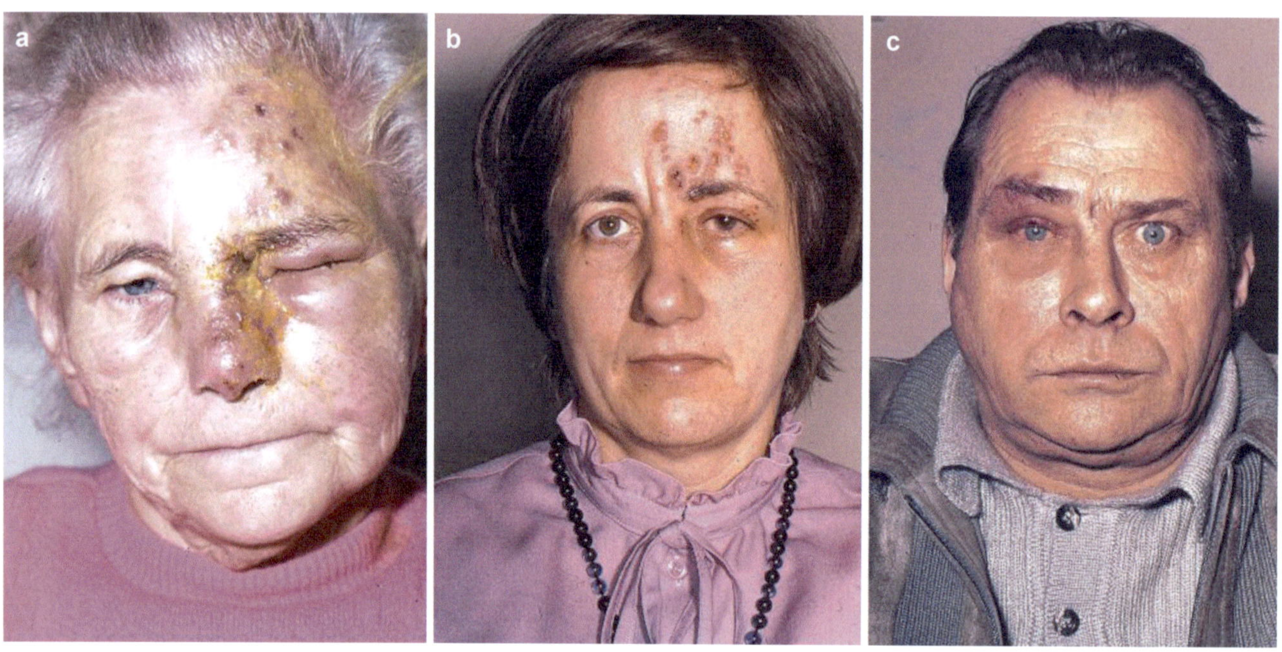

Center image (Reprinted from Sundmacher R. Varicella zoster virus (VZV) diseases of the anterior segment and the adnexes. In: Sundmacher R, editor. Color atlas of herpetic eye disease: a practical guide to clinical management. Heidelberg: Springer Verlag; 2008. p. 113–57. With permission from Springer Verlag)

Ultraviolet Keratitis

Ultraviolet Keratitis = Welder's keratitis + Snow Blindness → UV light causes death of corneal epithelial cells

Symptoms & Signs

- FB sensation
- Eye pain
- Tearing
- Photophobia
- Blepharospasm
- No visual changes
- Conjunctival injection
- Corneal edema – On slit lamp

Ultraviolet Keratitis = Usually a delay of 6–12 hours

Ultraviolet Keratitis = Diffuse, bilateral punctate lesions on cornea

Ultraviolet Keratitis Treatment = Patch for comfort + Cycloplegics + Analgesia

Corneal Abrasion, Laceration, and Ulcers

Corneal Abrasion

Corneal abrasion = Corneal scratch → Due to: Contact lenses, Fingernails, Dust, Other FB

Symptoms & Signs

- FB sensation
- Eye pain
- Tearing
- ± Photophobia
- No visual changes – Unless full thickness corneal laceration
- Mild corneal injection
- ± Subconjunctival hemorrhage
- Blepharospasm
- Lid swelling

Corneal abrasion = Relief of pain with topical anesthesia

Dx of Corneal abrasion = Irregular corneal defect → Appears green after fluorescein staining under cobalt blue light

Corneal abrasion Treatment = Cycloplegics (Decreases pain) + Topical antibiotics ± Topical NSAIDs (Does not impair healing) ± Patch for comfort

Corneal abrasion pitfalls = Metal FB causing abrasion (Consider intraocular FB) + Not examining under the lids (Retained FB; "Ice rink sign") + Dispensing topical anesthetics (Retards healing) + Patching eye abrasions due to organic matter (Increases infection risk)

Corneal Lacerations

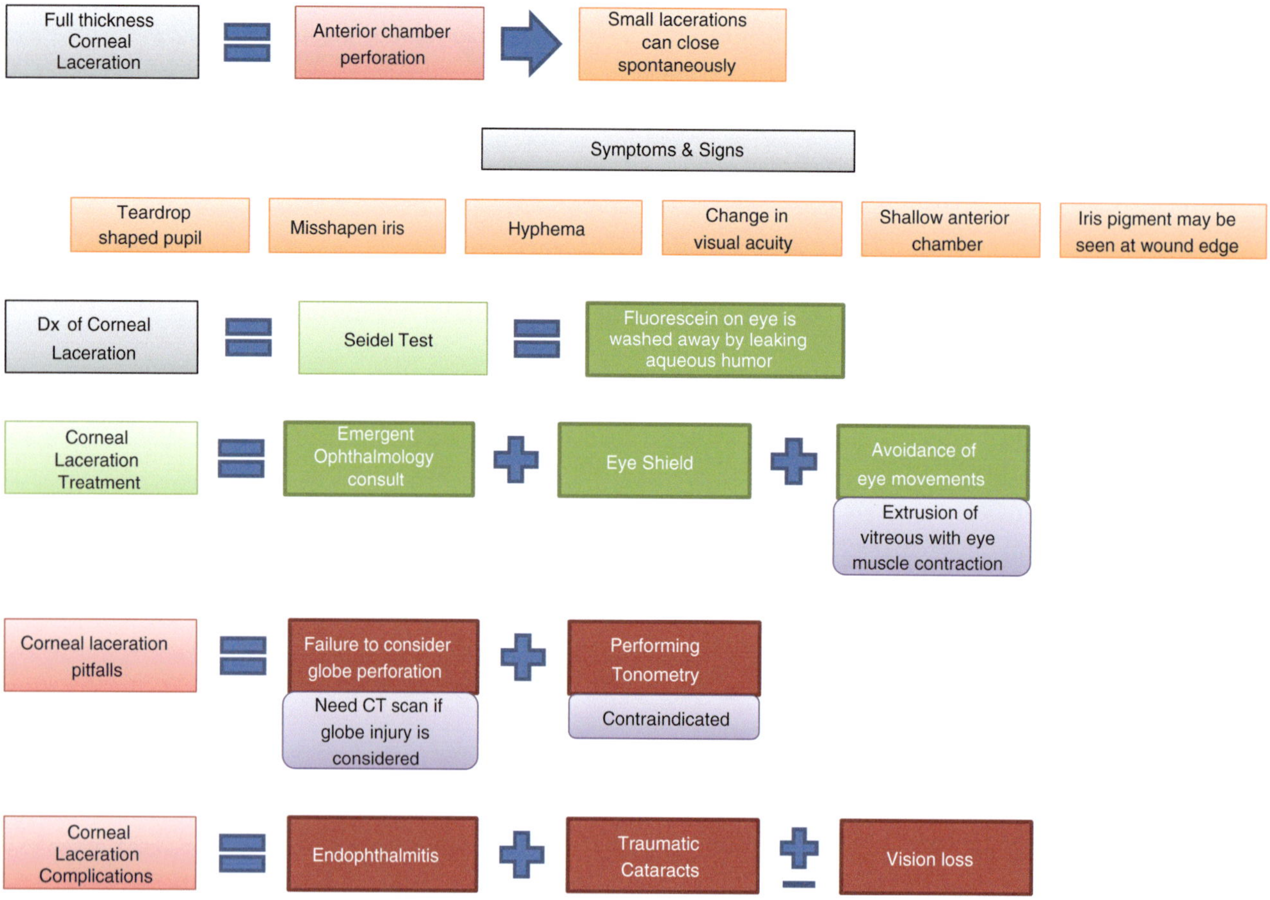

Corneal Ulcers

Corneal Ulcer = Infection of multiple layers of the cornea → Due to → Breaks in epithelial layer → Trauma; Infection; Dry eyes; Contact lens (Pseudomonas)

Symptoms & Signs

- FB sensation
- Eye pain
- Tearing
- ± Photophobia
- ± Subconjunctival hemorrhage
- Mild corneal injection
- No visual changes (Unless full thickness corneal laceration; Or ulcer at visual axis)
- Mucopurulent discharge
- Blepharospasm
- Lid swelling
- Associated iritis (Miotic pupil)

Dx of Corneal Ulcer = Round or irregular defect → Whitish on appearance → Slit Lamp May Show: Cells & Flare = Iritis, ± Hypopyon + Culture

Corneal Ulcer Treatment = Cycloplegics (Decrease pain) + Topical antibiotics + Ophthalmology consult

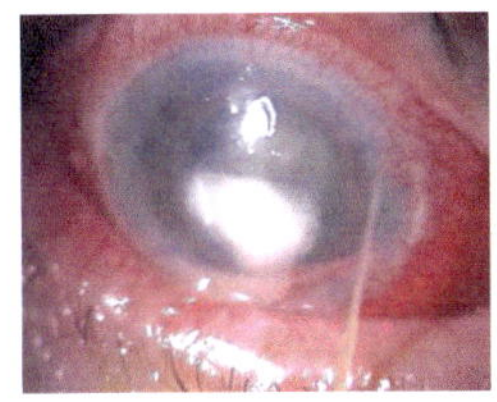

Corneal abrasion pitfalls = Patching eyes (Worsen *Pseudomonas* infection) + Not referring to Ophthalmology

Corneal Ulcer Complications = Synechiae + Glaucoma + Cataracts + Corneal perforation + Corneal scarring

Bottom right image (Reprinted from Heiligenhaus A, Heinz C, Schmitz K, Tappeiner C, Bauer D, Meller D. Amniotic membrane transplantation for the treatment of corneal ulceration in infectious keratitis. In: Reinhard T, Larkin F, editors. Cornea and external eye disease. Heidelberg: Springer Verlag; 2008. p. 15–36. With permission from Springer Verlag)

Corneal Foreign Bodies

Corneal Foreign Bodies = Usually superficial

Symptoms & Signs

- FB sensation
- Blurred vision
- Tearing
- Edema of lids
- Chemosis
- Photophobia
- No visual changes

Metallic FB = If present for prolonged period of time → Metal will diffuse into cornea = Rust ring

Corneal Foreign Body Treatment = Removal in ED or by Ophthalmology + Topical antibiotics ± Cycloplegics

Corneal Foreign Body Pitfalls = Failure to assess for globe penetration (Will see hyphema) + Failure to evert lid ("Ice rink" sign) + Failure to refer to ophthalmology when metallic FB removed (Rust may reaccumulate)

Uveitis and Iritis

Introduction

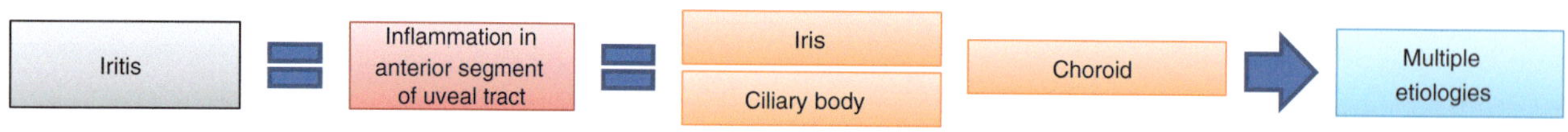

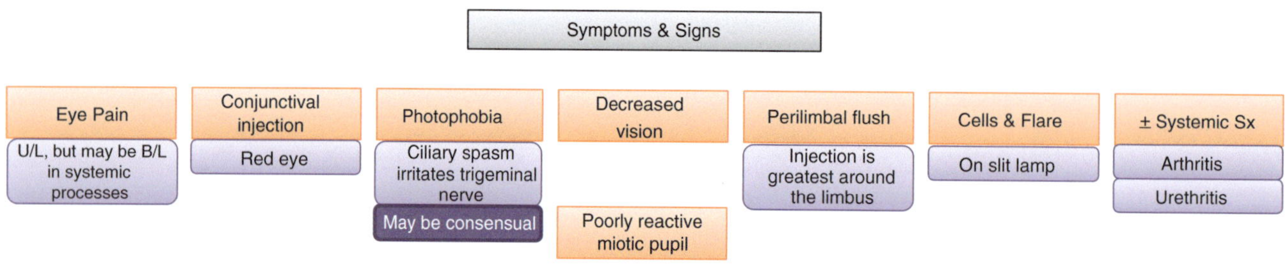

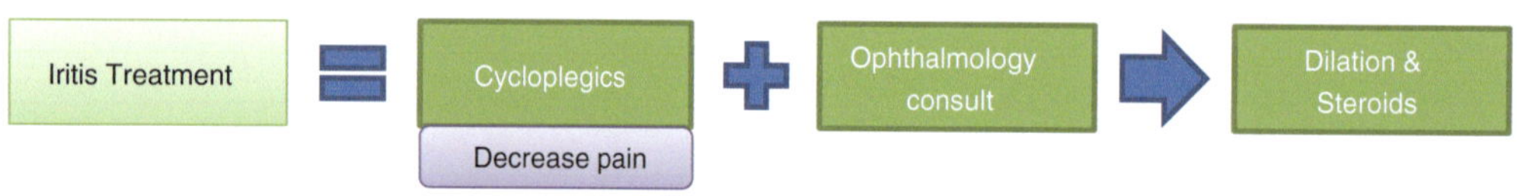

Differential Diagnosis of Iritis

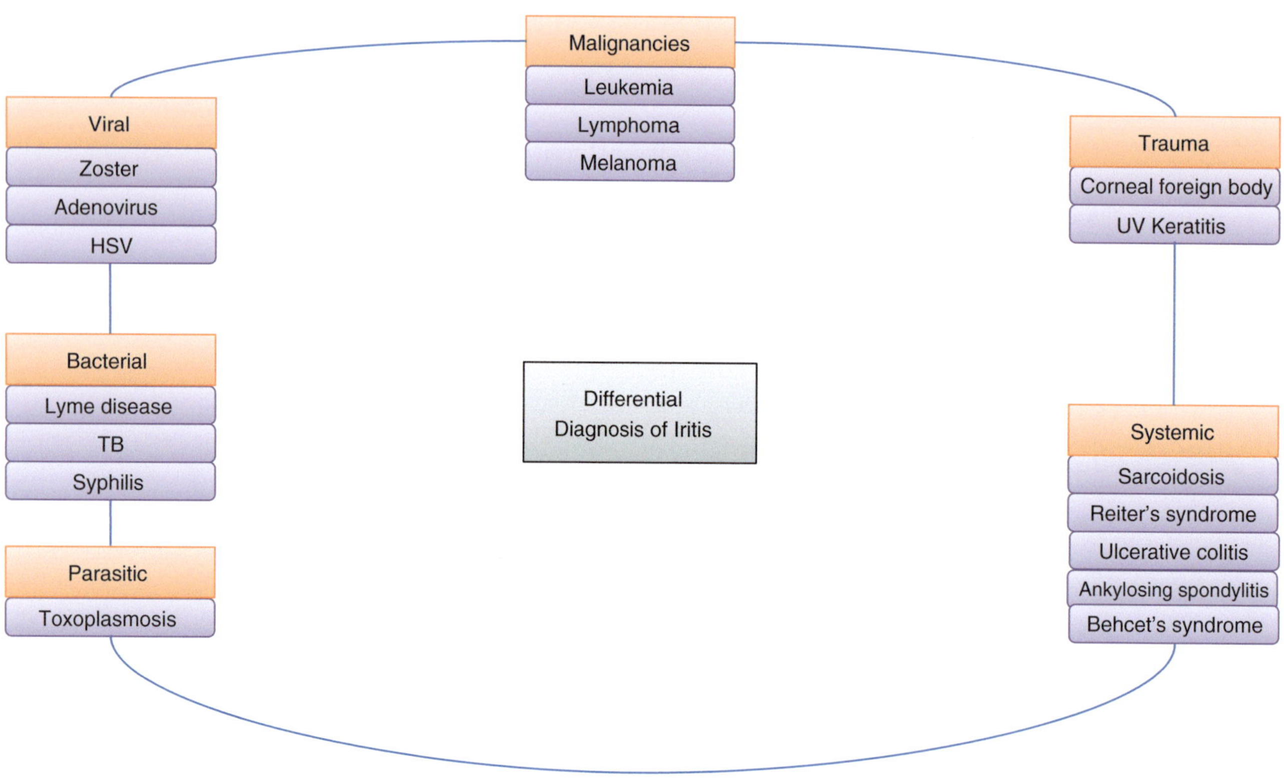

Vitreous and Intraocular Cavities

Endophthalmitis

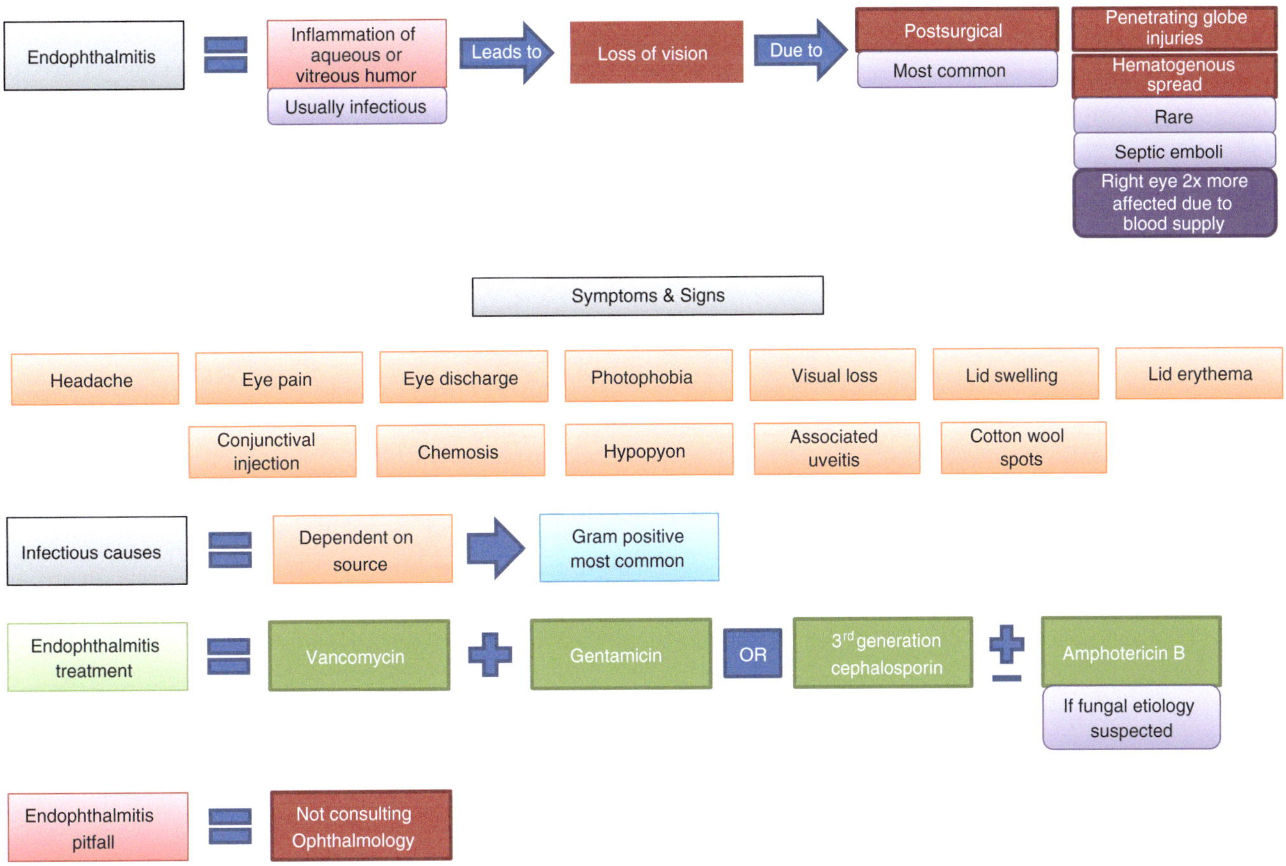

Vitreous Hemorrhage

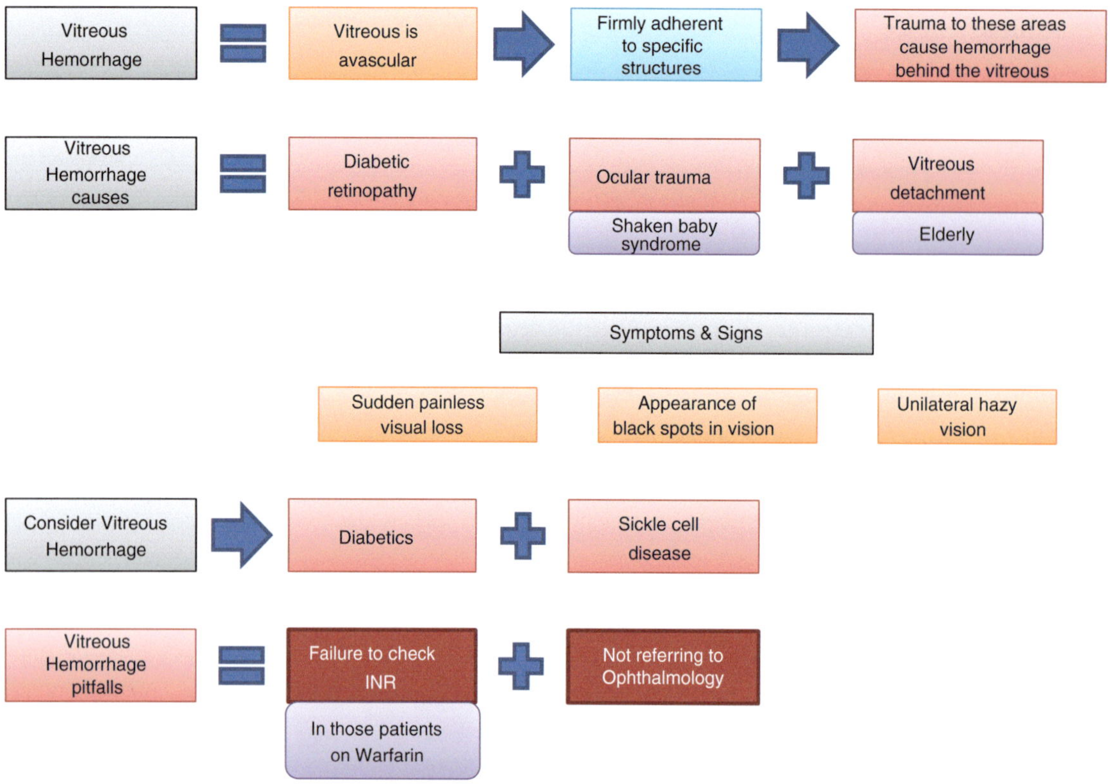

Retina

Central Retinal Artery Occlusion (CRAO)

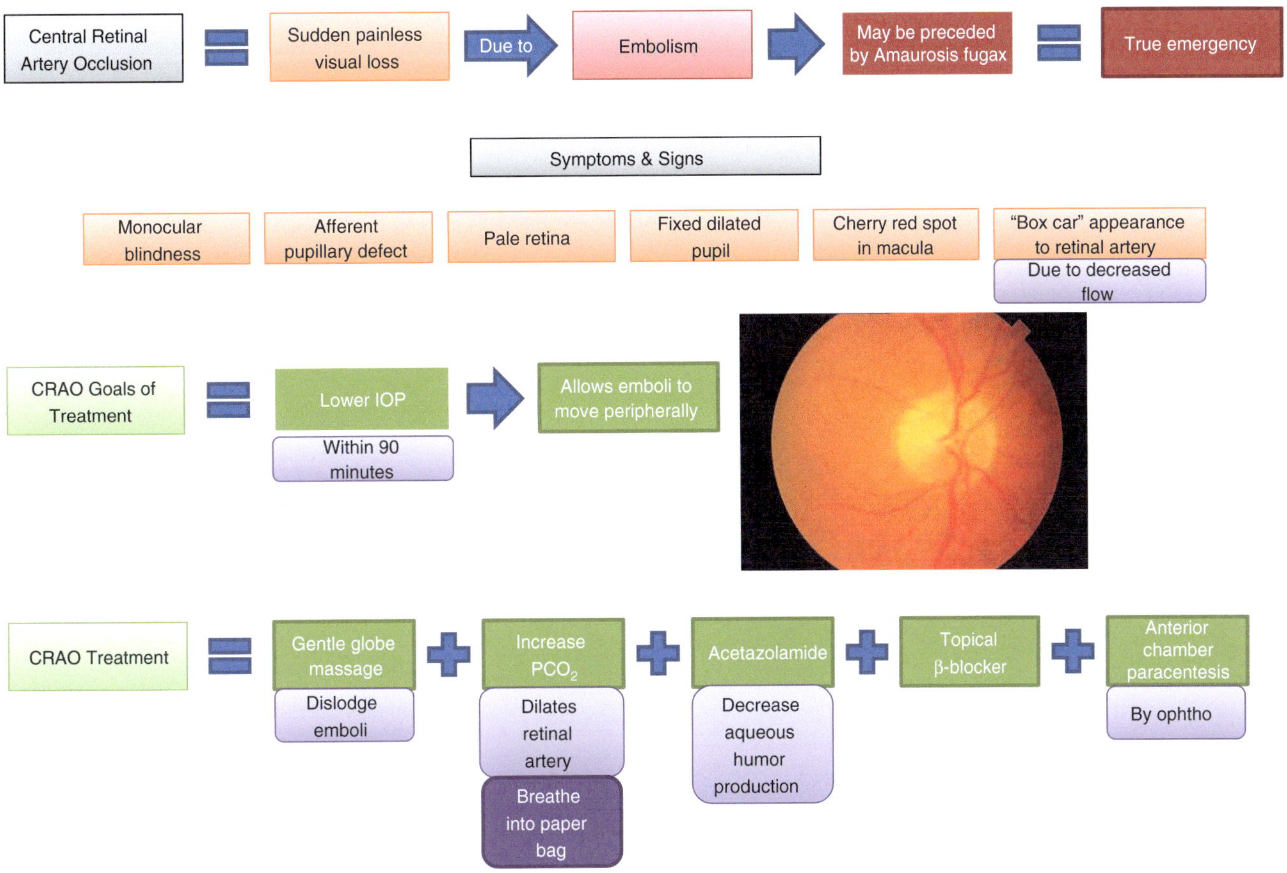

Center right image (Reprinted from Galloway NR, Amoaku WMK, Galloway PH, Browning AC. Systemic disease and the eye. In: Galloway NR, Amoaku WMK, Galloway PH, Browning AC, editors. Common eye diseases and their management. London: Springer Verlag; 2006. p. 165–78. With permission from Springer Verlag)

Etiologies of Central Retinal Artery Syndrome

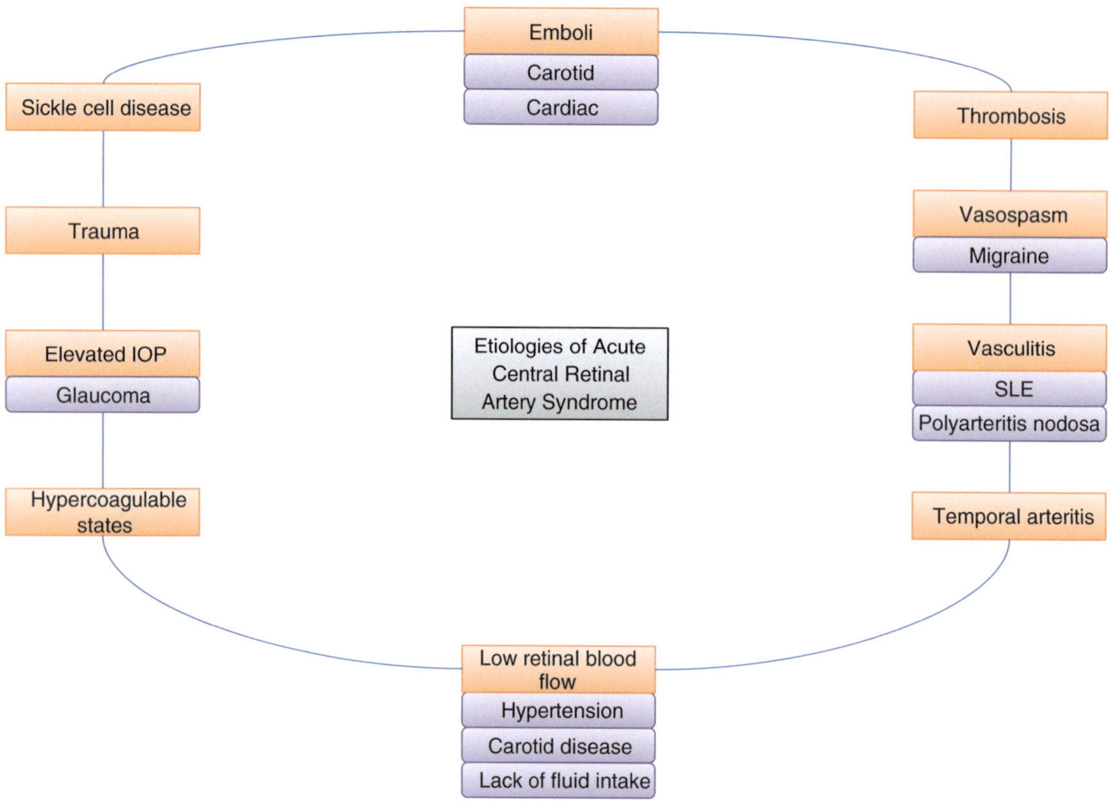

Central Retinal Vein Occlusion (CRVO)

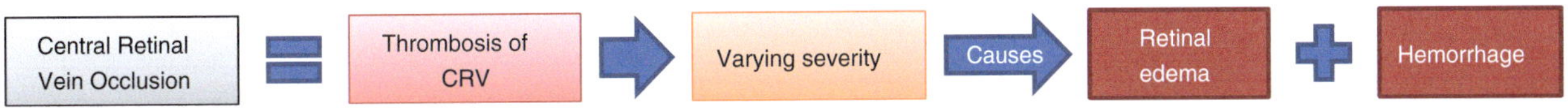

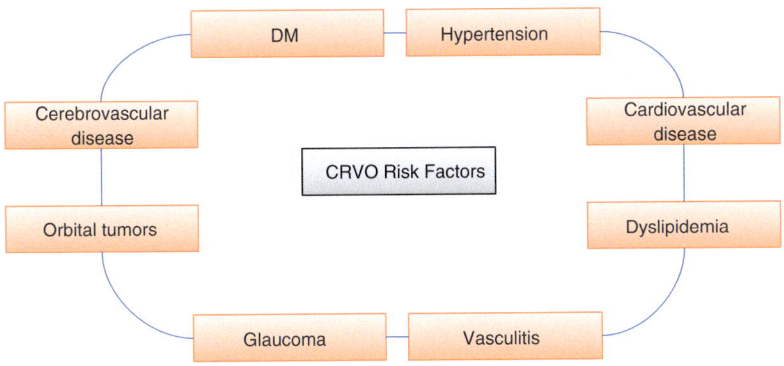

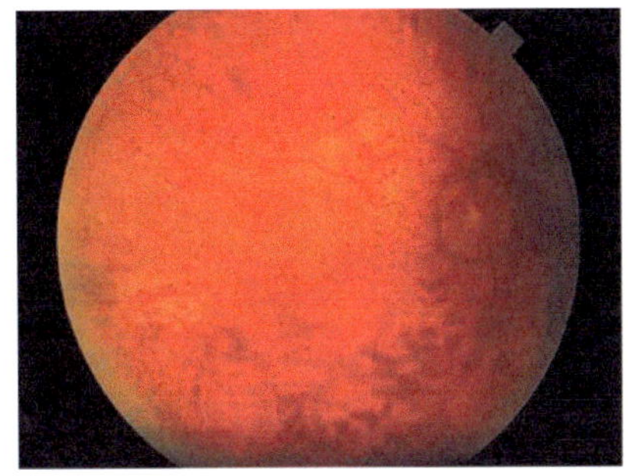

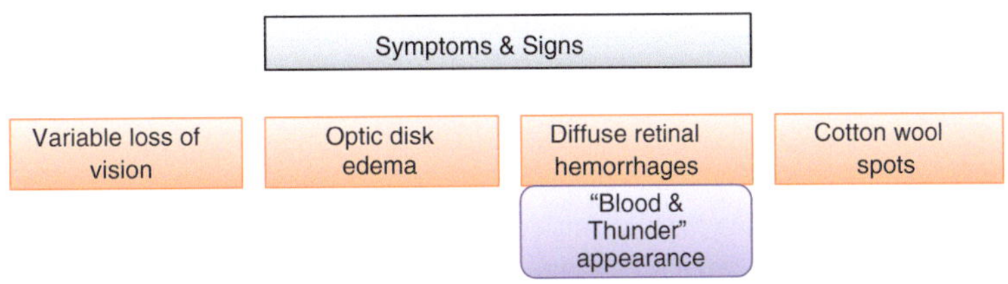

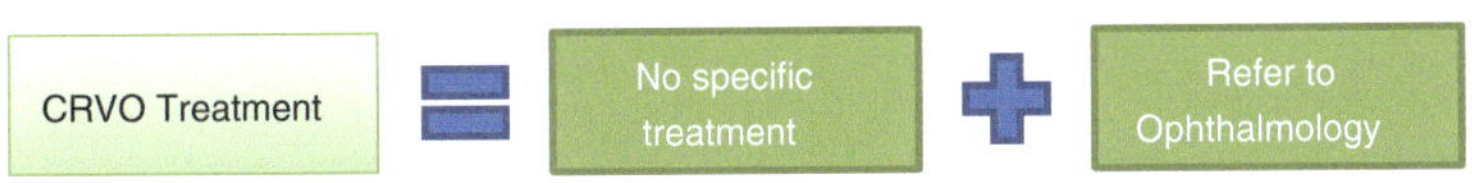

Center right image (Reprinted from Galloway NR, Amoaku WMK, Galloway PH, Browning AC. Systemic disease and the eye. In: Galloway NR, Amoaku WMK, Galloway PH, Browning AC, editors. Common eye diseases and their management. London: Springer Verlag; 2006. p. 165–78. With permission from Springer Verlag)

Retinal Detachment

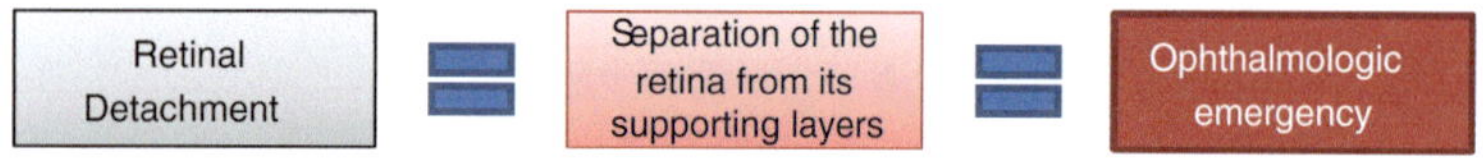

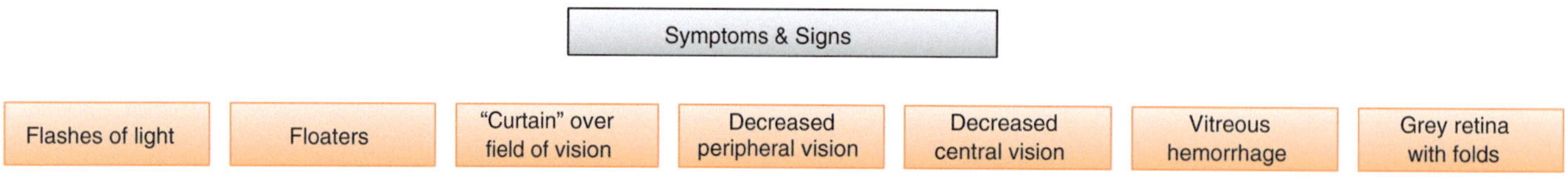

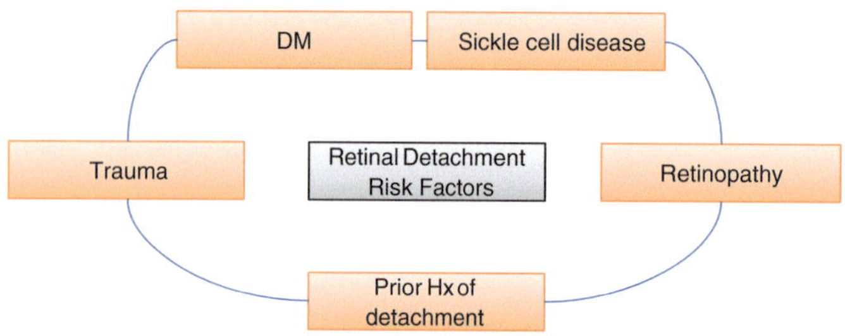

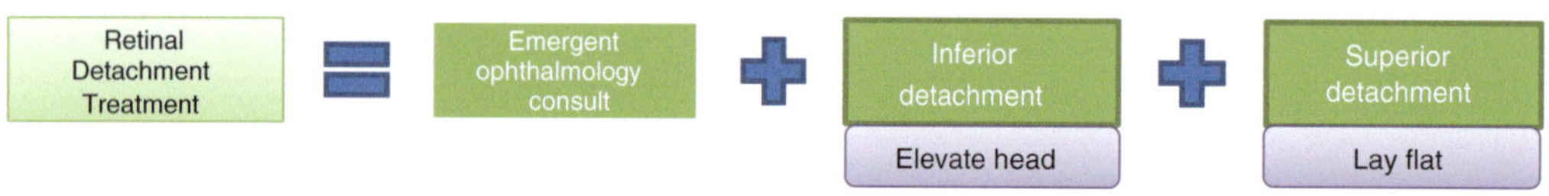

Optic Nerve

Optic Neuritis

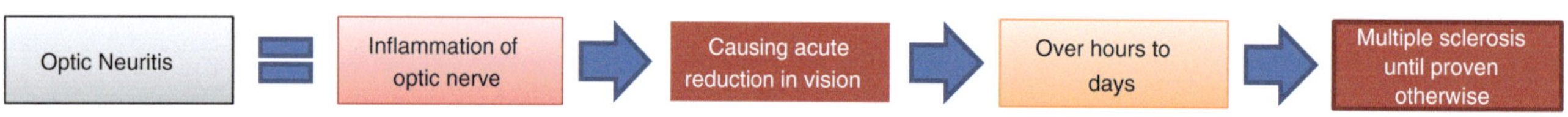

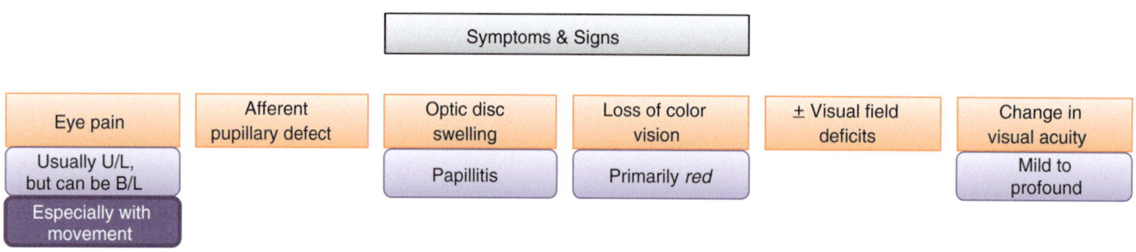

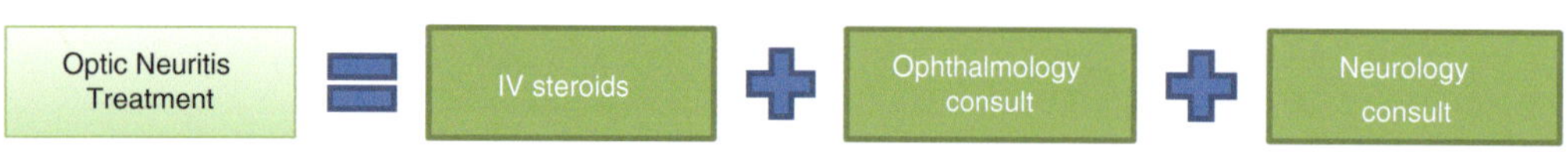

Papilledema and Pseudotumor Cerebri

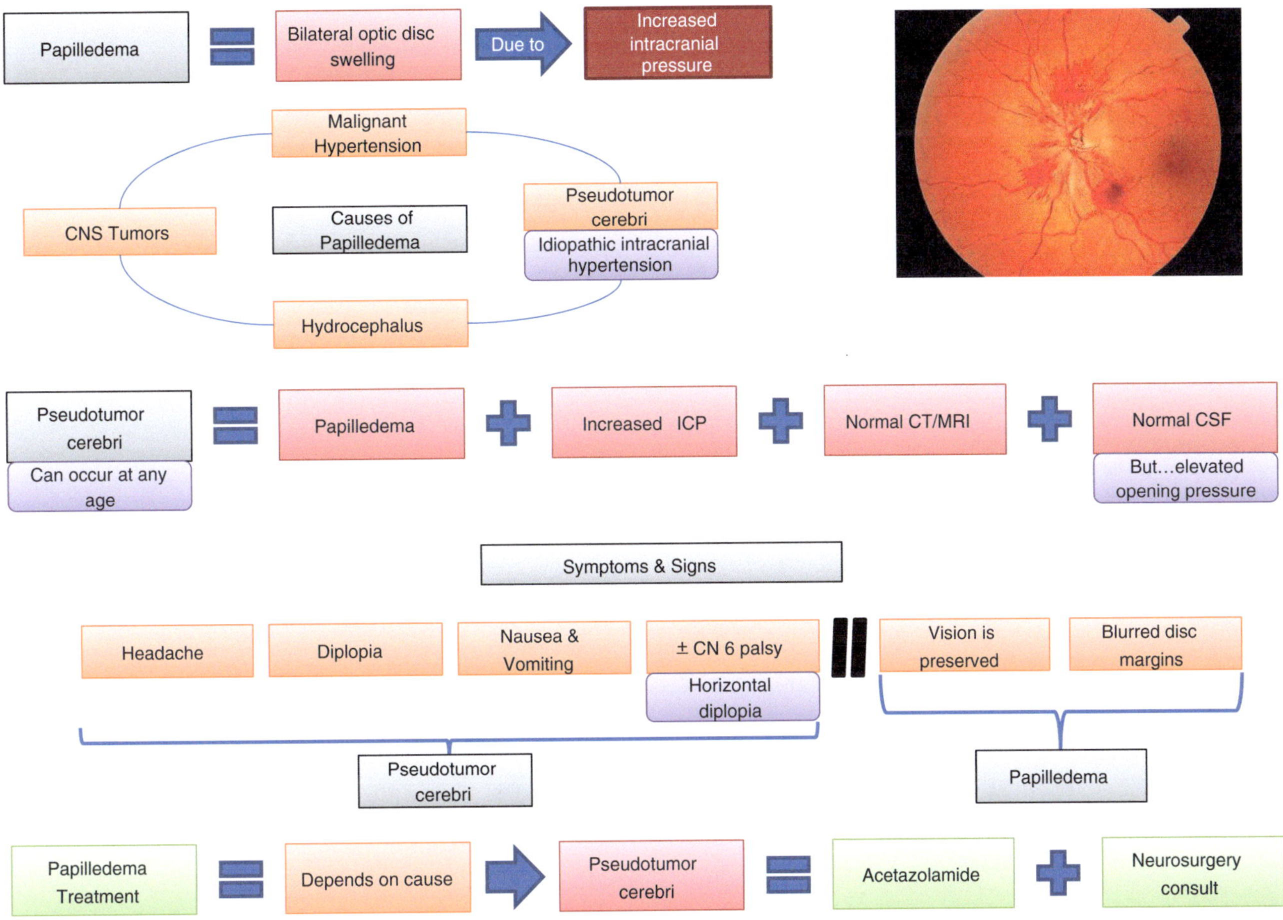

Top right image (Reprinted from Galloway NR, Amoaku WMK, Galloway PH, Browning AC. Neuro-ophthalmology. In: Galloway NR, Amoaku WMK, Galloway PH, Browning AC, editors. Common eye diseases and their management. London: Springer Verlag; 2006. p. 179–88. With permission from Springer Verlag)

Temporal Arteritis

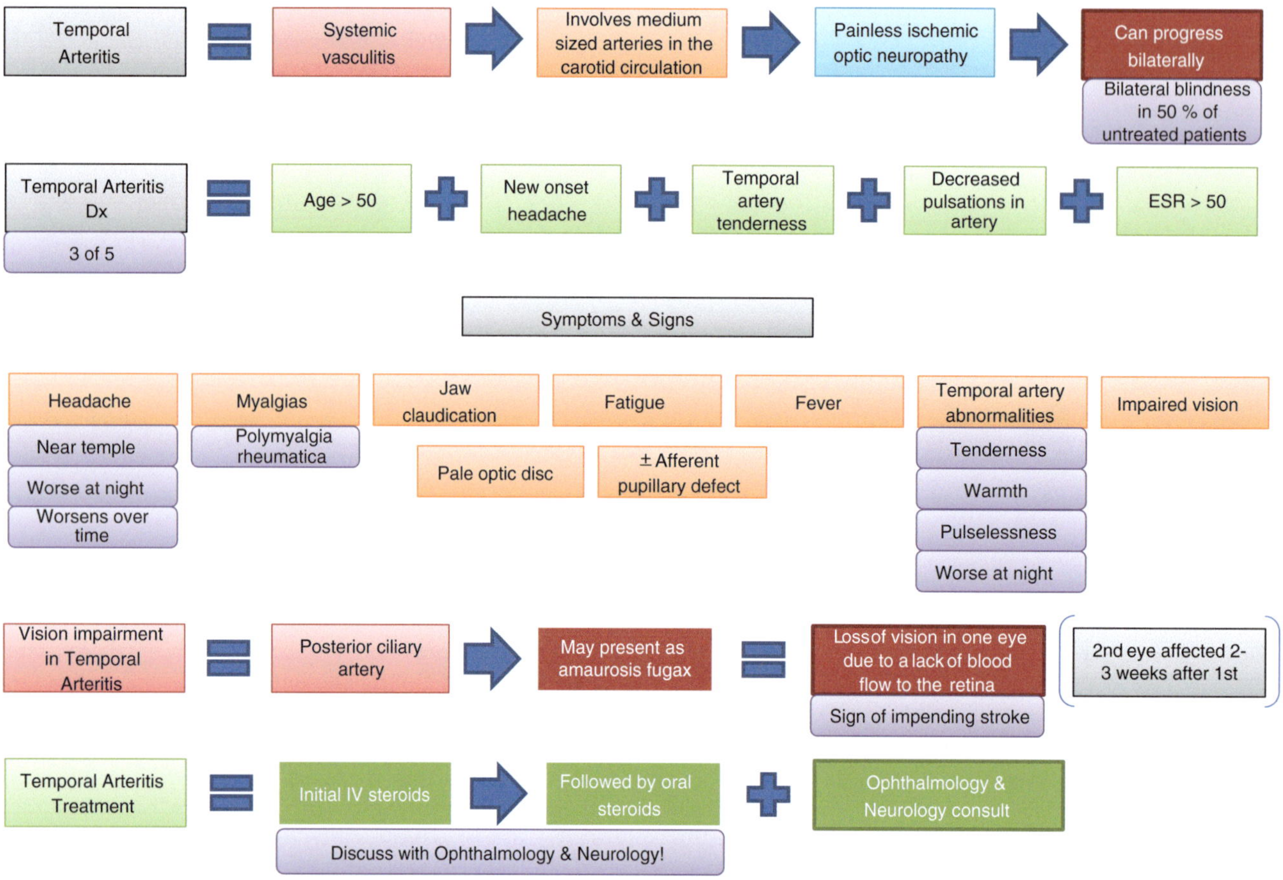

Glaucoma

Acute Angle-Closure Glaucoma

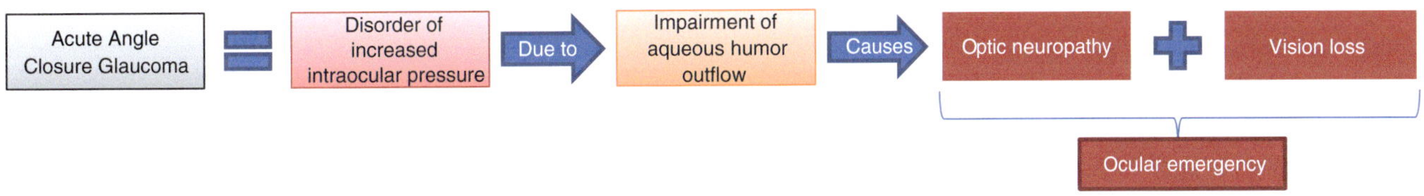

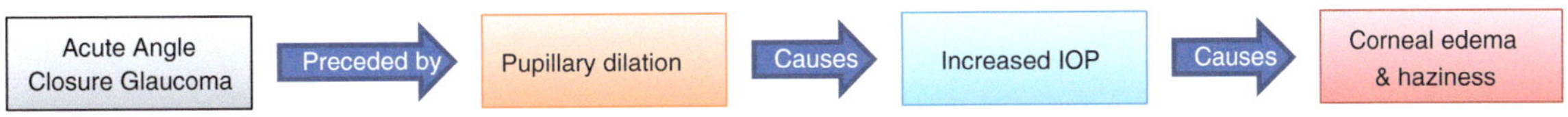

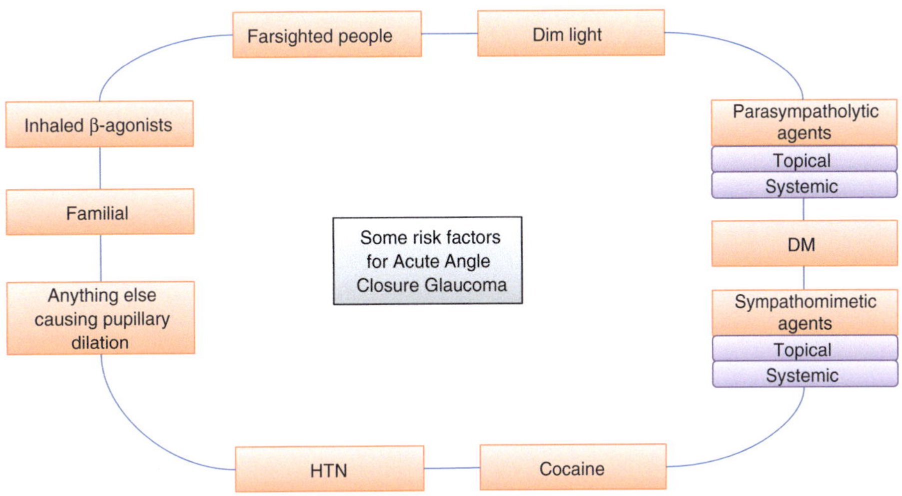

Acute Angle-Closure Glaucoma Symptoms and Signs

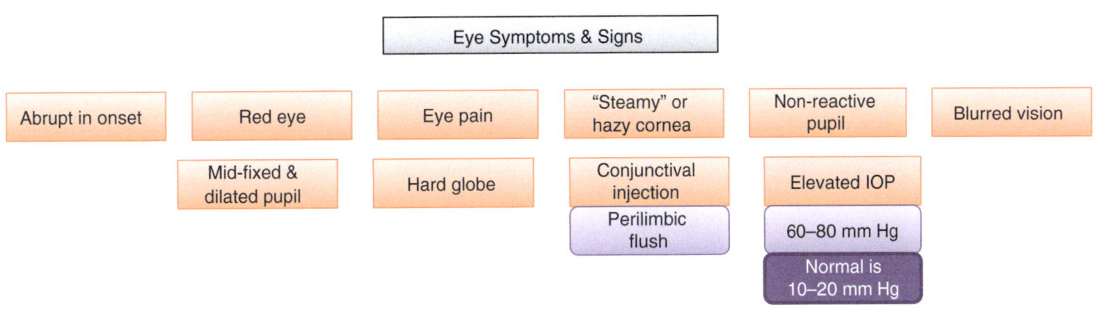

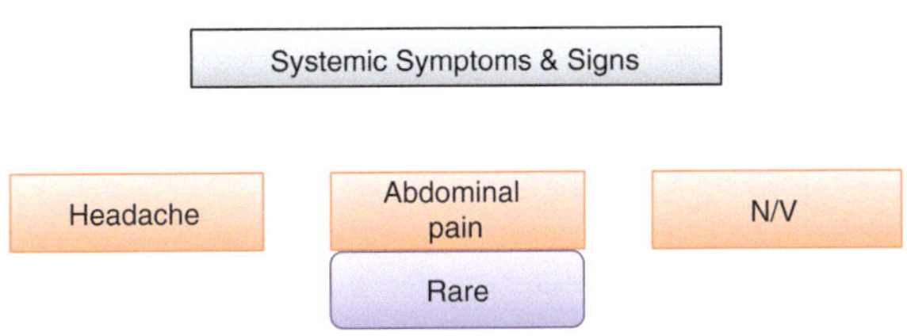

Acute Angle-Closure Glaucoma Treatment

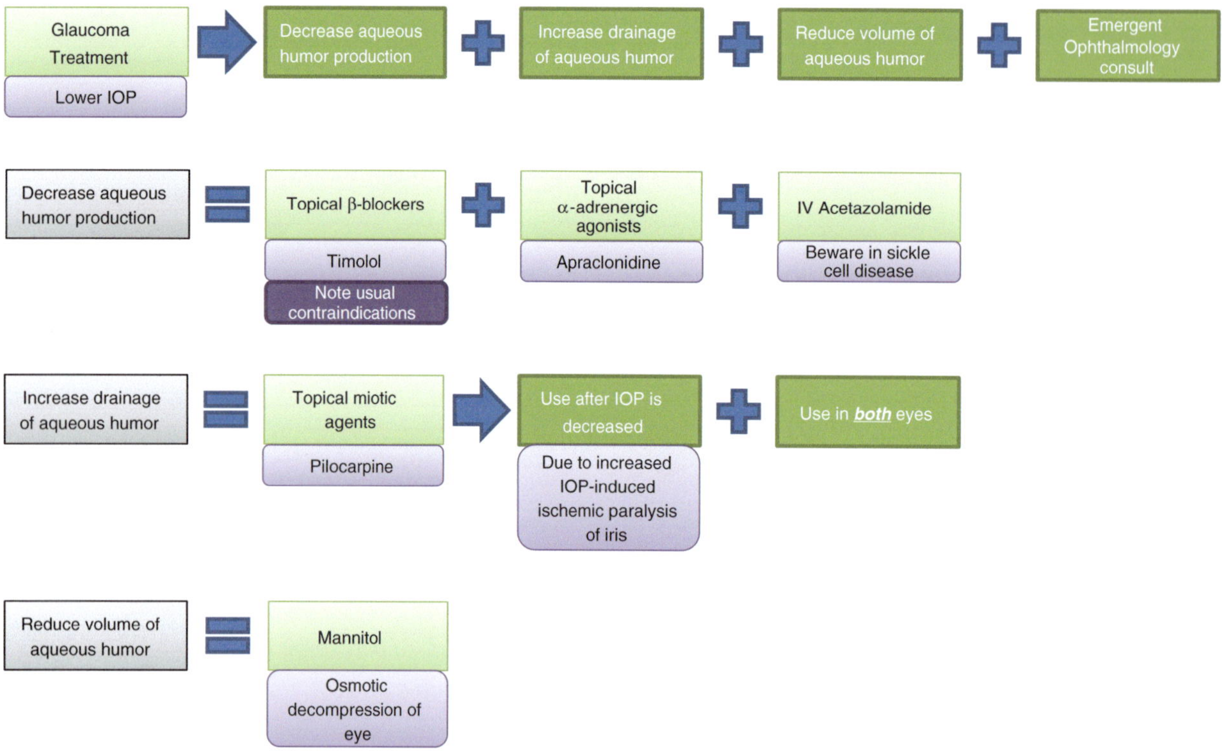

Trauma

Blunt Eye Trauma

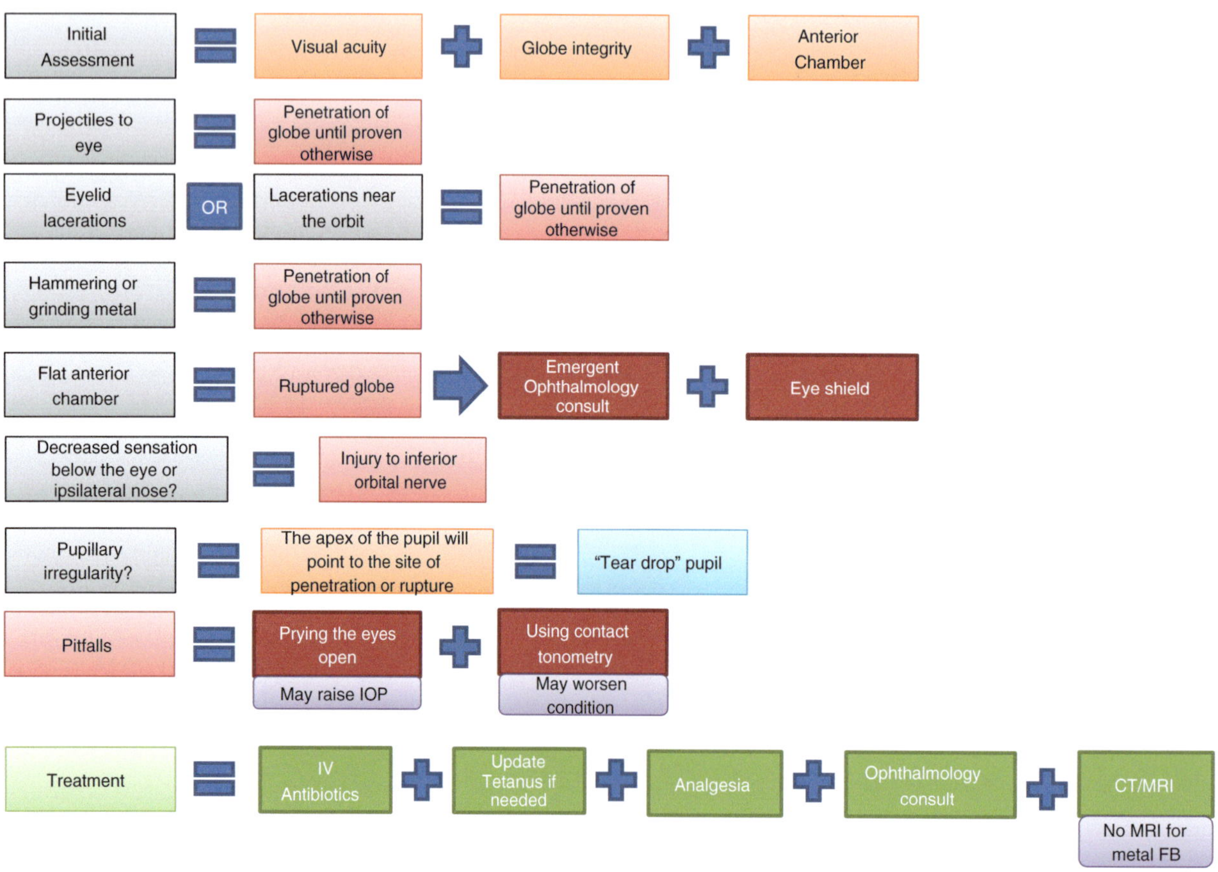

Signs and Symptoms of Blunt Ocular Trauma and Globe Rupture

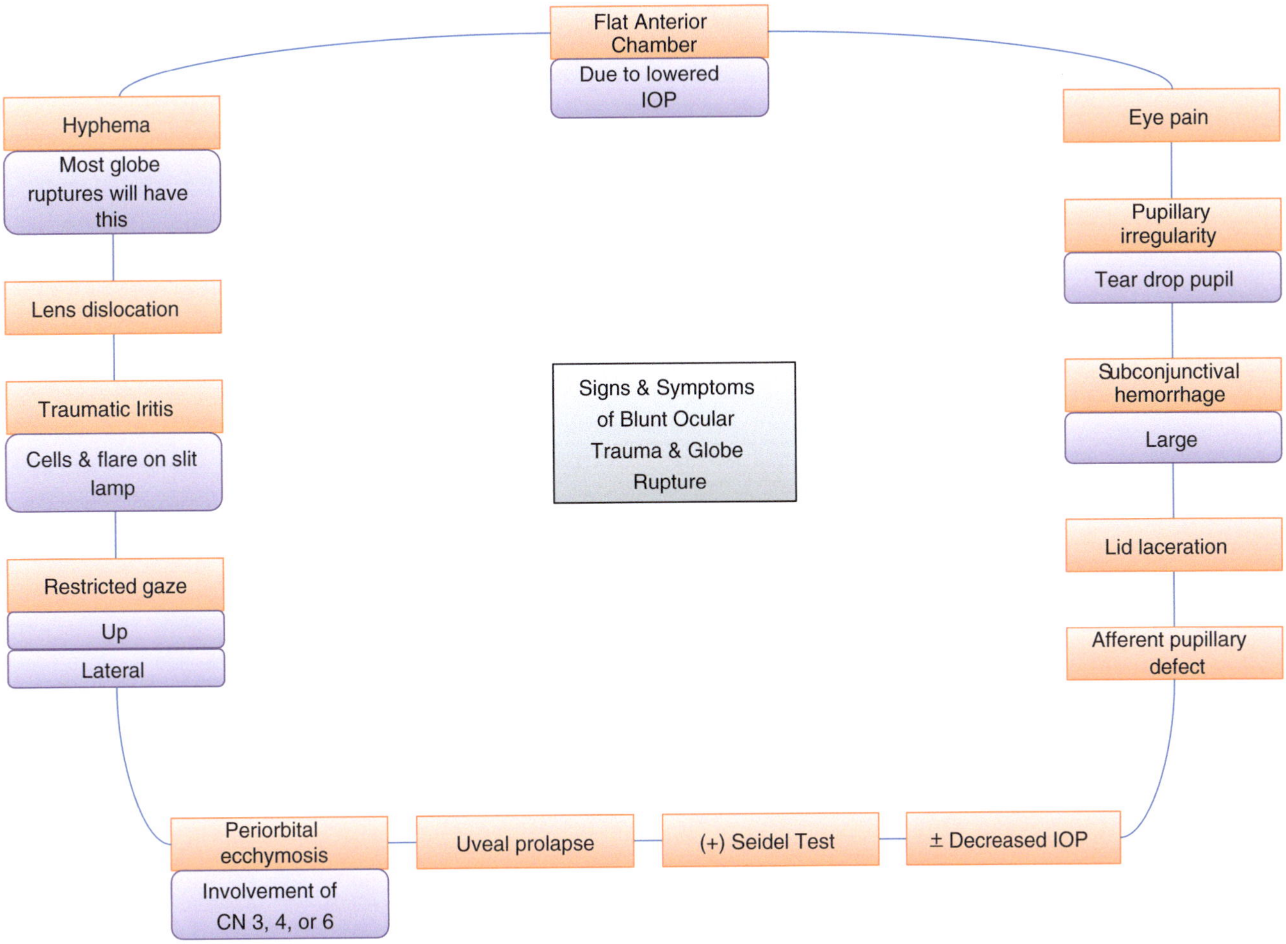

Hyphema

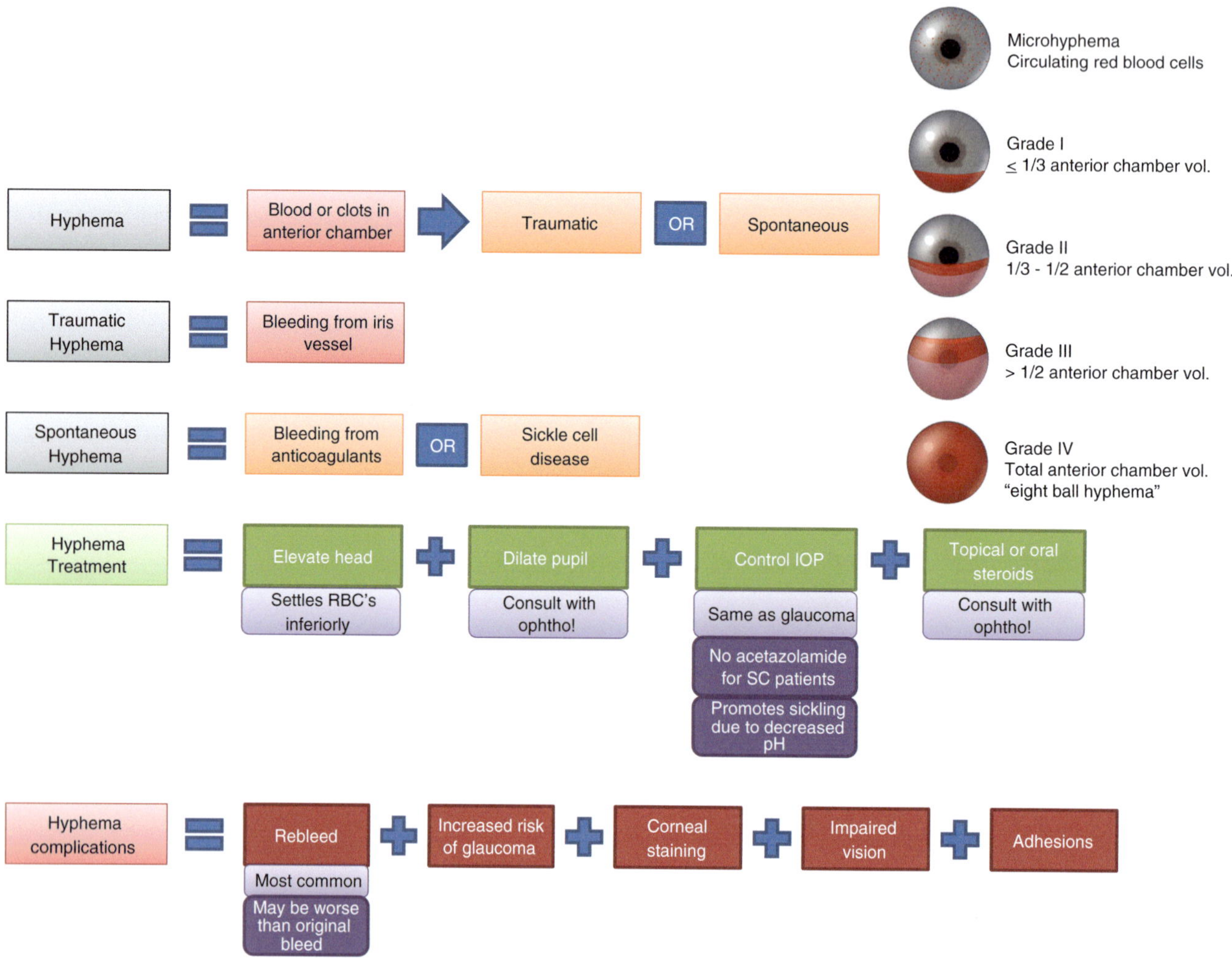
Microhyphema
Circulating red blood cells
Grade I
≤ 1/3 anterior chamber vol.
Grade II
1/3 - 1/2 anterior chamber vol.
Grade III
> 1/2 anterior chamber vol.
Grade IV
Total anterior chamber vol.
"eight ball hyphema"
Hyphema
Blood or clots in anterior chamber
Traumatic
OR
Spontaneous
Traumatic Hyphema
Bleeding from iris vessel
Spontaneous Hyphema
Bleeding from anticoagulants
OR
Sickle cell disease
Hyphema Treatment
Elevate head
Settles RBC's inferiorly
Dilate pupil
Consult with ophtho!
Control IOP
Same as glaucoma
No acetazolamide for SC patients
Promotes sickling due to decreased pH
Topical or oral steroids
Consult with ophtho!
Hyphema complications
Rebleed
Most common
May be worse than original bleed
Increased risk of glaucoma
Corneal staining
Impaired vision
Adhesions

Blow-Out Fractures

Sites for blow out fractures = Inferior wall into the maxillary sinus + Medial wall into the ethmoid sinus = Most common orbital wall fx = Caused by direct trauma to orbit

Medial wall fx → Subcutaneous emphysema = Orbital rupture into sinus or nose

Inferior wall fx = Contents of orbits through orbital floor = Restriction of upward gaze = Diplopia

Decreased sensation below the eye or ipsilateral nose? = Injury to inferior orbital nerve

Epistaxis + Eye Trauma − Nasal trauma = Blowout fx until proven otherwise

Dx of Blowout fracture = CT (Better) OR Water's view X-ray = Opacity in maxillary sinus = Blood or tissue in sinus

Isolated Blow Out − Entrapment = Referral for repair in 3-10 days

Treatment = PO Antibiotics + Update Tetanus if needed + Analgesia + Ophthalmology & Face consult + CT

Pitfalls = Not referring to ophthalmology & Face (All will need dilated exam) + Using contact tonometry (May worsen condition) + Not giving Abx

Retrobulbar Hematoma

Retrobulbar Hematoma = Bleeding behind orbit → Traumatic exophthalmos

Large hematoma → Increase in IOP → Acute glaucoma + Decreased blood flow to optic nerve & retina = Retinal ischemia

Symptoms & Signs

- Eye pain
- Proptosis
- Decreased vision
- Afferent pupillary defect

Penetration of globe NOT suspected = Measure IOP → Increased IOP (>40) = Lateral canthotomy + Medications to reduce IOP

Diagnosis = CT = Blood in *Tenon's capsule*

Chemical Burns

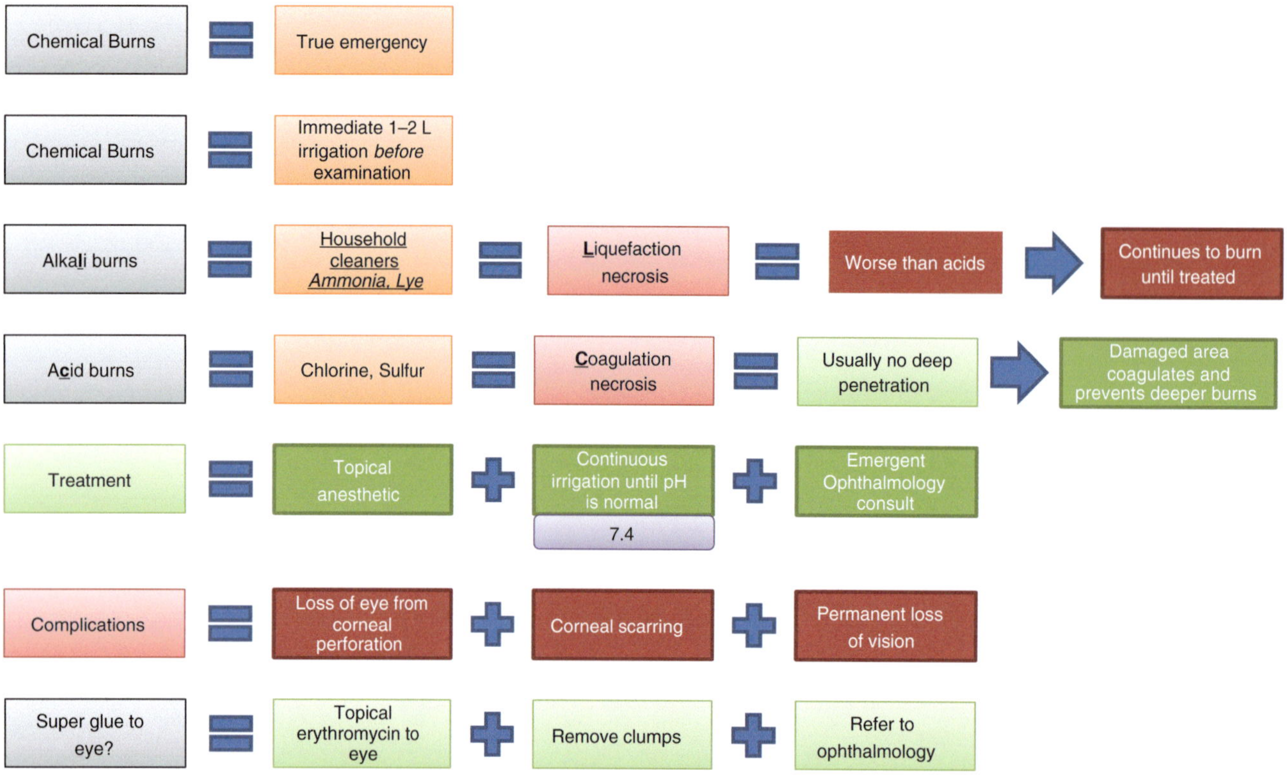

Lacerations to Refer

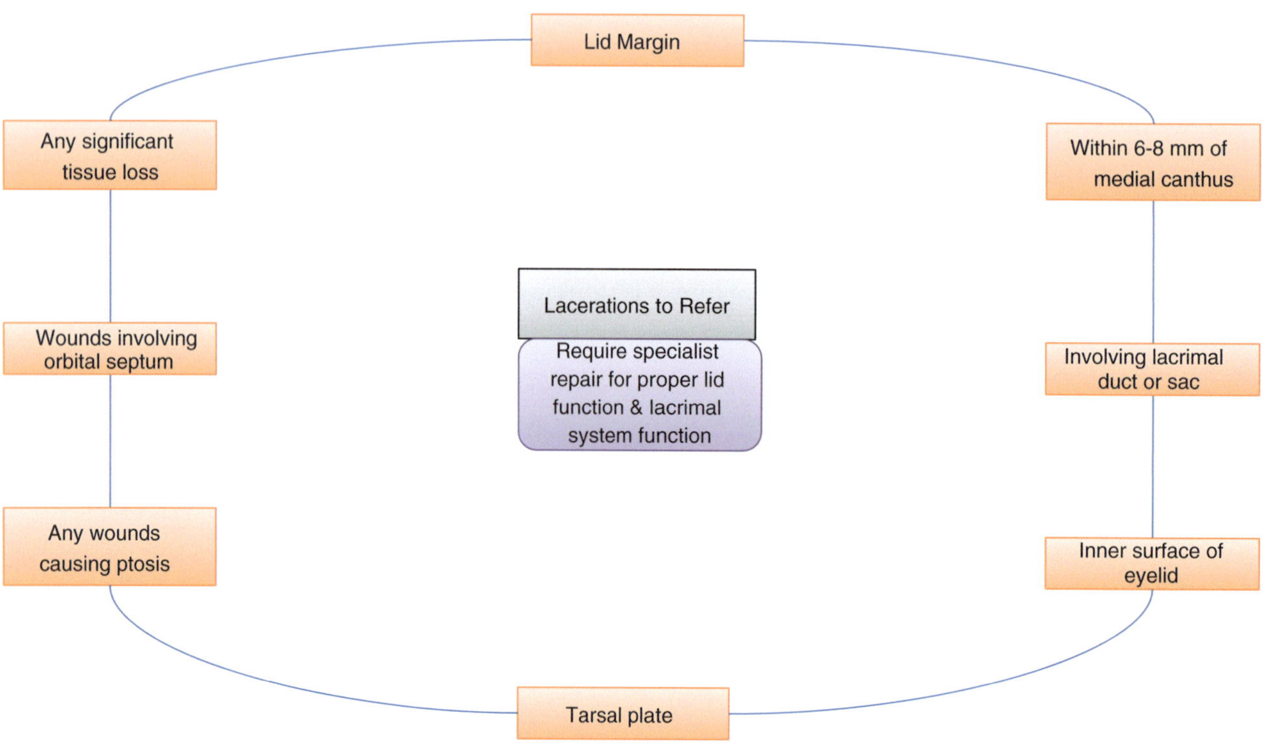

Toxicologic Emergencies

Matthew Ryan and Bobby Desai

Contents

General Approach to the Poisoned Patient ... 676

Data Interpretation ... 685

Toxidromes ... 687

Specific Toxins and Poisons ... 692

M. Ryan, MD, PhD • B. Desai, MD, MEd
Department of Emergency Medicine, University of Florida,
Gainesville, FL, USA
e-mail: bdesai@ufl.edu

B. Desai, B.R. Allen (eds.), *Nailing the Written Emergency Medicine Board Examination*,
DOI 10.1007/978-3-319-30838-8_13

General Approach to the Poisoned Patient

Primary Survey

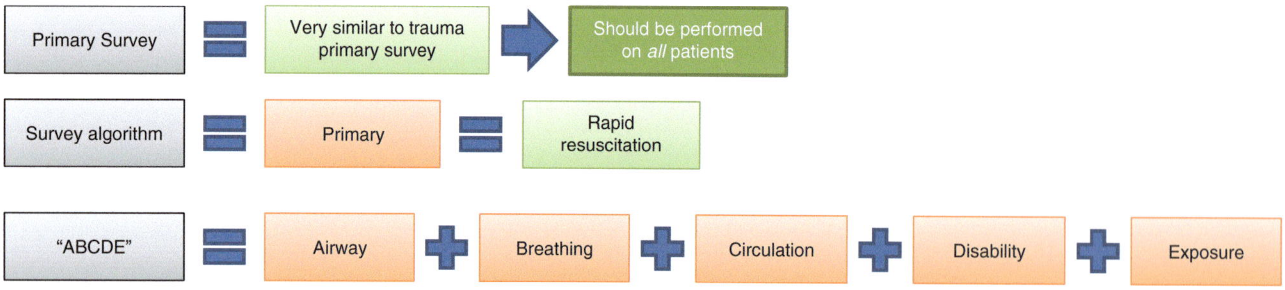

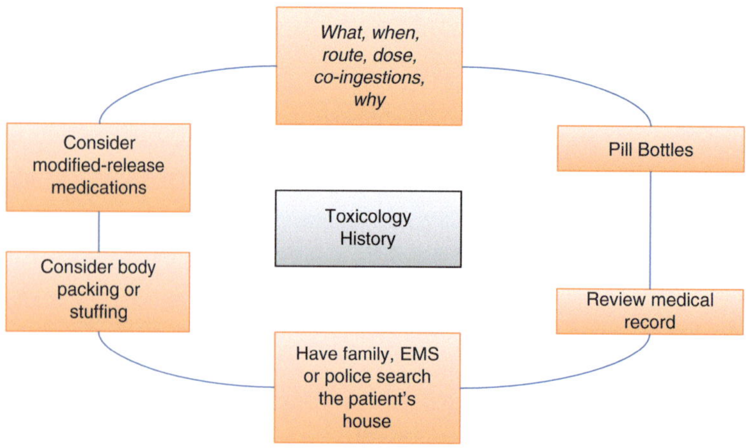

Airway Assessment

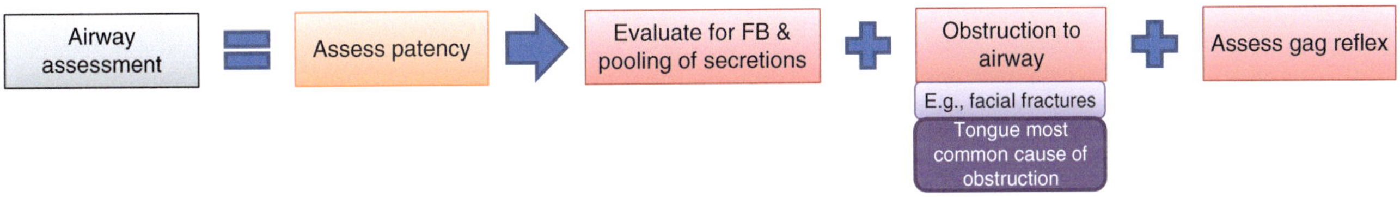

Breathing Assessment

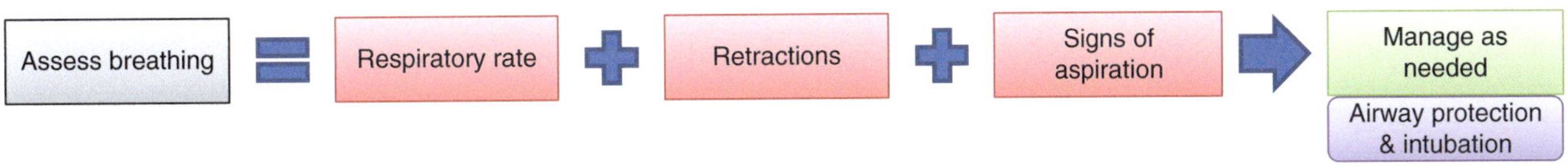

Circulation Assessment

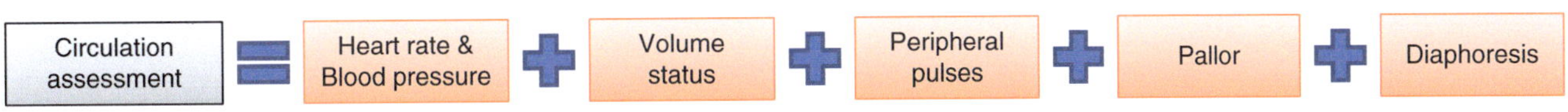

Disability Assessment

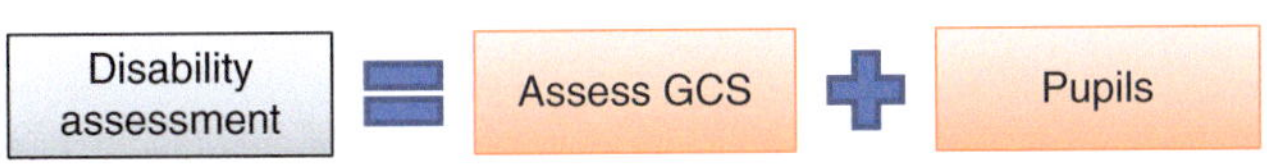

Exposure

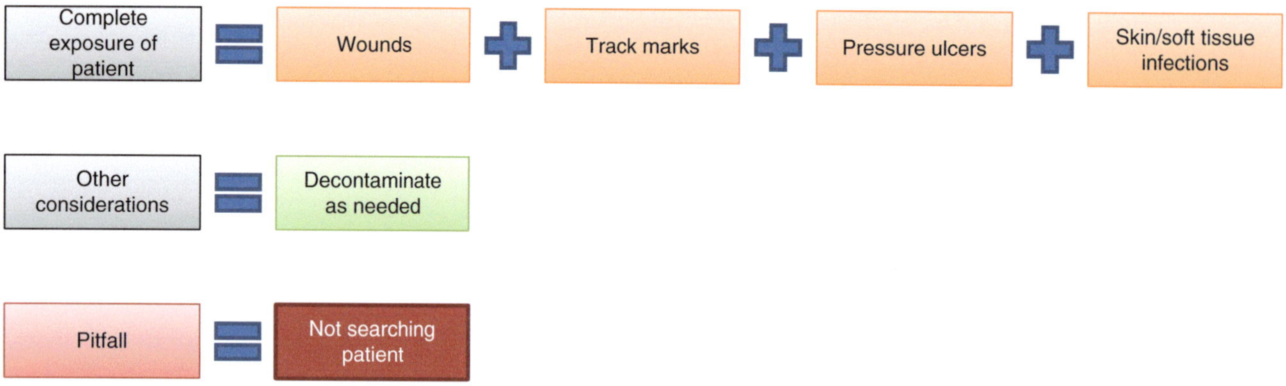

Primary Survey Adjuncts

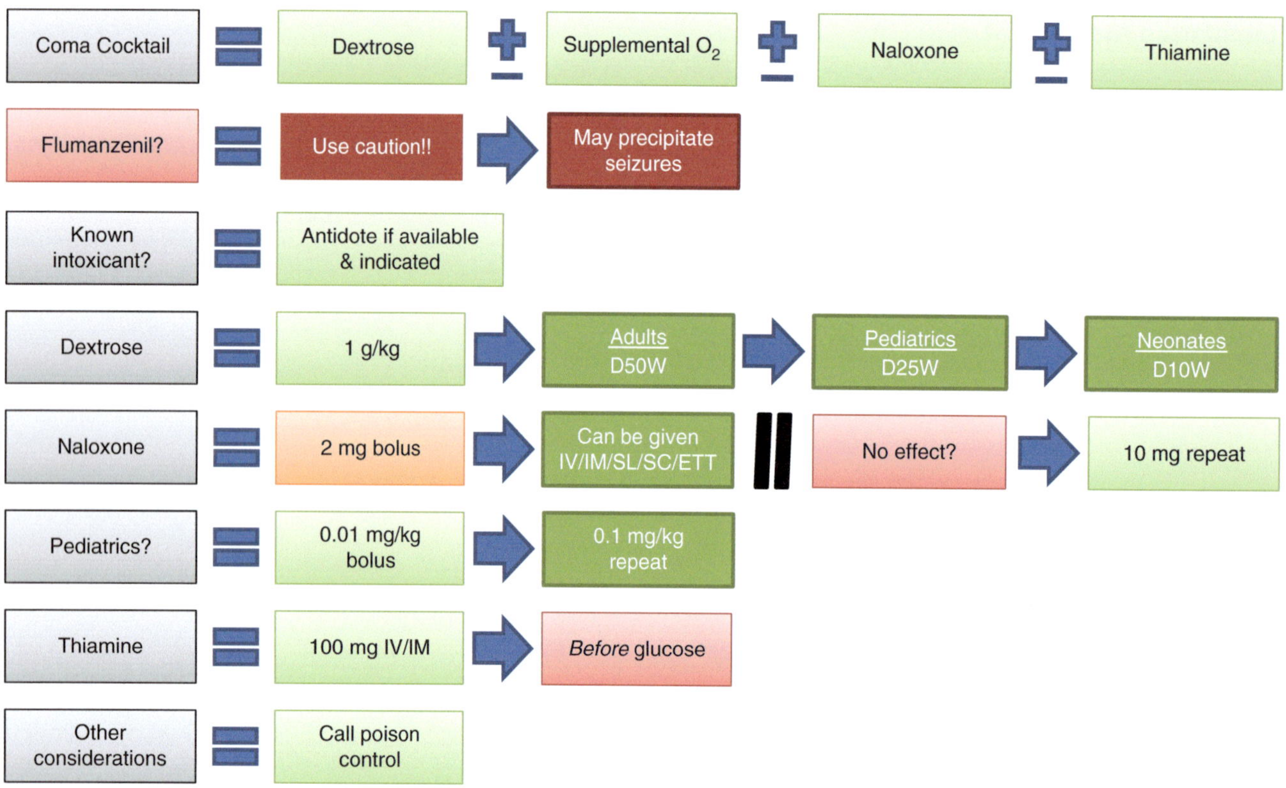

Laboratory Studies

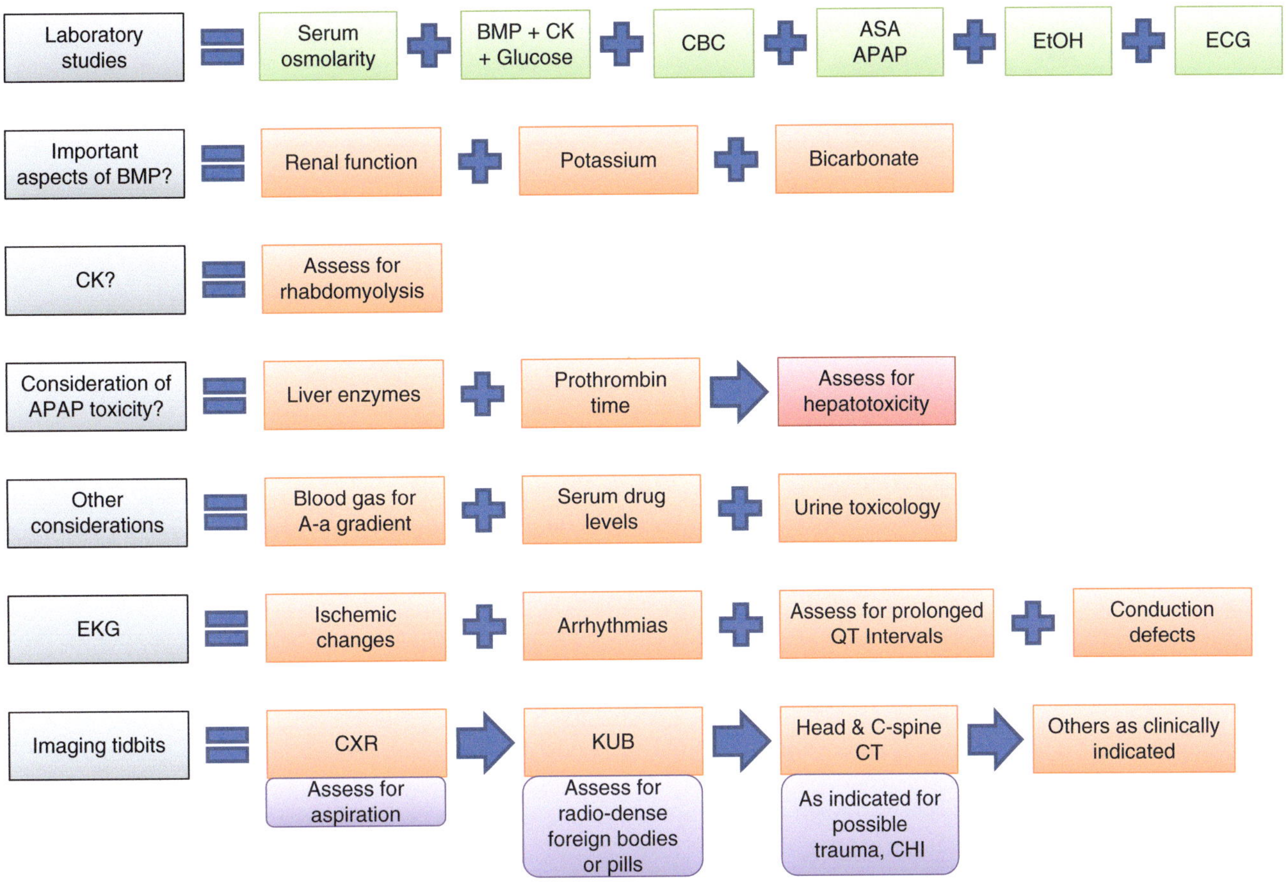

Toxicology Screens

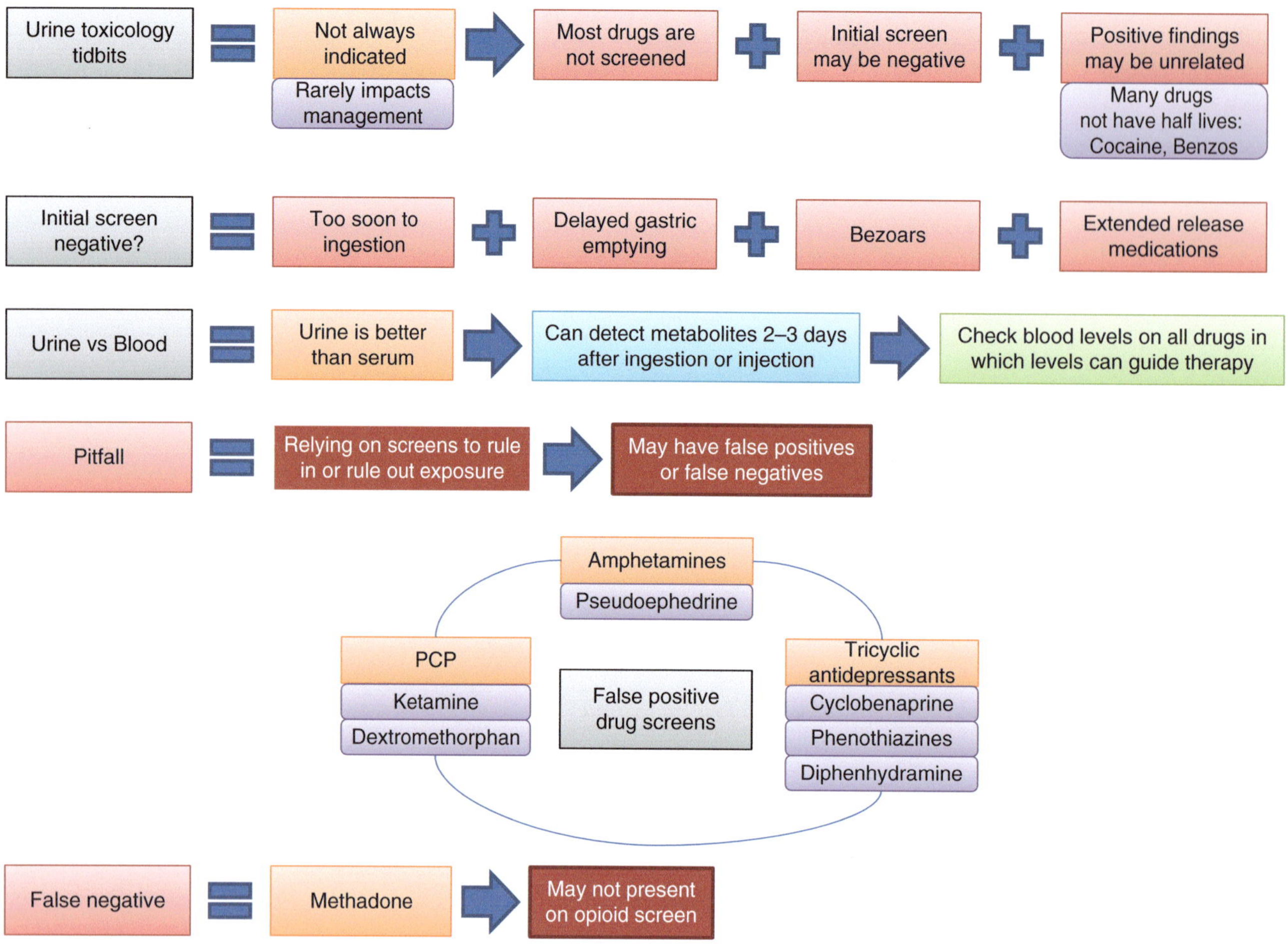

Urinalysis Tidbits

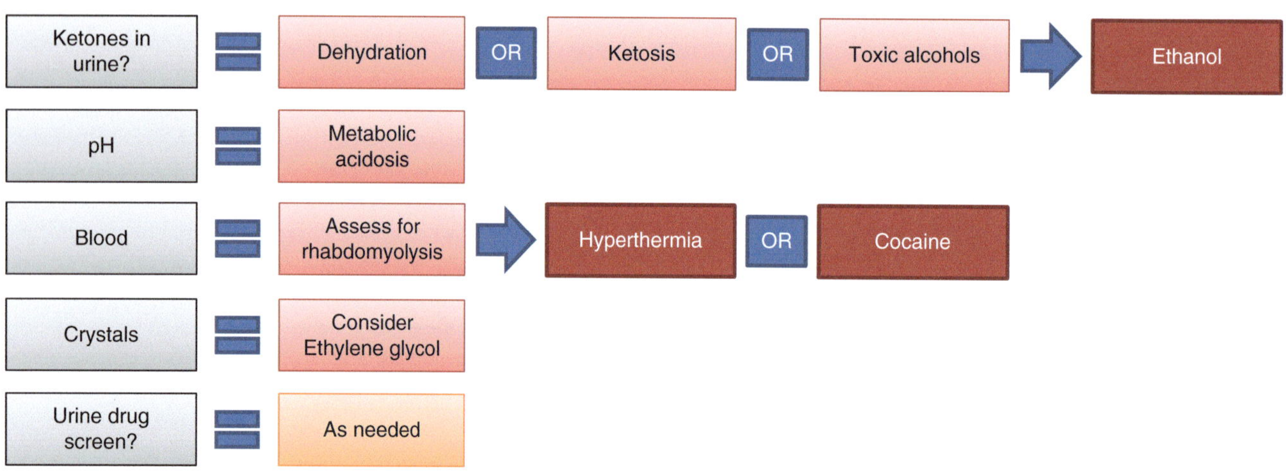

Secondary Survey and Adjuncts

Secondary Survey = Head to toe examination of patient + Specific antidotes for known ingestions

Physical exam features = Track marks + Pressure ulcers + Skin/Soft tissue infections + Skin popping + Check groin & axilla for sweat ("Toxicology handshake")

Other considerations? = Trauma? + Toxidromes? + Other Dx that mimic a toxic ingestion

Gastric lavage = No clinical trials to date have shown efficacy + Best performed within 1–2 hours of ingestion

Environmental exposure? = Shower or irrigation → Pesticides + Cutaneous exposure

Modified release medication or ingestion? = Whole bowel irrigation

Activated charcoal = Within 1 hour of ingestion → Must be awake & cooperative → Risk of aspiration

Elimination strategies = Alkalinization (TCA & ASA) + Forced saline diuresis + Dialysis

Charcoal Tidbits

Activated charcoal = 1st line for GI decontamination → Administer within 1 hour of ingestions → 1 g/kg → Massive overdose may require extra doses

Activated charcoal = Decreases enterohepatic recirculation → Prevents re-absorption of agent

Pitfall = Not effective for ionic or charged substances → Lithium, Bases, Acids, Heavy Metals

Medications that bind poorly: Lithium, Iron, Cyanide, Hydrocarbons, Alcohols, Acids, Alkali

Multidose Charcoal: Sustained release drugs, Theophylline, Phenobarbital, Carbamazepine, Salicylates

Contraindications = Caustics + Altered mental status + Ileus OR Obstruction

Pitfall = Using multidose cathartics → Cause electrolyte problems & dehydration

Other Methods of Drug Elimination

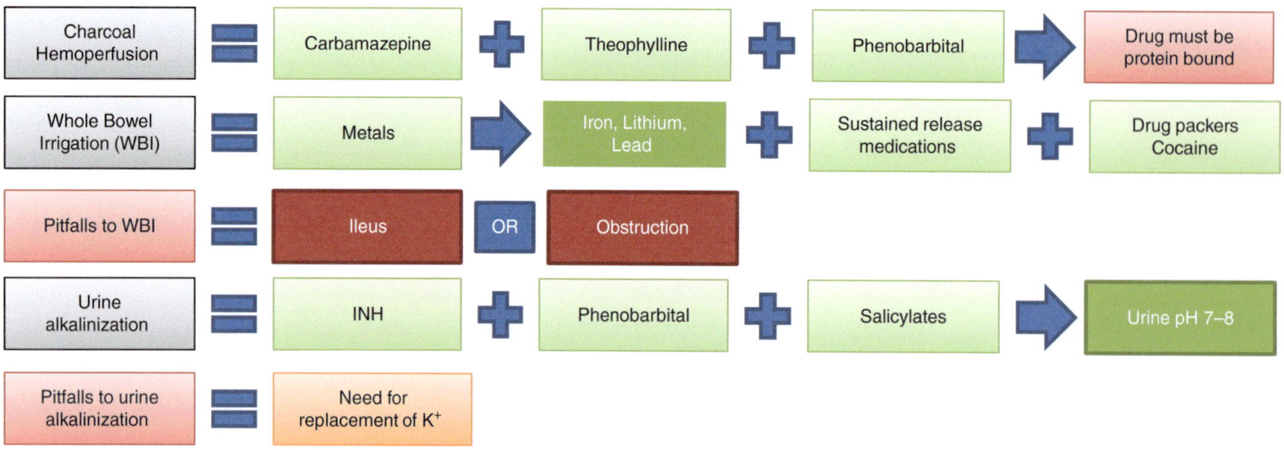

Dialysis Tidbits

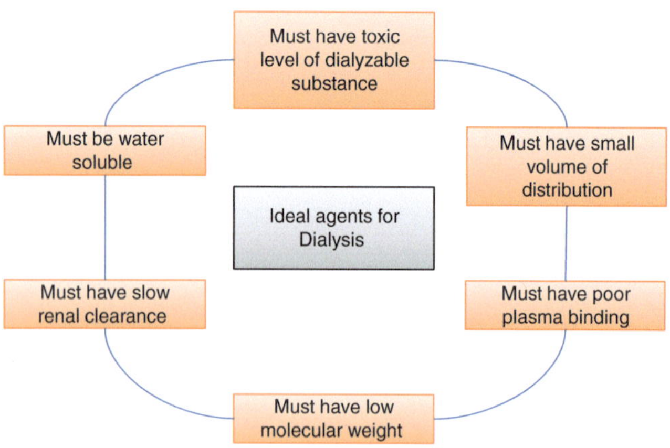

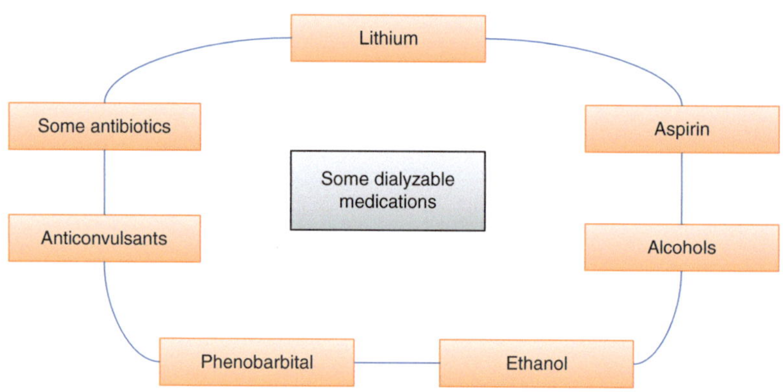

Toxins That Alter Thermoregulation or Cause Temperature Changes

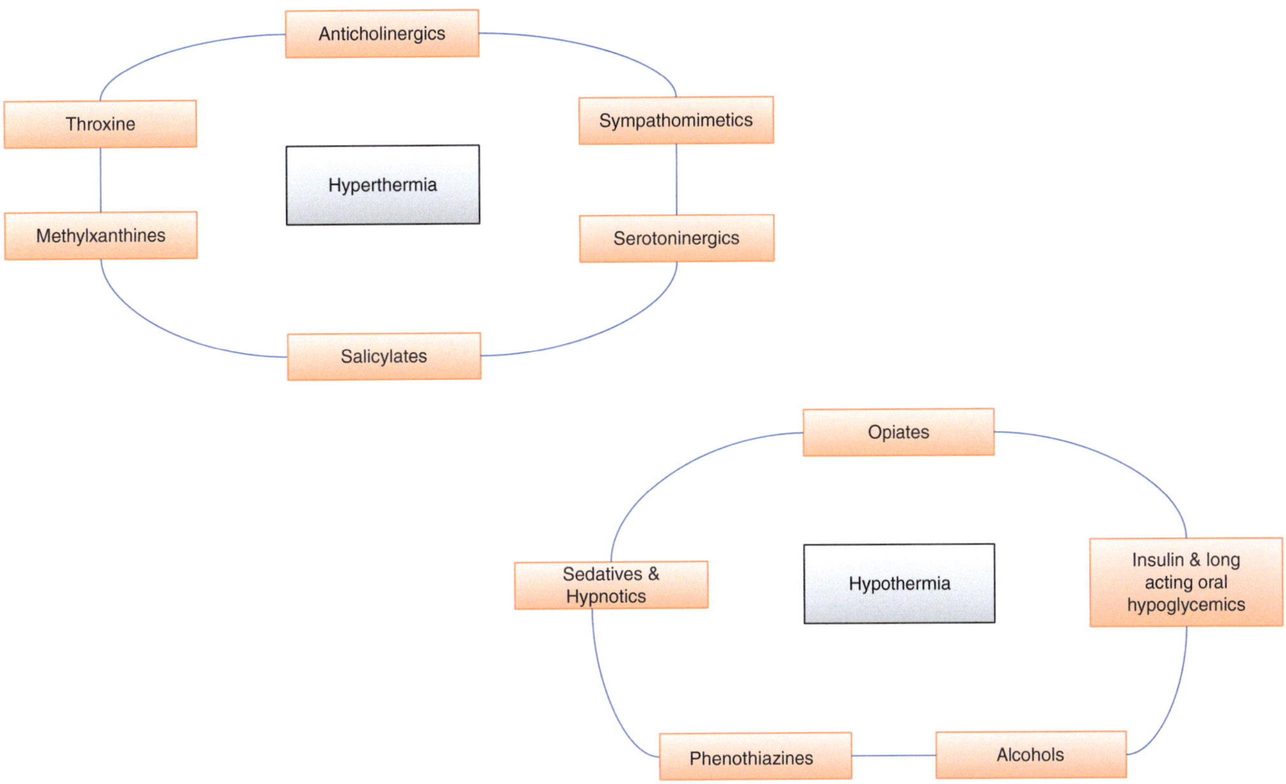

Toxins That Cause Hypoglycemia

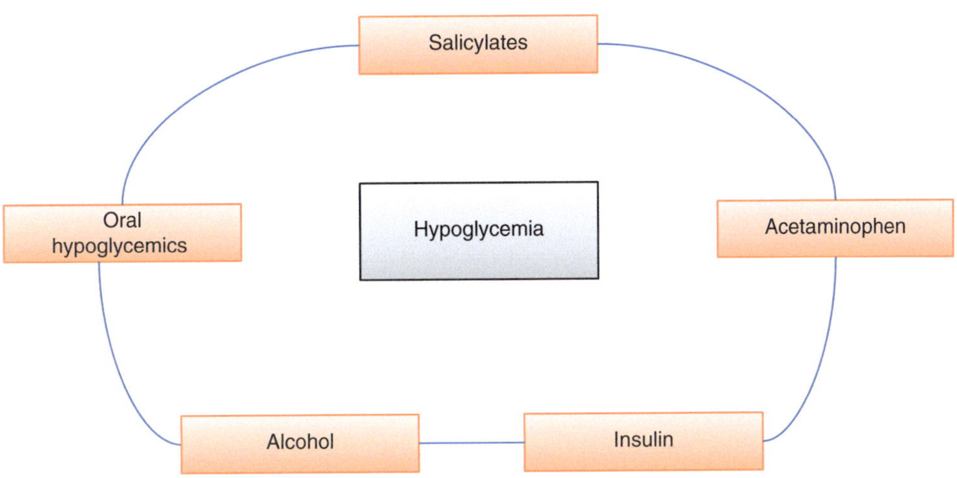

Select Antidotes

Agent/ Drug	Antidote
Acetaminophen	N-Acetylcysteine
Anticholinesterase	Atropine/Pralidoxime
Anticholinergics	Physostigmine
Benzodiazepines	Flumanezil
β-blockers	Glucagon
Calcium-channel blockers	Glucagon
Coumadin	Phytonadione
Cyanide	Amyl nitrate, Sodium nitrite, Sodium thiosulfate or Hydroxocobalamin
Digoxin	Digibind
Extrapyramidal symptoms	Diphenhydramine
Ethylene glycol	Fomepizole
Heparin	Protamine sulfate
Insulin reaction	Glucose
Iron	Deferoxamine
Lead	Dimercapol, EDTA
Narcotics	Naloxone
TCA's	Sodium bicarbonate

Overdose Odor Pearls

Odor	Agent
Burnt Almonds	Cyanide
Carrots	Water Hemlock
Fruity breath	Ethanol, Acetone, Isopropanol, Hydrocarbons
Garlic	Arsenic, arsenates
Glue	Toluene, Benzene, Polyaromatic hydrocarbons & other solvents
Pears	Chloral hydrate, Paraldehyde
Rotten eggs	Hydrogen Disulfide
Wintergreen	Topical Salicylate, e.g., Methyl Salicylate

Data Interpretation

Arterial-Alveolar Gradient

Arterial-alveolar Gradient = Difference between arterial versus alveoli oxygenation

Alveolar gas = Ambient gas minus what displaces it from the internal environment

P_AO_2 = Inspired O_2 − (CO_2 ÷ 0.8)

A-a gradient = P_AO_2 − P_aO_2

Normal A-a gradient? = (Age/4) + 4

Anion Gap

Anion gap = Measured cations − Measured anions

Anion gap = Sodium (Na^+) − (Chloride (Cl^-) + Bicarbonate (HCO_3^-))

Normal anion gap? = 10–15

Anion gap = Largely due to albumin

Lower anion gap = Malnourished + Chronically ill + Hypo-albuminemic pts

Anion gap = CAT MUDPILES

Toxins Associated with Anion Gap

Toxins	Tidbits
CO/CN	Inhibits oxidative phosphorylation
Ethanol (Alcohol)	Acidosis, Respiratory depression, Dehydration
Toluene	
Methanol	Formic acid
Uremia	
Diabetic Ketoacidosis	
Paraldehyde	Acetic and Chloracetic acid
Isoniazid	Lactic acidosis
Iron	Inhibits oxidative phosphorylation
Lactic acidosis	Sepsis
Ethylene glycol	Oxalic acid
Salicylates	Acidosis & Inhibits oxidative phosphorylation

Osmolar Gap

Osmolar Gap = Measured osmolality − Calculated osmolality

Normal osmolar gap? = −15 up to +10 (mean +2) → Usually < 10

Normal gap due to ? = Calcium + Lipids + Proteins

Differential diagnosis of osmolar gap = Increased protein OR Alcohols OR Hyperglycemia OR Ketosis OR Acidosis

Presence of osmolar gap? = Consider toxic alcohols OR AKA OR DKA OR Mannitol

Most common cause of gap? = Ethanol

Toxidromes

Anticholinergic Toxidrome

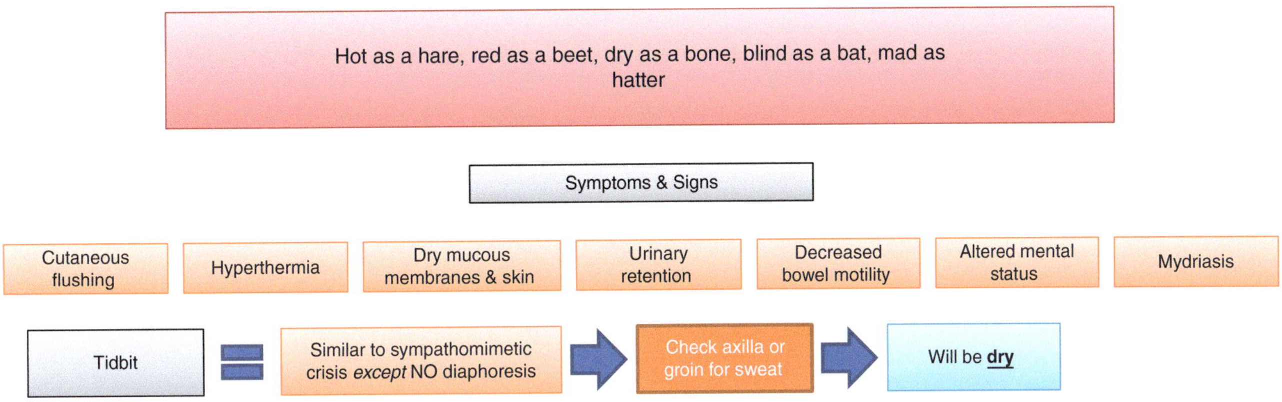

Anticholinergic Causes

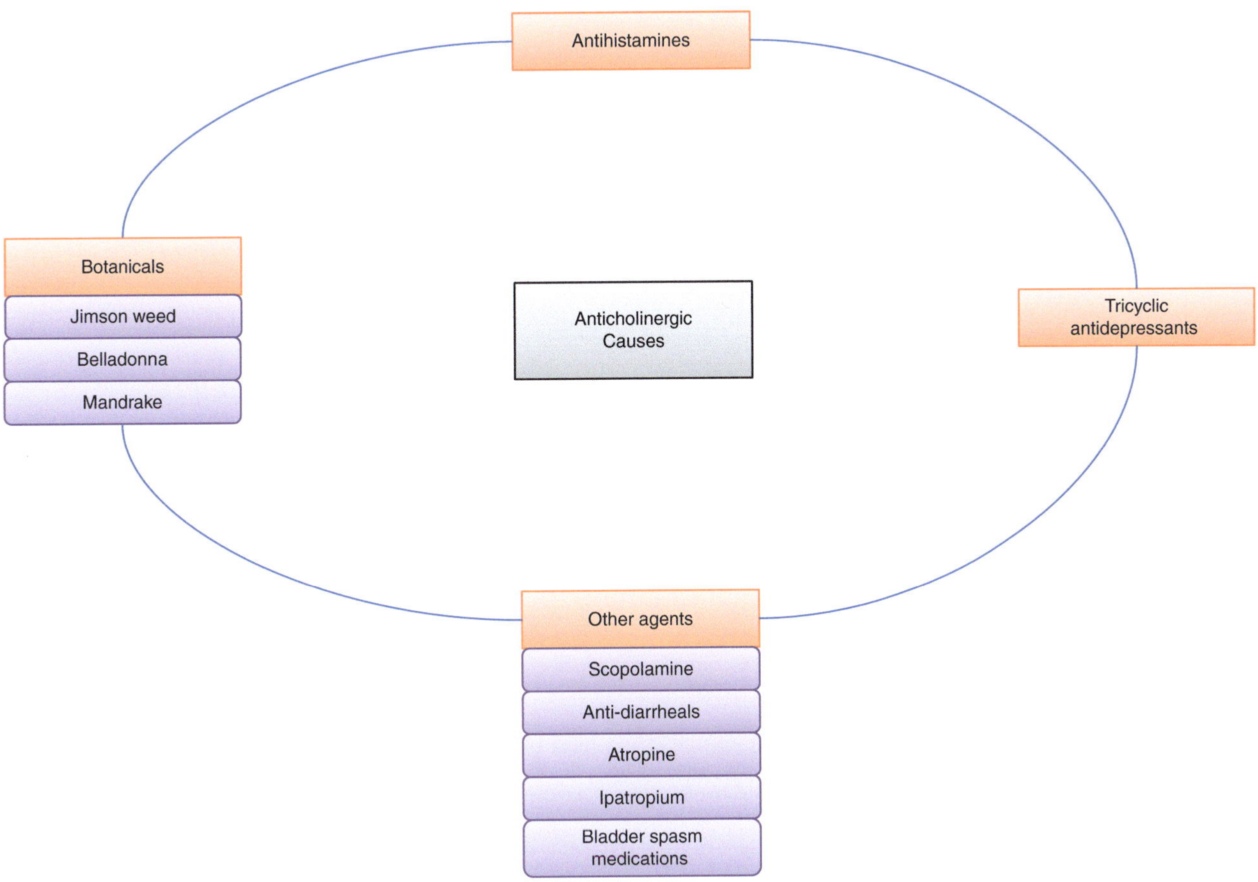

Anticholinergic Treatment Tidbits

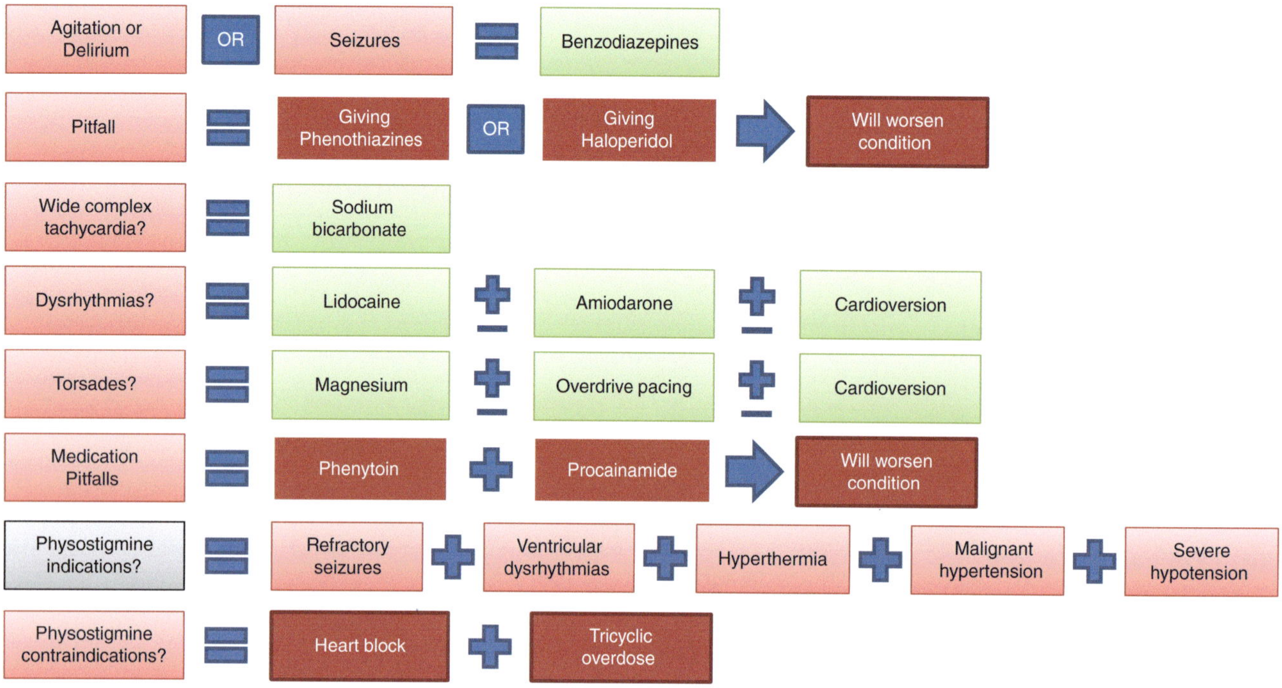

Cholinergic Toxidrome

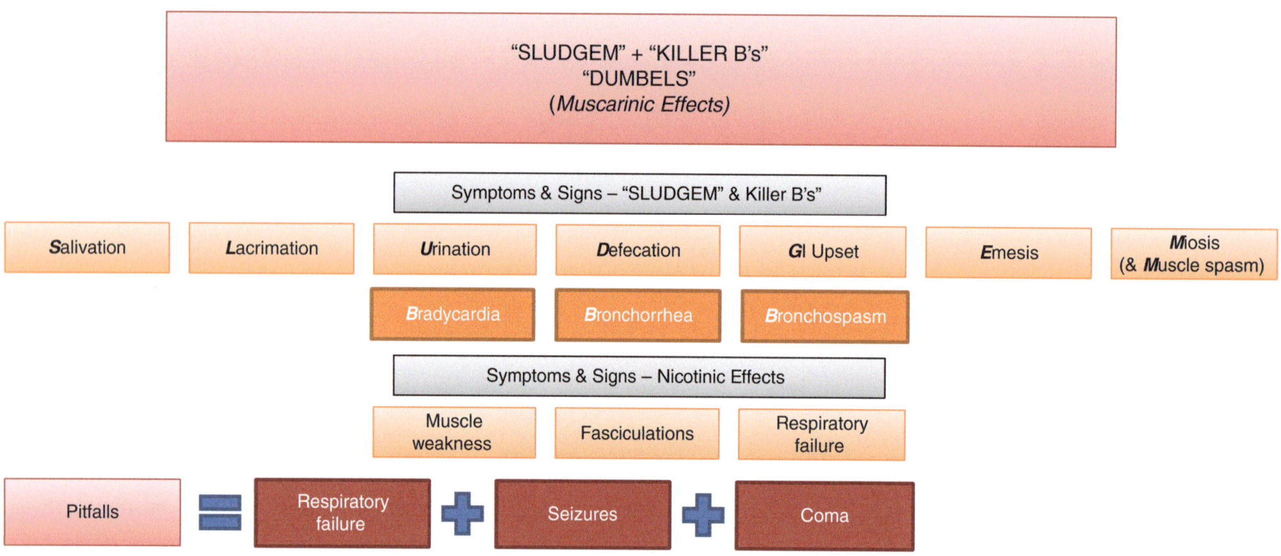

Cholinergic Causes

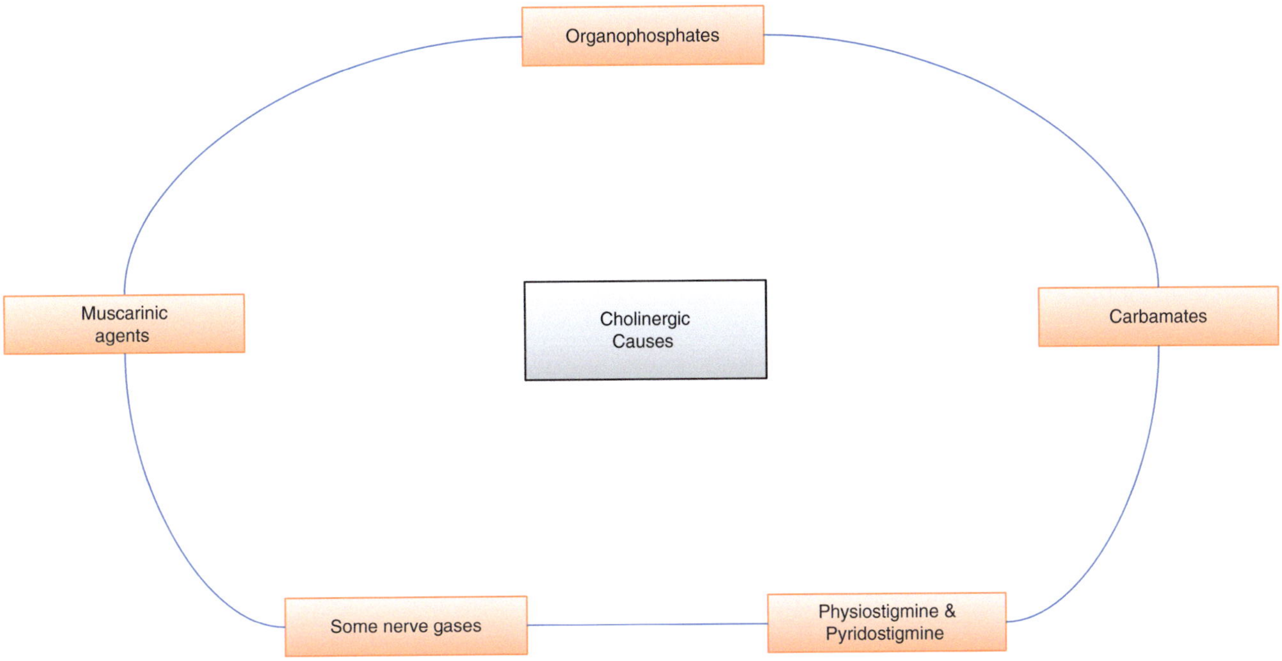

Opioid Toxidrome

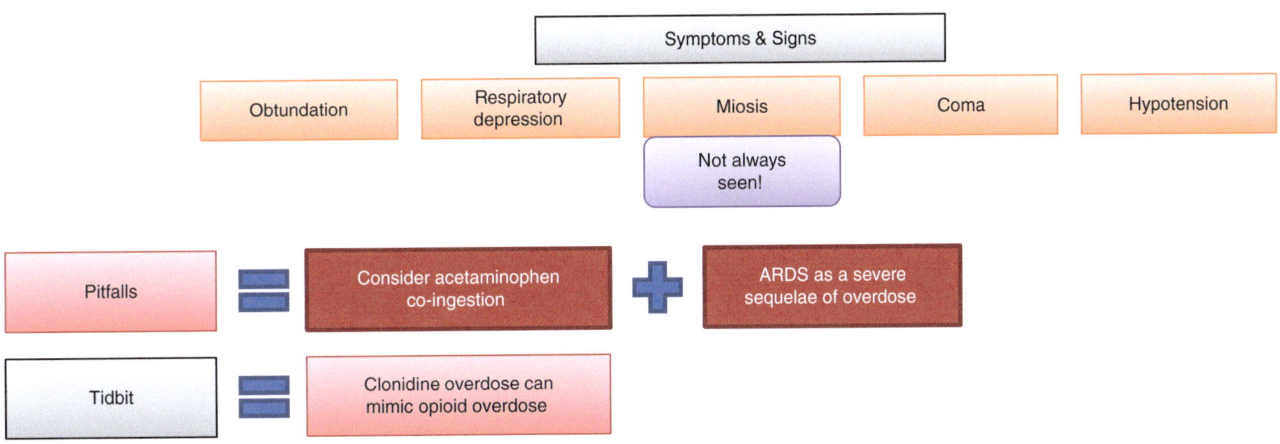

Common Opioids

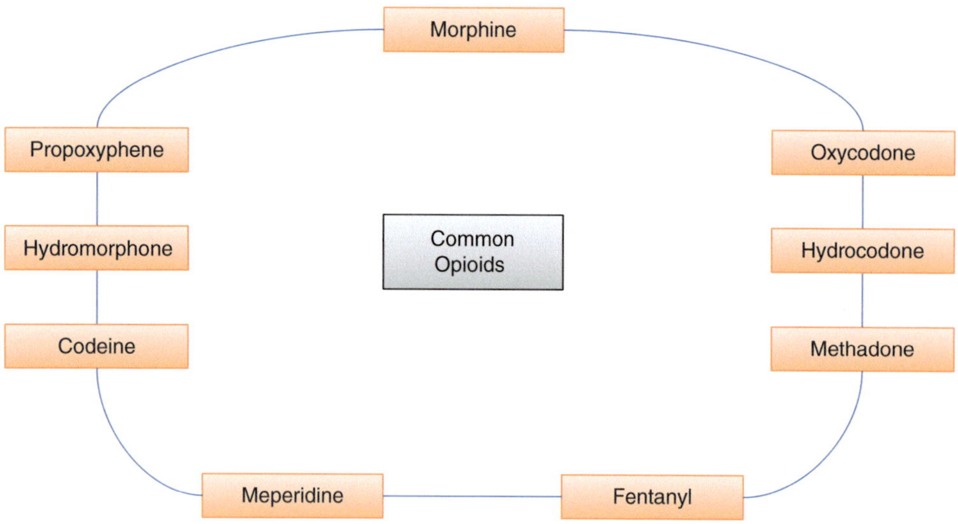

Sedative Toxidrome

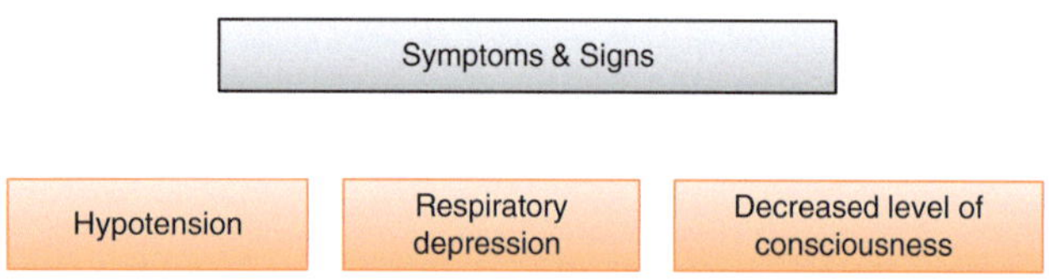

Considerations for Sedative Toxidrome

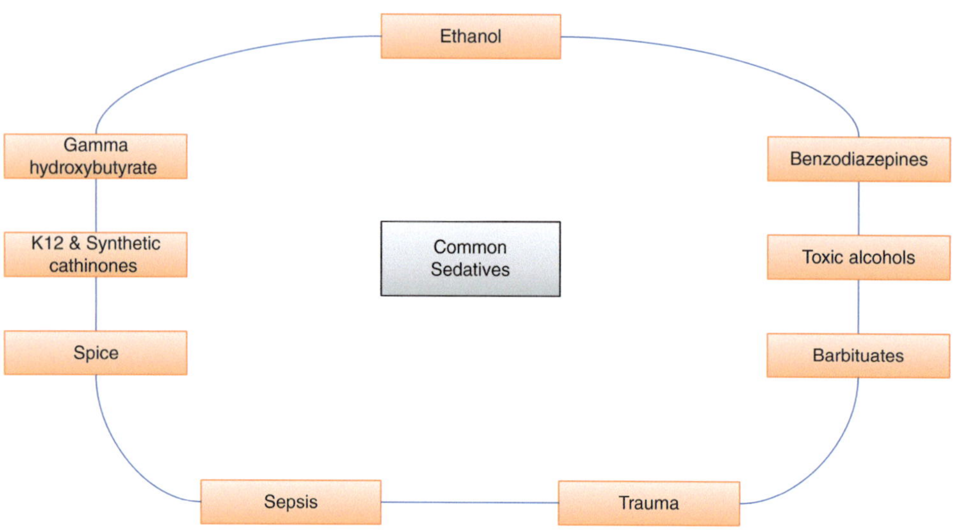

Sympathomimetic Toxidrome

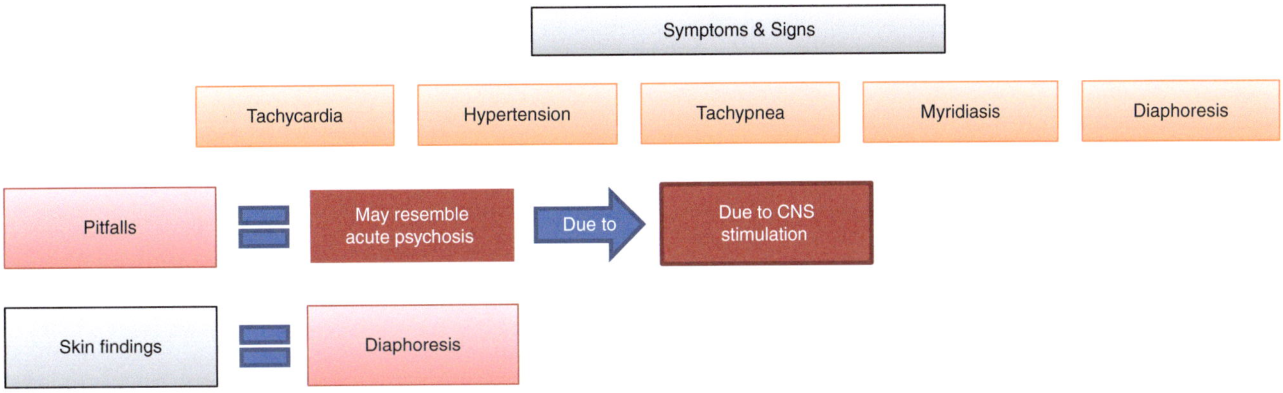

Sympathomimetic Agents

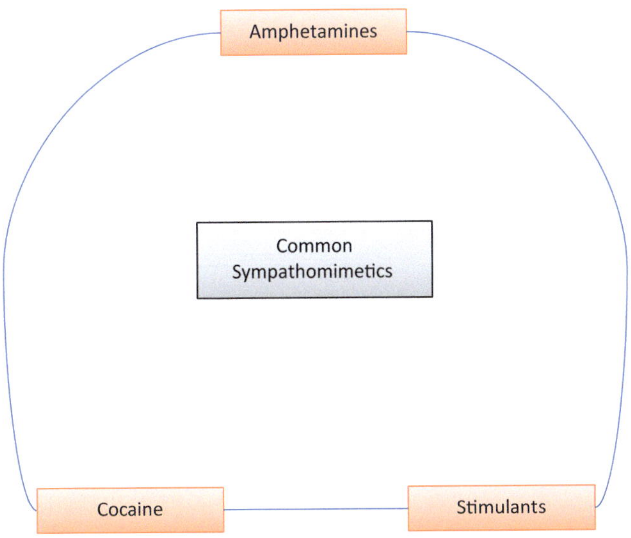

Withdrawal Symptoms

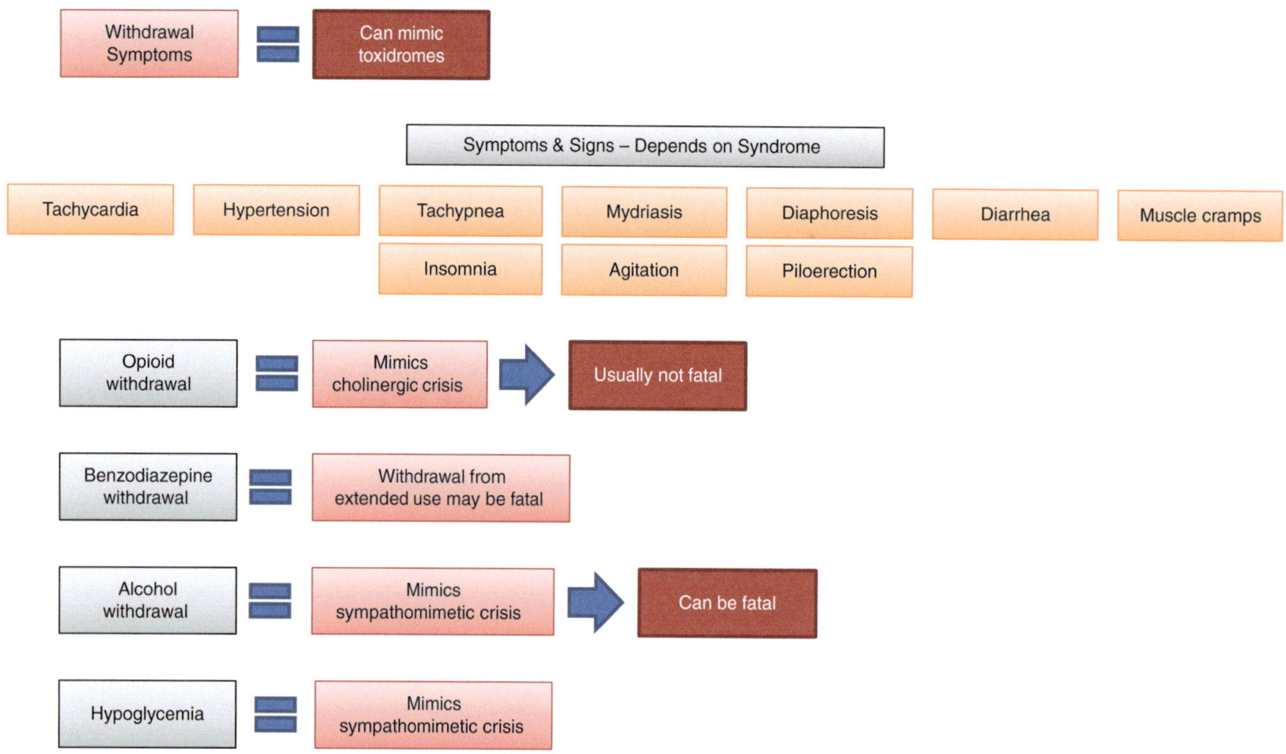

Specific Toxins and Poisons

Alcohols: Introduction

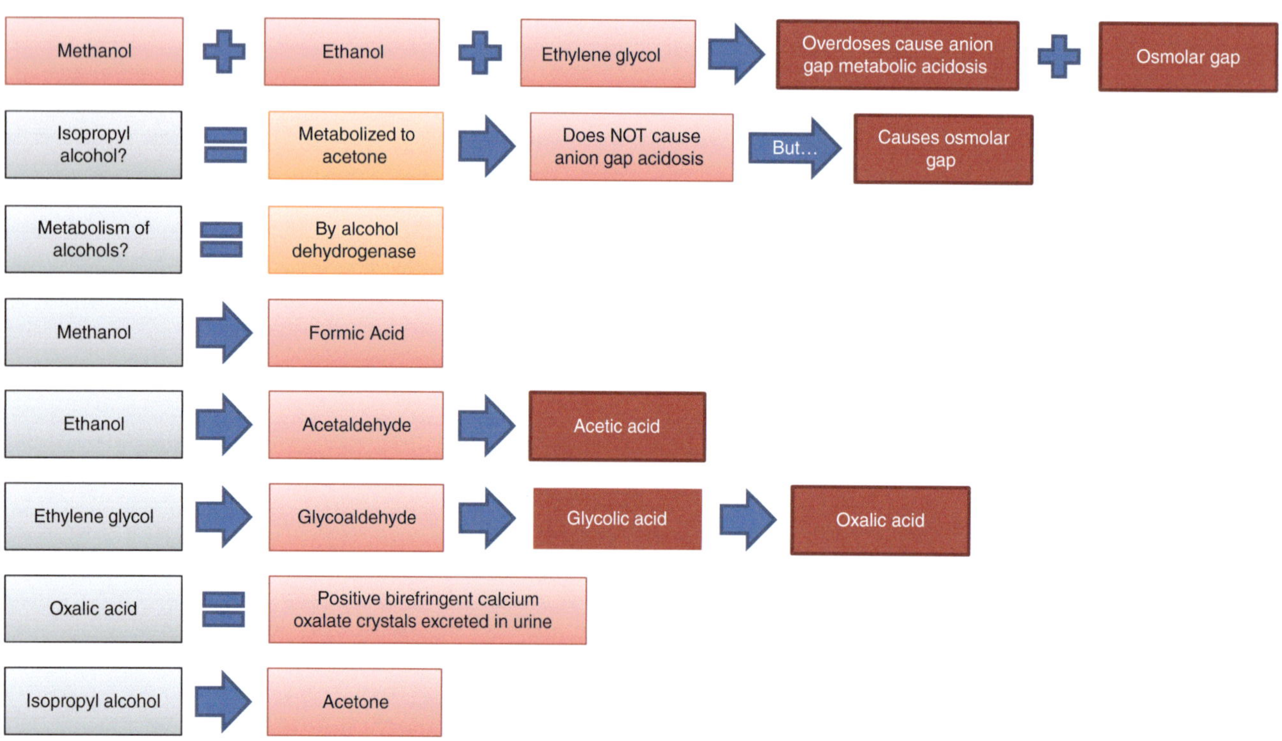

Alcohols: Methanol

Methanol = Solvent found in → Paint thinner / Gasoline additives / Windshield wiper fluid → Anion & Osmolar gap in OD

Methanol overdose = Can cause anion gap acidosis → From formic acid production

Formic acid effects = Toxic to retina → Snowstorm vision → Eventual blindness → May see disc hyperemia

Symptoms & Signs → May be delayed 12–18 hours

N/V | Seizures | Respiratory failure | Pancreatitis | Blindness

Initial Treatment = ABC's + IV Fluids + Repletion of Thiamine + Repletion of electrolytes & glucose

Agitation &/or seizures? = Benzodiazepines

Specific antidote? = Fomepizole → Inhibits conversion of methanol to formic acid → Allows methanol to be directly excreted unchanged by the kidneys

Other Treatment = Ethanol → Alcohol dehydrogenase preferentially metabolizes it over methanol & ethylene glycol

Indications for hemodialysis = Serum methanol > 25 mg/dL + Altered mental status + Metabolic acidosis + No response to standard therapy

Alcohols: Ethanol

Ethanol = Causes euphoria & disinhibition → In small to moderate amounts → Anion & Osmolar gap in OD

CNS Toxic Effects

Slurred speech | Decreased reflexes | Altered mental status | Obtundation | Coma | Death

Alcohol toxicity

Respiratory depression | Hypothermia | Hypotension | (Hypoglycemia → Alcoholic ketoacidosis)

Initial Treatment = ABC's + IV Fluids + Repletion of Thiamine + Repletion of electrolytes & glucose

Agitation &/or seizures? = Benzodiazepines

Indications for hemodialysis = Coma + Depressed vital signs + Significant overdose

Ethanol intoxication = Most require a period of observation and can be discharged when clinically sober

Ethanol Tidbits

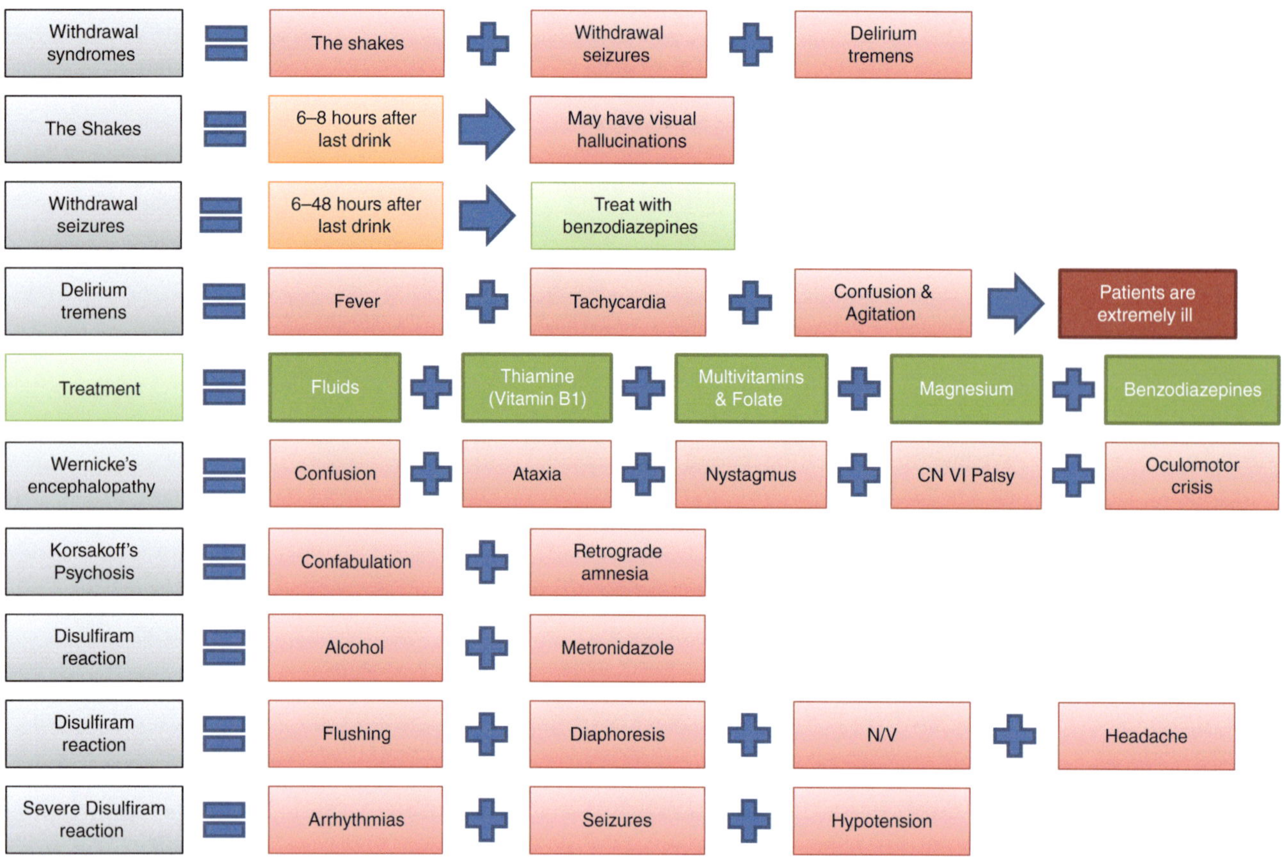

Alcohols: Ethylene Glycol

- Ethylene Glycol = Solvent found in → Antifreeze → Anion & Osmolar gap in OD
- Ethylene Glycol = Progressive toxin (Due to complex metabolite profile) → Early stages similar to ethanol intoxication → Later stages of toxicity leads to renal failure (Oxalic aciduria) + CNS deficits
- Ethylene Glycol Metabolism = Broken down by alcohol dehydrogenase → Oxalic acid + Glycolic acid
- Other laboratory abnormalities = Hypocalcemia + Renal failure (elevated BUN/Cr) + Hematuria
- Glycolic acid = Causes acidosis
- Oxalic acid = Precipitates with calcium to form calcium oxalate crystals
- Initial Treatment = ABC's + IV Fluids + Repletion of Thiamine + Repletion of electrolytes & glucose
- Agitation &/or seizures? = Benzodiazepines
- Specific antidote? = Fomepizole → Inhibits conversion of ethylene glycol to oxalic acid
- Treatment tidbits = Requires supplemental Pyridoxine & Thiamine → Both are consumed in the metabolism of ethylene glycol
- Indications for hemodialysis = High ethylene glycol level + Altered mental status + Metabolic acidosis + No response to standard therapy

Alcohols: Isopropyl Alcohol

- Isopropyl alcohol = Solvent found in → Rubbing alcohol → Overdose causes osmolar gap
- Metabolism = ½ metabolized to acetone → Rest excreted by lungs & kidney
- Isopropyl alcohol = Presents similar to ethanol toxicity → But…NO anion gap acidosis → Ketosis *is* present

Isopropyl alcohol toxicity:

- CNS depression
- Hemorrhagic gastritis
- Hypotension (may be severe)
- Pulmonary edema
- Hypoglycemia

- Initial Treatment = ABC's + IV Fluids + Repletion of Thiamine + Repletion of electrolytes & glucose
- Indications for hemodialysis = Serum level > 400 mg/dL + Altered mental status + Hypotension

Amphetamine Examples

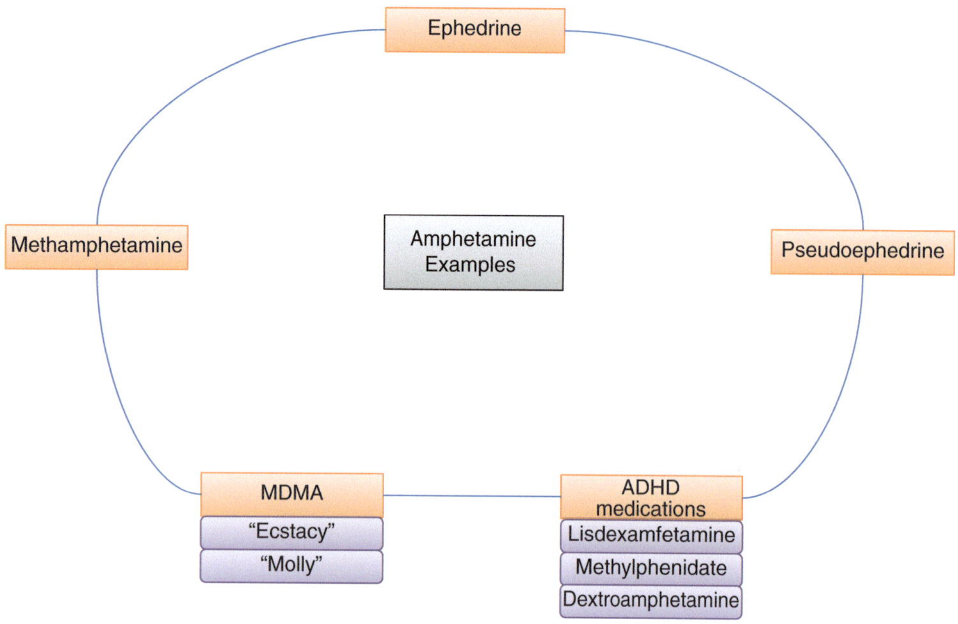

Amphetamines

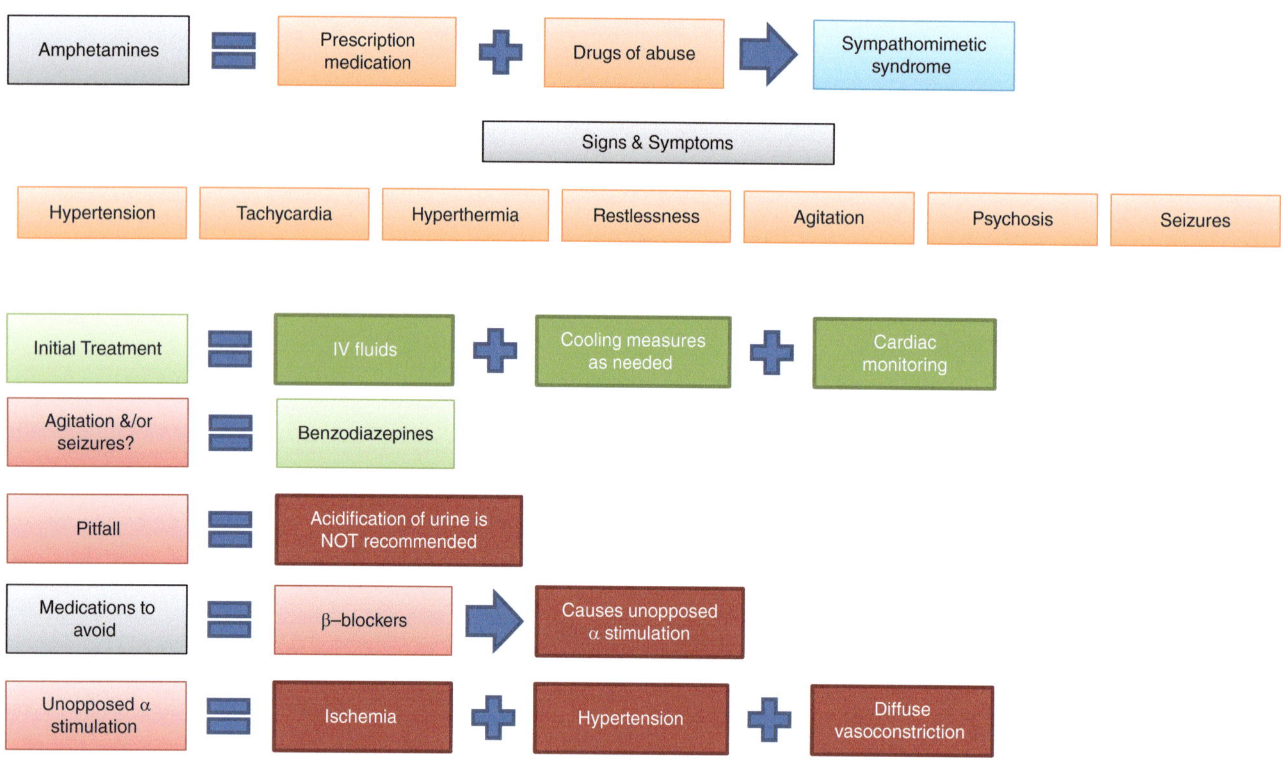

Analgesics: Acetaminophen

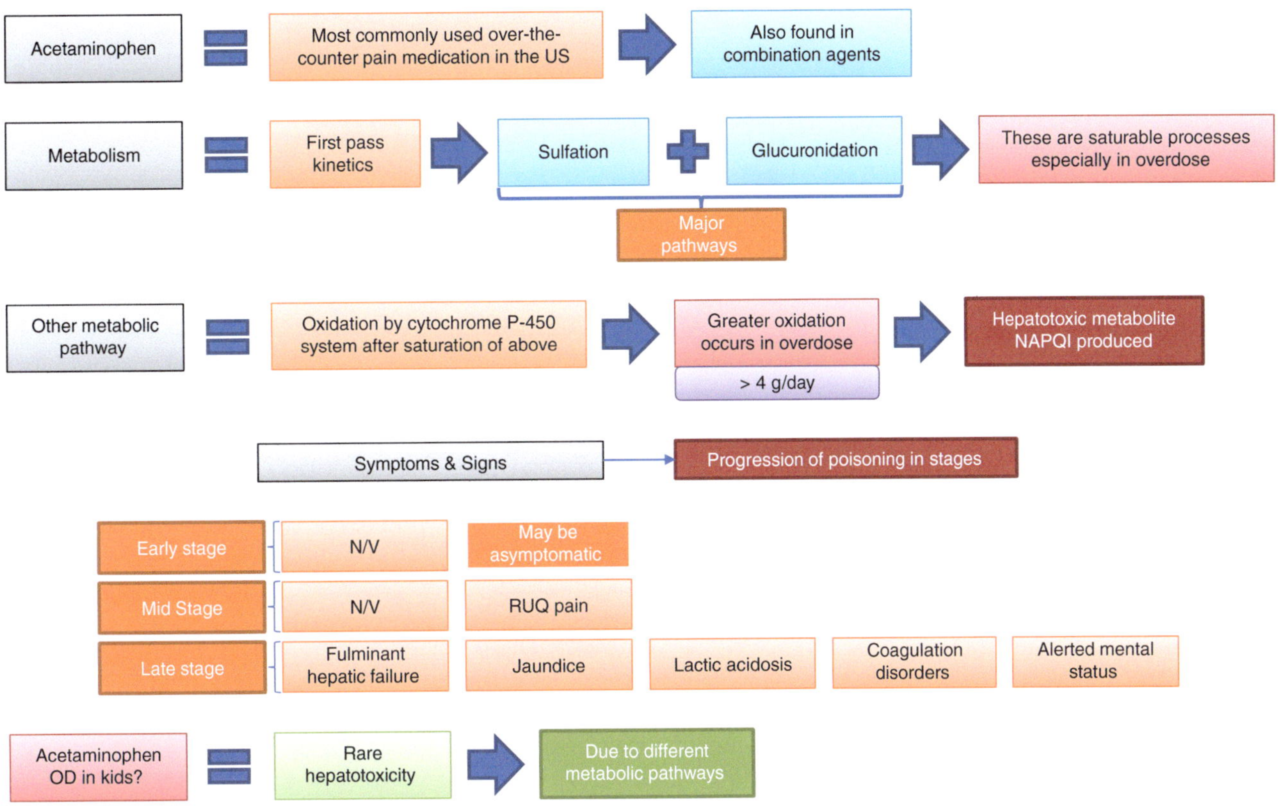

Rumack-Matthew Nomogram

Antidose dosing [=] Based on Rumack - Matthew Nomogram

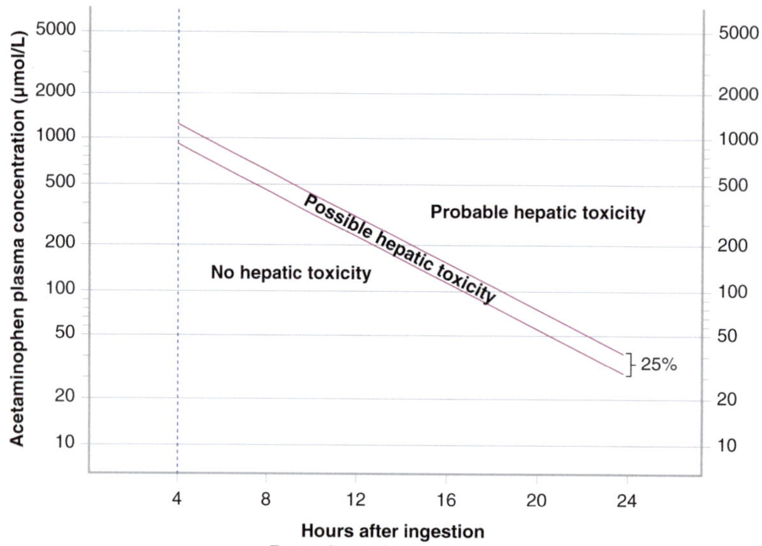

Rumack matthew nomogram

Tidbits [=] A level of > 150 mg/dL at the four level requires treatment with NAC [+] Treat multiple ingestions as a single ingestion initiated at the first ingestion

Nomogram pitfall [=] Less useful for delayed presentations > 24 hours or for modified-release formulations

Acetaminophen Overdose Treatment

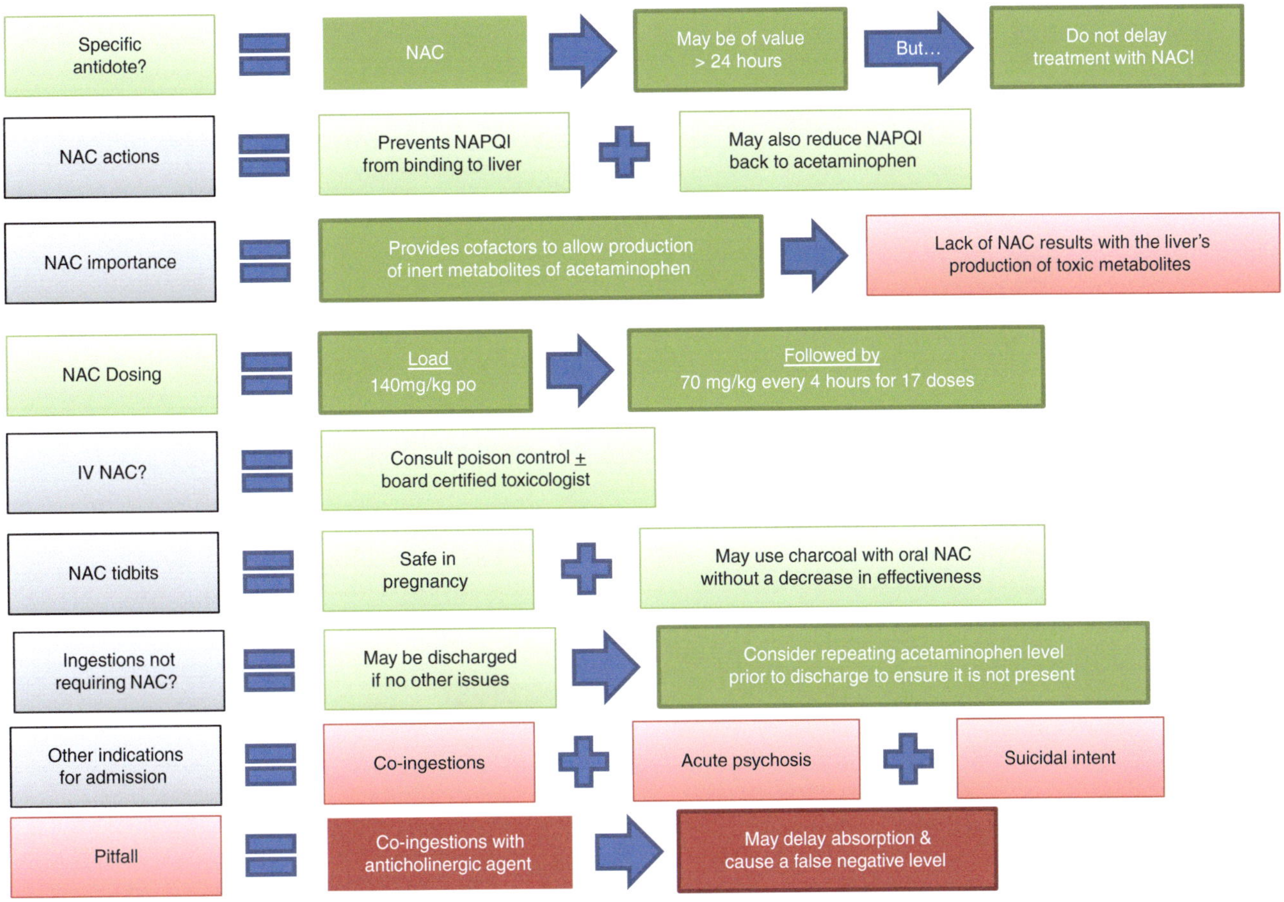

Salicylate Examples

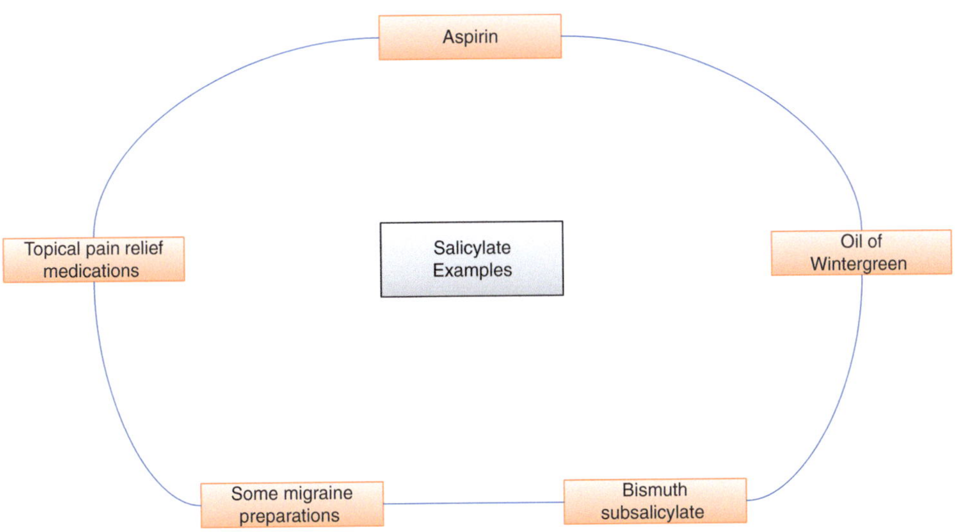

Analgesics: Salicylates

Salicylate overdose = Uncouples oxidative phosphorylation → Leads to metabolic and lactic acidosis

Classic finding = Anion gap metabolic acidosis + Respiratory alkalosis → Due to increased respiratory rate

Other Tidbits = Salicylate overdose alters glucose metabolism + Neutral salicylates can cross blood -brain barrier

Symptoms & Signs → Presentation is dose dependent

- < 150 mg/kg: N/V; GI upset; Sweating (esp. in kids)
- 150–300 mg/kg: N/V; Tachypnea (esp. in kids); AMS; Tinnitus
- >300 mg/kg (Severe): Altered mental status; Unstable vital signs; ARDS; Seizures; Dysrhythmias

Chronic poisoning = More CNS & Less GI symptoms → Level may not correlate with symptoms

Salicylate Overdose Treatment

Initial Treatment = ABC's + IV Fluids + O_2 + Cardiac monitor

Laboratory studies = Salicylate level + BMP + LFT + Glucose + CBC + ABG + ECG + Others as needed

Classic finding = Anion gap metabolic acidosis + Respiratory alkalosis

Other findings = Hypoglycemia + ↑ T3/T4 levels

Overdose within 1 hour? = Consider charcoal

Definitive treatment = Urinary alkalinization → 150 mEq $NaHCO_3$ in 1 L of D5W → Maintain urine output of 1–2 cc/kg/hr + Urine pH 7.5–8

Pitfall = Alkalinization will worsen hypokalemia → Replete electrolytes as needed

Indications for hemodialysis = Refractory or worsening symptoms + Worsening acid-base derangements + Unstable vital signs

Medication pitfall = Oil of wintergreen has high salicylate level → Very toxic

Nonsteroidal Anti-Inflammatory Agents

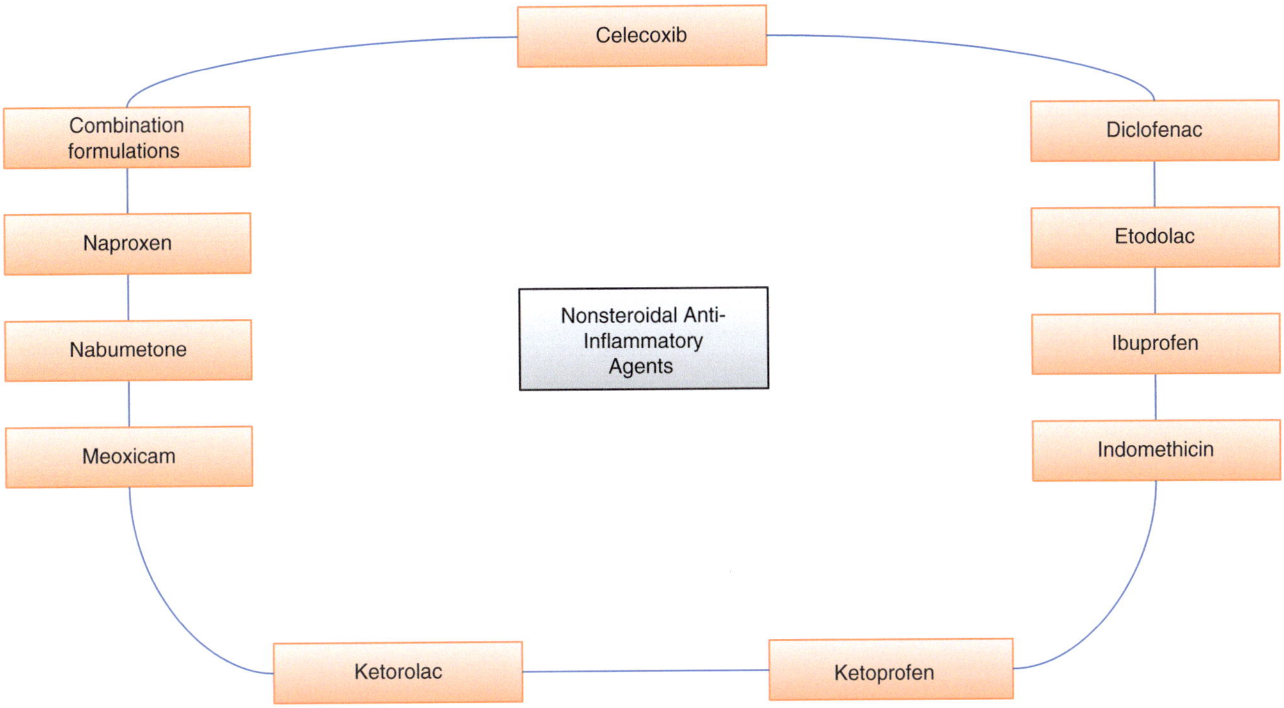

Analgesics: NSAIDs

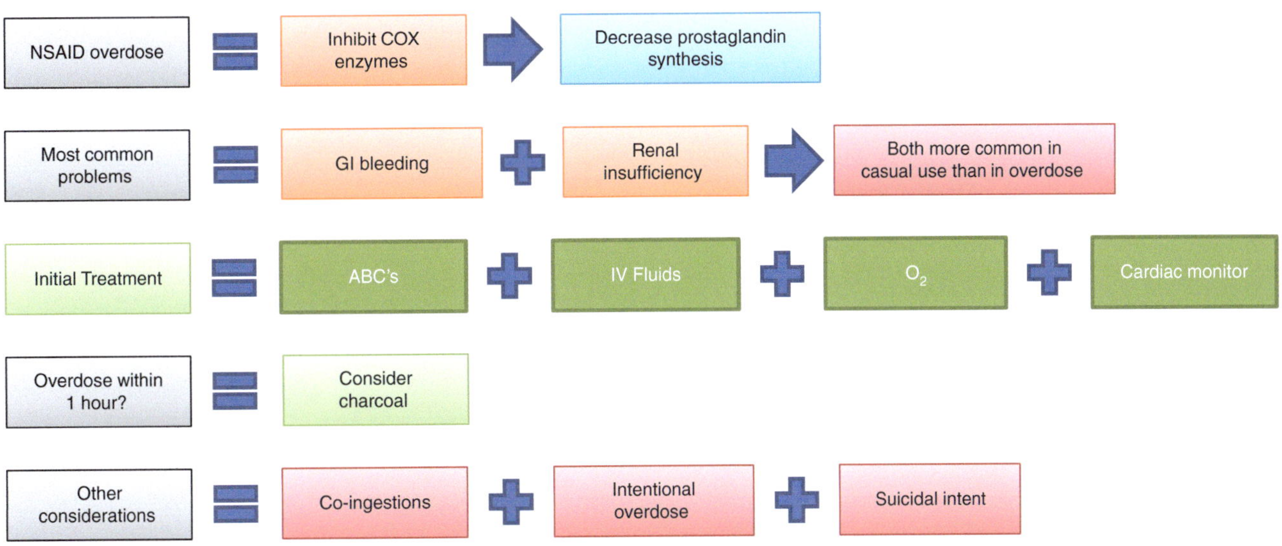

Anticonvulsants: Valproate

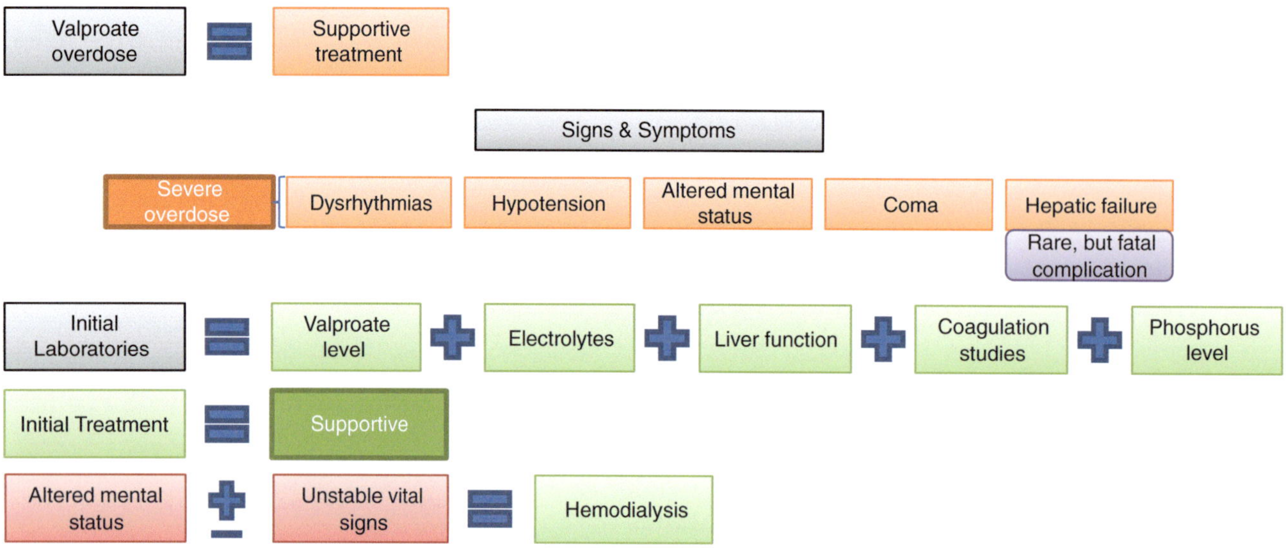

Anticonvulsants: Carbamazepine

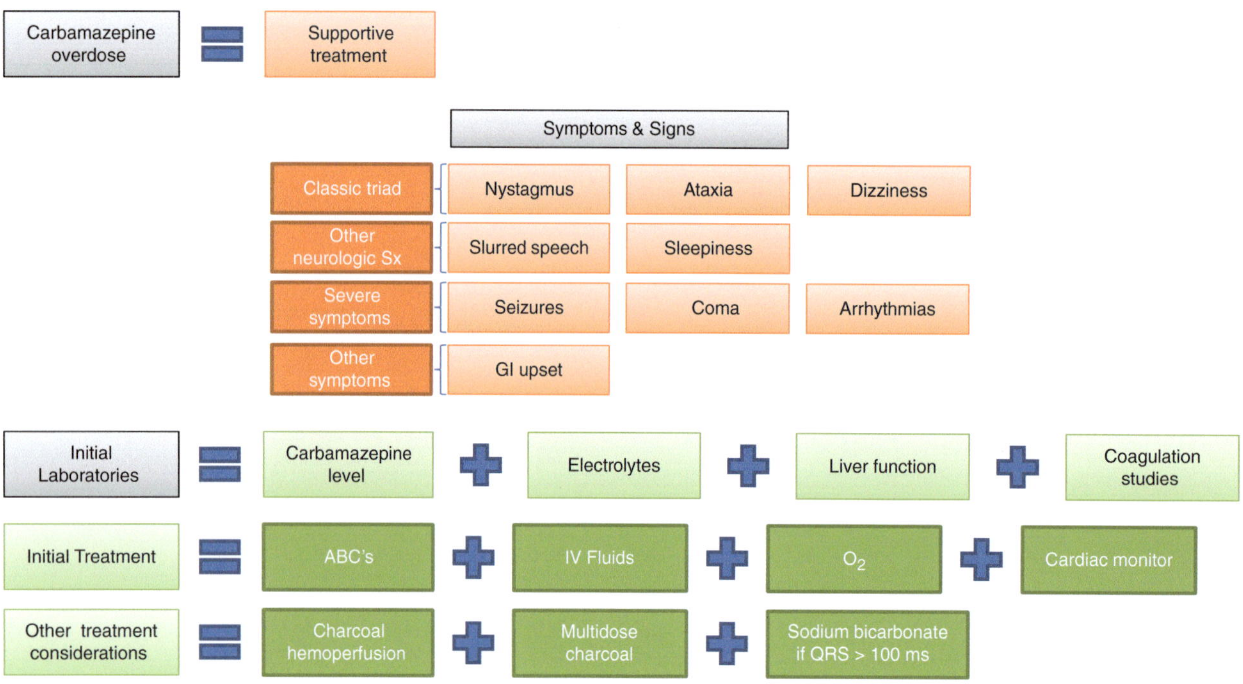

Anticonvulsants: Phenytoin and Fosphenytoin

Phenytoin mechanism = Blocks sodium channels → CNS & cardiac activity || Fosphenytoin is a pro-drug with a safer side effect profile

Considerations = Acute vs Chronic ingestion + Oral vs IV

IV Phenytoin = IV is more cardiovascular toxic + IV Phenytoin is diluted in propylene glycol which itself can cause hypotension & bradycardia

Symptoms & Signs

- Common Sx: Nystagmus (→ Vertical, horizontal or both), Ataxia, Dysarthria, Hyporeflexia, Hypotonia
- Severe: AMS, Seizures, Coma, Respiratory failure
- Cardiovascular: Hypotension, Bradycardia, Conduction delays, AV Blocks, Tachydysrhythmias

Initial Laboratories = Phenytoin level + Electrolytes + ECG + Others as needed

Initial Treatment = ABC's, O_2, Cardiac monitor + Activated charcoal → Decreases absorption & enhances elimination → Dialysis NOT useful

Seizures? = Benzodiazepines

Bradycardia? = Pacing OR Atropine

Antihistamines

Antihistamine examples = Diphenhydramine + Doxylamine → Central & peripheral action

Antihistamine overdose = Anticholinergic effects + Sodium channel blockade → QT prolongation

Initial Treatment = ABC's + IV Fluids + O_2 + Cardiac monitor

Definitive Treatment = Supportive

Agitation or psychosis? = Benzodiazepines → Avoid phenothiazines

Severe symptoms? = Consider physostigmine

Antimicrobials

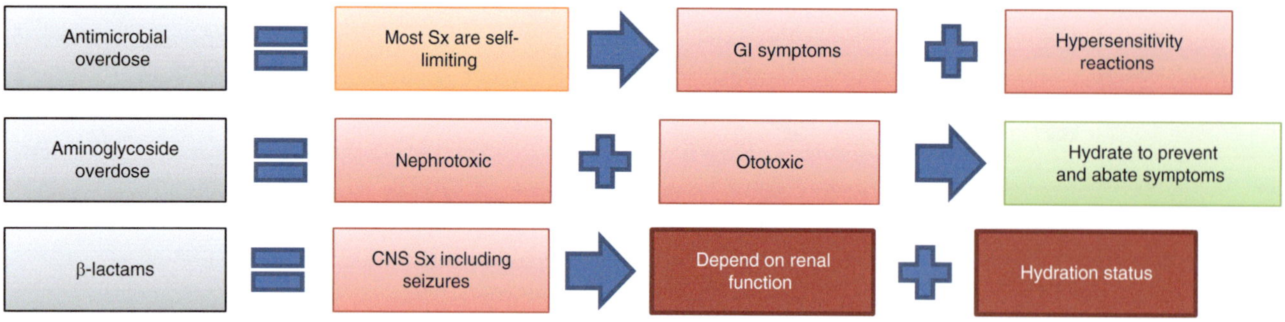

Isoniazid

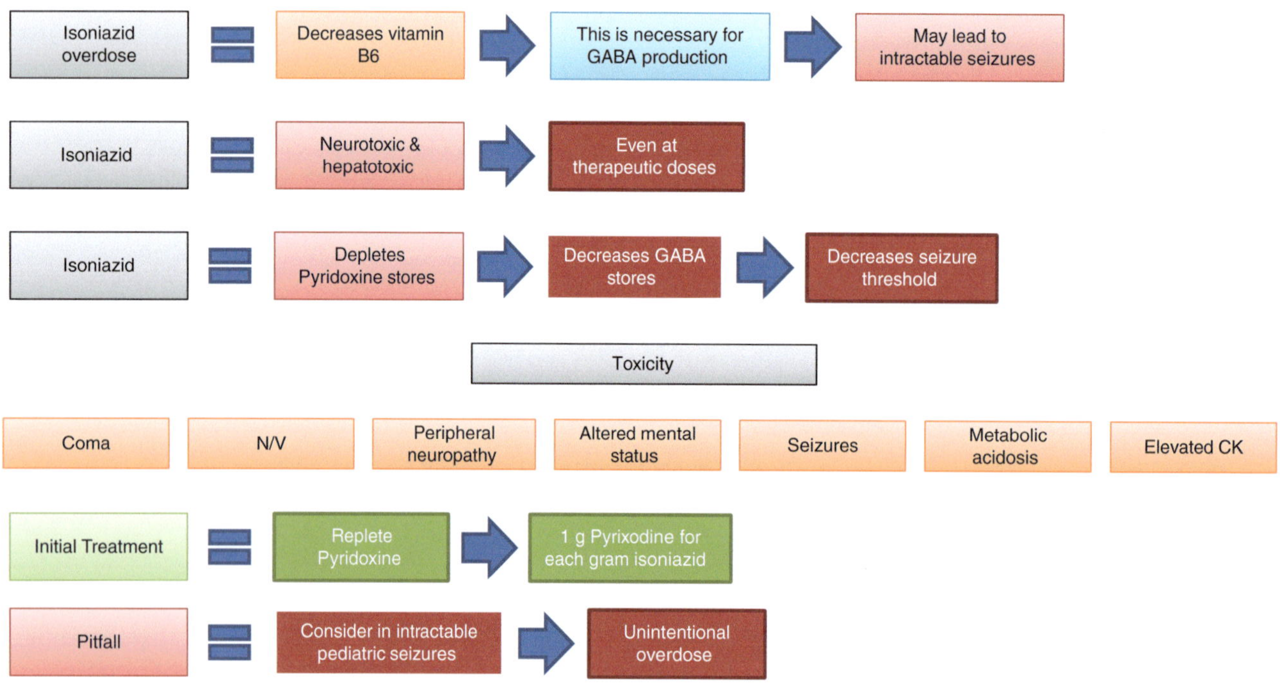

Cardiac Medications: β-Blockers

β-blockers = Binds to β_1 receptors of the myocardium → Blocks production of cAMP

β-blocker effects = Negative iotrope and chronotrope effects on heart + Vasoconstrictor + Causes bronchospasm + Hypoglycemia

Toxicity

Hypotension | Bradycardia | Conduction delays | Dysrhythmias | AV Block | Hypoglycemia

Initial Treatment = ABC's + IV Fluids + O_2 + Cardiac monitor

Specific Treatment = Glucagon 0.1 mg/kg bolus up to 10 mg/hr thereafter as a continuous infusion OR High dose insulin up to 2 mg/kg/hr & dextrose

Refractory hypotension? = Epinephrine infusion

High grade blocks? = Pacemaker

Pitfall = Topical medications can cause systemic toxicity

Cardiac Medications: Calcium Channel Blockers

Calcium Channel Blockers = Block the effects of Ca on smooth & cardiac muscle || Most common = Nifedipine/ Nicardipine + Diltiazem + Verapamil

Calcium Channel Blockers = Most common causes of death from cardiovascular drugs

Pitfall = Long acting formulations require at least 24 hours of continuous cardiac monitoring

Toxicity

Hypotension | Bradycardia | Conduction delays | Dysrhythmias

Initial Treatment = ABC's + IV Fluids + O_2 + Cardiac monitor

Specific Treatment = Calcium gluconate + Glucagon 0.1 mg/kg bolus up to 10 mg/hr thereafter as a continuous infusion OR High dose insulin up to 2 mg/kg/hr & dextrose

Refractory hypotension? = Epinephrine infusion

Bradycardia? = Atropine

Cardiac Medications: Clonidine

Clonidine = Centrally acting α2-agonist → Has some peripheral effects as well

Clonidine effects = Can cause opioid-like symptoms → Respiratory depression + Coma + Seizures + Miosis

Symptoms & Signs

- Central effects: Hypotension; Bradycardia
- Peripheral effects: Hypertension followed by hypotension
- CNS effects: Lethargy; Apnea; Miosis; Hyporeflexia
- Cardiac effects: AV blocks

Initial Treatment = ABC's + IV Fluids + O_2 + Cardiac monitor

Specific Treatment = Naloxone may be of some benefit → Greatest effect is on reversal of CNS depression

Refractory hypotension? = Pressors

Bradycardia? = Atropine

Clonidine withdrawal = Hypertension + Anxiety + Tachycardia + Sweating

Cardiac Medications: Digitalis

Digitalis = A cardiac glycoside that inhibits the Na-K-ATPase pump

Digitalis = Increases intracellular Na^+ → Increases Ca^{2+} in the sarcoplasm reticulum → K^+ leaks extracellularly → Increased cardiac contractility

Acute toxicity = Children or young adults → Accidental or intentional overdoses

Chronic toxicity = Older patients → Due to decreased renal excretion

Symptoms & Signs

- Acute toxicity: Dysrhythmias; N/V; Altered mental status; Visual changes; Hyperkalemia
- Dysrhythmias: SVT; AV Block; Bradycardia; Tachycardia; Ventricular tachycardia; PVC's (most common); PAT with block (Pathognomonic)
- Chronic toxicity: Decreased excretion; Generalized weakness; N/V; Dysrhythmias; Altered mental status

Digitalis Management and Treatment

Initial Treatment = ABC's + IV Fluids + O_2 + Cardiac monitor

Laboratory investigations = EKG + Electrolytes (May see elevated K^+) + Digitalis level + Others as needed

Specific Treatment = Digibind

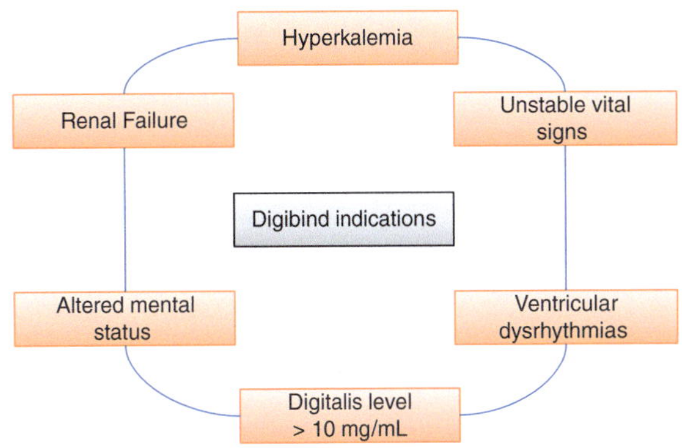

Amount? = Start with 5–10 vials initially → Discuss with poison control

Pitfall = Avoid repleting Potassium, Calcium and Magnesium

Replace Calcium? = May cause cardiac arrest in face of Dig Toxicity

Hyperkalemia? = Treat hyperkalemia with all other modalities (Fluids, glucose/insulin, sodium bicarbonate and enhanced GI elimination)

Ventricular dysrhythmia requiring cardioversion? = Use least amount of joules possible → Due to → Myocardial irritability → May lead to V. Fib

Carbon Monoxide (CO) Poisoning

CO Poisoning = Leading cause of toxic death → CO binds to hemoglobin, myoglobin & cytochrome A3 → Carboxyhemoglobin has an affinity for O_2 that is ***250 times*** > Hemoglobin

Pathophysiology → Shifts oxyhemoglobin dissociation curve to the ***left*** → Inhibits O_2 release from hemoglobin

Symptoms & Signs

Headache | Nausea | Confusion | Seizures | NO cyanosis

Diagnosis = Carboxyhemoglobin level → Pulse ox *not* reliable

Initial Treatment = ABC's + 100 % O_2 + Cardiac monitor ± Hyperbaric O_2

Half-life of CO = Room Air 320 minutes → 100 % O_2 90 minutes → Hyperbaric O_2 20 minutes

Neurologic sequelae? = Hyperbaric chamber

Pitfall = CO crosses the placenta + Fetal hemoglobin has high CO affinity + Not considering cyanide toxicity with smoke inhalation & acidosis

Caustic Agents: Acids

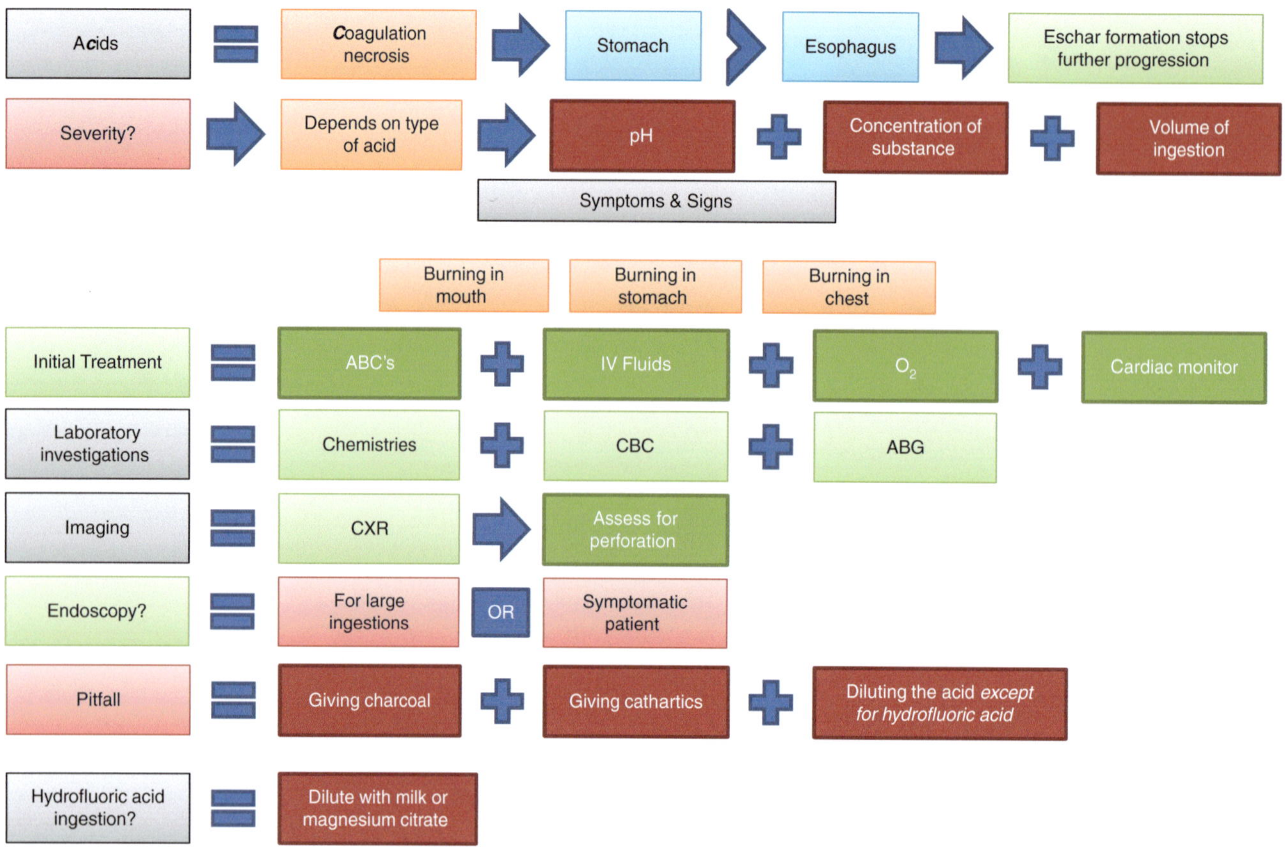

Specific Acid: Hydrogen Fluoride

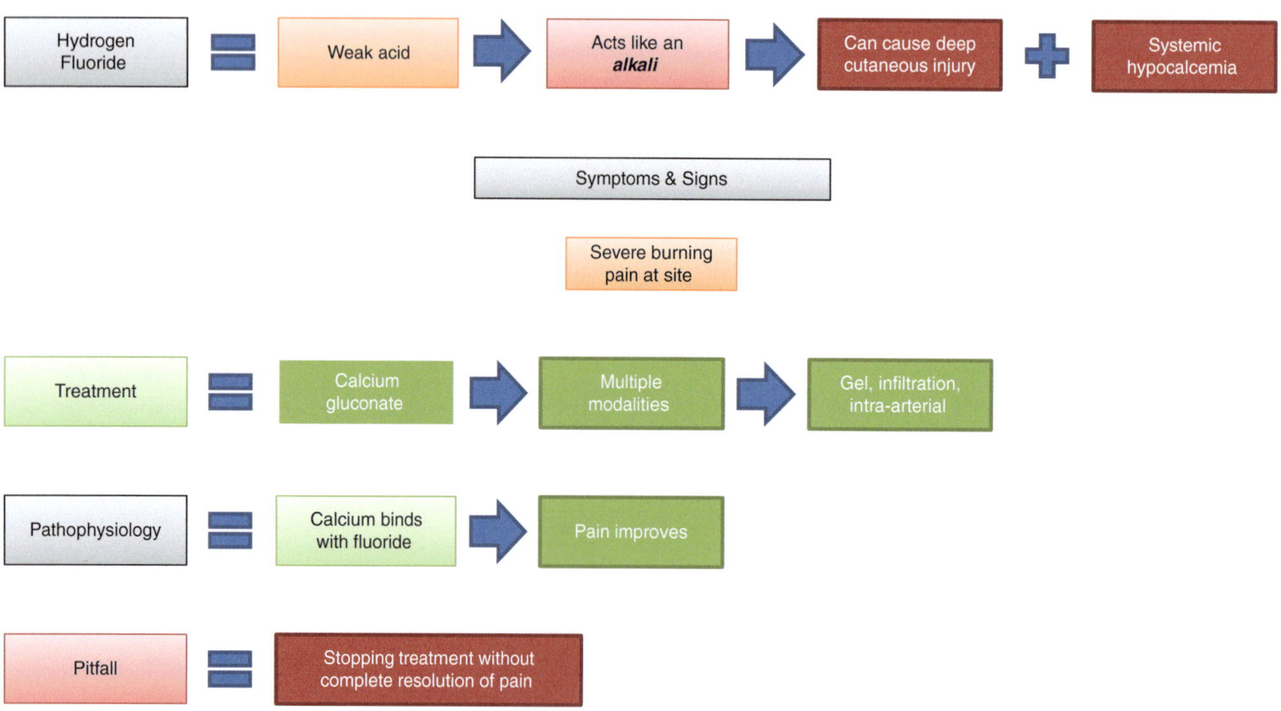

Caustic Agents: Alkali

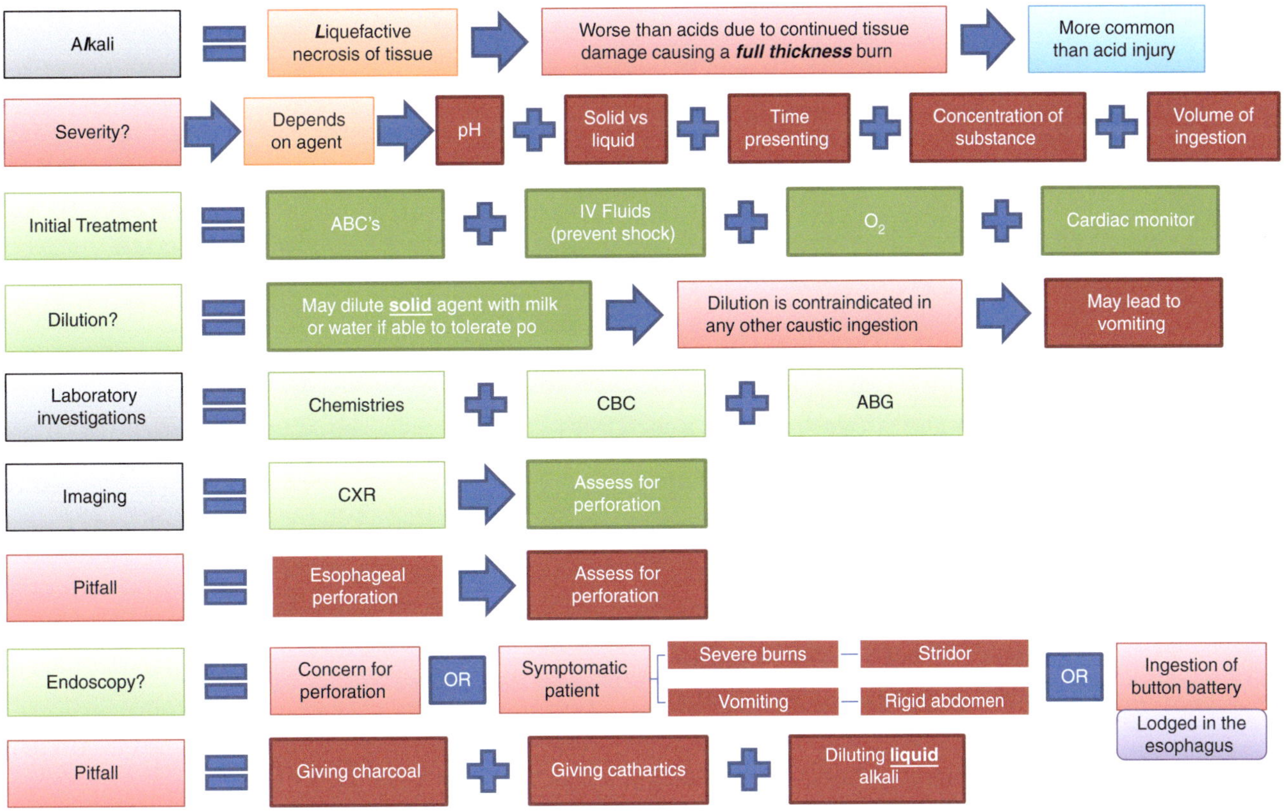

Chlorine

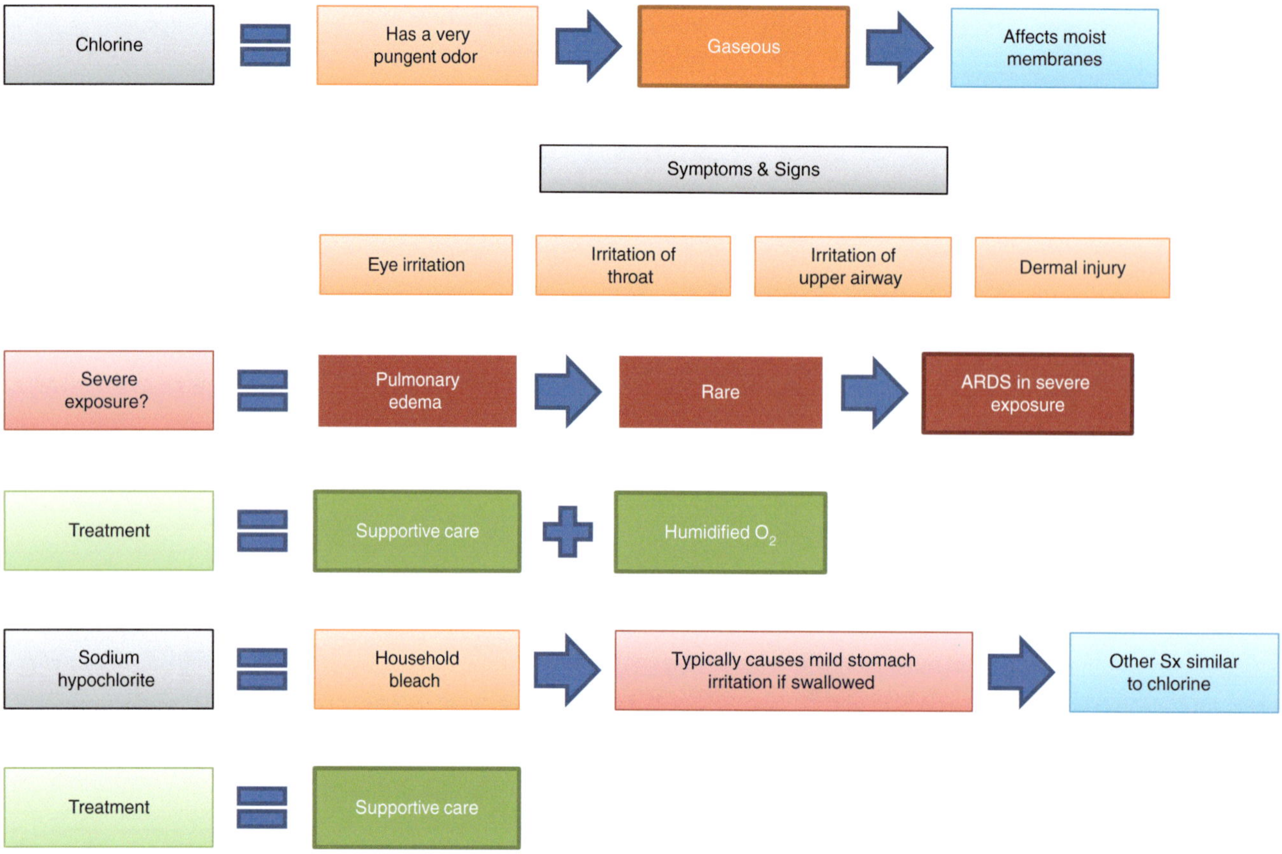
Chlorine
Has a very pungent odor
Gaseous
Affects moist membranes
Symptoms & Signs
Eye irritation
Irritation of throat
Irritation of upper airway
Dermal injury
Severe exposure?
Pulmonary edema
Rare
ARDS in severe exposure
Treatment
Supportive care
Humidified O_2
Sodium hypochlorite
Household bleach
Typically causes mild stomach irritation if swallowed
Other Sx similar to chlorine
Treatment
Supportive care

Cocaine

Cocaine = CNS and cardiac stimulant

Cocaine & Chest pain = Abnormal EKG may be seen → May be early repolarization → But if ST elevation? → Requires cardiology consult

Disposition = No EKG changes + Normal cardiac markers after 6–12 hours → May discharge

Symptoms & Signs

Agitation | Tachycardia | Hypertension

Initial Management = ABC's + O_2 + Cardiac monitor

Treatment = Benzodiazepines ± Nitroglycerin (for chest pain) → Avoid Haloperidol

Hyperthermia? = Cooling blankets + Evaporative cooling

Medications to avoid = β–blockers + Labetalol → May increase cardiac ischemia

Medications to avoid = Lidocaine → May increase seizure activity

Cocaine Tidbits

Body packers = Transporters → Whole bowel irrigation until all packets pass → May have positive plain film

Body stuffers = Ingestors attempting to avoid detection → Observe until asymptomatic

Symptoms in any? = Admit if symptomatic for continued medical & potential surgical management

Cyanide and Nitriles

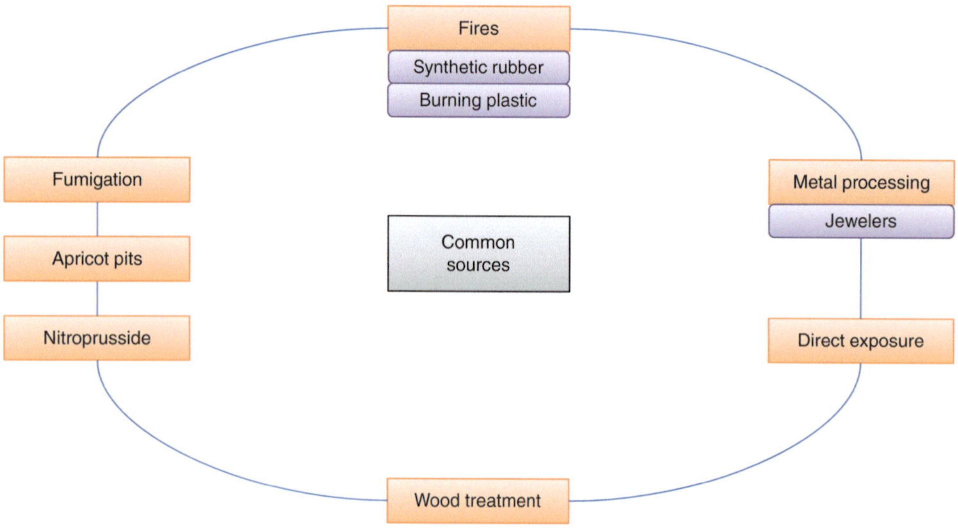

Cyanide

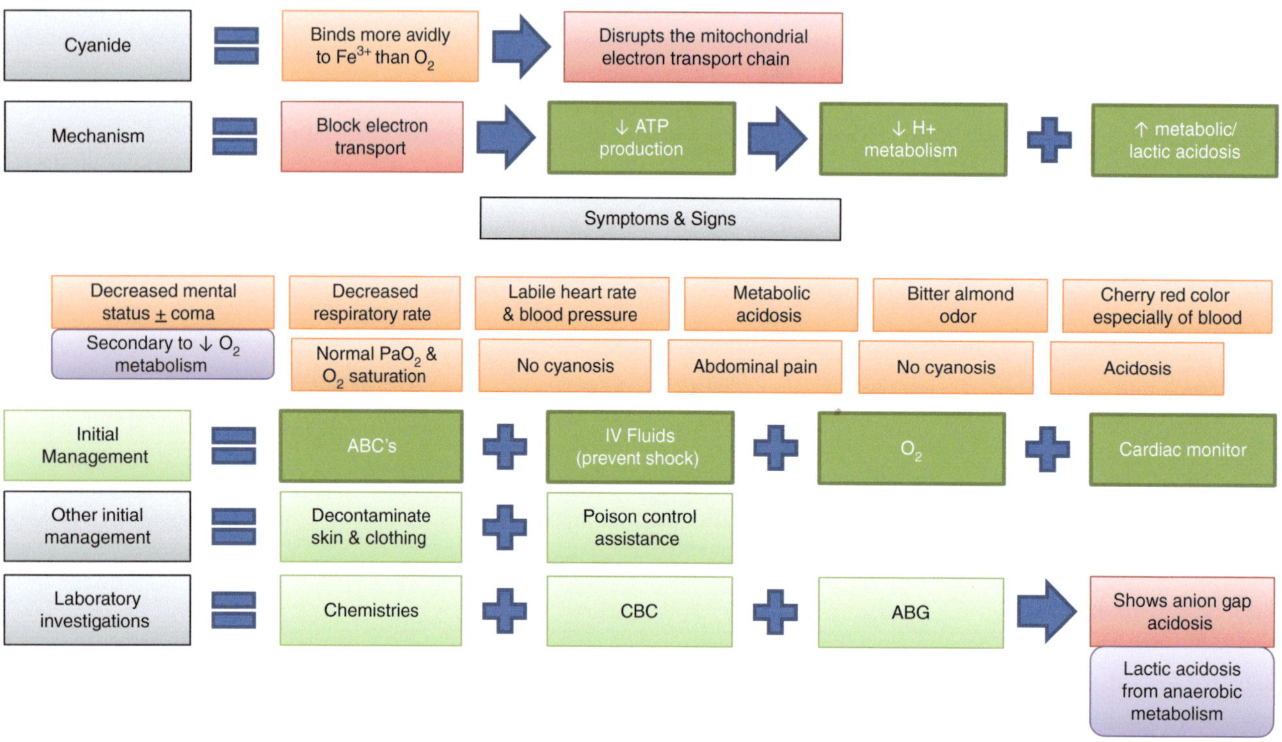

Cyanide Treatment

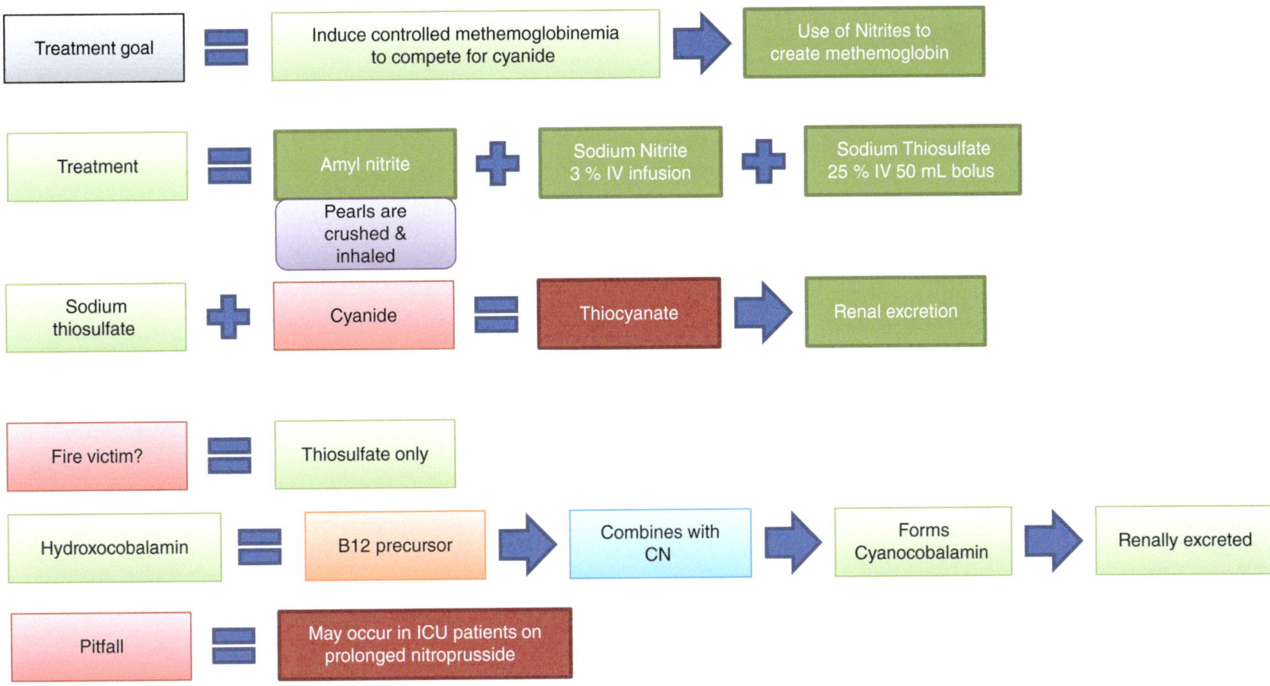

Hallucinogens

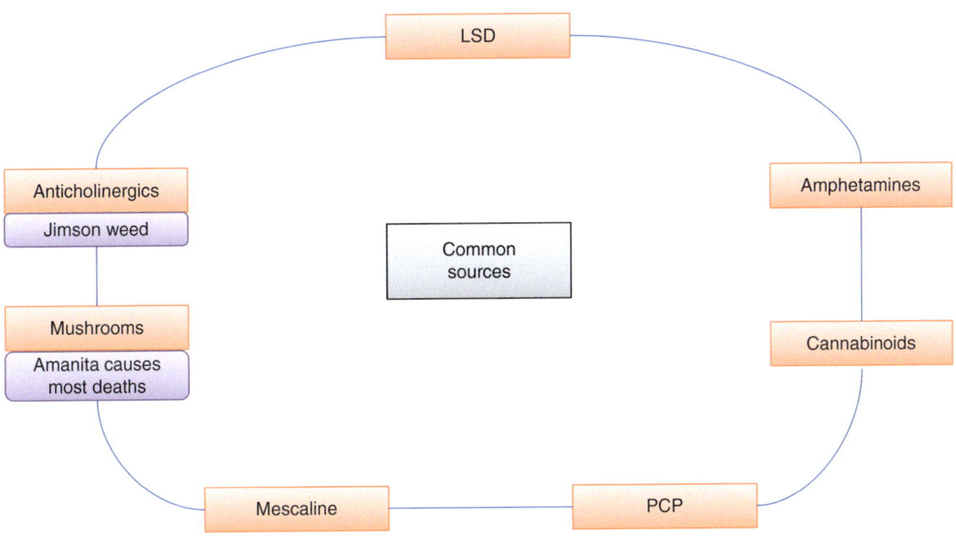

Hallucinogens

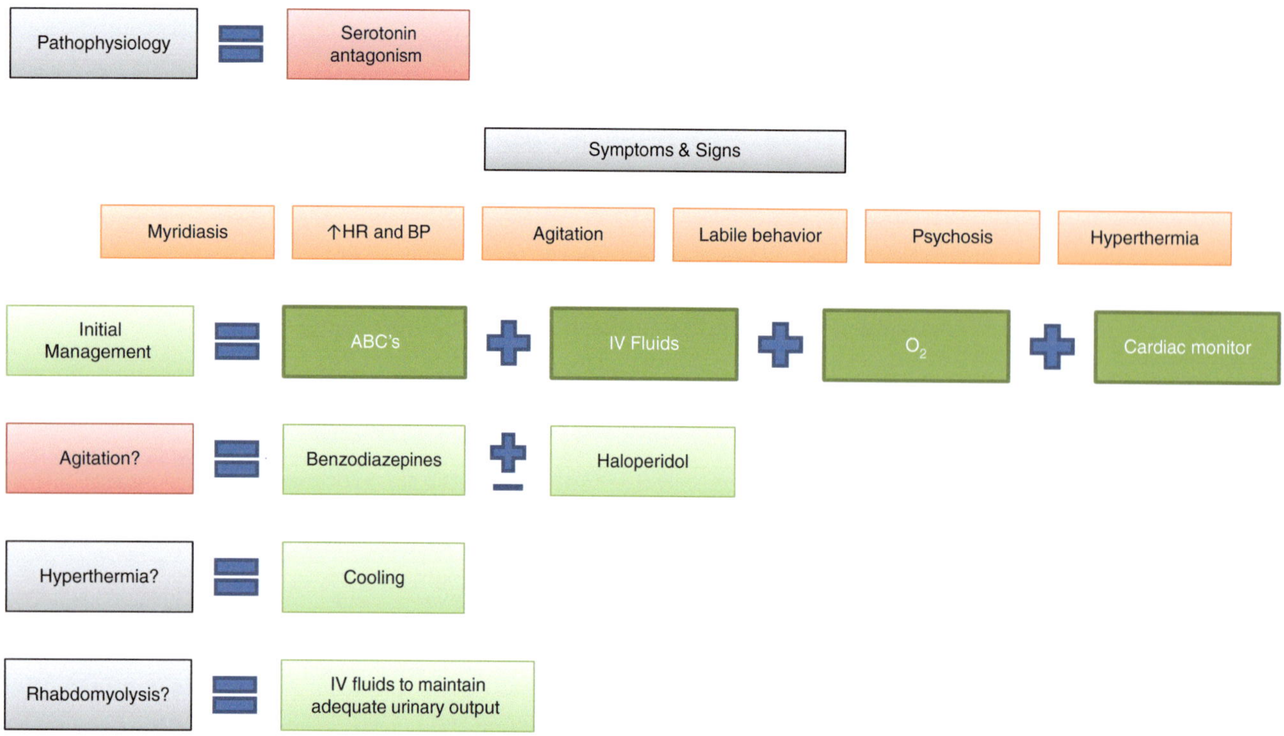

Phencyclidine (PCP)

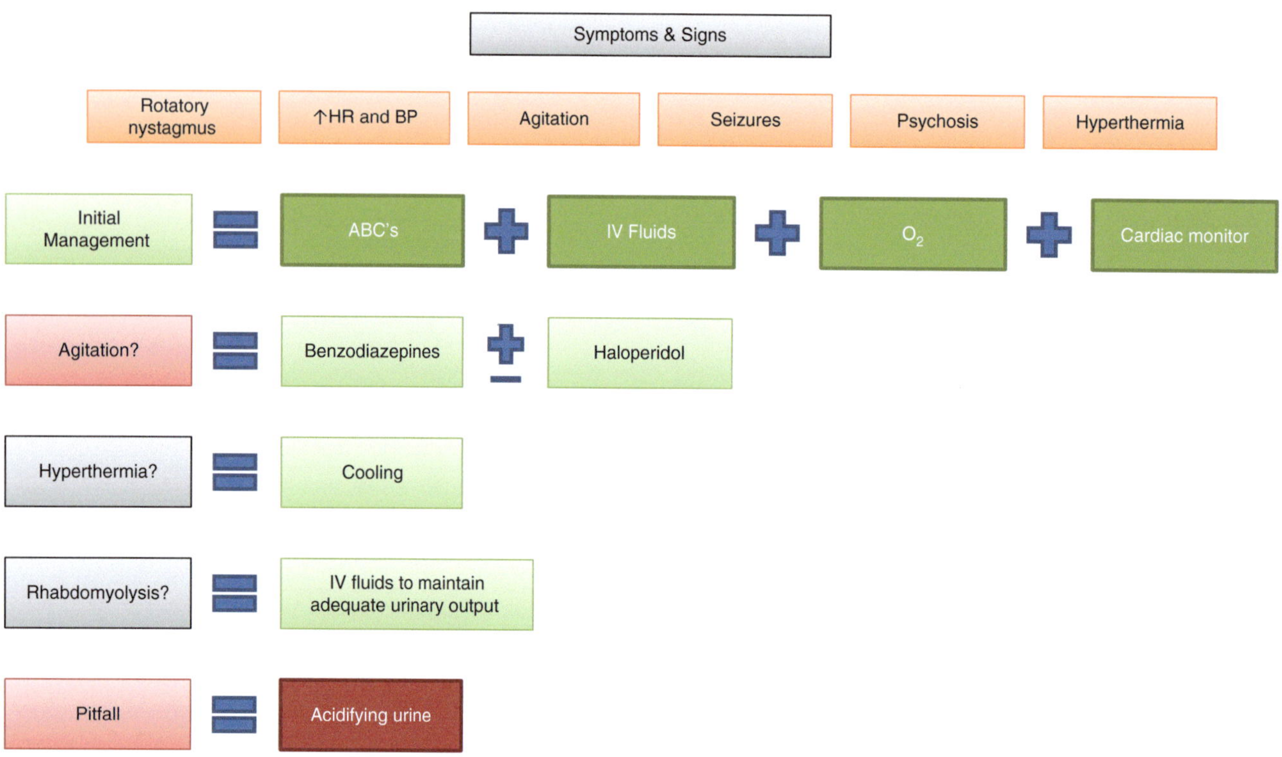

Metals and Metalloids

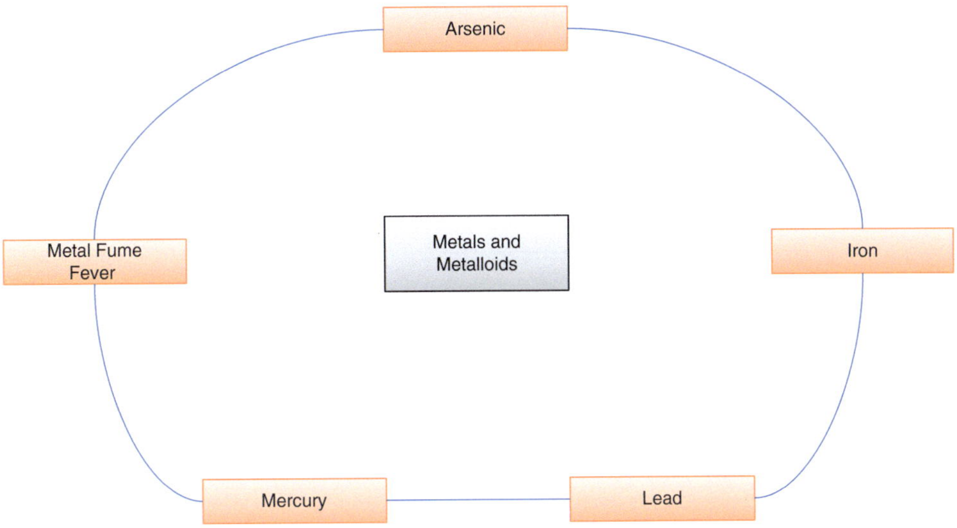

Arsenic

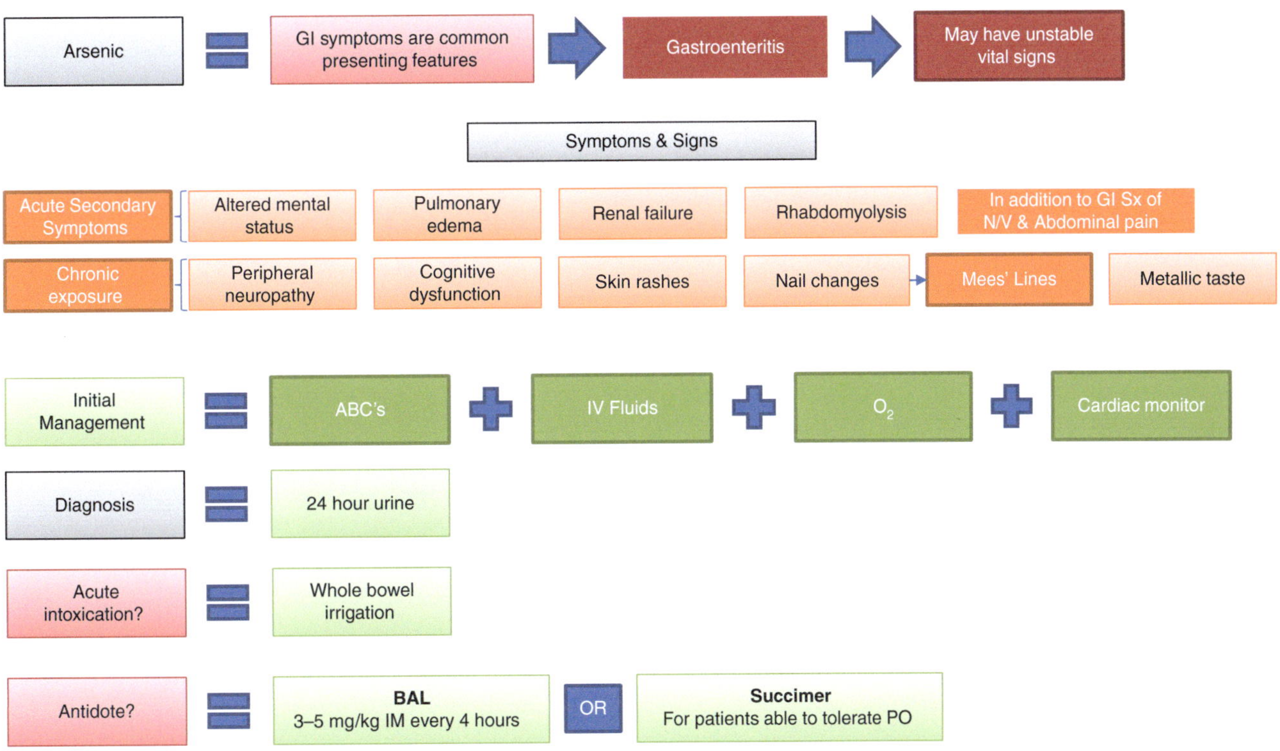

Iron

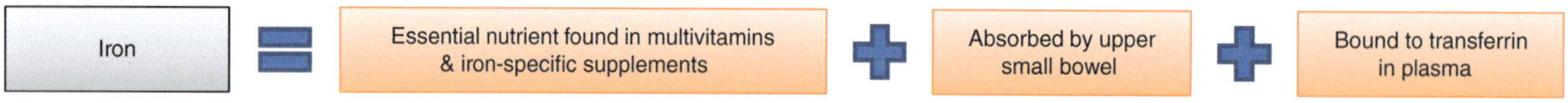

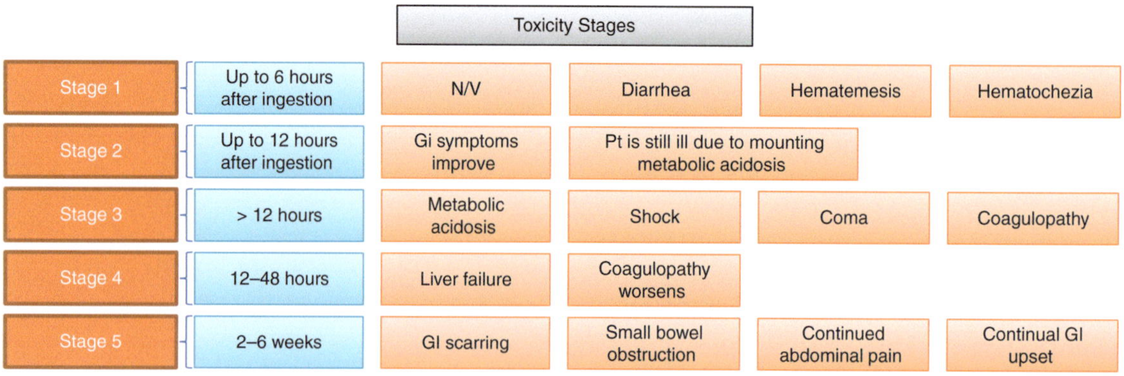

Iron Treatment and Management

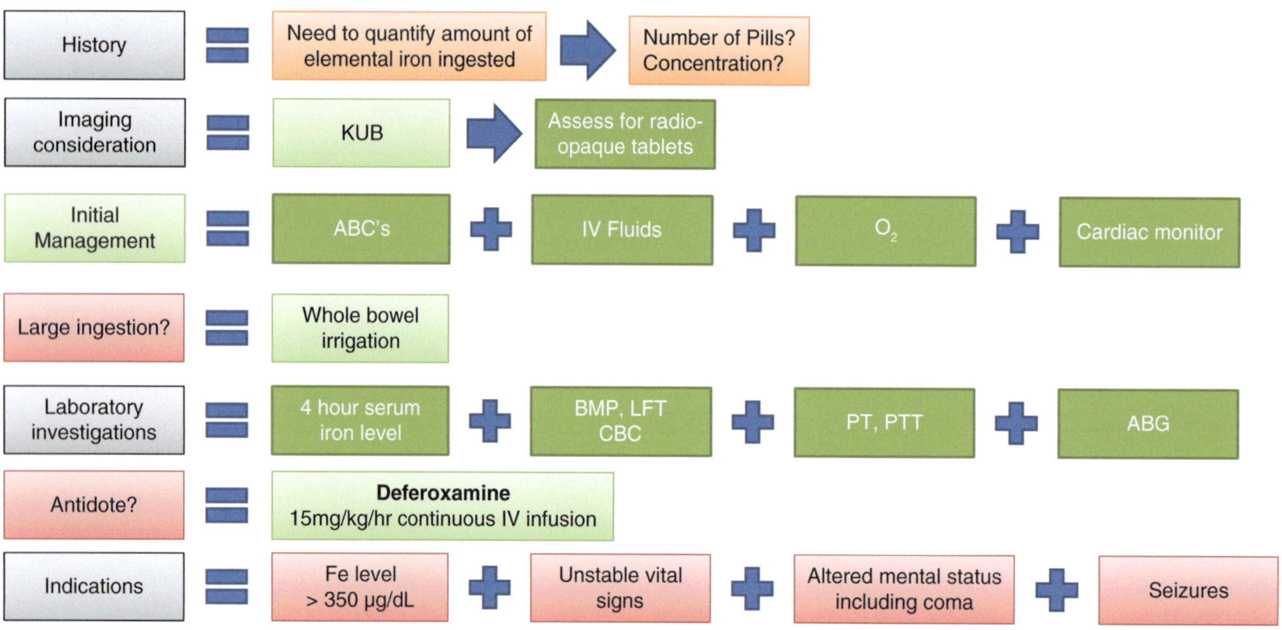

Lead

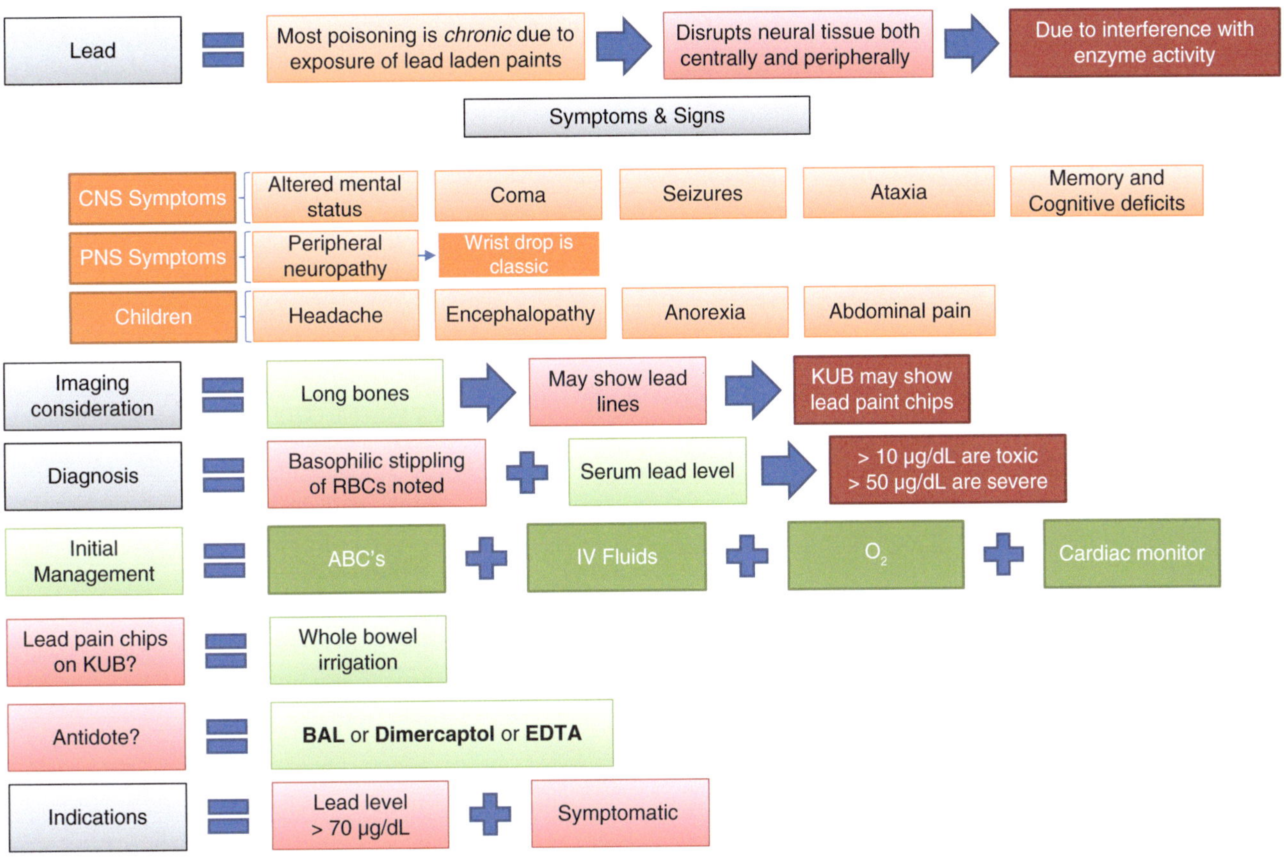
Lead
Most poisoning is chronic due to exposure of lead laden paints
Disrupts neural tissue both centrally and peripherally
Due to interference with enzyme activity
Symptoms & Signs
CNS Symptoms
Altered mental status
Coma
Seizures
Ataxia
Memory and Cognitive deficits
PNS Symptoms
Peripheral neuropathy
Wrist drop is classic
Children
Headache
Encephalopathy
Anorexia
Abdominal pain
Imaging consideration
Long bones
May show lead lines
KUB may show lead paint chips
Diagnosis
Basophilic stippling of RBCs noted
Serum lead level
> 10 μg/dL are toxic
> 50 μg/dL are severe
Initial Management
ABC's
IV Fluids
O_2
Cardiac monitor
Lead pain chips on KUB?
Whole bowel irrigation
Antidote?
BAL or Dimercaptol or EDTA
Indications
Lead level > 70 μg/dL
Symptomatic

Mercury

Mercury = Toxicity depends on amount, type, & route of exposure → Metallic mercury has no effects if ingested, but severe effects if injected or inhaled

Symptoms & Signs

- CNS Symptoms: Altered mental status; Depression; Memory loss; Ataxia
- GI Symptoms: Abdominal pain; N/V
- Renal symptoms: Acute tubular necrosis

Diagnosis = 24 hour urine collection

Antidote? = **BAL** 3–5 mg/kg IM every 4 hours OR **Succimer** 10 mg/kg PO every 8 hours

Child swallowed thermometer mercury? = This mercury is inert → Not absorbed by GI tract

Metal Fume Fever

Metal Fume Fever = Cause from breathing in fumes secondary to welding → Can result from the preparation of coinage metals: copper, silver and gold

Symptoms & Signs

- Flu-like Symptoms: URI symptoms; F/C; Nausea; Malaise; Myalgias; Headaches

Treatment = Supportive

Hydrocarbons

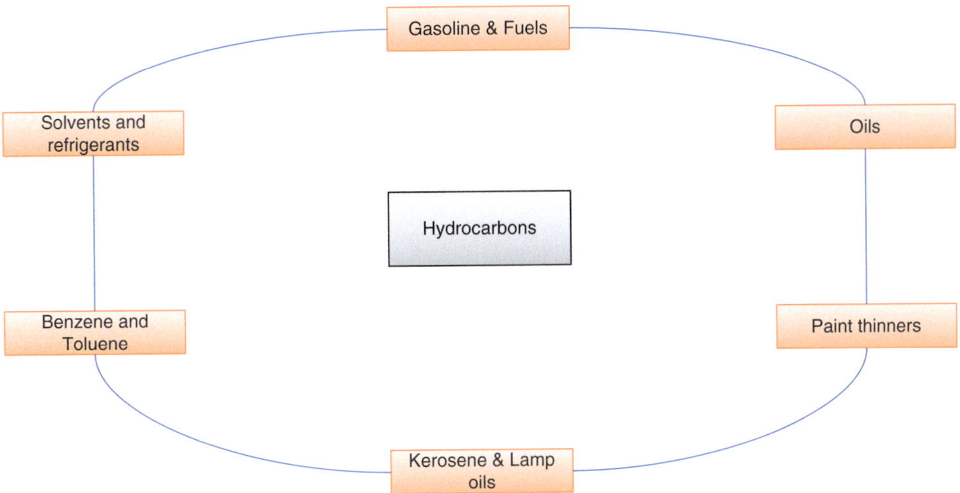

Hydrocarbons: Introduction

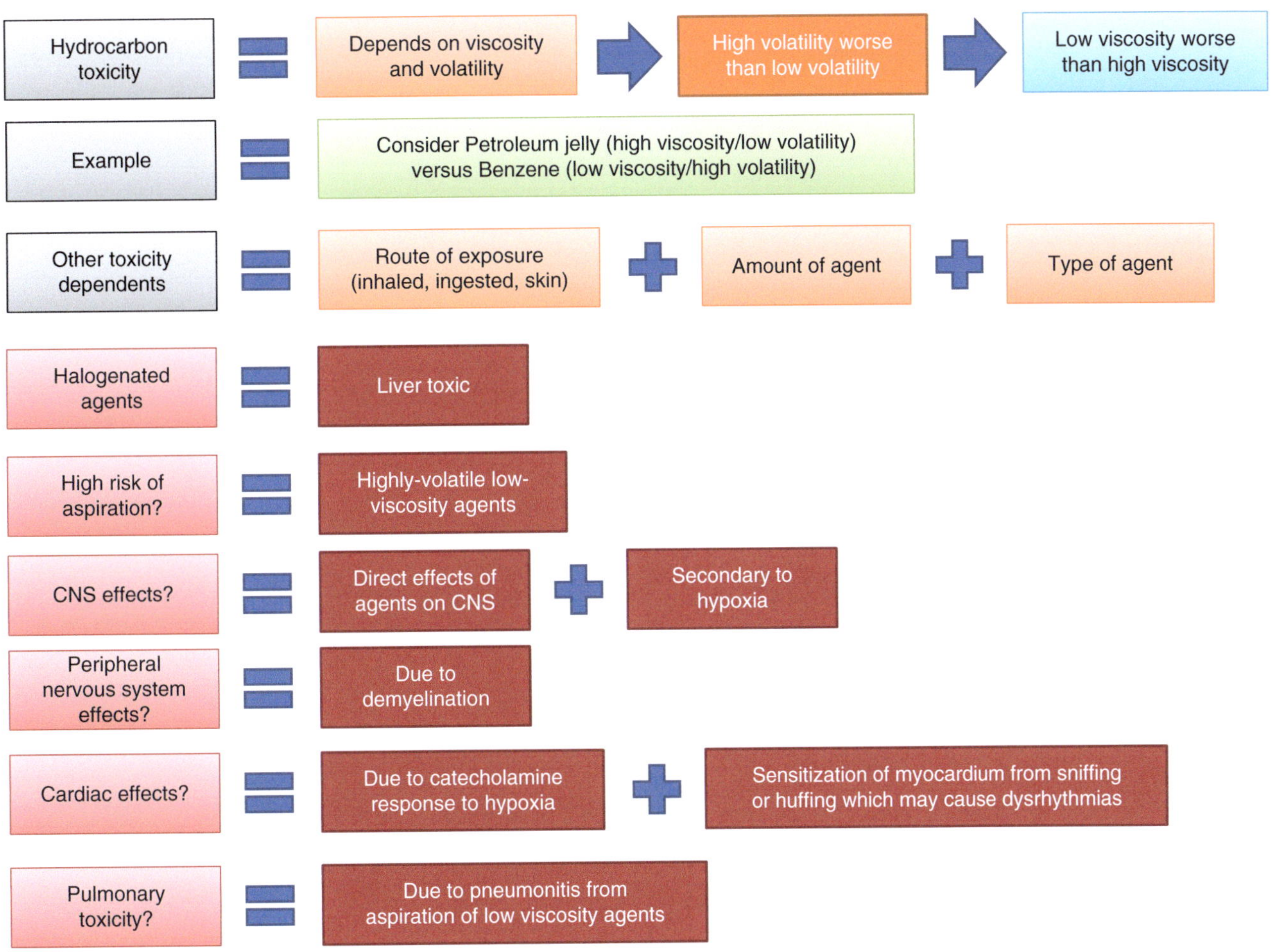

Hydrocarbon: Treatment and Management

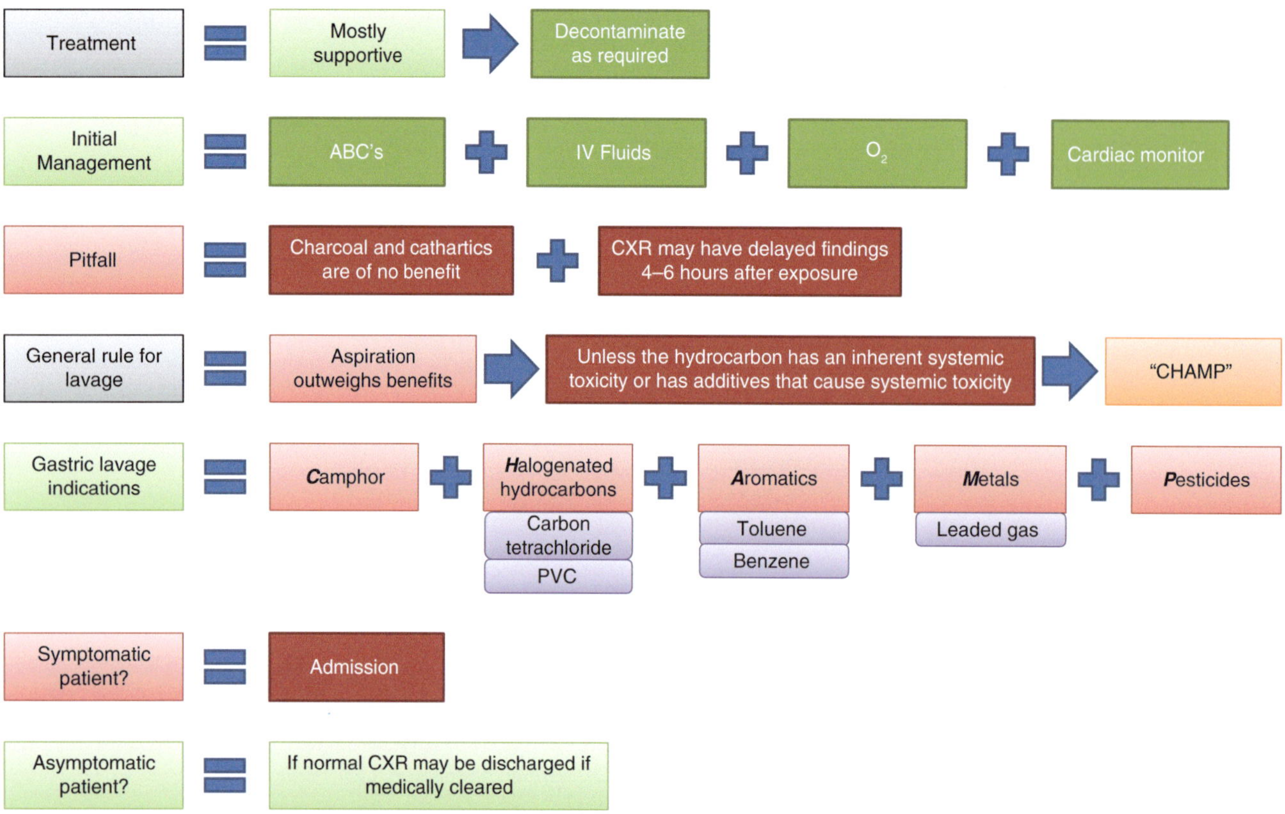

Hypoglycemic Agents

Hypoglycemic Agents = Concern when Glucose < 60 mg/dL OR Patient is symptomatic

Short acting agent? = Replete glucose with IV & oral modalities + Give a meal (e.g., turkey and cheese sandwich which contains protein, carbohydrates and fat + D/C if asymptomatic after observation

Long acting agents = Sulfonylureas → May cause serious symptoms → Requires admission

Risk factors for sulfonylurea toxicity = Old or young + Alcohol use + Liver or kidney insufficiency + Poor nutrition + Use of β-blockers

Sulfonylurea Toxicity

Altered mental status | Unstable vital signs | Continuous hypoglycemia despite treatment

Initial Management = ABC's + IV Fluids + O_2 + Cardiac monitor

Initial treatment = IV bolus of D50

No effect or continued Sx? = IV infusion D5NS + Every 1–2 hour blood glucose → 2 mg/kg D25 for children 2 mg/kg D10 for neonates

May consider = Glucagon ± D10 drip ± Gastric decontamination

Non-sulfonylureas? = No hypoglycemia ‖ Metformin? = May cause lactic acidosis

Lithium

Lithium = Used to treat manic depression → Small therapeutic window → Most pts under long term therapy will develop toxicity at some time

Lithium tidbits = Excreted by kidneys → Hypovolemia or hyponatremia will increase toxicity

Symptoms & Signs

- Early CNS Symptoms: Fatigue, Confusion, Tremor
- CNS Symptom progression: Altered mental status → Ataxia
- Late CNS Symptoms: Clonus, Rigidity, Seizures, Coma
- Renal Symptoms: Diabetes insipidus, Polyuria, Decreased ability to concentrate urine
- GI Symptoms: N/V, Diarrhea, Anorexia
- Cardiac Symptoms: QT Prolongation, Arrhythmias
- Skin Symptoms: Maculopapular rash

Lithium Toxicity Treatment

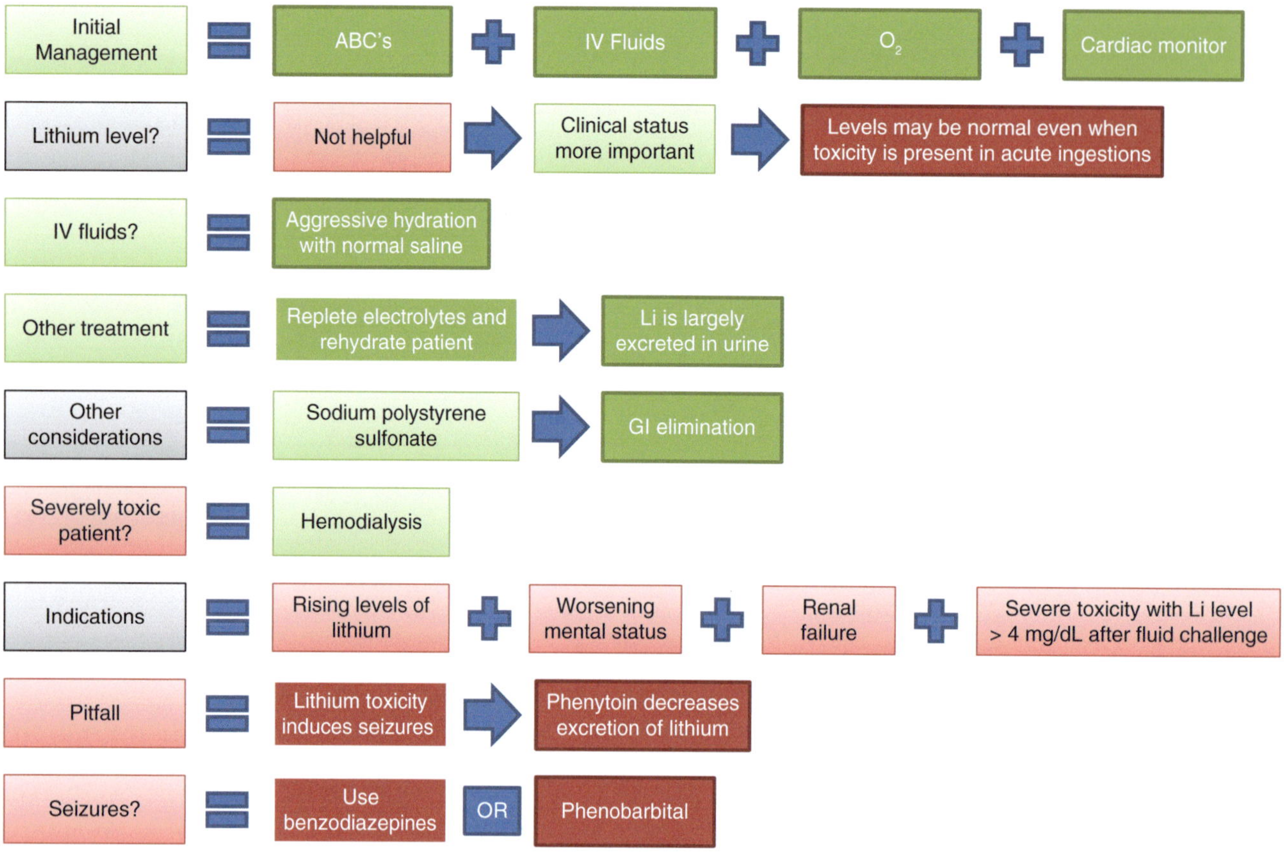

Monoamine Oxidase Inhibitor (MAOI) Overdose

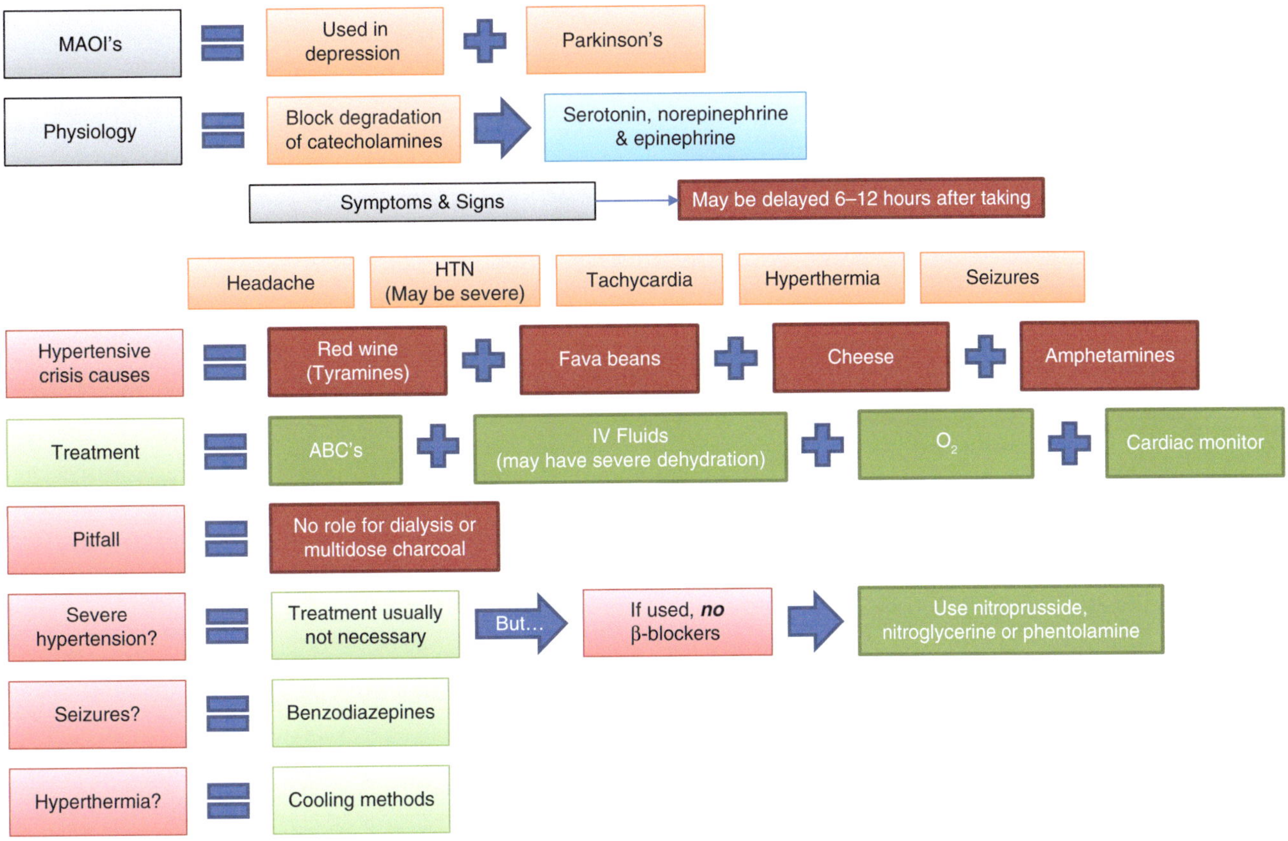

Mushrooms: *Amanita*

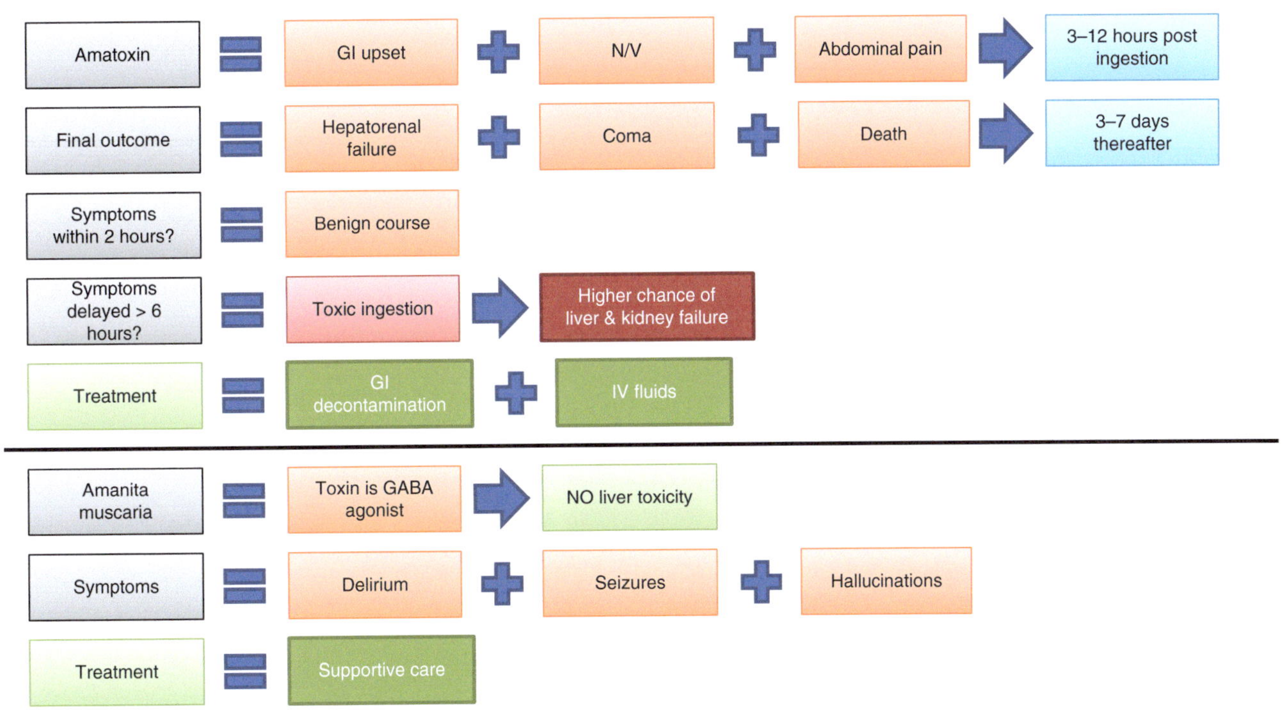

Mushrooms: Others

Gyromitrins = Hydrazine used as a fuel & propellant

Gyromitrins = N/V + Seizures + Hepatorenal failure → 6–12 hours post ingestion

Treatment = GI decontamination + Supportive care + Benzodiazepines & Pyridoxine for seizures

---

Muscarines = Muscarinic effects → DUMBELS + Psychoactive

Treatment = GI decontamination + Supportive care + Atropine for “Killer B’s” → Bradycardia, Bronchorrhea, Bronchospasm

---

Corpines = N/V + Cutaneous flushing + Tachycardia → Due to increased acetaldehyde production

Treatment = Supportive

Narcotics

Toxidromes = Overdose + Withdrawal

Symptoms & Signs

- Overdose: Obtundation, Miosis, Respiratory depression
- Respiratory complications: Respiratory depression, Decreased cough reflex, Aspiration pneumonia, Septic emboli, Pulmonary edema
- Withdrawal: Similar to cholinergic crisis → Yawning, Piloerection

Antidote? = Naloxone → 2 mg initial dose and up to 10 mg if no response → Continuous infusion = ½ the dose given to elicit response given each hour

Pitfall = Half lives of narcotics is variable → **Methadone**, **Modified-release morphine** & **Oxycodone** have long half-lives and may require repeated dosing of Naloxone and continuous infusion

Higher doses of naloxone = Propoxyphene, Methadone, Fentanyl, Codeine

Complications = Bacterial endocarditis + Skin & Soft tissue infections + Rhabdomyolysis

IVDA Bacterial endocarditis = Right sided *Staph aureus* + Left sided *Pseudomonas* → *S. aureus* most common overall

Skin & Soft tissue infections = Look for sites of injection, track marks & retained foreign bodies → Abscess at injection site or distal to site (CNS)

Organophosphates (OP) and Carbamates

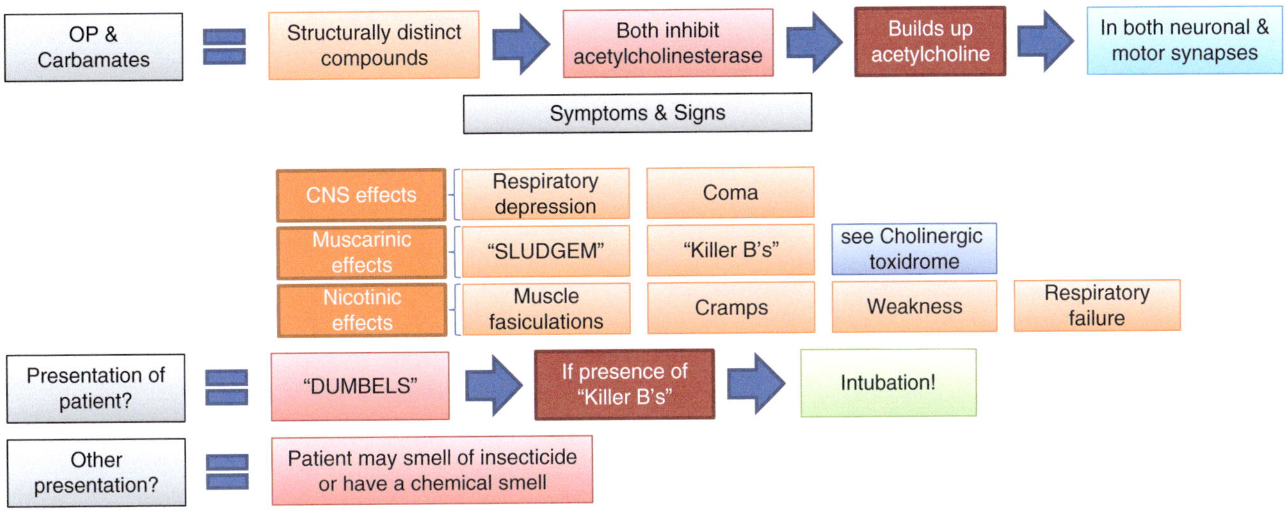

Treatment and Management

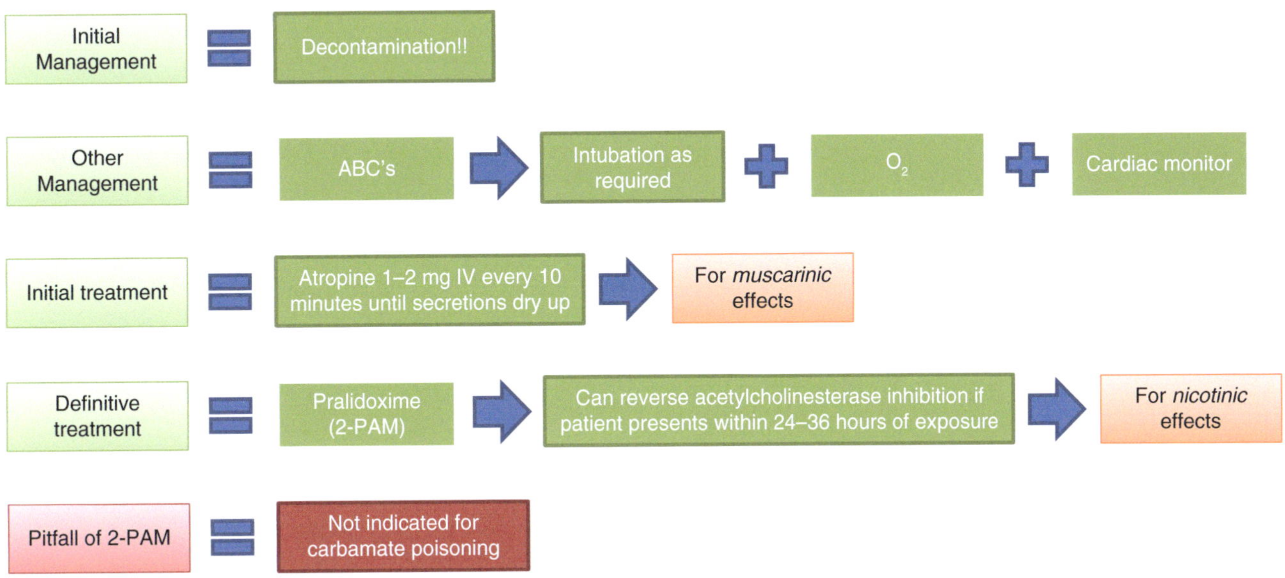

Phenothiazines

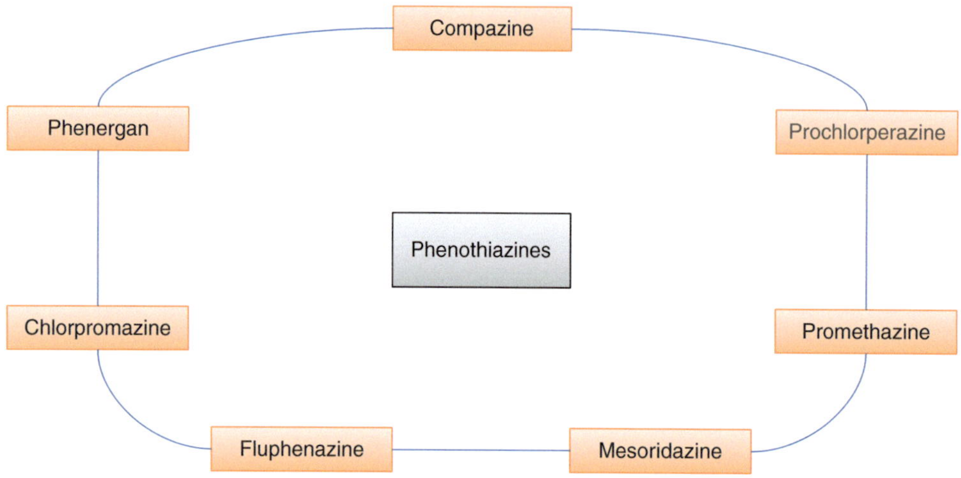

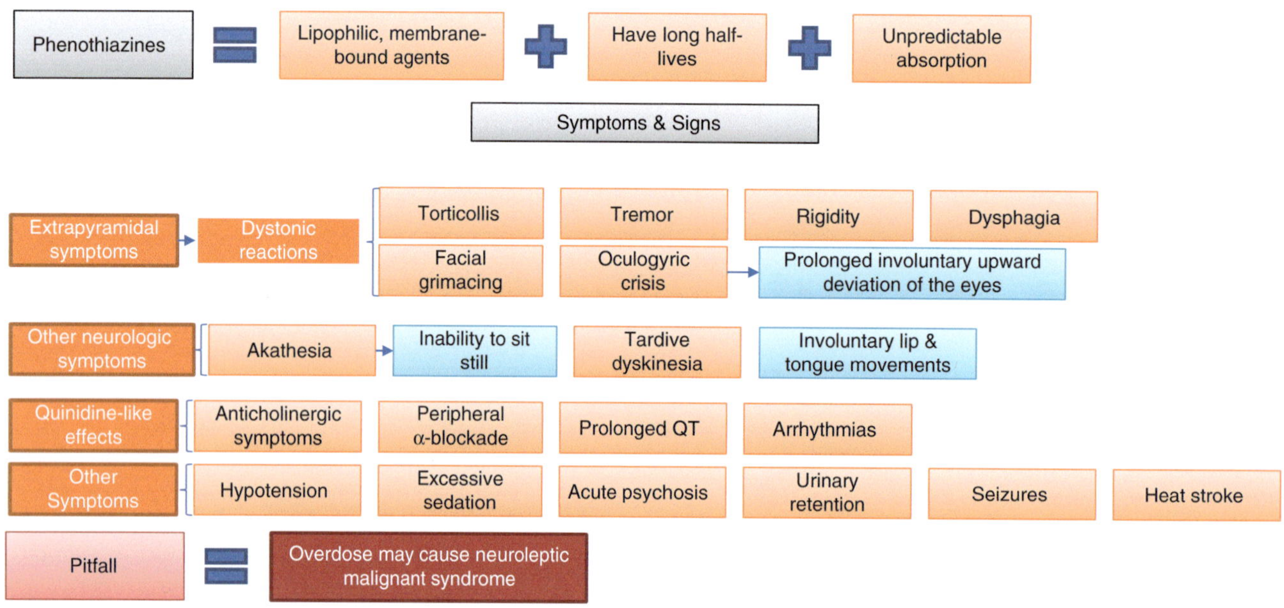

Treatment and Management

Initial Management = ABC's + IV Fluids + O_2 + Cardiac monitor

Extrapyramidal symptoms? = Diphenhydramine OR Benztropine

Seizures? = Benzodiazepines

Dysrhythmias? = Sodium bicarbonate ± Lidocaine

Other considerations = Consider GI decontamination

Neuroleptic Malignant Syndrome (NMS)

NMS = Rare syndrome + Not related to doses of medications ingested → May occur due to dopamine antagonism *or* lack of dopamine agonists

Symptoms & Signs

- CNS effects: Altered mental status; Rigidity; Opisthotonus; Opisthotonus
- Constitutional symptoms: Severe hyperthermia
- Cardiovascular effects: Tachycardia; Hypertension

Laboratory abnormalities = ↑CK, ↑WBC, ↑BUN/Cr, ↑LFTs, metabolic acidosis

Treatment = Control fever + Benzodiazepines + Consider Dantrolene + Consider Bromocriptine

- Control fever: Cooling blankets; Cool IV fluids; Medications may not be effective

Need to intubate? = Use nondepolarizing agent

Serotonin syndrome comparison = Serotonin syndrome occurs soon after starting medications + Rigidity is *greater* in NMS → Except in lower extremities where in serotonin syndrome it is greater

Serotonin Syndrome

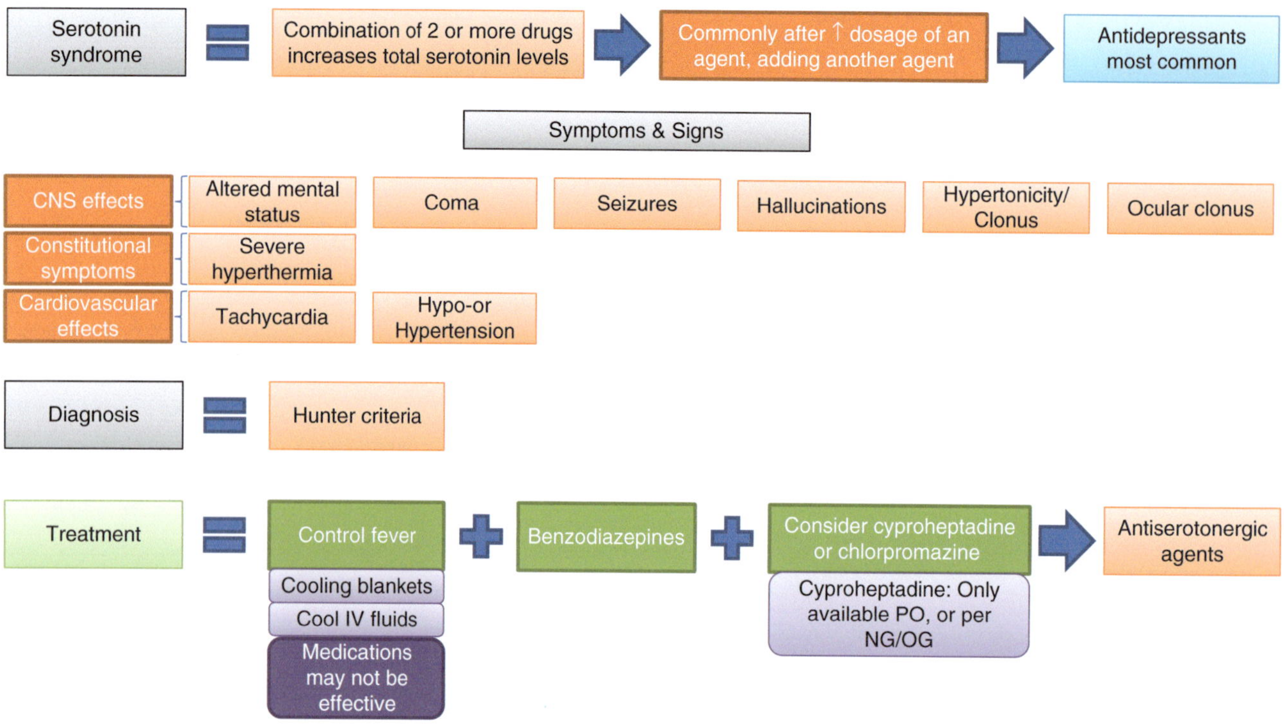

Hunter Criteria for Serotonin Syndrome

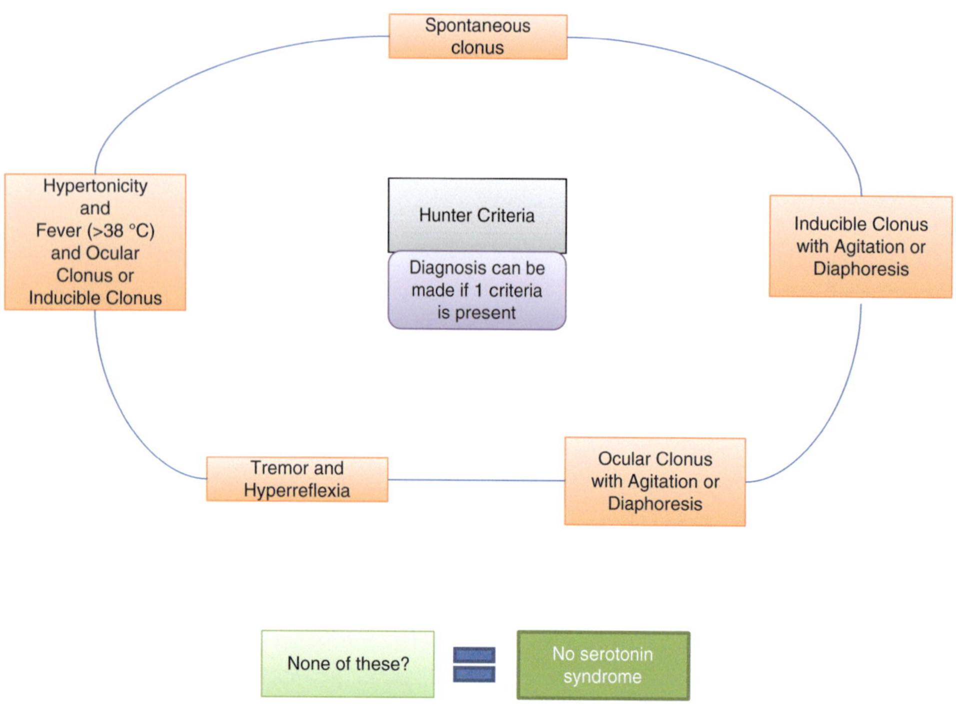

Agents Causing Serotonin Syndrome

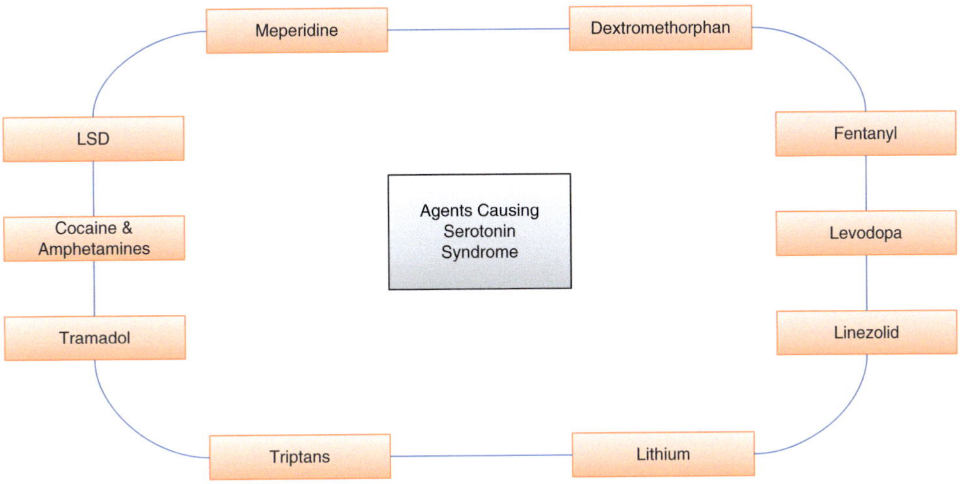

Sedative-Hypnotics: Barbiturates

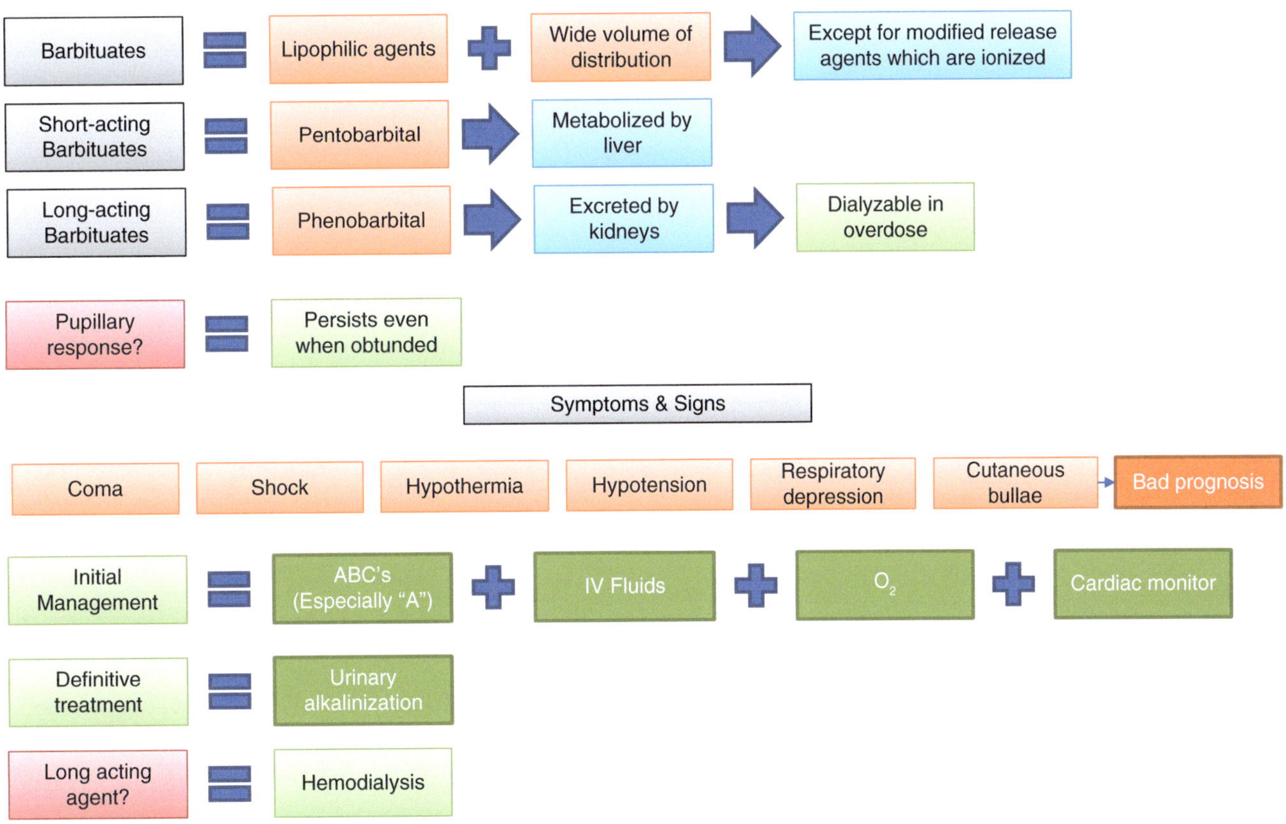

Sedative-Hypnotics: Benzodiazepines

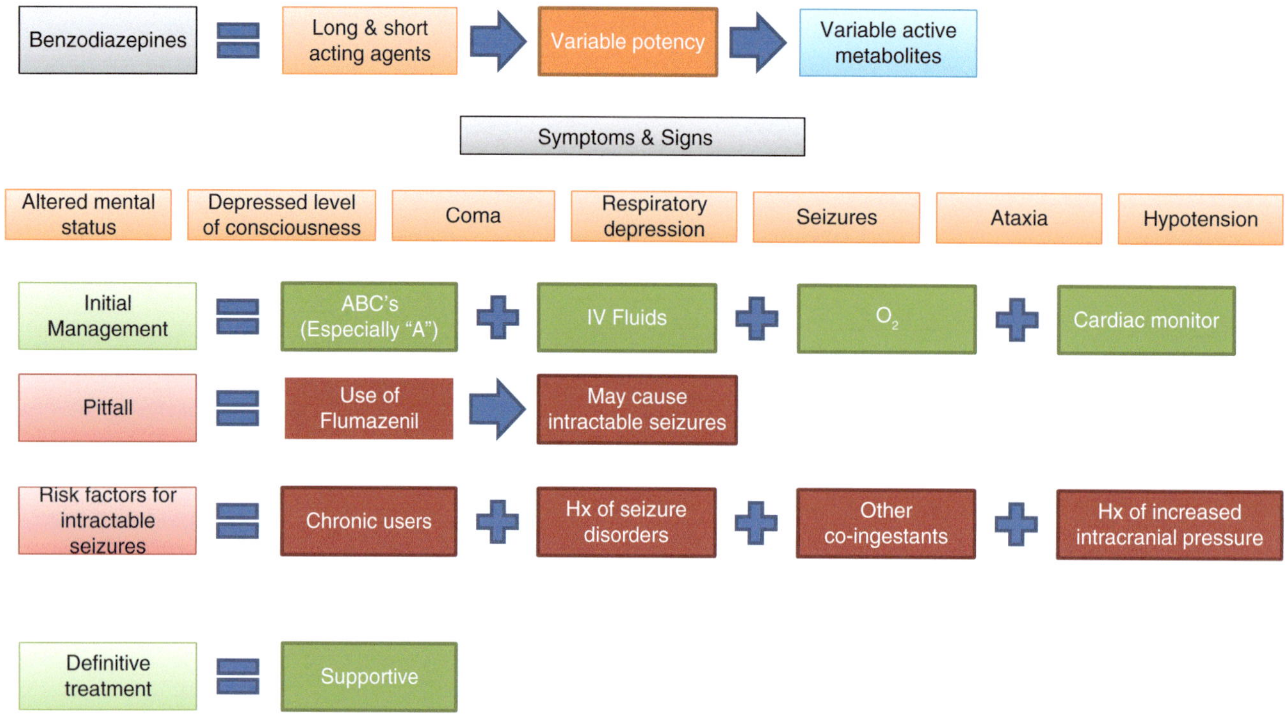

Sedative-Hypnotics: Gamma-Hydroxybutyrate (GHB)

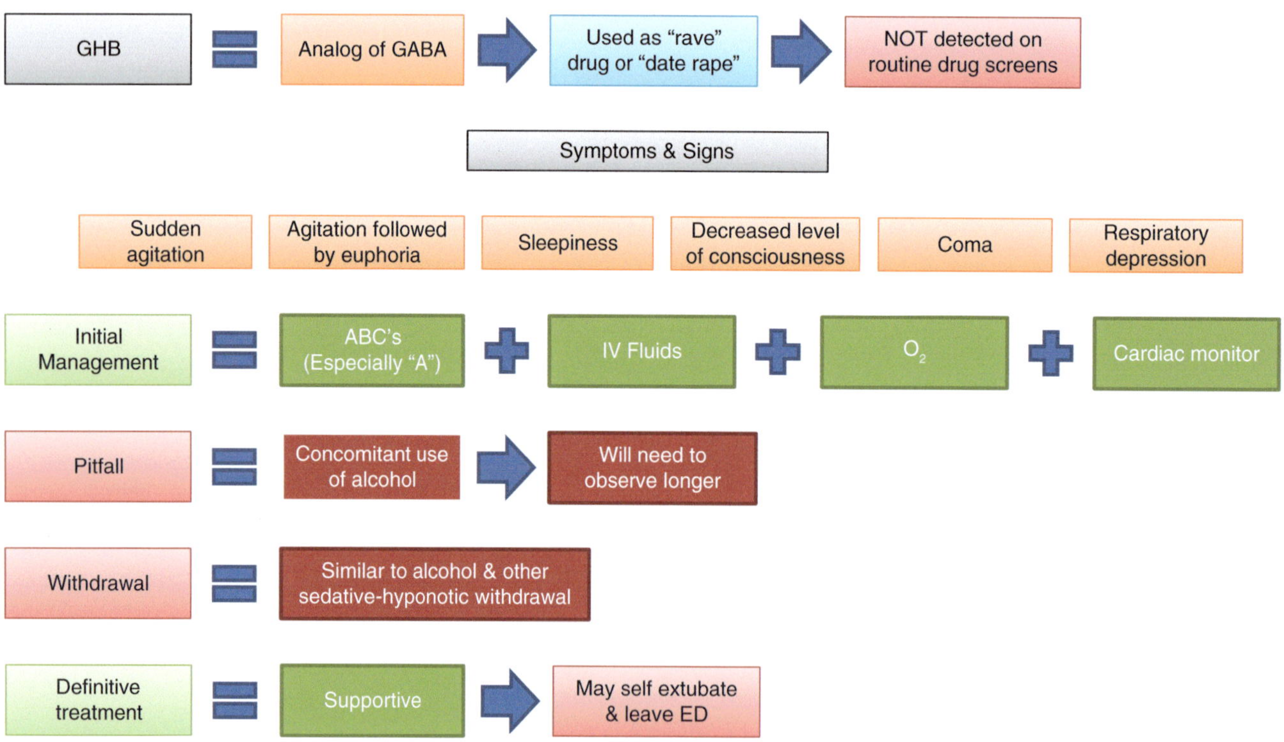

Strychnine Toxicity

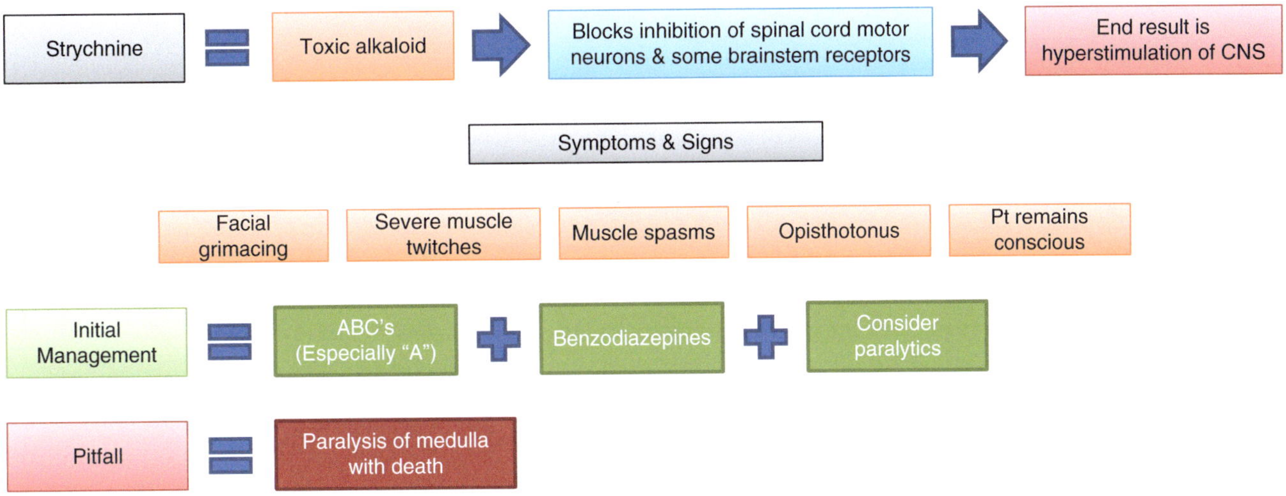

Tricyclic Antidepressants (TCA)

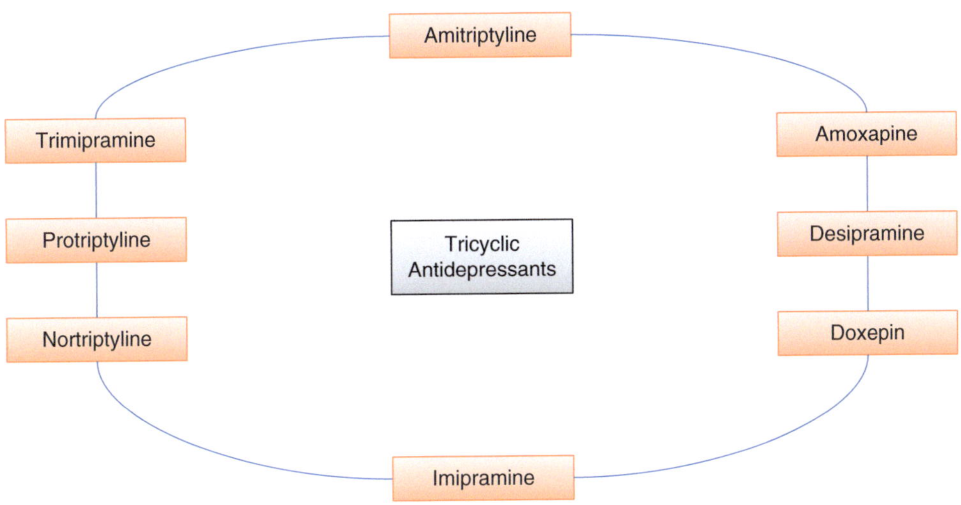

Tricyclic Antidepressants (TCA)

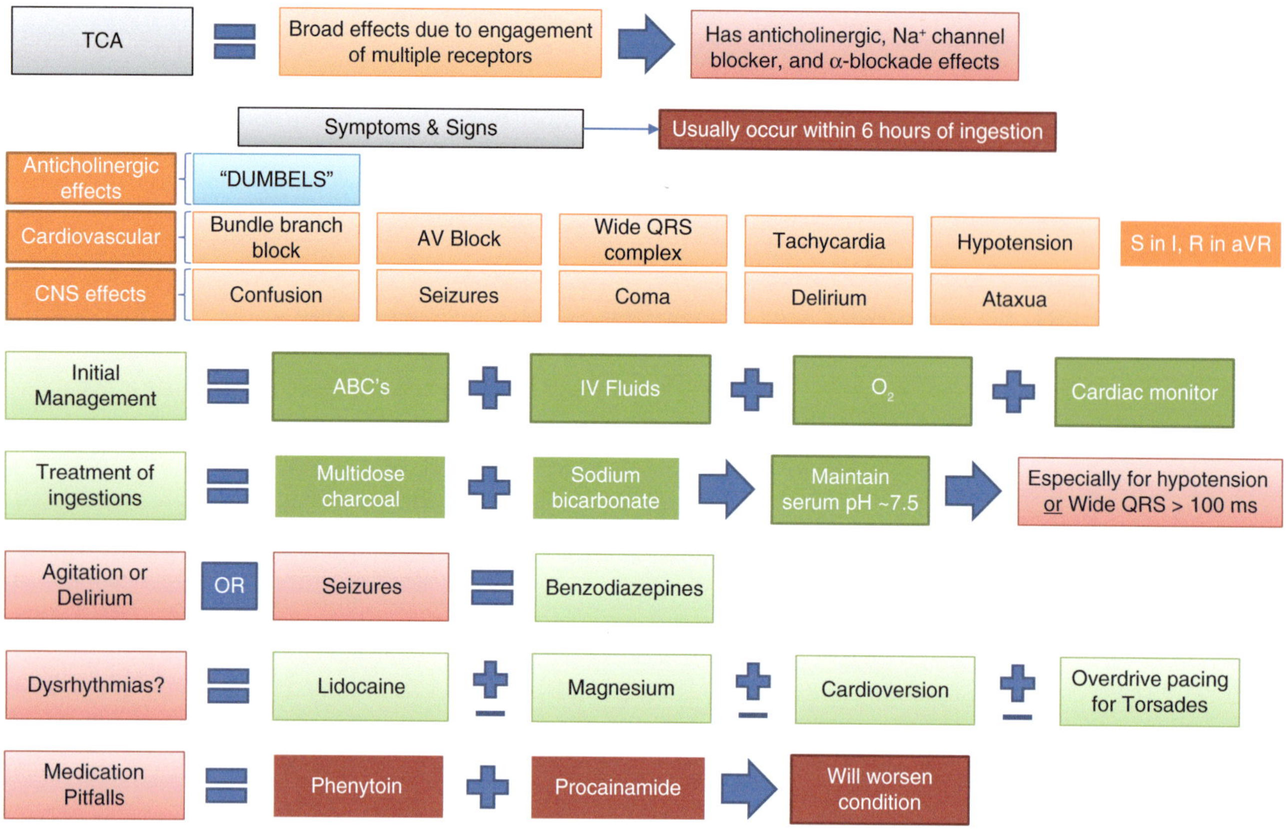

Xanthines

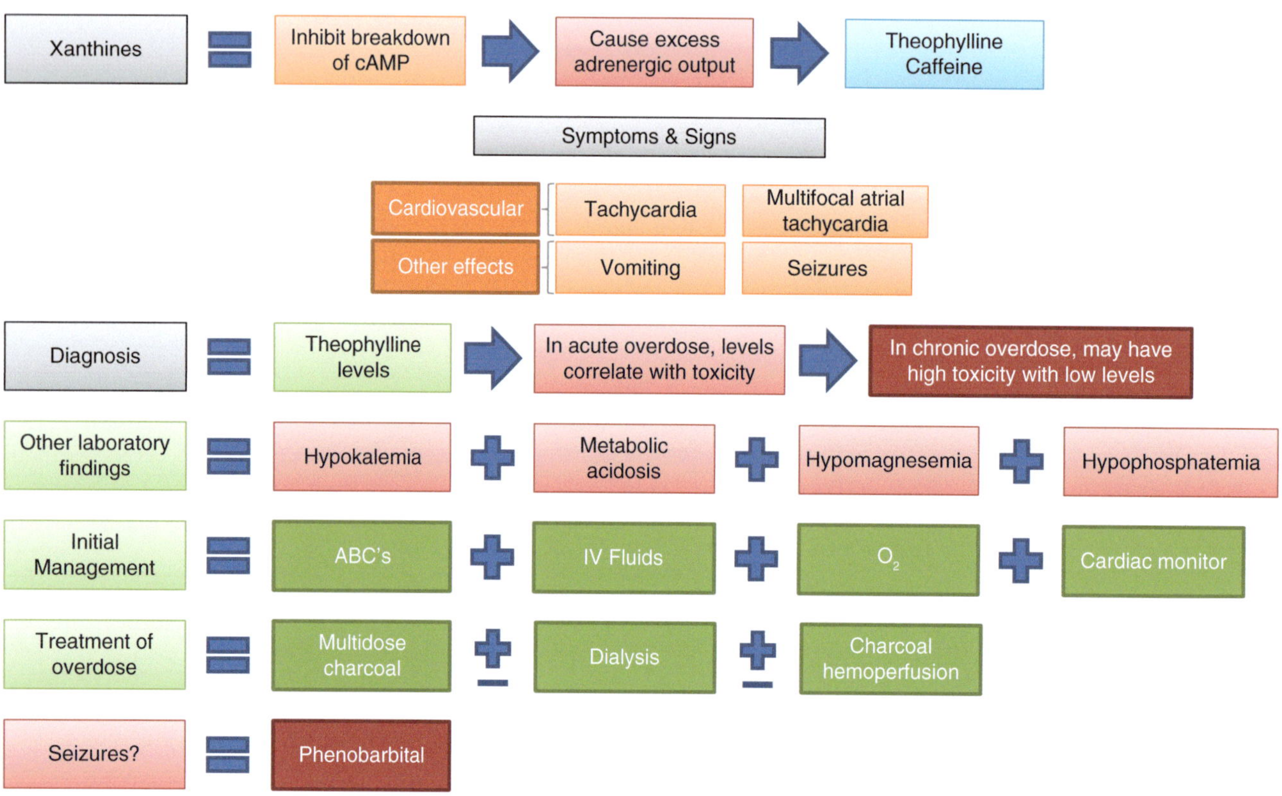

Malignant Hyperthermia

Malignant Hyperthermia = Hypermetabolism involving skeletal muscle → Triggered by inhalation anesthetics & succinylcholine → Inherited disorder

Pathophysiology = Calcium released from sarcoplasmic reticulum of skeletal muscle and causes a hypermetabolicstate after exposure to triggering agents

Symptoms & Signs

Muscle rigidity | Muscle stiffness | Hyperthemia (> 40.5 °C) | Tachypnea | Tachycardia | Rhabdomyolysis | Mottled skin

Some laboratory findings = Acidosis + Hyperkalemia + Myoglobinuria

Initial Management = ABC's + IV Fluids + O_2 + Cardiac monitor

Further Management = Discontinue affecting agent + Dantrolene + Cooling of patient

Dantrolene = Interferes with muscle contraction → Lowers temperature

Complications = DIC + Cardiac failure + Renal failure

Orthopedic Emergencies

Bobby Desai

Contents

Tidbits 736
The Hand 738
Fractures and Dislocations of the Wrist 750
The Forearm 756
The Elbow 760
The Humerus and Shoulder 766
Nontraumatic Hip Disorders 777
The Femur 781
The Knee 782
The Leg 791
The Ankle 795
The Foot 797
Osteomyelitis 800
Thoracic and Lumbar Pain 801
Rheumatologic Emergencies 808

B. Desai, MD, MEd
Department of Emergency Medicine, University of Florida,
Gainesville, FL, USA
e-mail: bdesai@ufl.edu

B. Desai, B.R. Allen (eds.), *Nailing the Written Emergency Medicine Board Examination*,
DOI 10.1007/978-3-319-30838-8_14

Tidbits

Growing Bone Anatomy

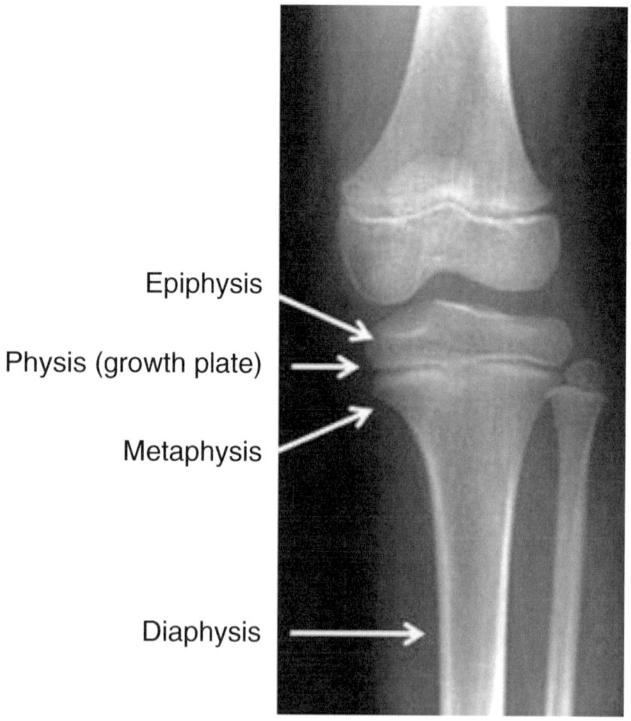

Center image (Reprinted from Abdelgawad A, Naga O. Introduction to orthopedic nomenclature. In: Abdelgawad A, Naga O, editors. Pediatric orthopedics: a handbook for primary care physicians. New York: Springer; 2014. p. 1–14. With permission from Springer Science + Business Media)

Salter-Harris Fractures

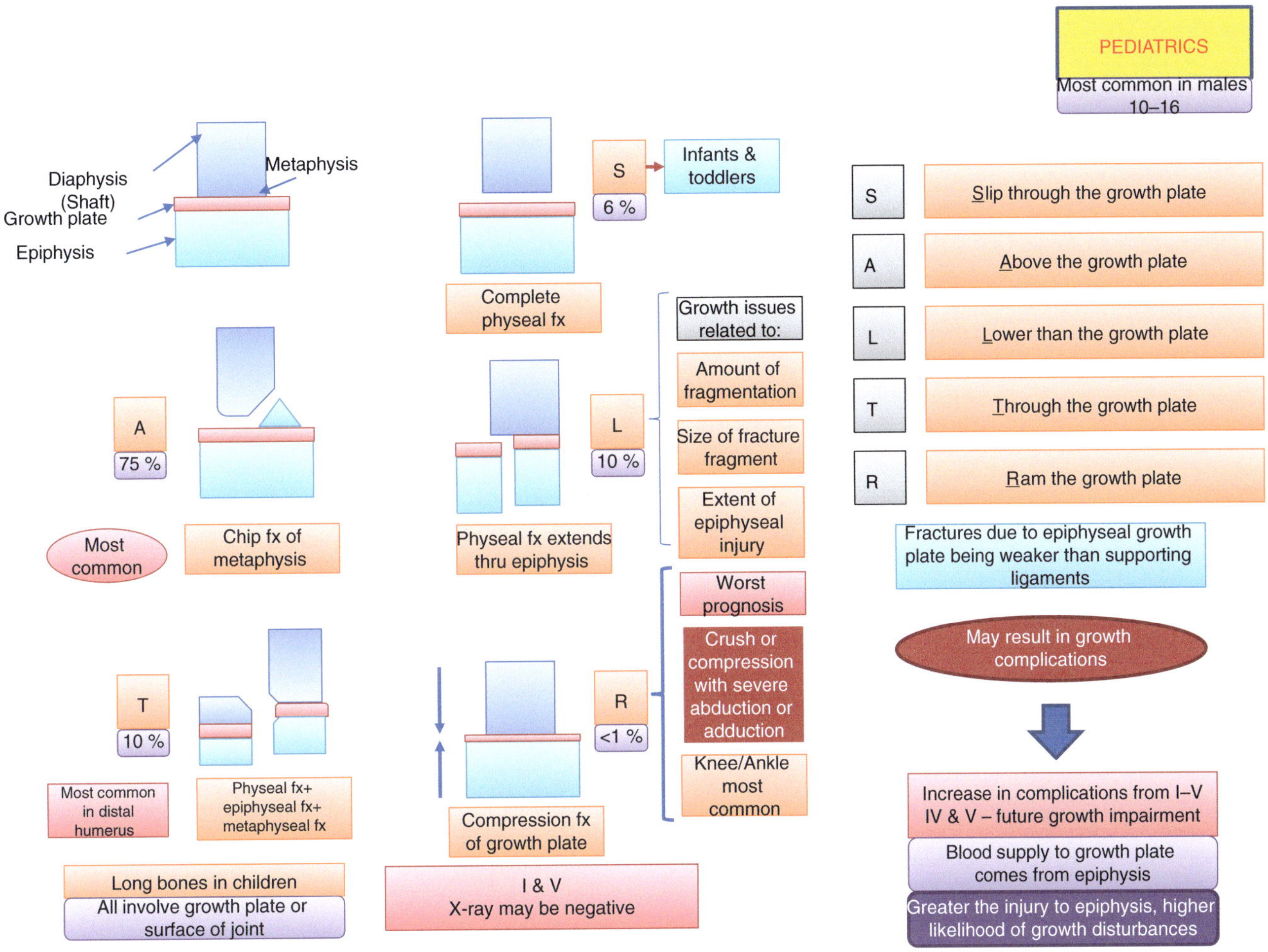

The Hand

Nerves of the Hand

Sensory

- **Radial**: Dorsal web space between index finger & thumb
- **Median**: Thumb, index, long and ½ of ring finger
- **Ulnar**: ½ of little & ring fingers

Recurrent Median Nerve
Pure motor nerve to thenar muscles

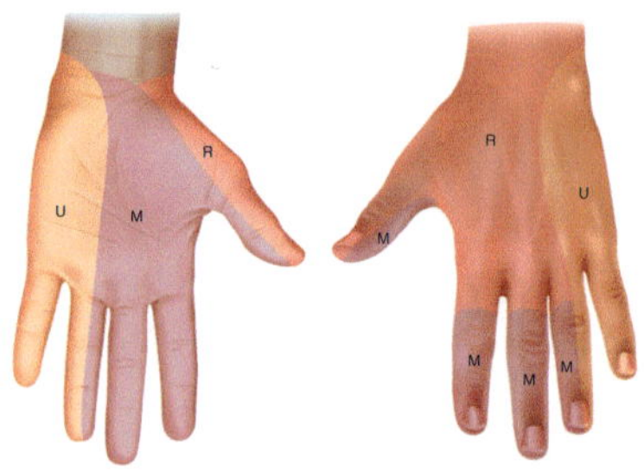

Motor

- **Radial**: Finger/Wrist extension
- **Median**: Flexion of index & middle fingers + Thumb opposition
- **Ulnar**: Finger adduction & abduction + flexion of ring & little fingers

Dorsal branch of Radial Nerve
Pure sensory

DrCuMa

- ***D*rop Hand = *R*adial**
- ***C*law Hand = *U*lnar**
- **Finger *A*pposition = *M*edian**

Amputation of the Digit (Look in Trauma)

Initial management = Place digit in plastic bag in water → But… Do NOT place digit directly on ice! → Clean & sharp wounds have best prognosis

Indications for Reimplantation

- Multiple digits
- Thumb
  - Better prognosis proximal to IP joint
- Single digit between PIP & DIP
- Metacarpal (Palm) area
- Wrist or Forearm
- Consider any part for reimplantation in a child

Hand Infections

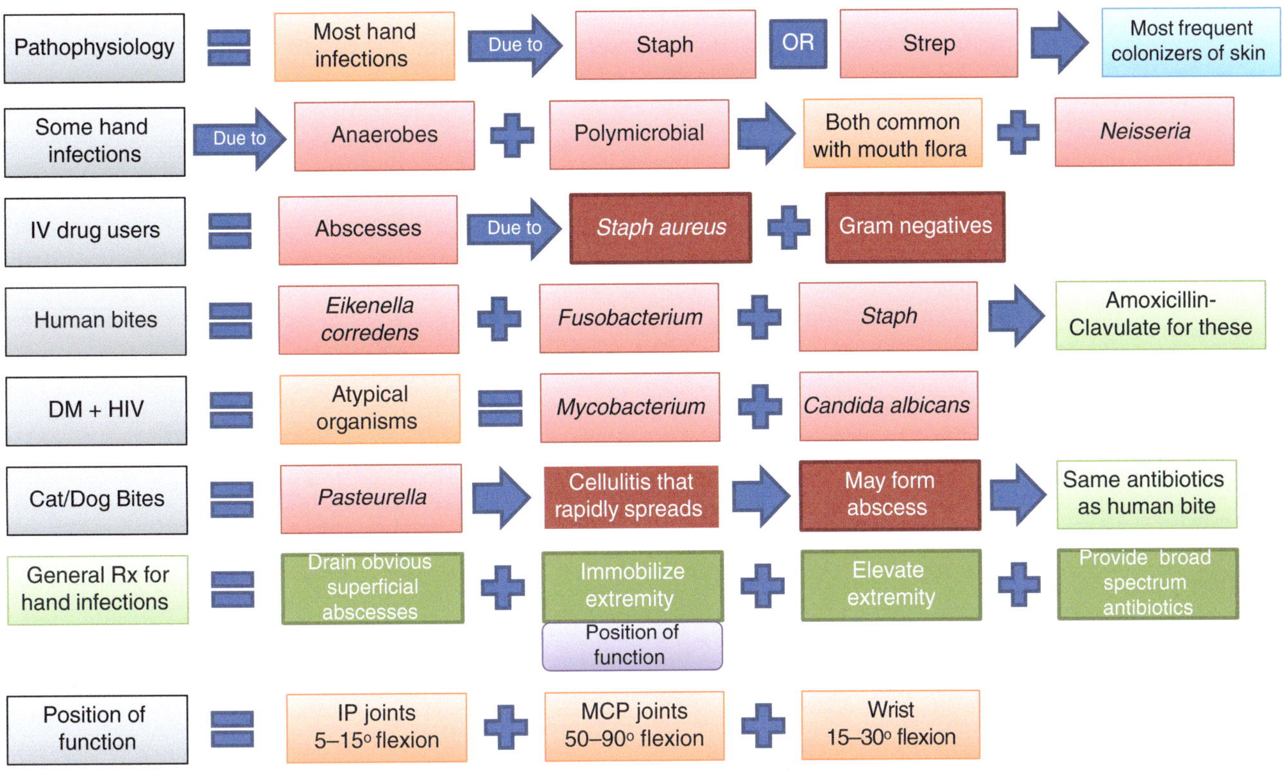

Felon

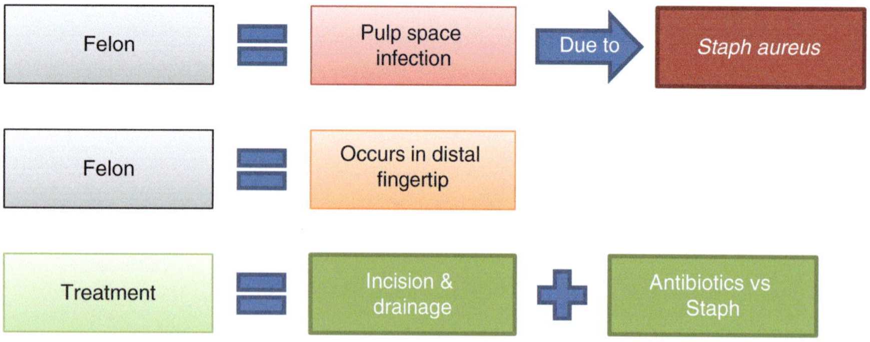

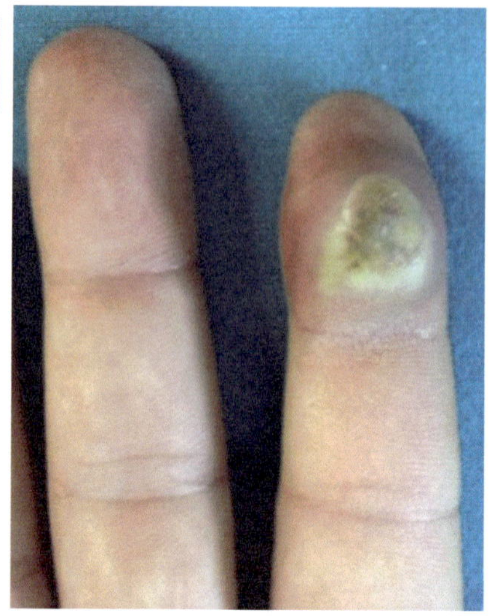

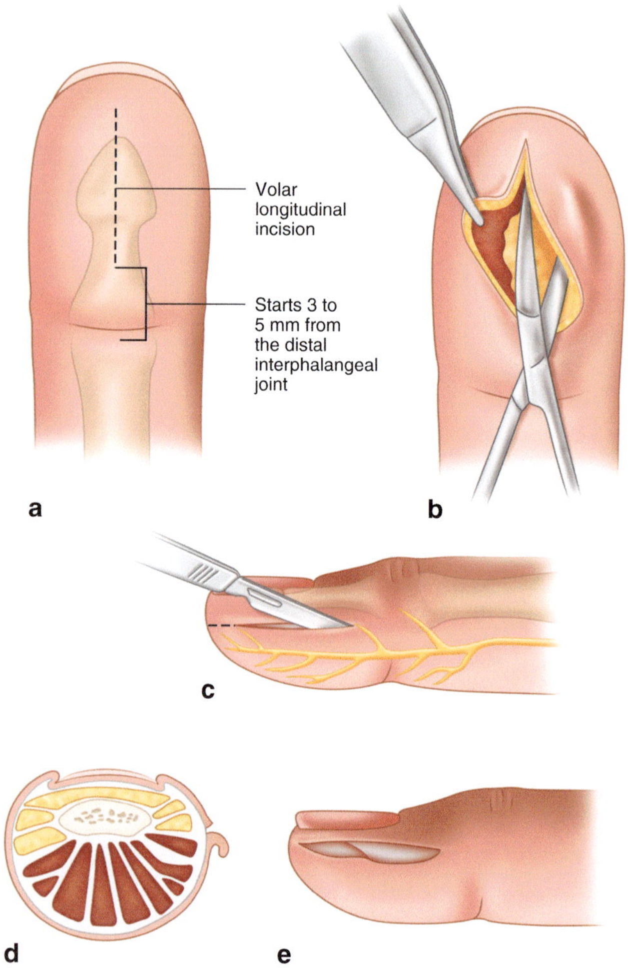

Top right image (Reprinted from Dailana ZH, Rigopoulos N. Infections of the hand. In: Bentley G, editor. European surgical orthopaedics and traumatology. Heidelberg: Springer Verlag; 2014. p. 2009–31. With permission from Springer Verlag)

Paronychia

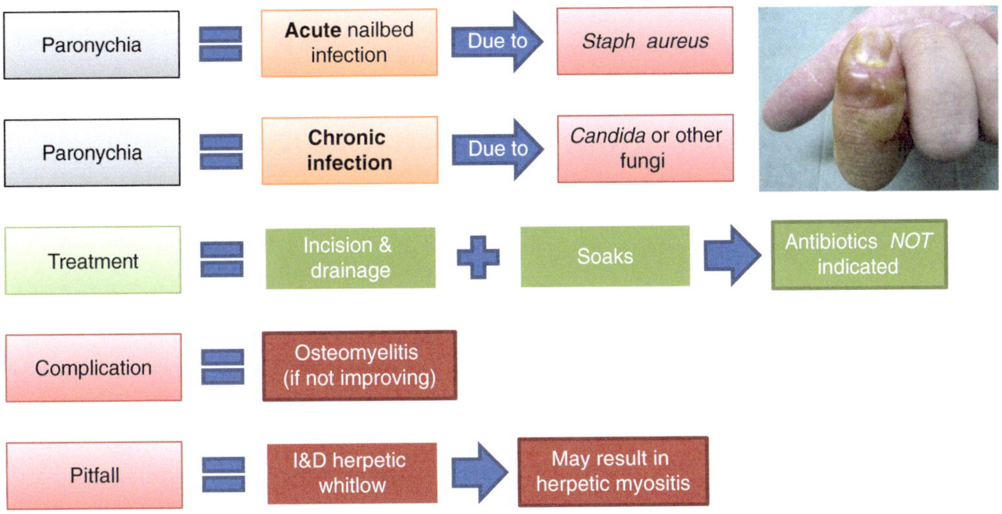

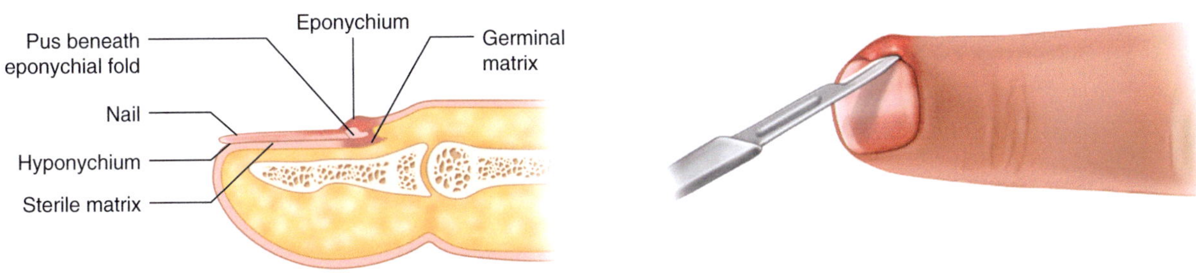

Top right image (Reprinted from Dailana ZH, Rigopoulos N. Infections of the hand. In: Bentley G, editor. European surgical orthopaedics and traumatology. Heidelberg: Springer Verlag; 2014. 2009–31. With permission from Springer Verlag)

Collar Button Abscess

Collar Button Abscess = Infection of hand → Spreads → Between metacarpals → Erupts dorsally → Palmar aponeurosis presents volar extension

Collar Button Abscess = Dorsal & volar abscess connected by a tract → Due to → Foreign body OR Splinter

Treatment = Incision & drainage + Antibiotics → Urgent orthopedic consultation

Flexor Tenosynovitis

Flexor Tenosynovitis = Surgical emergency → Failure to Dx will result in loss of both digit & hand function → Due to → Penetrating trauma → *Staph* most common; May have anaerobes

Diagnosis = Kanavel's signs

Kanavel's signs = Tenderness over flexor tendon sheath + Symmetric finger swelling + Pain with passive extension + Flexed posture of digit

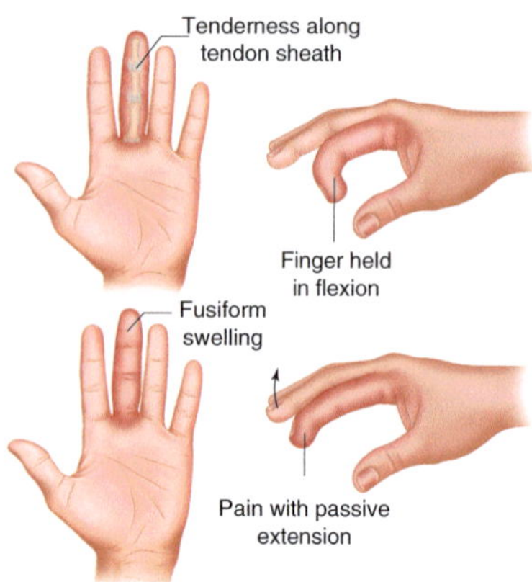

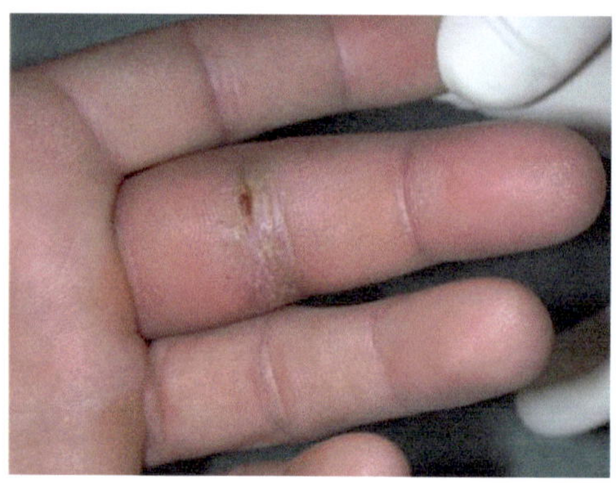

Treatment = IV antibiotics + Surgical I&D

Bottom right image (Reprinted from Dailana ZH, Rigopoulos N. Infections of the hand. In: Bentley G, editor. European surgical orthopaedics and traumatology. Heidelberg: Springer Verlag; 2014. p. 2009–31. With permission from Springer Verlag)

Sporotrichosis

Sporotrichosis = Fungal infection with skip lesions → Due to → *Sporothrix schenckii* → Occurs in Rose gardeners

Treatment = Itraconazole OR Supersaturated potassium iodide

Boutonniere Deformity

Boutonneire Deformity = Central slip extensor hood disruption near PIP joint — Due to → Forced flexion at PIP joint

Boutonneire Deformity = Lateral bands of extensor hood split to become PIP flexors

Boutonneire Deformity = May have concomitant avulsion fracture

Treatment = Splint PIP in extension

Boutonneire deformity

PIP flexion + DIP extension

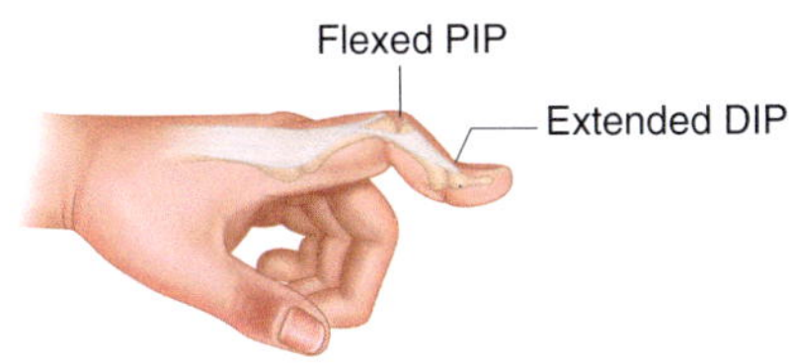

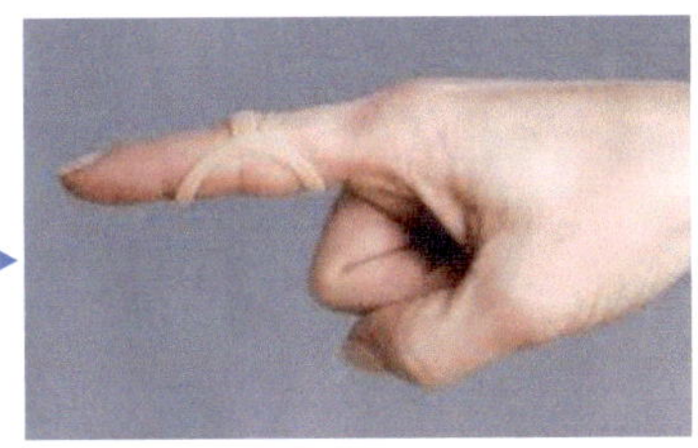

Mallet Finger

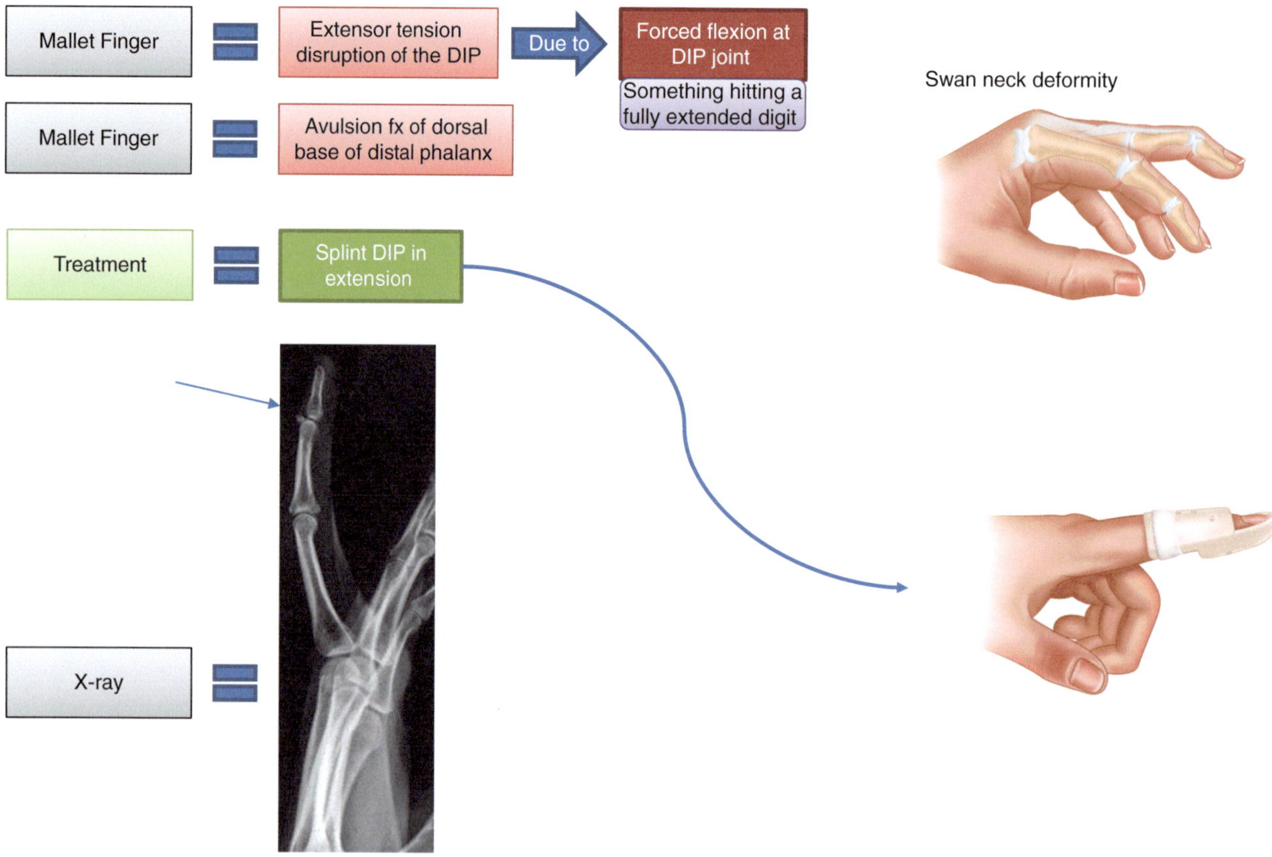

Bottom left image (Reprinted from Almusa E, Peterson II WM, Bianchi S, Jacob D, Hoffman D. Radiological investigations. In: Chick G, editor. Acute and chronic finger injuries in ball sports. Paris: Springer Verlag; 2013. p. 89–124. With permission from Springer Verlag)

Gamekeeper's (Skier's) Thumb

Gamekeeper's Thumb = Injury to ulnar collateral ligament of thumb MCP → Due to → Forced radial abduction of MCP joint

Ulnar collateral ligament = Important for grasp & pincher function of thumb

Gamekeeper's Thumb = May have concomitant avulsion fracture

X-ray =

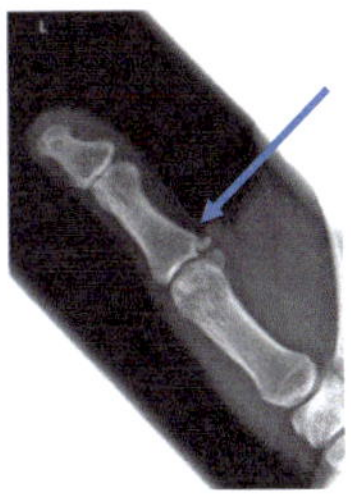

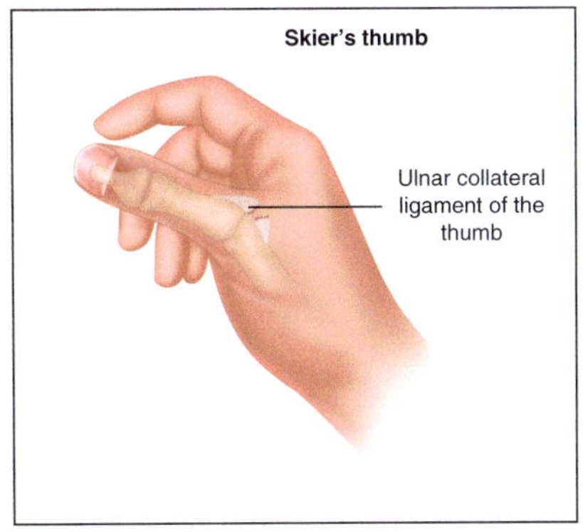

Treatment = Partial tear → Thumb spica splint || Complete tear → Surgery

Pitfall = Chronic instability of thumb

Complication = >40° radial angulation indicates complete rupture = Surgical consultation

Bull rider's Thumb = RCL injury

Center left image (Reprinted from Almusa E, Peterson II WM, Bianchi S, Jacob D, Hoffman D. Radiological investigations. In: Chick G, editor. Acute and chronic finger injuries in ball sports. Paris: Springer Verlag; 2013. p. 89–124. With permission from Springer Verlag)

Herpetic Whitlow

Herpetic Whitlow = Viral infection of distal finger → Due to → Herpes simplex → Due to → Contact with oral herpetic infection

Adults = HSV 2 || Children = Associated with gingivostomatitis HSV-1

Symptoms & Signs

- Burning
- Pruritis
- Red, tender lesion
- Vesicular bullae
- Potential induration of finger

Pitfall = Mistaken for felon → DO NOT I&D!

Treatment = Usually self limited → Consider antiviral agents

De Quervain's Tenosynovitis

De Quervain's Tenosynovitis = Excessive use of thumb or wrist → Due to → Tenosynovitis of extensor pollicis brevis & abductor pollicislongus

Pain = Radial aspect of wrist radiating to thumb or wrist

Diagnosis = Painful ROM of thumb + Pain over distal radial styloid + Positive Finkelstein's test

Treatment = Immobilize thumb & wrist with splint + Anti-inflammatory medications

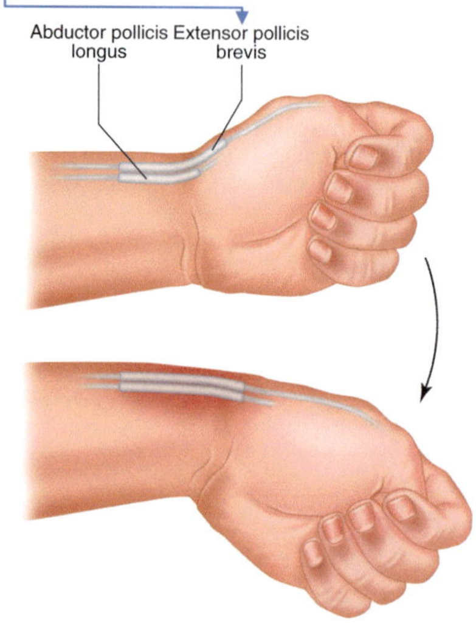

Carpal Tunnel Syndrome

Carpal Tunnel Syndrome = Polyneuropathy → Due to → Entrapment of median nerve in the carpal tunnel → Causing Sx

Paresthesias = Long finger + Index finger + Radial aspect of ring finger + Palmar aspect of thumb

Other Sx = Radiation of pain to forearm & shoulder + Waking up at night with burning pain + Tingling in hand + Numbness with prolonged flexed hand

Etiology = Overuse, CHF, Hypothyroidism, Pregnancy, Renal disease, Rheumatoid arthritis

Diagnosis = Tinel's sign → Tapping over the median nerve + Phalen's sign (More sensitive & specific) → Flexing wrist for 1 min

Treatment = Volar splint + NSAIDs ± Referral to hand surgeon

Fractures of the Hand: Phalanx

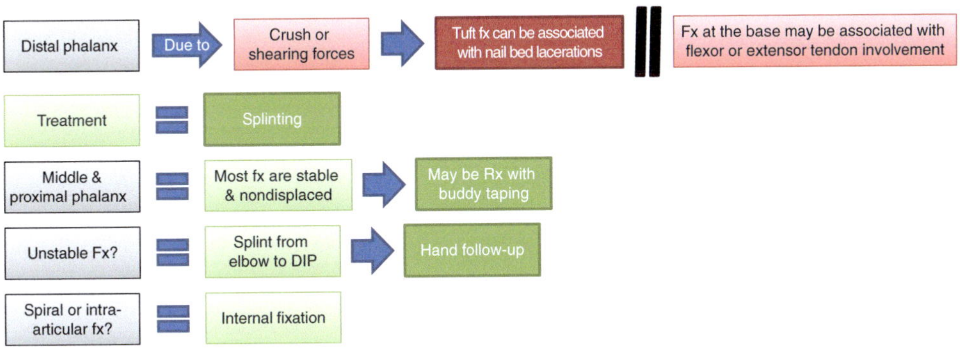

Fractures of the Hand: Metacarpals

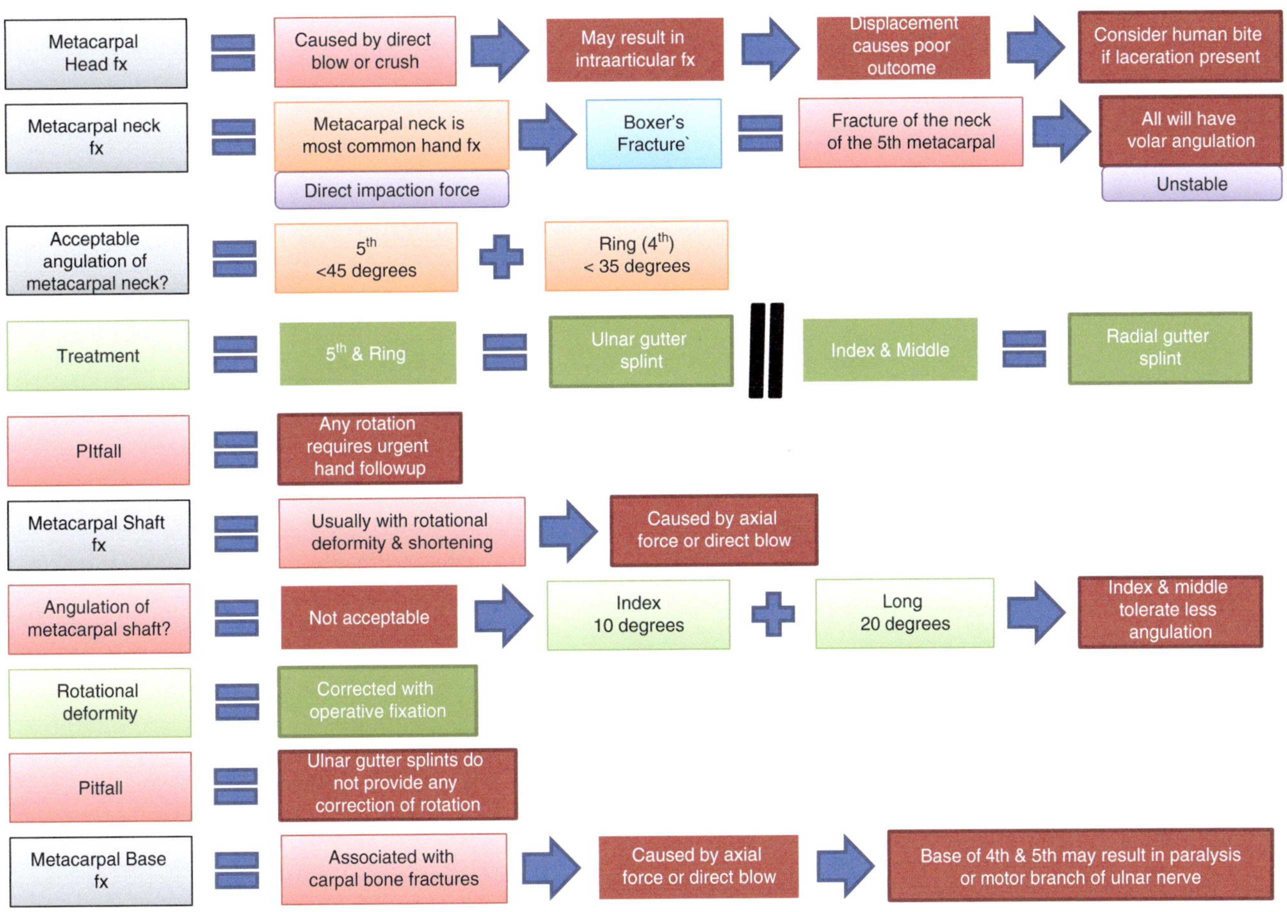

Special Fractures of the Metacarpals

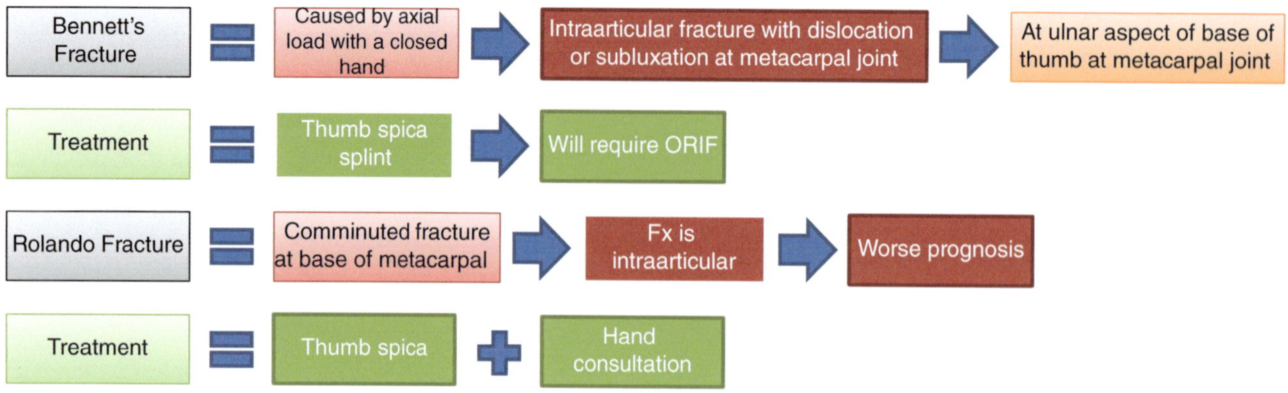

Finger Dislocation

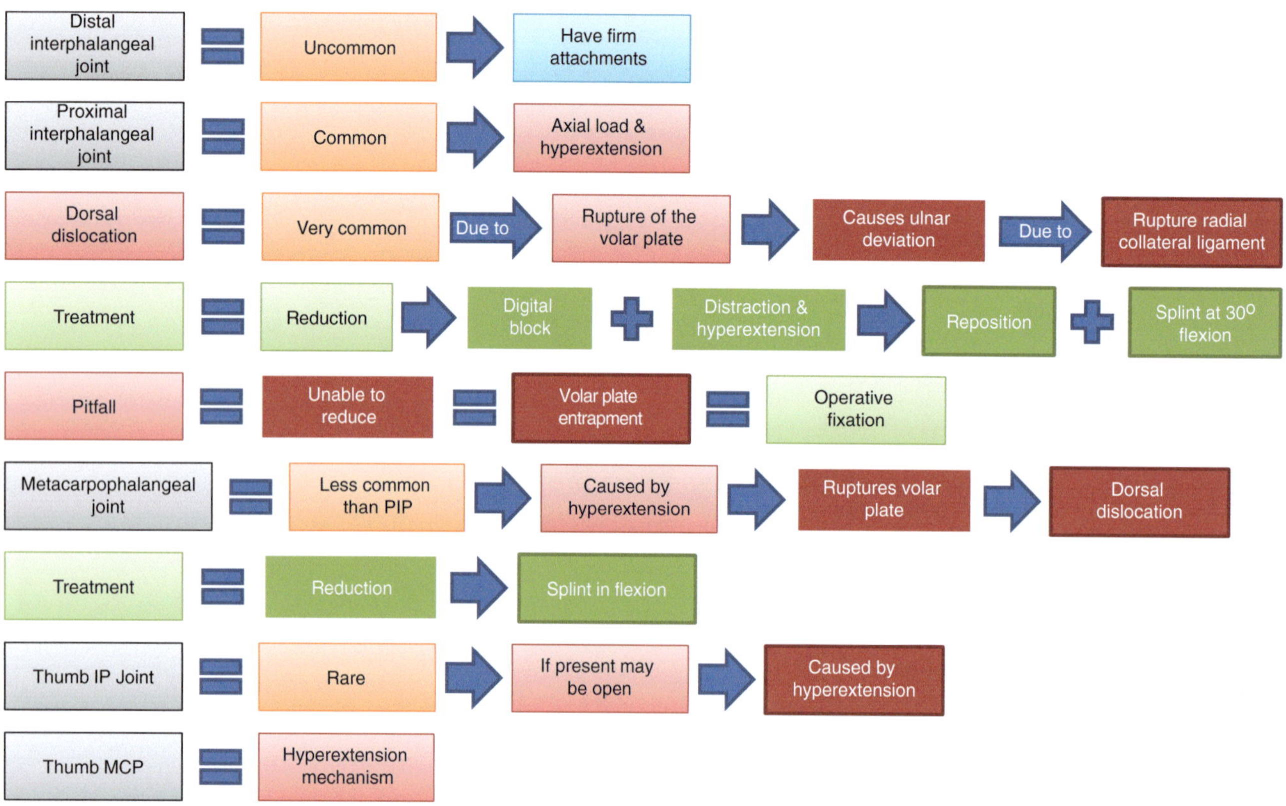

High-Pressure Injection Injury

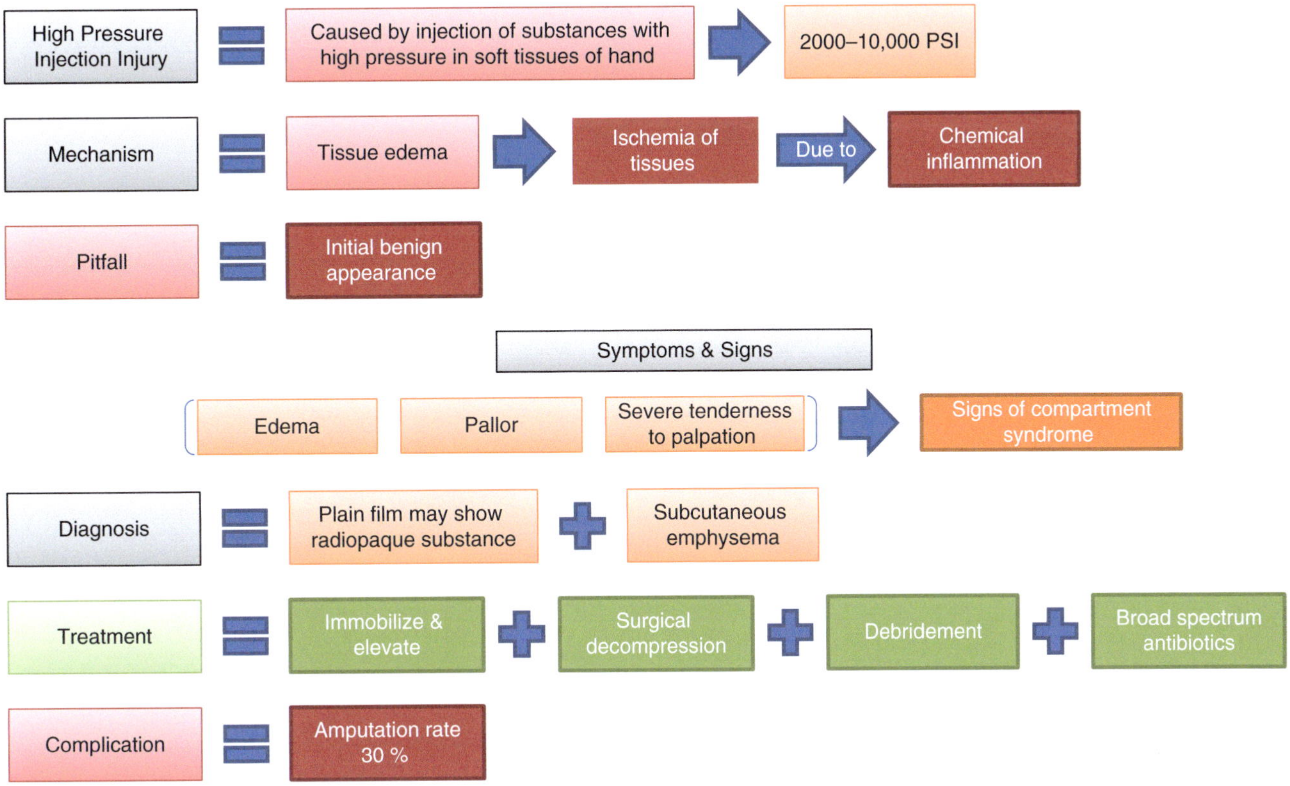

Fractures and Dislocations of the Wrist

Colles' Fracture

Colles' Fracture = Most common fx in adults > 50 → Due to → Fall on outstretched hand

Colles' Fracture = Distal radial metaphysis fx → Dorsal angulation = "Dinner fork deformity" → May have fx of ulnar styloid

Diagnosis = Plain film → Lateral view has best view of angulation

X-ray =

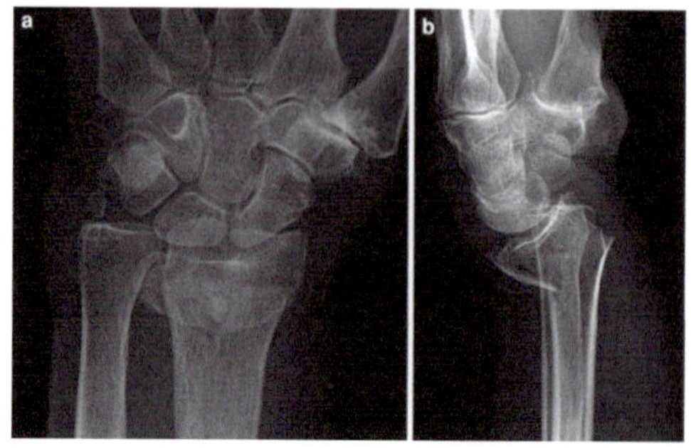

Treatment = Closed reduction + Sugar tong splint

Unstable fx? = > 20° of angulation + Involvement of joint + Significant comminution + > 1 cm of shortening

Complications = Malunion + Median nerve injury + Joint instability + Arthritis

Center right image (Reprinted from Raby N. Imaging of wrist trauma. In: Davies AM, Grainger AJ, James SJ, editors. Imaging of the hand and wrist. Heidelberg: Springer Verlag; 2013. p. 141–69. With permission from Springer Verlag)

Smith's Fracture

Smith's Fracture = "Reverse Colles'" → ue to → Fall or direct blow on dorsum of hand

Smith's Fracture = Distal radial metaphysis fx → Volar angulation = "Garden spade deformity"

Diagnosis = Plain film → Lateral view has best view of angulation

X-ray =

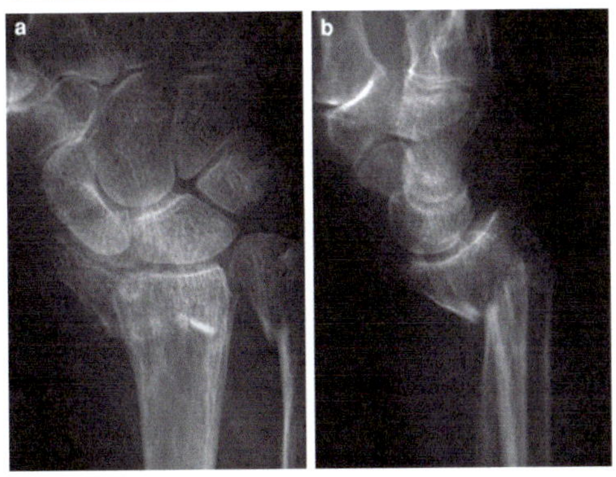

Treatment = Closed reduction + Sugar tong splint

Associations = Median nerve injury + Flexor tendon injury

Complications = Same as Colles'

Center image (Reprinted from Raby N. Imaging of wrist trauma. In: Davies AM, Grainger AJ, James SJ, editors. Imaging of the hand and wrist. Heidelberg: Springer Verlag; 2013. p. 141–69. With permission from Springer Verlag)

Scaphoid Fracture

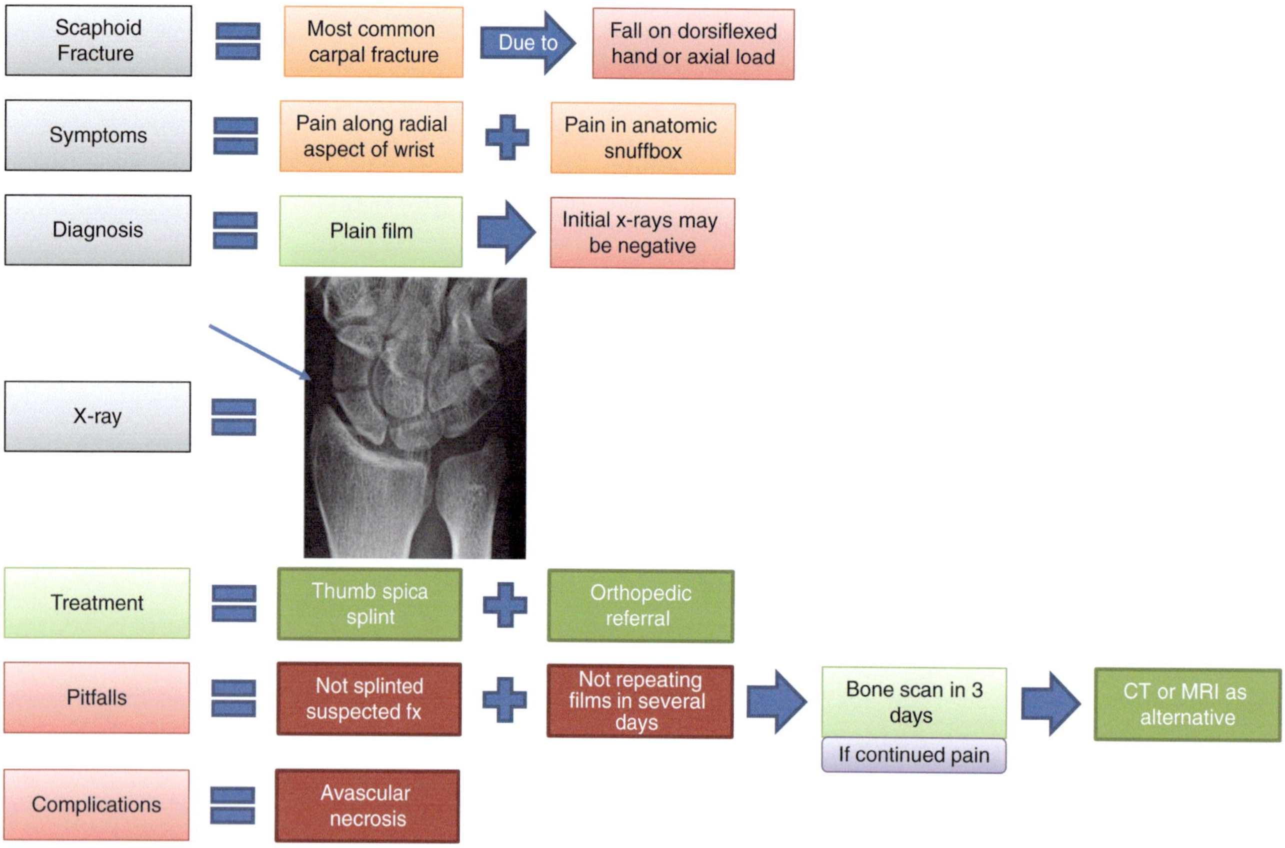

Center image (Reprinted from Raby N. Imaging of wrist trauma. In: Davies AM, Grainger AJ, James SJ, editors. Imaging of the hand and wrist. Heidelberg: Springer Verlag; 2013. p. 141–69. With permission from Springer Verlag)

Triquetral Fracture

Triquetrum Fracture = 2nd most common carpal fracture → May be an avulsion fx

Symptoms = Pain along dorsum of wrist distal to ulnar styloid + Pain to flexion

Diagnosis = Plain film

X-ray =

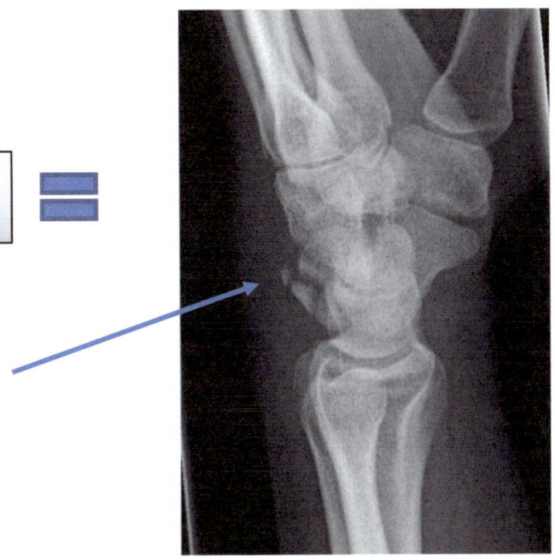

Treatment = Splint + Orthopedic referral

Center bottom image (Reprinted from Raby N. Imaging of wrist trauma. In: Davies AM, Grainger AJ, James SJ, editors. Imaging of the hand and wrist. Heidelberg: Springer Verlag; 2013. p. 141–69. With permission from Springer Verlag)

Other Hand Fracture Tidbits

Lunate Fracture = Occurs with other carpal injuries → Due to → Fall on outstretched hand

Pitfall = Risk of avascular necrosis

Diagnosis = Plain film → May be difficult to isolate lunate from other carpals

Treatment = Splint + Orthopedic referral

Avascular necrosis = Kienbock disease = Lunate collapse + Osteoarthritis + Decreased grip + Chronic pain

Scapholunate Dissociation

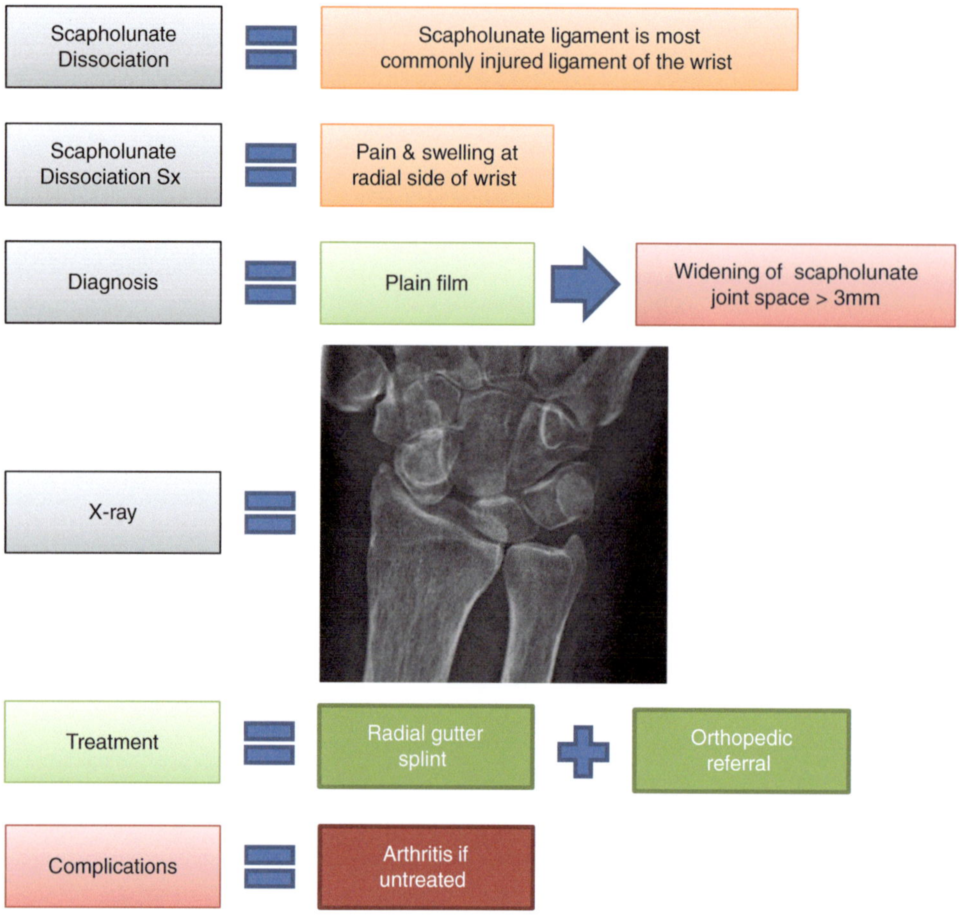

Center image (Reprinted from Raby N. Imaging of wrist trauma davies. In: Davies AM, Grainger AJ, James SJ, editors. Imaging of the hand and wrist. Heidelberg: Springer Verlag; 2013. p. 141–69. With permission from Springer Verlag)

Perilunate and Lunate Dislocations

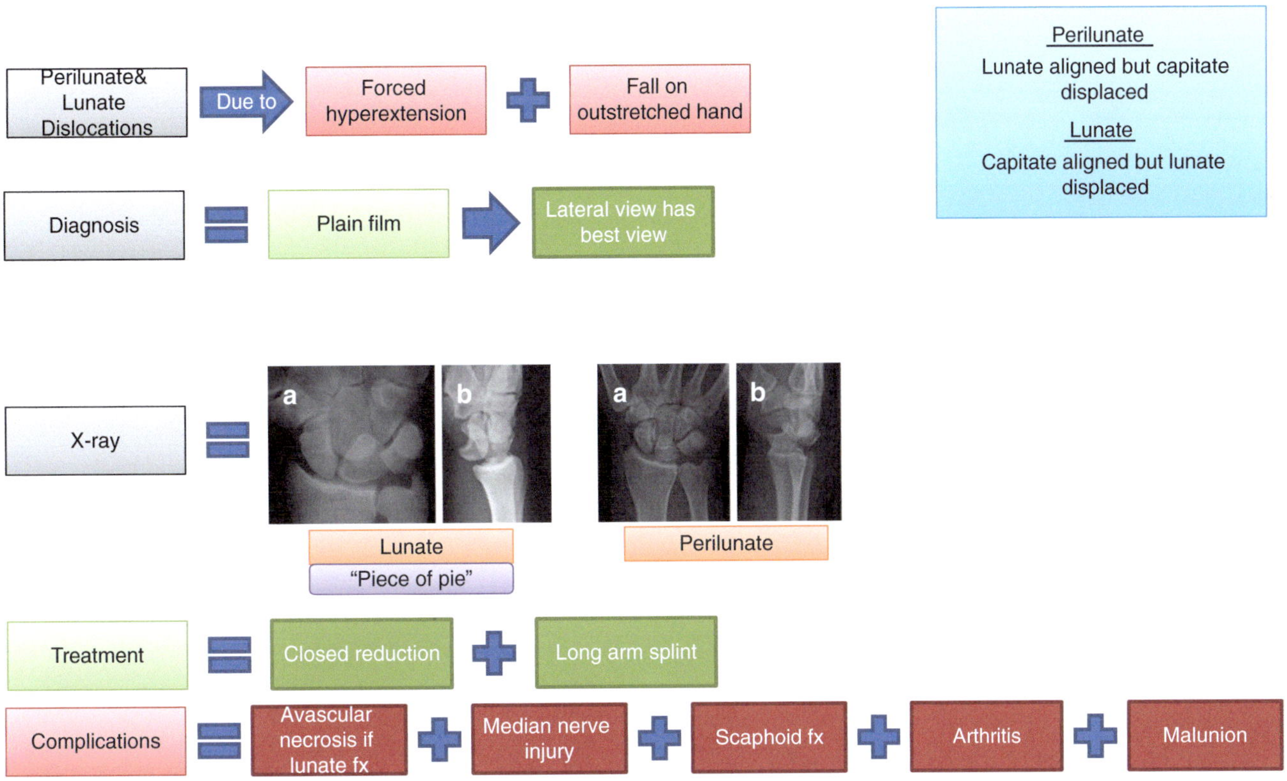

Center left image (Reprinted from Raby N. Imaging of wrist trauma davies. In: Davies AM, Grainger AJ, James SJ, editors. Imaging of the hand and wrist. Heidelberg: Springer Verlag; 2013. p. 141–69. With permission from Springer Verlag)
Center right image (Reprinted from Raby N. Imaging of wrist trauma davies. In: Davies AM, Grainger AJ, James SJ, editors. Imaging of the hand and wrist. Heidelberg: Springer Verlag; 2013. p. 141–69. With permission from Springer Verlag)

The Forearm

Ulnar Nightstick Fracture

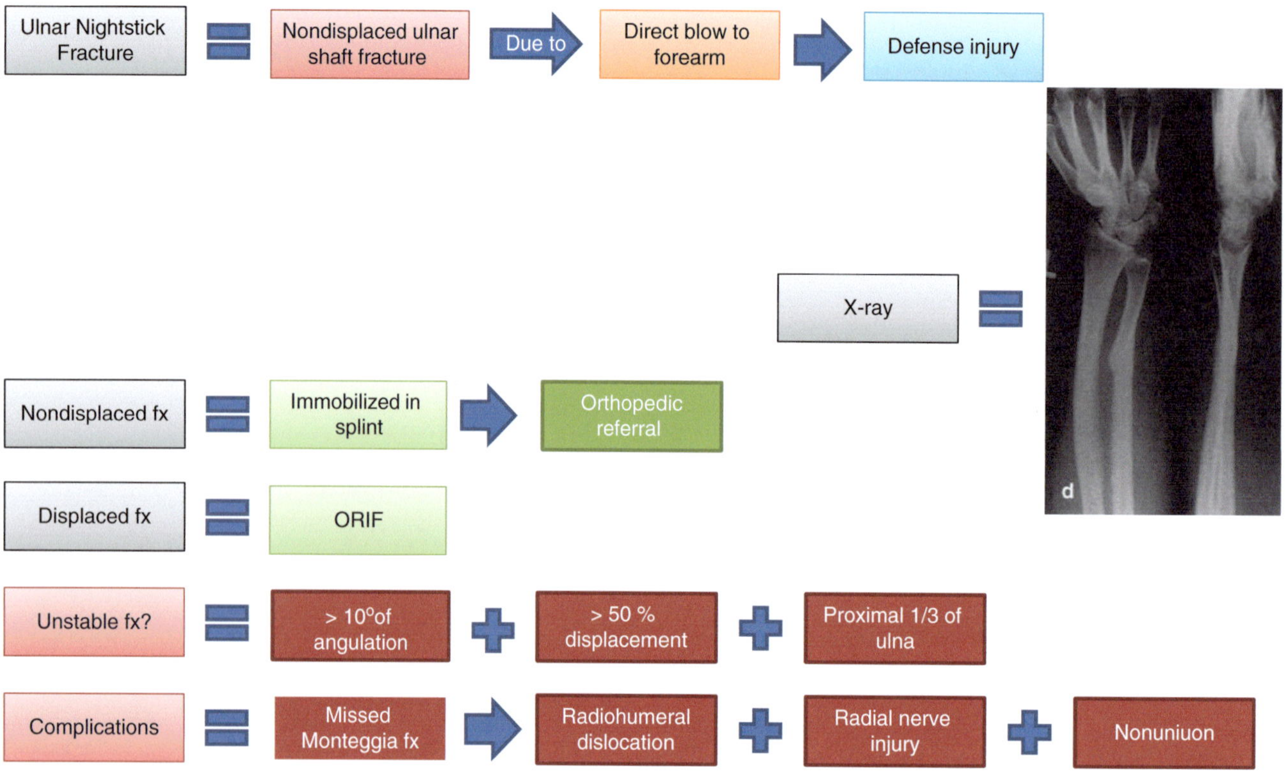

Center right image (Reprinted from De Boeck H, Haentjens P, Handelberg F, Casteleyn PP, Opdecam P. Treatment of isolated distal ulnar shaft fractures with below-elbow plaster cast. Arch Orthop Trauma Surg. 1996;115(6):316–20. With permission from Springer Verlag)

Galeazzi Fracture

Galeazzi Fracture = Fx of distal 1/3 of radial shaft + Dislocation of distal radioulnar joint → Due to: Fall on outstretched hand OR Direct blow

Galeazzi Fracture = Usually displaced

Symptoms = Local tenderness & swelling over distal radius & wrist

Diagnosis = Plain film

MUGR

Monteggia – **U**lna

Galeazzi - **R**adius

X-ray =

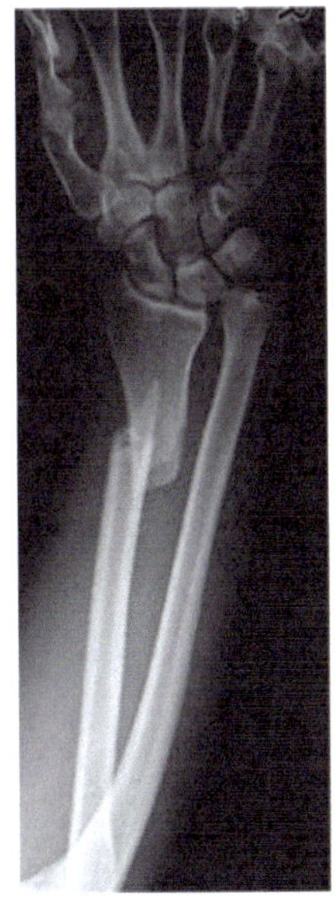

Treatment = ORIF + Sugar tong splint

Complications = Malunion + Ulnar nerve injury

Lower right image (Reprinted from Haugstvedt JR. Galeazzi's fracture and Essex-Lopresti injuries: dislocation fractures of the forearm. In: Hove LM, Lindau T, Hølmer P, editors. Distal radius fractures: current concepts. Heidelberg: Springer Verlag; 2014. p. 391–401. With permission from Springer Verlag)

Monteggia Fracture

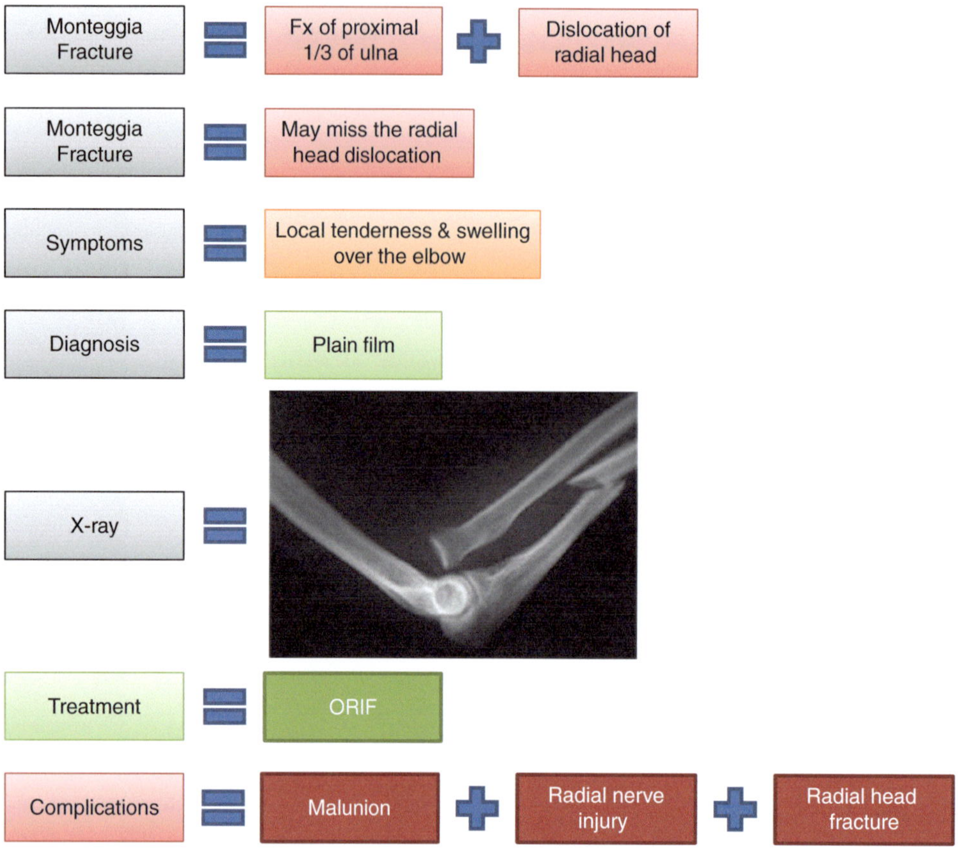

Bottom center image (Reprinted from Casado-Sanz E, Barco R, Antuña SA. Complex fractures of the proximal humerus. In: Rodríguez-Merchán EC, Rubio-Suárez JC, editors. Complex fractures of the limbs. Zug: Springer International Publishing; 2014. p. 1–8. With permission from Springer International Publishing)

Both Ulna and Radius Fractures

Both Ulna & Radius Fractures = Requires significant force → Are usually displaced → Due to → MVC, Fall from height

Symptoms = Local tenderness & swelling over the forearm

Diagnosis = Plain film

X-ray =

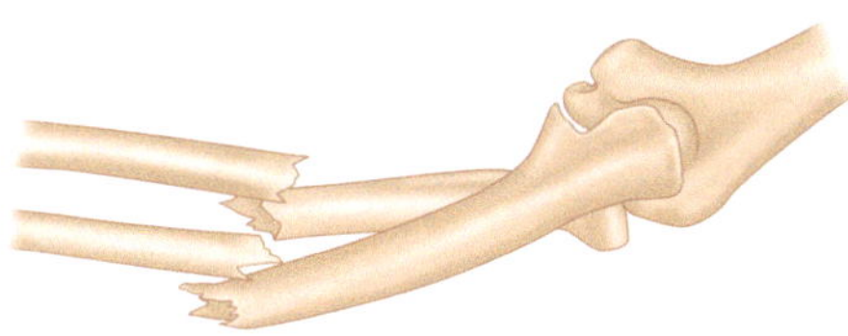

Treatment = Adults: ORIF → Children → Greenstick: Immobilization ‖ Other fx in kids: ORIF

Complications = Inability to supinate & pronate + Neurovascular injury + Compartment syndrome + Non-or malunion + Osteomyelitis

Volkmann's Ischemic Contracture

Volkmann's Ischemic Contracture → Due to → Decreased circulation to the forearm → Typically from unrecognized or delayed treatment of compartment syndrome → Caused by compressive states

Volkmann's Ischemic Contracture = Pronation of forearm + Flexion of wrist & digits + Paralysis of intrinsic muscles

Symptoms & Signs

Pain | Swelling & edema of digits | Paresthesias

Causes = Elbow fracture + Forearm fractures + Inappropriately tight casts

Pitfall = Damage is irreversible in 6 hours = Need for prompt recognition & treatment

Cast + Pain + Numbness = Removal of cast

The Elbow

Soft Tissue Injuries

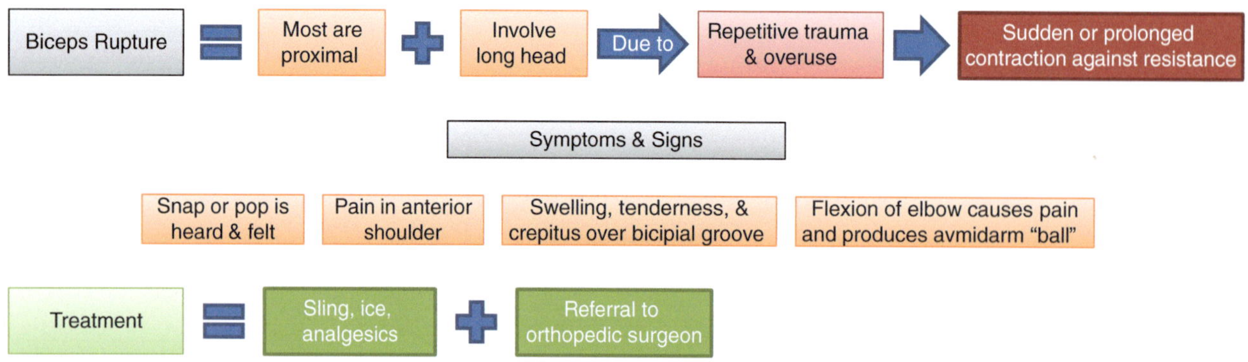

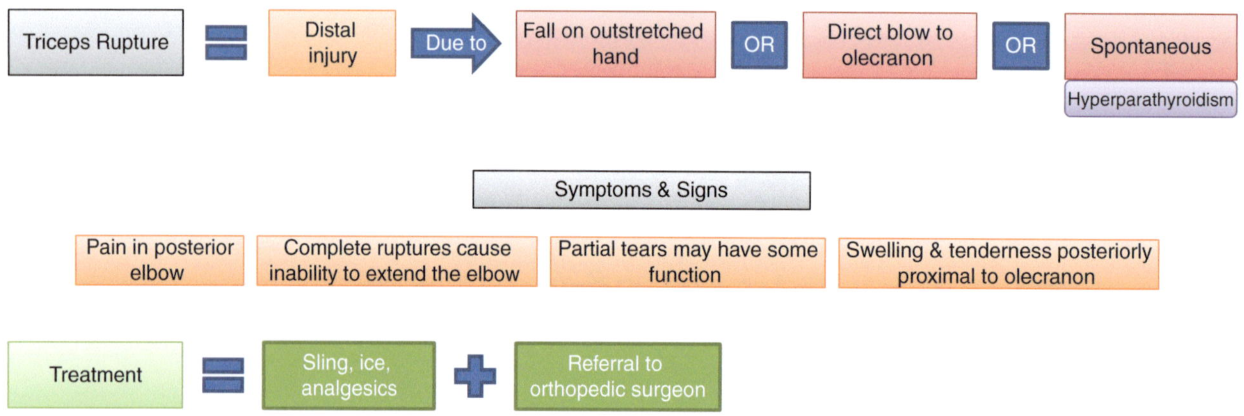

Bursitis

Bursitis = Acute or chronic inflammation of bursa → Olecranon in elbow + Prepatellar in knee → Due to → Repetitive trauma

Pitfall = Not recognizing septic bursitis

Septic bursitis = Abrupt onset of swollen, hot, red & tender area

Diagnosis = Aspiration of fluid → Both diagnostic & therapeutic || Some may need open debridement

Organisms = MRSA + Strep

Treatment non-septic = RICE + NSAID's

Treatment septic = PO vs IV antibiotics → Depends on clinical condition

Epicondylitis

Lateral Epicondylitis = "Tennis elbow" → Due to → Overuse of forearm extensors

Symptoms & Signs

- Tenderness of lateral epicondyle
- Pain on forced extension & supination of forearm against resistance

Treatment = RICE + Anti-inflammatories + Immobilization

Medial Epicondylitis = "Golfer's elbow" → Due to → Overuse of forearm flexors

Symptoms & Signs

- Tenderness of medial epicondyle
- Pain on forced flexion & pronation of forearm, wrist & digits against resistance

Treatment = Sling, ice, analgesics + Anti-inflammatories + Immobilization

Complication = Ulnar neuropathy

Nursemaid's Elbow

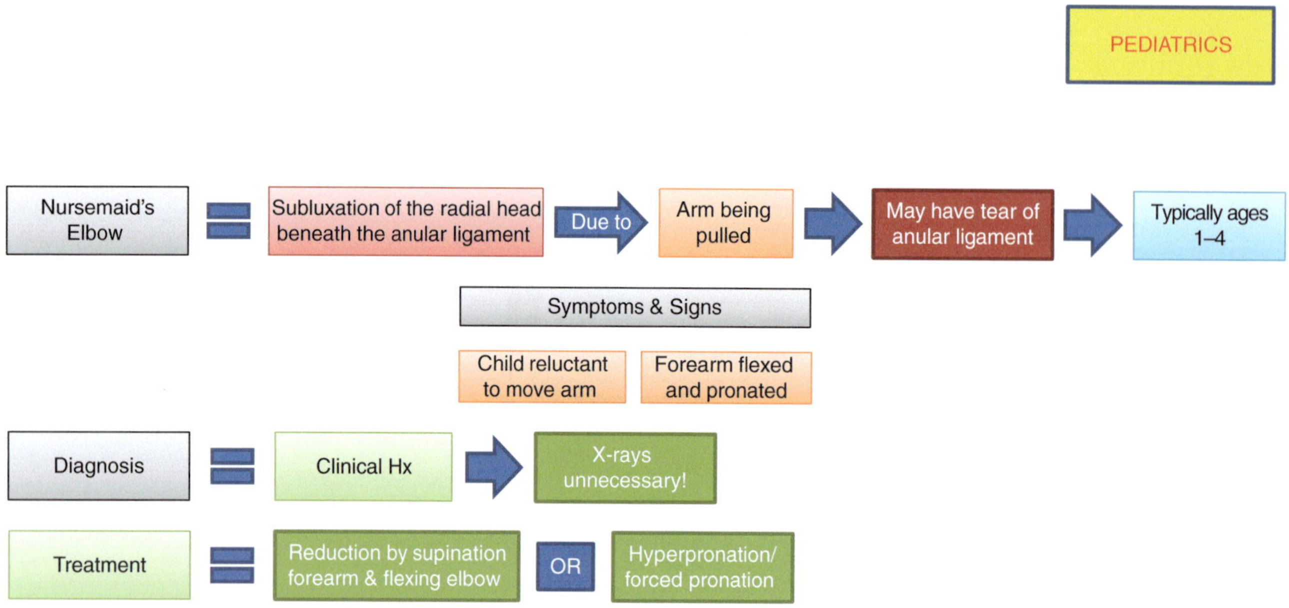

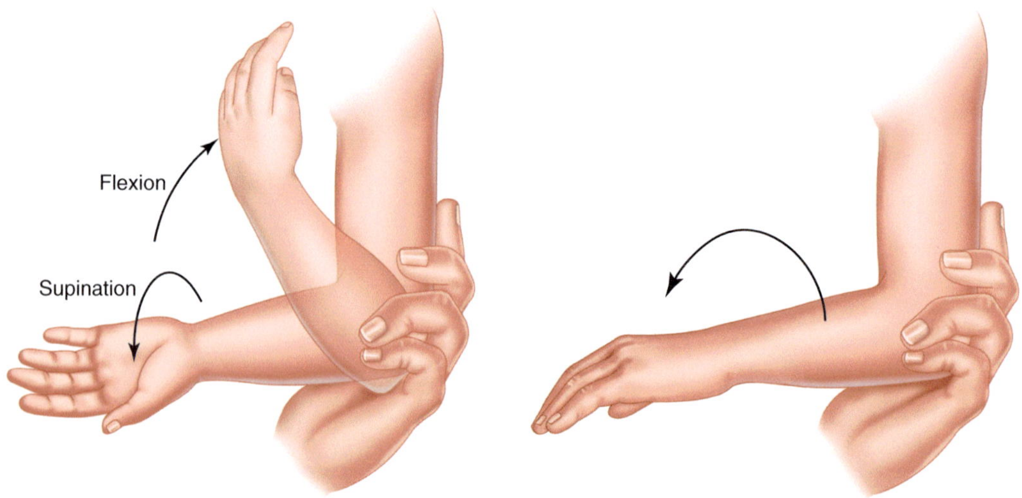

Supination-flexion

Hyperpronation

Elbow Dislocation

Elbow dislocation = Vast majority (90%) are posterior → Due to → Fall on outstretched hand

Elbow dislocation = Pt presents with elbow in 45° flexion → Must assess neurovascular status = Brachial artery (Most common arterial injury) + Ulnar nerve (Most common nerve injury) / Radial nerve / Median nerve

Consider Arterial injury? = No radial pulse + Open dislocation = Arteriogram

X-ray =

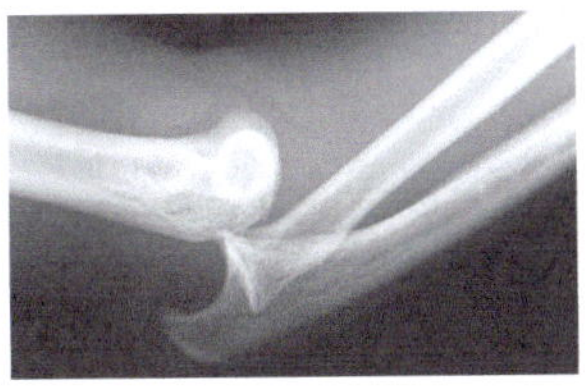

→ Children may have associated medial epicondyle fx || Coronoid process fx? = Unstable

Treatment = Closed reduction → Longitudinal traction of wrist & forearm + Long arm posterior splint + Orthopedic consultation

Pitfalls = Hyperextension → Causes bleeding from arterial injury

Complications = Malunion + Median nerve injury + Joint instability + Arthritis

Left center image (Reprinted from Spina V, Baldini L. Imaging of the elbow. In: Celli A, Celli L, Morrey BF, editors. Treatment of elbow lesions: new aspects in diagnosis & surgical techniques. Milan: Springer Verlag; 2008. p. 21–38. With permission from Springer Verlag)

Elbow Fracture Tidbits

Elbow Fractures = Radial head + Proximal ulna + Distal humerus

Radiologic signs = Anterior fat pad → A small one may be seen normally → Large one is abnormal = "Sail sign"

Radiologic signs = Posterior fat pad → Never normal

Posterior fat pad = Intraarticular hemorrhage OR Intracapsular hemorrhage OR Occult radial head fx OR Gout, synovitis or other infections

Anterior humeral line test = Picks up occult supracondylar fx → In normal imaging, the anterior aspect of the humerus bisects middle 1/3 of capitellumon the lateral view

Radial Head Fracture

Radial Head Fracture = Most common fx of the elbow / Most common occult fx in adults — Due to → Fall on outstretched hand → Radial head is driven into the capitellum → May have additional injury

May have additional injury:
- Capitellum fx
- Coronoid fx
- Olecranon fx
- Elbow dislocation
- MCL injury
- Avulsion fx of medial epicondyle

Symptoms & Signs: Lateral elbow pain; Lateral elbow swelling; Tenderness of radial head; Pain with passive rotation of forearm

Diagnosis = Plain film → Look for fat pads

X-ray =

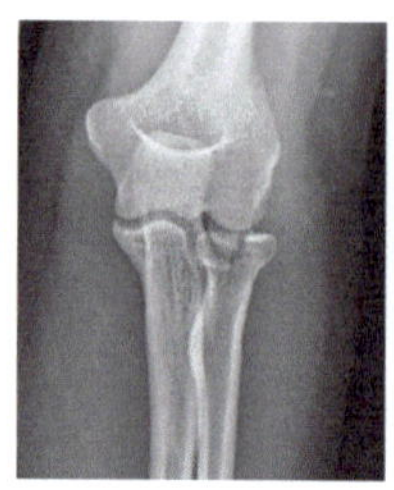

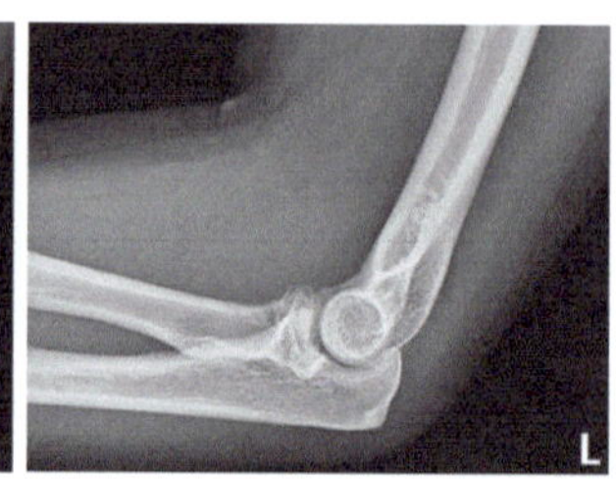

Treatment Non-displaced = Immobilization + RICE

Displaced Fx OR Decreased ROM = Surgical repair

Complications = Restricted elbow ROM + Chronic pain

Right center image (Reprinted from Daneshvar P, Pollock JW, Athwal GS. Fractures and dislocations of the proximal ulna and radial head. In: Antuña S, Barco R, editors. Essentials in elbow surgery. London: Springer Verlag; 2014. p. 61–89. With permission from Springer Verlag)

Right image (Reprinted from Daneshvar P, Pollock JW, Athwal GS. Fractures and dislocations of the proximal ulna and radial head. In: Antuña S, Barco R, editors. Essentials in elbow surgery. London: Springer Verlag; 2014. p. 61–89. With permission from Springer Verlag)

Supracondylar Fracture

Supracondylar Fracture = Most common fx of the elbow in children → Extension type (>95 %) (Posterior displacement) OR Flexion type (<5 %) (Anterior displacement)

Extension type = Fall on outstretched hand || Flexion type = Direct force anteriorly to a flexed elbow

Symptoms & Signs

- Edema around elbow
- Tenderness of elbow
- Prominent olecranon
- Depression proximal to elbow
- ± medial or lateral displacement

Diagnosis = Plain film

X-ray =

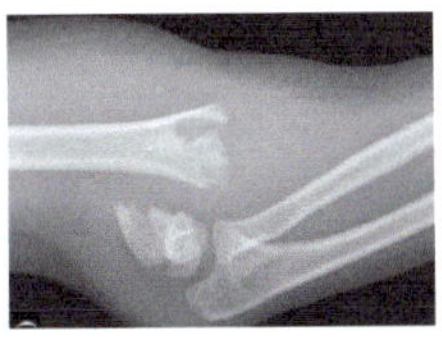

Treatment Displaced fx = Reduction + Emergent orthopedic consultation

Complications = Brachial artery injury (Vascular compromise) + Nerve injury (Median, Radial) + Compartment syndrome + Eventual Volkmann's contracture

Left center image (Reprinted from Abdelgawad A, Enes Kanlic. Orthopedic trauma. In: Abdelgawad A, Naga O, editors. Pediatric orthopedics: a handbook for primary care physicians. New York: Springer; 2014. p. 409–83. With permission from Springer Science + Business Media)

The Humerus and Shoulder

Proximal Humerus Fracture

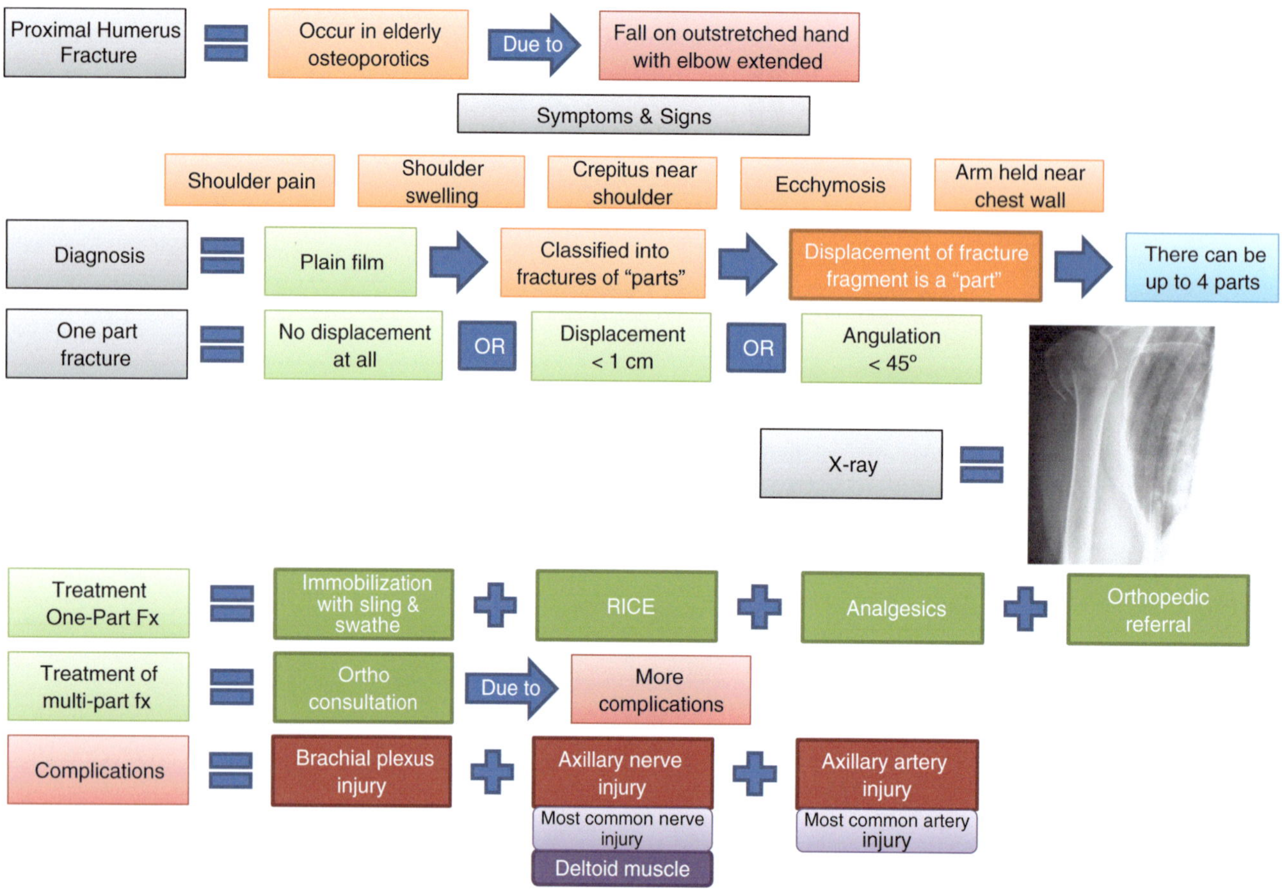

Right center image (Reprinted from Erhardt JB, Roderer G, Grob K, Forster TN, Stoffel K, Kuster MS. Early results in the treatment of proximal humeral fractures with a polyaxial locking plate. Arch Orthop Trauma Surg. 2009;129(10):1367–74. With permission from Springer Science + Business Media)

Humerus Shaft Fracture

Humerus Shaft Fracture = Occur in elderly osteoporotics & young men → Due to → Fall on outstretched hand = Spiral fx + Direct blow = Transverse fx

Most commonly in middle 1/3 of humerus

Symptoms & Signs

Localized tenderness | Arm swelling | Arm pain | Abnormal mobility | Crepitus on palpation | May have shortening with displaced fx

Diagnosis = Plain film → Displacement of fx fragments is common → Due to → Actions of various muscles

X-ray =

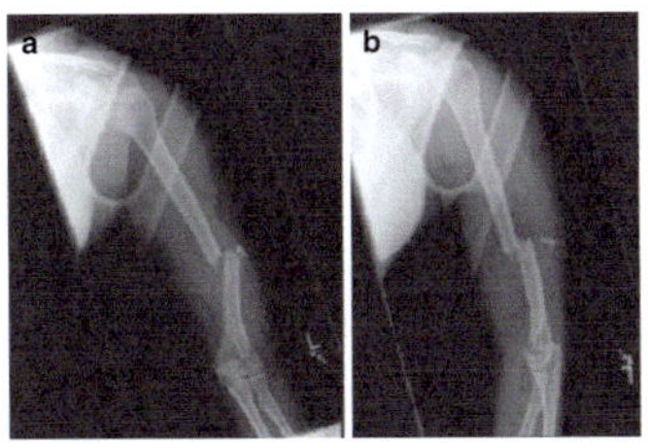

Treatment = Immobilization with sling & swathe + RICE + Analgesics + Orthopedic referral

Complications = Brachial artery or vein injury + Radial, median or ulnar nerve injury → Radial is most common nerve injury = Wrist drop & decreased sensation at dorsal thumb-index web space

Left center image (Reprinted from Ristevski B, Hall J. Humeral shaft fractures. In: Sethi MK, editor. Orthopedic traumatology: an evidence-based approach. New York: Springer Science. 2014. p. 129–40. With permission from Springer Science + Business Media)

Nontraumatic Shoulder Pain

Nontraumatic Shoulder Pain = Intrinsic causes + Extrinsic causes

Extrinsic causes = Referred pain → Heart | Gallbladder | Spleen | Lungs | Liver | Neck

Intrinsic causes = Rotator cuff tendinitis + Impingement syndrome + Adhesive capsulitis

Rotator cuff tendinitis = Secondary to repetitive over head use of arm → Active ROM painful & limited + Passive ROM is full & impeded → Impingement syndrome can occur

Rotator cuff = Supraspinatus + Infraspinatus + Teres minor + Subscapularis

Treatment = Immobilization for comfort → Rotator cuff strengthening exercises + RICE + Analgesics

Adhesive capsulitis = After long period of immobilization → Painful & limited ROM → Both active & passive

Sternoclavicular Injuries

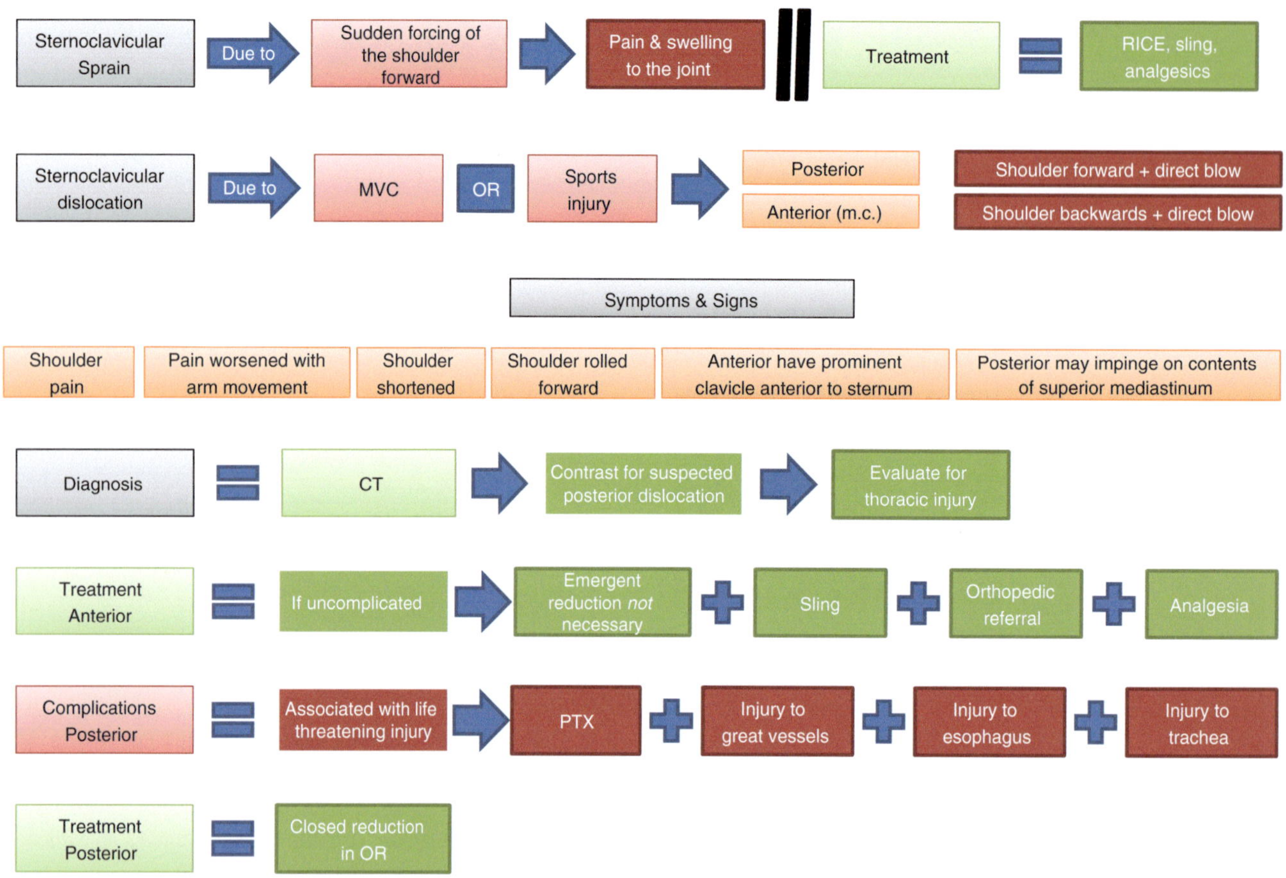

Acromioclavicular (AC) Injuries

Acromioclavicular Sprain → Due to → Direct trauma to AC joint → Fall with arm adducted

Diagnosis = Clinical

Symptoms & Signs

- Shoulder pain
- Tender at AC joint
- Painful to move arm across body

Type	Injury	Imaging
Type 1	Sprain of AC ligament	Normal
Type 2	AC rupture, coracoclavicular (CC) ligament sprain	Clavicle 25–50 % above acromion
Type 3	AC rupture, CC rupture	AC joint dislocated 100 %, CC interspace widened up to 100 %
Type 4	All supporting structures ruptured	Appear similar to 2 & 3

Types 5 & 6 have AC dislocation, gross deformity and have potential for multiple associated injuries

Treatment Types 1 & 2 = Immobilization with sling & swathe + RICE + Analgesics + Orthopedic referral

Treatment Types 3–6 = Severe injury → Orthopedic evaluation → Surgical repair

Clavicle Fracture

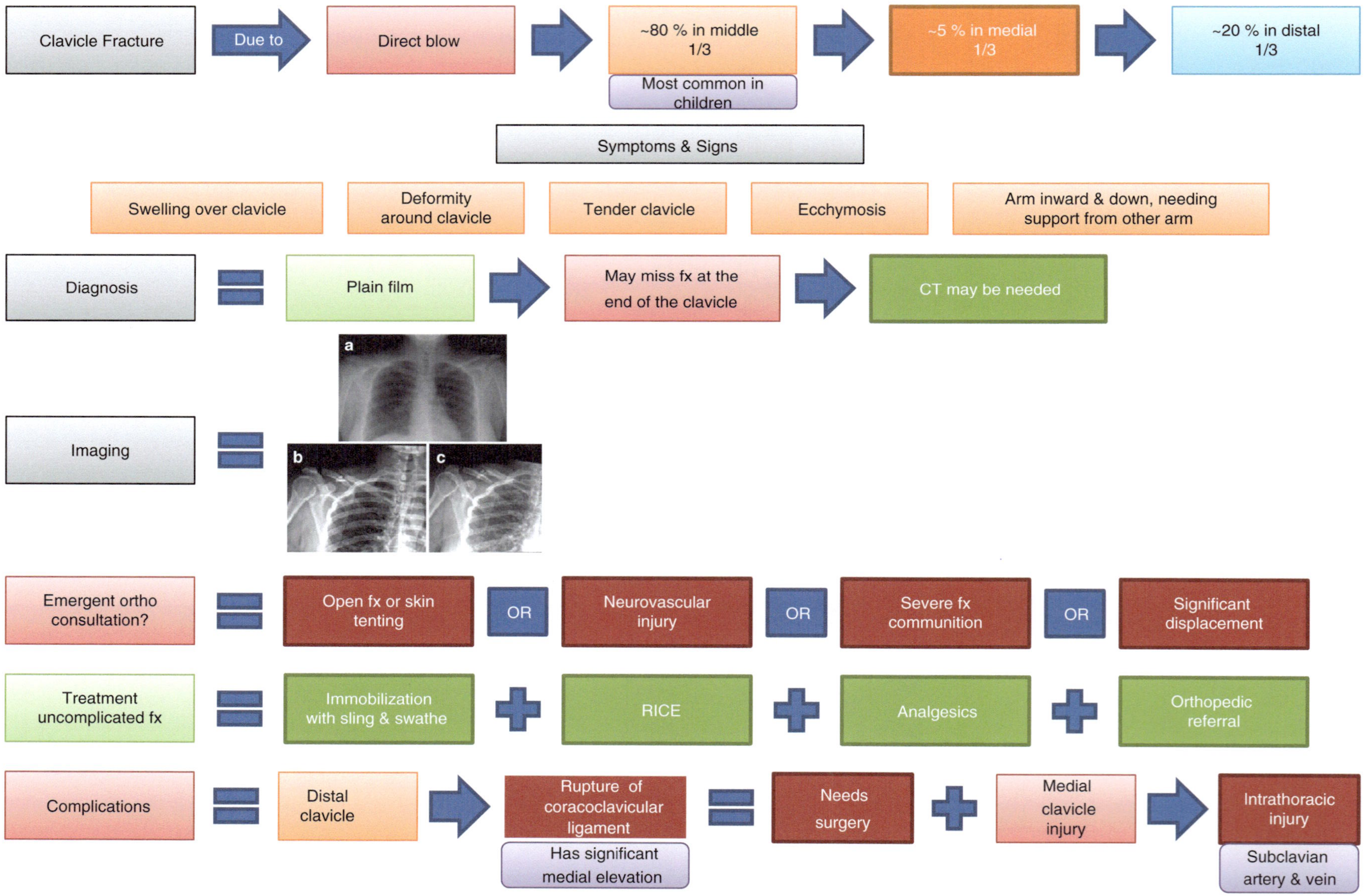

Left center image (Reprinted from Geddes CR, McKee MD. Clavicle fractures. In: Sethi MK, editor. Orthopedic traumatology: an evidence-based approach. New York: Springer Science. 2014. p. 87–102. With permission from Springer Science + Business Media)

Scapula Fracture

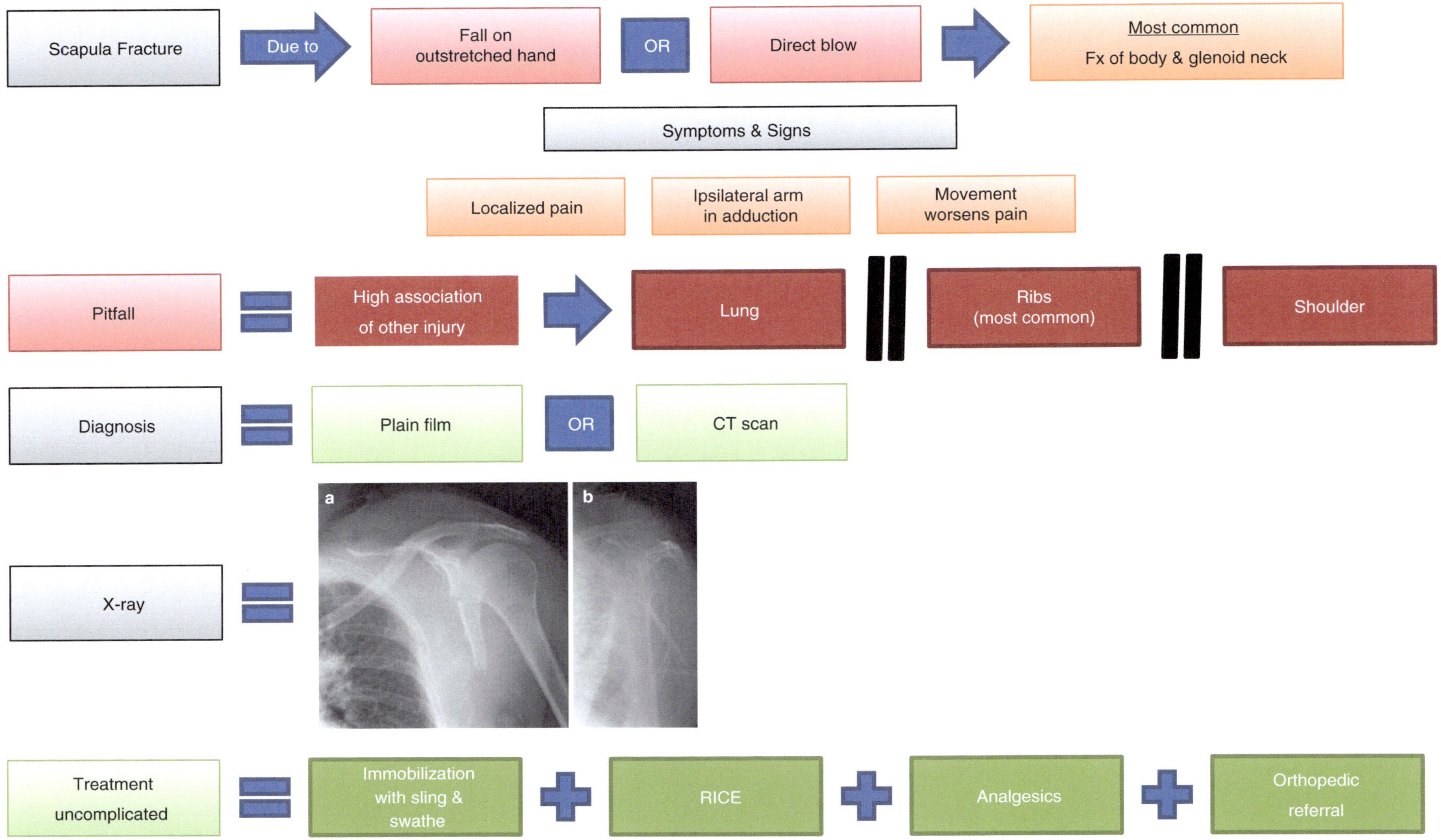

Bottom center image (Reprinted from Cole PA, Hill BW. Scapula fractures. In: Sethi MK, editor. Orthopedic traumatology: an evidence-based approach. New York: Springer Science. 2014. p. 71–86. With permission from Springer Science + Business Media)

Shoulder Dislocations: Anterior

Shoulder dislocations = Anterior 99 % + Posterior <1 % + Inferior = Luxatio erecta

Anterior Shoulder dislocations = Subcoracoid (most common) + Subglenoid + Subclavicular + Intrathoracic

- Subcoracoid (most common): Anterior to glenoid & inferior to coracoid
- Subglenoid: Inferior & anterior to glenoid
- Subclavicular: Medial to coracoid below the clavicle
- Intrathoracic: Between the ribs & thoracic cavity

Mechanism = Indirect blow to arm → Arm is abducted, extended & externally rotated

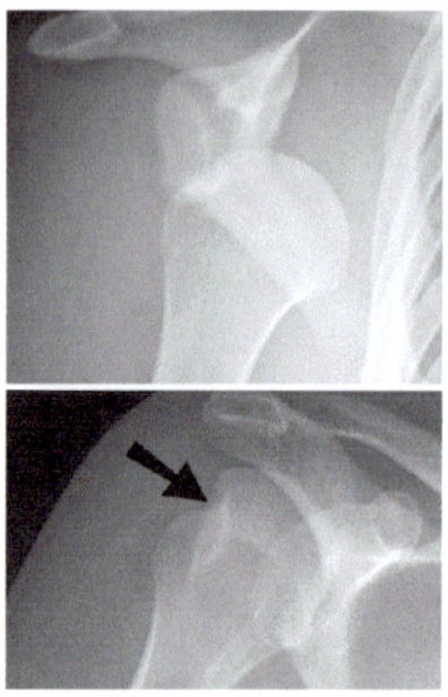

Anterior d/l with Hill-Sach's deformity (bottom)

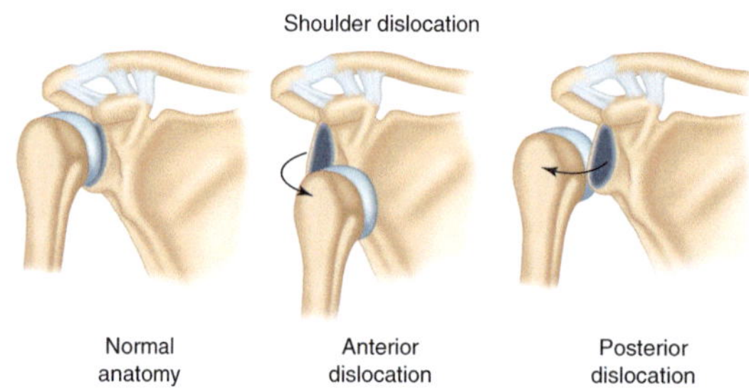

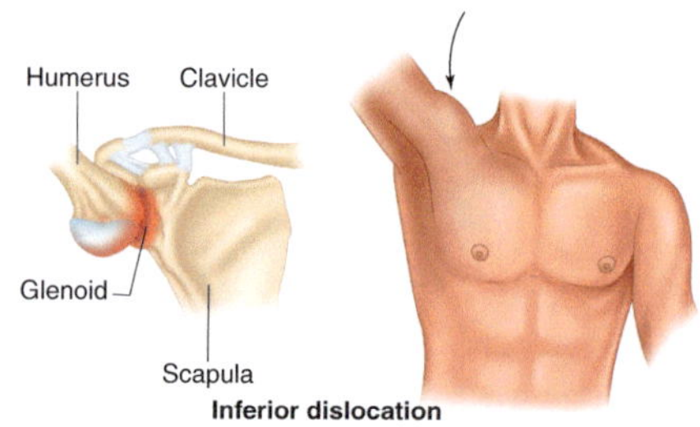

Symptoms & Signs

- Arm in abduction & external rotation
- Resists abduction & internal rotation
- Potential axillary nerve injury

Bottom left image (Reprinted from Missiroli C, Singh A. Emergencies of the biliary tract. In: Singh A, editor. Emergency radiology: Imaging of acute pathologies. New York: Springer Science; 2013. p. 11–25. With permission from Springer Science + Business Media)

Diagnosis and Treatment: Anterior

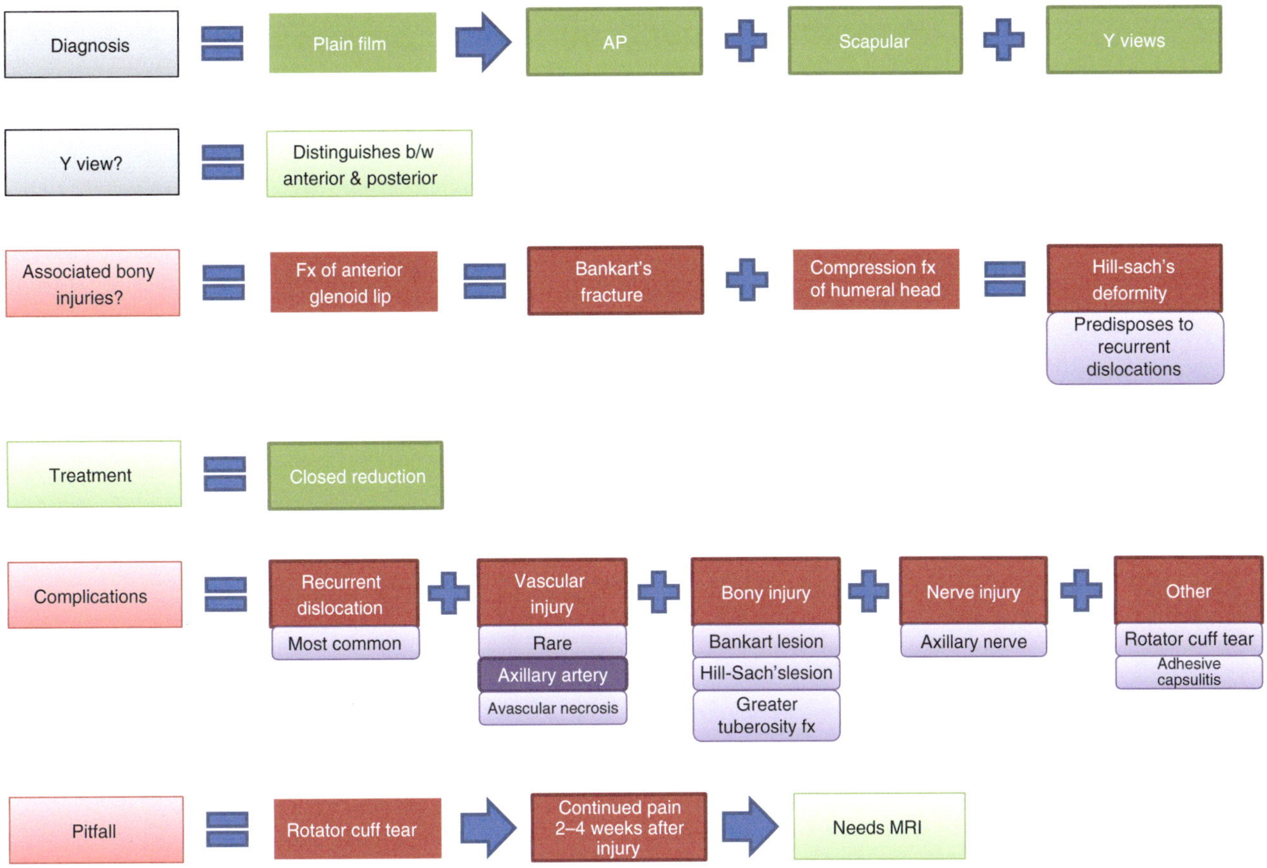

Shoulder Dislocations: Posterior

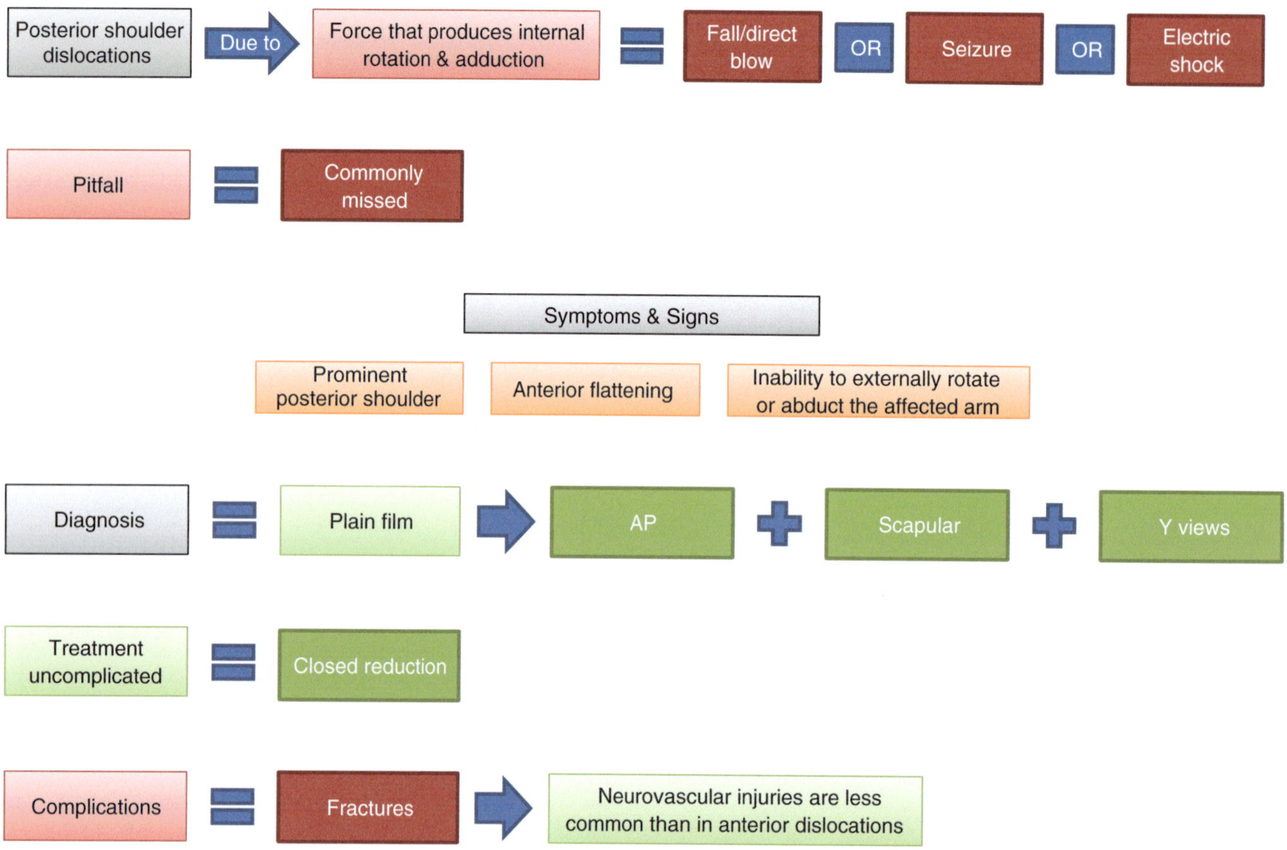

Shoulder Dislocations: Inferior

Inferior shoulder dislocation = Luxatio erecta → Due to → Hyperabduction force → Tearing inferior capsule → Pushing humeral head inferiorly

Symptoms & Signs

- Humerus is fully abducted
- Arm raised with hand above head
- Elbow is flexed
- Ecchymosis
- Arm held near chest wall

Diagnosis = Plain film

Treatment = Closed reduction + RICE + Analgesics + Orthopedic referral

Complications = Proximal humerus fx + Rotator cuff injuries (All patients will have this) + Severe soft tissue injury + Inability to reduce (Will need surgery)

Rotator Cuff Injuries

Rotator Cuff Injuries = Typically 40–50 years of age → Due to → Tear of SITS muscles → Partial tear is more common

SITS Muscles = ***S***upraspinatus + ***I***nfraspinatus + ***T***eres Minor + ***S***ubscapularis

Symptoms & Signs

- Muscle weakness
- Atrophy
- Decreased abduction
- Decreased external rotation
- Arm held near chest wall

Diagnosis = Clinical → MRI may be needed

Most common muscle injury? = Supraspinatus

Muscles of Rotator Cuff

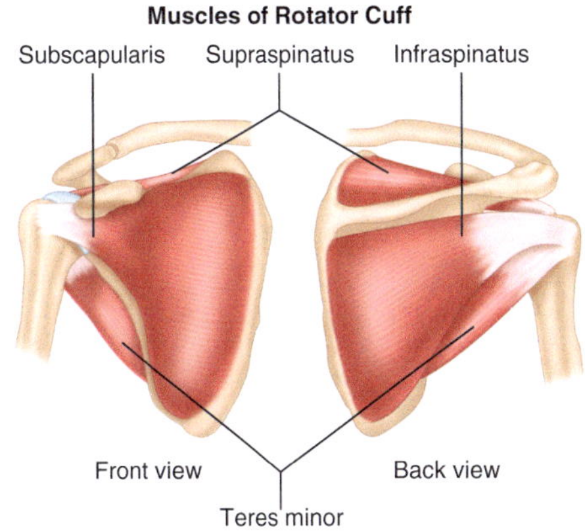

Thoracic Outlet Syndrome (TOS)

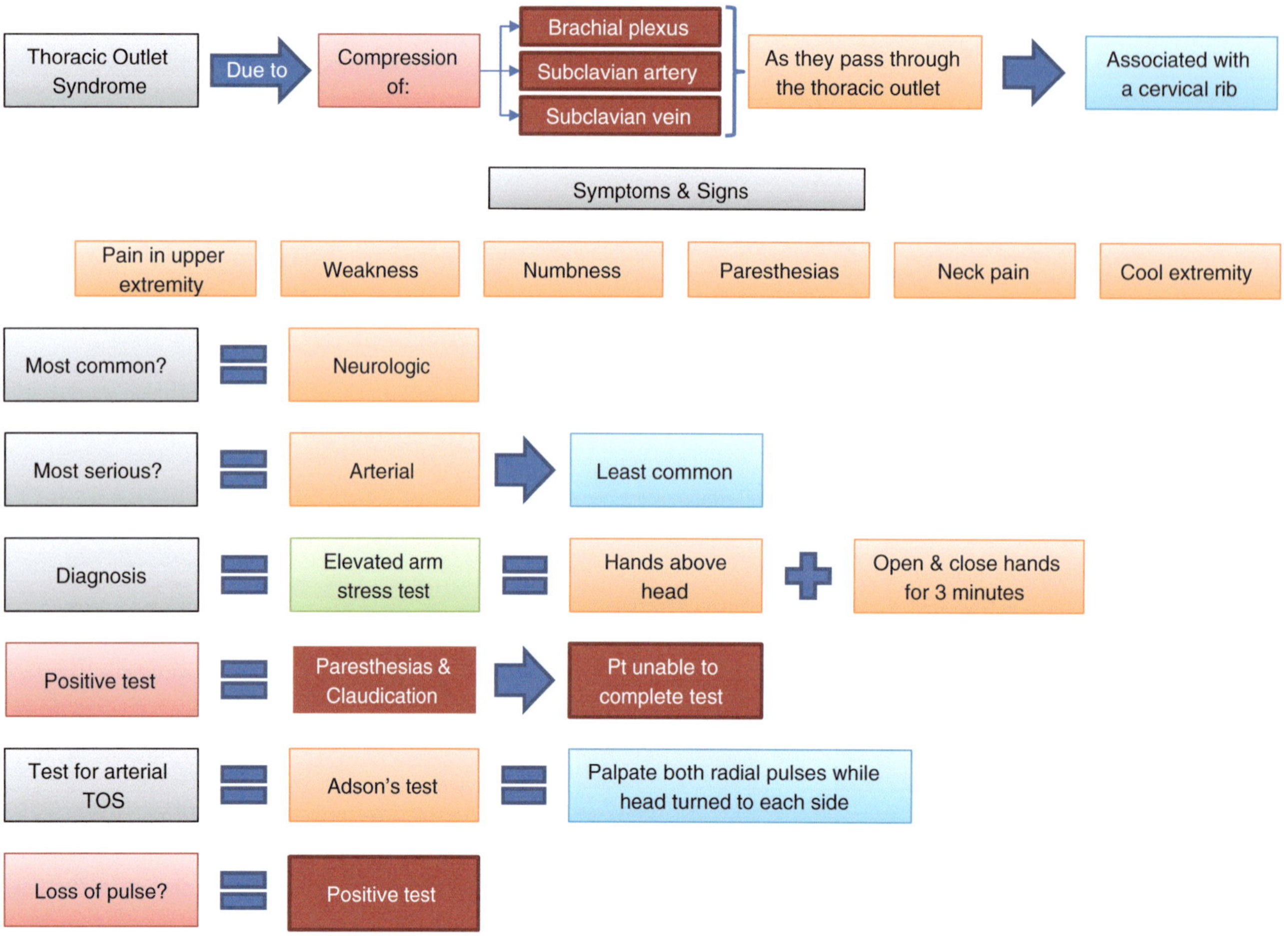

Nontraumatic Hip Disorders

Legg-Calve-Perthes Disease

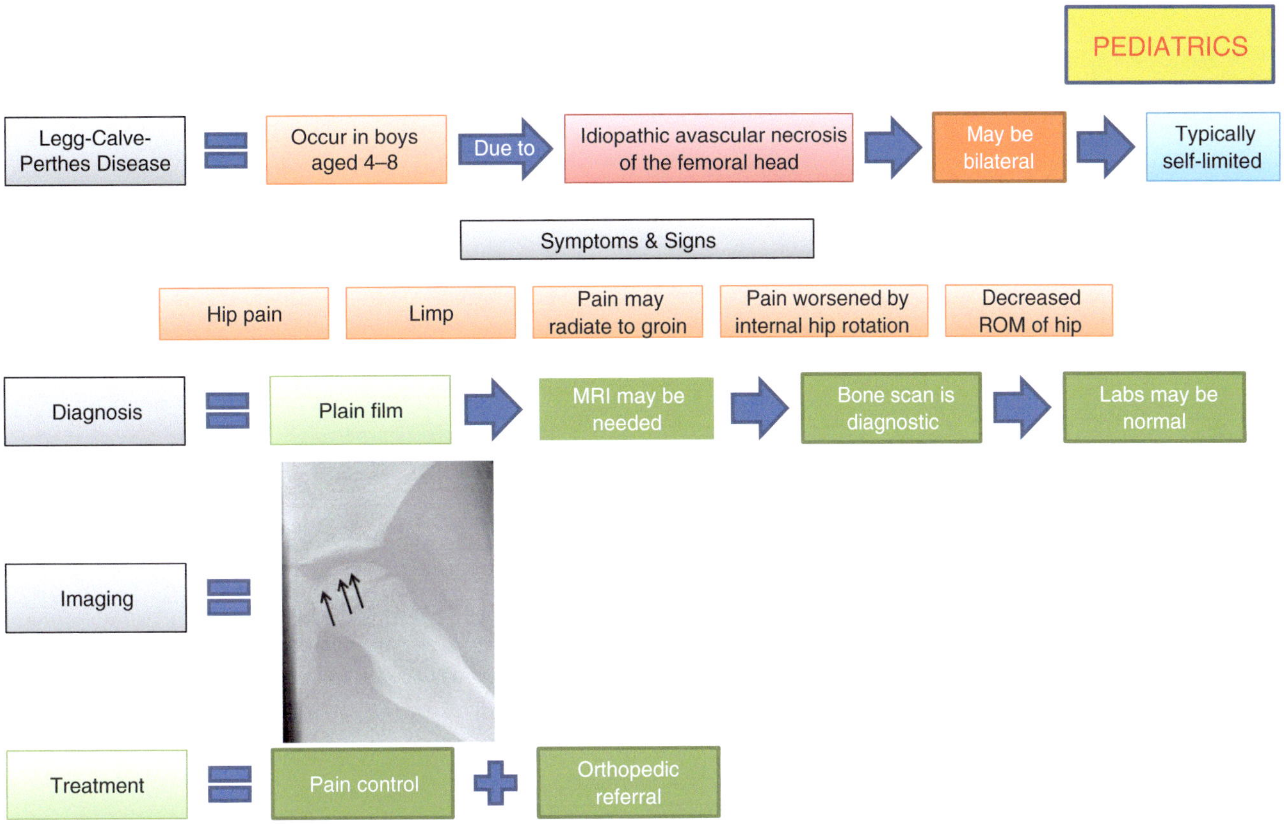

Left center image (Reprinted from Abdelgawad A, Naga O. The hip. In: Abdelgawad A, Naga O, editors. Pediatric orthopedics: a handbook for primary care physicians. New York: Springer; 2014. p. 85–116. With permission from Springer Science + Business Media)

Slipped Capital Femoral Epiphysis

PEDIATRICS

Slipped Capital Femoral Epiphysis = Occur in obese boys aged 10–16 → Unknown cause → May be bilateral → Typically self-limited

Slipped Capital Femoral Epiphysis = Most common cause of hip disability in adolescents

Symptoms & Signs

- Hip pain
- Limp
- Pain may radiate to groin
- Pain worsened by internal hip rotation
- Decreased ROM of hip

Diagnosis = Plain film → Frog leg view → "Melting ice cream cone"

Imaging =

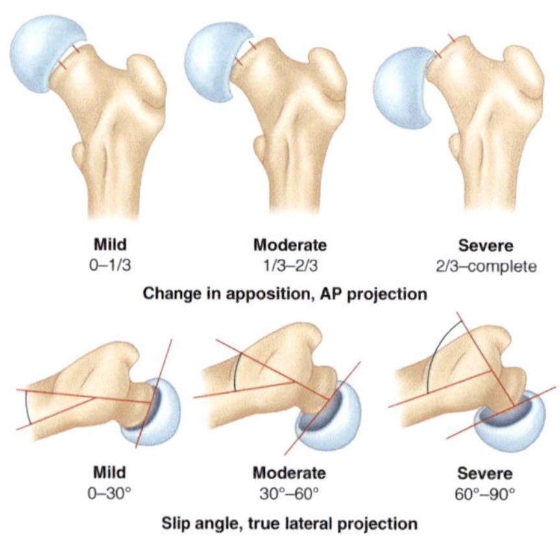

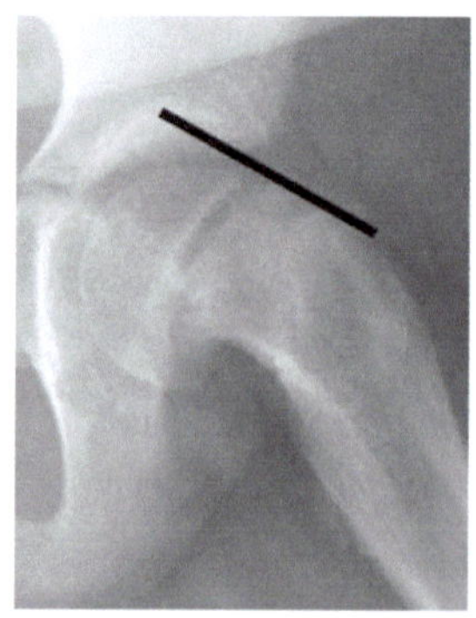

Treatment = No weight bearing + ORIF

Right center image (Reprinted from Abdelgawad A, Naga O. The hip. In: Abdelgawad A, Naga O, editors. Pediatric orthopedics: a handbook for primary care physicians. New York: Springer; 2014. p. 85–116. With permission from Springer Science + Business Media)

Septic Arthritis

PEDIATRICS

Septic arthritis = Occur in all age ranges → Most common cause of painful hip in *infants* → Hip & knee most common → Usually from hematogenous spread

Organisms = *Salmonella* (Sickle cell) + *S. aureus* (Most common) + *H. influenza* + *N. gonorrhoeae* (Adolescents) + Strep spp + Gram negatives

Symptoms & Signs → May be subtle!

- Pseudoparalysis — Infants
- Fever, Localizing signs, Refusal to ambulate — Older children
- Erythema
- Hip tenderness
- Decreased ROM of hip

Plain films = Frequently nondiagnostic early → May see widening of joint spaces → Fat lines may be displaced

Ultrasound = May see joint effusion

Diagnosis = Arthrocentesis + Labs → May see elevated WBC & CRP

Treatment = IV antibiotics + Joint drainage by orthopedics

Septic Arthritis Tidbits

Septic arthritis mechanisms = Hematogenous spread + Direct extension

Newborn causes = *Staphylococcus aureus* + Group B Streptococcus + *Neisseria* + Enterobacter

Children = *Staphylococcus aureus* + *Streptococcus pyogenes* + *Streptococcus pneumoniae* + *Hemophilus influenzae* + Other Gram (-) bacilli

Young sexually active adults = *Staphylococcus aureus* + *Streptococcus* + *Neisseria*

Direct extension = *Staphylococcus aureus* most common

Sickle cell disease = *Salmonella*

Joint prosthesis = Early *Staphylococcus* + Late Gram (-)'s

IV Drug Users = Involves axial skeleton → *Pseudomonas*

Toxic Synovitis

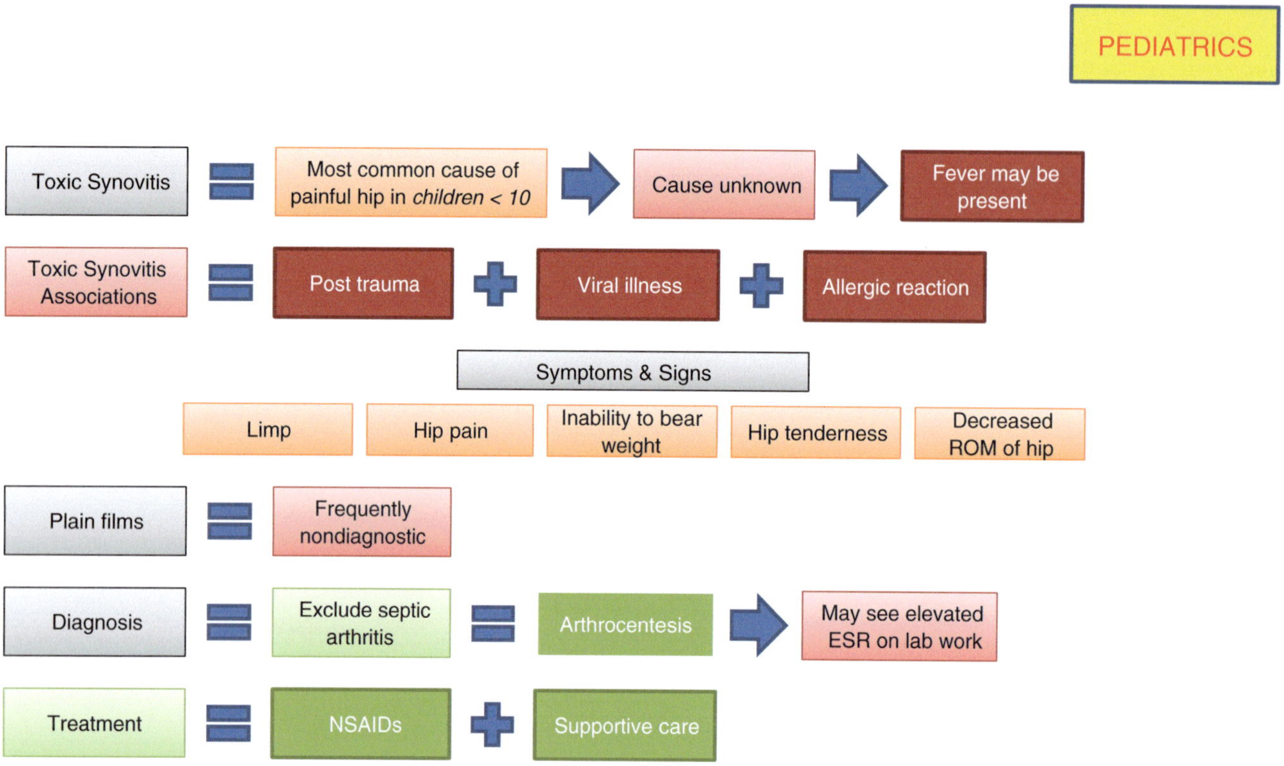

The Femur

Femoral Shaft Fracture

Femoral Shaft Fracture = Occur in younger patients → Due to → High energy trauma → MVC + Falls

Fx types due to direct trauma = Transverse (most common) OR Oblique or spiral oblique fx OR Comminuted

Pathologic fx → Due to → Primary bone tumors → Osteogenic sarcoma OR Metastases → Breast, lung, prostate

Symptoms & Signs

Shortening of leg | Leg deformity | Leg swelling | Severe pain | Inability to bear weight

Diagnosis = Plain film

Imaging =

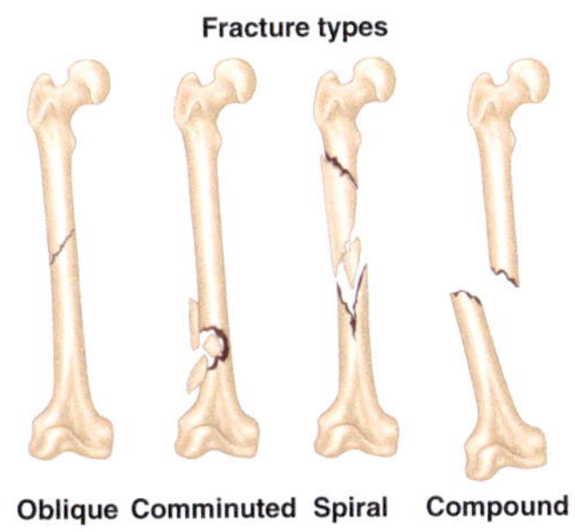

Treatment = Traction splint & Ortho consult → But… → Not for open fracture with contaminated ends OR Potential for sciatic injury = These need ORIF!

Complications = Neurovascular injury + Fat emboli + Hemorrhage + Post traumatic arthritis

The Knee

The Knee Tidbits

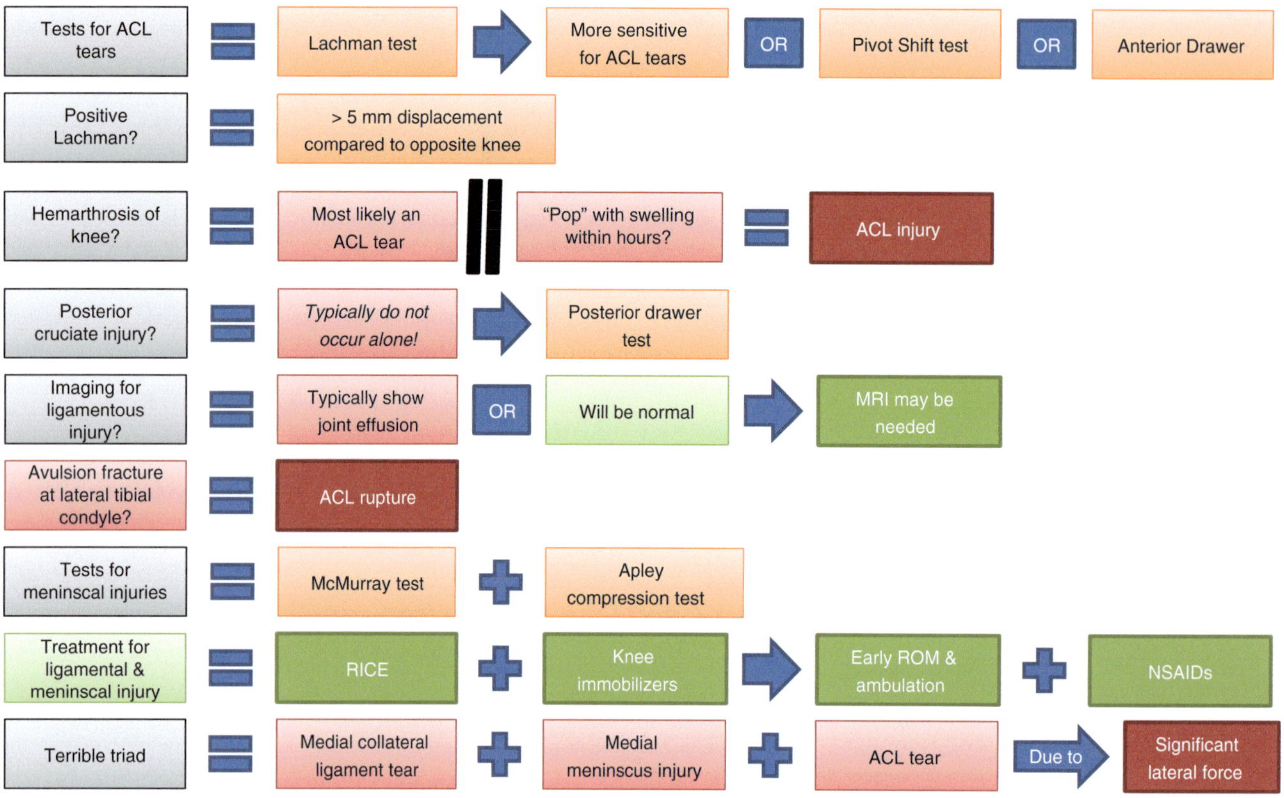

Ottawa Knee Rules

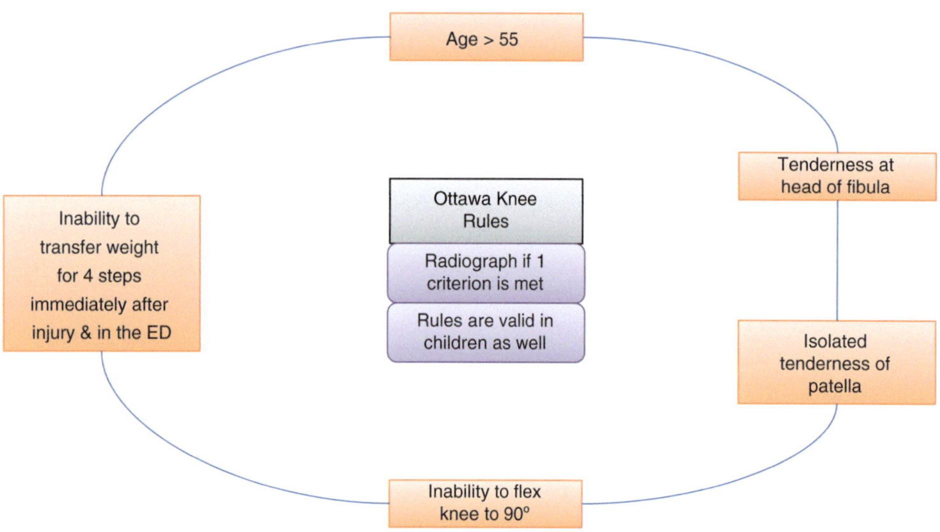

Patellar Fractures

Patellar Fractures → Due to → Typically a direct blow → Transverse fx most common → More likely to be displaced + Associated with extensor mechanism disruption

Symptoms & Signs

- Local patella tenderness
- Knee swelling
- Knee effusion
- Ecchymosis

Diagnosis = Plain film

X-ray =

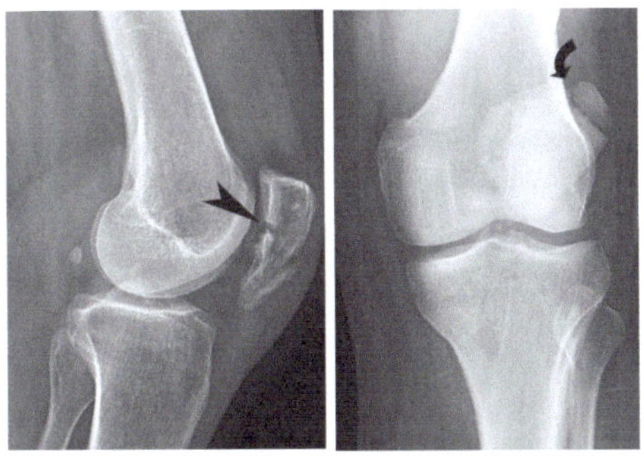

Treatment non-displaced = Knee Immobilizer + RICE + Analgesics + Orthopedic referral

Surgical treatment? = Displacement > 3mm OR Open fracture OR Severe comminution OR Rupture of extensor mechanism

Left center image (Reprinted from Kaewlai R, Singh A. Lower extremity trauma. In: Singh A, editor. Emergency radiology: imaging of acute pathologies. New York: Springer Science; 2013. p. 277–98. With permission from Springer Science + Business Media)
Center image (Reprinted from Kaewlai R, Singh A. Lower extremity trauma. In: Singh A, editor. Emergency radiology: imaging of acute pathologies. New York: Springer Science; 2013. p. 277–98. With permission from Springer Science + Business Media)

Patellar Dislocation

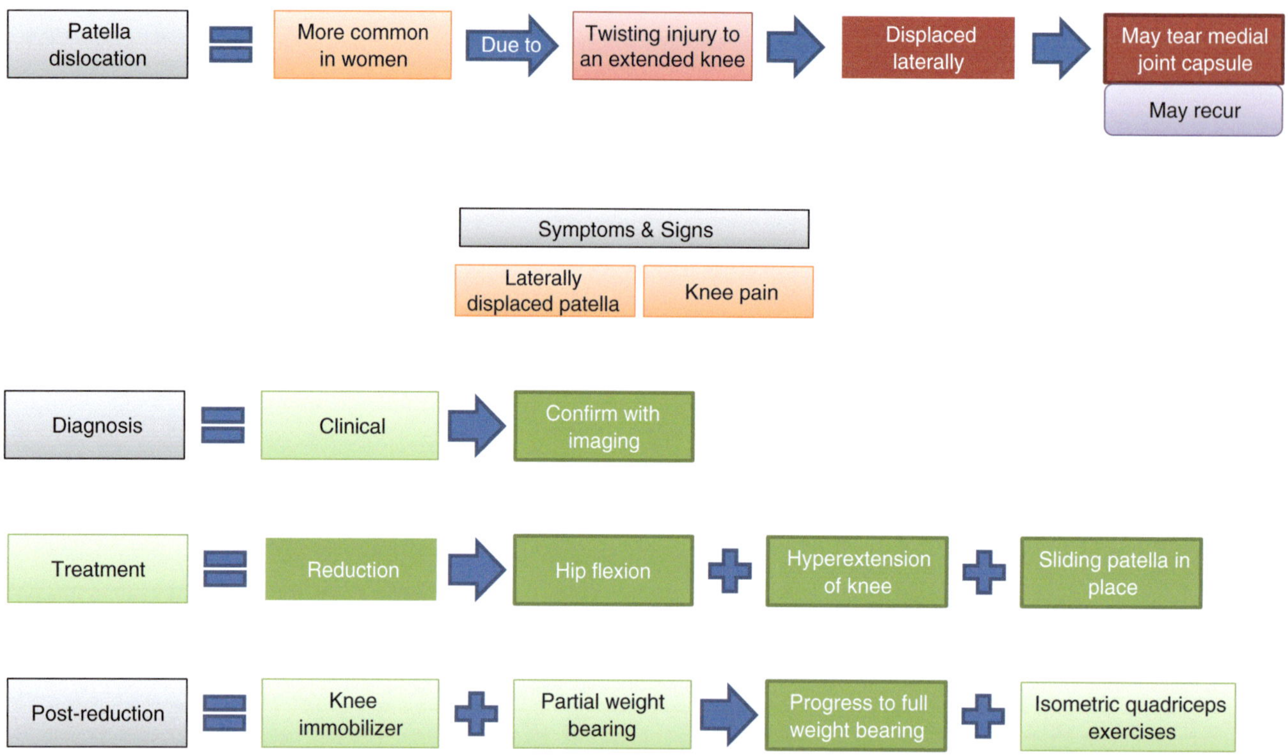

Tibial Plateau Fractures

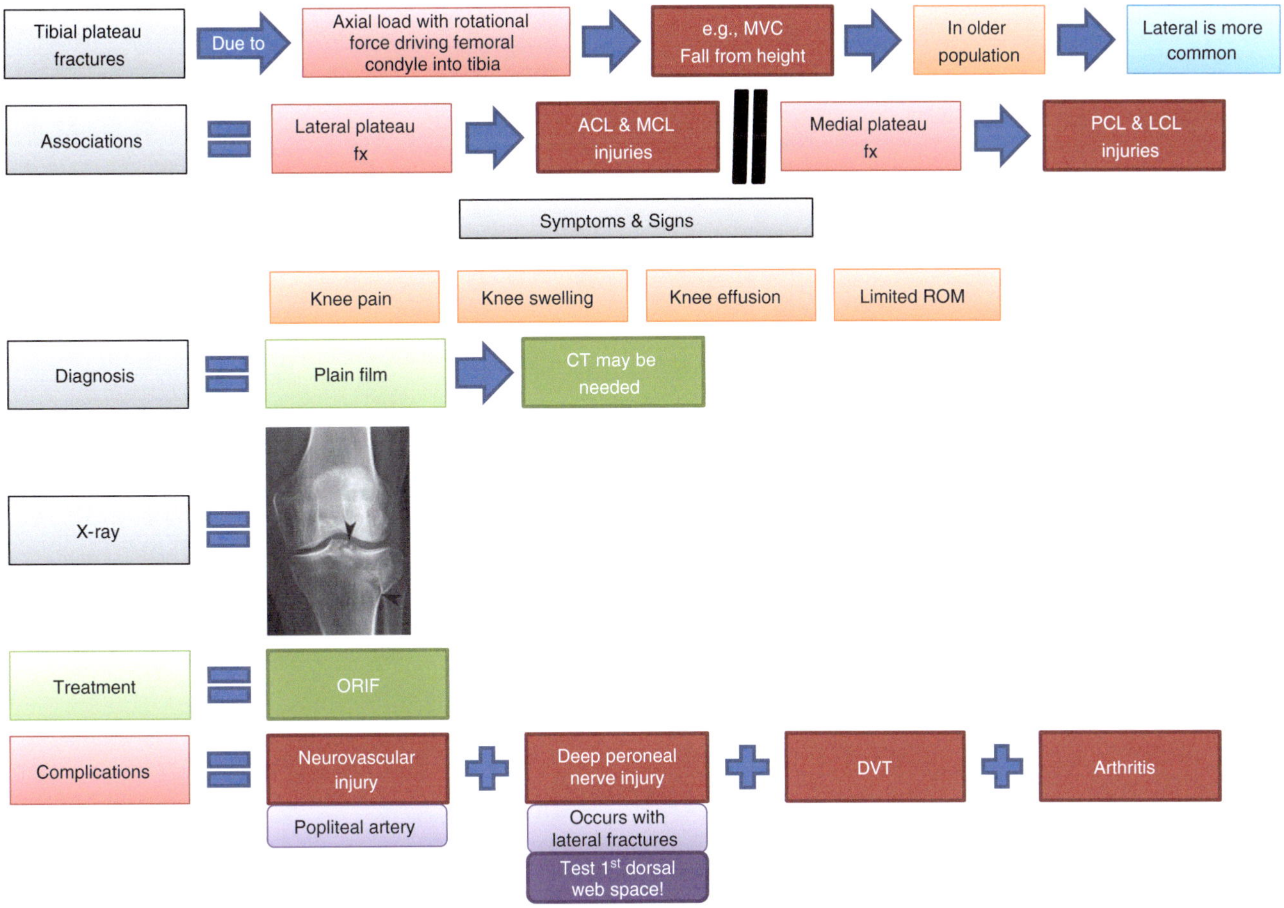

Left center image (Reprinted from Kaewlai R, Singh A. Lower extremity trauma. In: Singh A, editor. Emergency radiology: imaging of acute pathologies. New York: Springer Science; 2013. p. 277–98. With permission from Springer Science + Business Media)

Knee Dislocation

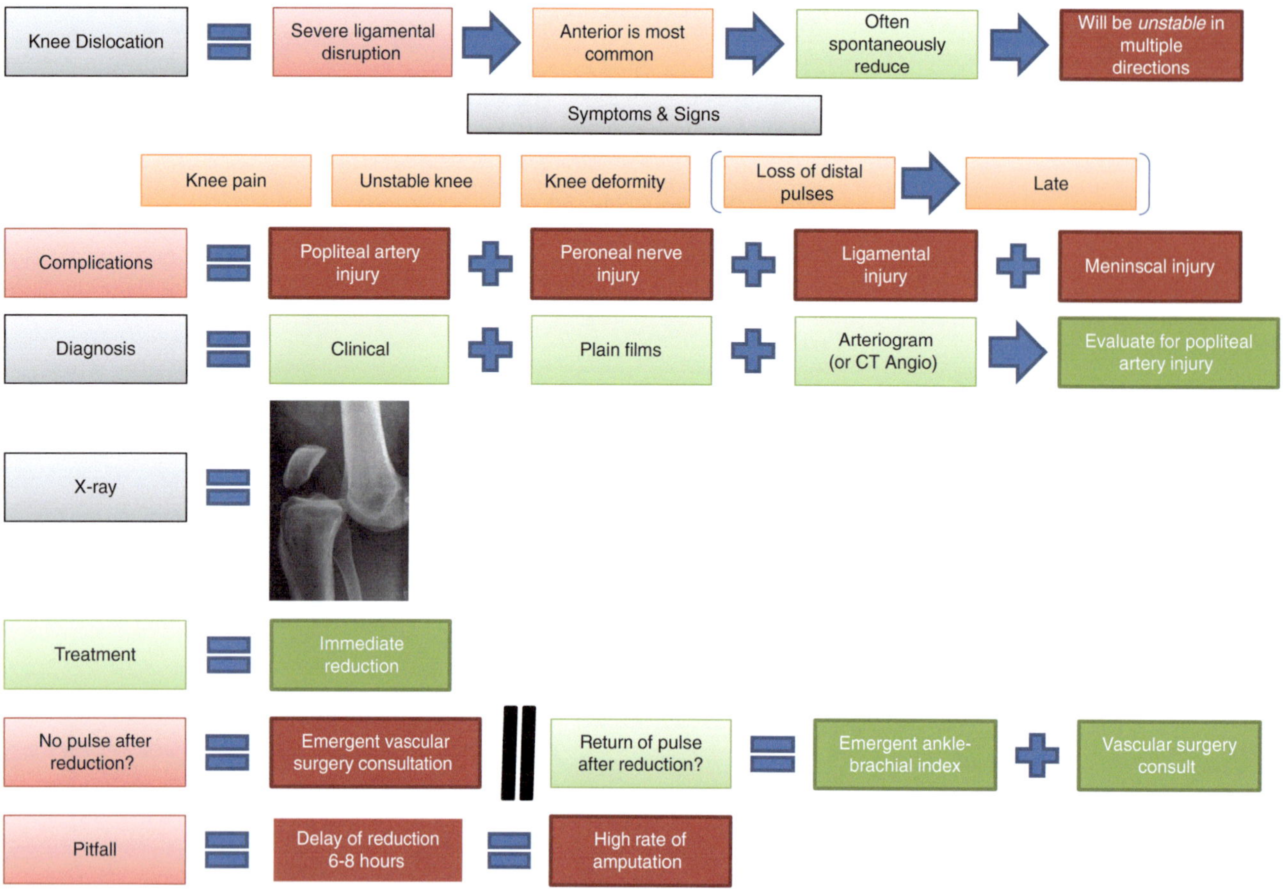

Left center image (Reprinted from Kaewlai R, Singh A. Lower extremity trauma. In: Singh A, editor. Emergency radiology: imaging of acute pathologies. New York: Springer Science; 2013. p. 277–98. With permission from Springer Science + Business Media)

Tendon Rupture: Quadriceps and Patella

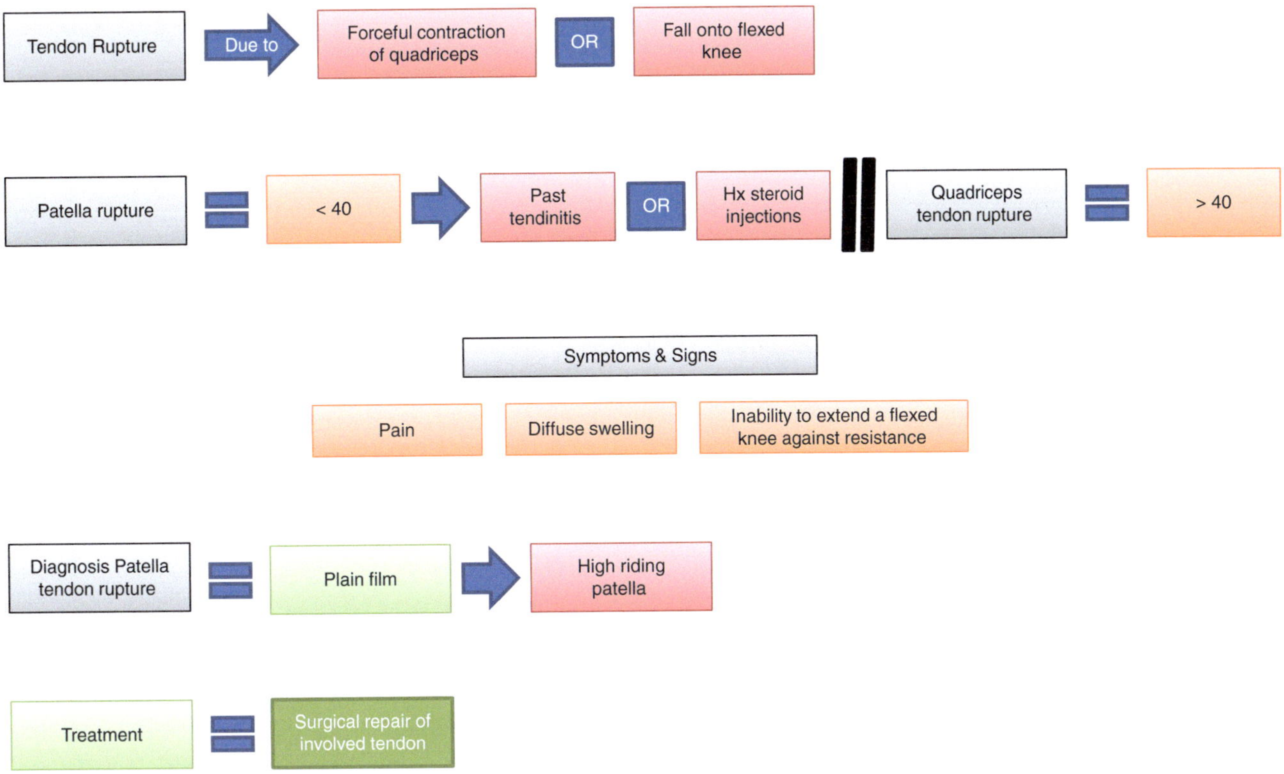

Osteochondritis Dissecans

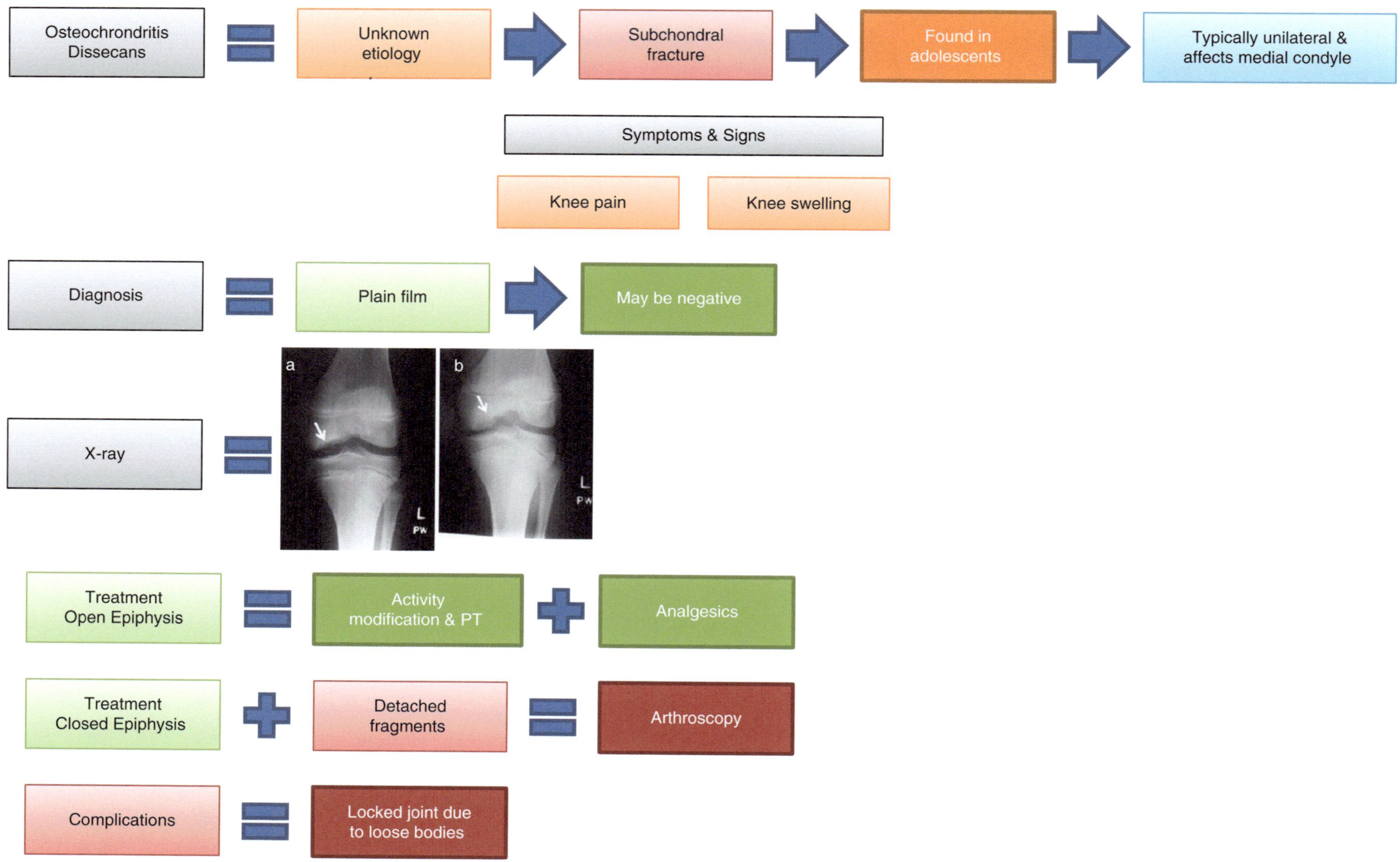

Left center image (Reprinted from Abdelgawad A, Naga O. The knee/leg. In: Abdelgawad A, Naga O, editors. Pediatric orthopedics: a handbook for primary care physicians. New York: Springer; 2014. p. 117–56. With permission from Springer Science + Business Media)

Osgood-Schlatter Disease

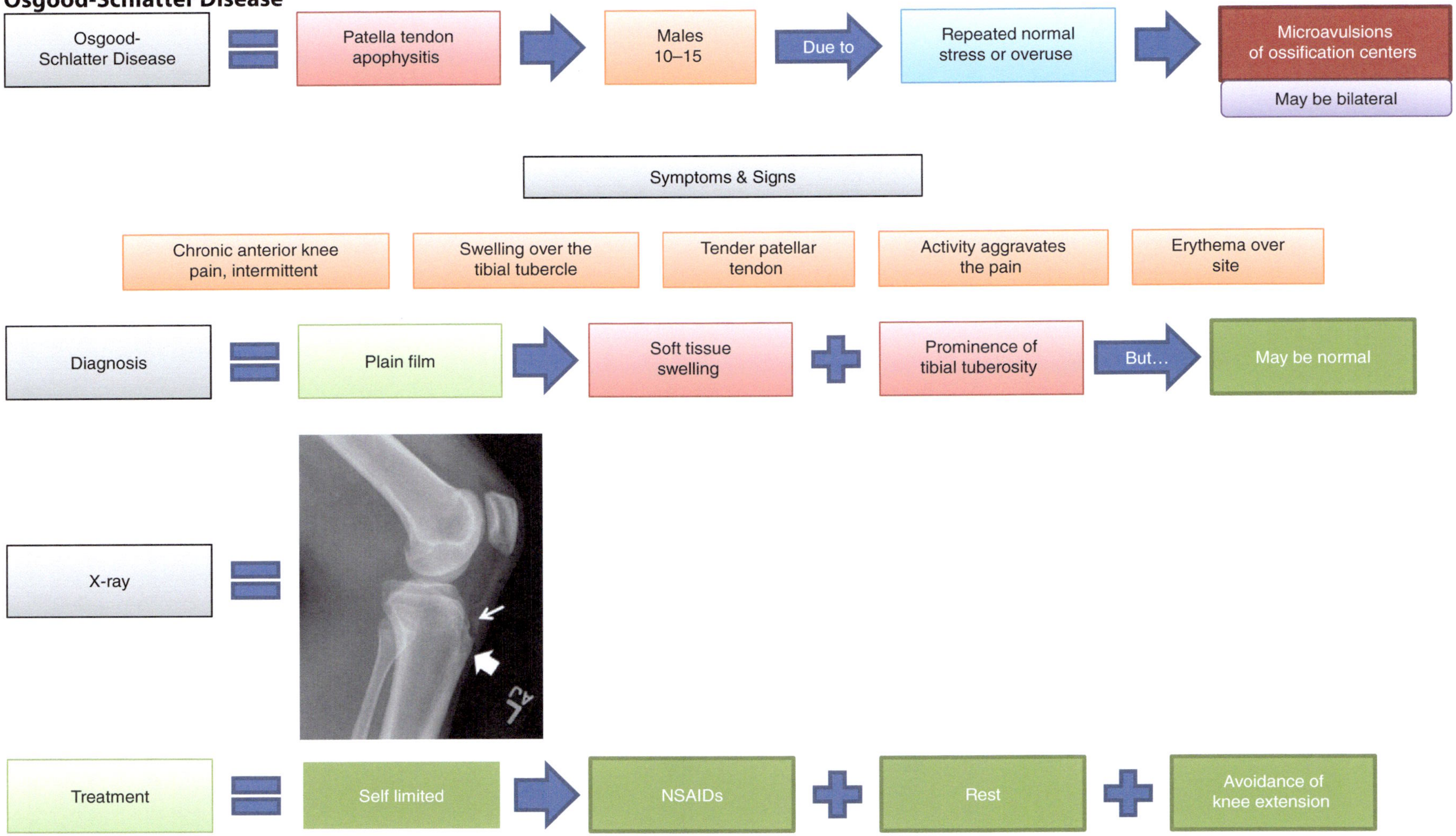

Left center image (Reprinted from Abdelgawad A, Naga O. The knee/leg. In: Abdelgawad A, Naga O, editors. Pediatric orthopedics: a handbook for primary care physicians. New York: Springer; 2014. p. 117–56. With permission from Springer Science + Business Media)

Baker's Cyst

Baker's Cyst = Inflammation of gastrocnemius bursa → May mimic thrombophlebitis

Symptoms & Signs

- Painful knee
- Painful calf
- Swollen knee
- Swollen calf
- Tender at popliteal fossa

Diagnosis = Ultrasound

Imaging =

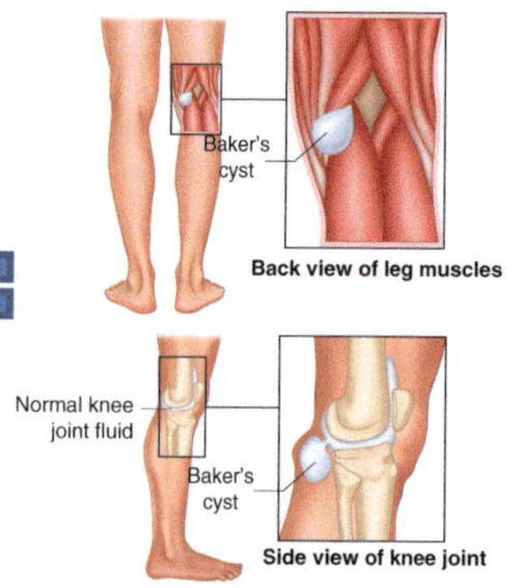

Treatment = RICE + Analgesics

The Leg

Tibial Shaft Fractures

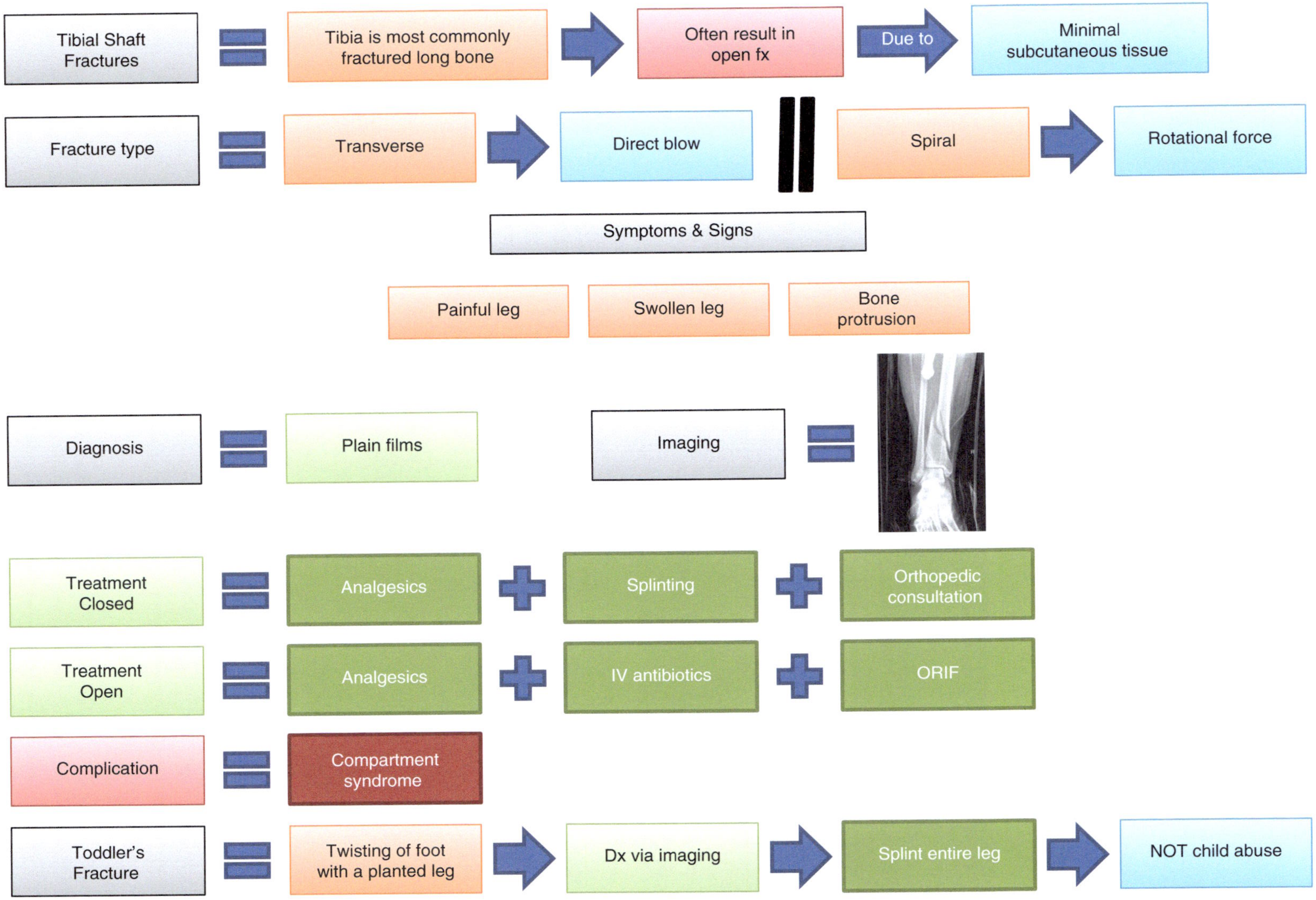

Left center image (Reprinted from Lichte P, Pape H-C. Tibial shaft fractures. In: Oestern HJ, Trentz O, Uranues S, editors. Bone and joint injuries: trauma surgery III. Heidelberg: Springer Verlag; 2014. p. 341–46. With permission from Springer Verlag)

Compartment Syndrome

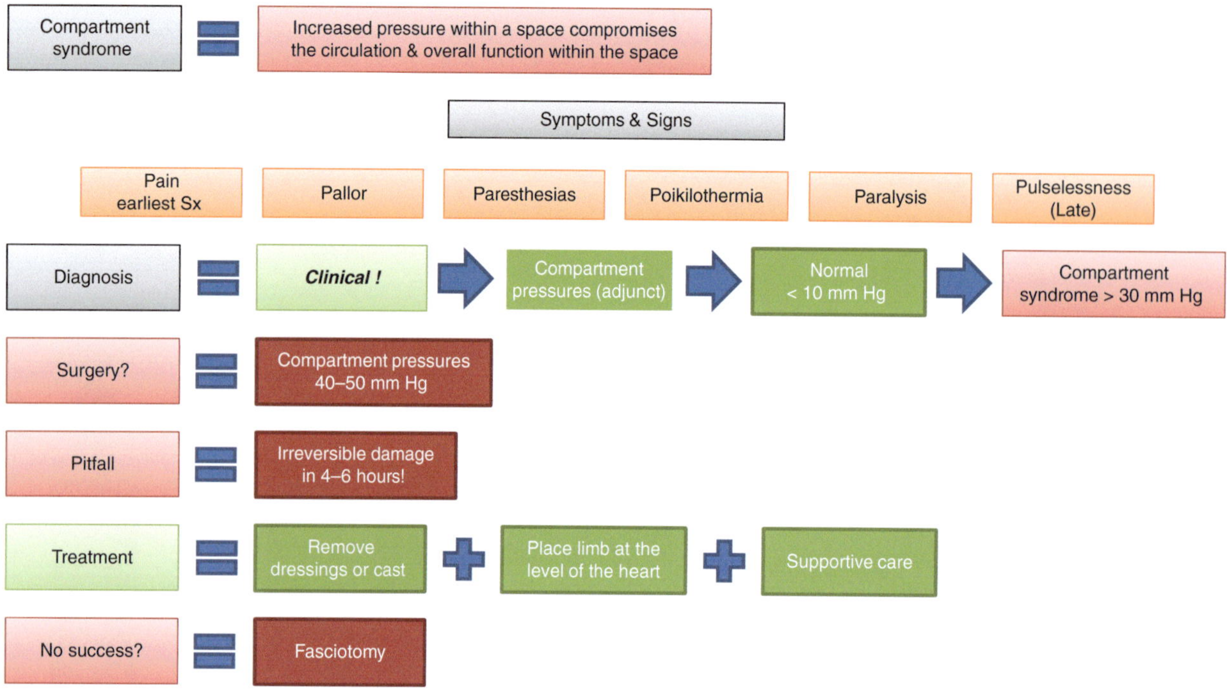

Causes of Compartment Syndrome

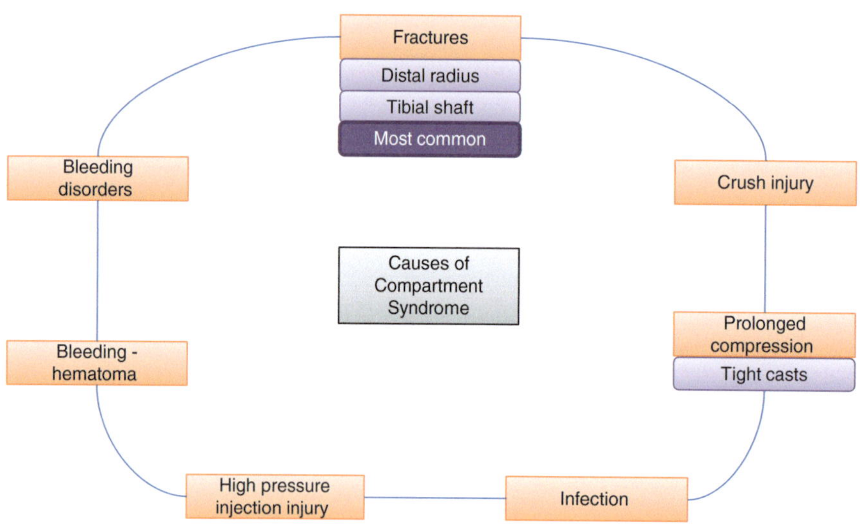

Pilon (Tibial Plafond) Fracture

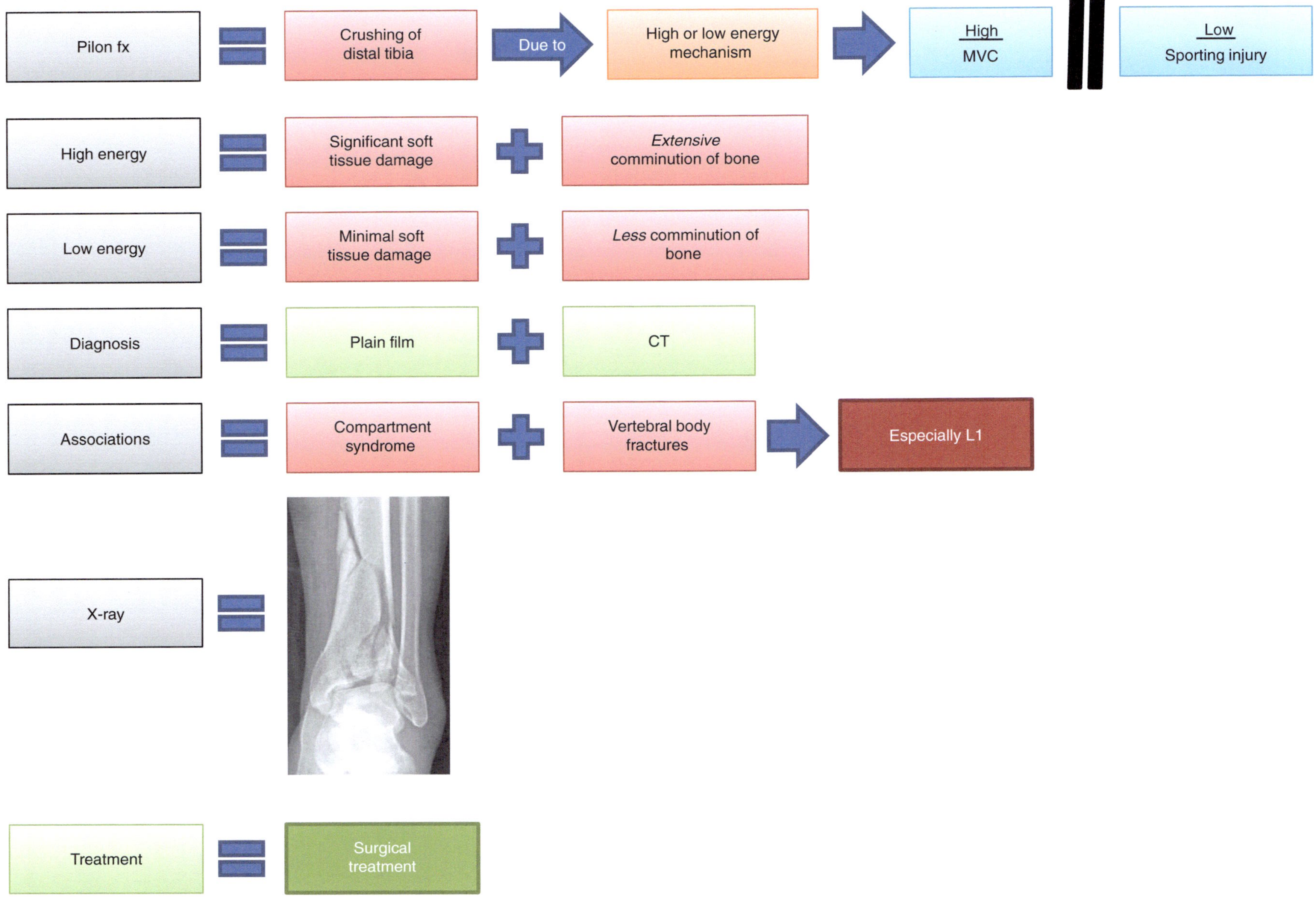

Bottom center image (Reprinted from Kaewlai R, Singh A. Lower extremity trauma. In: Singh A, editor. Emergency radiology: imaging of acute pathologies. New York: Springer Science; 2013. p. 277–98. With permission from Springer Science + Business Media)

Fibula Fracture

Maisonneuve fx → Due to → External rotation of the foot → Medial malleolus or deltoid ligament injury + Interosseous membrane tear + Proximal fibula fx

Any medial ankle swelling & pain after trauma = Maisonneuve fx until proven otherwise!

Treatment = Eventual Surgery

Treatment = 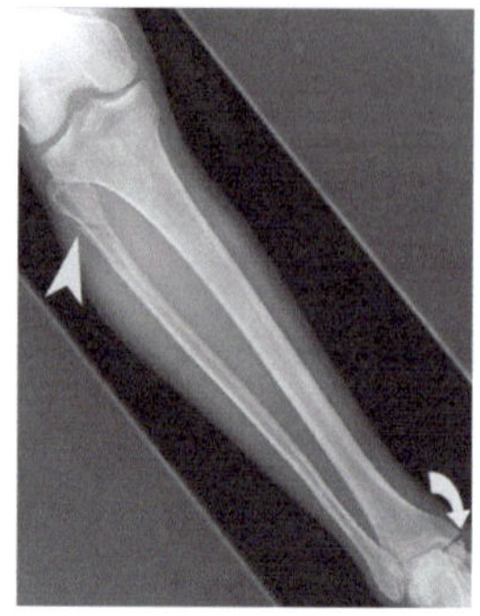

Pitfall = May be missed on plain film

Midshaft fibula fx = Associated with tibia fx → Isolated injury can occur

Intact tibia? = Knee immobilizer OR Elastic bandage for distal fx

Right center image (Reprinted from Kaewlai R, Singh A. Lower extremity trauma. In: Singh A, editor. Emergency radiology: imaging of acute pathologies. New York: Springer Science; 2013. p. 277–98. With permission from Springer Science + Business Media)

Achilles Tendon Rupture

Achilles Tendon = Largest & strongest tendon in the body → Typical pt is a middle aged man → Sudden eccentric force applied to a dorsiflexed foot

Risk factors = Older age + Prior Quinolone use + Prior steroid use

Symptoms & Signs

Sudden pain

Calf swelling

Feel/hear a "pop"

Inability to palpate tendon

Noticeable defect 2–6 cm proximal to calcaneus

Unable to stand on toes

Diagnosis = Thompson test → Failure of foot to plantar flex when calf if squeezed → Radiographs unnecessary → Consider MRI or US

US is operator dependent

Treatment = Short leg cast → Foot slightly plantar flexed + Orthopedic referral

Gastrocnemius Rupture

Gastrocnemius Rupture = Same mechanism → "Push off" → Medial head is most commonly injured

Diagnosis = Thompson test is *negative* → Foot *does* plantar flex when calf if squeezed = Achilles is intact → Consider MRI

Treatment = Short leg cast → Foot slightly plantar flexed + Orthopedic referral

The Ankle

Ankle Sprains

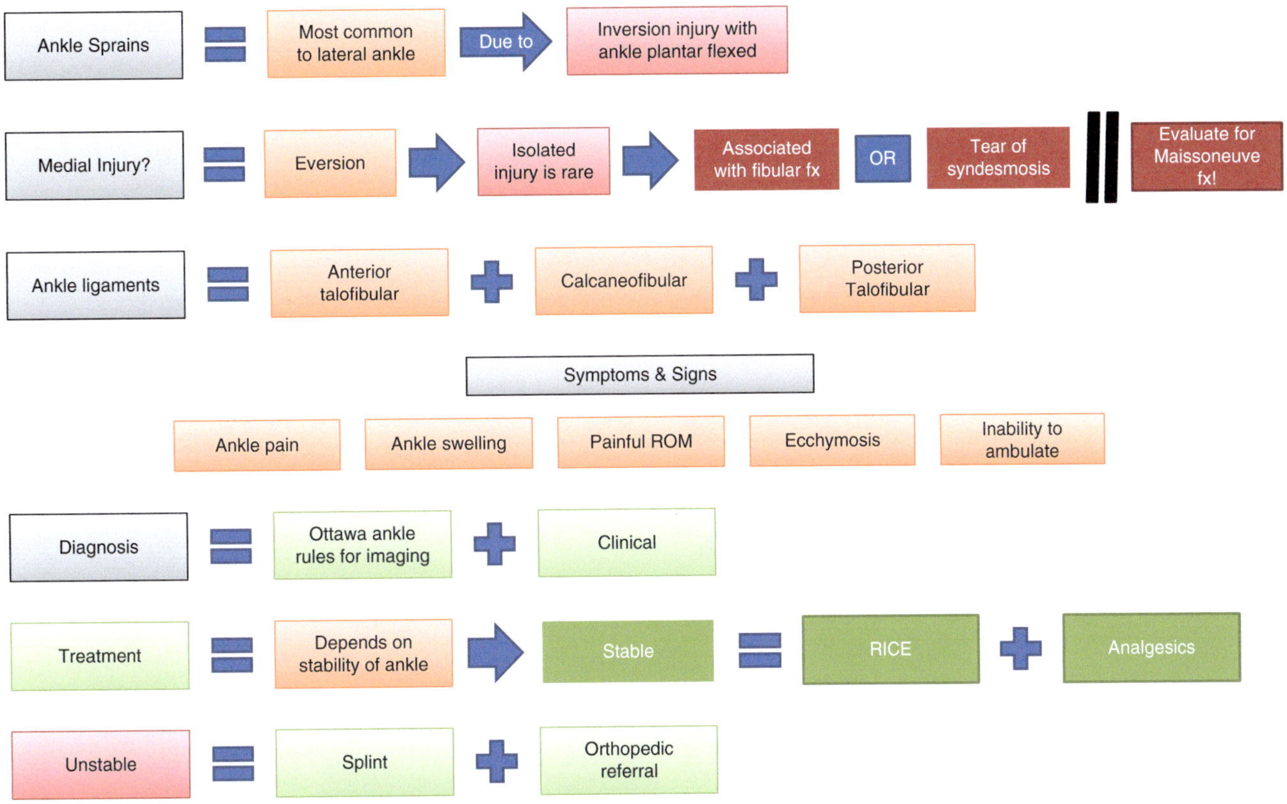

Ottawa Ankle Rules

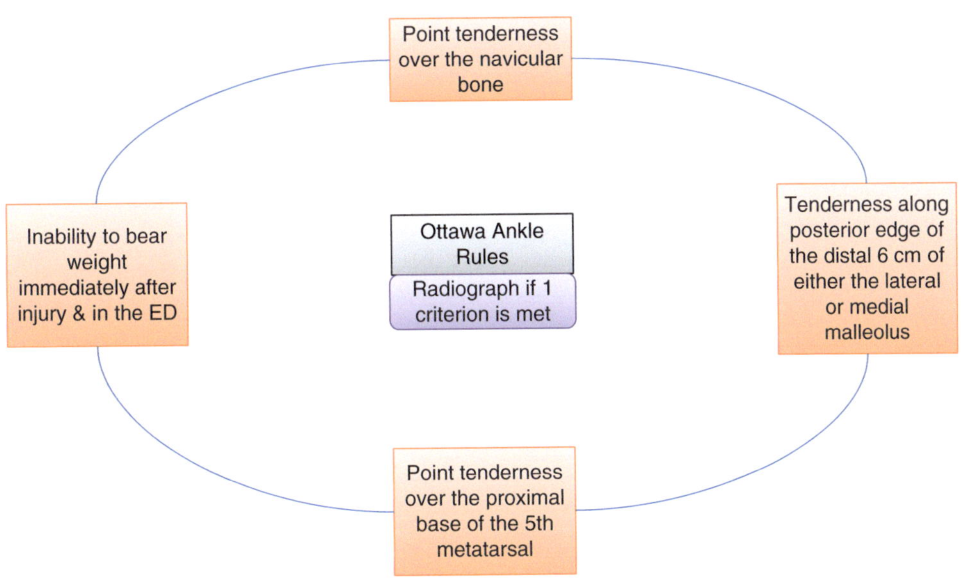

Ankle Dislocations

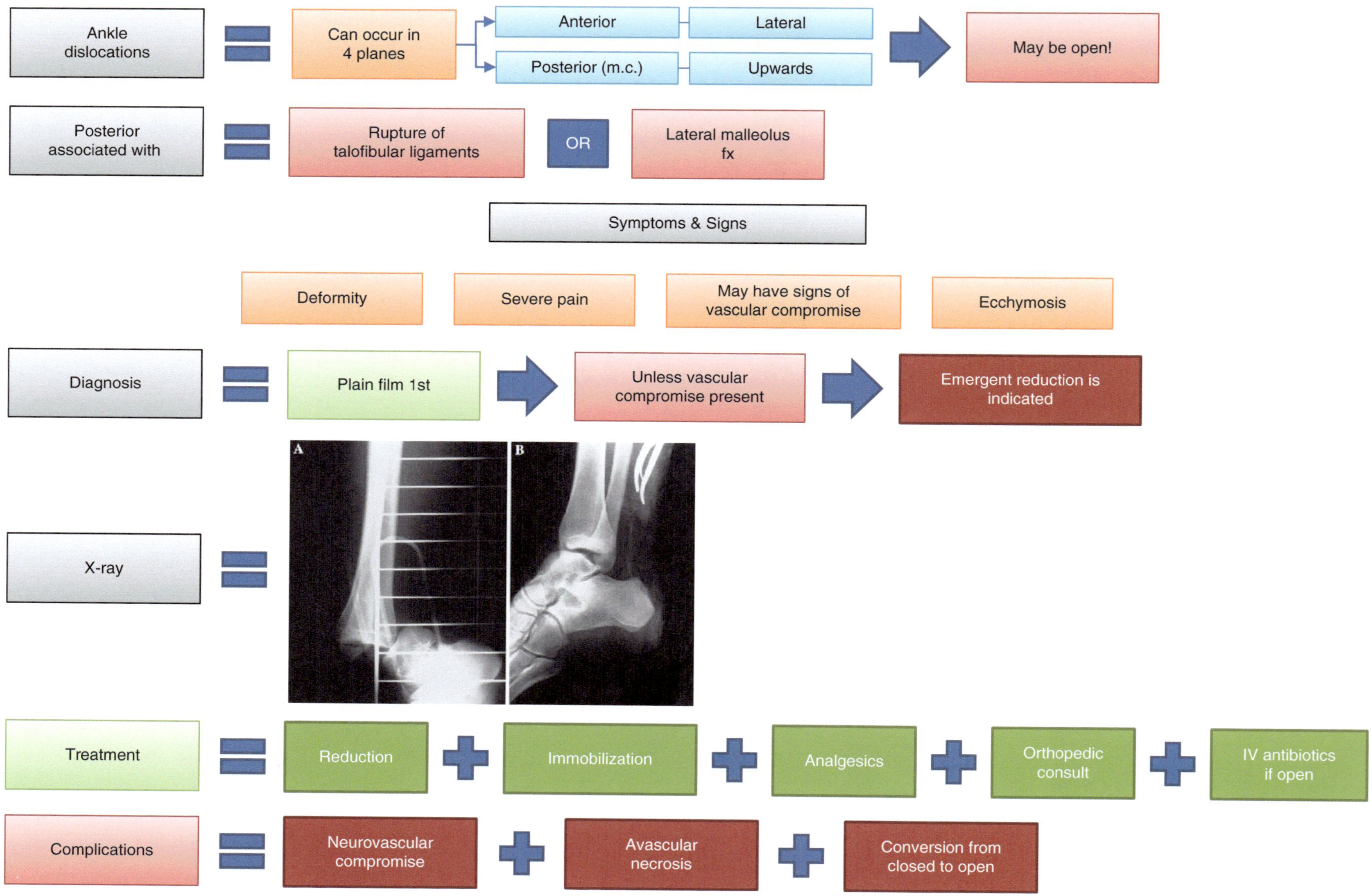

Left center image (Reprinted from Ríos-Luna A, Villanueva-Martínez, M, Fahandezh-Saddi H, Pereiro J, Martín-García A. Isolated dislocation of the ankle: two cases and review of the literature. Eur J Orthop Surg Traumatol. 2007;17(4):403–7. With permission from Springer Verlag)

The Foot

Calcaneal Fractures

Calcaneus Fractures = Require a large compressive force → Due to → Fall from height → Associated injuries are common

Associated injuries = Lumbosacral fx + Injury to other extremities + Injury to other calcaneus + GU & renal injuries

Symptoms & Signs

Foot pain | Foot swelling | Tender hindfoot | Ecchymosis | Low back pain

Diagnosis = Plain film lateral view → Bohler's angle may be reduced with fx → Normal 20-40 degrees → CT may be needed

Imaging & Boehler's angle =

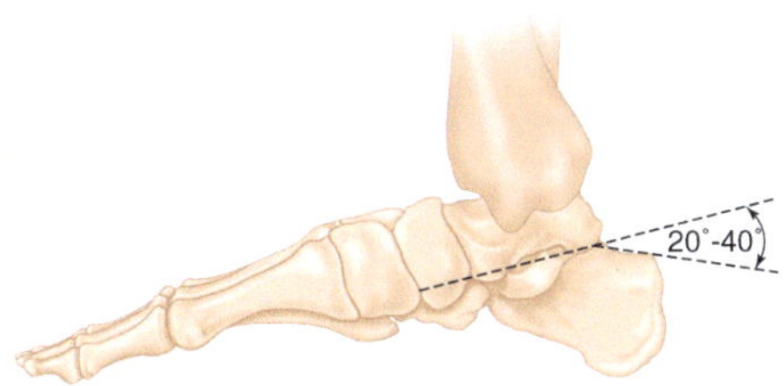

Bohler's angle

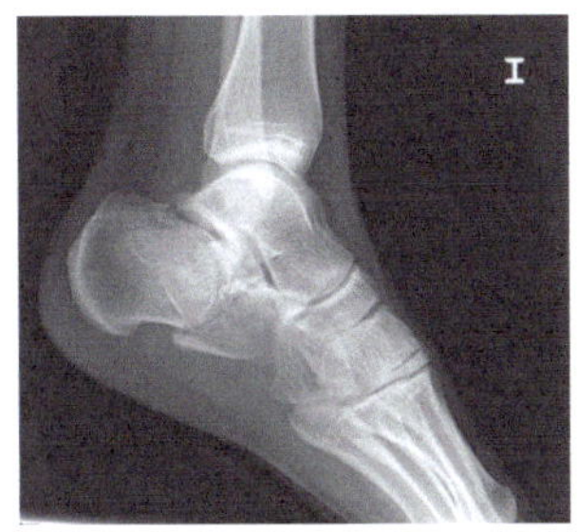

Treatment = Immobilization → Posterior splint + Analgesics + Orthopedic referral

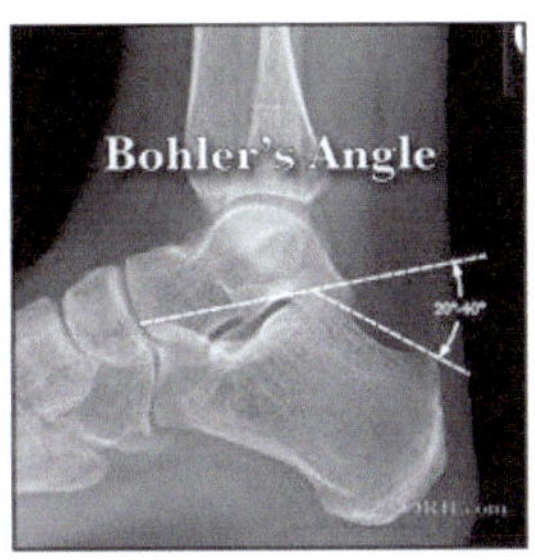

Right center image (Reprinted from García-Rey E. Complex fractures of the calcaneus. In: Rodríguez-Merchán EC, Rubio-Suarez JC, editors. Complex fractures of the limbs. Zug: Springer International Publishing; 2014. p. 95–9. With permission from Springer International Publishing)

Lisfranc Injuries

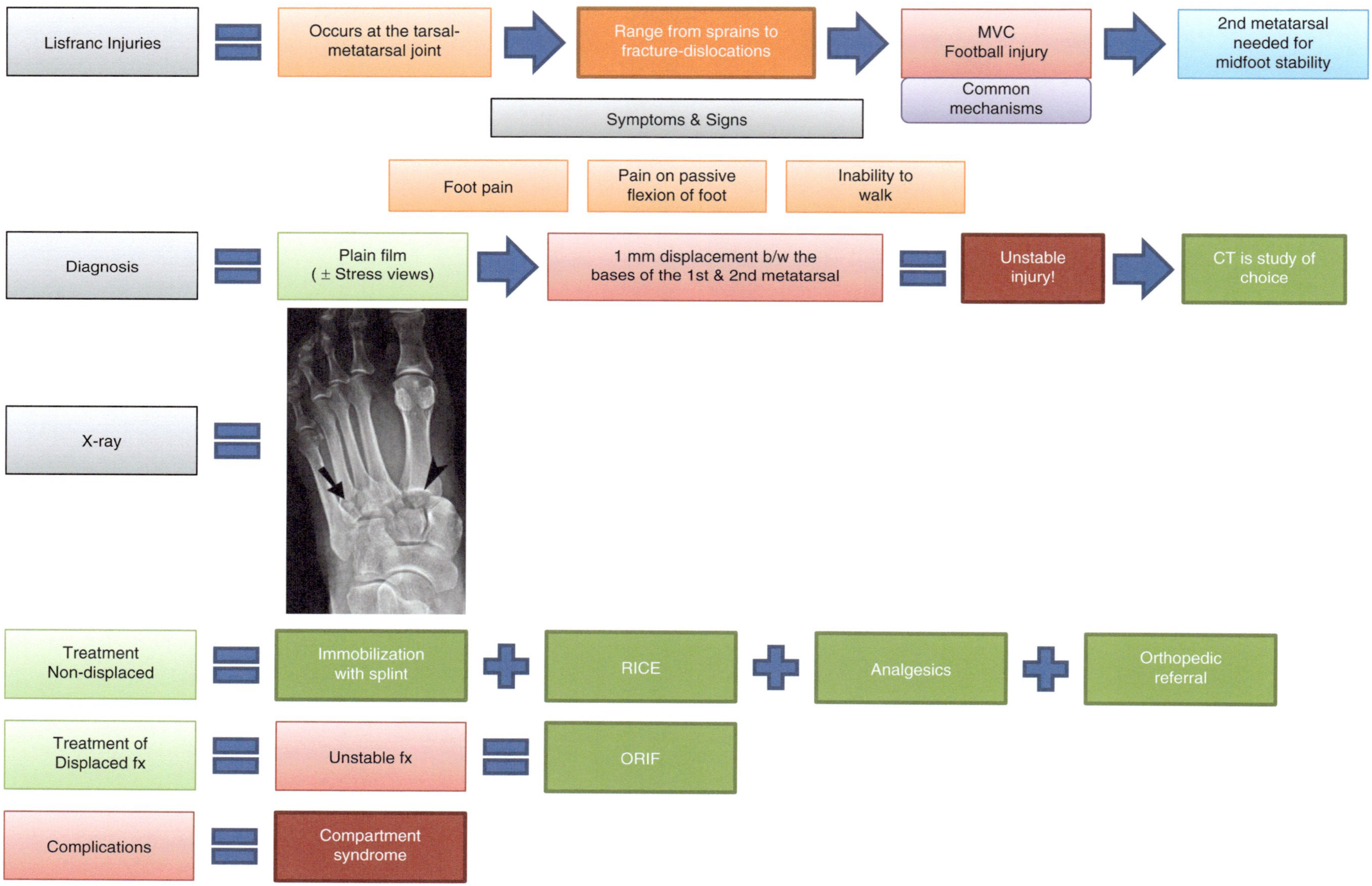

Left center image (Reprinted from Kaewlai R, Singh A. Lower extremity trauma. In: Singh A, editor. Emergency radiology: imaging of acute pathologies. New York: Springer Science; 2013. p. 277–98. With permission from Springer Science + Business Media)

Metatarsal Fractures

5th Metatarsal Fracture = 3 forms → Styloid fx proximal to the joint + Jones Fracture + Diaphyseal stress fractures

Jones Fracture = Transverse fx at proximal diaphysis → Common in athletes that run & jump → Has high incidence of nonunion → Treatment is ORIF

Dancer's Fracture = Avulsion fx of 5th metatarsal base → Near attachment of peroneus brevis → Inversion injury → Treatment is cast shoe

Imaging =

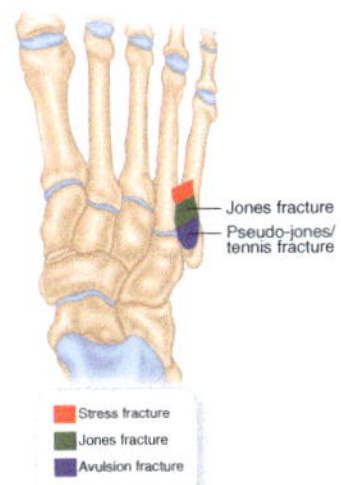

Diagnosis = Plain film

Other metatarsal fx tidbits → Displacement 3–4 mm OR > 10 degree angulation = ORIF

March fracture = Stress fx of 2nd metatarsal → Repeated pushing off

Tarsal Tunnel Syndrome

Tarsal Tunnel Syndrome = Entrapment neuropathy → Posterior tibial nerve → Motor to foot muscles + Sensory to bottom of foot

Associations = Nighttime foot pain + Has a Tinel's sign as well for aid in diagnosis

Treatment = Analgesia + Walking boot

Complication = Claw toe

Osteomyelitis

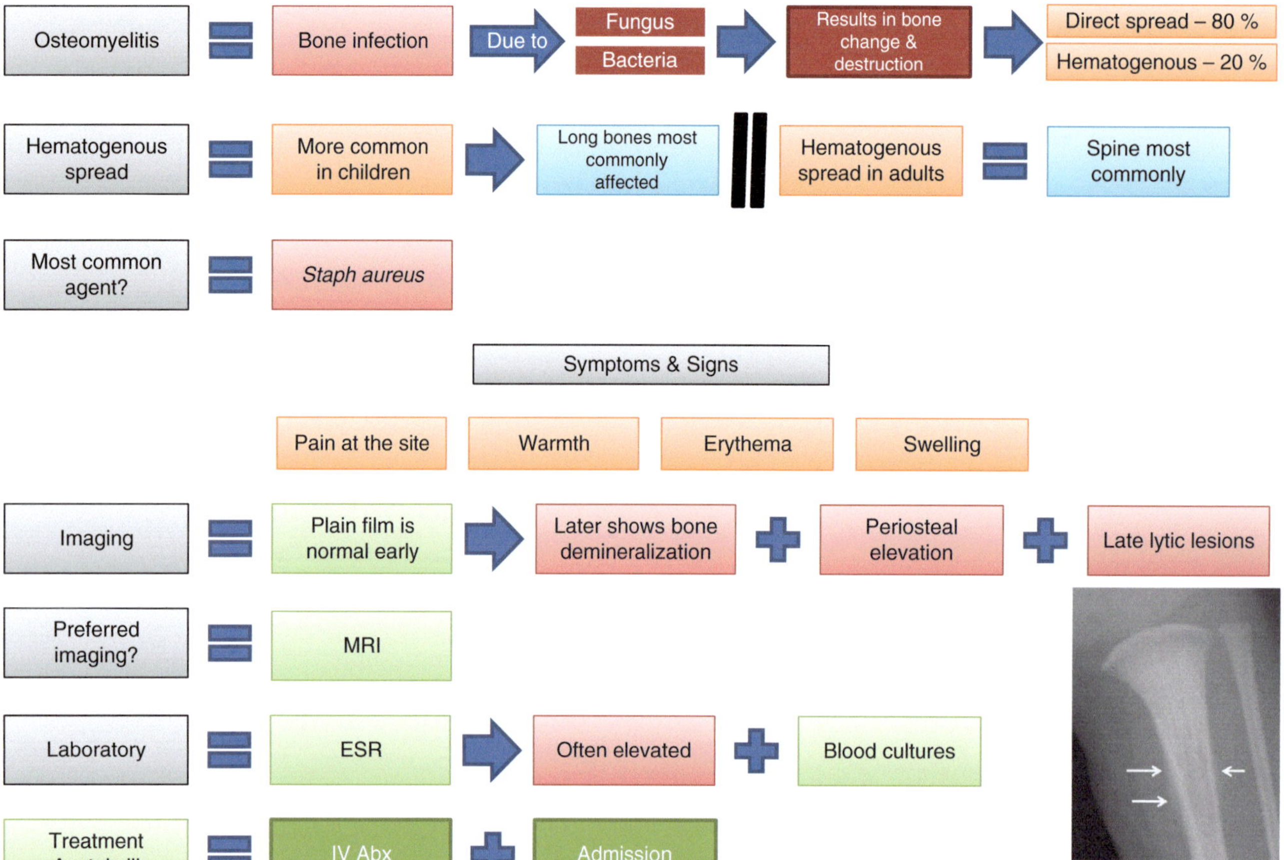

Bottom right image (Reprinted from Abdelgawad A, Naga O. Musculoskeletal infections. In: Abdelgawad A, Naga O, editors. Pediatric orthopedics: a handbook for primary care physicians. New York: Springer; 2014. p. 561–84. With permission from Springer Science + Business Media)

Risk Factors and Likely Agents for Osteomyelitis

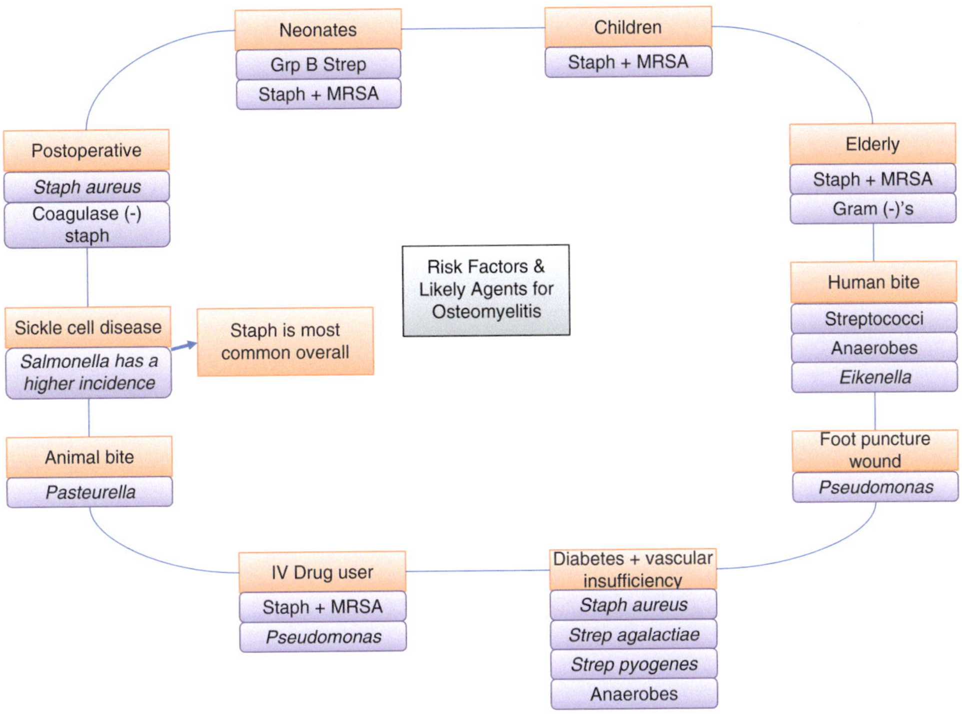

Thoracic and Lumbar Pain

Back Pain Tidbits

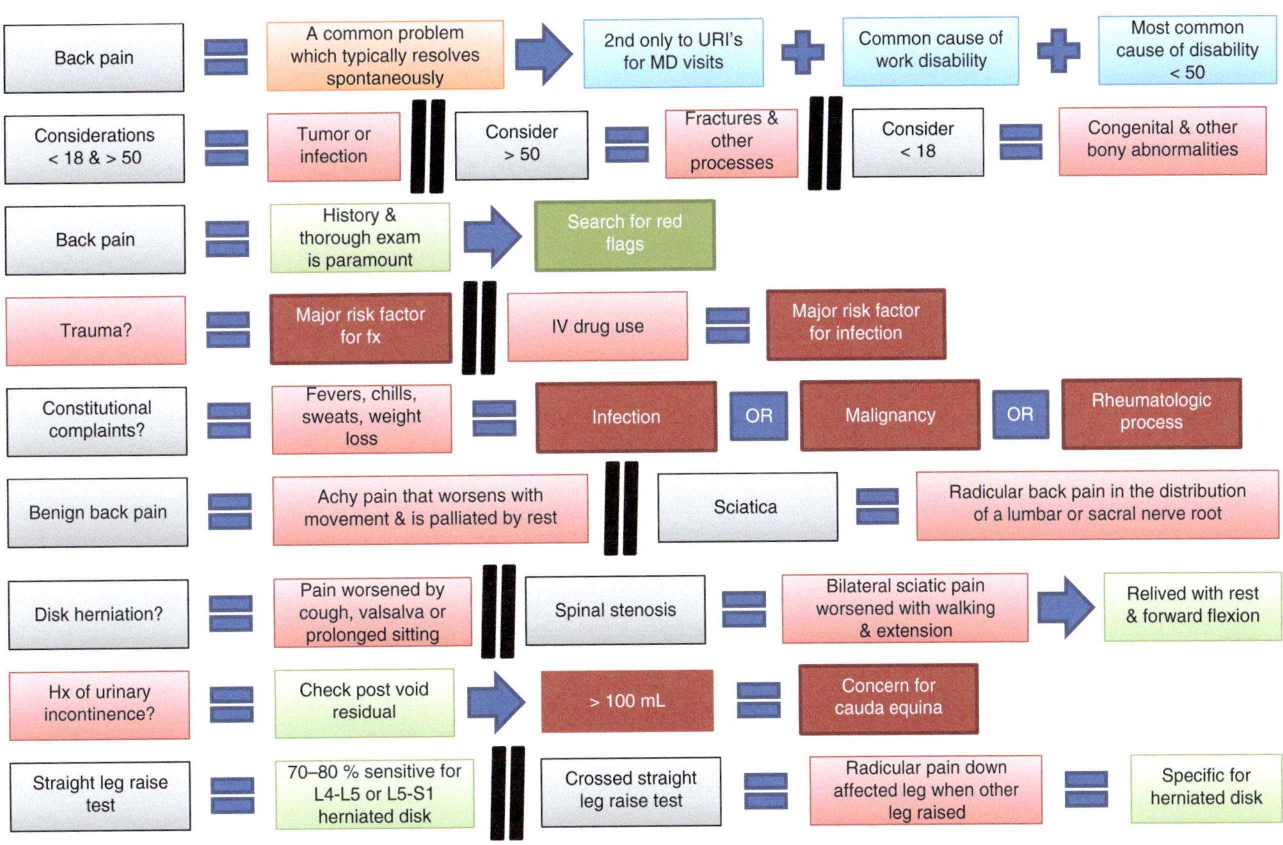

Red Flags

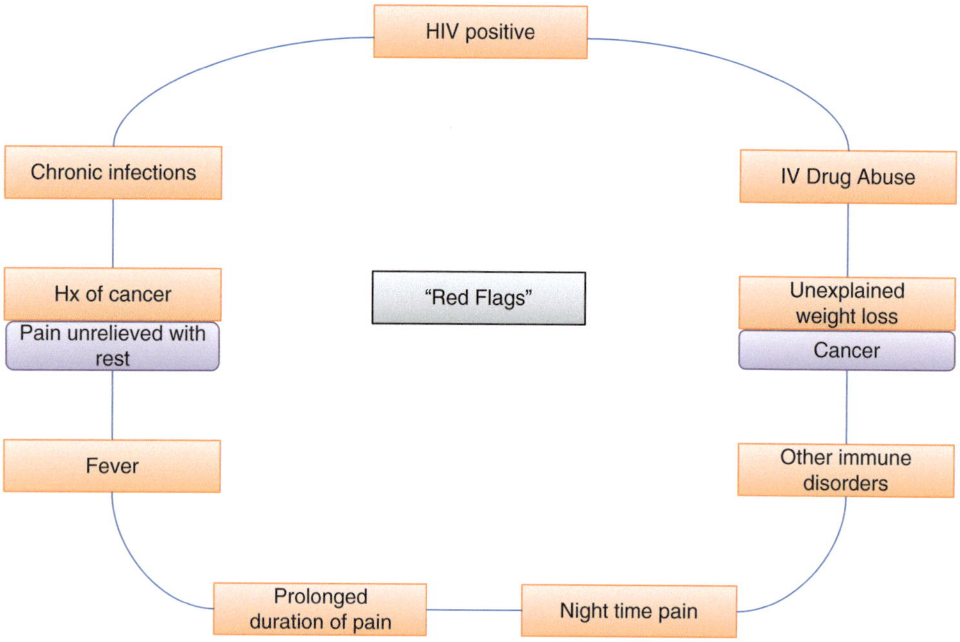

Back Pain Workup

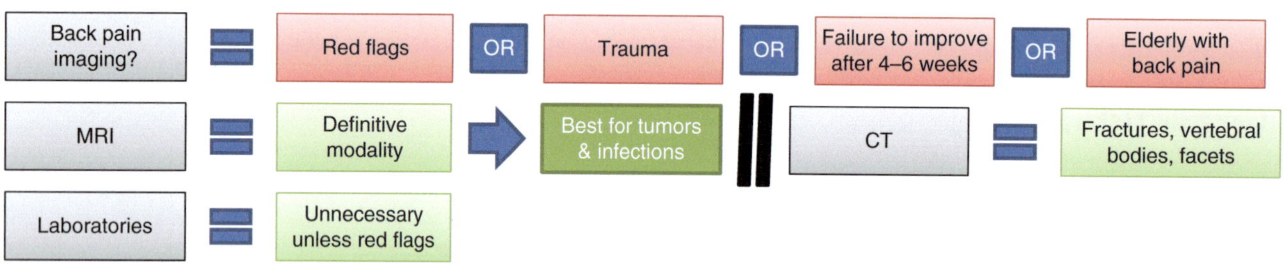

Lumbar Strain/Nonspecific Back pain

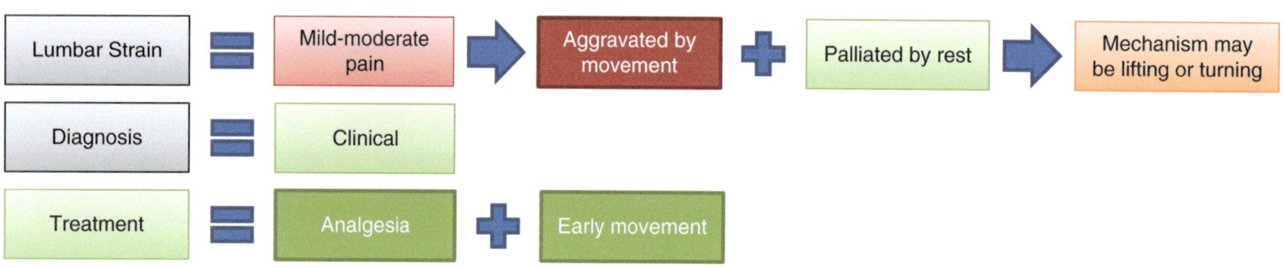

Disk Herniation

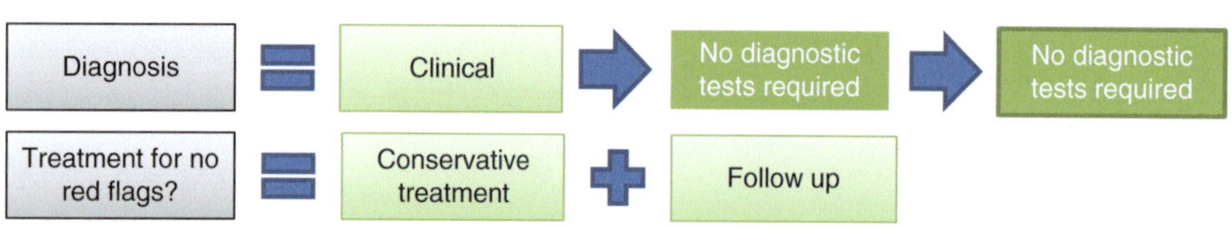

Spinal Stenosis

Spinal Stenosis = More common in elderly → Due to → Narrowing of lumbar canal → May have facet hypertrophy + Ligamentum flavum thickening

Spinal Stenosis = May have associated sciatica → Other physical findings may be absent

Symptoms & Signs

- Low back pain worsened with standing & extension of spine
- Pain relieved with rest & forward flexion
- (Neurogenic claudication)
- Low back & lower extremity pain with walking

Diagnosis = CT OR MRI

Treatment = Analgesia, NSAIDs + Leg exercises + Physical therapy + Epidural steroids

Ankylosing Spondylitis

Ankylosing Spondylitis = Autoimmune arthritis → Affects spine & pelvis → Associated with HLA-B27 + May be Trauma & infection

Ankylosing Spondylitis = Pts < 40 + Males 3:1

Symptoms & Signs

- Waking with low back pain & stiffness that improves with activity
- Malaise
- Fatigue

Diagnosis = Thorough Hx + Imaging → Sacroiliitis + "Bamboo spine"

Treatment = NSAIDs + Referral to rheumatology

Cauda Equina Syndrome

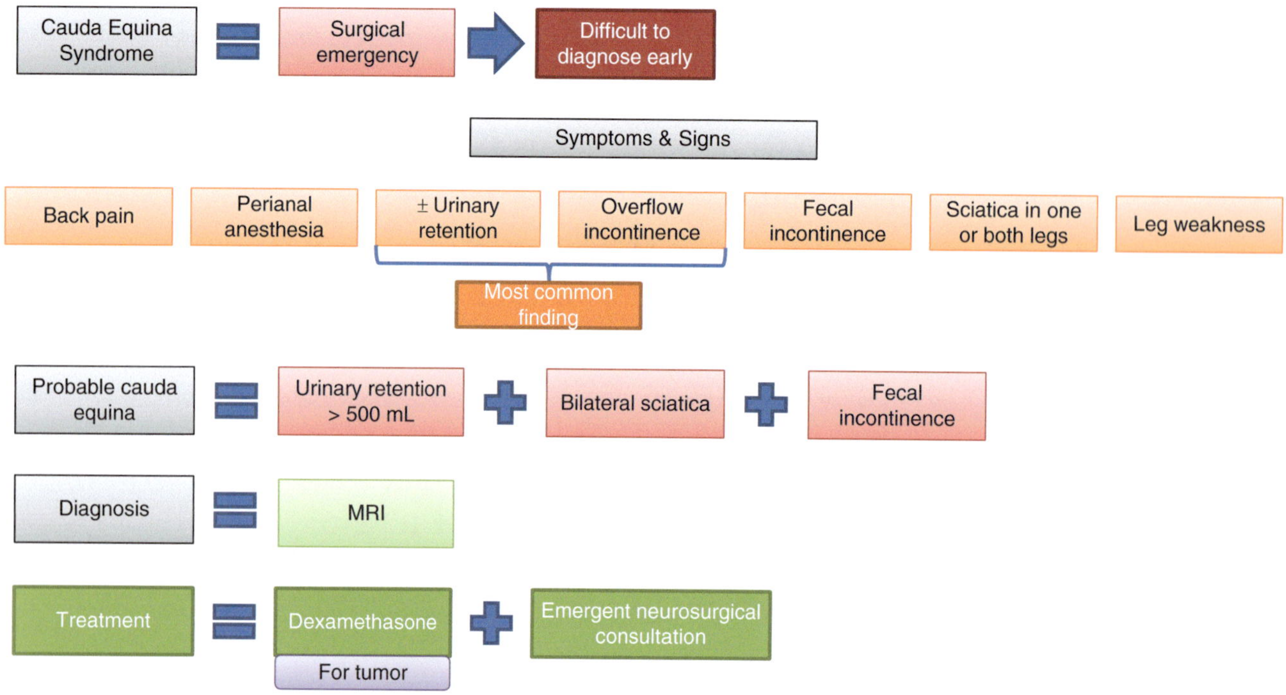

Causes of Cauda Equina

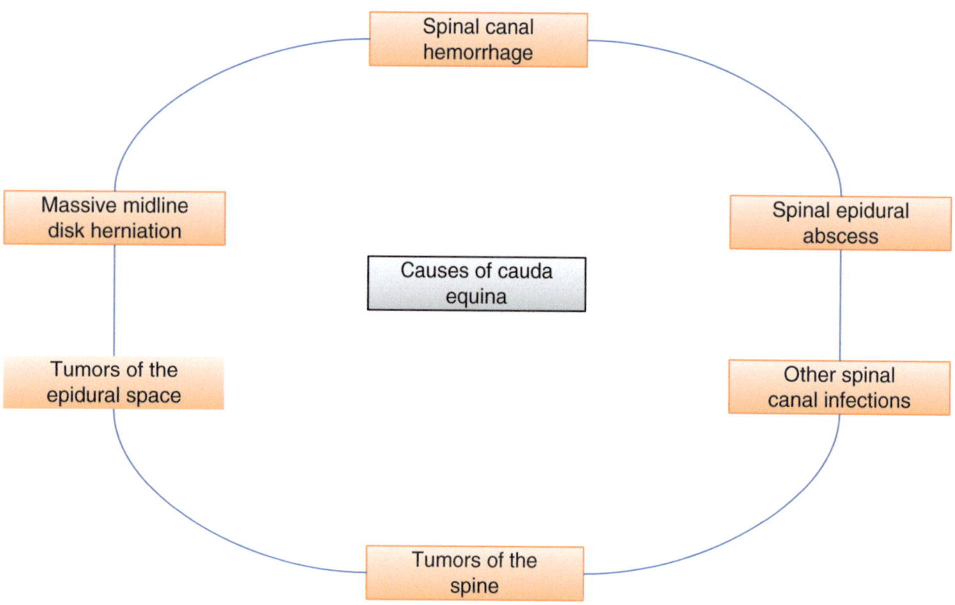

Transverse Myelitis

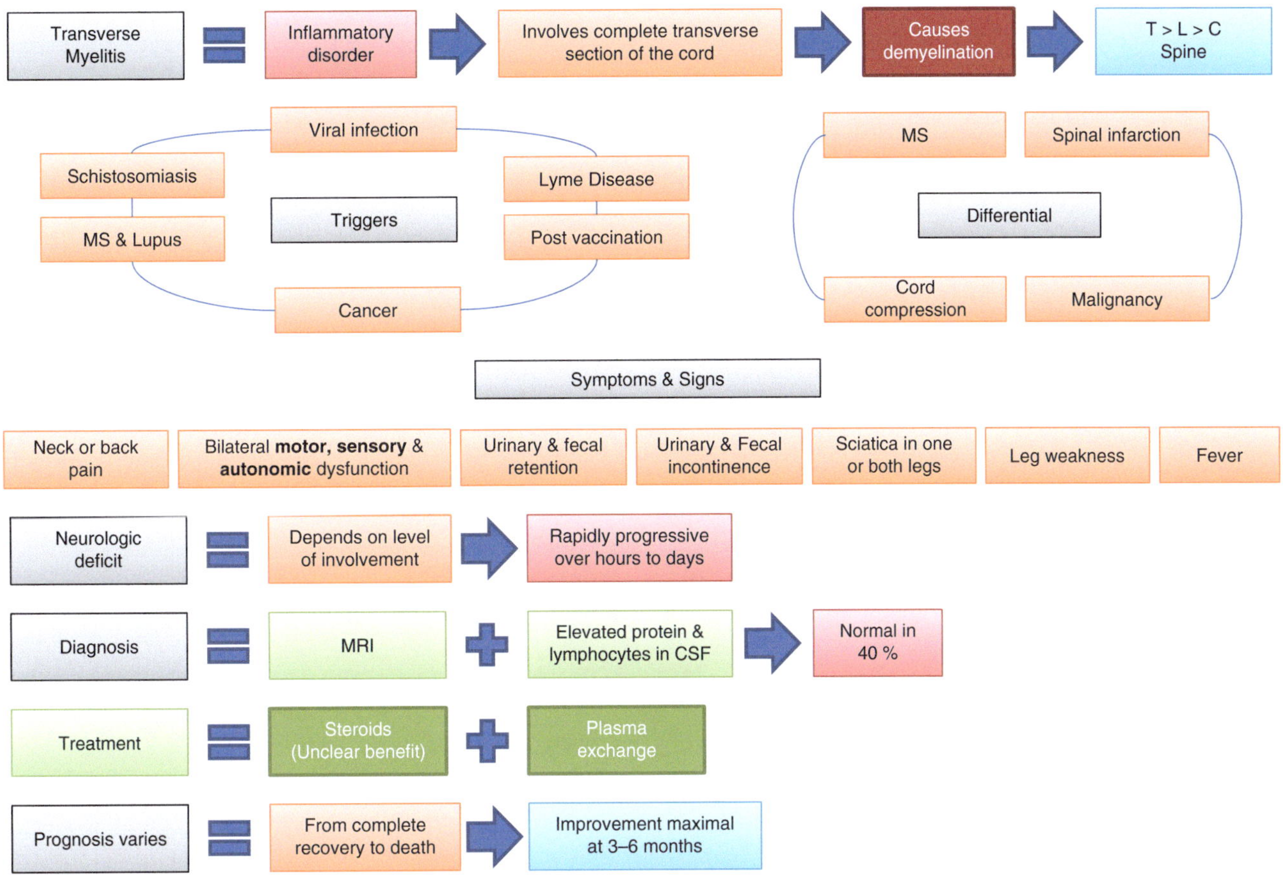

Spinal Infections

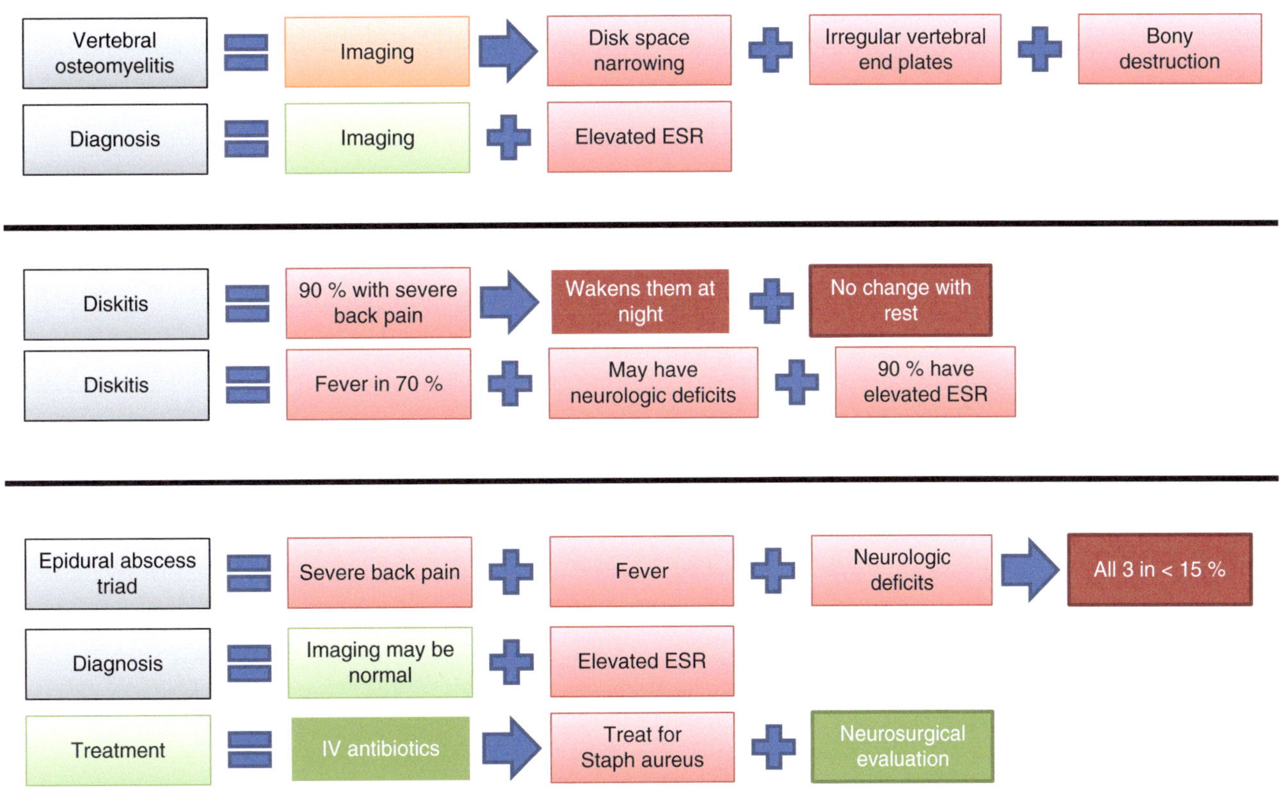

Diskitis

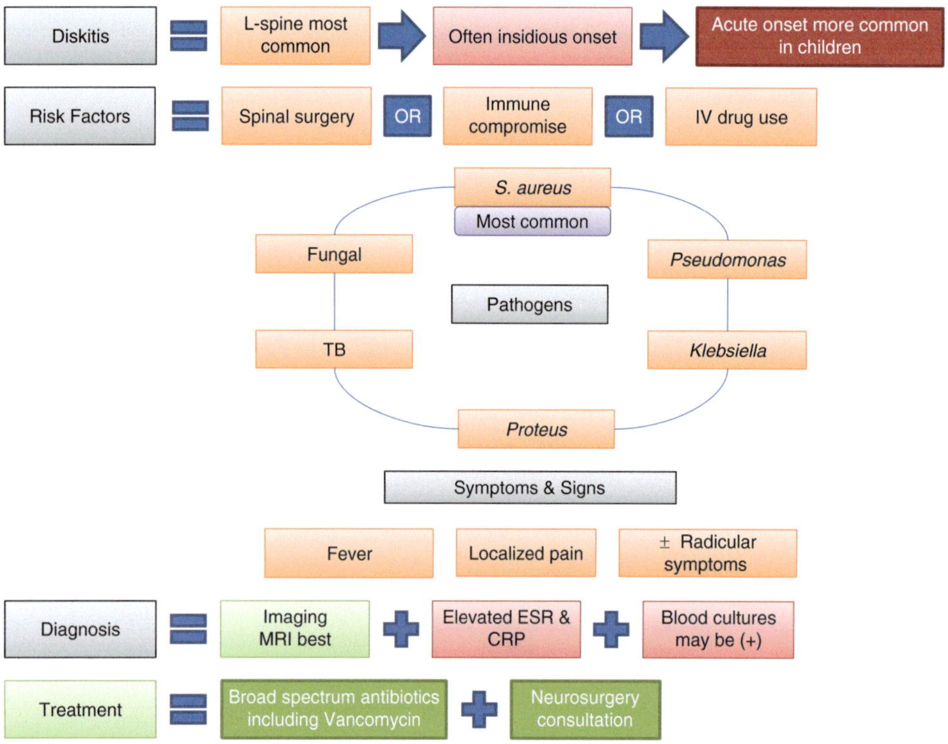
Diskitis
L-spine most common
Often insidious onset
Acute onset more common in children
Risk Factors
Spinal surgery
OR
Immune compromise
OR
IV drug use
S. aureus
Most common
Fungal
Pseudomonas
Pathogens
TB
Klebsiella
Proteus
Symptoms & Signs
Fever
Localized pain
± Radicular symptoms
Diagnosis
Imaging MRI best
Elevated ESR & CRP
Blood cultures may be (+)
Treatment
Broad spectrum antibiotics including Vancomycin
Neurosurgery consultation

Spinal Epidural Abscess

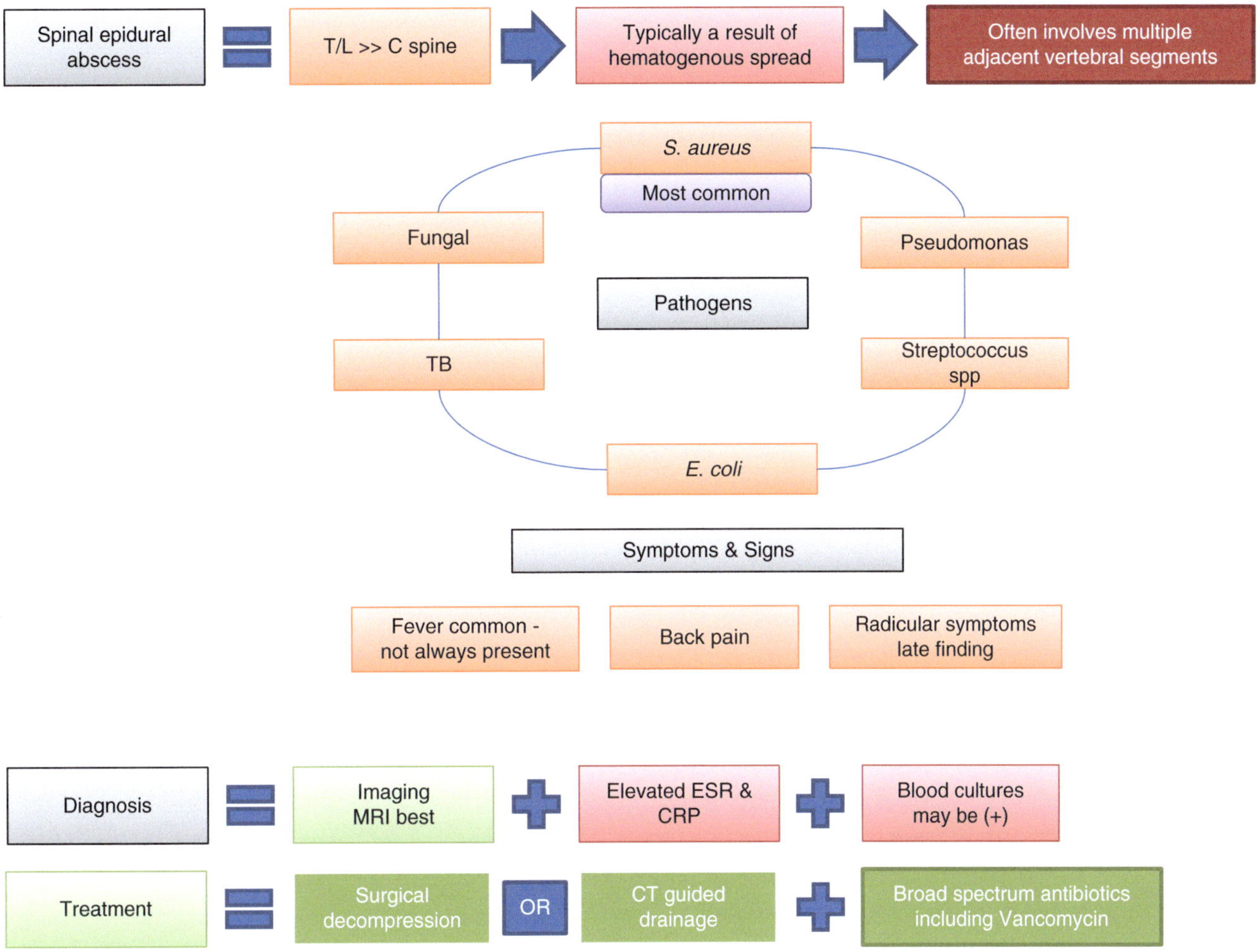

Risk Factors for Epidural Abscess

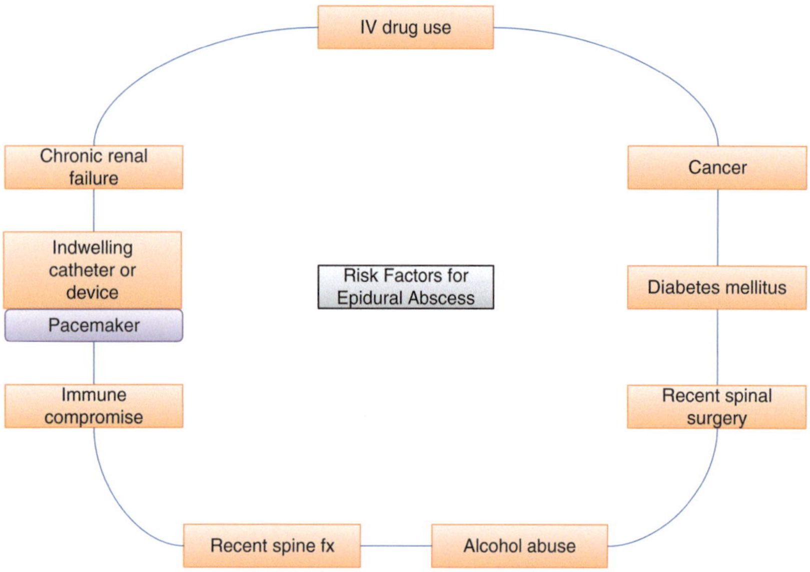

Rheumatologic Emergencies

Joint Fluid Analysis

	Normal	Non-Inflammatory	Inflammatory	Septic
Clarity	Transparent	Transparent	Translucent to opaque	Opaque
Color	Clear	Yellow tinged	Yellow tinged	Yellow to green
WBC (per mm^3)	< 200	200–2000	2,000–50,000	>50,000
PMN's (%)	< 25	< 25	≥ 50	≥ 75
Culture	Negative	Negative	Negative	Often positive
Crystals	None	None	None or multiple	None
Conditions		Osteoarthritis	Gout, pseudogout, Lupus	Staph, GC

Joint Fluid Tidbits

Testing includes = Cell count + Gram stain + Culture + Crystals

Most important test = Cell count → Distinguishes between inflammatory, non-inflammatory & septic conditions

Other considerations = Protein + Glucose → Glucose may be low in Septic arthritis & Rheumatoid arthritis

Gout and Pseudogout

Gout = Precipitation of uric acid crystals → Due to → Overproduction of uric acid due to multiple causes OR Decreased renal excretion

Pseudogout = Precipitation of calcium pyrophosphate crystals → May be idiopathic OR Associated with hypercalcemia

Gout = Needle shaped crystals + Non-specific imaging

Pseudogout = Rhomboid shaped crystals + Chondrocalcinosis

Chondrocalcinosis = Radiographic densities in cartilage due to deposition of calcium pyrophosphate crystals

Treatment = NSAID's → Steroids for severe cases

Rheumatoid Arthritis

Rheumatoid arthritis flare = Joint edema + Increased arthralgias → Labs show elevated CRP & ESR

Treatment = NSAID's + Steroids

Rheumatoid arthritis pitfalls = Have cervical instability → Especially at C1–C2 → Beware even minor trauma in this group of patients

Treatment with disease modifying agents = Predispose to serious bacterial infections

Tidbit = Felty syndrome = Rheumatoid arthritis + Neutropenia + Enlarged spleen

Antiphospholipid Syndrome

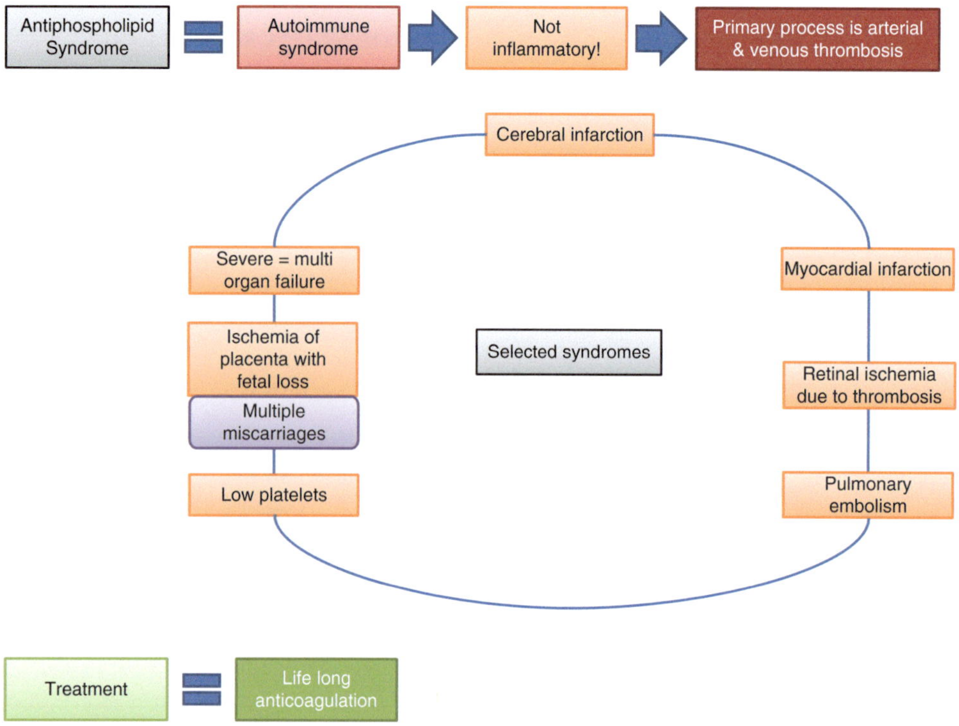

Systemic Lupus Erythematosus (SLE) Tidbits

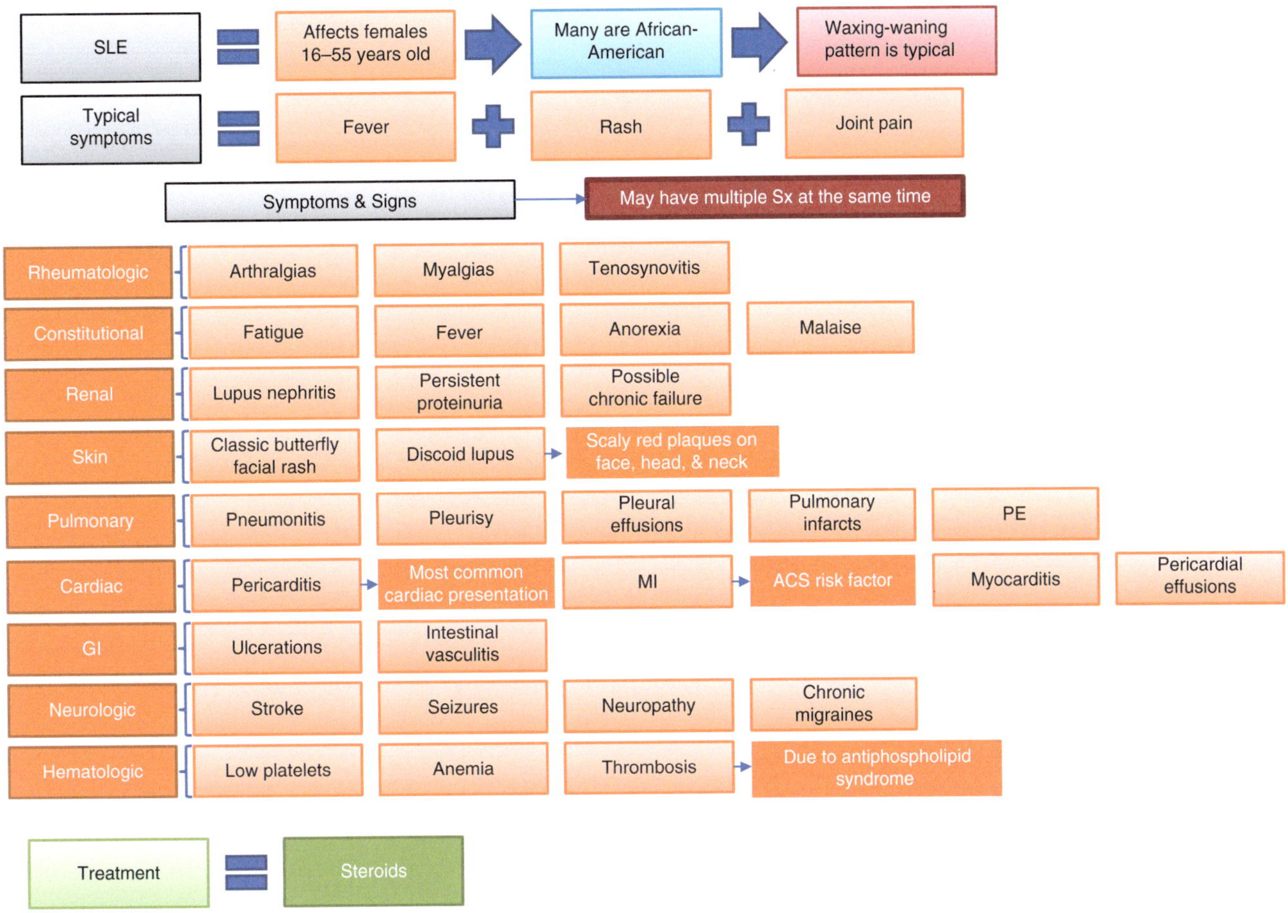

Trauma

Henry Young II and Bobby Desai

Contents

Introduction 814

Spinal Injuries 826

Spinal Cord Injuries 830

Penetrating Neck Injury 835

Chest Trauma 838

Abdominal Trauma 847

Pelvis and Hip Trauma 852

Extremity Injuries 856

Trauma in Special Populations 858

H. Young II, MD
Department of Emergency Medicine, UF Health at the University of Florida, Gainesville, FL, USA

B. Desai, MD, MEd (✉)
Department of Emergency Medicine, University of Florida, Gainesville, FL, USA
e-mail: bdesai@ufl.edu

B. Desai, B.R. Allen (eds.), *Nailing the Written Emergency Medicine Board Examination*,
DOI 10.1007/978-3-319-30838-8_15

Introduction

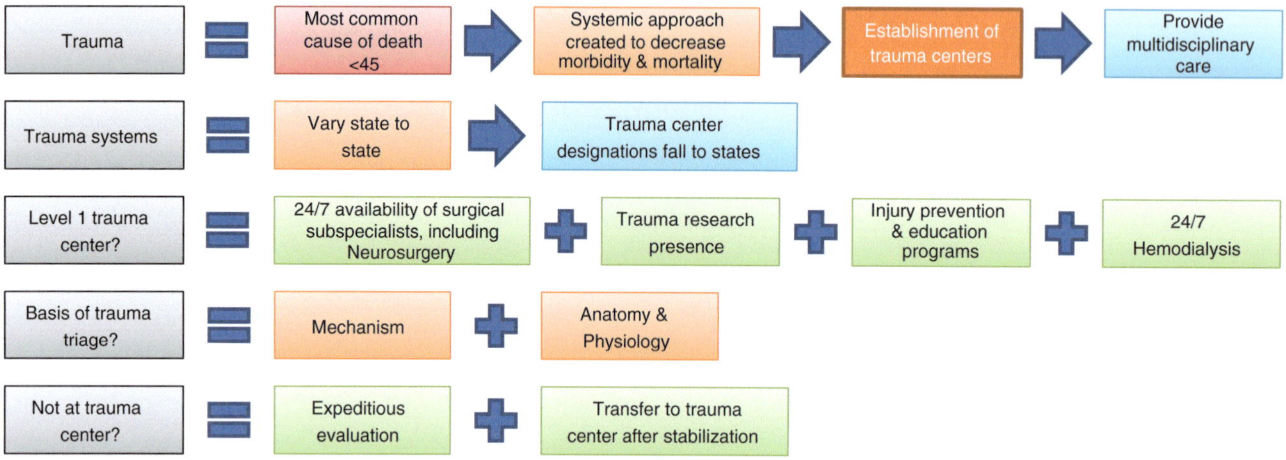

Primary Survey

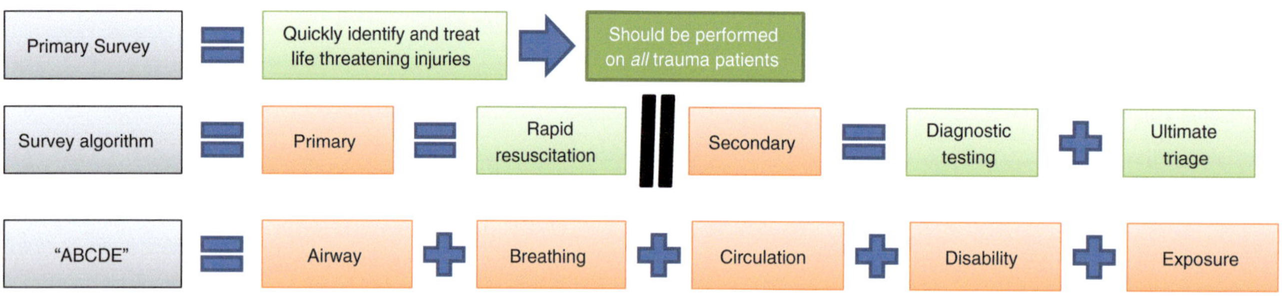

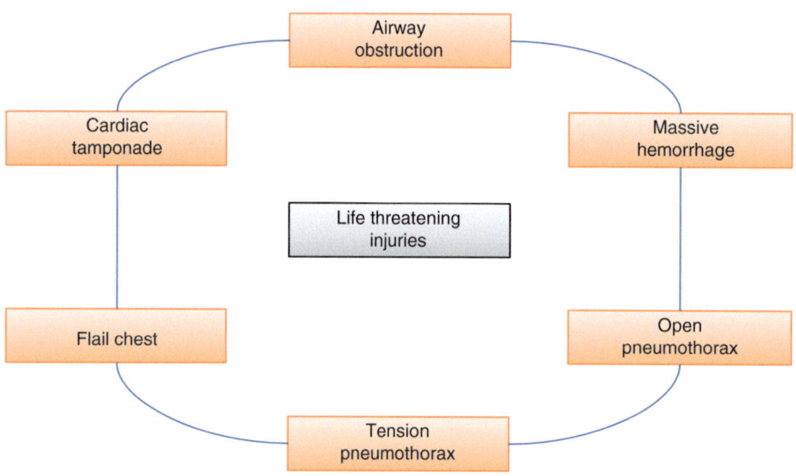

Airway Assessment

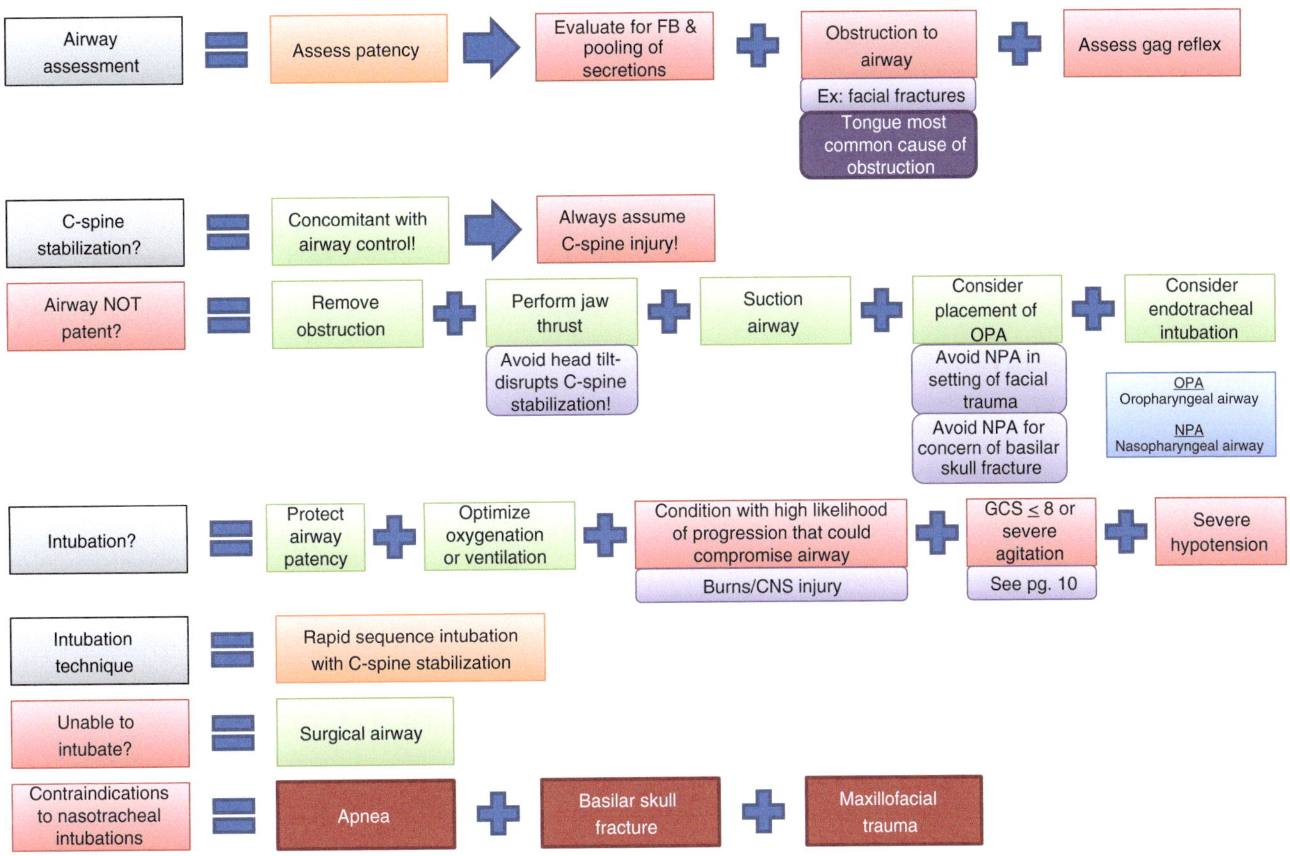

Breathing Assessment

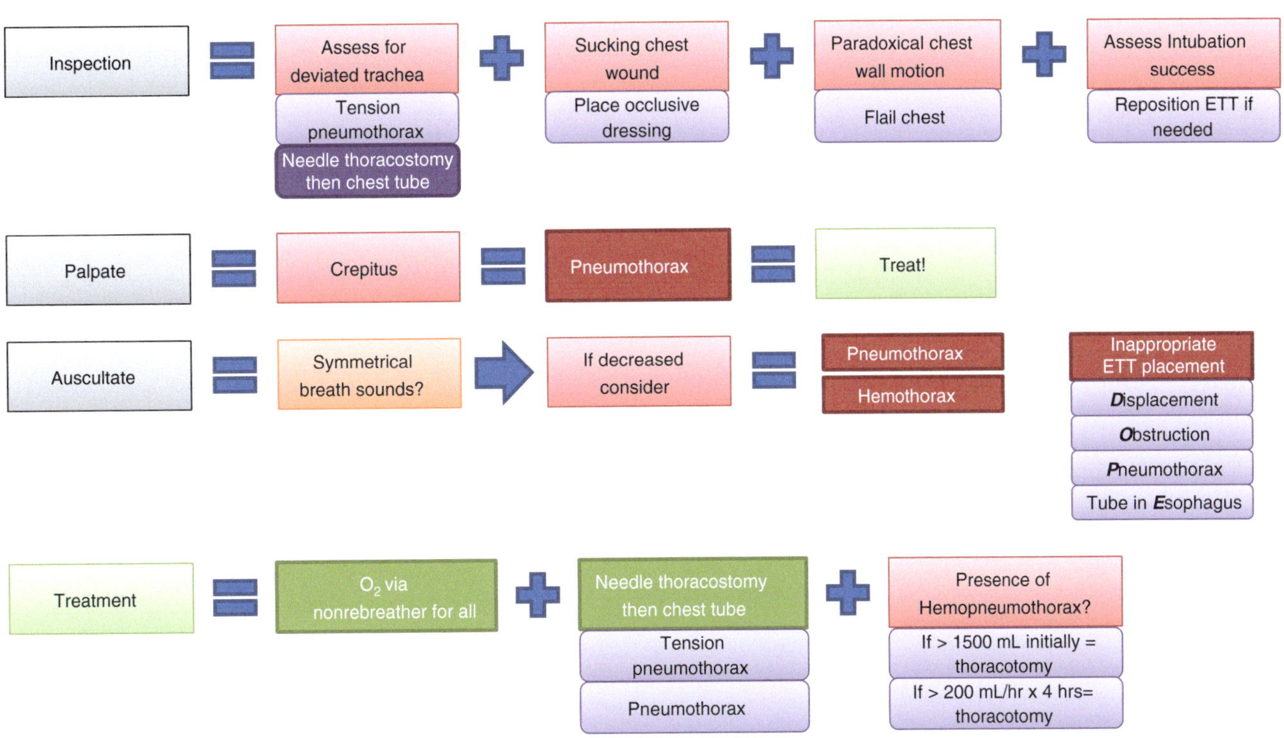

Circulation Assessment

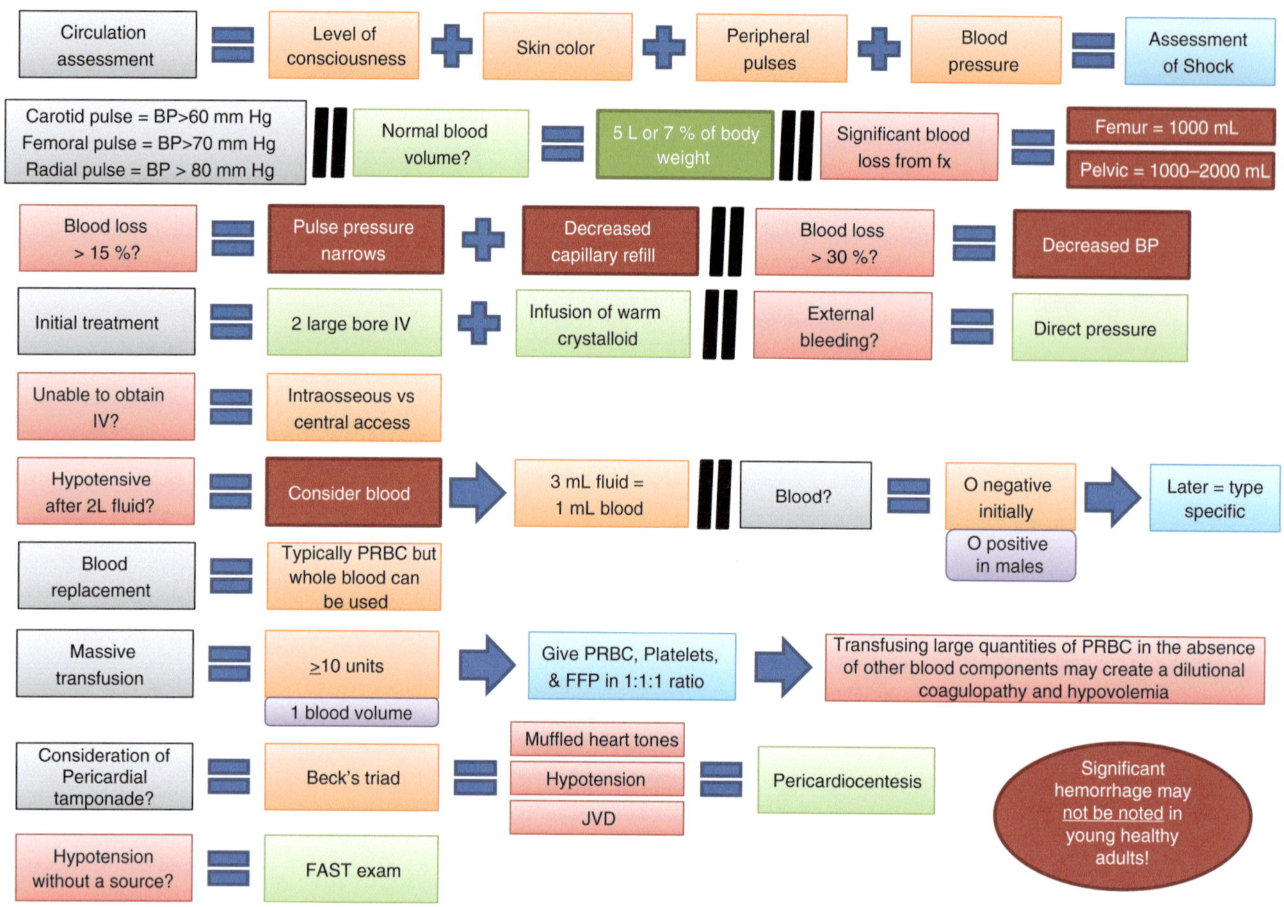

Classification of Hemorrhage

	Blood loss	Cardiovascular	Neurologic	Skin	Renal
Class I	< 15 % < 750 ml	HR normal or slightly increased; BP normal	Normal or slightly anxious	Warm, pink, normal capillary refill	Normal output
Class II	15–30 % 750-1500ml	**Tachycardia**, BP normal	irritable, confused, **combative**	Cool, mottling, delayed capillary refill	Oliguria, increased spec. gravity
Class III	30–40 % 1500-2000ml	Significant **tachycardia**, thready pulse, **hypotension**, metabolic acidosis	Lethargic, diminished pain response	Cool, mottling, pallor, prolonged capillary refill	Oliguria, elevated BUN
Class IV	>40 % >2000ml	Severe tachycardia & hypotension, thready central pulse	Lethargic, coma	Cold extremities, pallor, **cyanosis**	**Anuria**

Disability Assessment

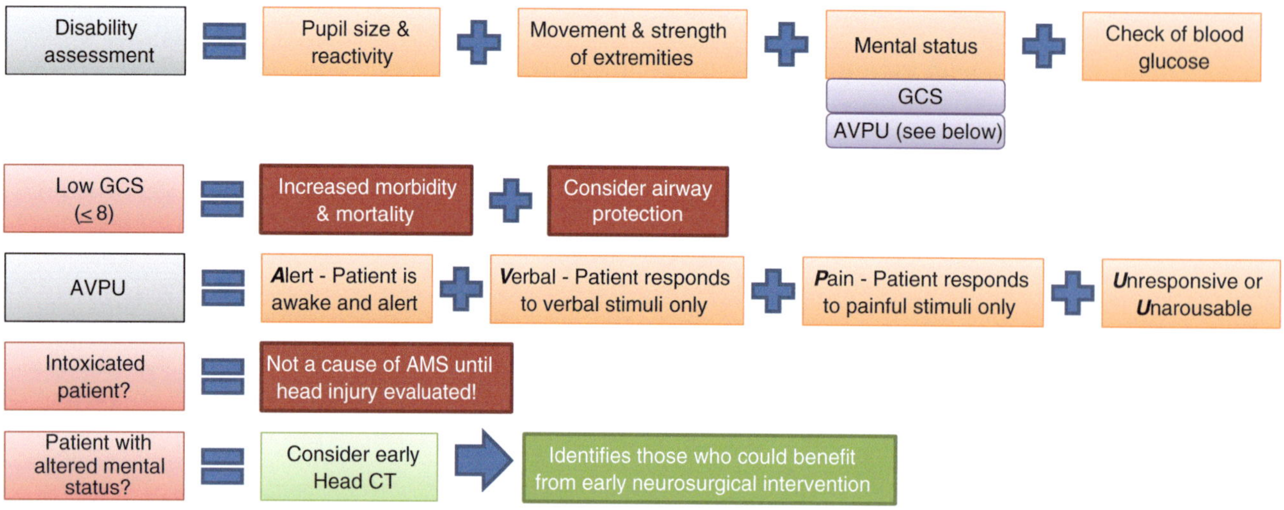

GCS

Eye opening	Best verbal	Best motor
4-Spontaneous	5-Oriented/converses	6-Obeys
3-Verbal command	4-Disoriented/converses	5-Localizes pain
2-Pain	3-Inappropriate words	4-Withdraw to stim
1-No response	2-Incomprehensible	3-Abn ext/decert
	1-No response	2-Abn ext/decer
		1-No response

Center bottom image (Reprinted from Allen B, Ganti L, Desai B. Trauma and ATLS. In: Allen B, Ganti L, Desai B, editors. Quick hits in emergency medicine. New York: Springer Science; 2013. p. 37–45. With permission from Springer Science + Business Media)

Exposure

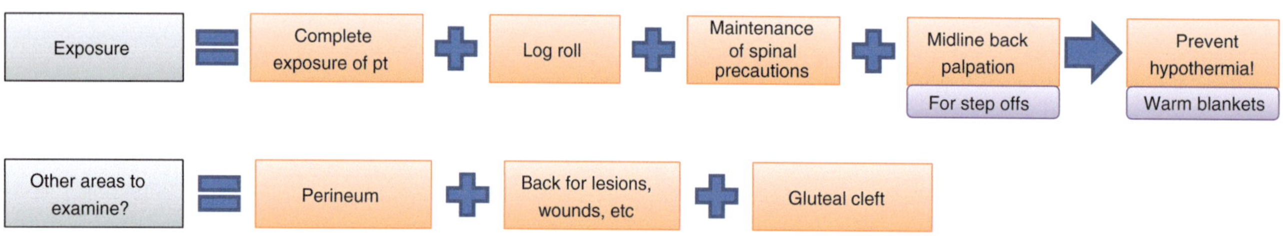

Secondary Survey

Secondary Survey = Head to toe examination of patient → Identify as many injuries as possible + AMPLE Hx + FAST exam + Consultations as needed

AMPLE Hx = **A**llergies, **M**edications, **P**MH, Time of **L**ast meal, **E**vents of injury

AMPLE considerations = Mechanism of injury + Blood loss at scene + Damage at scene + Tetanus status + Pregnancy?

Secondary Survey Labs = BMP + Glucose + CBC + Type & screen + EtOH + Pregnancy + Urine drug screen

Secondary Survey Imaging = CXR + Pelvis + Extremities as needed

Multi-system trauma? = Consider CT's of chest, abdomen/pelvis

Traumatic Arrest and ED Thoracotomy

Absolute indication = Penetrating chest trauma + Signs of life (Pre-hospital or ED) + Cardiac activity in ED

Signs of life = Palpable pulse or blood pressure OR Pupil reactivity OR Organized cardiac rhythm OR Purposeful movement OR Respiratory effort

Liberal indications = (Abdominal trauma + Cardiac activity → Requiring cross clamping of aorta to get to OR) OR Blunt chest trauma with loss of vital signs in ED

Return of spontaneous circulation? = Operating room

Pitfalls? = Must open pericardium vertically → Avoids phrenic nerve + Inadvertent cross clamping of esophagus

Head Trauma Introduction

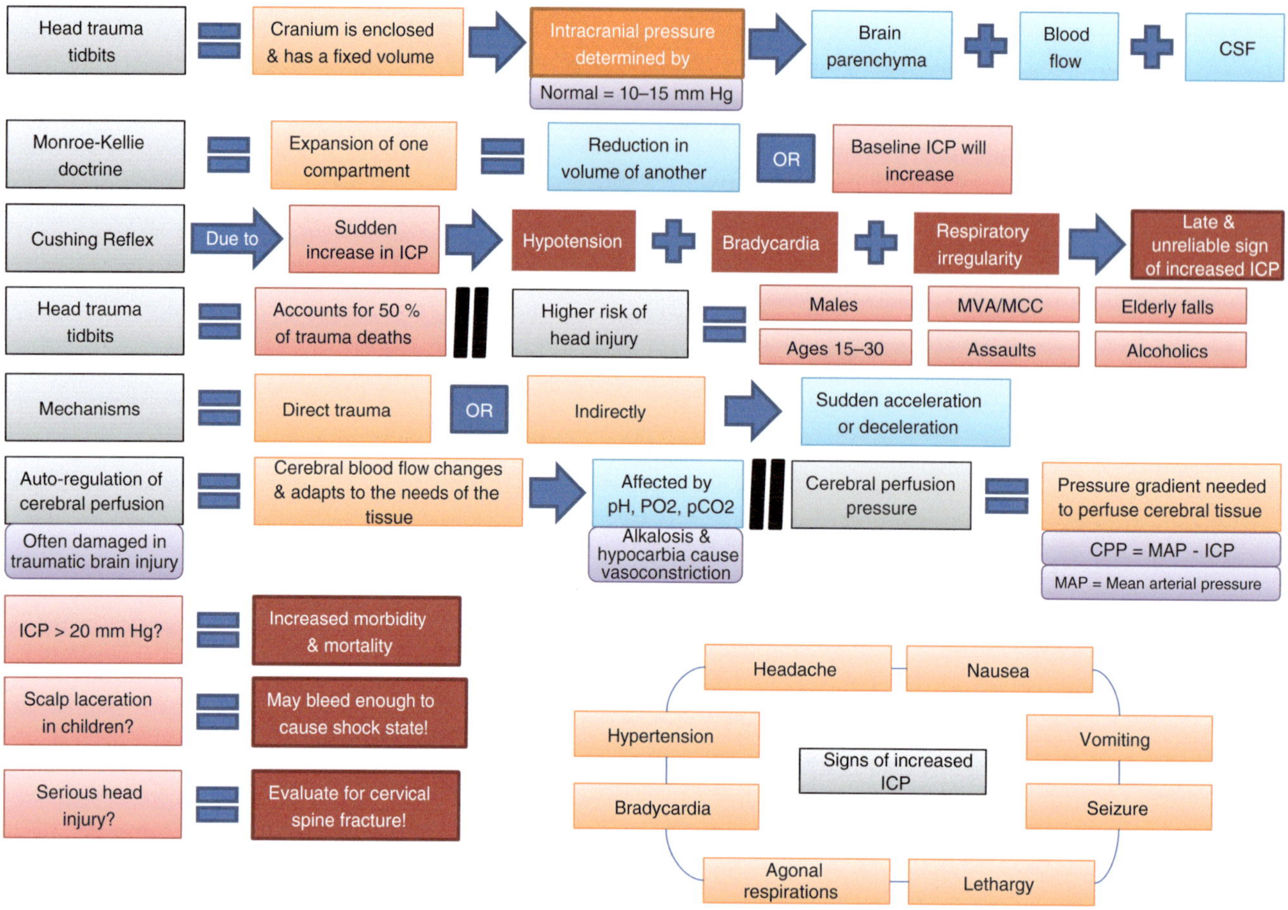

Brain Herniation

- Brain herniation = Due to increased ICP
- Brain herniation syndromes → Uncal transtentorial (Most common) + Central transtentorial + Cerebellotonsilar + Upward Posterior Fossa
- Uncal herniation = Uncus of the temporal lobe herniates inferiorly through the tentorium (Due to mass effect from edema or hemorrhage) = Fixed & dilated pupil (Compression of parasympathetic fibers of 3rd cranial nerve) + Contralateral motor paralysis (Compression of cerebral peduncle; Compression of ipsilateral corticospinal tract) → Occasionally opposite corticospinal tract is compressed (Ipsilateral hemiplegia)
- Brainstem compression? = Coma

Central transtenorial herniation (Earliest sign is CN 6 palsy):
- Bilateral pinpoint pupils
- Bilateral Babinski's sign
- Increased muscle tone

Upward transtentorial herniation:
- Conjugate downward gaze
- Pinpoint pupils
- Absence of vertical eye movements

Cerebellotonsillar herniation (Cerebellar tonsils herniate thru the foramen magnum):
- Pinpoint pupils
- Flaccid paralysis
- Sudden death
- Respiratory arrest

Treatment of Elevated ICP

- Elevated ICP? = Elevate head of bed to 30° → Increase CSF outflow from skull base
- Elevated ICP? = Maintain PCO_2 at 35–40 mm Hg + O2 saturation > 95 % ‖ Mechanically ventilated? = Maintenance of appropriate sedation (Agitation increases ICP)
- Elevated ICP? = Avoid hypotension → Decreases cerebral perfusion
- Other treatment = Prevention of seizures (Seizures increase ICP) + Mannitol (Osmotic agent than can lower ICP; 30 min. onset, lasts 6 hours; 1 g/kg) → Beware in hypotension!
- Hyperventilation? = Recommended for brief periods in the event of impending herniation
- GCS < 8 = Consider invasive monitoring + Intubation

Traumatic Seizures

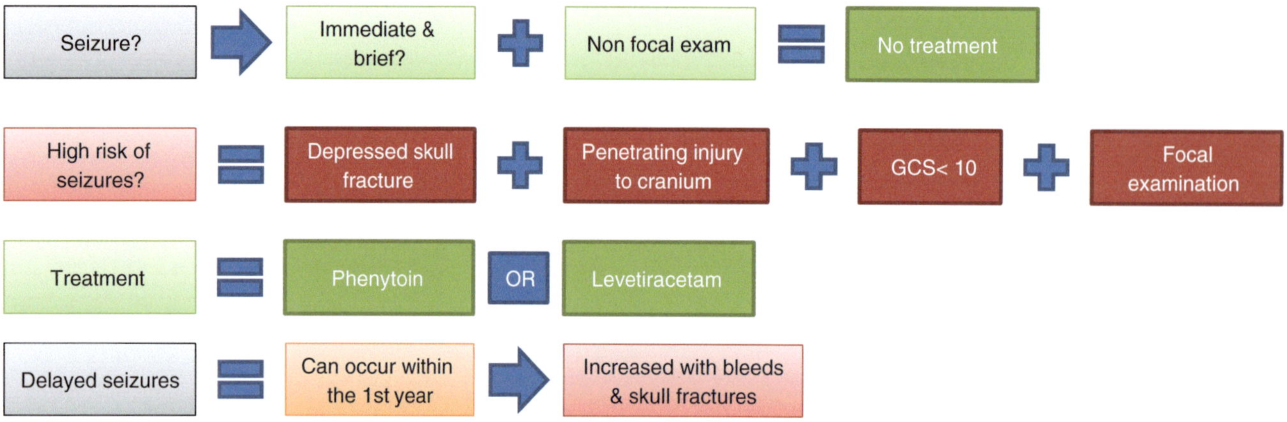

Mild Traumatic Brain Injury (TBI)

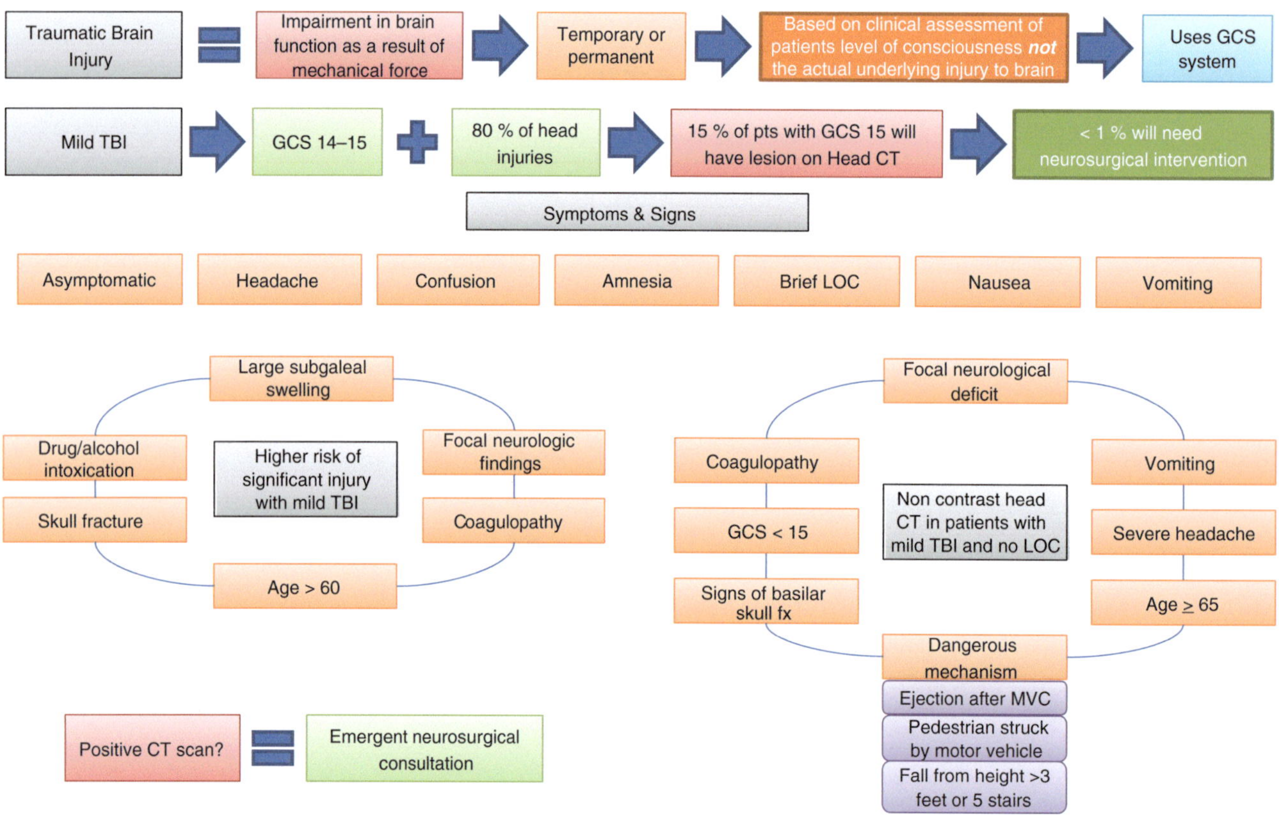

Moderate and Severe TBI

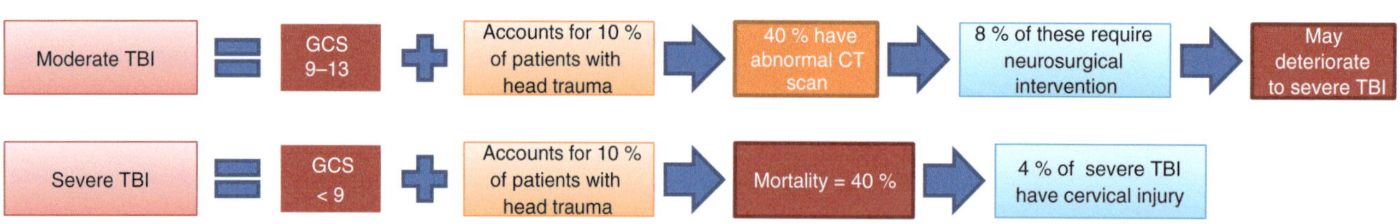

Cerebral Contusions

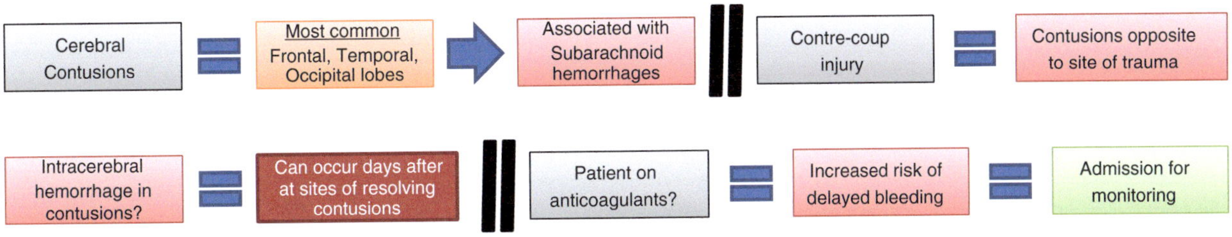

Concussion

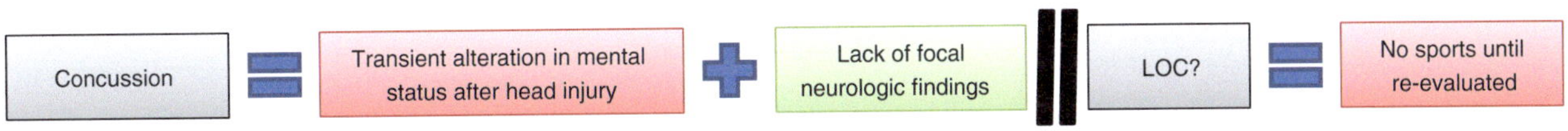

Second Impact Syndrome

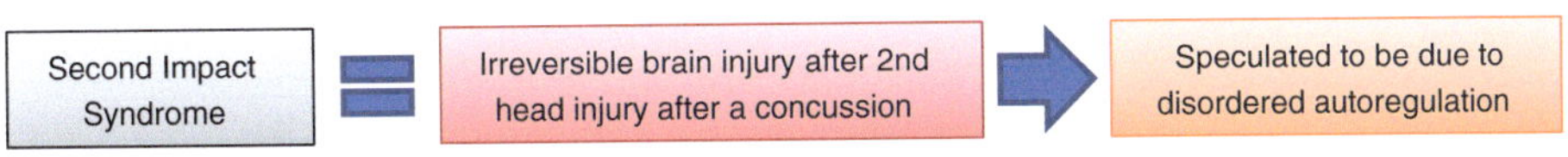

Postconcussive Syndrome

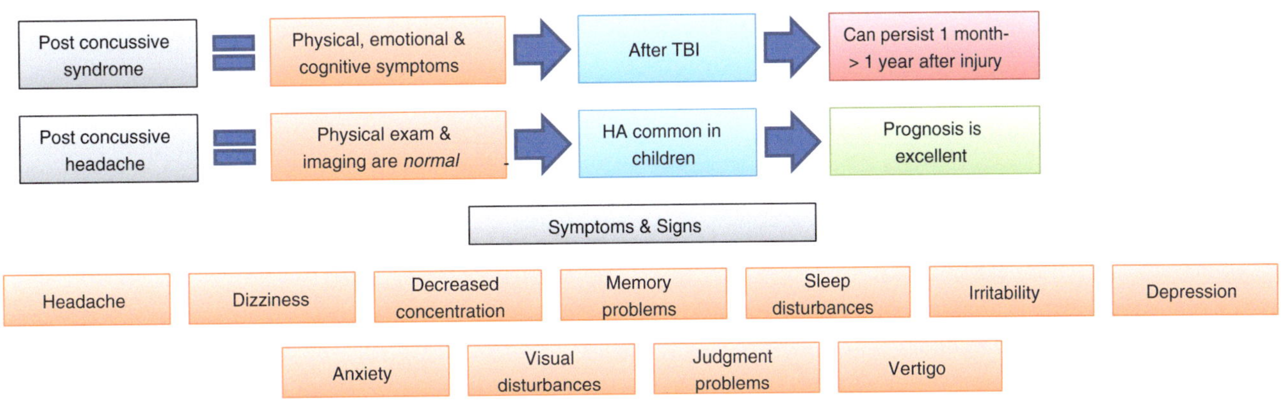

Basilar Skull Fracture

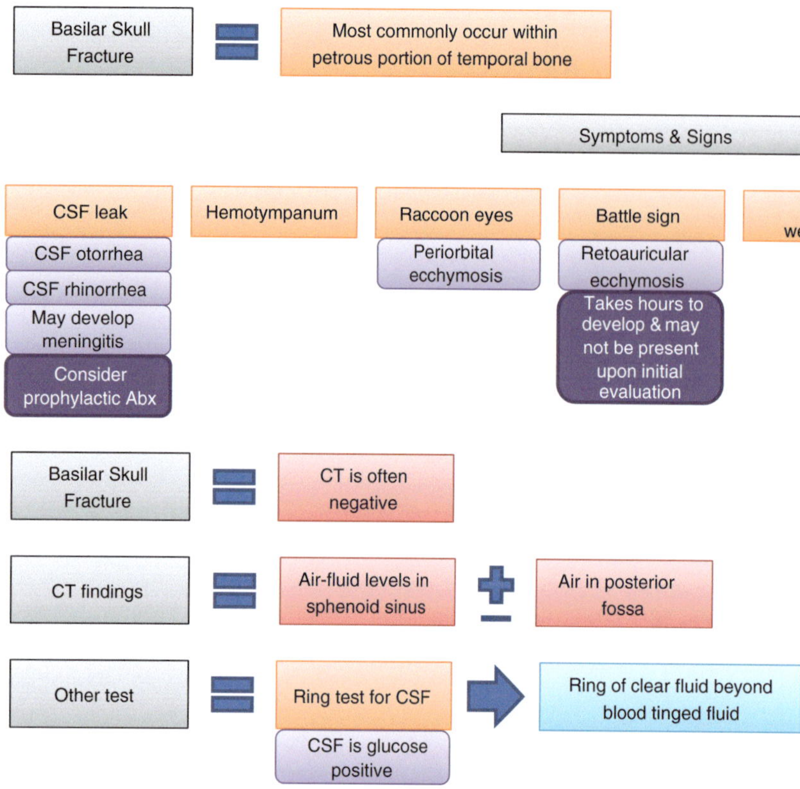

Skull Fracture

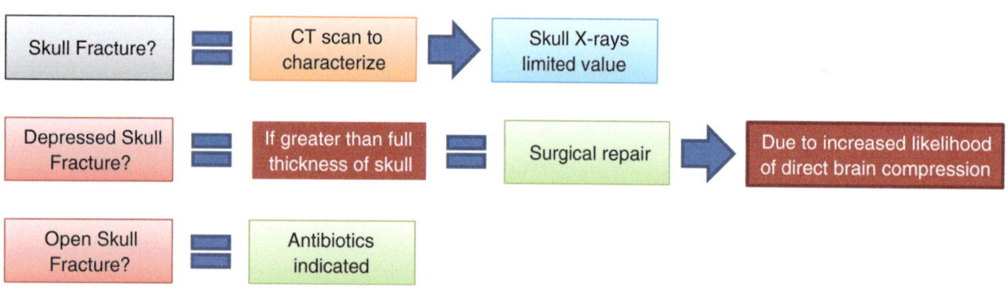

Intracranial Hemorrhage

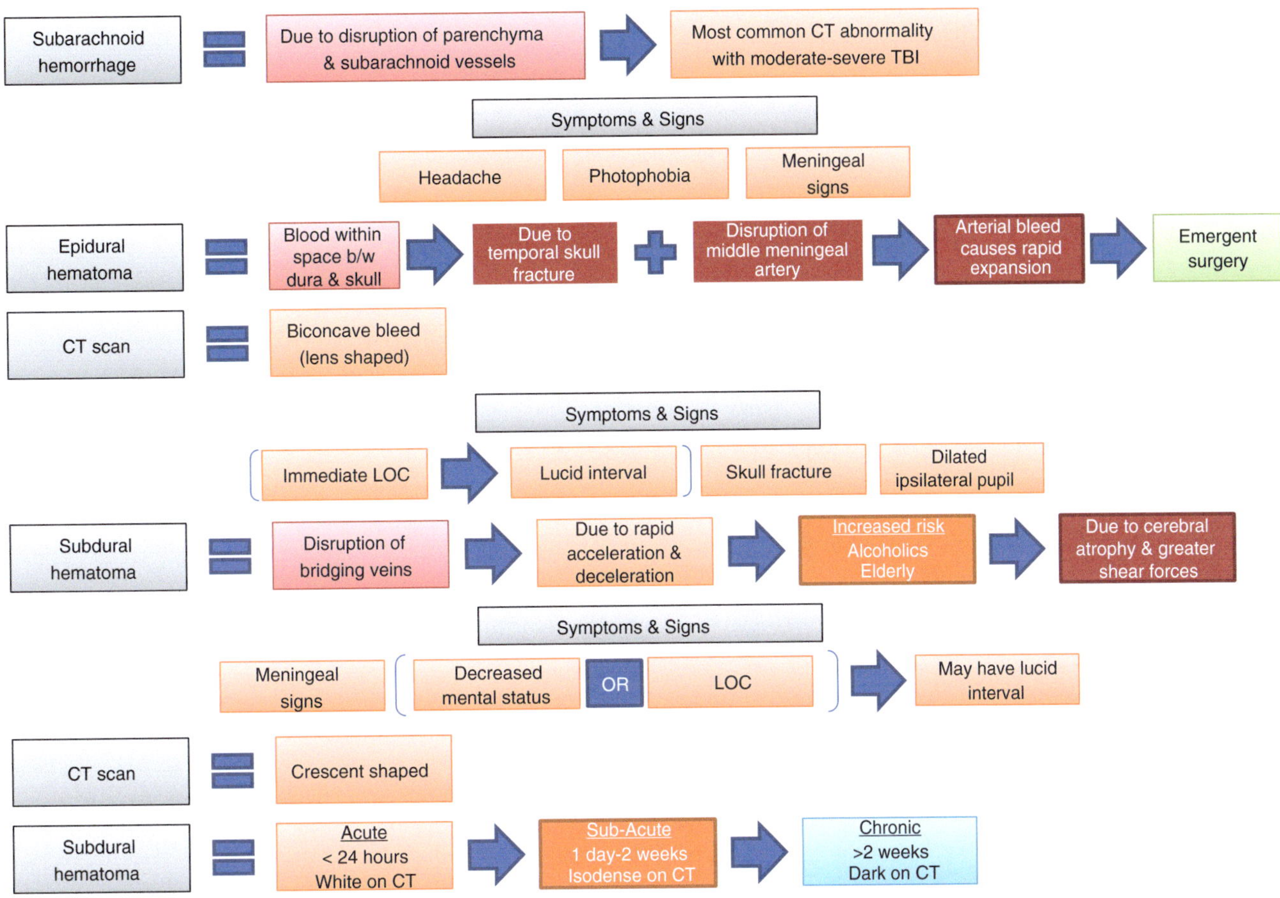

Pediatric Head Trauma

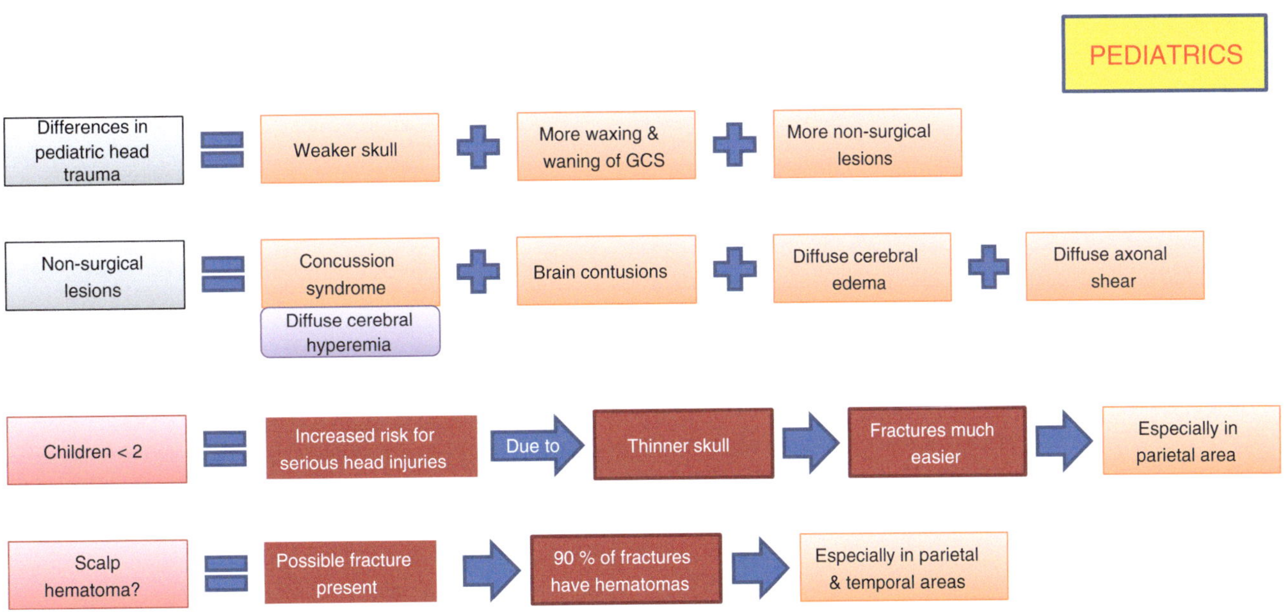

Spinal Injuries

Spinal Injury Introduction

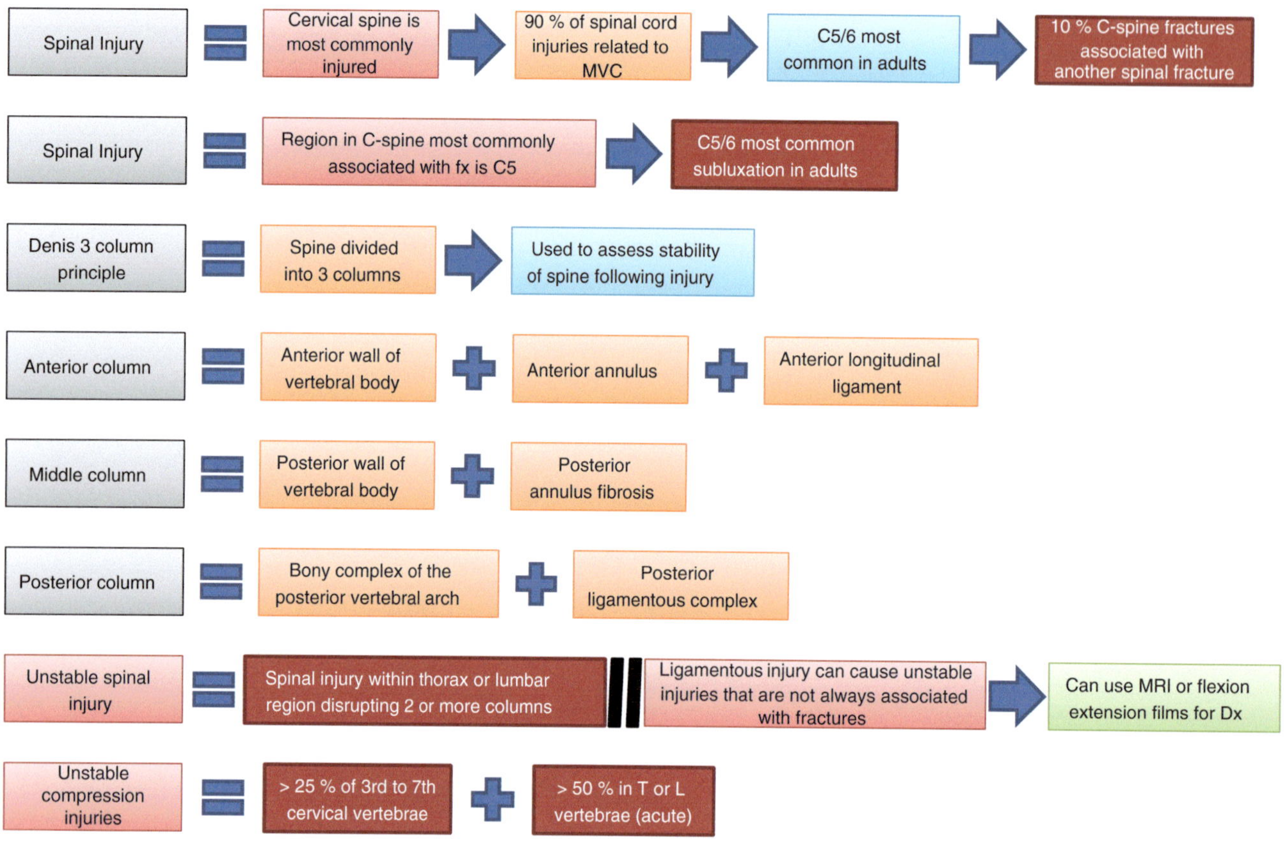

Cervical Spine Clearance

Imaging for Cervical clearance = Not always needed → Clinical criteria that can be used = NEXUS + Canadian C-spine rule

Canadian C-spine rule = Better sensitivity + Better specificity → Apply to those that are unlikely to have significant cervical injury + To those pts who are awake and alert

NEXUS criteria

Failure to meet any 1 = need for imaging

- No posterior midline tenderness
- No intoxication
- No distracting injury
- Normal level of consciousness
- No focal neurologic deficits

} 99 % sensitive

Low risk by either criteria? = Thorough neurologic exam + Full exam of C-spine + Active ROM of C-spine

Distracting injury OR Intoxication OR Altered mental status = NO clearance!

Cervical Spine Evaluation

PEDIATRICS

Anatomy (4 lines) = Anterior longitudinal + Posterior longitudinal + Spinolaminar + Spinous process

Important measurements on plain films = Predental space → Peds < 5 mm, Adults < 3 mm + Prevertebral space → 6 mm at C2, 22 mm at C6

Imaging tidbits = X-rays = 3 views → AP, Lateral, & Odontoid → Must see ALL 7 vertebrae on film + Top of T1

20 % C-spine injuries occur at C7

Imaging tidbits = Plain films miss 15 % of injuries + Negative plain films do not rule out injury!

Plain film inadequate? = CT

CT instead of plain film? = Age > 65 + High risk mechanism + Those receiving CT of other areas + Suspected head trauma or AMS

Pseudosubluxation

Pseudosubluxation = Pediatric C-spine → Common below 8 years of age → Typically occurs C2 on C3 → 2–3 mm anterior misalignment

Pseudosubluxation = *Normal* alignment of the spinolaminar line

Stable Cervical Fractures

Type of Fracture	Mechanism	Tidbits
Wedge Fracture	Flexion	May be unstable if loss of >50 % of vertebral height
Clay Shoveler's Fracture	Flexion against contracted posterior muscles	Most common at C7 Can occur at C6 & T1
Transverse Process Fracture	Flexion	
Unilateral Facet	Flexion & Rotation	Disruption of posterior ligament complex "Bow-Tie" deformity on lateral X-Ray Is potentially unstable
Burst Fracture	Vertical compression	Becomes unstable if fracture fragments enter spinal canal
Isolated fractures of articular pillar & vertebral body	Vertical compression	
Posterior Neural Arch of C1	Hyperextension	Stable when isolated Arch may be congenitally absent

Unstable Cervical Fractures

Jefferson Bit Off A Hangman's Thumb

Type of Fracture	Mechanism	Tidbits
C1 Burst Fracture (Jefferson Fracture)	Axial load with vertical compression (Diving injury)	Lateral masses of C1 are displaced outward
Bilateral facet dislocation	Flexion	High incidence of spinal cord injuries May see > 5mm subluxation
Odontoid Type II or III	Flexion or Extension	See next page
Atlantoaxial or Atlanto-occipital (or Any Fx/dislocation)	Atlantoaxial or Atlanto-occipital = Flexion or extension	Atlantoaxial C1/2 disruption Rheumatoid arthritis or ankylosing spondylitis
Hangman's Fracture	Extension	Bilateral Fx of pedicles of C2 with forward movement of C2 on C3
Teardrop fractures	Flexion or Extension	Flexion? = extreme flexion with complete ligamentous disruption Extension? = Hyperextension; Associated with central cord syndrome; anterior longitudinal ligament avulses inferior part of vertebral body

Odontoid Fractures

Odontoid Fractures = Increase in prevertebral space → 3 types → Most common cervical fracture in children → Atlanto-dens interval 5 mm in pediatrics 3 mm in adults

Type 1 = Stable → Avulsion at tip of dens

Type 2 = Most common → Unstable → At the junction of odontoid & body of C2

Type 3 = Unstable → Fracture at base of dens

Thoracolumbar Fractures

Thoracic spine = Not injured as frequently as C or L spine → Due to → Increased rigidity → But… → Higher incidence of cord injury → Due to → Narrower spinal canal

Minor thoracolumbar fx = Transverse process fx + Spinous process fx + Pars Interarticularis → Part of vertebra located between the inferior & superior articular processes of the facet joint

Type of Fracture	Mechanism	Tidbits
Wedge Compression Fracture	Flexion	
Flexion-distraction Fracture	Flexion with compression of anterior elements and distraction of posterior elements	
Translational Fracture	Shear	
Chance Fracture	Flexion around an anterior axis associated with lap belt	Horizontal fracture & is UNSTABLE due to disruption of posterior ligament Usually at L1 or L2 Beware Bowel, Spleen & Liver injury!! Ileus may occur
Burst Fracture	Vertical compression	L1> L2> T12 Disruption of anterior & middle columns = Unstable fracture Unstable if > 50 % loss of height Consider calcitonin spray for Rx

Spinal Cord Injuries

Spinal Cord Syndromes

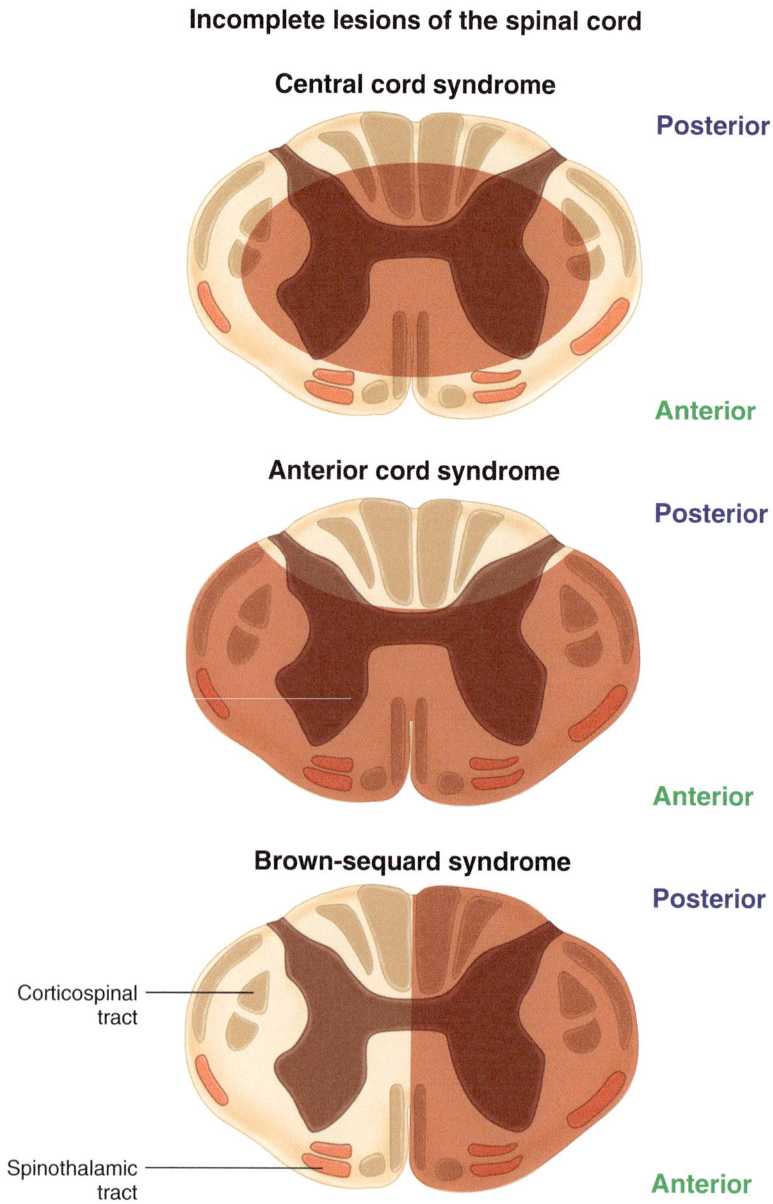

Incomplete Spinal Cord Injury

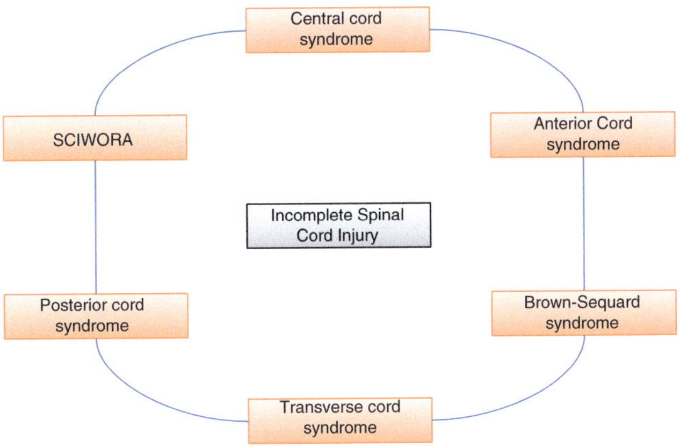

Central Cord Syndrome

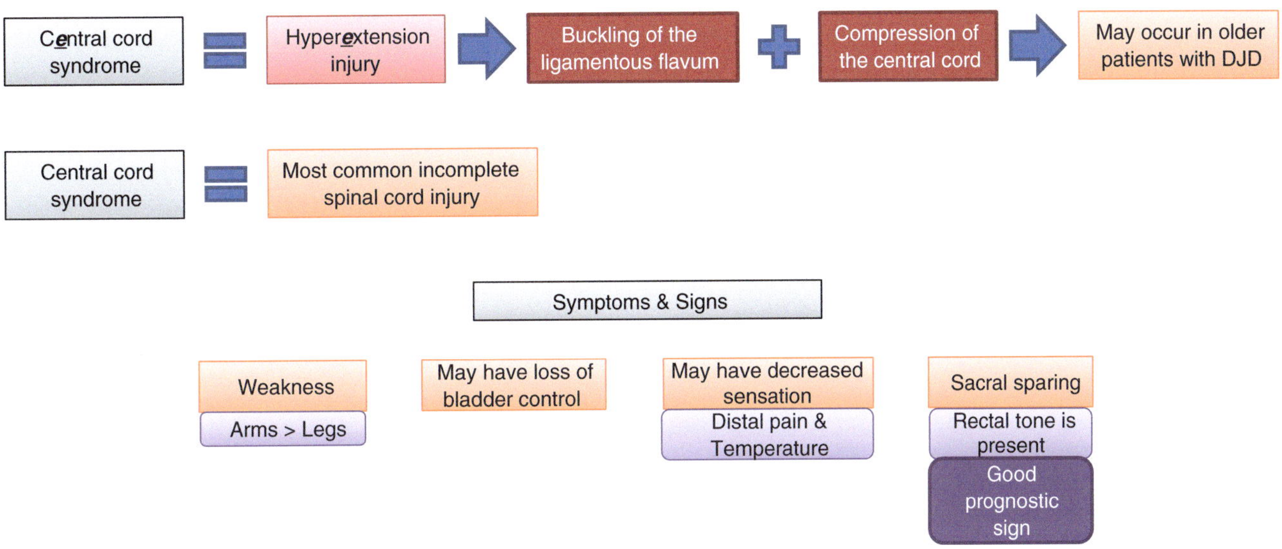

Anterior Cord Syndrome

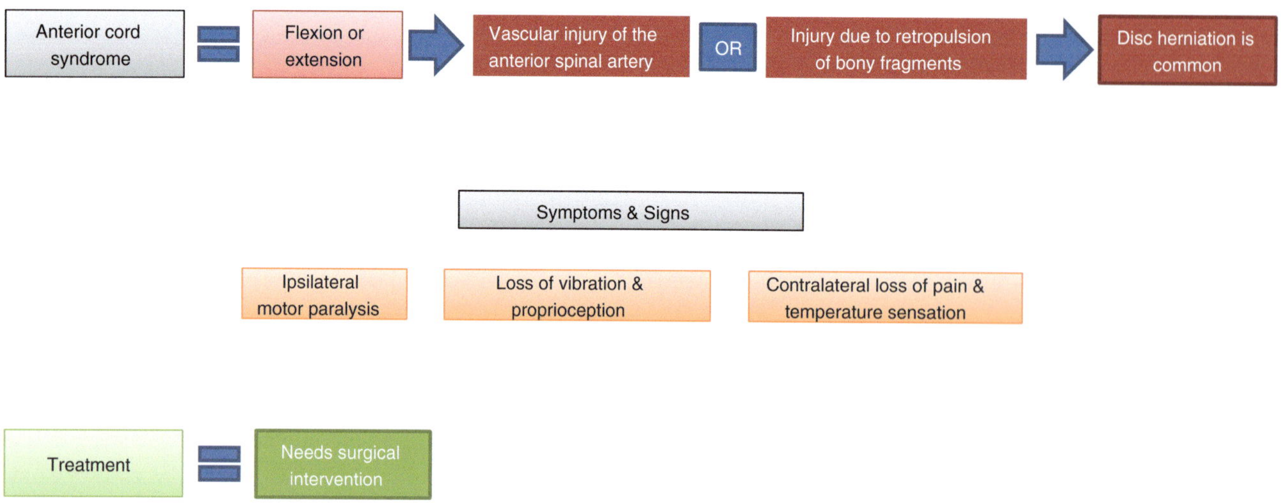

Brown-Sequard Syndrome

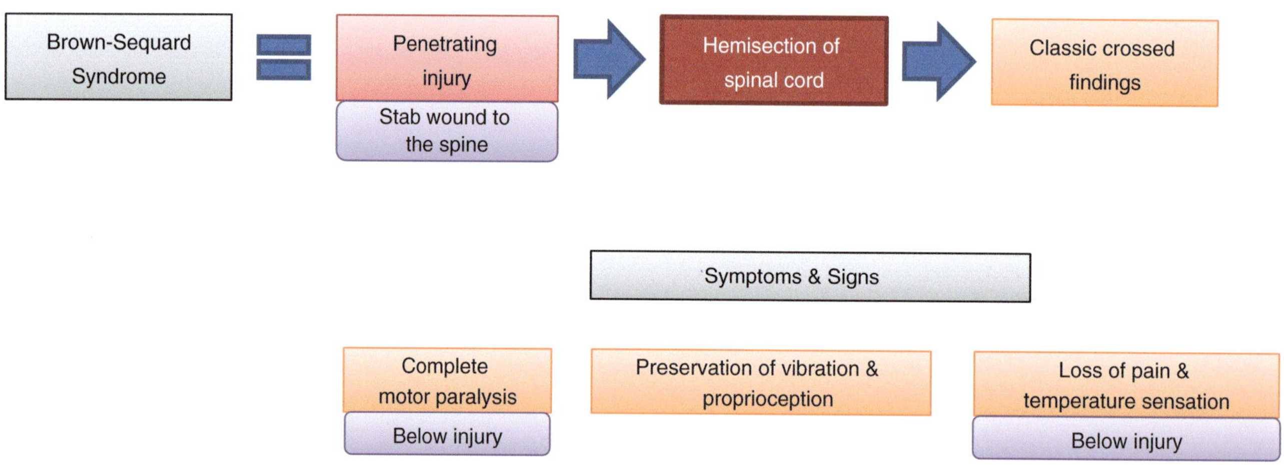

Transverse Cord Syndrome

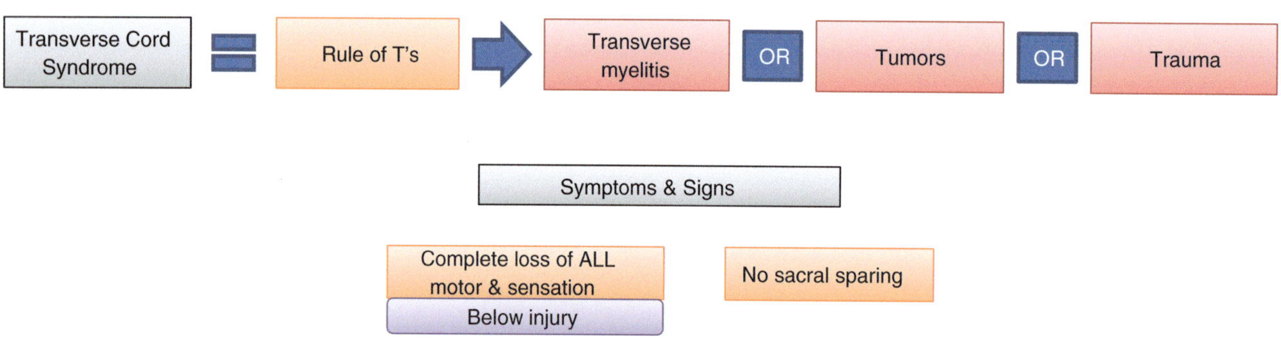

Posterior Cord Syndrome

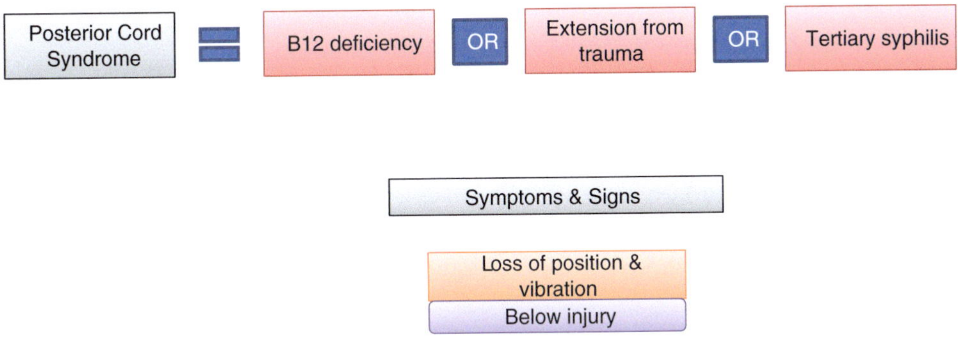

SCIWORA

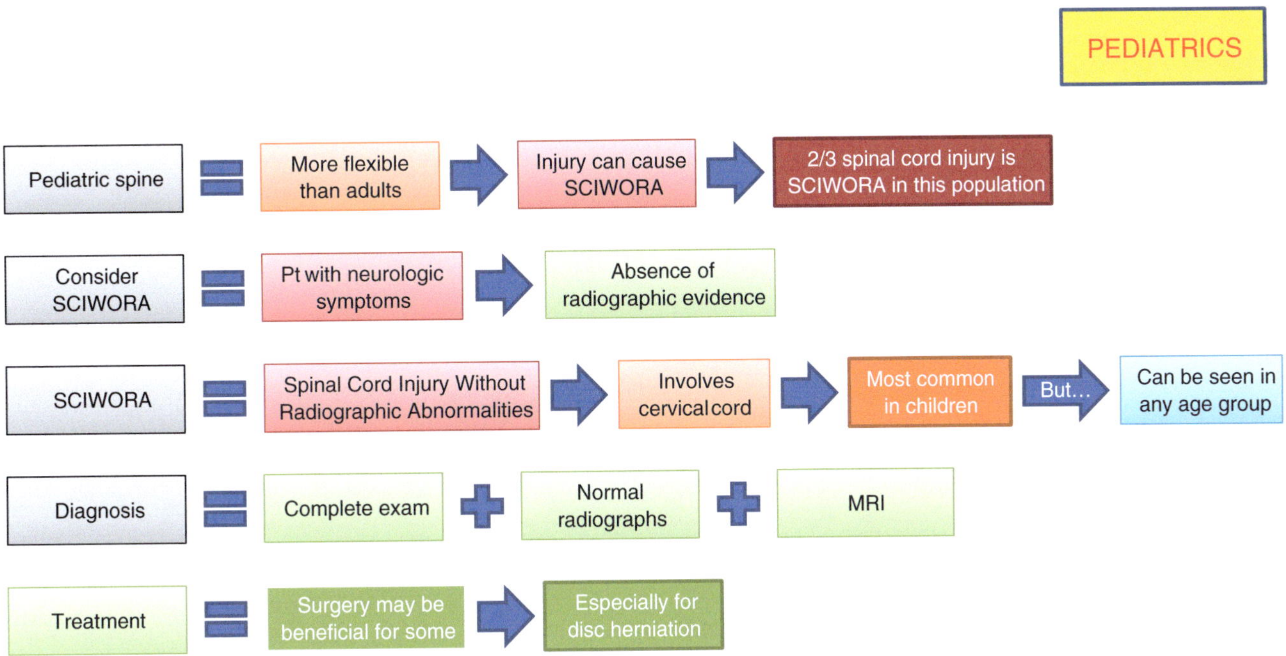

Spinal Shock

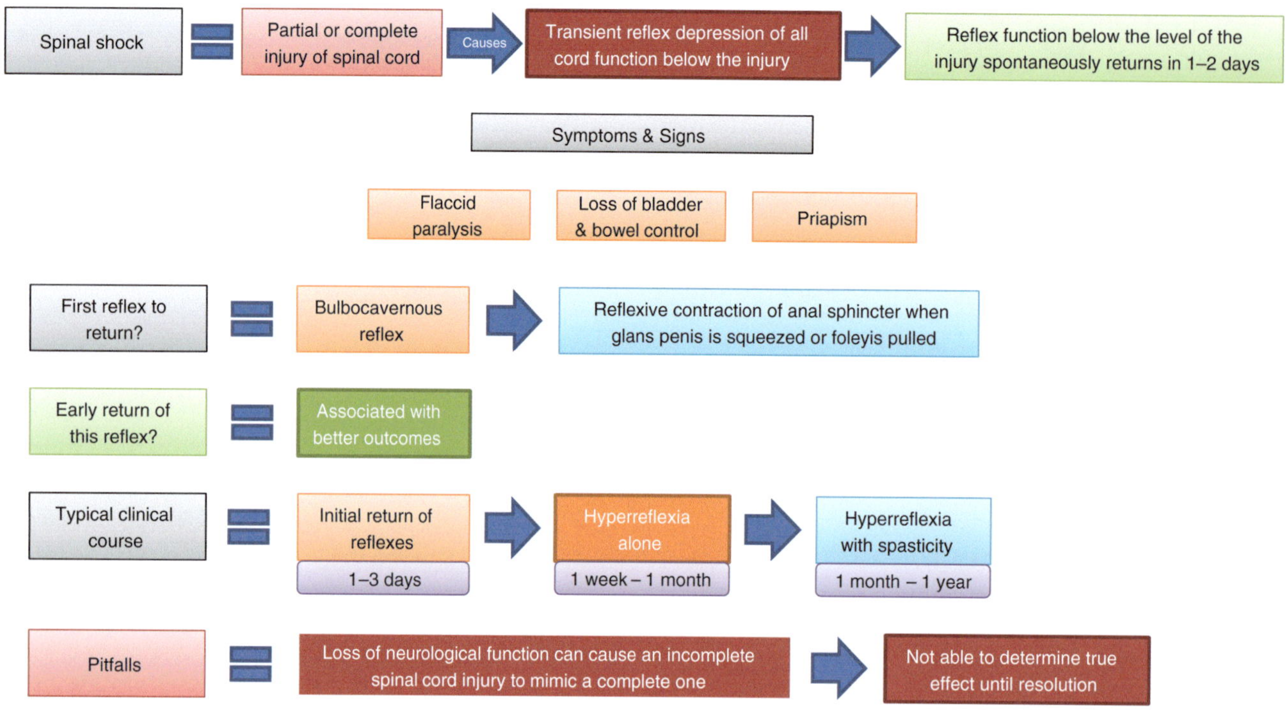

Neurogenic Shock

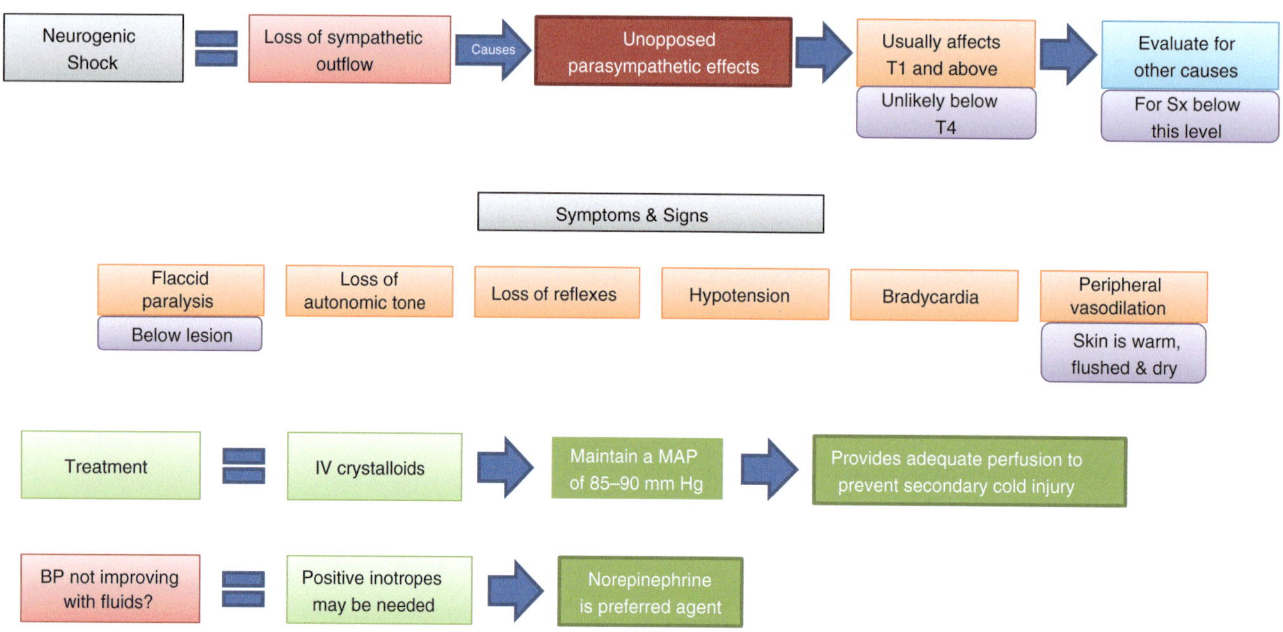

Penetrating Neck Injury

Penetrating Neck Injury Introduction

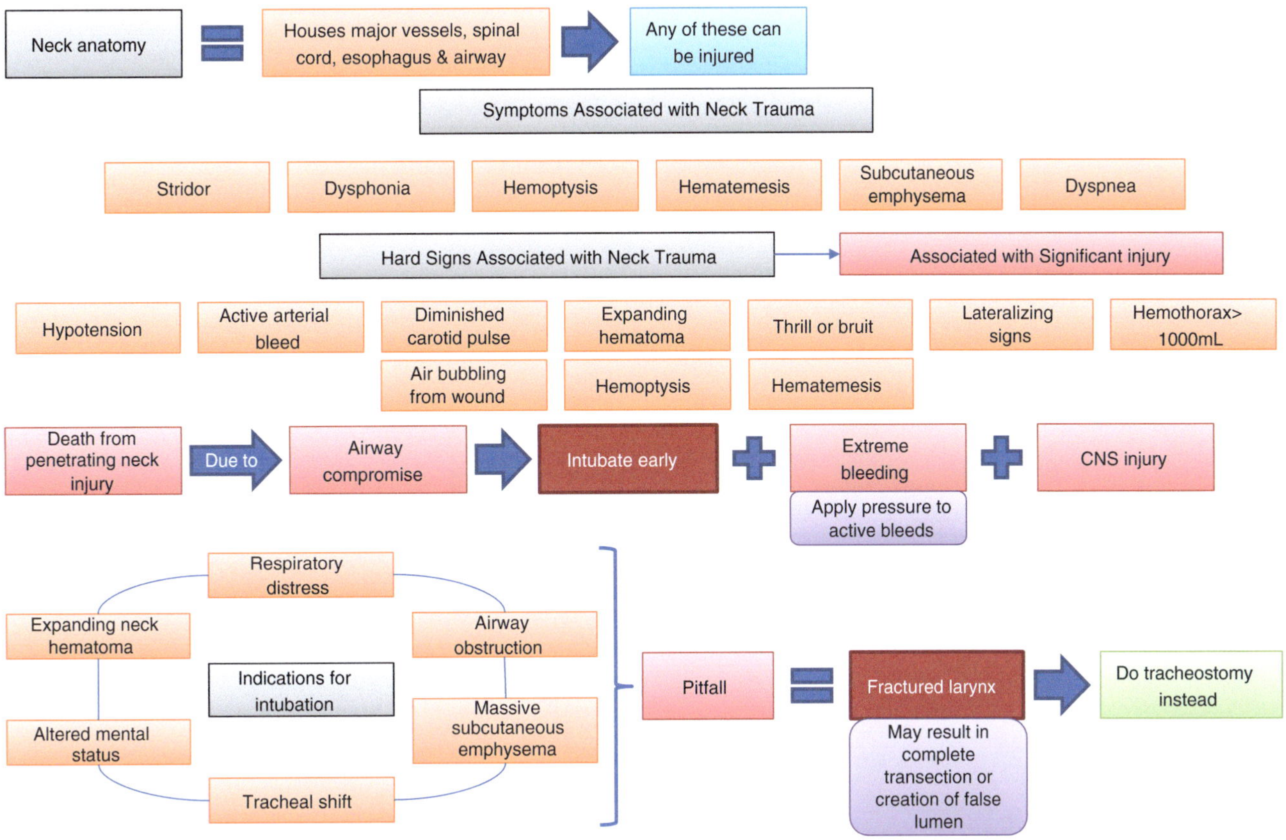

Zones of the Neck

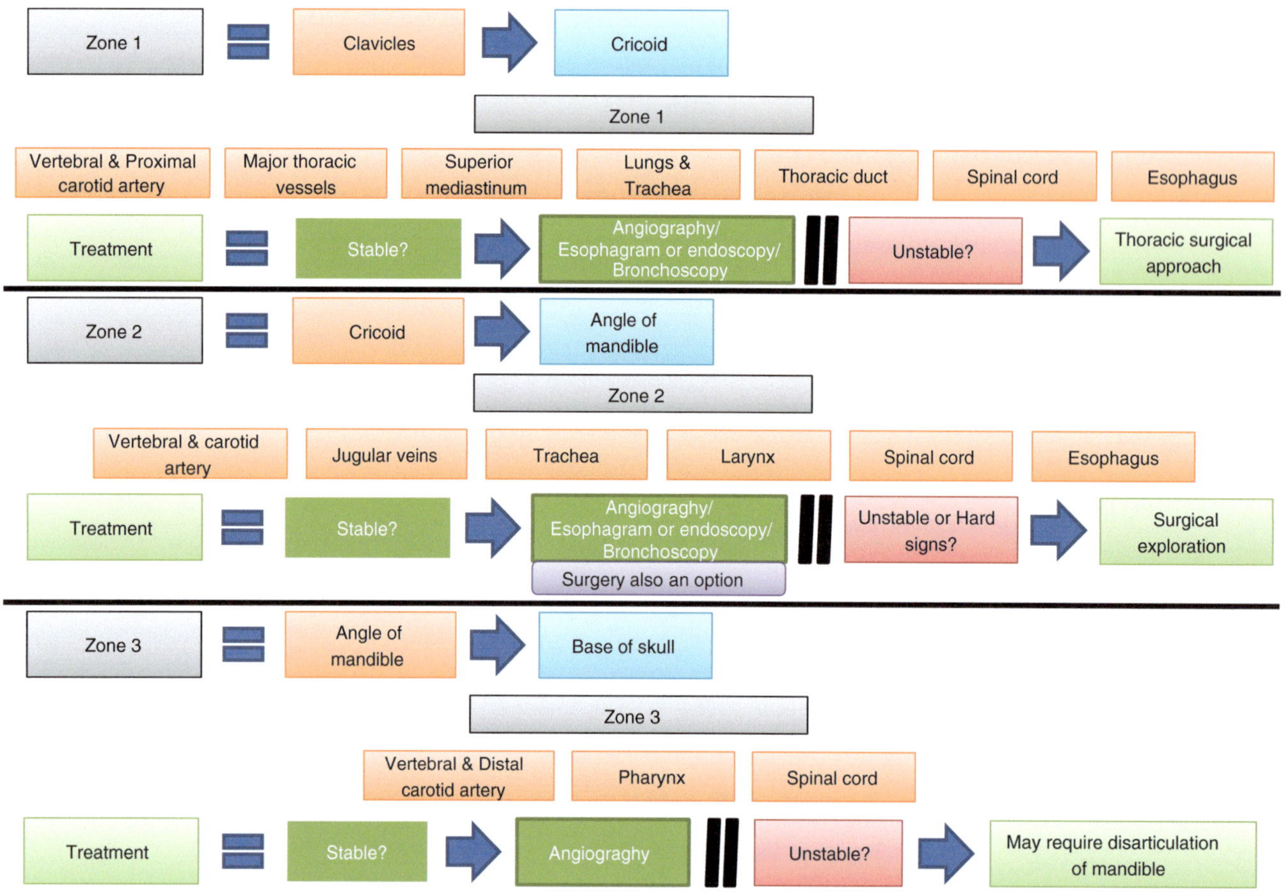

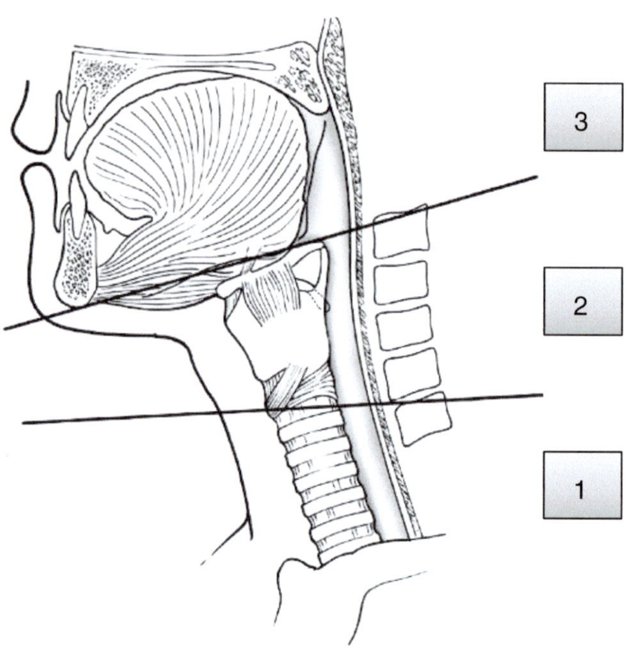

Center image (Reprinted from Ustin J. Access to the neck in penetrating trauma. In: Velmahos GC, Degiannis E, Doll D, editors. Penetrating trauma. Heidelberg: Springer Verlag; 2012. p. 37–45. With permission from Springer Verlag)

General Treatment of Penetrating Neck Trauma

Violation of the platysma? = Emergent surgical consultation → But… → Do not explore at bedside! → Any vascular injuries need proximal & distal control → NO blind clamping!

Active bleeding? = Apply direct pressure → No blind clamping!

NO violation of the platysma? + Minor neck trauma + No signs of structural damage to nerves or major vessels = Careful closure in ED + D/C after 4-6 hours of observation

Diagnostic tools = CT scan of neck ± chest ± Plain radiographs of chest & C-spine

Pitfall? = Air embolism → May be fatal

Airway Embolism = Classic machinery murmur

Treatment = Trendelenburg + Left lateral decubitus position → Prevents migration of air bubble

Pharynx Trauma

Larynx trauma see ENT

Pharynx Trauma = Blunt or penetrating trauma → Same with esophageal trauma

Symptoms & Signs

- Hematemesis
- Odynophagia
- SQ emphysema
- Pneumomediastinal air
- Retropharyngeal air

Diagnosis = Cervical soft tissue plain films (If stable to leave ED) + Consider endoscopy + Consider esophageal imaging

Treatment = NPO + Broad spectrum antibiotics

Blunt Neck Trauma

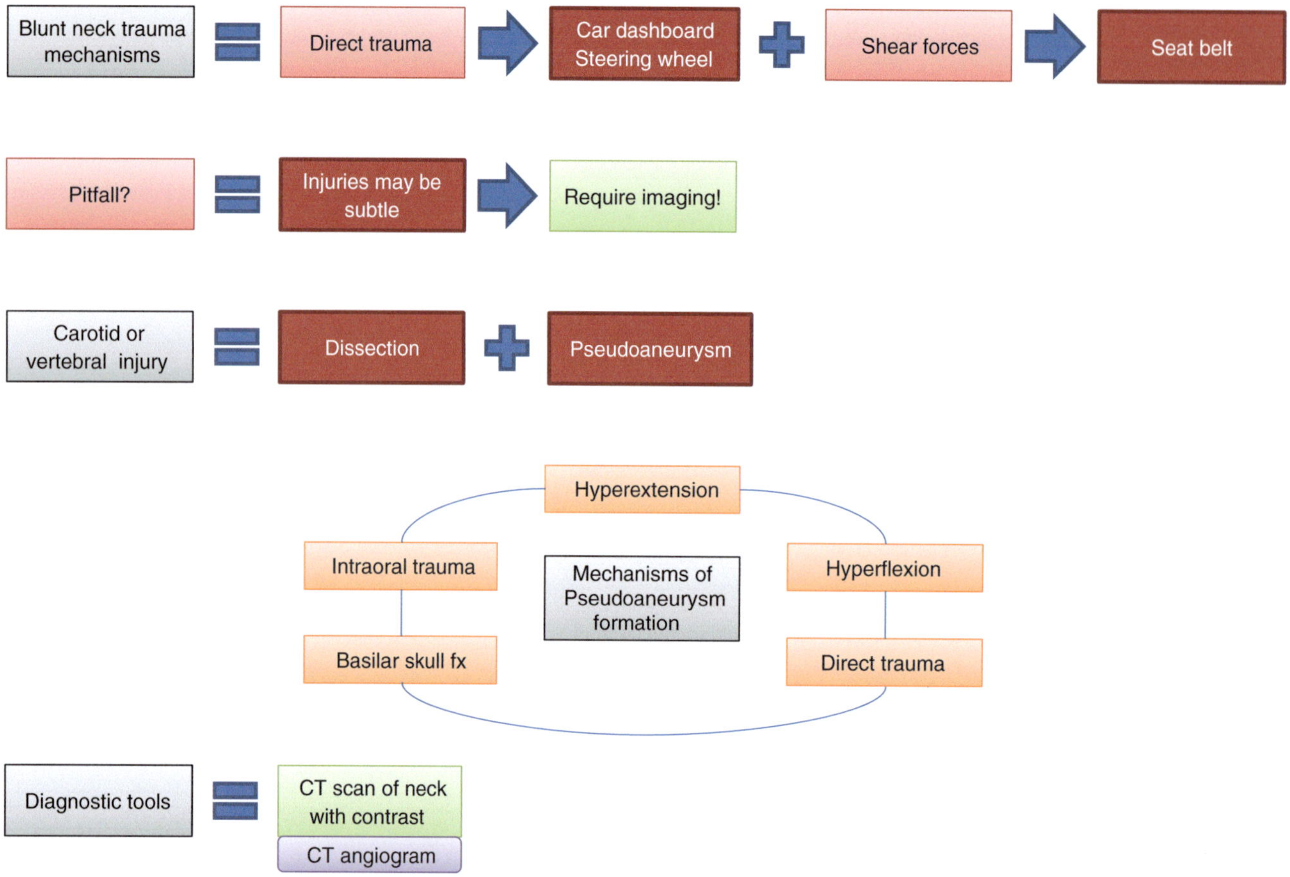

Chest Trauma

Chest Trauma Tidbits

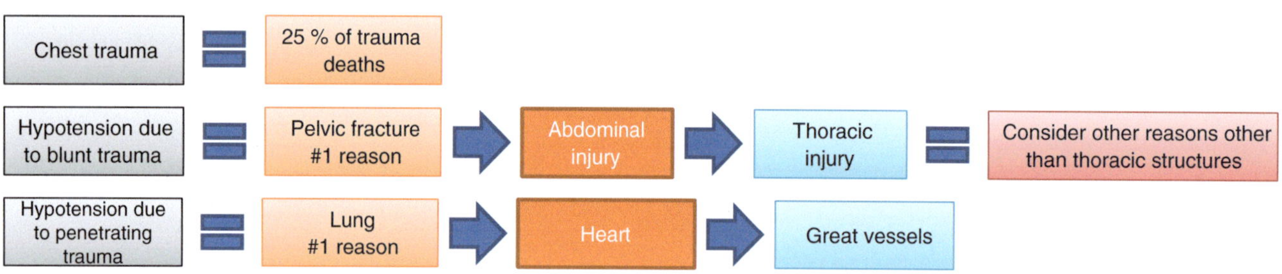

Pneumomediastinum (PM)

PM = Air within the mediastinum → Injury to air containing structures in thoracic cavity || No trauma? = Ruptured alveoli

Air containing structures = Pharynx + Larynx + Trachea + Major bronchi + Esophagus

Spontaneous? = Valsalva + Restraints with combative pts + Mechanical ventilation + Sneezing + Ruptured bleb

Signs = Subcutaneous emphysema + Hamman's sign → Crunching sound over heart during systole

Diagnosis = CT scan ± (Contrast esophagram OR Endoscopy → For evaluation of esophageal injury)

Pneumothorax (PTX)

Pneumothorax = Accumulation of air within pleural space

Symptoms & Signs

- Ipsilateral decreased or absent breath sounds
- Hyperresonance to percussion
- Subcutaneous emphysema
- Chest pain
- Dyspnea

Subcutaneous emphysema + No PTX on CXR = PTX until proven otherwise! → Findings can be delayed by 4–6 hrs! → Repeat CXR if Sx persist

Diagnosis = CXR (Expiratory) ± Ultrasound ± CT

CXR findings = Ipsilateral decreased lung markings + Subcutaneous emphysema + Ipsilateral low lateral diaphragm (Deep sulcus) → Decubitus CXR has higher sensitivity than upright CXR

Ultrasound = As accurate as CT + Supine US has higher negative predictive value than CXR

Pneumothorax Treatment

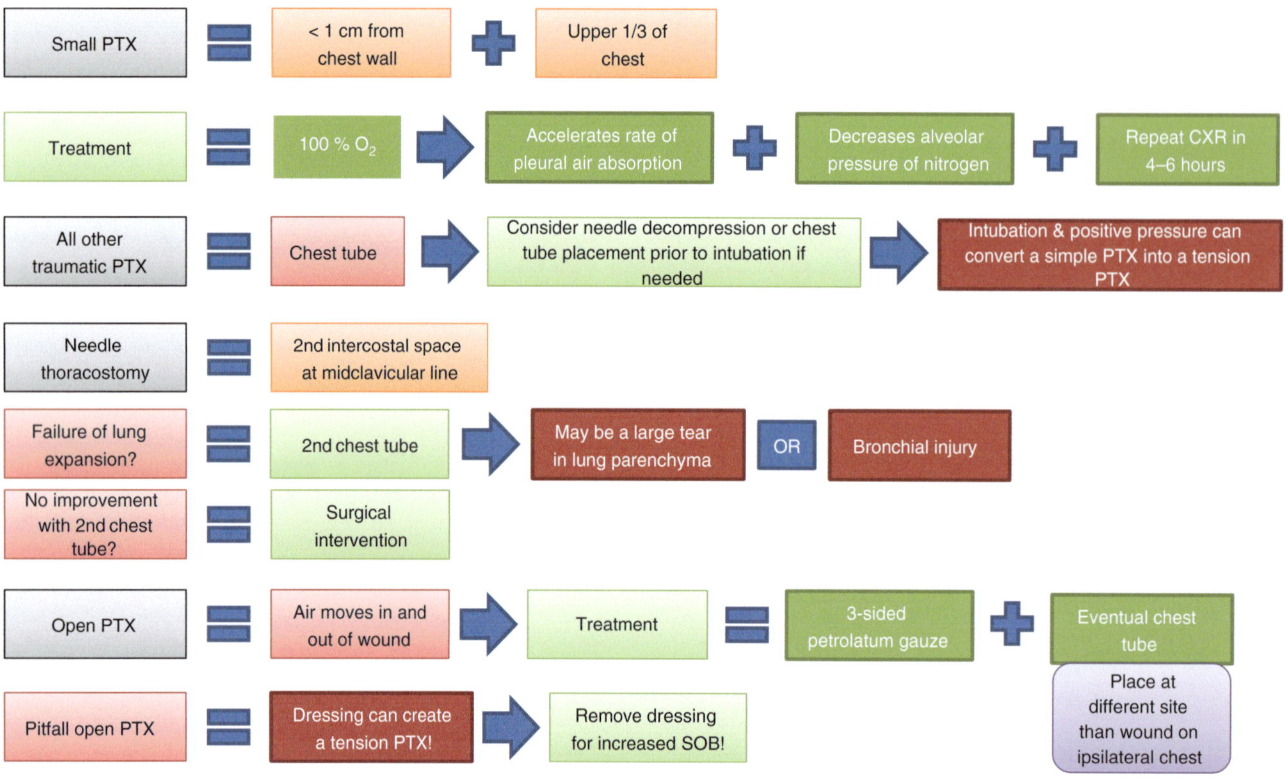

Tension Pneumothorax

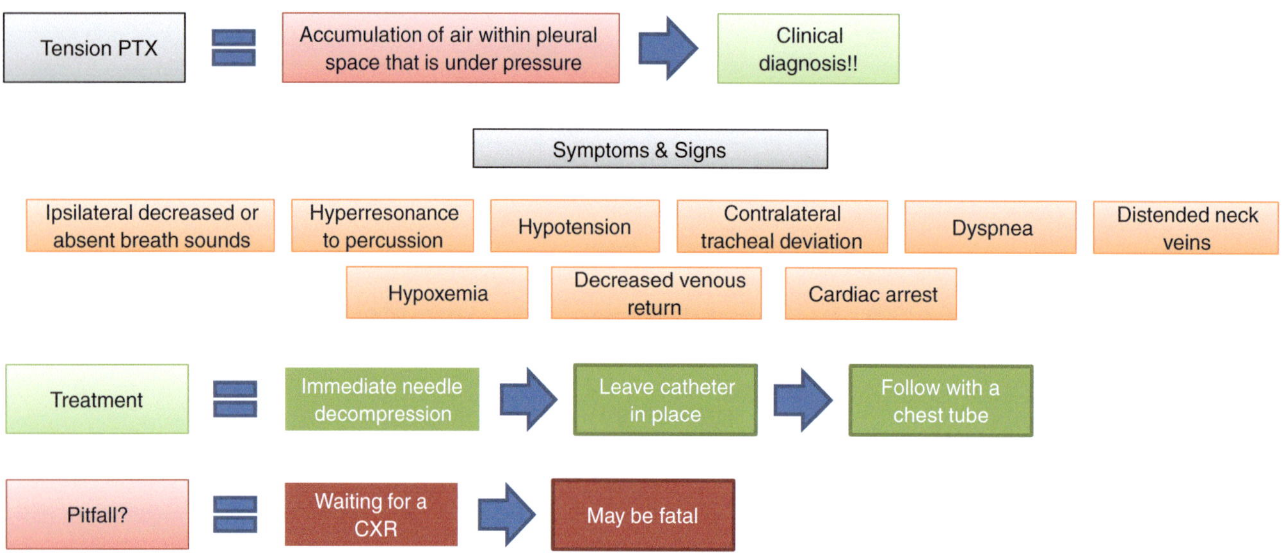

Hemothorax

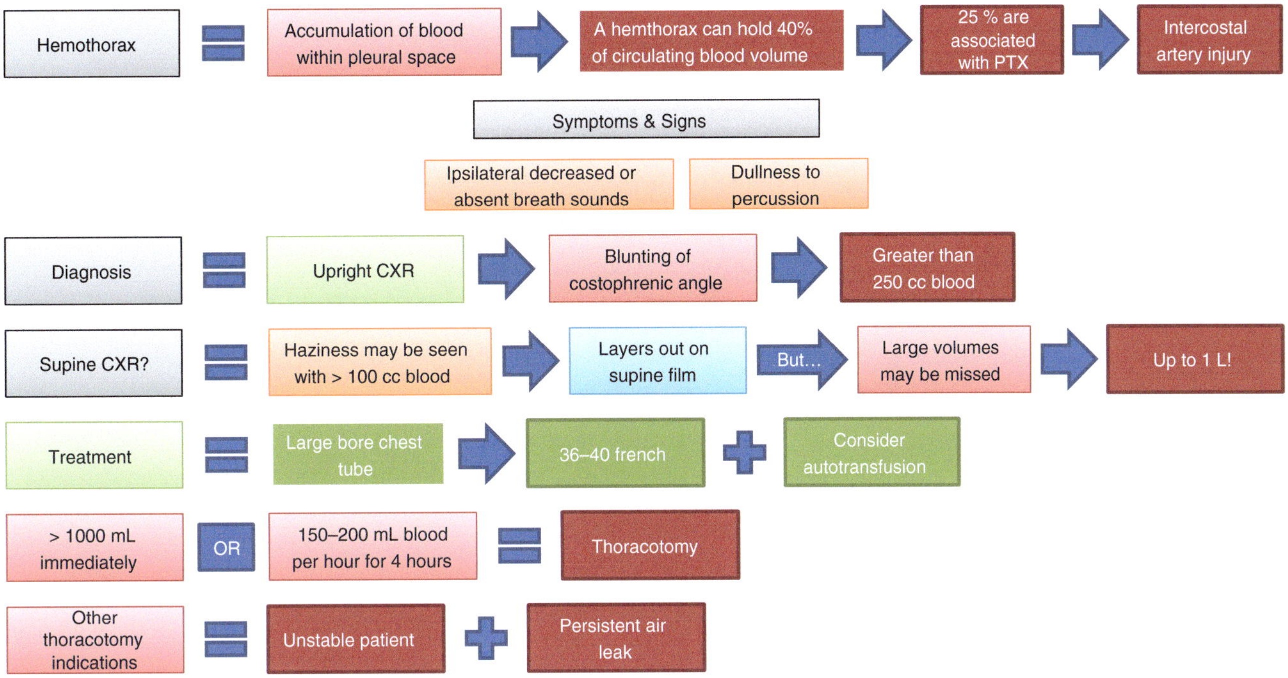

Rib Fractures

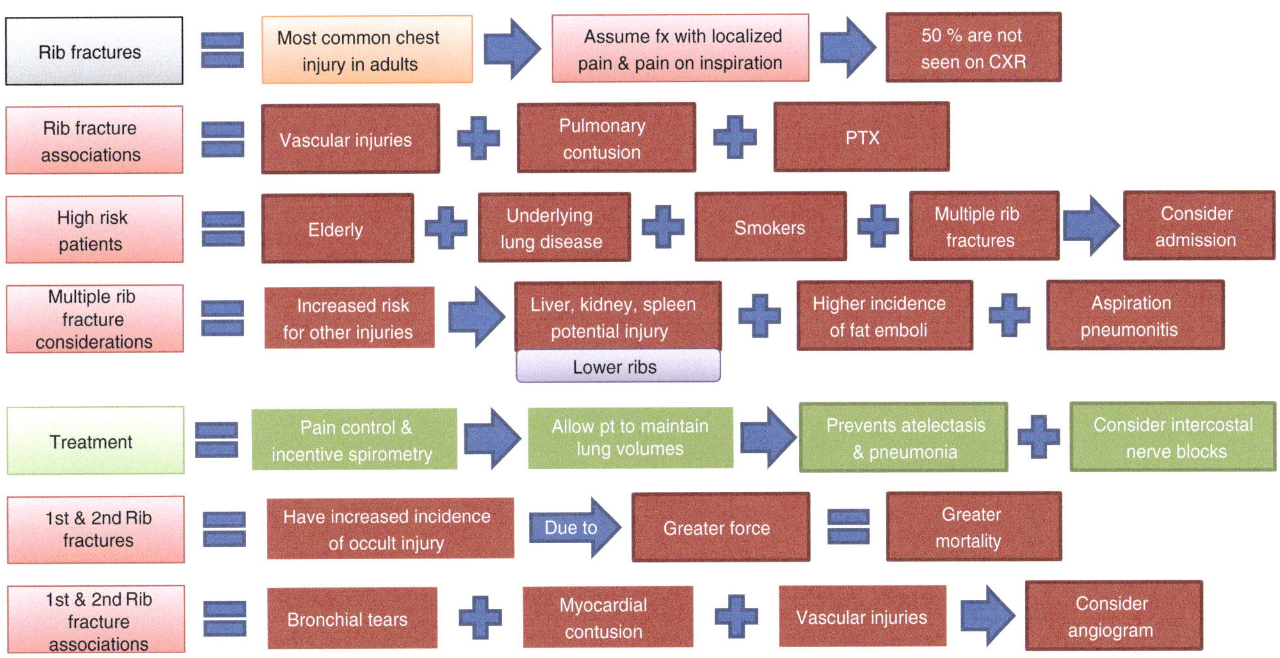

Flail Chest

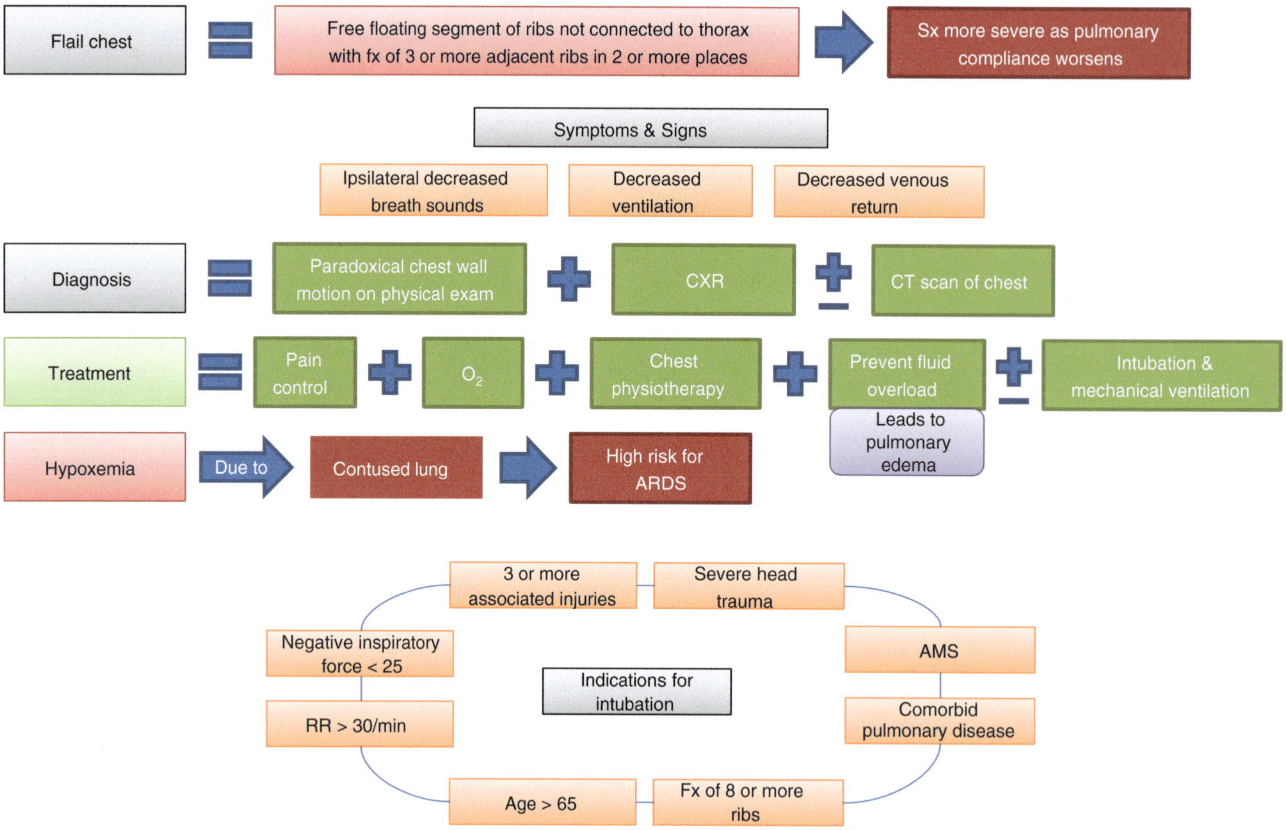

Sternal Fracture

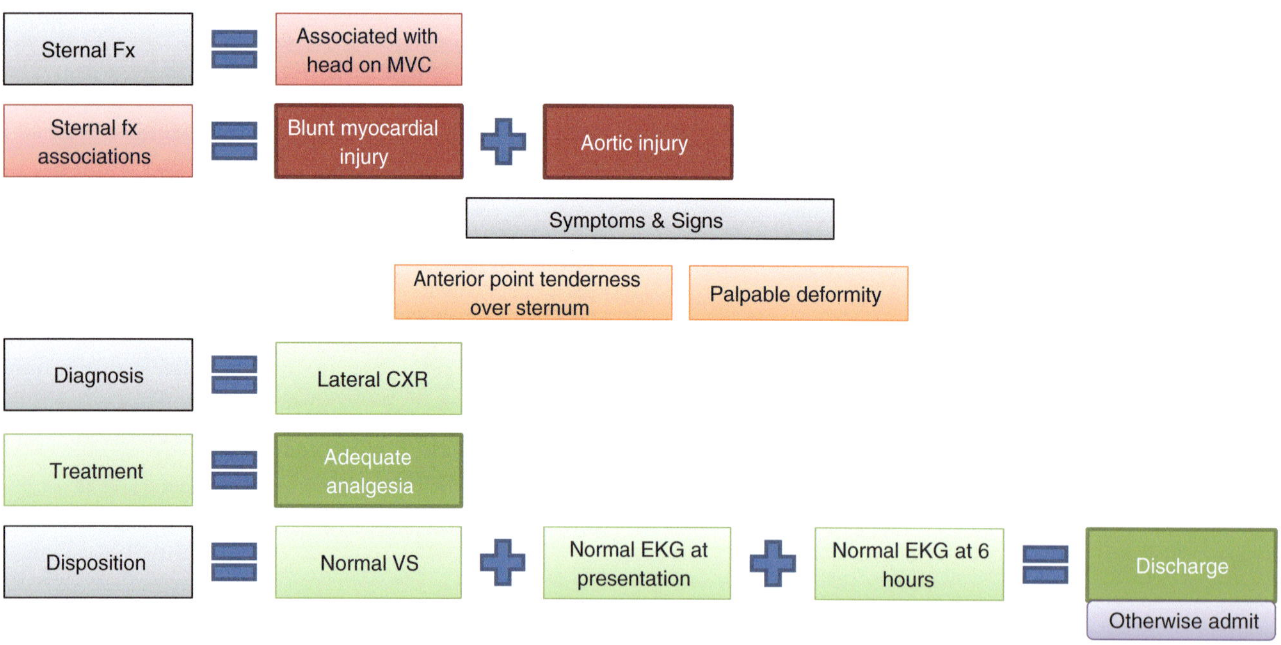

Pulmonary Contusion

Pulmonary contusion = Direct damage to lung → Leads to → Hemorrhage + Edema → Associated with flail chest

Pitfall = Secondary insult → Due to → Fluid administration during resuscitation (Beware aggressive fluid resuscitation) + Development of edema in unaffected lung due to reflex shunting of blood

Pulmonary contusion = Most common significant chest injury in children → Due to → Elasticity of chest wall

Symptoms & Signs

Decreased compliance of lung | Hemoptysis (common) | Hypoxemia

Diagnosis = CXR OR CT → CT is more accurate

CXR findings = Opaque patches of lung OR Patchy alveolar infiltrates → May be delayed up to 6 hours

Treatment = Analgesia + Pulmonary toilet + Respiratory support → Consider PEEP & permissive hypercapnia

Consider intubation = If > 28 % of lung affected → 1 lobe = 18 % total lung volume

Severe contusion? = Decubitus position → Uninjured lung down → Enhances ventilation & perfusion

Tracheobronchial Injuries

Tracheobronchial Injuries = Associated with shear forces → Due to → Deceleration → Typically occurs within 2cm of the carina → High mortality with rupture

Continuous bubbling in chest tube? = Bronchopleural fistula

Symptoms & Signs

Chest pain | Dyspnea | Hamman's crunch | Hypoxemia | Hemoptysis | Subcutaneous emphysema

Diagnosis = CXR + CT → CT is more accurate

CXR findings = PTX OR Pneumomediastinum + Rib fractures

Treatment = Oxygenation + Ventilation + Chest tube

Cardiac Trauma

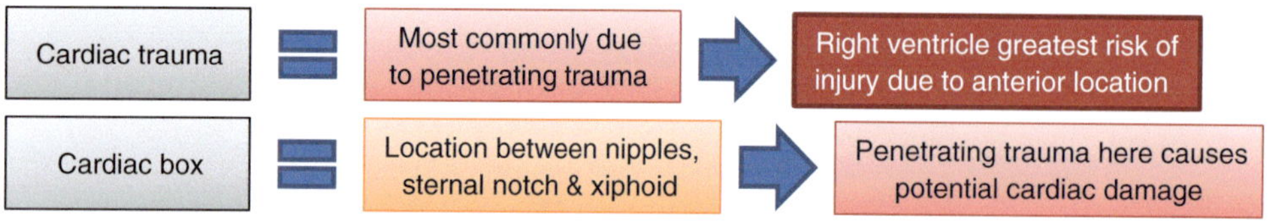

Cardiac Tamponade

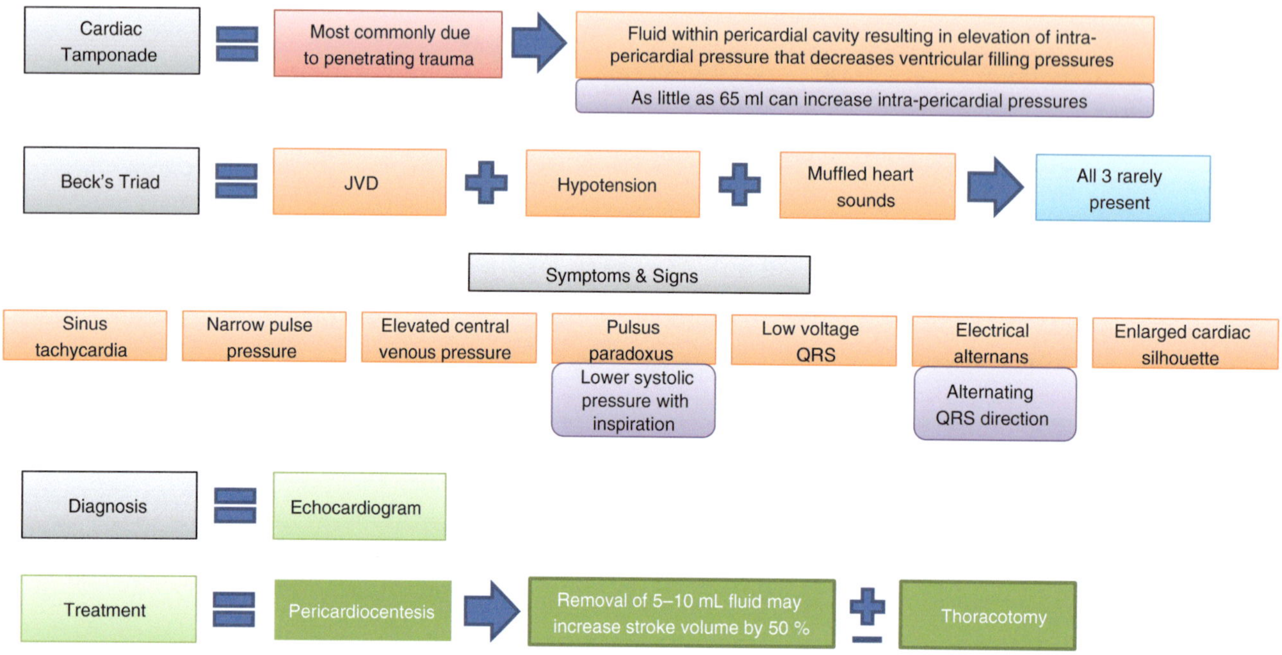

Cardiac Contusion

Cardiac contusion = Blunt myocardial injury → 20 % MVC deaths due to this

Mechanisms = Blast injury + Direct precordial impact + Deceleration or torsion → Causes tear in heart at point of fixation
- Right atrium
- Vena cava

Symptoms & Signs
- Chest pain
- Tachycardia
- Arrhythmia

Injuries =
- Wall rupture: 90 % die at scene
- Valve injuries: Aortic most common
- Contusion: RV most common
- Septal rupture
- Coronary artery thrombosis
- Coronary artery laceration
- Pericardial injury

Diagnosis = No definitive screening tests → EKG + Monitoring + Troponin 4–6 hrs post injury + Consider echocardiogram (Wall motion defects)

Treatment = O_2 to maintain PaO_2 >80 + IVF & pressors (Hypotensive pts)

Complications = Post-trauma pericarditis + VSD + Valve defects + Ventricular aneurysm + Tamponade

Commotio cordis = 2nd most common cause of death in young athletes → Sudden death due to blunt trauma to chest → Caused by impact to chest wall 10-30 milliseconds before T wave that induces ventricular fibrillation

Commotio cordis = Associated with baseball, hockey, & lacrosse + Football – Direct blow to sternum

Traumatic Aortic Injury (TAI)

Traumatic Aortic Injury (TAI) = 90 % with blunt trauma & TAI die at scene → 50 % of the rest die within 24 hours → Mechanism = Deceleration / High speed side impact / Penetrating trauma

Most common region injured = Proximal descending aorta ‖ Survivors who reach ED → Have tear at ligamentum arteriosum

Symptoms & Signs
- Unequal BP in extremities: Elevated BP in UE, Decreased in LE
- Intrascapular bruits or murmurs: Harsh systolic murmur
- Retrosternal chest pain
- Pulse difference b/w UE & LE
- Dysphagia
- Dyspnea
- Stridor

Diagnosis = CXR + CT – angio scan ± Transesophageal echo

Treatment = Maintain systolic BP < 120 mm Hg + Heart rate of 60 bpm + Avoid Valsalva + Surgery

CXR Findings Suggestive of Aortic Injury

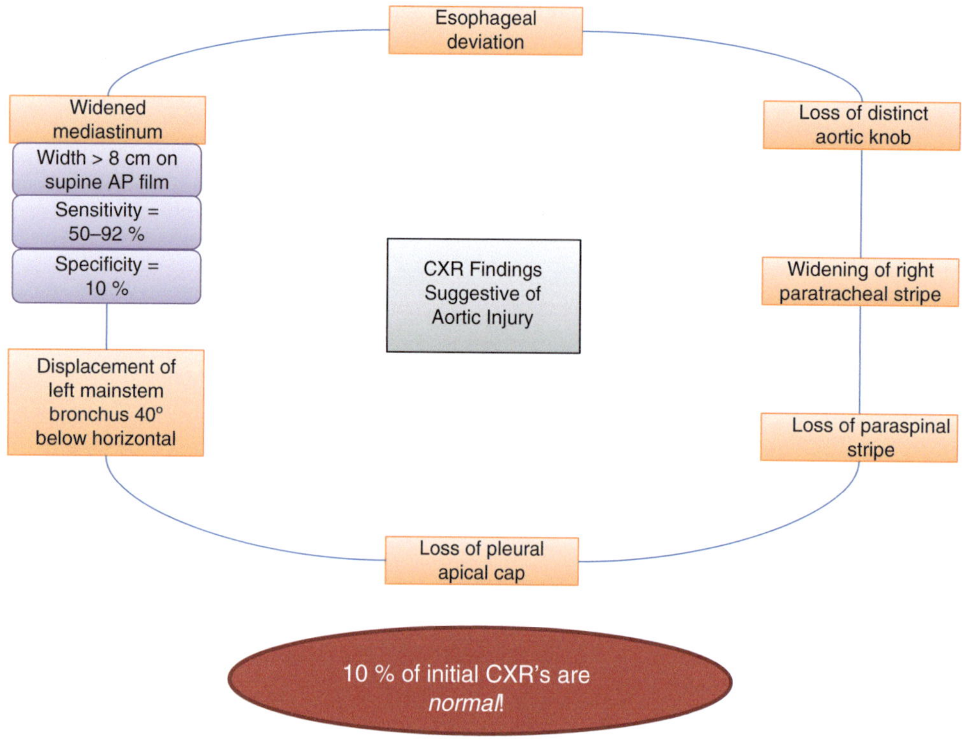

Diaphragmatic Injury

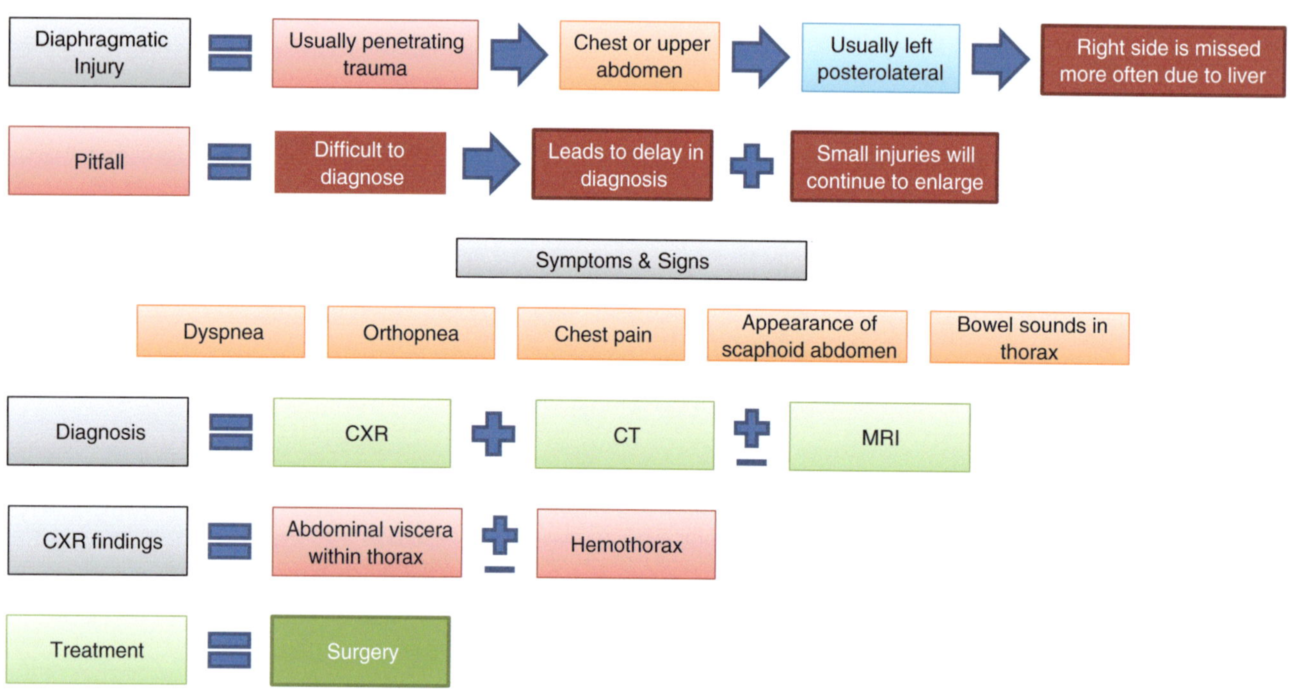

Abdominal Trauma

Abdominal Trauma Introduction

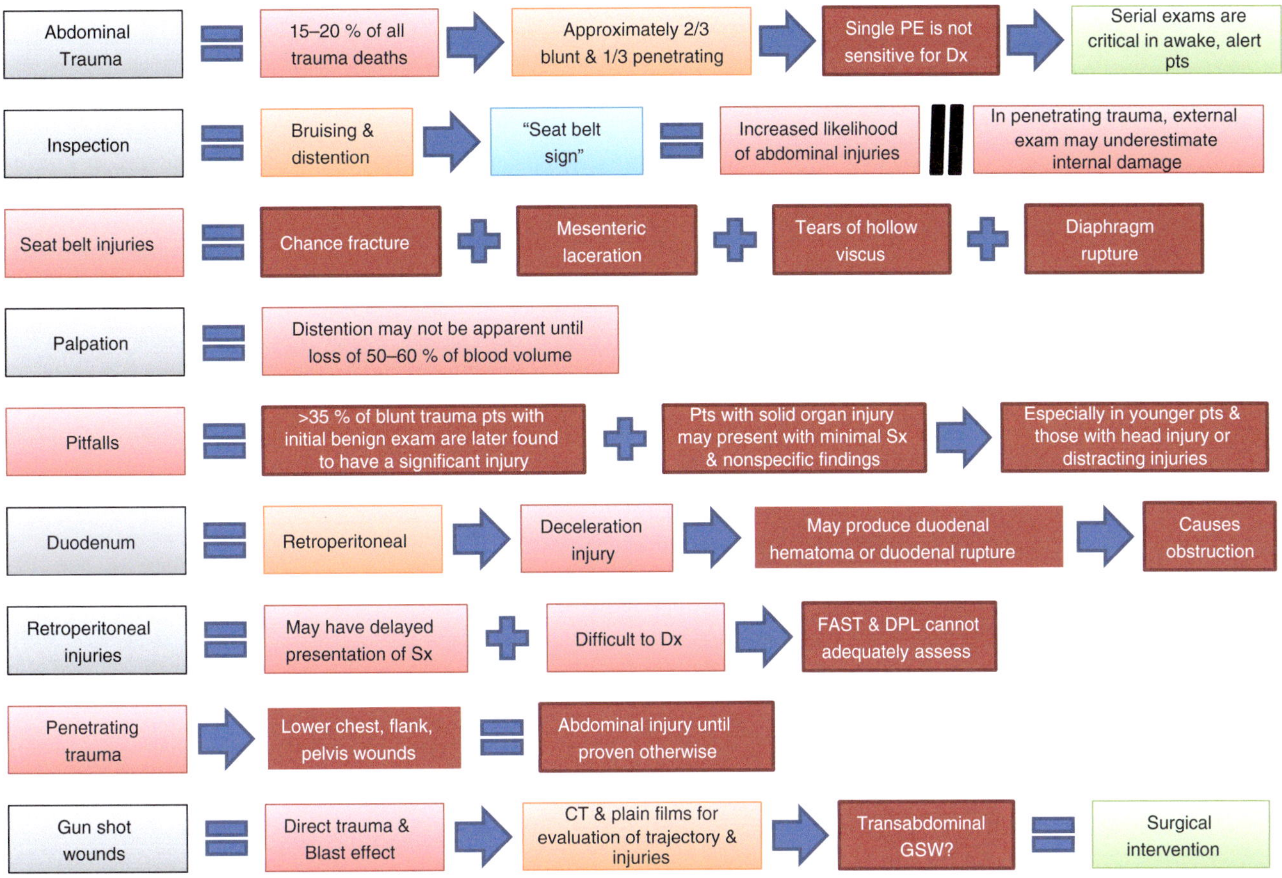

Penetrating Abdominal Trauma

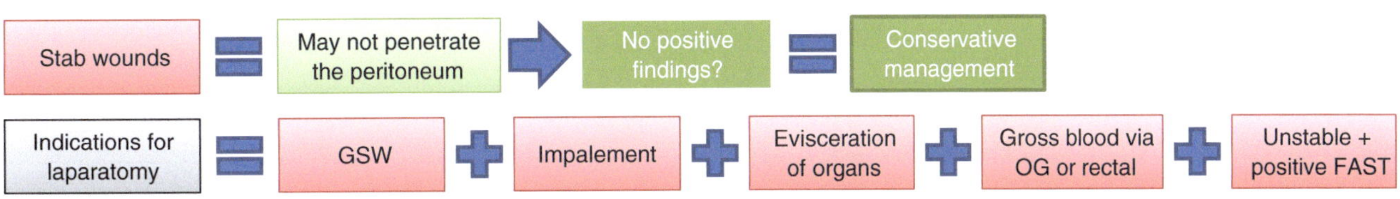

Abdominal Signs

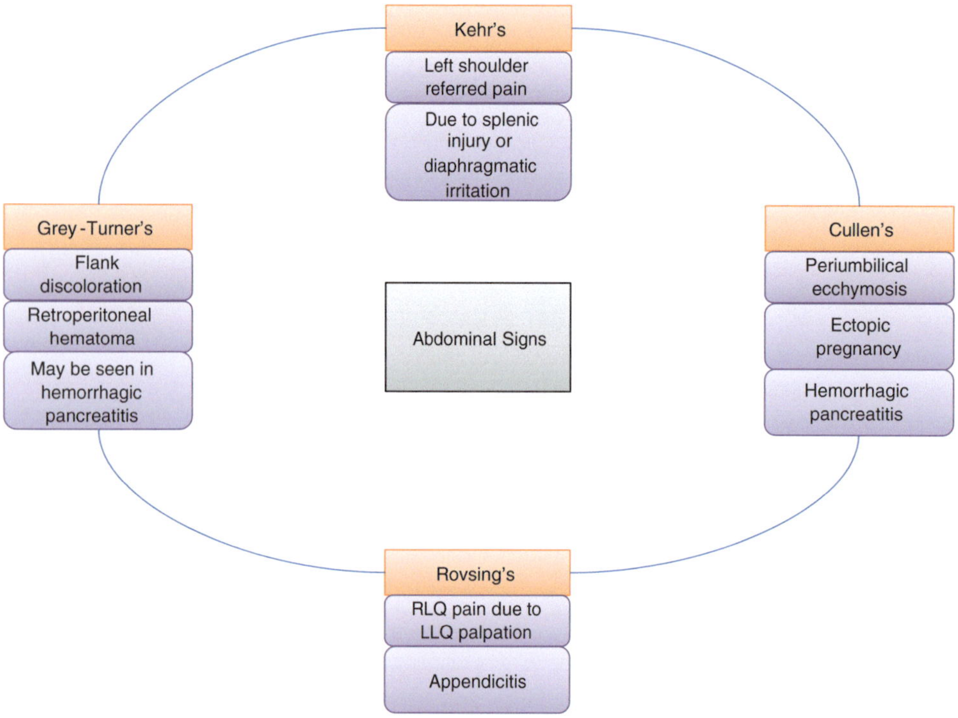

Abdominal Trauma Imaging

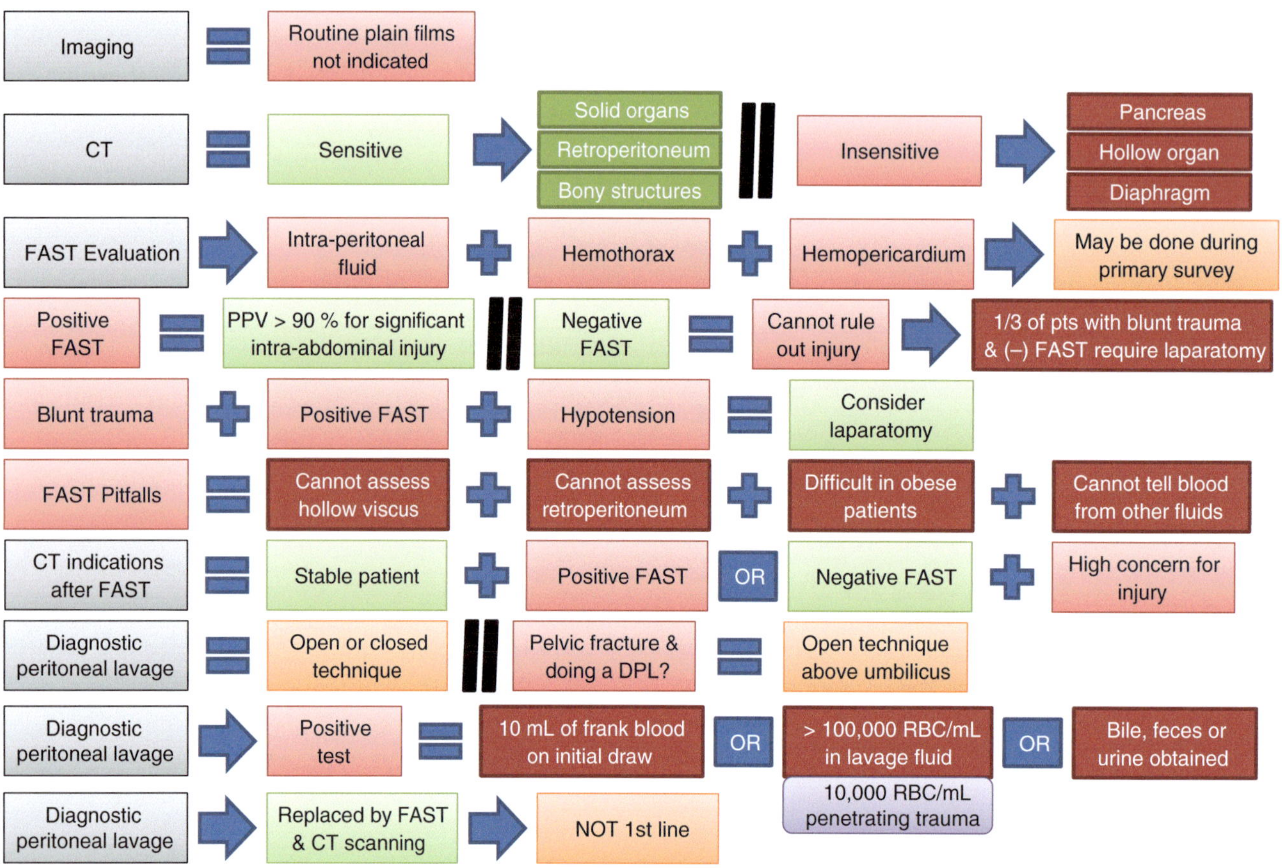

Spleen and Liver Trauma

Solid organ injury with blunt trauma = Spleen most commonly injured → Also consider with left lower rib injuries || Solid organ injury penetrating trauma = Liver most common

Symptoms & Signs

- LUQ pain – Spleen
- Kehr's sign – Spleen
- R shoulder pain – Liver
- RUQ pain – Liver
- Shock – For both

Diagnosis = CT

Treatment = Depending on extent of injury may consider non-operative management

After splenectomy = Appropriate vaccinations Due to Risk of encapsulated organism sepsis → *S.pneumoniae* + *Neisseria meningitidis*

Pancreas/Stomach/Duodenum/Intestine Trauma

Pancreas = Commonly injured in *blunt* trauma → Deceleration injury + Steering wheel injury + Bicycle handlebar (Also duodenum)

Pain = May be delayed Due to Retroperitoneal location

Diagnosis = CT

Treatment = Depends on extent of injury

Stomach & Duodenum = Commonly injured in *penetrating* trauma → Duodenal injury associated with liver injury

Small intestine = Commonly injured in *penetrating* trauma → May have multiple locations of injury → Sx may be delayed + Associated with lumbar spine injuries

Large intestine = Typically *transverse* colon injured Due to Location

Diagnosis of hollow viscus injuries = May be difficult

Penetrating Flank and Buttock Injuries

Penetrating Flank & Buttock Injuries = Consider rectal exam → Look for gross blood & rectal tone || Blood on exam? = Bowel injury until proven otherwise

GSW to flank entering peritoneum? = Laparatomy

Wound to flank + Hemodynamically stable? = Triage based on CT results

Unstable pt? = Surgical consultation + Antibiotics for anaerobic & Gram (–) coverage

Stable pt + No CT evidence of injury = Observation for 6 hours

Diagnosis = CT + U/A + CBC + Type & screen

Possible bowel injury? = CT with oral & rectal contrast

Kidney Injuries

Kidney injuries = Present in 10 % of pts with abdominal trauma || Higher risk with → Flank bruising; Lower rib fx; Hematuria

Mechanism = Compression + Deceleration + Penetrating trauma

Gross hematuria? = Renal injury until proven otherwise!

Absence of ANY hematuria? = Does NOT exclude renal injury!

Pt with renal injury? = 80 % will have other injuries → Skeletal OR Visceral

Blunt trauma + Gross hematuria + Suspicion for renal trauma + Deceleration injuries + Multiple trauma = Imaging (CT)

Penetrating trauma to flank or abdomen + Hematuria = Imaging (CT) || Suspicion of renal vascular injury? = Angiogram

Type of CT? = Contrast enhanced CT → Early extravasation = Ongoing hemorrhage

Delayed CT scan? = CT done 10 minutes after contrast → Extravasation from kidney, ureter or bladder = Genitourinary injury

Pitfall = Renal vascular injury → Associated with multiple trauma → May not have hematuria → Must revascularize within 12 hours

Genitourinary Injuries: Bladder and Ureter Injury

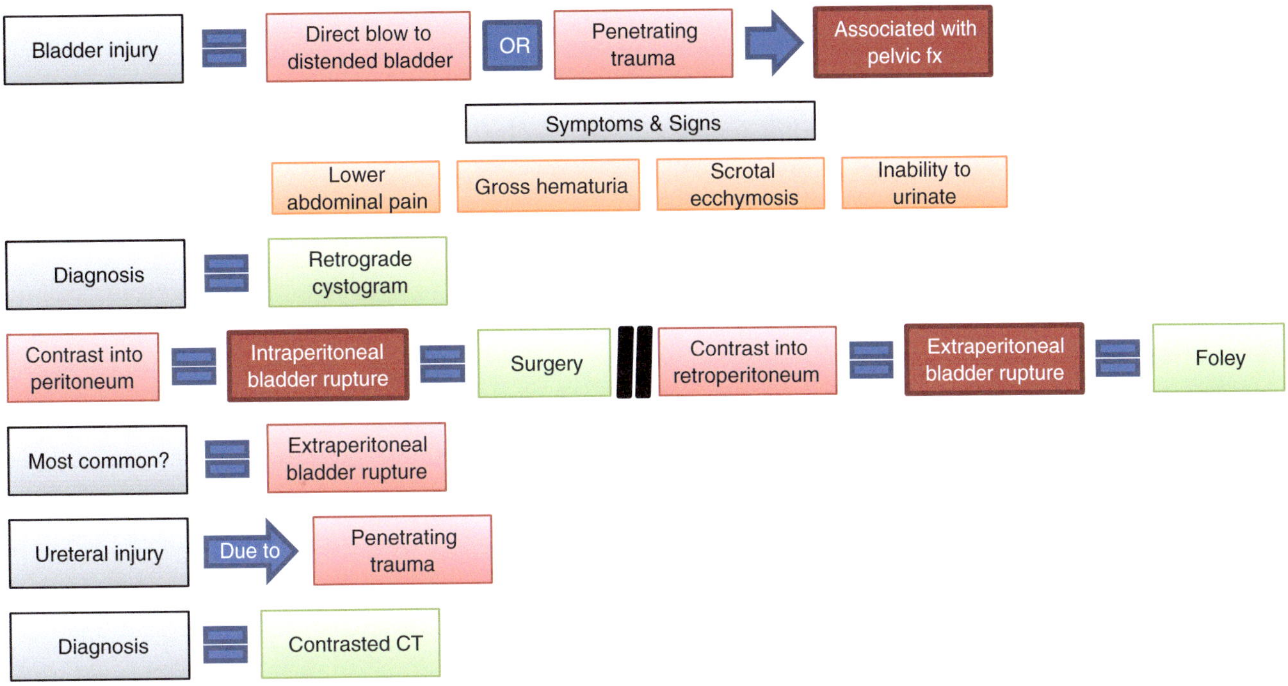

Genitourinary Injuries: Urethral Injury

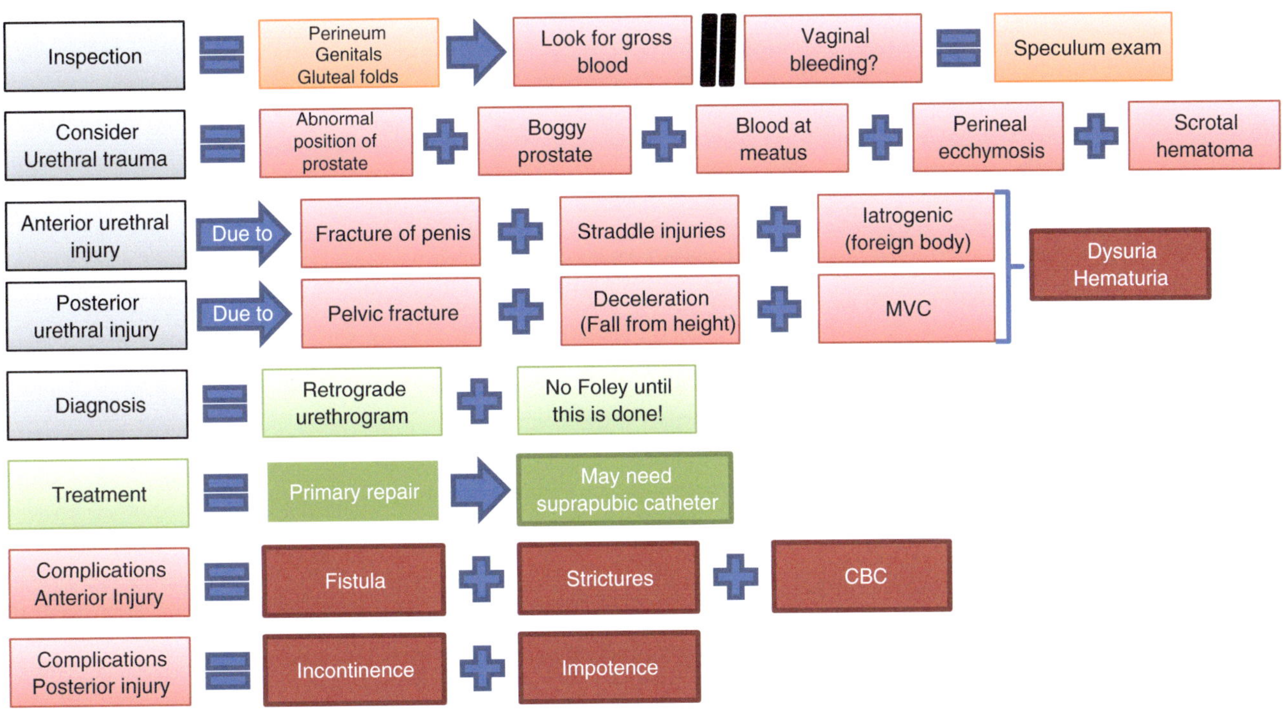

Genitourinary Injuries: Testicular Injury

Testicular injury = Most common in blunt or straddle injury

Symptoms & Signs

- Hematuria
- Scrotal pain
- Scrotal ecchymosis
- Scrotal edema

Diagnosis = Ultrasound ± Nuclear scan

Complications = Infertility + Abscess + Hydrocele

Pelvis and Hip Trauma

Introduction

Pelvis Trauma = Requires significant force → Associated with multiple trauma || Mortality of all pelvic fx = 5 %

Mechanisms = MVC + Fall from height + Pedestrian vs MVC

Pelvic fx associations = Significant hemorrhage + Neurologic injury → Due to → Close proximity to major vessels & nerves = Iliac vessels, Lumbar plexus, Sacral plexus

Diagnosis = Radiographs ± CT scan

Young-Burgees Classification System = Based on mechanism → Can predict likelihood of severe hemorrhage

Three Types = Major ring fx + Acetabular fx + Avulsion & Single bone fx

Symptoms & Signs

- Tenderness to palpation of pelvis
- Pelvis instability with lateral compression of iliac crests
- Pelvis instability with posterior compression at pubic symphysis
- Perineal lacerations – Open fx
- Destot's sign – Hematomas over scrotum or inguinal ligament
- Earle's sign – Ability to palpate pelvic fracture line on rectal exam

Major Ring Fractures

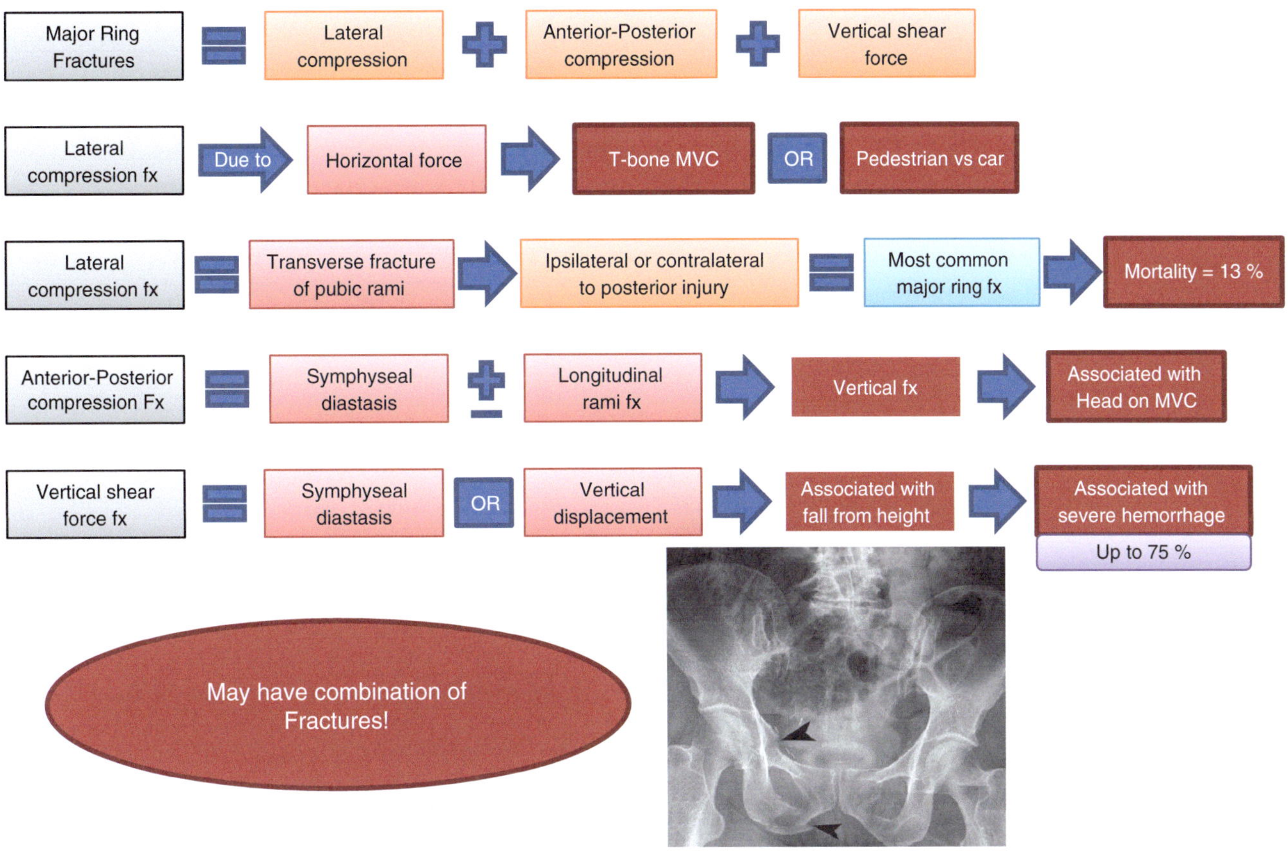

Center bottom image (Reprinted from Kaewlai R, Singh A. Lower extremity trauma. In: Singh A, editor. Emergency radiology: imaging of acute pathologies. New York: Springer Science; 2013. p. 277–98. With permission from Springer Science + Business Media)

Acetabular and Avulsion/Single Bone Fx

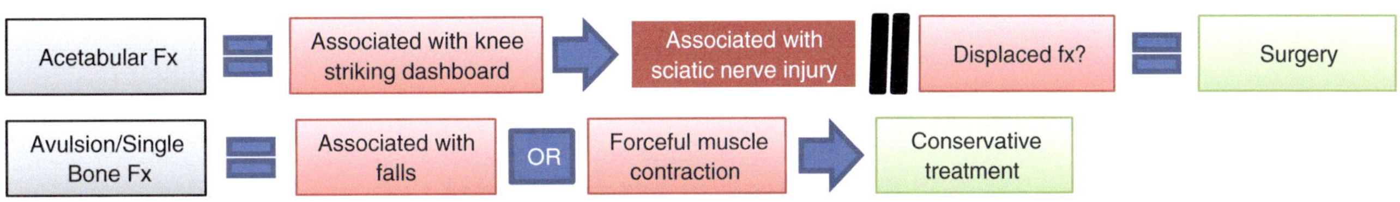

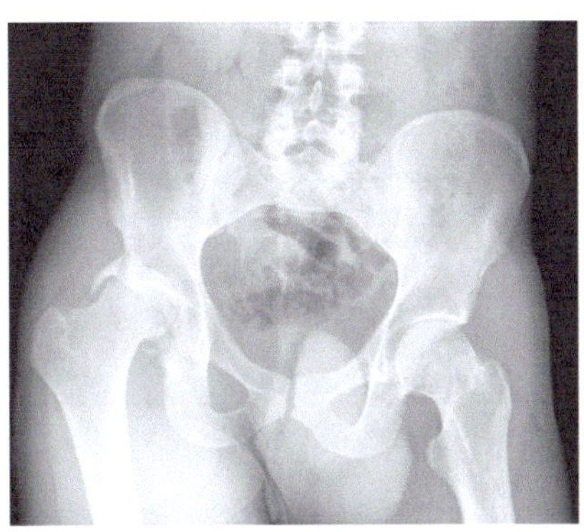

Center image (Reprinted from Zamora-Carrera E, Rubio-Suarez JC. Complex fractures of the acetabulum. In: Rodríguez-Merchán EC, Rubio-Suarez JC, editors. Complex fractures of the limbs. Zug: Springer International Publishing; 2014. p. 51–60. With permission from Springer International Publishing)

Pelvic Radiograph Tidbits

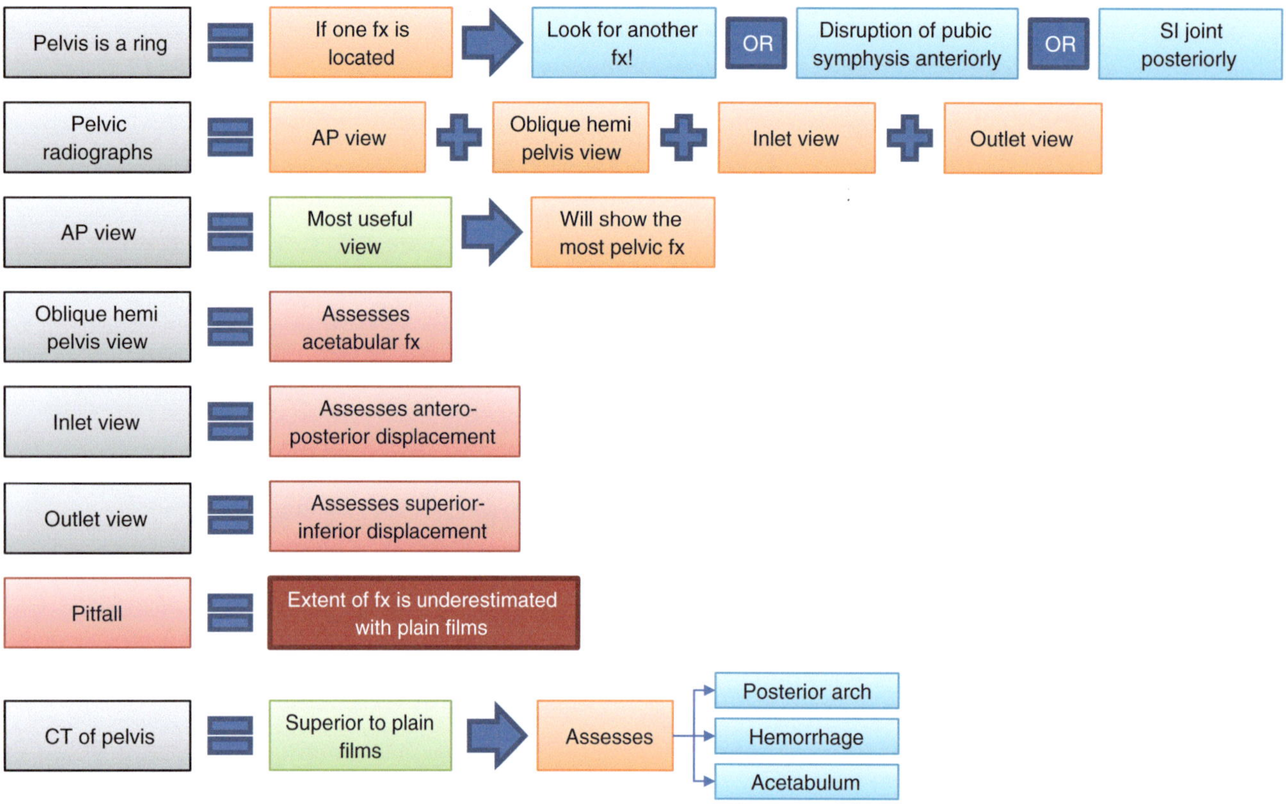

Treatment of Pelvic Fractures

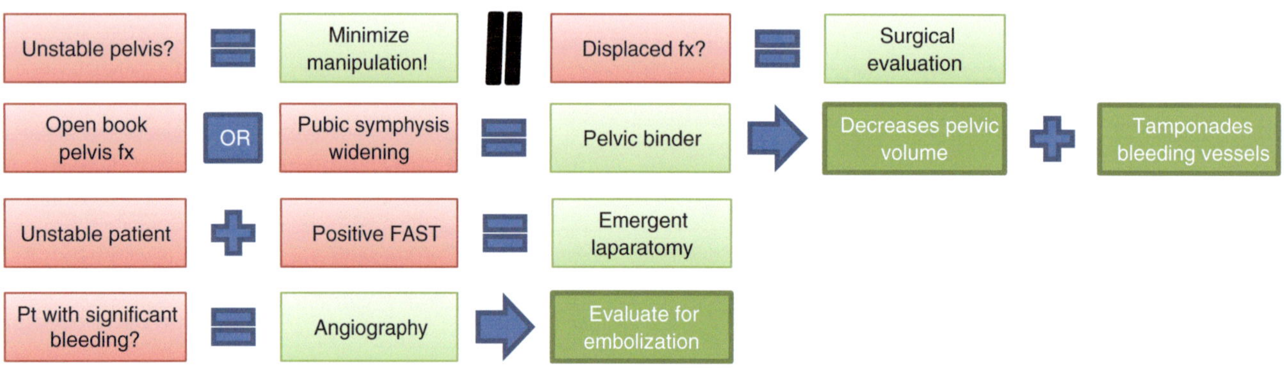

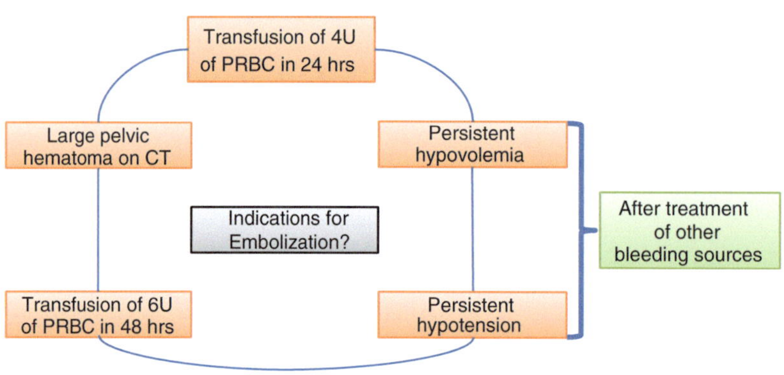

Complications of Pelvic Fractures

Urethral injury → Clinical suspicion = Retrograde urethrogram → Prior to Foley catheter

Vaginal laceration → Associated with anterior pelvic fx → Bimanual exam for females with pelvic fx → Blood on exam? = Speculum exam

Other complications = Rectal injuries + (Nerve root injuries → May be delayed)

Hip Dislocation Introduction

Hip Dislocations = 3 types → Anterior + Central + Posterior

Anterior hip dislocation = Anterior force + Medial force + Abducted leg

Central hip dislocation = Direct trauma through acetabulum

Posterior hip dislocation = Force directed posteriorly through a flexed knee = Most common hip dislocation → Associated with acetabular fractures

Posterior hip dislocation Due to → Head on MVC → Flexed knee strikes dashboard

Patient's extremity? = Shortened + Internally rotated + A***D***ducted

Diagnosis = Plain radiographs ± CT

Treatment = Adequate analgesia + Closed reduction

Complications Posterior hip dislocation = Avascular necrosis of femoral head → From prolonged dislocation

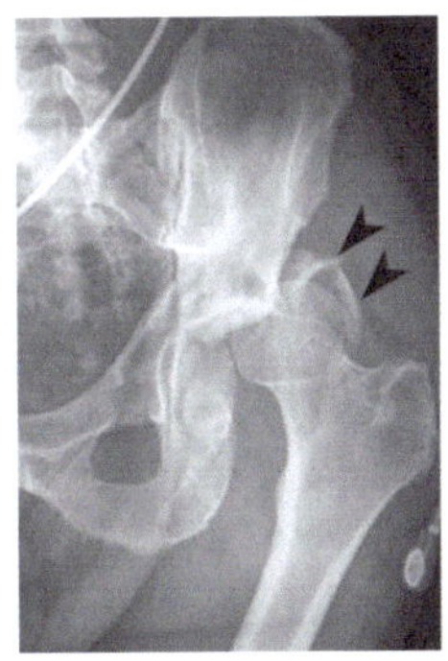

Bottom right image (Reprinted from Kaewlai R, Singh A. Lower extremity trauma. In: Singh A, editor. Emergency radiology: imaging of acute pathologies. New York: Springer Science; 2013. p. 277–98. With permission from Springer Science + Business Media)

Extremity Injuries

Introduction

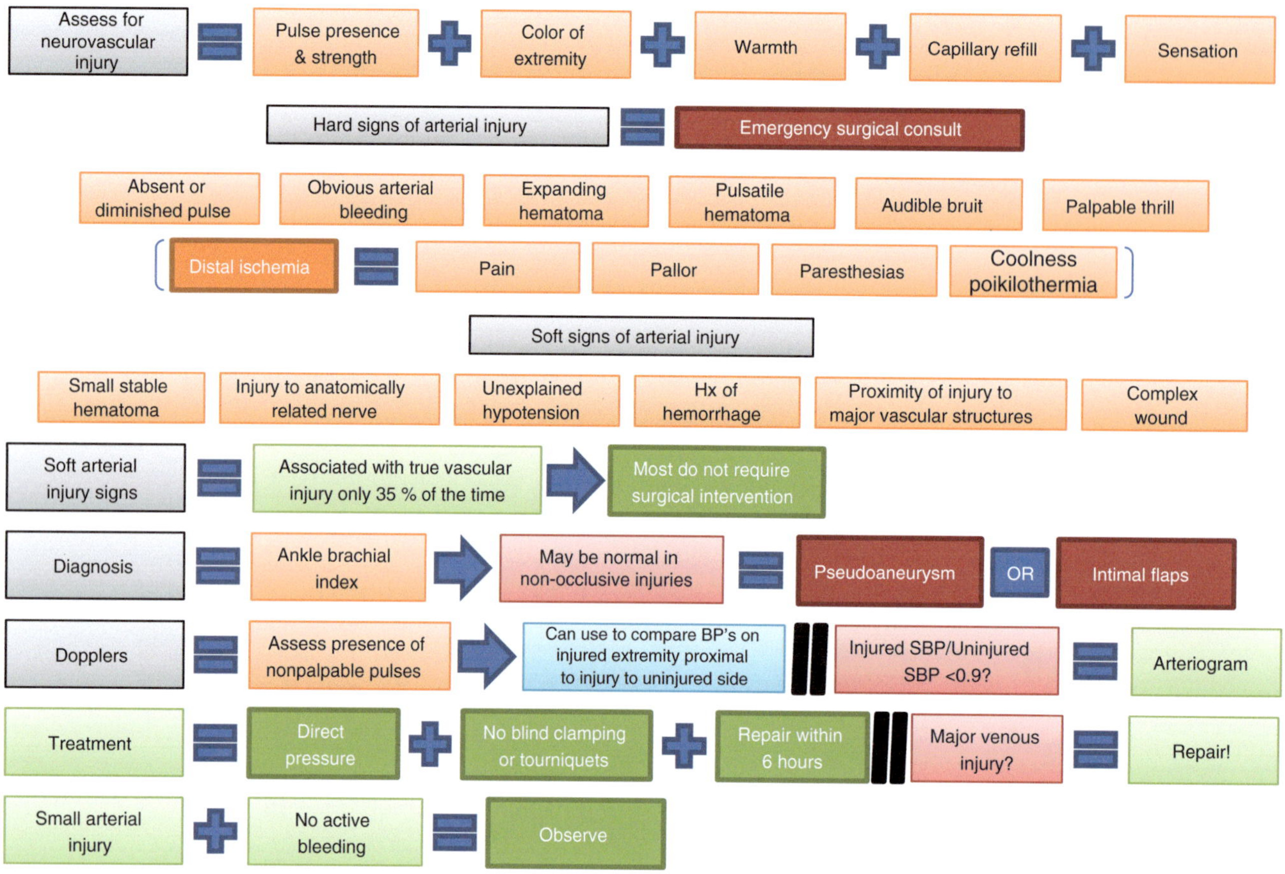

Amputations

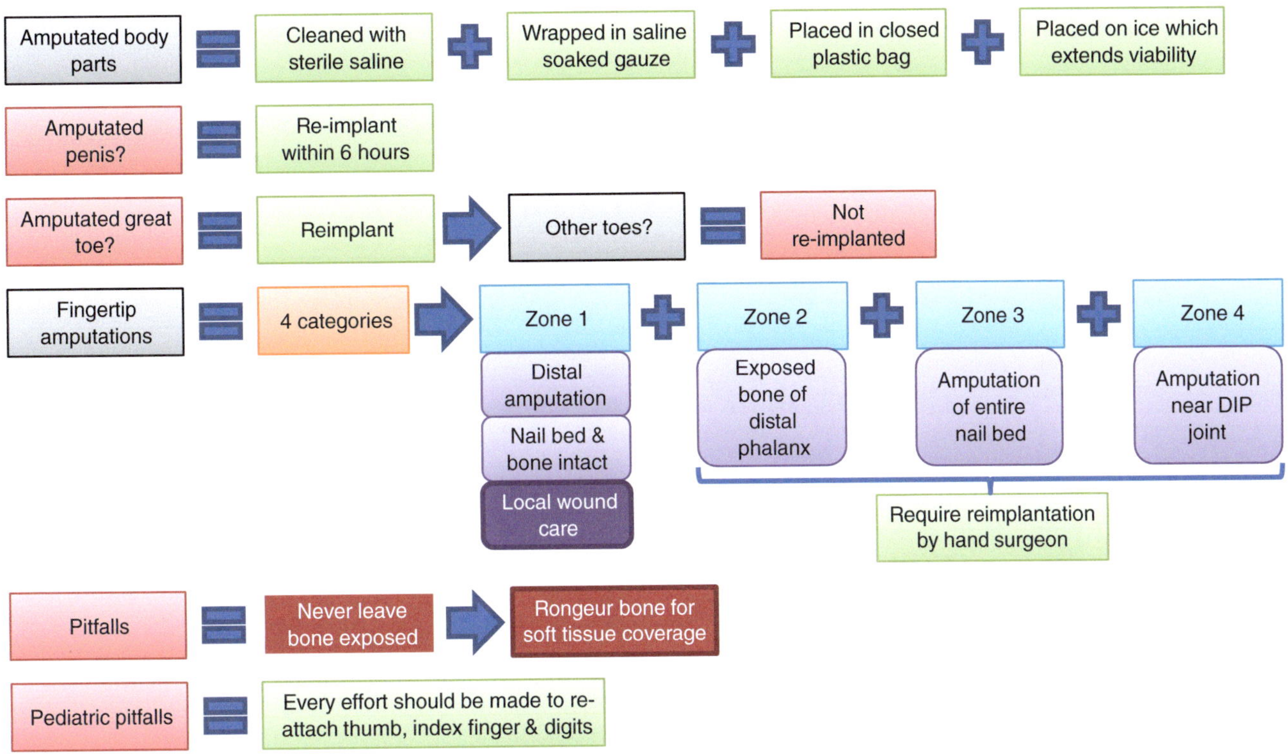

Trauma in Special Populations

Pediatric Trauma

Pediatric Trauma Tidbits

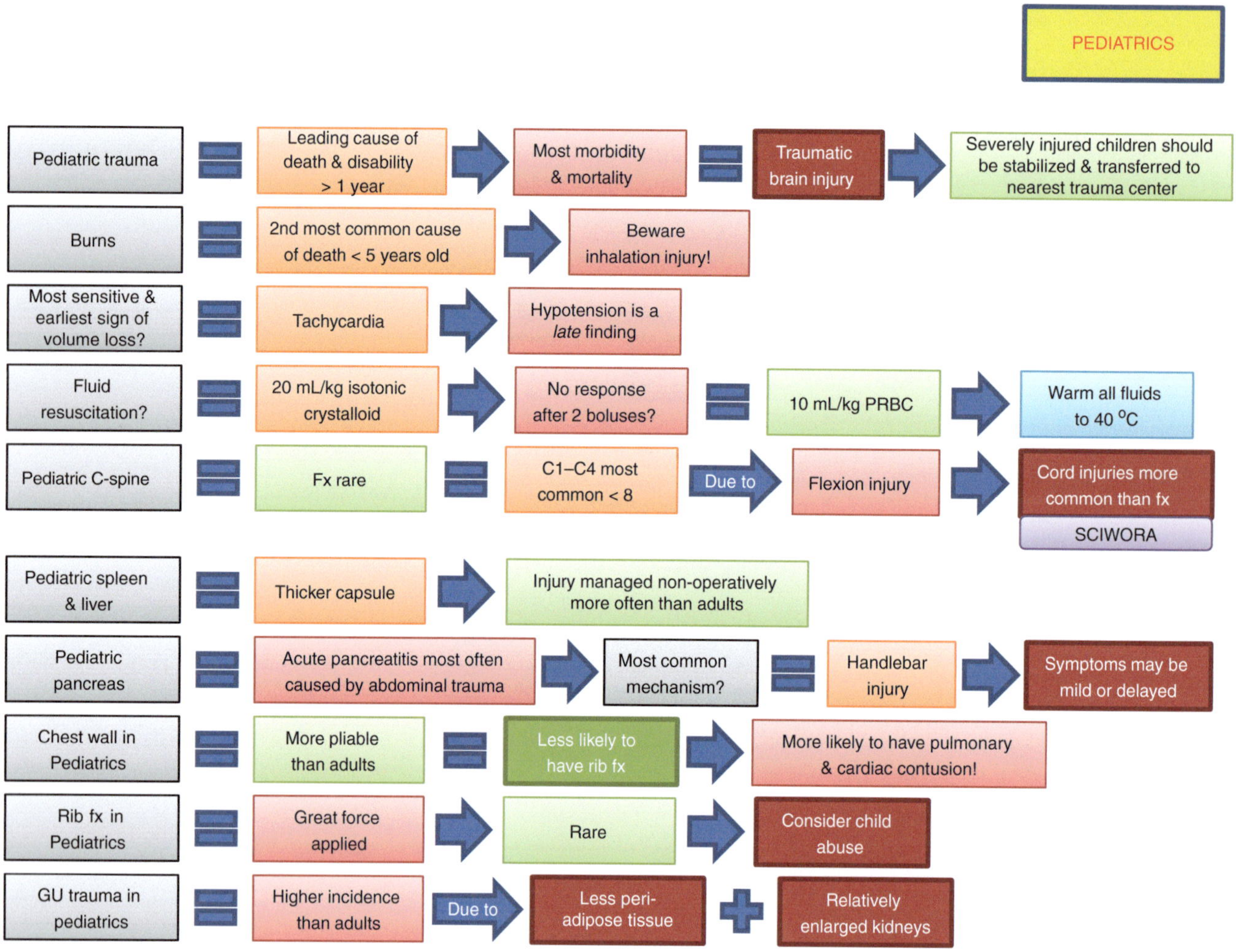

Pediatric Trauma Airway and Breathing

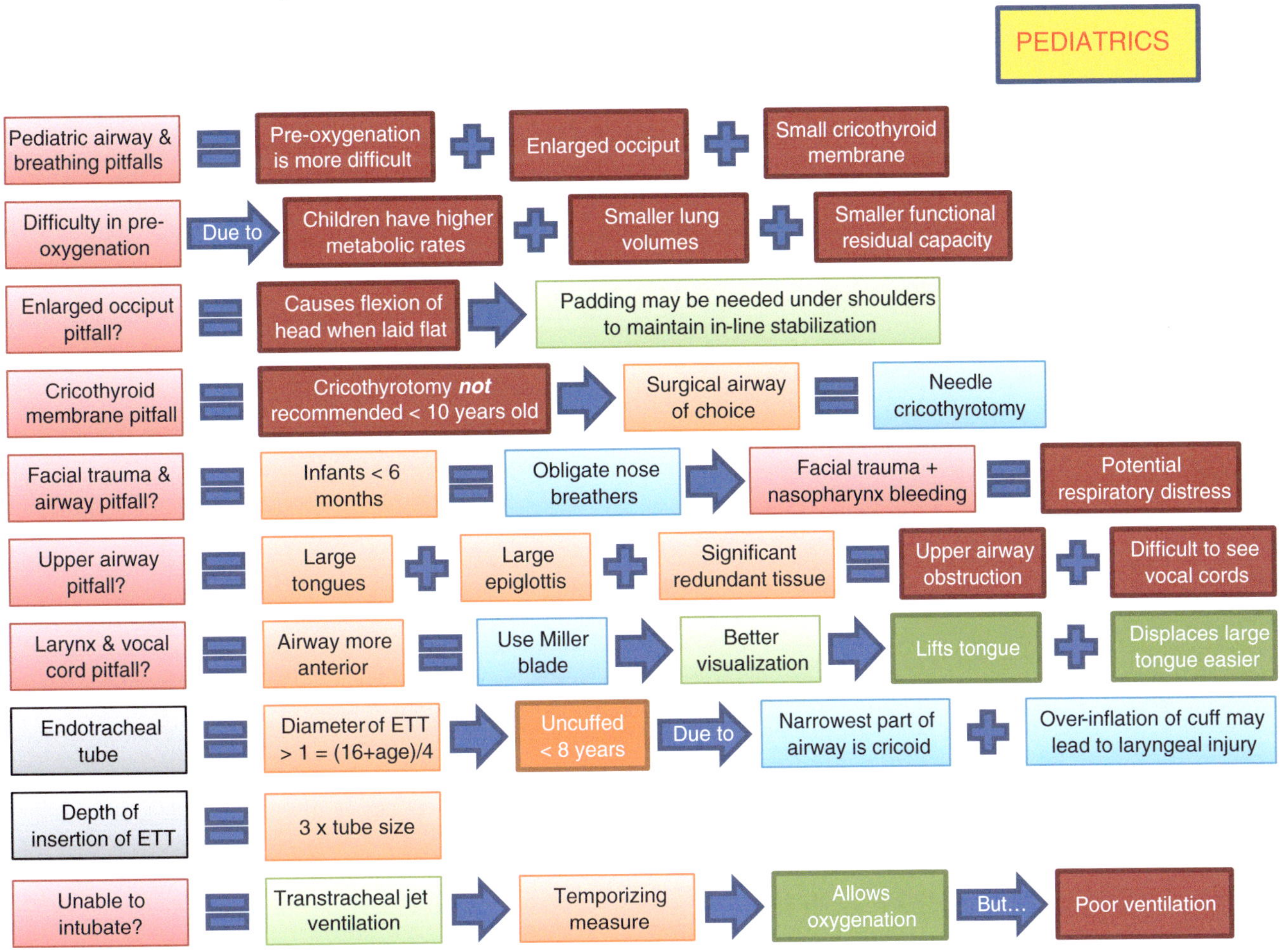

Indications for Transfer to Pediatric Trauma Center

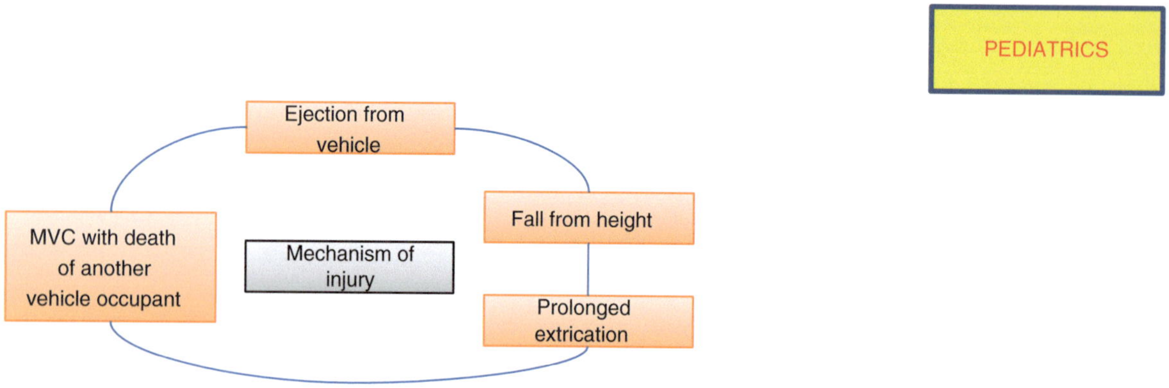

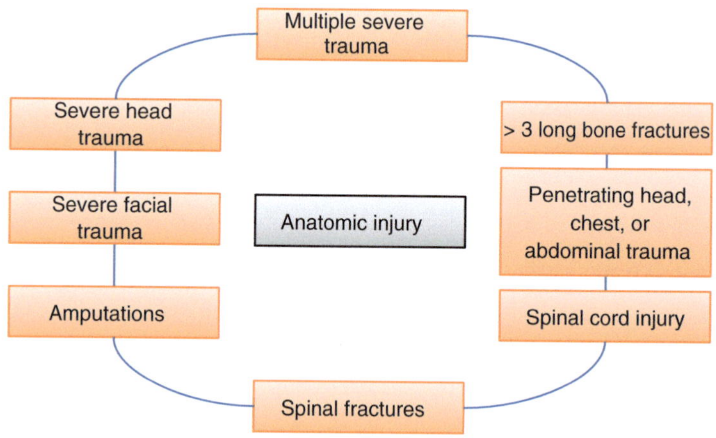

Nonaccidental Trauma

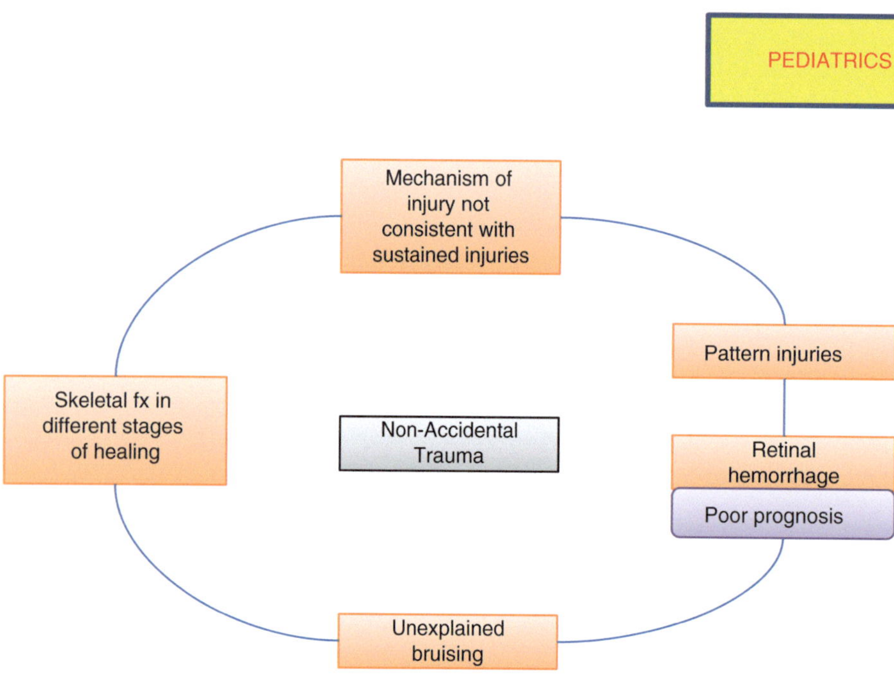

Child Abuse

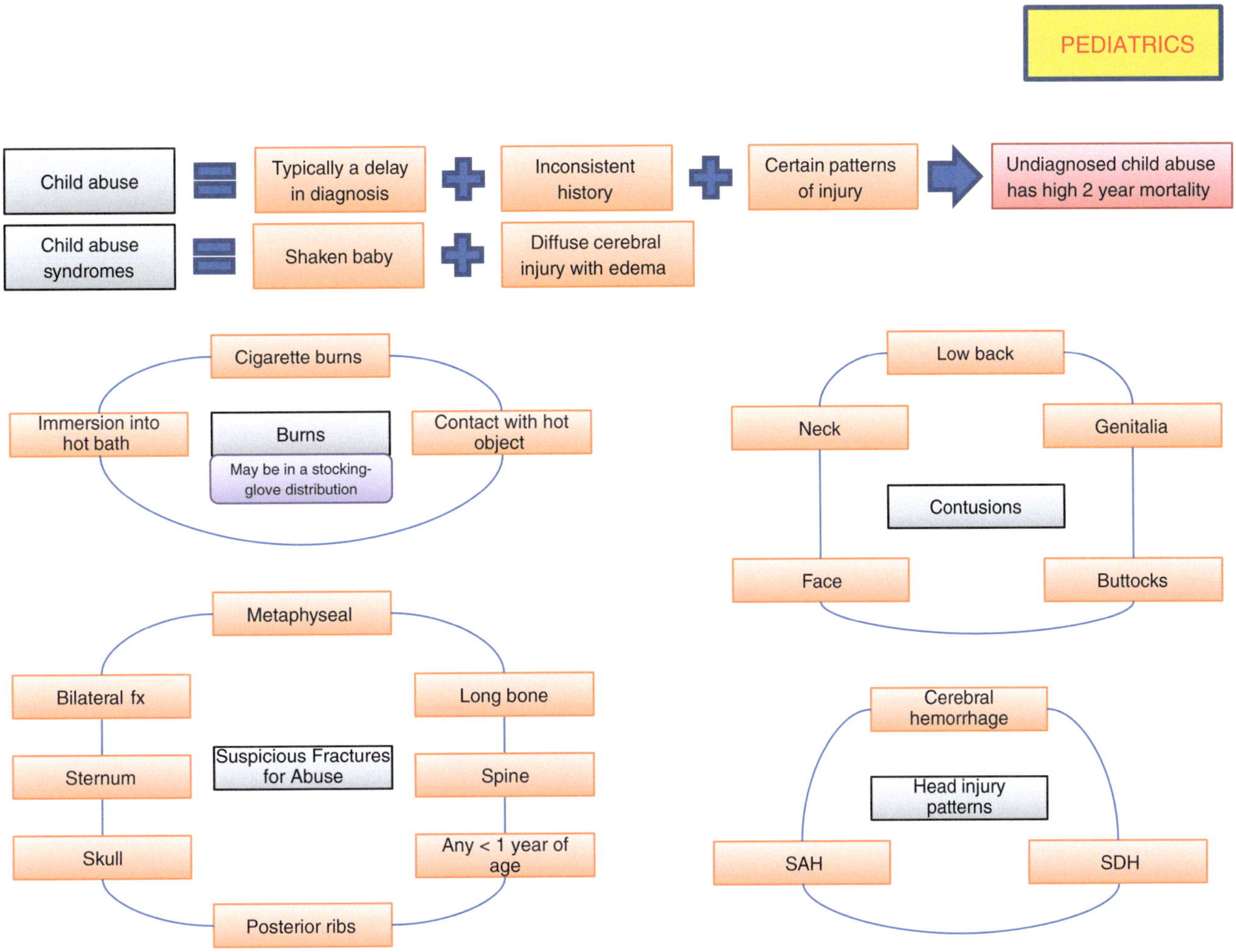
PEDIATRICS
Child abuse
Typically a delay in diagnosis
Inconsistent history
Certain patterns of injury
Undiagnosed child abuse has high 2 year mortality
Child abuse syndromes
Shaken baby
Diffuse cerebral injury with edema
Cigarette burns
Immersion into hot bath
Burns
May be in a stocking-glove distribution
Contact with hot object
Low back
Neck
Genitalia
Contusions
Face
Buttocks
Metaphyseal
Bilateral fx
Long bone
Sternum
Suspicious Fractures for Abuse
Spine
Skull
Any < 1 year of age
Posterior ribs
Cerebral hemorrhage
Head injury patterns
SAH
SDH

Geriatric Trauma

Geriatric Trauma Introduction

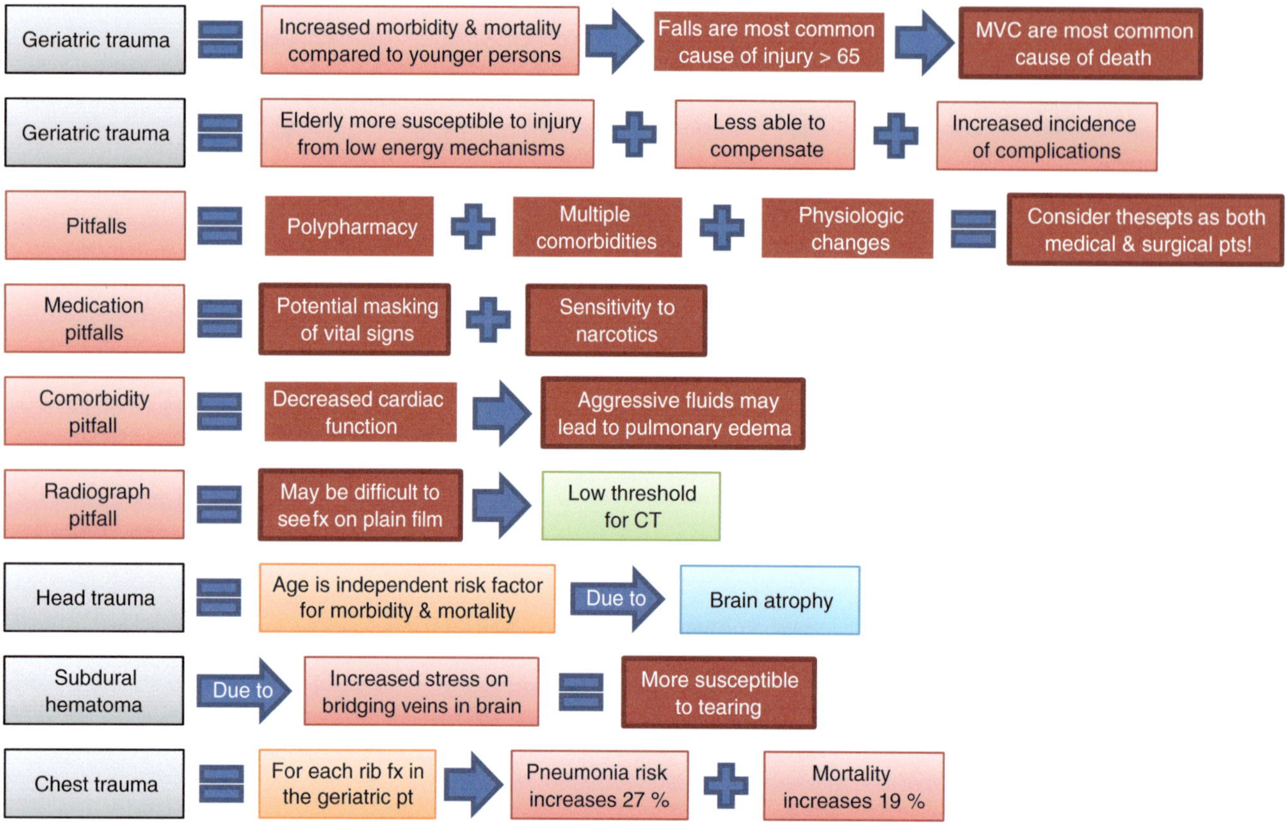

Trauma in Pregnancy

Introduction

Trauma = Leading cause of non-obstetric morbidity & mortality in pregnancy → Most common blunt trauma = MVC; Most common penetrating trauma = GSW

Pitfall = Physiologic changes = Difficult to interpret VS

Vital signs = Heart rate increase 10–20 blm + Blood pressure decreases 10–15 mm Hg

Physiologic anemia = Blood volume increases + RBC mass increases to a lesser degree → Pitfall = Pt may lose 35 % of blood volume before manifesting signs of shock

Supine hypotension syndrome = When a pregnant female is supine → Compresses inferior vena cava = Decrease in venous return = Tilt pt to left 30 degrees

Anatomic pitfalls = Bladder ascends to abdomen in 3rd trimester = Increases risk of injury || Most common cause of abdominal hemorrhage = Splenic injury

Uterine rupture? = Fetal mortality of 100 % → Not common → Late 2nd–3rd trimester

Risk factors for rupture? = Prior C-section + VBAC

Symptoms & Signs of uterine rupture

- Loss of uterine contour
- Shock
- Abdominal pain
- Fetal demise
- Able to palpate fetal parts

Complications of trauma = Preterm labor + Abruptio placenta → See OB/GYN

Maternal-Fetal Well-Being

Fetal well being = Depends on maternal stability & survival

Emergent C-section? = 75 % fetal survival rate → At ≥ 26 weeks + Presence of fetal heart tones + Procedure done at 1st sign of fetal distress

CPR & emergent C-section? = Continue CPR during procedure + As well as for a short time after the procedure

Perimortem C-section? = Only after optimal resuscitation + ≥ 23 weeks + Done within 5 minutes of maternal death

Burns

Burn Classification

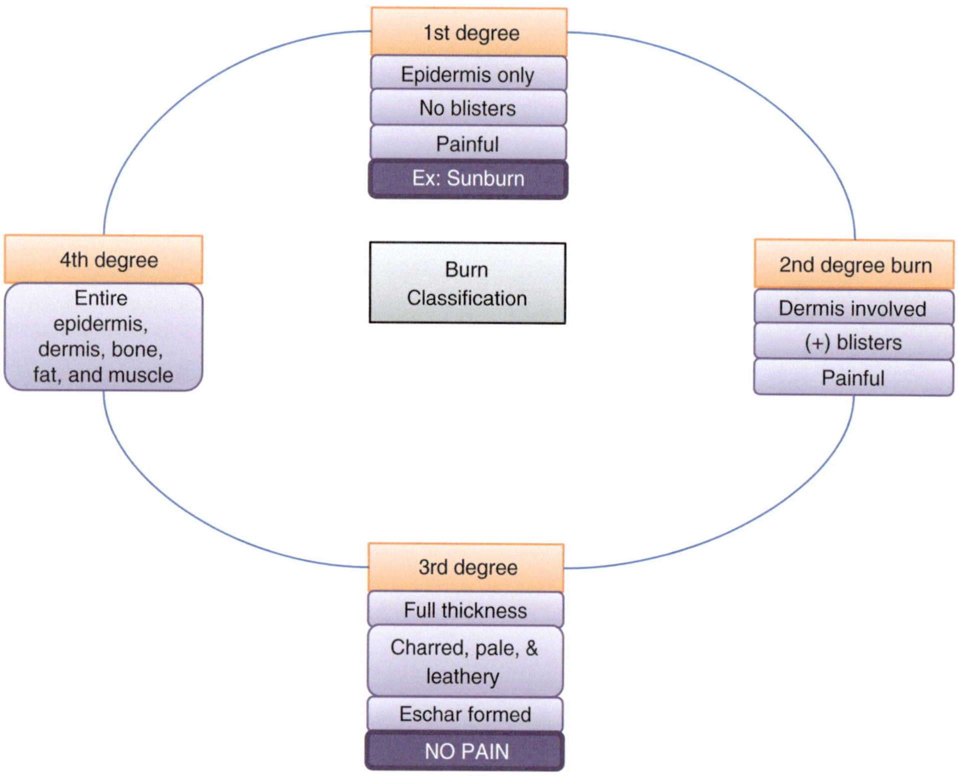

Burn Tidbits

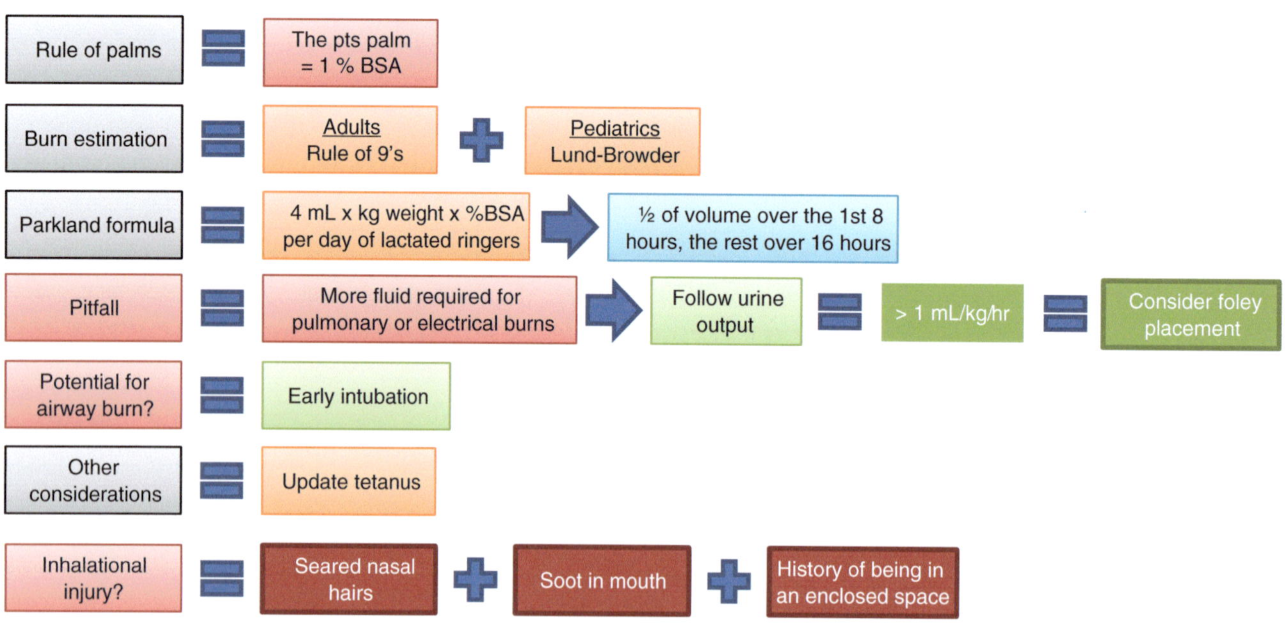

Burn Estimation

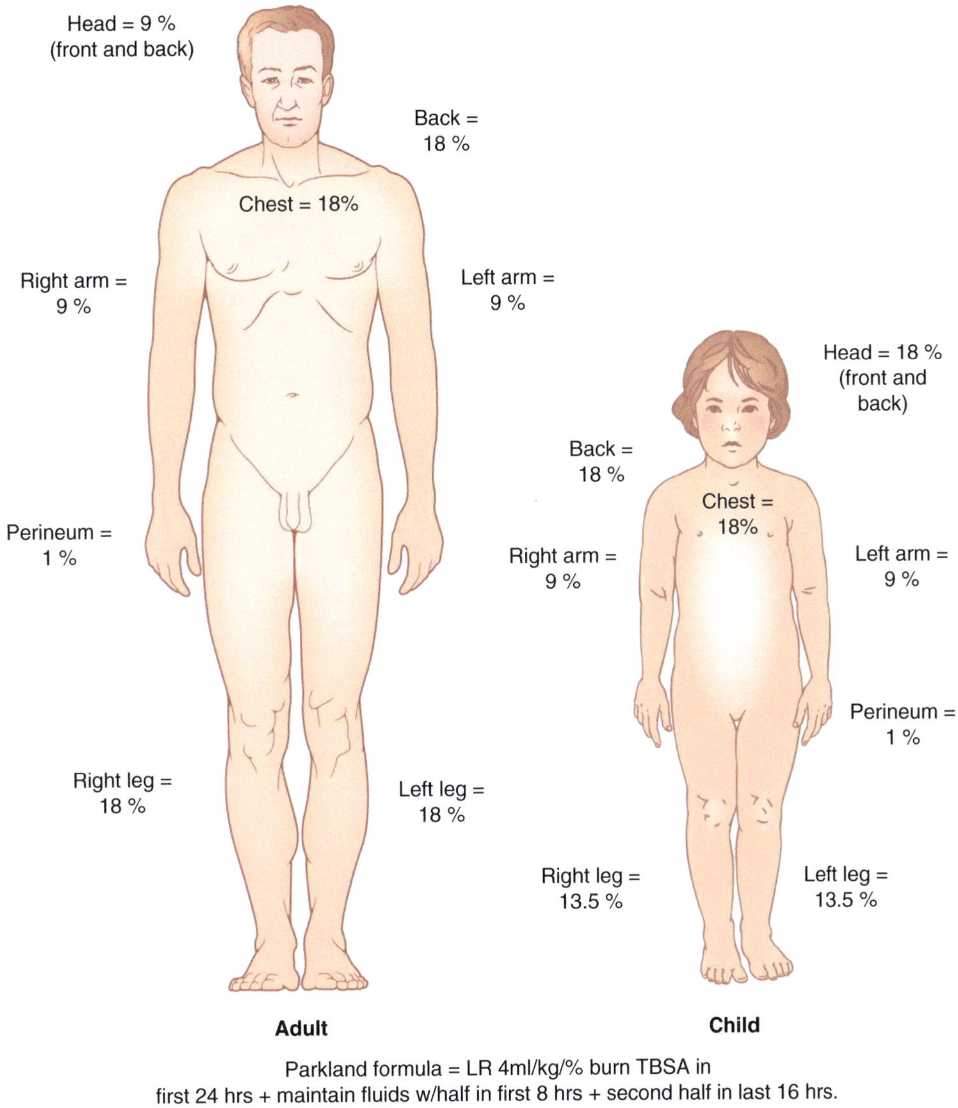

Center image (Reprinted from Allen B, Ganti L, Desai B. Trauma and ATLS. In: Allen B, Ganti L, Desai B, editors. Quick hits in emergency medicine. New York: Springer Science; 2013. p. 37–45. With permission from Springer Science + Business Media)

Indications for Transfer to Burn Center

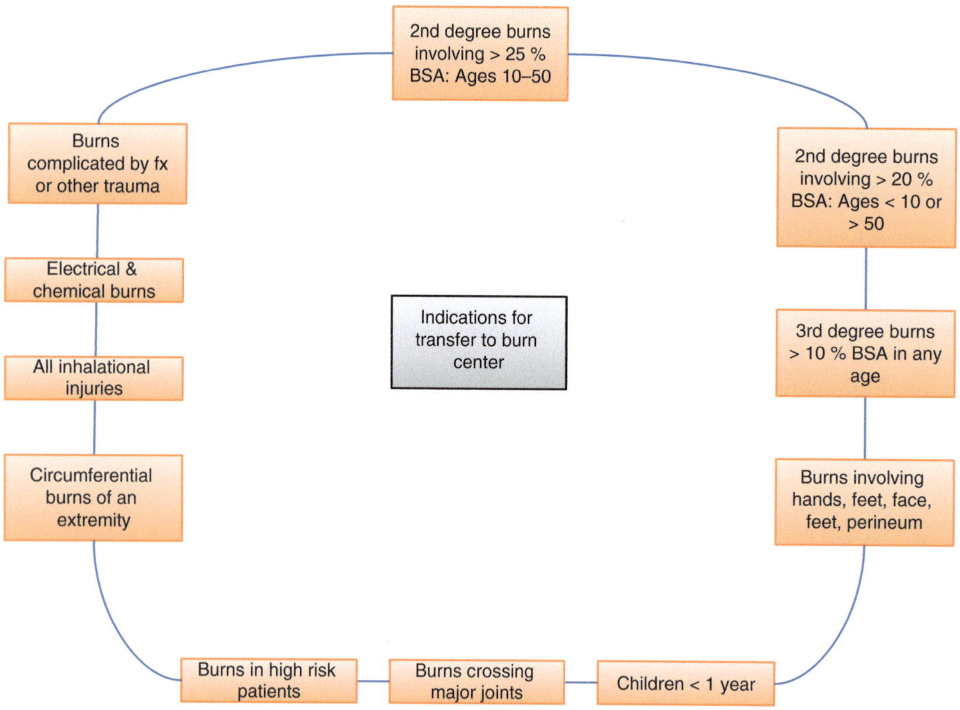

Burn Complications

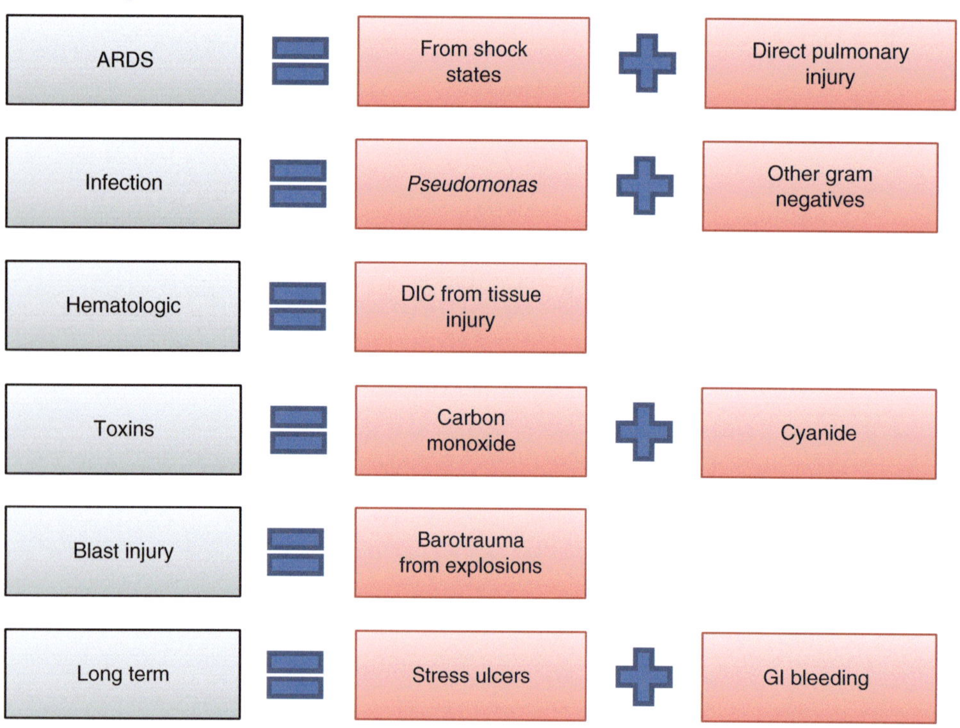

Escharotomy

Escharotomy indications	=	Full thickness chest wall burns	+	Full thickness circumferential limb burns
Limb burn indications?	=	Vascular insufficiency	→	Poor pulses & capillary refill
Chest wall indications?	=	Inadequate chest rise		
Technique	=	Cut along sides on the long axis	→	Avoid vasculature!
Chest technique	=	Chest wall box		
Tidbits	=	Will have a "popping" sensation as the tissues expand after cutting	+	Will have minimal bleeding

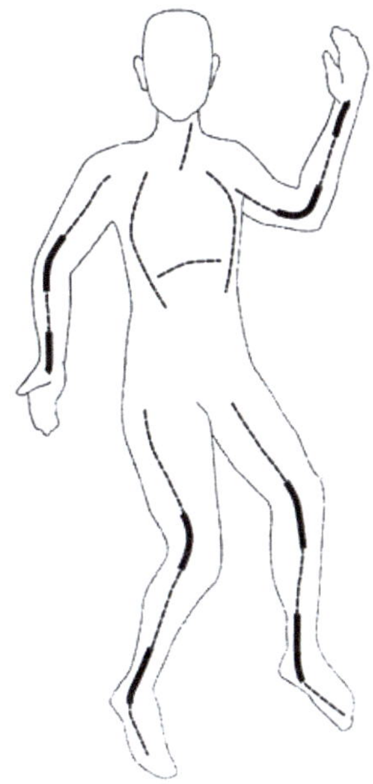

Center right image (Reprinted from Sjöberg F. Pre-hospital, fluid and early management, burn wound evaluation. In: Jeschke MG, Kamolz L-P, Sjöberg F, Wolf SE, editors. Handbook of burns: acute burn care volume 1. Vienna: Springer-Verlag/Wien; 2012. p. 105–16. With permission from Springer-Verlag/Wien)

Blast Injuries

Blast Injury Classification

Type I	=	Pulse pressure	→	Barotrauma effects		
Type II	=	Flying debris	→	Penetrating trauma		
Type III	=	Person is thrown from pulse wave	→	Deceleration impact		
Type IV	=	Toxic gas	±	Radiation	±	Burns
CNS Symptoms	=	LOC	→	Concussion	+	Air emboli from ruptured arteries
Ear injuries	=	TM rupture	+	Ossicle injury		
GI injury	=	Rupture of hollow viscus				
Pulmonary injury	=	Pneumothorax				

Index

A
AAA. *See* Abdominal aortic aneurysm (AAA)
Abdominal and pelvic pain, nonpregnant patient
  endometriosis, 624
  leiomyomas, 625
  ovarian/adnexal torsion, 624
  ovarian cysts, 623
Abdominal aortic aneurysm (AAA)
  description, 64
  diagnosis, 66
  general, 64
  signs, 65
  symptoms, 65
  treatment, 66
Abdominal trauma
  abdominal signs, 848
  bladder and ureter injury, 851
  imaging, 848
  kidney injuries, 850
  pancreas/stomach/duodenum/intestine trauma, 849
  penetrating, 847
  penetrating flank and buttock injuries, 850
  spleen and liver trauma, 849
  testicular injury, 852
  urethral injury, 851
Abnormal vaginal bleeding, 625
Abortions, 630
Abruptio placentae, 633
Abuse/neglect/violence
  ED staff/patient safety, 612
  elder abuse, 611
  intimate partner violence, 611
  sexual assault, 612
AC. *See* Allergic conjunctivitis (AC)
Acalculous cholecystitis, 227
Accelerated idioventricular rhythm (AIVR)
  description, 21
  EKG changes, 21
  treatment, 21
Acetaminophen, 697
  overdose treatment, 699
  Rumack-Matthew nomogram, 698
Achilles tendon rupture, 794
Acquired hemolytic anemia, 330
ACS. *See* Acute coronary syndrome (ACS)
Acute angle-closure glaucoma
  symptoms and signs, 669
  treatment, 670
Acute appendicitis
  appendicitis confounders, 247
  description, 246
  diagnosis, 248
  symptoms and signs, 247
  treatment, 248
Acute bronchitis, 149
Acute chest syndrome, 326
Acute constipation, etiologies of, 187
Acute COPD exacerbation causes, 145
Acute coronary syndrome (ACS)
  angina pectoris, 3
  atypical chest pain, 5
  causes, 4
  cocaine and chest pain, 5
  description, 2
  initial therapy, 17
  pathophysiology, 4
  physical exam, 3
  Prinzmetal's/variant angina, 6, 7
  stable and unstable angina, 6
Acute diverticulitis. *See* Diverticulitis
Acute hemolytic transfusion reaction
  description, 317
  laboratory investigations, 318
Acute ischemic stroke treatment, 561
Acute limb ischemia
  clinical diagnosis, 88
  clinical features, 87
  description, 87
  diagnosis, 88
  treatment, 88
Acute mastoiditis, 475
Acute mountain sickness, 536
Acute myocardial infarction (AMI)
  complications, 22
  conduction disturbances, 23
  description, 7
  EKG, 8
  reperfusion, 18, 19
  rhythm abnormalities, 23
Acute necrotizing ulcerative gingivitis (ANUG), 491
Acute periodic paralysis, 595
Acute renal failure
  in children, 263
  description, 262
  glomerular disease causes, 267
  interstitial disease causes, 266
  intrinsic renal failure, 265
  laboratory investigations, 272
  macroscopic urine, 272
  microthrombosis, 270
  postrenal failure, 270–271
  prerenal failure, 264

B. Desai, B.R. Allen (eds.), *Nailing the Written Emergency Medicine Board Examination*,
DOI 10.1007/978-3-319-30838-8

Acute renal failure (*cont.*)
  radiocontrast-induced nephropathy, 269
  RIFLE criteria, 263
  tubular disease causes, 268
  urinalysis, 273
  vascular/related disease, 269
Acute respiratory distress syndrome (ARDS)
  causes, 173
  description, 172
Addictive behavior and withdrawal
  alcohol withdrawal, 614
  benzodiazepine withdrawal, 614
  cocaine/sympathomimetic withdrawal, 616
  opiate withdrawal, 615
  substance abuse/dependence, 613
  THC withdrawal, 616
ADH-related diseases
  diabetes insipidus, 434–436
  SIADH, 431–433
Adrenal insufficiency and crisis
  adrenal hormones, 423
  causes of primary, 424
  causes of secondary, 425
  clinical features, 426
  disposition, 428
  laboratory abnormalities and testing considerations, 427
  treatment, 427
Adult status epilepticus management, 569
AF. *See* Atrial fibrillation (AF)
AFL. *See* Atrial flutter (AFL)
Airway
  rapid sequence intubation, 179
  tracheostomy and bleeding, 181
  tracheostomy and respiratory distress, 180
Airway foreign body (AFB), 507
AIVR. *See* Accelerated idioventricular rhythm (AIVR)
Akathisia, 599
Alcoholic ketoacidosis
  clinical features, 402
  description, 401
  diagnosis, 403
  disposition, 404
  pathophysiology, 402
  treatment, 403
Alcohols
  description, 692
  ethanol, 693–694
  ethylene glycol, 695
  isopropyl alcohol, 695
  methanol, 693
Alcohol withdrawal, 614
Allergic conjunctivitis (AC), 652
Allergic rhinitis, 480
Allergic transfusion reaction, 319
ALTE. *See* Apparent life-threatening events (ALTE)
Altered mental status
  description, 556
  in hemodialysis, 286
AMI. *See* Acute myocardial infarction (AMI)
Amnesia, 603
Amniotic fluid embolism, 635
Amphetamine, 696
Amyotrophic lateral sclerosis, 600
Anal fissures, 258
Analgesics
  acetaminophen, 697–699
  NSAIDs, 701
  salicylate, 699–700
Anemia
  causes, 310
  classification, 312
  description, 310
  high MCV (macrocytic), 312
  low MCV (microcytic), 312
  normal MCV (normocytic), 313
  specific labs, 311
  symptoms and signs, 311
  treatment, 313
Angina pectoris, 3
Angioedema, 364, 496
Anion gap, 685
Ankle
  dislocations, 796
  Ottawa rules, 795
  sprains, 795
Ankylosing spondylitis, 803
Anorectal abscess, 259
Anorectal emergencies
  anal fissures, 258
  anorectal abscess, 259
  hemorrhoids, 257–258
  rectal prolapse, 259
Anorexia, 607
Anovulatory bleeding, 626
Anterior circulation stroke, 559
Anterior cord syndrome, 832
Anterior MI, 10
  specifics, 12
Anthrax, 550
Antibiotic-associated diarrhea, 197
Anticholinergics, 141
Anticholinergic toxidromes
  causes, 687
  treatment, 688
Anticoagulants
  heparin, 341
  warfarin, 339–340
Anticonvulsants
  carbamazepine, 702
  phenytoin and fosphenytoin, 703
  valproate, 702
Antidotes, 684
Antihistamines, 703
Antimicrobials, 704
Antiphospholipid syndrome, 810
Antisocial personality disorders, 610
Anxiety
  description, 606
  disorders, 607
Aortic dissection
  anatomy, 67
  classification, 69
  clinical features, 69
  description, 67
  diagnosis, 70
  management, 71
  pathophysiology, 68
  risk factors, 68
  special circumstance, 71
Aortic regurgitation
  causes, 39
  CXR, 41
  description, 39
  diagnosis, 40
  symptoms, 40
  treatment, 41

Aortic stenosis
- description, 37
- diagnosis, 38
- treatment, 38

Apathetic thyrotoxicosis, 422
Aphthous stomatitis, 498
Aplastic crisis, sickle cell anemia, 327
Apparent life-threatening events (ALTE)
- causes, 182
- description, 181

Appendicitis confounders, 247
ARDS. *See* Acute respiratory distress syndrome (ARDS)
Arsenic, 715
Arterial-alveolar gradient, 133, 685
Arterial gas embolism, 529
Arteries and affected areas, 9
Ascending cholangitis, 227
Aspiration
- description, 166
- management, 167

Asthma
- anticholinergics, 141
- β-agonists, 141
- clinical features, 139
- description, 138
- leukotriene modifiers, 141
- magnesium, 141
- methylxanthines, 141
- peak flow, 140
- risk factors for death, 140
- severe asthma management, 142
- steroids, 141
- triggering agents, 139

Atrial fibrillation (AF)
- description, 105
- EKG changes, 106
- treatment, 107
- WPW syndrome, 112–113

Atrial flutter (AFL)
- EKG changes, 106
- treatment, 107
- WPW syndrome, 112–113

Atypical chest pain, 5
Auricular hematoma, 476
Automatic implantable cardioverter, 91

B

Babesiosis, 372
Bacillus cereus, 194
Back pain, 801
Back pain workup, 802
Bacterial conjunctivitis, 649
Bacterial diarrhea
- description, 190
- pathogens
  - *B. cereus,* 194
  - *Campylobacter,* 192
  - *C. perfringens,* 194
  - *E. coli,* 191
  - *Salmonella,* 191
  - *Shigella,* 191
  - *Staphylococcus,* 193
  - *Vibrio,* 193
  - *Yersinia,* 192

Bacterial keratitis, 654
Bacterial meningitis, 575
Bacterial tracheitis, 489
Bacterial vaginosis (BV), 621
β-agonists, 141
Baker's cyst, 790
Barbituates, 729
Barotitis externa, 527
Barotitis interna, 527
Barotitis media, 526
Barotrauma of ascent, 528
Barotrauma of ascent treatment, 530
Bartholin cyst and abscess, 622
Basilar skull fracture, 824
β-blockers, 705
Bees/wasps, 518
Bell's palsy, 593
Benign paroxysmal positional vertigo (BPPV), 510
Benzodiazepines, 730
Benzodiazepine withdrawal, 614
Bilirubin evaluation, 220
Biological agents and toxins, 549
Biological weapons, 548
- anthrax, 550
- plague, 551
- selected biological agents and toxins, 549
- smallpox, 551
- toxins, 552

Bipolar disorder, 605
Bites
- bees/wasps, 518
- black widow envenomation, 519
- brown recluse envenomation, 519
- mammalian bites, 520–523

Black widow envenomation, 519
Bladder and ureter injury, 851
Blast injuries, 867
Bleeding
- from heparin, 341
- and tracheostomy, 181
- from warfarin, 340

Blepharitis, 643
Blood pressure definitions, 72
Blow out fractures, 673
Blunt eye trauma, 670
Blunt neck trauma, 838
Blunt ocular trauma and globe rupture, 671
Bone anatomy, 736
Borderline personality disorders, 610
Boutonniere deformity, 743
Bowel obstruction
- causes, 234
- description, 234
- diagnosis, 235–236
- pathophysiology, 235
- symptoms and signs, 235
- treatment, 236

Bowel perforation
- description, 245
- diagnosis, 246
- treatment, 246

BPPV. *See* Benign paroxysmal positional vertigo (BPPV)
Brain abscess, 580
Brain herniation, 821
Branchial cleft cysts, 494
Bronchiolitis
- bronchopulmonary dysplasia, 151
- description, 150
- disposition, 151
- RSV management, 150

Bronchopulmonary dysplasia, 151

Brown recluse envenomation, 519
Brown-Sequard syndrome, 832
Brugada syndrome, 127–128
Bulimia nervosa, 608
Bullous myringitis, 474
Bullous pemphigoid, 354
Burns
  classification, 864
  complications, 866
  escharotomy, 867
  estimation, 865
  indications, 866

C
Calcaneal fractures, 797
Calcium, 445
  hypercalcemia, 448–450
  hypocalcemia, 446–448
Calcium channel blockers, 705
Campylobacter, 192
Candida vaginitis, 622
Candidiasis, 497
Carbamazepine, 702
Carbon monoxide (CO) poisoning, 707
Cardiac contusion, 845
Cardiac markers, 16
Cardiac medications
  β-blockers, 705
  calcium channel blockers, 705
  clonidine, 706
  digitalis, 706–707
Cardiac syncope, 78
Cardiac tamponade, 844
  causes, 62
  clinical features, 63
  description, 62
  treatment, 63
Cardiac trauma, 844
Cardiomyopathy (CM)
  dilated, 51–53
  general/description, 50
  hypertrophic, 53–54
  restrictive, 55–56
Carotid/vertebral artery dissection, 593
Carpal tunnel syndrome, 746
Cat bites and scratches, 523
Cauda equina syndrome, 804
Cauliflower ear, 476
Caustic agents
  acids, 708
  alkali, 709
Cavernous sinus thrombosis, 506
Central cord syndrome, 831
Central pontine myelinolysis, 433
Central retinal artery occlusion (CRAO), 663
Central retinal vein occlusion (CRVO), 665
Central vertigo
  cerebellar infarction and hemorrhage, 514
  migraine-related vertigo, 516
  multiple sclerosis, 515
  symptoms, 509
  vertebral artery dissection, 515
  vertebrobasilar insufficiency, 515
  Wallenberg syndrome, 514
Cerebellar infarction, 514, 561
Cerebellopontine angle tumors, 513
Cerebral contusions, 823
Cerebral edema, 400
Cerebrovascular accidents
  acute ischemic stroke treatment, 561
  anterior circulation stroke, 559
  cerebellar infarction, 561
  intracranial hemorrhage management, 564
  IV tPA exclusions, 562
  lacunar infarction, 560
  relative exclusions for IV tPA, 562
  spontaneous intracranial hemorrhage, 563
  stroke and TIA, 558
  stroke mimics, 557
  tPA complications, 563
  vertebrobasilar infarction, 560
Cervical cancer, 628
Cervical spine clearance, 827
Cervical spine evaluation, 827
Chalazion, 642
Chancroid, 306
Chemical burns, 674
Chemical weapons, 552
  nerve agents, 553
  vesicants, 553
Chest pain
  atypical, 5
  and cocaine, 5
Chest trauma, 838
  cardiac contusion, 845
  cardiac tamponade, 844
  cardiac trauma, 844
  CXR findings of aortic injury, 846
  diaphragmatic injury, 846
  flail chest, 842
  hemothorax, 841
  pneumomediastinum, 839
  pneumothorax, 839–840
  pulmonary contusion, 843
  rib fractures, 841
  sternal fracture, 842
  tracheobronchial injuries, 843
  traumatic aortic injury, 845
Children, acute renal failure in, 263. *See also* Pediatrics
Chlamydia, 302
Chlamydophila pneumoniae, 160
Chlorine, 710
Cholesteatoma, 475
Cholinergic toxidromes, 688–689
Chronic constipation, etiologies of, 188
Chronic obstructive pulmonary disease (COPD)
  acute bronchitis, 149
  acute COPD exacerbation causes, 145
  description, 143
  diagnostics, 145
  exacerbation disposition, 148
  exacerbation management, 146
  intubation, indications, 147
  NIPPV indications and contraindications, 146
  pathophysiology, 144
  permissive hypercapnia, 148
  ventilator management and pitfalls, 147
Chronic renal failure
  and end-stage renal disease, 277
  nephrotic syndrome, 278–279
  polycystic kidney disease, 280
  renal tubular acidosis, 279
  uremia, 280–282

Ciguatera, 195
Clonidine, 706
Clostridium difficile, 198
Clostridium perfringens, 194
Cluster headache, 584
CM. *See* Cardiomyopathy (CM)
CNS infections
  meningitis, 573–578
  typical CSF characteristics, 572
Cocaine
  and chest pain, 5
  description, 711
  sympathomimetic withdrawal, 616
Cold injury pathophysiology, 543
Collar button abscess, 742
Colles' fracture, 750
Coma testing, 557
Compartment syndrome, 792
Complicated *vs.* uncomplicated UTI, 289
Concussion, 823
Congestive heart failure
  causes of, 25
  diagnosis, 28
  diastolic heart failure, 26
  pathophysiology, 24
  systolic heart failure, 25
  treatment, 29, 30
Conjunctivitis, 648
  allergic, 652
  bacterial, 649
  EKC, 651
  ophthalmia neonatorum, 650
  subconjunctival hemorrhage, 652
  viral, 651
Constipation
  description, 187
  diagnosis, 188
  etiologies, 187–188
  symptoms and signs, 187
  treatment, 189
COPD. *See* Chronic obstructive pulmonary disease (COPD)
Cornea, 653–657
Corneal abrasion, 657
Corneal foreign bodies, 659
Corneal lacerations, 658
Corneal ulcers, 659
Cranial nerves, 638
Crohn's disease
  description, 253
  diagnosis, 254
  extraintestinal manifestations, 254
  symptoms and signs, 253
  treatment, 255
Croup, 489
Cryoprecipitate, 317
Cryptosporidium, 197
Cushing's Syndrome. *See* Hyperadrenalism
Cyanide and nitriles, 712–713
Cyanosis, 134
Cytomegalovirus, 373

D
Dacryoadenitis, 644
Dacryocystitis, 644
D-Dimer, 83
Decompression sickness, 530
Decubitus ulcers, 386
Deep venous thrombosis (DVT)
  clinical features, 81
  diagnosis, 81
  disposition, 86
Defibrillator nomenclature, 91
Delayed transfusion reaction, 319
Delirium *vs.* dementia, 601
Dental emergencies
  ANUG, 491
  dental trauma, 493
  ellis fractures, 492
  gingival hyperplasia, 492
  odontogenic infections, 490
  periodontal pathology, 491
  periostitis and alveolar osteitis and post-extraction bleeding, 490
Dental trauma, 493
De Quervain's tenosynovitis, 746
Dermatophyte infections, 362
Diabetes insipidus (DI)
  causes of central DI, 434
  causes of nephrogenic DI, 435
  clinical features, 435
  laboratory abnormalities and testing considerations, 436
  treatment and disposition, 436
Diabetes mellitus (DM)
  about hormones, 393
  insulin pump, 394
  types of insulin, 394
Diabetic ketoacidosis (DKA)
  bicarbonate, 400
  causes of, 395
  cerebral edema, 400
  clinical features, 397
  complications, 400
  diagnosis, 398
  differential diagnosis, 399
  disposition, 401
  precipitants, 398
  treatment, 399
Dialysis disequilibrium, 286
Diaphragmatic injury, 846
Diarrhea
  antibiotic-associated, 197
  bacterial, 190
  C. difficile, 198
  description, 189
  pseudomembranous enterocolitis, 198
  viral, 190
Diastolic heart failure, 26
DIC. *See* Disseminated intravascular coagulation (DIC)
Digitalis
  description, 706–707
  EKG changes, 100
Dilated cardiomyopathy
  clinical features, 52
  description, 51
  treatment, 53
Disk herniation, 802
Diskitis, 806
Disseminated intravascular coagulation (DIC)
  clinical features, 336
  description, 336
  etiologies, 335
  laboratory findings, 337
  treatment, 337

Diverticulitis
  description, 248
  diagnosis, 250
  risk factors, 249
  symptoms and signs, 249
  treatment, 250
Dog bites, 523
Drowning, 538–539
Drug rash/eruption, 356
Dysbarism
  arterial gas embolism, 529
  barotitis externa, 527
  barotitis interna, 527
  barotitis media, 526
  barotrauma of ascent, 528
  barotrauma of ascent treatment, 530
  decompression sickness, 530
  nitrogen narcosis, 529
  pulmonary barotrauma, 529
  recompression therapy, 531
  sinus barotrauma, 528
Dyshemoglobinemias
  clinical features, 322
  methemoglobin, 321
  methemoglobinemia
    drugs causing, 321
    types, 322
  treatment, 322
Dysphagia, 199
Dysrhythmias
  atrial fibrillation and atrial flutter, 105–107
  junctional escape rhythm, 102–103
  multifocal atrial tachycardia, 108–109
  premature ventricular contractions, 109–110
  supraventricular tachycardia, 103–105
  ventricular fibrillation, 117–118
  ventricular tachycardia, 115–117
  Wolff-Parkinson-White syndrome, 111–114
Dystonic reaction and chorea, 598

E
Ear
  acute mastoiditis, 475
  auricular hematoma, 476
  bullous myringitis, 474
  cauliflower ear, 476
  cholesteatoma, 475
  hearing loss, 469–471
  malignant otitis externa, 472–473
  otalgia, 468
  otitis externa, 472
  otitis media, 474
  perichondritis, 471
  tinnitus, 469
  tympanic membrane perforation, 477
Early repolarization, predicting factors, 11
Eastern coral snake envenomation, 525
Eclampsia, 632
E. coli, 191
Ectopic pregnancy, 629
Eczema, 358
Edema of upper airway
  angioedema, 496
  uvular edema, 496
ED staff/patient safety, 612
Ehrlichiosis, 371
Eighth cranial nerve lesions, 513
EKG
  in AMI, 8
  changes related to
    electrolytes and metabolic conditions, 96–99
    medications, 100–101
  and emergent reperfusion, 12
  MI predicting factors, 11
  ventricular aneurysm predicting factors, 22
Elbow
  bursitis, 761
  dislocation, 763
  epicondylitis, 761
  fracture, 764
  nursemaid's elbow, 762
  radial head fracture, 764
  soft tissue injuries, 760
  supracondylar fracture, 765
Elder abuse, 611
Electrical injuries
  description, 531
  lightning injury, 533–534
  management, 532
Electrolyte complications, of ESRD, 282
Electrolytes and acid-base
  calcium, 445–450
  magnesium, 450–453
  metabolic acidosis, 458–462
  metabolic alkalosis, 462–463
  metabolic derangements, 456–457
  phosphorus, 453–456
  potassium, 441–444
  respiratory acidosis, 463–464
  respiratory alkalosis, 464–465
  sodium, 437–440
Ellis fractures, 492
Emergency dialysis, indications for, 283
Emergency pacing, 89
Emergent reperfusion and EKG, 12
Empyema, 175
Encephalitis
  causes, 579
  description, 578
  diagnosis and management, 579
Endometriosis, 624
Endometritis, 636
Endophthalmitis, 661
End organ and other syndromes, 73–74
End-stage renal disease (ESRD), 277
Entamoeba histolytica, 196
ENT emergencies
  airway foreign body, 507
  causes of trismus, 505
  cavernous sinus thrombosis, 506
  post-tonsillectomy bleeding, 504
  Ramsay Hunt syndrome, 506
  trigeminal neuralgia, 505
Epidemic keratoconjunctivitis (EKC), 651
Epididymitis, 299
Epiglottitis, 486
Epistaxis, 478–479
Erysipelas, 503
Erythema multiforme, 350
Erythema nodosum, 357
Escharotomy, 867
Esophageal emergencies
  dysphagia, 199

transfer dysphagia, 199–201
transport dysphagia, 202–204
Esophageal foreign bodies
caustic ingestions, 209
description, 207
diagnosis and treatment, 208
symptoms and signs, 207
Esophageal perforation
causes, 205
description, 204
diagnosis and treatment, 206
symptoms and signs, 206
Esophagitis, 211
Ethanol, 693–694
Ethylene glycol, 695
Exacerbation disposition, asthma, 148
Exacerbation management, asthma, 146
Exfoliative dermatitis, 355
External eye
lids, 642–644
periorbital and orbital cellulitis, 645–647
Extremity injuries
amputations, 857
description, 856
Exudates, 174
Eye movements, 638
Eye muscles, 638

F
Facial cellulitis, 503
Facial fractures
frontal and zygoma fractures, 482
mandible fractures, 483
midface fractures, 483
Facial infections
erysipelas, 503
facial cellulitis, 503
impetigo, 504
Factitious disorders, 609
Febrile nonhemolytic reaction, 318
Febrile seizures, 570–571
Felon, 740
Femoral shaft fracture, 781
FFP. *See* Fresh frozen plasma (FFP)
Fibula fracture, 794
Finger dislocation, 748
First-degree heart block (1° HB)
description, 120
EKG changes, 121
treatment, 121
Fitz-Hugh-Curtis syndrome, 619
Flail chest, 842
Flexor tenosynovitis, 742
Foot
calcaneal fractures, 797
lisfranc injuries, 798
metatarsal fractures, 799
tarsal tunnel syndrome, 799
Forearm
Galeazzi fracture, 757
Monteggia fracture, 758
ulna and radius fractures, 759
ulnar nightstick fracture, 756
Volkmann's ischemic contracture, 759
Foreskin disorders
glans penis and, 296
traumatic penis and, 296
Fractures, 747
Fresh frozen plasma (FFP), 316
Frontal and zygoma fractures, 482
Fungal meningitis, 578

G
Gallbladder
acalculous cholecystitis, 227
ascending cholangitis, 227
description, 226
diagnosis, 228
pathophysiology, 227
symptoms and signs, 228
treatment, 229
Gamekeeper's thumb, 745
Gamma-hydroxybutyrate, 730
Gastrocnemius rupture, 794
Generalized skin rashes and disorders
angioedema, 364
bullous pemphigoid, 354
dermatophyte infections, 362
drug rash/eruption, 356
eczema, 358
erythema multiforme, 350
erythema nodosum, 357
exfoliative dermatitis, 355
pemphigus vulgaris, 353
pityriasis rosea, 361
psoriasis, 359
seborrheic dermatitis, 360
SJS and TEN, 351
skin cancers, 365
SSSS, 352
tinea versicolor, 363
Genital warts, 308
GERD
description, 210
symptoms and signs, 210
treatment, 211
Geriatric trauma, 862
Gestational trophoblastic disease, 631
Giardia, 196
GI bleeding
LGIB (*see* Lower GI bleeding (LGIB))
terminology, 214
UGIB (*see* Upper GI bleeding (UGIB))
Gingival hyperplasia, 492
Glans penis and foreskin disorders, 296
Glaucoma, 669–670
Glomerular disease, causes, 267
Gonorrhea, 303
G6PD deficiency, 329
Granuloma inguinale, 307
Graves disease, 416
Grief reaction, 605
Guillain-Barre syndrome, 595
Gynecologic oncology
cervical cancer, 628
ovarian cancer, 627
uterine cancer, 627

H
Haemophilus influenzae, 158
Hallucinogens, 713–714

Hand
  Boutonniere deformity, 743
  carpal tunnel syndrome, 746
  collar button abscess, 742
  De Quervain's tenosynovitis, 746
  felon, 740
  finger dislocation, 748
  flexor tenosynovitis, 742
  Gamekeeper's thumb, 745
  herpetic whitlow, 745
  high-pressure injection injury, 749
  infections, 739
  Mallet finger, 744
  nerves, 738
  paronychia, 741
  sporotrichosis, 742
Hand-foot-mouth disease, 381
Headache syndromes
  carotid/vertebral artery dissection, 593
  classification, 581
  cluster headache, 584
  CNS tumors, 586
  headache red flags, 581
  hydrocephalus, 587–588
  migraine, 582–583
  post-lumbar puncture headache, 585
  pseudotumor cerebri, 586
  subarachnoid hemorrhage, 591–592
  tension headache, 583
  toxic metabolic headache, 585
  trigeminal neuralgia, 584
  venous sinus thrombosis, 591
  ventricular shunt headache, 589
  VP shunt complications, 589–590
Head trauma, 820
Hearing loss, 469
  causes of, 470
  medications and drugs, 471
Heart blocks
  first-degree heart block, 120–121
  left bundle branch block, 118–119
  right bundle branch block, 119–120
  second-degree type 1 heart block, 122–123
  second-degree type 2 heart block, 123–125
  third-degree heart block, 125–126
Heart failure
  clinical features and presentation, 27
  congestive (*see* Congestive heart failure)
  left *vs.* right, 26
Heart failure preserved ejection fraction. *See* Diastolic heart failure
Heart failure reduced ejection fraction. *See* Systolic heart failure
Heat dissipation *vs.* generation, 540
Heat stroke, 542
HELLP syndrome, 633
Hemangiomas, 387
Hematuria, causes, 292
Hemodialysis (HD)
  altered mental status, 286
  complications, 284
  dialysis disequilibrium, 286
  emergency dialysis, indications for, 283
  hemorrhagic complications, 285
  hypotension during, 285
  infectious complications, 284
  peritoneal dialysis, 287
Hemolytic anemias
  acquired hemolytic anemia, 330
  hemolytic uremic syndrome, 332
  hereditary
    G6PD deficiency, 329
    hereditary spherocytosis, 329
  microangiopathic hemolytic anemia, 331
  thrombotic thrombocytopenic purpura, 331
Hemolytic uremic syndrome (HUS), 332
Hemophilia
  description, 338
  treatment, 338
Hemoptysis, 134–135
Hemorrhage, 514
Hemorrhoids
  description, 257
  risk factors, 258
Hemostasis tests
  activated partial thromboplastin time, 324
  bleeding time, 323
  prothrombin time, 324
Hemothorax, 841
Henoch-Schonlein Purpura, 382
Heparin
  bleeding from, 341
  description, 341
Heparin-induced thrombocytopenia (HIT), 341
Hepatic encephalopathy, 225
Hepatitis
  hepatic encephalopathy, 225
  hepatitis A, 223
  hepatitis B, 223
  hepatitis C, 224
  hepatitis D, 224
  hepatitis E and G, 224
  indications for hospitalization, 222
  laboratory abnormalities, 222
  symptoms and signs, 221
  toxic, 225
Hepatitis A, 223
Hepatitis B, 223
Hepatitis C, 224
Hepatitis D, 224
Hepatitis E and G, 224
Hereditary spherocytosis, 329
Hernias
  description, 242
  diagnosis, 244
  inguinal, 242
  treatment, 244
  ventral, 243
Herpangina, 498
Herpes Simplex, 305
Herpes Zoster, 374
Herpes Zoster ophthalmicus, 656
Herpetic whitlow, 745
Hiccups, 176
High-altitude cerebral edema, 536
High-altitude illness, 535
  acute mountain sickness, 536
  high-altitude cerebral edema, 536
  high-altitude pulmonary edema, 537
High-altitude pulmonary edema, 537
High MCV (macrocytic), 312
High-pressure injection injury, 749
Hip dislocation, 855
Hirschsprung's disease, 239
Histrionic personality disorders, 610
HIT. *See* Heparin-induced thrombocytopenia (HIT)

Hordeolum, 642
HSV infections, 497
HSV keratitis, 655
Humerus and shoulder
  acromioclavicular injuries, 769
  anterior dislocations, 772
  clavicle fracture, 770
  diagnosis and treatment, 773
  inferior dislocations, 775
  nontraumatic pain, 767
  posterior dislocations, 774
  proximal fracture, 766
  rotator cuff injuries, 775
  scapula fracture, 771
  shaft fracture, 767
  sternoclavicular injuries, 768
  thoracic outlet syndrome, 776
HUS. *See* Hemolytic uremic syndrome (HUS)
Hydrocarbons
  description, 719
  treatment and management, 720
Hydrocephalus
  description, 587
  normal pressure, 588
  pediatric, 588
Hyperacute T waves, 10
Hyperadrenalism
  clinical features, 428
  disposition, 429
  laboratory abnormalities and testing considerations, 429
  treatment, 429
Hypercalcemia
  causes of, 449
  description, 448
  diagnosis, 450
  EKG changes, 98
  symptoms and signs, 449
  treatment, 450
Hypercapnia, 133
Hyperglycemia
  effects of, 396
  systemic effects of, 397
Hyperkalemia
  causes of, 443
  diagnosis, 444
  EKG changes, 97
  symptoms and signs, 444
  treatment, 444
Hypermagnesemia
  causes of, 452
  diagnosis, 453
  symptoms and signs, 453
  treatment, 453
Hypernatremia
  causes of, 440
  description, 439
  symptoms, 440
  treatment, 440
Hyperosmolar hyperglycemic nonketotic syndrome (HHNS)
  clinical features, 405
  diagnosis, 406
  disposition, 406
  pathophysiology, 404
  precipitating factors, 405
  treatment, 406
Hyperphosphatemia
  causes of, 455
  diagnosis, 456
  treatment, 456
Hypertension
  blood pressure definitions, 72
  description, 631
  end organ and other syndromes, 73–74
  hypertensive emergencies, 72
  medication effects, 74–75
  pulmonary, 76
  severe asymptomatic hypertension, 75
  side effects, 74–75
Hypertensive emergencies, 72
Hyperthyroidism
  causes of, 416, 417
  clinical features, 417
  description, 415
  Graves disease, 416
Hypertrophic cardiomyopathy
  clinical features, 54
  description, 53
  treatment, 54
Hyphema, 672
Hypocalcemia
  causes of, 447
  description, 446
  diagnosis, 448
  EKG changes, 97
  symptoms and signs, 447
  treatment, 448
Hypoglycemia
  agents for glucose control, 390
  clinical features, 391
  description, 683
  differential diagnosis, 392
  treatment, 392
Hypoglycemic agents, 721
Hypokalemia
  causes of, 442
  description, 441
  diagnosis, 443
  EKG changes, 96
  symptoms and signs, 442
  treatment, 443
Hypomagnesemia
  causes of, 451
  description, 450
  diagnosis, 452
  EKG changes, 98
  symptoms and signs, 451
  treatment, 452
Hyponatremia
  causes of, 438
  causes of hypotonic hyponatremia, 439
  description, 437
  diagnosis, 438
  treatment, 438
Hypophosphatemia
  causes of, 454
  diagnosis, 455
  symptoms and signs, 454
  treatment, 455
Hypotension, during hemodialysis, 285
Hypothermia
  description, 545
  EKG changes, 96
  manifestations, 546
  treatment, 546

Hypothyroidism
  causes of, 409
  clinical features, 410
  specific clinical features, 410
Hypoxemia, 132
Hypoxia, 132

I
Iatrogenic pneumothorax, 136
Idiopathic intracranial hypertension. *See* Pseudotumor cerebri
Idiopathic thrombocytopenic purpura (ITP), 334
Ileus, 233
Impetigo, 504
Incomplete spinal cord injury, 831
Infectious diseases and associated skin lesions
  babesiosis, 372
  cytomegalovirus, 373
  ehrlichiosis, 371
  hand-foot-mouth disease, 381
  Henoch-Schonlein purpura, 382
  Herpes Zoster, 374
  Kawasaki's disease, 383
  leptospirosis, 369
  lyme disease, 368
  malaria, 376
  measles, 378
  meningococcemia, 367
  Molluscum contagiosum, 375
  rocky mountain spotted fever, 370
  roseola infantum, 379
  rubella, 377
  scarlet fever, 384
  varicella, 380
Infective endocarditis
  acute *vs.* subacute, 43
  clinical findings, 45
  description, 42
  diagnosis, 46
  left-sided *vs.* right-sided endocarditis, 44
  organisms, 44–45
  pathophysiology, 43
  prophylaxis, 47
  treatment, 46
Inferior MI, 14
Inferior MI specifics, 13
Inferior-posterior MI, 14
Inguinal hernias, 242
Interstitial disease, causes, 266
Intimate partner violence, 611
Intracranial hemorrhage, 564, 825
Intraoral and tongue lesions
  leukoplakia, 499
  oral cancer, 500
  strawberry tongue, 499
Intrinsic renal failure, 265
Intubation
  indications, 147
  rapid sequence intubation, 179
Intussusception
  description, 236–237
  diagnosis, 237
  treatment, 238
Iron, 716
Irritable bowel syndrome, 257
Isoniazid, 704
Isopropyl alcohol, 695
ITP. *See* Idiopathic thrombocytopenic purpura (ITP)
IV tPA exclusions, 562

J
Jellyfish stings, 524
Junctional escape rhythm (JER)
  description, 102
  EKG changes, 102
  treatment, 103

K
Kawasaki's disease, 383
Keratitis, 653
  bacterial, 654
  Herpes Zoster ophthalmicus, 656
  HSV, 655
  ultraviolet, 657
Kidney injuries, 850
Kidney stones
  diagnosis and treatment, 293–294
  stone admission criteria, 294
Klebsiella pneumoniae, 159
Knee
  Baker's cyst, 790
  dislocation, 786
  Osgood-Schlatter disease, 789
  osteochondritis dissecans, 788
  Ottawa rules, 782
  patellar dislocation, 784
  patellar fractures, 783
  tendon rupture, 787
  tibial plateau fractures, 785

L
Labyrinthitis, 512
Lacerations, 674
Lactic acidosis, 460
Lacunar infarction, 560
Lambert-Eaton myasthenic syndrome, 597
Larynx trauma, 495
Lead, 717
Left bundle branch block (LBBB)
  description, 118
  EKG changes, 119
Left-sided *vs.* right-sided endocarditis, 44
Left ventricular assist devices (LVAD)
  coding, 95
  complications, 95
  description, 94
  echo findings, 95
  EKG, 95
  emergencies, 94
  patient assessment, 94
Left *vs.* right heart failure, 26
Leg
  Achilles tendon rupture, 794
  compartment syndrome, 792
  fibula fracture, 794
  gastrocnemius rupture, 794
  pilon fracture, 793
  tibial shaft fractures, 791
Legg-Calve-Perthes disease, 777
Leiomyomas, 625
Leptospirosis, 369

Lesions, 307
Leukoplakia, 499
Leukotriene modifiers, 141
LGV. *See* Lymphogranuloma venereum (LGV)
Lids
  blepharitis, 643
  chalazion, 642
  dacryoadenitis, 644
  dacryocystitis, 644
  hordeolum, 642
Lightning injury, 533–534
Lisfranc injuries, 798
Lithium, 721–722
Liver
  bilirubin evaluation, 220
  description, 219
  hepatitis (*see* Hepatitis)
  neonatal jaundice, 221
  spontaneous bacterial peritonitis, 226
Localized cold injuries, 543–544
Lower GI bleeding (LGIB)
  causes, 217, 218
  description, 217
  diagnosis and treatment, 218
  disposition, 219
Low MCV (microcytic), 312
Ludwig's angina, 488
Lumbar strain, 802
Lung abscess, 17, 172
LVAD. *See* Left ventricular assist devices (LVAD)
Lyme disease, 368
Lymphangiomas, 388
Lymphogranuloma venereum (LGV), 306

M
Macroscopic urine, 272
Magnesium
  description, 141
  hypermagnesemia, 452–453
  hypomagnesemia, 450–452
MAHA. *See* Microangiopathic hemolytic anemia (MAHA)
Major depression, 604
Major ring fractures, 853
Malaria, 376
Male genital emergencies
  epididymitis and orchitis, 299
  foreskin disorders
    glans penis and, 296
    traumatic penis and, 296
  priapism, 297
  prostatitis, 300
  scrotal disorders, 295
  testicular torsion, 298
  urethritis, 300
  urinary retention, 301
Malignancy, complications of
  adrenal insufficiency, 347
  airway obstruction, 343
  febrile neutropenia, 348
  hypercalcemia, 346
  hyperviscosity syndrome, 348
  pathologic fractures from bone metastases, 344
  pericardial effusion and tamponade, 344
  SIADH, 346
  spinal cord compression, 345
  superior vena cava syndrome, 345
  tumor lysis syndrome, 347
Malignant hyperthermia, 733
Malignant otitis externa (MOE), 472–473
Malingering, 609
Mallet finger, 744
Mammalian bites
  cat bites and scratches, 523
  description, 520
  dog bites, 523
  rabies, 521–522
Mandible fractures, 483
Marine envenomation
  eastern coral snake envenomation, 525
  jellyfish stings, 524
  pit viper envenomation, 525
  snake bites, 524
  stingray stings, 524
Massive blood transfusion, 315
Mastitis, 636
MAT. *See* Multifocal atrial tachycardia (MAT)
Measles, 378
Mediastinal masses, 178
Mediastinitis, 176
Meniere's disease, 511
Meningitis
  bacterial, 575
  description, 573
  empiric antibiotic treatment, 577
  evaluation, 577
  fungal, 578
  prophylaxis, 576
  risk factors, 576
  viral, 574
Meningococcemia, 367
Mercury, 718
Mesenteric ischemia
  description, 251
  diagnosis, 252
  risk factors, 251
  symptoms and signs, 252
  treatment, 252
Metabolic acidosis
  abnormal anion gap without acid-base disturbance, 458
  anion gap, 458
  causes of anion gap, 459
  effects, 461
  lactic acidosis, 460
  non-anion gap causes, 461
  treatment, 462
Metabolic alkalosis
  causes of, 463
  description, 462
  effects, 463
  treatment, 463
Metabolic derangements
  description, 456
  history and physical, 457
  laboratory investigations, 457
Metal fume fever, 718
Metatarsal fractures, 799
Methanol, 693
Methemoglobin (MHb), 321
Methemoglobinemia
  drugs causing, 321
  types, 322
Methylxanthines, 141
Microangiopathic hemolytic anemia (MAHA), 331

Microthrombosis, causes, 270
Midface fractures, 483
Migraine
 description, 582
 treatment, 583
Migraine-related vertigo, 516
Mild traumatic brain injury (TBI), 822
Minor/moderate heat illness, 541
Miscellaneous skin-related disorders
 decubitus ulcers, 386
 hemangiomas, 387
 lymphangiomas, 388
 venous stasis ulcers, 385
Mitral regurgitation
 description, 33
 diagnosis, 34
 symptoms, 34
 treatment, 35
Mitral stenosis
 description, 32
 diagnosis, 32
 treatment, 33
Mitral valve prolapse
 description, 35
 diagnosis, 36
 treatment, 36
Moderate and severe TBI, 822
Molluscum contagiosum, 375
Monoamine oxidase inhibitor (MAOI) overdose, 723
Movement disorders
 akathisia, 599
 dystonic reaction and chorea, 598
 Parkinson's disease, 599
 tardive dyskinesia, 599
Multifocal atrial tachycardia (MAT)
 description, 108
 EKG changes, 108
 treatment, 109
Multiple sclerosis, 515, 594
Munchausen's syndrome, 609
Mushrooms, 723–724
Myasthenia gravis
 Lambert-Eaton myasthenic syndrome, 597
 precipitants, 596
 treatment, 597
Mycoplasma pneumoniae, 160
Myocarditis
 clinical features, 58
 description, 56
 infectious causes, 57
 treatment, 58
Myxedema coma
 description, 411
 differential diagnosis, 413
 disposition, 414
 precipitating factors, 412
 treatment, 414

N
Narcissistic personality disorders, 610
Narcotics, 724
Nasal fractures, 480
Neck, 494
Neck masses
 branchial cleft cysts, 494
 larynx trauma, 495
 neck, 494
 thyroglossal duct cysts, 495
Necrotizing enterocolitis, 186
Necrotizing infections, 488
Neonatal jaundice, 221
Neonatal seizures, 571
Nephrotic syndrome
 causes, 279
 description, 278
Nerve agents, 553
Neurogenic shock, 834
Neuroleptic malignant syndrome (NMS), 727
Neuromuscular disorders
 acute periodic paralysis, 595
 Guillain-Barre syndrome, 595
 multiple sclerosis, 594
 myasthenia gravis, 596–597
 tick paralysis, 595
Neuro-ophthalmology
 cranial nerves, 638
 eye movements, 638
 eye muscles, 638
 sympathetic chain and Horner's syndrome, 639
Neuropathies, 600
NIPPV indications and contraindications, 146
Nitrogen narcosis, 529
Nonaccidental trauma, 860
Non-cardiogenic pulmonary edema, 30
Nonsteroidal anti-inflammatory agents (NSAIDs), 701
Nontraumatic hip disorders
 Legg-Calve-Perthes disease, 777
 septic arthritis, 779
 slipped capital femoral epiphysis, 778
 toxic synovitis, 780
Non-ulcer-forming processes, 302
Normal MCV (normocytic), 313
Normal pressure hydrocephalus, 588
Nose
 allergic rhinitis, 480
 epistaxis, 478–479
 nasal fractures, 480
 sinusitis, 481

O
Obsessive-compulsive disorder, 607
Obstetrics
 abortions, 630
 abruptio placentae, 633
 amniotic fluid embolism, 635
 eclampsia, 632
 ectopic pregnancy, 629
 endometritis, 636
 gestational trophoblastic disease, 631
 HELLP syndrome, 633
 hypertension, 631
 mastitis, 636
 peripartum cardiomyopathy, 636
 placenta previa, 634
 postpartum hemorrhage, 635
 preeclampsia, 632
 preterm birth and premature rupture of membranes, 634
 RhoGAM, 630
 umbilical cord prolapse, 635
Odontogenic infections, 490
Odontoid fractures, 829
Ophthalmia neonatorum, 650
Opiate withdrawal, 615
Opioid toxidromes, 689–690

Optic nerve
  optic neuritis, 666
  papilledema and pseudotumor cerebri, 667
Optic neuritis, 666
Oral cancer, 500
Orchitis, 299
Organic acute psychosis etiologies medical conditions, 602
Organic acute psychosis etiologies medications/drugs, 602
Organic *vs.* functional psychosis, 603
Organophosphates (OP) and carbamates, 725
Orthostatic syncope, 78
Osgood-Schlatter disease, 789
Osmolal gap, causes, 466
Osmolar gap, 686
Osteomyelitis, 800, 801
Otalgia, 468
Otitis externa (OE), 472
Otitis media (OM), 474
Ottawa rules
  ankle, 795
  knee, 782
Ovarian/adnexal torsion, 624
Ovarian cancer, 627
Ovarian cysts, 623
Overdose odor pearls, 684
Ovulatory bleeding, 626

P
Pacemakers
  automatic implantable cardioverter, 91
  emergency pacing, 89
  failure, 93
  malfunctions, 92
  nomenclature, 90
Packed red blood cells (PRBC), 314
Pancreas/stomach/duodenum/intestine trauma, 849
Pancreatitis
  causes, 229
  complications, 230
  diagnosis, 231
  Ranson's criteria, 232
  symptoms and signs, 231
  treatment, 232
Papilledema and pseudotumor cerebri, 667
Parkinson's disease, 599
Paronychia, 741
Pediatric gastroenterology, 186
Pediatrics
  apparent life-threatening events, 181–182
  head trauma, 825
  hydrocephalus, 588
  sudden infant death syndrome, 183
Pediatric trauma, 858
  airway and breathing, 859
  child abuse, 861
  indications, 860
  nonaccidental trauma, 860
Pelvic inflammatory disease (PID)
  admission criteria, 619
  complications, 619
  diagnosis and treatment, 618
Pelvis and hip trauma, 852
  acetabular and avulsion/single bone Fx, 853
  complications, 855
  hip dislocation, 855
  major ring fractures, 853
  pelvic radiograph, 854
  treatment, 854
Pemphigus vulgaris, 353
Penetrating abdominal trauma, 847
Penetrating flank and buttock injuries, 850
Penetrating neck injury, 835
  blunt neck trauma, 838
  general treatment, 837
  pharynx trauma, 837
  zones of neck, 836
Peptic ulcer disease (PUD)
  causes, 212
  complications, 214
  description, 212
  diagnosis and treatment, 213
  gastritis, 212
  pathophysiology, 212
  symptoms and signs, 213
Pericarditis
  causes, 59
  clinical features and diagnosis, 60
  EKG changes, 61
  infectious causes, 59
  treatment, 61
Perichondritis, 471
Perilymph fistula, 512
Periodontal pathology, 491
Periorbital and orbital cellulitis
  complications, 647
  description, 645
  postseptal cellulitis, 647
  preseptal cellulitis, 646
Periostitis and alveolar osteitis and post-extraction bleeding, 490
Peripartum cardiomyopathy, 636
Peripheral polyneuropathies, 600
Peripheral vertigo
  BPPV, 510
  cerebellopontine angle tumors, 513
  eighth cranial nerve lesions, 513
  labyrinthitis, 512
  Meniere's disease, 511
  perilymph fistula, 512
  posttraumatic vertigo and post-concussive syndrome, 513
  symptoms, 509
  vestibular neuronitis, 511
Peritoneal dialysis, 287
Peritonsillar abscess (PTA), 485
Permissive hypercapnia, 148
Personality disorders, 610
Pertussis
  complications, 152
  description, 152
  treatment, 153
Pharyngitis and tonsillitis, 484
Pharynx trauma, 837
Phencyclidine (PCP), 714
Phenothiazines, 726–727
Phenytoin and fosphenytoin, 703
Pheochromocytoma
  clinical features, 429
  diagnosis, 430
  treatment and disposition, 430
Phosphorus
  description, 453
  hyperphosphatemia, 455–456
  hypophosphatemia, 454–455
PID. *See* Pelvic inflammatory disease (PID)
Pilon fracture, 793
Pit viper envenomation, 525

Pityriasis rosea, 361
Placenta previa, 634
Plague, 551
Platelet disorders
  description, 333
  disseminated intravascular coagulation, 335–337
  idiopathic thrombocytopenic purpura, 334
Platelet transfusion, 316
Pleural effusions
  description, 173
  empyema, 175
  exudates, 174
  hiccups, 176
  mediastinal masses, 178
  mediastinitis, 176
  pneumoconioses, 177
  sarcoid, 177
  superior vena cava syndrome, 178
  transudates, 174
Pneumoconioses, 177
Pneumocystis jirovecii, 161
Pneumomediastinum, 137, 839
Pneumonia
  aspiration, 166, 167
  classification, 153
  C. pneumoniae, 160
  cultures and treatment, 164
  cystic fibrosis, 165
  disposition, 163
  fungal PNA etiologies, 162
  H. influenzae, 158
  K. pneumoniae, 159
  Legionella, 160
  M. pneumoniae, 160
  P. aeruginosa, 158
  pathogens in HIV, 162
  pathophysiology, 154
  pediatric pneumonia, 156
  P. jirovecii, 161
  S. aureus, 159
  special considerations, 155
  in special patients, 164
  S. pneumoniae, 157
  treatment, 154
  zoonotic PNA etiologies, 161
Pneumothorax
  description, 839–840
  diagnosis and management, 136
  iatrogenic, 136
  pneumomediastinum, 137
  spontaneous, 135
Poisoned patient
  airway assessment, 677
  antidotes selection, 684
  breathing assessment, 677
  charcoal, 681
  circulation assessment, 677
  dialysis, 682
  disability assessment, 677
  exposure, 678
  laboratory studies, 679
  methods of drug elimination, 682
  overdose odor pearls, 684
  primary survey, 676
  primary survey adjuncts, 678
  secondary survey and adjuncts, 681
  toxicology screens, 680
  toxins, 683
  urinalysis, 680
Polycystic kidney disease, 280
Postconcussive syndrome, 823
Posterior cord syndrome, 833
Posterior infarction, 16
Post-lumbar puncture headache, 585
Postpartum hemorrhage, 635
Postrenal failure
  causes, 271
  description, 270
Postseptal cellulitis, 647
Post-tonsillectomy bleeding, 504
Posttraumatic vertigo and post-concussive syndrome, 513
Potassium
  hyperkalemia, 443–444
  hypokalemia, 441–443
PRBC. *See* Packed red blood cells (PRBC)
Preeclampsia, 632
Premature ventricular contractions (PVCs)
  description, 109
  EKG changes, 110
  treatment, 110
Prerenal failure
  causes, 264
  description, 264
Preseptal cellulitis, 646
Preterm birth and premature rupture of membranes (PROM), 634
Priapism, 297
Prinzmetal's angina
  description, 6
  predicting factors, 7
Prostatitis, 300
Protozoan pathogens
  Cryptosporidium, 197
  E. histolytica, 196
  Giardia, 196
Pseudomembranous enterocolitis, 198
Pseudomonas aeruginosa, 158
Pseudosubluxation, 828
Pseudotumor cerebri, 586
Psoriasis, 359
Psychiatric emergencies
  amnesia, 603
  anorexia, 607
  anxiety, 606–607
  bipolar disorder, 605
  bulimia nervosa, 608
  delirium *vs.* dementia, 601
  factitious disorders, 609
  grief reaction, 605
  major depression, 604
  malingering, 609
  Munchausen's syndrome, 609
  obsessive-compulsive disorder, 607
  organic acute psychosis etiologies medical conditions, 602
  organic acute psychosis etiologies medications/drugs, 602
  organic *vs.* functional psychosis, 603
  personality disorders, 610
  schizophrenia, 606
  somatoform disorders, 608
  suicide, 604
PUD. *See* Peptic ulcer disease (PUD)
Pulmonary barotrauma, 529
Pulmonary contusion, 843
Pulmonary embolism (PE)
  anticoagulation treatment, 85

basic tests, 82
clinical features, 80
CT angiography, 83
description, 79
disposition, 86
embolectomy, 86
fibrinolysis, 85
massive and less severe, 85
pretest probability, 82
pulmonary angiography, 84
venography, 84
venous ultrasound, 84
VQ scanning, 84
Pulmonary hypertension, 76
Pupil abnormalities, 640
PVCs. *See* Premature ventricular contractions (PVCs)
Pyloric stenosis
description, 238
diagnosis, 239
treatment, 239

R

Rabies, 521–522
Radiation, 548
Radiocontrast-induced nephropathy, 269
Ramsay Hunt syndrome, 506
Ranson's criteria, 232
Rapid sequence intubation, 179
RBBB. *See* Right bundle branch block (RBBB)
Reactivation tuberculosis, 169
Recompression therapy, 531
Rectal prolapse, 259
Red flags, 802
Renal transplant, 295
Renal tubular acidosis, 279
Respiratory acidosis
causes of, 464
description, 463
treatment, 464
Respiratory alkalosis
causes of, 465
description, 464
treatment, 465
Respiratory distress and tracheostomy, 180
Restrictive cardiomyopathy
clinical features, 55
description, 55
treatment, 56
Retina
central retinal artery occlusion, 663
central retinal vein occlusion, 665
etiologies of central retinal artery syndrome, 664
retinal detachment, 666
Retinal detachment, 666
Retrobulbar hematoma, 673
Retropharyngeal abscess, 487
Rewarming methods, 547
Rewarming physiology, 547
Rhabdomyolysis
causes, 274
clinical features, 275
complications, 276
description, 274
diagnosis, 275
treatment, 276
Rheumatic heart disease
description, 48
diagnosis, 48
treatment, 49
Rheumatologic emergencies
antiphospholipid syndrome, 810
gout and pseudogout, 809
joint fluid, 809
joint fluid analysis, 808
rheumatoid arthritis, 809
systemic lupus erythematosus, 811
RhoGAM, 630
Rib fractures, 841
RIFLE criteria, 263
Right bundle branch block (RBBB)
description, 119
EKG changes, 120
Right ventricular infarction, 15
Rocky mountain spotted fever, 370
Roseola infantum, 379
Rubella, 377

S

Salicylate, 699–700
Salivary gland disorders
sialolithiasis, 502
suppurative parotitis, 502
viral parotitis, 501
Salmonella, 191
Salter-Harris fractures, 737
Sarcoid, 177
SBP. *See* Spontaneous bacterial peritonitis (SBP)
Scarlet Fever, 384
Schizophrenia, 606
SCIWORA, 833
Scombroid, 195
Scrotal disorders, 295
Seborrheic dermatitis, 360
Second-degree type 1 Heart Block (2° type 1 HB)
description, 122
EKG changes, 122
treatment, 123
Second-degree type 2 Heart Block (2° type 2 HB), 125
description, 123
EKG changes, 124
treatment, 124
Second impact syndrome, 824
Sedative-hypnotics
barbituates, 729
benzodiazepines, 730
gamma-hydroxybutyrate, 730
Seizures
adult status epilepticus management, 569
causes of, 566
definitions, 565
disposition, 570
febrile, 570–571
focal classification, 566
generalized classification, 565
mimics, 567
neonatal, 571
recurrent seizure evaluation, 568
routine first seizure evaluation, 568
vs. syncope, 567
Serotonin syndrome
agents, 729
Hunter criteria, 728

Severe asthma management, 142
Severe asymptomatic hypertension, 75
Sexual assault, 612
Sexually transmitted diseases
- chancroid, 306
- chlamydia, 302
- genital warts, 308
- gonorrhea, 303
- granuloma inguinale, 307
- Herpes Simplex, 305
- lesions, 307
- lymphogranuloma venereum, 306
- non-ulcer-forming processes, 302
- syphilis, 304
- *Trichomoniasis,* 303
- ulcer-forming processes, 301

Sgarbossa Criteria, 13
Shigella, 191
SIADH. *See* Syndrome of inappropriate antidiuretic hormone secretion (SIADH)
Sialolithiasis, 502
Sickle cell anemia, 325
- acute chest syndrome, 326
- aplastic crisis, 327
- description, 325
- infectious complications, 328
- neurologic complications, 328
- splenic sequestration, 327
- vaso-occlusive crisis, 326

SIDS. *See* Sudden infant death syndrome (SIDS)
Sinus barotrauma, 528
Sinusitis, 481
SJS and TEN, 351
Skin cancers, 365
Skull fracture, 824
Smallpox, 551
Smith's fracture, 751
Snake bites, 524
Sodium
- hypernatremia, 439–440
- hyponatremia, 437–439

Soft tissue lesions
- aphthous stomatitis, 498
- candidiasis, 497
- herpangina, 498
- HSV infections, 497

Somatoform disorders, 608
Specific toxins and poisons
- alcohols, 692–695
- amphetamine, 696
- analgesics, 697–701
- anticonvulsants, 702–703
- antihistamines, 703
- antimicrobials, 704
- arsenic, 715
- cardiac medications, 705–707
- caustic agents, 708, 709
- chlorine, 710
- cocaine, 711
- cyanide and nitriles, 712–713
- hallucinogens, 713–714
- hydrocarbons, 719–720
- hydrogen fluoride, 708
- hypoglycemic agents, 721
- iron, 716
- isoniazid, 704
- lead, 717
- lithium, 721–722
- malignant hyperthermia, 733
- mercury, 718
- metal fume fever, 718
- monoamine oxidase inhibitor overdose, 723
- mushrooms, 723–724
- narcotics, 724
- neuroleptic malignant syndrome, 727
- organophosphates and carbamates, 725
- phencyclidine, 714
- phenothiazines, 726–727
- sedative-hypnotics, 729–730
- serotonin syndrome, 728–729
- strychnine, 731
- tricyclic antidepressants, 731–732
- xanthines, 732

Spinal cord injuries
- anterior cord syndrome, 832
- Brown-Sequard syndrome, 832
- central cord syndrome, 831
- incomplete spinal cord injury, 831
- neurogenic shock, 834
- posterior cord syndrome, 833
- SCIWORA, 833
- spinal cord syndromes, 830
- spinal shock, 834
- transverse cord syndrome, 832

Spinal cord syndromes, 830
Spinal disorders, 600
Spinal epidural abscess, 807, 808
Spinal infections, 805
Spinal injuries, 826
- cervical spine clearance, 827
- cervical spine evaluation, 827
- odontoid fractures, 829
- pseudosubluxation, 828
- stable cervical fractures, 828
- thoracolumbar fractures, 829
- unstable cervical fractures, 828

Spinal shock, 834
Spinal stenosis, 803
Spleen and liver trauma, 849
Splenic sequestration, 327
Spontaneous bacterial peritonitis (SBP), 226
Spontaneous intracranial hemorrhage, 563
Spontaneous pneumothorax, 135
Sporotrichosis, 742
SSSS. *See* Staphylococcal scalded skin syndrome (SSSS)
Stable angina, 6
Stable cervical fractures, 828
Staphylococcal scalded skin syndrome (SSSS), 352
Staphylococcus, 193
Staphylococcus aureus, 159
Sternal fracture, 842
Steroids, 141
Stingray stings, 524
Strawberry tongue, 499
Streptococcus pneumoniae, 157
Stroke and TIA, 558
Stroke mimics, 557
Strychnine, 731
ST-segment elevation, causes of, 9
Subarachnoid hemorrhage (SAH)
- description, 591
- diagnosis, 592
- treatment, 592

Subconjunctival hemorrhage, 652

Submersion, 538–539
Substance abuse/dependence, 613
Sudden infant death syndrome (SIDS), 183
Suicide, 604
Superior vena cava (SVC) syndrome, 178
Suppurative parotitis, 502
Supraventricular tachycardia (SVT)
  description, 103
  EKG changes, 104
  treatment, 104, 105
Sympathetic chain and Horner's syndrome, 639
Sympathomimetic toxidromes, 691
Syncope
  cardiac, 78
  causes, 77
  description, 77
  evaluation, 79
  vasovagal and orthostatic syncope, 78
Syndrome of inappropriate antidiuretic hormone secretion (SIADH)
  causes of, 431
  central pontine myelinolysis, 433
  clinical features, 432
  laboratory abnormalities and testing considerations, 432
  treatment and disposition, 433
Syphilis, 304
Systolic heart failure, 25

T

Tardive dyskinesia, 599
Tarsal tunnel syndrome, 799
TB. *See* Tuberculosis (TB)
Temperature-related illness
  cold injury pathophysiology, 543
  heat dissipation *vs.* generation, 540
  heat stroke, 542
  hypothermia, 545–546
  localized cold injuries, 543–544
  minor/moderate heat illness, 541
  predisposing factors, 540
  radiation, 548
  rewarming methods, 547
  rewarming physiology, 547
Temporal arteritis, 668
Tension headache, 583
Testicular injury, 852
Testicular torsion, 298
Tetanus, 554
Tetralogy of Fallot, 129
THC withdrawal, 616
Third-degree heart block (3° HB)
  description, 125
  EKG changes, 126
  treatment, 126
Thoracic and lumbar pain
  ankylosing spondylitis, 803
  back pain, 801
  back pain workup, 802
  cauda equina syndrome, 804
  disk herniation, 802
  diskitis, 806
  lumbar strain, 802
  red flags, 802
  spinal epidural abscess, 807, 808
  spinal infections, 805
  spinal stenosis, 803
  transverse myelitis, 805
Thoracic outlet syndrome (TOS), 776
Thoracolumbar fractures, 829
Throat/neck/upper airway infections
  bacterial tracheitis, 489
  croup, 489
  epiglottitis, 486
  Ludwig's angina, 488
  necrotizing infections, 488
  peritonsillar abscess, 485
  pharyngitis and tonsillitis, 484
  retropharyngeal abscess, 487
Thromboembolism, risk factors, 80
Thrombolysis, absolute and relative contraindications, 342
Thrombolytic therapy
  complications, 20
  successful, 20
Thrombotic thrombocytopenic purpura (TTP), 331
Thyroglossal duct cysts, 495
Thyroid disorders, 407
Thyroid hormones, 407
Thyroid storm
  diagnosis, 420
  differential diagnosis, 419
  disposition, 421
  precipitating factors, 418
  specific clinical features, 418
  treatment, 421
Tibial shaft fractures, 791
Tick paralysis, 595
Tinea versicolor, 363
Tinnitus, 469
Torsades De Pointes, 99
Toxic hepatitis, 225
Toxic megacolon, 256
Toxic metabolic headache, 585
Toxidromes
  anticholinergic, 687–688
  cholinergic, 688–689
  opioid, 689–690
  sedative, 690
  sympathomimetic, 691
  withdrawal symptoms, 692
Toxins, 552
  associated with anion gap, 686
  ciguatera, 195
  hypoglycemia, 683
  scombroid, 195
  that alter thermoregulation/cause temperature changes, 683
tPA complications, 563
Tracheobronchial injuries, 843
Tracheostomy
  and bleeding, 181
  and respiratory distress, 180
Transfer dysphagia
  description, 199
  localized causes, 201
  neuromuscular causes, 200
Transfusion therapy
  complications
    acute hemolytic transfusion reaction, 317–318
    allergic transfusion reaction, 319
    delayed transfusion reaction, 319
    febrile nonhemolytic reaction, 318
    infectious complications, 320
  cryoprecipitate, 317
  fresh frozen plasma, 316
  massive blood transfusion, 315
  packed red blood cells, 314
  platelet transfusion, 316

Transport dysphagia
  description, 202
  motor causes, 204
  obstructive causes, 203
Transudates, 174
Transverse cord syndrome, 832
Transverse myelitis, 805
Trauma
  abdominal, 847–852
  airway assessment, 815
  basilar skull fracture, 824
  blast injuries, 867
  blunt eye, 670
  blunt ocular trauma and globe rupture, 671
  brain herniation, 821
  breathing assessment, 815
  burns, 864–867
  cerebral contusions, 823
  chest (*see* Chest trauma)
  circulation assessment, 816
  classification of hemorrhage, 817
  concussion, 823
  disability assessment, 818
  elevated ICP, 821
  exposure, 818
  extremity injuries, 856–857
  geriatric, 862
  head trauma, 820
  hyphema, 672
  intracranial hemorrhage, 825
  mild TBI, 822
  moderate and severe TBI, 822
  pediatric, 858–861
  pediatric head trauma, 825
  pelvis and hip, 852–855
  penetrating neck injury, 835–838
  postconcussive syndrome, 823
  pregnancy, 863
  primary survey, 814
  secondary survey, 819
  second impact syndrome, 824
  skull fracture, 824
  spinal cord injuries, 830–834
  spinal injuries, 826–829
  traumatic arrest and ED thoracotomy, 819
  traumatic seizures, 822
Traumatic aortic injury, 845
Traumatic penis and foreskin disorders, 296
Traumatic seizures, 822
Trichomoniasis, 303, 621
Tricyclic antidepressants (TCA), 731–732
  EKG changes, 101
Trigeminal neuralgia, 505, 584
Triggering agents, 139
Trismus, 505
Troponin elevation, reasons for, 17
TTP. *See* Thrombotic thrombocytopenic purpura (TTP)
Tuberculosis (TB), 168
  diagnosis, 171
  initial evaluation, 170
  pathophysiology, 169
  PPD and CXR, 170
  presentation, 170
  reactivation, 169
  treatments and side effects, 171
Tubular disease, causes, 268
Tympanic membrane perforation, 477

U
Ulcerative colitis
  description, 256
  diagnosis, 257
  irritable bowel syndrome, 257
  toxic megacolon, 256
  treatment, 257
Ulcer-forming processes, 301
Ultraviolet keratitis, 657
Umbilical cord prolapse, 635
Unstable angina, 6
Unstable cervical fractures, 828
Upper GI bleeding (UGIB)
  description, 215
  diagnosis and treatment, 216
  disposition, 216
  symptoms and signs, 215
Uremia
  cardiovascular complications of, 280
  gastrointestinal complications of, 282
  hematologic complications of, 281
  neurologic complications of, 281
Urethral injury, 851
Urethritis, 300
Urinalysis, 273
Urinary retention, 301
Urinary tract infections (UTI)
  clinical features, 290
  complicated *vs.* uncomplicated, 289
  description, 288
  diagnosis, 291
Uterine cancer, 627
UTI. *See* Urinary tract infections (UTI)
Uveitis and iritis, 660
Uvular edema, 496

V
Valproate, 702
Valvular emergencies
  aortic regurgitation, 39–41
  aortic stenosis, 37–38
  mitral regurgitation, 33–35
  mitral stenosis, 32–33
  mitral valve prolapse, 35–36
  new murmur, 31
Variant angina. *See* Prinzmetal's angina
Varicella, 380
Vascular/related disease, 269
Vaso-occlusive crisis, sickle cell anemia, 326
Vasovagal syncope, 78
Venous sinus thrombosis, 591
Venous stasis ulcers, 385
Ventilator management and risks, 147
Ventral hernias, 243
Ventricular aneurysm, predicting factors on EKG, 22
Ventricular fibrillation (VF)
  description, 117
  EKG changes, 118
Ventricular shunt headache, 589
Ventricular tachycardia (VT)
  description, 115
  EKG changes, 115
  EKG features, 116
  treatment, 117
Vertebral artery dissection, 515
Vertebrobasilar infarction, 560

Vertebrobasilar insufficiency, 515
Vertigo
central (*see* Central vertigo)
description, 508
peripheral (*see* Peripheral vertigo)
Vesicants, 553
Vestibular neuronitis, 511
VF. *See* Ventricular fibrillation (VF)
Vibrio, 193
Viral conjunctivitis, 651
Viral diarrhea, 190
Viral meningitis, 574
Viral parotitis (Mumps), 501
Visual field deficits, 641
Vitreous and intraocular cavities
endophthalmitis, 661
vitreous hemorrhage, 662
Vitreous hemorrhage, 662
Volkmann's ischemic contracture, 759
Volvulus
description, 240
diagnosis, 241
malrotation with, 241
treatment, 242
Vomiting, 186
Von Willebrand's disease (VWD), 339
VP shunt complications, 589–590
VT. *See* Ventricular tachycardia (VT)
Vulvovaginitis
bacterial vaginosis, 621
bartholin cyst and abscess, 622
candida vaginitis, 622
description, 620
trichomoniasis, 621

W
Wallenberg Syndrome, 514
Warfarin
bleeding from, 340
description, 339
skin necrosis from, 340
Wernicke's encephalopathy, 601
Wolff-Parkinson-White (WPW) syndrome
atrial fibrillation/flutter, 112–113
atrioventricular reentry tachycardias, 112–113
description, 111
EKG changes in sinus rhythm, 112
treatment, 114
Wrist
Colles' fracture, 750
perilunate and lunate dislocations, 755
scaphoid fracture, 752
scapholunate dissociation, 754
Smith's fracture, 751
triquetral fracture, 753

X
Xanthines, 732

Y
Yersinia, 192

MIX
Papier aus verantwortungsvollen Quellen
Paper from responsible sources
FSC® C105338

If you have any concerns about our products,
you can contact us on
ProductSafety@springernature.com

In case Publisher is established outside the EU,
the EU authorized representative is:
Springer Nature Customer Service Center GmbH
Europaplatz 3, 69115 Heidelberg, Germany

Printed by Libri Plureos GmbH
in Hamburg, Germany